W9-CCV-937

ICD-10-PCS

The complete official code set

Codes valid from October 1, 2020
through September 30, 2021

2021

optum360coding.com

Notice

ICD-10-PCS: The Complete Official Code Set is designed to be an accurate and authoritative source regarding coding and every reasonable effort has been made to ensure accuracy and completeness of the content. However, Optum360 makes no guarantee, warranty, or representation that this publication is accurate, complete, or without errors. It is understood that Optum360 is not rendering any legal or other professional services or advice in this publication and that Optum360 bears no liability for any results or consequences that may arise from the use of this book. Please address all correspondence to:

Optum360
2525 Lake Park Blvd
Salt Lake City, UT 84120

Our Commitment to Accuracy

Optum360 is committed to producing accurate and reliable materials. To report corrections, please visit www.optum360coding.com/accuracy or email accuracy@optum.com. You can also reach customer service by calling 1.800.464.3649, option 1.

Copyright

Made in the USA
ISBN 978-1-62254-545-2 (Spiral)
ISBN 978-1-62254-547-6 (Softbound)

Acknowledgments

Marianne Randall, CPC, *Product Manager*
Karen Schmidt, BSN, *Technical Director*
Anita Schmidt, BS, RHIA, AHIMA-approved ICD-10-CM/PCS Trainer, *Subject Matter Expert*
Karen Krawzik, RHIT, CCS, AHIMA-approved ICD-10-CM/PCS Trainer, *Subject Matter Expert*
Leanne Patterson, CPC, *Subject Matter Expert*
LaJuana Green, RHIA, CCS, *Subject Matter Expert*
Stacy Perry, *Manager, Desktop Publishing*
Tracy Betzler, *Senior Desktop Publishing Specialist*
Hope M. Dunn, *Senior Desktop Publishing Specialist*
Katie Russell, *Desktop Publishing Specialist*
Kate Holden, *Editor*

Anita Schmidt, BS, RHIA, AHIMA-approved ICD-10-CM/PCS Trainer

Ms. Schmidt has expertise in ICD-10-CM/PCS, DRG, and CPT with more than 15 years' experience in coding in multiple settings, including inpatient, observation, and same-day surgery. Her experience includes analysis of medical record documentation, assignment of ICD-10-CM and PCS codes, and DRG validation. She has conducted training for ICD-10-CM/PCS and electronic health record. She has also collaborated with clinical documentation specialists to identify documentation needs and potential areas for physician education. Most recently she has been developing content for resource and educational products related to ICD-10-CM, ICD-10-PCS, DRG, and CPT. Ms. Schmidt is an AHIMA-approved ICD-10-CM/PCS trainer and is an active member of the American Health Information Management Association (AHIMA) and the Minnesota Health Information Management Association (MHIMA).

Karen Krawzik, RHIT, CCS, AHIMA-approved ICD-10-CM/PCS Trainer

Ms. Krawzik has expertise in ICD-10-CM, ICD-9-CM, CPT/HCPCS, DRG, and data quality and analytics, with more than 30 years' experience coding in multiple settings, including inpatient, observation, ambulatory surgery, ancillary, and emergency room. She has served as a DRG analyst and auditor of commercial and government payer claims, as a contract administrator, and worked on a team providing enterprise-wide conversion of the ICD-9-CM code set to ICD-10. More recently, she has been developing print and electronic content related to ICD-10-CM and ICD-10-PCS coding systems, MS-DRGs, and HCCs. Ms. Krawzik is credentialed by the American Health Information Management Association (AHIMA) as a Registered Health Information Technician (RHIT) and a Certified Coding Specialist (CCS) and is an AHIMA-approved ICD-10-CM/PCS trainer. She is an active member of AHIMA and the Missouri Health Information Management Association.

Contents

What's New for 2021

The Centers for Medicare and Medicaid Services is the agency charged with maintaining and updating ICD-10-PCS. CMS released the most current revisions, a summary of which may be found on the CMS website at https://www.cms.gov/medicare/icd-10/2021-icd-10-pcs.

Due to the unique structure of ICD-10-PCS, a change in a character value may affect individual codes and several code tables.

Change Summary Table

2020 Total	New Codes	Revised Titles	Deleted Codes	2021 Total
77,559	544	0	0	78,103

ICD-10-PCS Code FY 2021 Totals, By Section

Medical and Surgical	67,655
Obstetrics	304
Placement	861
Administration	1,336
Measurement and Monitoring	421
Extracorporeal or Systemic Assistance and Performance	51
Extracorporeal or Systemic Therapies	46
Osteopathic	100
Other Procedures	78
Chiropractic	90
Imaging	2,973
Nuclear Medicine	463
Radiation Therapy	2,087
Physical Rehabilitation and Diagnostic Audiology	1,380
Mental Health	30
Substance Abuse Treatment	59
New Technology	169
Total	78,103

ICD-10-PCS Table Changes Highlights

- Device value of Radioactive element added to root operation table of Insertion in several body systems, including:
  — Central Nervous System and Cranial Nerves
  — Peripheral Nervous
  — Lymphatic and Hemic
  — Ear, Nose, Sinus
  — Mouth and Throat
  — Gastrointestinal
  — Hepatobiliary System and Pancreas
  — Endocrine
  — Urinary
  — Female Reproductive
  — Male Reproductive
- New row added to root operation table of Bypass in the Heart and Great Vessels body system for Percutaneous bypass of left atrium to right atrium with synthetic substitute

- New row added to root operation table Fragmentation capturing body part values Pulmonary Trunk, Pulmonary Artery, Right/Left and Pulmonary Vein, Right/Left
- New root operation table of Fragmentation added in the Upper Arteries, Lower Arteries, Upper Veins and Lower Veins body systems
- New rows added to root operation table of Supplement in the Heart and Great Vessels body system
- Qualifier values added to root operation table Bypass in the Hepatobiliary System and Pancreas and Anatomical Regions, General body systems
- Device value of Other device added to root operation table Insertion in the Subcutaneous Tissue and Fascia body system
- Body part values of Lumbar Vertebra, Sacrum, Acetabulum, Right/Left and Coccyx added to root operation table of Removal in the Lower Bones body system
- Device value of Internal Fixation Device, Sustained Compression added to root operation table Fusion in the Upper Joints and Lower Joints body systems
- New root operation table of Transplantation added to Male Reproductive body system
- Approach values of Via Natural and Artificial Opening and Via Natural or Artificial Opening Endoscopic added for body part Pelvic Cavity in the Anatomical Regions, General body system
- Approach values of Open and Percutaneous Endoscopic added to root operation table of Extraction for body part Products of Conception, Ectopic in the Obstetrics body system
- Substance value of Hematopoietic Stem/Progenitor Cells, Genetically Modified and qualifier value of Autologous added to root operation table of Transfusion for Peripheral Vein and Central Vein body system/region in the Administration section
- Qualifier value of High Nasal Flow/Velocity added to root operation Assistance in the Extracorporeal or Systemic Assistance and Performance section
- New root operation table of Other Imaging added to Hepatobiliary System and Pancreas and Anatomical Regions body systems in the Imaging section
- Isotope value of Cesium 131 (Cs-131) added to Brachytherapy tables in the Radiation Therapy section for the following body systems:
  — Central and Peripheral Nervous System
  — Lymphatic and Hematologic
  — Eye
  — Ear, Nose, Mouth, and Throat
  — Respiratory
  — Gastrointestinal
  — Hepatobiliary System and Pancreas
  — Endocrine
  — Breast
  — Urinary
  — Female Reproductive
  — Male Reproductive
  — Anatomical Regions

- Modality qualifier of Intraoperative Radiation Therapy (IORT) added to Other Radiation table in the Central and Peripheral Nervous body system in the Radiation Therapy section
- Many new substances and devices added to the New Technology tables — see New Definitions Addenda — Device and Substance Definitions for more information

New Definitions Addenda

Section Ø — Medical and Surgical
Root Operation

ICD-10-PCS Value	Definition	
Supplement	Delete	Includes/Examples: Herniorrhaphy using mesh, free nerve graft, mitral valve ring annuloplasty, put a new acetabular liner in a previous hip replacement
	Add	Includes/Examples: Herniorrhaphy using mesh, mitral valve ring annuloplasty, put a new acetabular liner in a previous hip replacement

Section Ø — Medical and Surgical
Body Part

ICD-10-PCS Value	Definitions	
Abdominal Sympathetic Nerve	Add	Renal nerve
Hand Bursa and Ligament, Right Hand Bursa and Ligament, Left	Delete	Scapholunate ligament
Wrist Bursa and Ligament, Right Wrist Bursa and Ligament, Left	Add	Scapholunate ligament

Section Ø — Medical and Surgical
Device

ICD-10-PCS Value	Definition	
Add Internal Fixation Device, Sustained Compression for Fusion in Lower Joints	Add	DynaNail Mini®
	Add	DynaNail®
Add Internal Fixation Device, Sustained Compression for Fusion in Upper Joints	Add	DynaNail Mini®
	Add	DynaNail®
Intraluminal Device, Branched or Fenestrated, One or Two Arteries for Restriction in Lower Arteries	Delete	Cook Zenith AAA Endovascular Graft
	Delete	Zenith AAA Endovascular Graft
	Add	Cook Zenith® Fenestrated AAA Endovascular Graft
	Add	Zenith® Fenestrated AAA Endovascular Graft
Intraluminal Device, Branched or Fenestrated, Three or More Arteries for Restriction in Lower Arteries	Delete	Cook Zenith AAA Endovascular Graft
	Delete	Zenith AAA Endovascular Graft
	Add	Cook Zenith® Fenestrated AAA Endovascular Graft
	Add	Zenith® Fenestrated AAA Endovascular Graft
Synthetic Substitute	Add	Barricaid® Annular Closure Device (ACD)
	Add	Corvia IASD®
	Add	IASD® (InterAtrial Shunt Device), Corvia
	Add	InterAtrial Shunt Device IASD®, Corvia
	Add	V-Wave Interatrial Shunt System

Section 3 — Administration
Substance

ICD-10-PCS Value	Definition	
Add Hematopoietic Stem/Progenitor Cells, Genetically Modified	Add	OTL-101

Section B — Imaging
Type

ICD-10-PCS Value	Definition	
Add Other Imaging	Add	Definition: Other specified modality for visualizing a body part.

Section X — New Technology
Root Operation

ICD-10-PCS Value	Definition	
Add Supplement	Add	Definition: Putting in or on biological or synthetic material that physically reinforces and/or augments the function of a portion of a body part.

Section X – New Technology Approach

ICD-10-PCS Value		Definition	
Add	Via Natural or Artificial Opening	Add	Definition: Entry of instrumentation through a natural or artificial external opening to reach the site of the procedure.

Section X — New Technology Device/Substance/Technology

ICD-10-PCS Value		Definition	
Add	Atezolizumab Antineoplastic	Add	TECENTRIQ®
Add	Brexanolone	Add	ZULRESSO™
Add	Brexucabtagene Autoleucel Immunotherapy	Add	Brexucabtagene Autoleucel
Add	Cefiderocol Anti-infective	Add	FETROJA®
Add	Ceftolozane/Tazobactam Anti-infective	Add	ZERBAXA®
Add	Durvalumab Antineoplastic	Add	IMFINZI®
Add	Eculizumab	Add	Soliris®
Add	Esketamine Hydrochloride	Add	SPRAVATO™
Add	Lefamulin Anti-infective	Add	XENLETA™
Add	Lisocabtagene Maraleucel Immunotherapy	Add	Lisocabtagene Maraleucel
Add	Mineral-based Topical Hemostatic Agent	Add	Hemospray® Endoscopic Hemostat
Add	Nerinitide	Add	NA-1 (Nerinitide)
Add	Omadacycline Anti-infective	Add	NUZYRA™
Add	Synthetic Substitute, Mechanically Expandable (Paired) in New Technology	Add	SpineJack® system

List of Updated Files

2021 Official ICD-10-PCS Coding Guidelines

- New guidelines B3.18 and B5.2b added in response to public comment
- Guidelines B3.1b and B3.10c revised in response to public comment and internal review
- Downloadable PDF

2021 ICD-10-PCS Code Tables and Index (Zip file)

- Code tables for use beginning October 1, 2020
- Downloadable PDF: file name is pcs_2021.pdf
- Downloadable xml files for developers: file names are icd10pcs_tables_2021.xml, icd10pcs_index_2021.xml, icd10pcs_definitions_2021.xml

- Accompanying schema for developers: file names are icd10pcs_tables.xsd; icd10pcs_index.xsd; icd10pcs_definitions.xsd

2021 ICD-10-PCS Codes File (Zip file)

- ICD-10-PCS codes file is a simple format for nontechnical uses, containing the valid FY 2021 ICD-10-PCS codes and their long titles.
- File is in text file format: file name is icd10pcs_codes_2021.txt
- Accompanying documentation for codes file: file name is icd10pcsCodesFile.pdf
- Codes file addenda in text format: file name is codes_addenda_2021.txt

2021 ICD-10-PCS Order File (Long and Abbreviated Titles) (Zip file)

- ICD-10-PCS order file is for developers, provides a unique five-digit "order number" for each ICD-10-PCS table and code, as well as a long and abbreviated code title.
- ICD-10-PCS order file name is icd10pcs_order_2021.txt
- Accompanying documentation for tabular order file: file name is icd10pcsOrderFile.pdf
- Tabular order file addenda in text format: file name is order_addenda_2021.txt

2021 ICD-10-PCS Final Addenda (Zip file)

- Addenda files in downloadable PDF: file names are tables_addenda_2021.pdf; index_addenda_2021.pdf; definitions_addenda_2021.pdf
- Addenda files also in machine-readable text format for developers: file names are tables_addenda_2021.txt; index_addenda_2021.txt; definitions_addenda_2021.txt

2021 ICD-10-PCS Conversion Table (Zip file)

- ICD-10-PCS code conversion table is provided to assist users in data retrieval, in downloadable Excel spreadsheet: file name is icd10pcs_conversion_table_2021.xlsx
- Conversion table also in machine-readable text format for developers: file name is icd10pcs_conversion_table_2021.txt
- Accompanying documentation for code conversion table: file name is icd10pcsConversionTable.pdf

Introduction

ICD-10-PCS: The Complete Official Code Set is your definitive coding resource for procedure coding in acute inpatient hospitals. In addition to the official ICD-10-PCS Coding System Files, revised and distributed by the Centers for Medicare and Medicaid Services (CMS), Optum360's coding experts have incorporated Medicare-related coding edits and proprietary features, such as coding tools and appendixes, into a comprehensive and easy-to-use reference.

This manual provides the most current information that was available at the time of publication. For updates to official source documents that may have occurred after this manual was published, please refer to the following:

- **CMS International Classification of Disease, 10th Revision, Procedural Coding System (ICD-10-PCS):**

    https://www.cms.gov/medicare/icd-10/2021-icd-10-pcs

- **CMS Inpatient Prospective Payment System Proposed Rule, FY2021**

    https://www.cms.gov/medicare/acute-inpatient-pps/fy-2021-ipps-proposed-rule-home-page

- **CMS Inpatient Prospective Payment System Proposed Rule, FY 2021 - Proposed, version 38, MS-DRG Grouper software, Definitions Manual files and Medicare Code Editor (MCE) files**

    https://www.cms.gov/Medicare/Medicare-Fee-for-Service-Payment/AcuteInpatientPPS/MS-DRG-Classifications-and-Software

- **American Hospital Association (AHA) Coding Clinics**

    https://www.codingclinicadvisor.com/

ICD-10-PCS Code Structure

ICD-10-PCS has a seven-character alphanumeric code structure. Each character contains up to 34 possible values. Each value represents a specific option for the general character definition. The 10 digits Ø–9 and the 24 letters A–H, J–N, and P–Z may be used in each character. The letters O and I are not used so as to avoid confusion with the digits Ø and 1. An ICD-10-PCS code is the result of a process rather than as a single fixed set of digits or alphabetic characters. The process consists of combining semi-independent values from among a selection of values, according to the rules governing the construction of codes.

	Section	Body System	Root Operation	Body Part	Approach	Device	Qualifier
Characters:	1	2	3	4	5	6	7

A code is derived by choosing a specific value for each of the seven characters. Based on details about the procedure performed, values for each character specifying the section, body system, root operation, body part, approach, device, and qualifier are assigned. Because the definition of each character is also a function of its physical position in the code, the same letter or number placed in a different position in the code has a different meaning.

The seven characters that make up a complete code have specific meanings that vary for each of the 17 sections of the manual.

Procedures are then divided into sections that identify the general type of procedure (e.g., Medical and Surgical, Obstetrics, Imaging). The first character of the procedure code always specifies the section. The second through seventh characters have the same meaning within each section, but may mean different things in other sections. In all sections, the third character specifies the general type of procedure performed (e.g., Resection, Transfusion, Fluoroscopy), while the other characters give additional information such as the body part and approach.

In ICD-10-PCS, the term *procedure* refers to the complete specification of the seven characters.

Number of Codes in ICD-10-PCS

The table structure of ICD-10-PCS permits the specification of a large number of codes on a single page. At the time of this publication, there are 78,103 codes in the 2021 ICD-10-PCS.

ICD-10-PCS Manual

Index

Codes may be found in the index based on the general type of procedure (e.g., resection, transfusion, fluoroscopy), or a more commonly used term (e.g., appendectomy). For example, the code for percutaneous intraluminal dilation of the coronary arteries with an intraluminal device can be found in the Index under *Dilation*, or a synonym of *Dilation* (e.g., angioplasty). The Index then specifies the first three or four values of the code or directs the user to see another term.

Example:

> **Dilation**
> > Artery
> > > Coronary
> > > > One Artery Ø27Ø

Based on the first three values of the code provided in the Index, the corresponding table can be located. In the example above, the first three values indicate table Ø27 is to be referenced for code completion.

The tables and characters are arranged first by number and then by letter for each character (tables for ØØ-, Ø1-, Ø2-, etc., are followed by those for ØB-, ØC-, ØD-, etc., followed by ØB1, ØB2, etc., followed by ØBB, ØBC, ØBD, etc.).

Note: The Tables section must be used to construct a complete and valid code by specifying the last three or four values.

Tables

The tables in ICD-10-PCS provide the valid combination of character values needed to build a unique procedure code. Each table is preceded by the first three characters of the code, along with their descriptions. In the Medical and Surgical section, for example, the first three characters contain the name of the section (character 1), the body system (character 2), and the root operation performed (character 3).

Listed underneath the first three characters is a table comprising four columns and one or more rows. The four columns in the table specify the last four characters needed to complete the ICD-10-PCS code. Depending on the section, the labels for each column may be different. In the Medical and Surgical section, they are labeled body part (character 4), approach (character 5), device (character 6), and qualifier (character 7). Each row in the table specifies the valid combination of values for characters 4 through 7.

Table 1: Row from table Ø27

Ø	Medical and Surgical
2	Heart and Great Vessels
7	Dilation

7 Dilation Definition: Expanding an orifice or the lumen of a tubular body part

Explanation: The orifice can be a natural orifice or an artificially created orifice. Accomplished by stretching a tubular body part using intraluminal pressure or by cutting part of the orifice or wall of the tubular body part.

Body Part Character 4	Approach Character 5	Device Character 6	Qualifier Character 7
Ø Coronary Artery, One Artery 1 Coronary Artery, Two Arteries 2 Coronary Artery, Three Arteries 3 Coronary Artery, Four or More Arteries	Ø Open 3 Percutaneous 4 Percutaneous Endoscopic	4 Intraluminal Device, Drug-eluting 5 Intraluminal Device, Drug-eluting, Two 6 Intraluminal Device, Drug-eluting, Three 7 Intraluminal Device, Drug-eluting, Four or More D Intraluminal Device E Intraluminal Device, Two F Intraluminal Device, Three G Intraluminal Device, Four or More T Intraluminal Device, Radioactive Z No Device	6 Bifurcation Z No Qualifier

For instance, table 1 above shows the first row from table Ø27 in ICD-10-PCS. The values Ø27 specify the section *Medical and Surgical (Ø)*, the body system *Heart and Great Vessels (2)*, and the root operation *Dilation (7)*. As shown, the root operation (Dilation) is also accompanied by its corresponding definition and explanation. Note, a definition of the root operation is provided for every table in ICD-10-PCS; however, an explanation may not always be applicable.

In total, this single row can be used to construct 240 unique procedure codes. The valid codes shown in table 2 (below) are constructed using the body part (character 4) value of Ø, Coronary artery, one artery, combined with all valid approach (character 5) values, device (character 6) values, and a qualifier (character 7) value of Z, No Qualifier.

Table 2: Code titles for dilation of one coronary artery (Ø27Ø)

Code	Title
Ø27ØØ4Z	Dilation of Coronary Artery, One Artery with Drug-eluting Intraluminal Device, Open Approach
Ø27ØØ5Z	Dilation of Coronary Artery, One Artery with Two Drug-eluting Intraluminal Devices, Open Approach
Ø27ØØ6Z	Dilation of Coronary Artery, One Artery with Three Drug-eluting Intraluminal Devices, Open Approach
Ø27ØØ7Z	Dilation of Coronary Artery, One Artery with Four or More Drug-eluting Intraluminal Devices, Open Approach
Ø27ØØDZ	Dilation of Coronary Artery, One Artery with Intraluminal Device, Open Approach
Ø27ØØEZ	Dilation of Coronary Artery, One Artery with Two Intraluminal Devices, Open Approach
Ø27ØØFZ	Dilation of Coronary Artery, One Artery with Three Intraluminal Devices, Open Approach
Ø27ØØGZ	Dilation of Coronary Artery, One Artery with Four or More Intraluminal Devices, Open Approach
Ø27ØØTZ	Dilation of Coronary Artery, One Artery with Radioactive Intraluminal Device, Open Approach
Ø27ØØZZ	Dilation of Coronary Artery, One Artery, Open Approach
Ø27Ø34Z	Dilation of Coronary Artery, One Artery with Drug-eluting Intraluminal Device, Percutaneous Approach
Ø27Ø35Z	Dilation of Coronary Artery, One Artery with Two Drug-eluting Intraluminal Devices, Percutaneous Approach
Ø27Ø36Z	Dilation of Coronary Artery, One Artery with Three Drug-eluting Intraluminal Devices, Percutaneous Approach
Ø27Ø37Z	Dilation of Coronary Artery, One Artery with Four or More Drug-eluting Intraluminal Devices, Percutaneous Approach
Ø27Ø3DZ	Dilation of Coronary Artery, One Artery with Intraluminal Device, Percutaneous Approach
Ø27Ø3EZ	Dilation of Coronary Artery, One Artery with Two Intraluminal Devices, Percutaneous Approach
Ø27Ø3FZ	Dilation of Coronary Artery, One Artery with Three Intraluminal Devices, Percutaneous Approach
Ø27Ø3GZ	Dilation of Coronary Artery, One Artery with Four or More Intraluminal Devices, Percutaneous Approach
Ø27Ø3TZ	Dilation of Coronary Artery, One Artery with Radioactive Intraluminal Device, Percutaneous Approach
Ø27Ø3ZZ	Dilation of Coronary Artery, One Artery, Percutaneous Approach
Ø27Ø44Z	Dilation of Coronary Artery, One Artery with Drug-eluting Intraluminal Device, Percutaneous Endoscopic Approach
Ø27Ø45Z	Dilation of Coronary Artery, One Artery with Two Drug-eluting Intraluminal Devices, Percutaneous Endoscopic Approach
Ø27Ø46Z	Dilation of Coronary Artery, One Artery with Three Drug-eluting Intraluminal Devices, Percutaneous Endoscopic Approach
Ø27Ø47Z	Dilation of Coronary Artery, One Artery with Four or More Drug-eluting Intraluminal Devices, Percutaneous Endoscopic Approach
Ø27Ø4DZ	Dilation of Coronary Artery, One Artery with Intraluminal Device, Percutaneous Endoscopic Approach
Ø27Ø4EZ	Dilation of Coronary Artery, One Artery with Two Intraluminal Devices, Percutaneous Endoscopic Approach
Ø27Ø4FZ	Dilation of Coronary Artery, One Artery with Three Intraluminal Devices, Percutaneous Endoscopic Approach
Ø27Ø4GZ	Dilation of Coronary Artery, One Artery with Four or More Intraluminal Devices, Percutaneous Endoscopic Approach
Ø27Ø4TZ	Dilation of Coronary Artery, One Artery with Radioactive Intraluminal Device, Percutaneous Endoscopic Approach
Ø27Ø4ZZ	Dilation of Coronary Artery, One Artery, Percutaneous Endoscopic Approach

Table 3: Rows from table ØØH

Ø   **Medical and Surgical**
Ø   **Central Nervous System and Cranial Nerves**
H   **Insertion**   Definition: Putting in a nonbiological appliance that monitors, assists, performs, or prevents a physiological function but does not physically take the place of a body part
Explanation: None

Body Part Character 4		Approach Character 5	Device Character 6	Qualifier Character 7

Ø Brain
   Cerebrum
   Corpus callosum
   Encephalon
		Ø Open	**1** Radioactive Element
			2 Monitoring Device
			3 Infusion Device
			4 Radioactive Element, Cesium-131 Collagen Implant
			M Neurostimulator Lead
			Y Other Device
				Z No Qualifier

Ø Brain
   Cerebrum
   Corpus callosum
   Encephalon
		3 Percutaneous
		4 Percutaneous Endoscopic
			1 Radioactive Element
			2 Monitoring Device
			3 Infusion Device
			M Neurostimulator Lead
			Y Other Device
				Z No Qualifier

6 Cerebral Ventricle
   Aqueduct of Sylvius
   Cerebral aqueduct (Sylvius)
   Choroid plexus
   Ependyma
   Foramen of Monro (intraventricular)
   Fourth ventricle Interventricular foramen (Monro)
   Left lateral ventricle
   Right lateral ventricle
   Third ventricle
	E Cranial Nerve
	U Spinal Canal
	   Epidural space, spinal
	   Extradural space, spinal
	   Subarachnoid space, spinal
	   Subdural space, spinal
	   Vertebral canal
	V Spinal Cord
		Ø Open
		3 Percutaneous
		4 Percutaneous Endoscopic
			1 Radioactive Element
			2 Monitoring Device
			3 Infusion Device
			M Neurostimulator Lead
			Y Other Device
				Z No Qualifier

Table 3, is split into three rows; values of characters must all be selected from within the same row of the table. Rows 1 and 2 have the same body part (character 4) value of Ø Brain and the same qualifier value (character 7) of Z No Qualifier. However, the approach (character 5) values are not the same for these two rows, and there is one additional device (character 6) value in row 1 that is not included in row 2. As shown in row 1, body part value Brain (Ø) with device value Radioactive Element, Cesium-131 Collagen Implant (4) can only be used with approach value Open (Ø). In other words, code ØØHØ34Z would be invalid as the approach value 3 is only applicable to row 2 and the device value 4 is only applicable to row 1. It would be inappropriate to build a code for body part Ø if all of the values are not contained in its own row.

Note: In this manual, there are instances in which some tables due to length must be continued on the next page. Each section must be used separately and value selection must be made within the same row of the table.

Character Meanings

In each section, each character has a specific meaning, and this character meaning remains constant within that section. Character meaning tables have been provided at the beginning of each body system in the Medical and Surgical section (Ø) and the Obstetric section (1) to help the user identify the character members available within that section. These tables have purple headers, unlike the official code tables that have green headers and **SHOULD NOT** be used to build a PCS code. Following is an excerpt of a character meaning table.

Table 4: Rows from Central Nervous System and Cranial Nerves - Character Meanings Table

Operation–Character 3	Body Part–Character 4	Approach–Character 5	Device–Character 6	Qualifier–Character 7
1 Bypass	Ø Brain	Ø Open	Ø Drainage Device	Ø Nasopharynx
2 Change	1 Cerebral Meninges	3 Percutaneous	1 Radioactive Element	1 Mastoid Sinus
5 Destruction	2 Dura Mater	4 Percutaneous Endoscopic	2 Monitoring Device	2 Atrium
7 Dilation	3 Epidural Space, Intracranial	X External	3 Infusion Device	3 Blood Vessel
8 Division	4 Subdural Space, Intracranial		4 Radioactive Element, Cesium-131 Collagen Implant	4 Pleural Cavity
9 Drainage	5 Subarachnoid Space, Intracranial		7 Autologous Tissue Substitute	5 Intestine
B Excision	6 Cerebral Ventricle		J Synthetic Substitute	6 Peritoneal Cavity
C Extirpation	7 Cerebral Hemisphere		K Nonautologous Tissue Substitute	7 Urinary Tract
D Extraction	8 Basal Ganglia		M Neurostimulator Lead	8 Bone Marrow
F Fragmentation	9 Thalamus		Y Other Device	9 Fallopian Tube
H Insertion	A Hypothalamus		Z No Device	A Subgaleal space
J Inspection	B Pons			B Cerebral Cisterns

Sections

Procedures are divided into sections that identify the general type of procedure (e.g., Medical and Surgical, Obstetrics, Imaging). The first character of the procedure code always specifies the section.

The sections are listed below:

Medical and Surgical section
Ø   Medical and Surgical

Medical and Surgical-related sections
1   Obstetrics
2   Placement
3   Administration
4   Measurement and Monitoring
5   Extracorporeal or Systemic Assistance and Performance
6   Extracorporeal or Systemic Therapies
7   Osteopathic
8   Other Procedures
9   Chiropractic

Ancillary Sections
B   Imaging
C   Nuclear Medicine
D   Radiation Therapy
F   Physical Rehabilitation and Diagnostic Audiology
G   Mental Health
H   Substance Abuse Treatment

New Technology Section
X   New Technology

Medical and Surgical Section (Ø)

Character Meaning

The seven characters for Medical and Surgical procedures have the following meaning:

Character	Meaning
1	Section
2	Body System
3	Root Operation
4	Body Part
5	Approach
6	Device
7	Qualifier

The Medical and Surgical section constitutes the vast majority of procedures reported in an inpatient setting. Medical and Surgical procedure codes all have a first character value of Ø. The second character indicates the general body system (e.g., Mouth and Throat, Gastrointestinal). The third character indicates the root operation, or specific objective, of the procedure (e.g., Excision). The fourth character indicates the specific body part on which the procedure was performed (e.g., Tonsils, Duodenum). The fifth character indicates the approach used to reach the procedure site (e.g., Open). The sixth character indicates whether a device was left in place during the procedure (e.g.,

Synthetic Substitute). The seventh character is qualifier, which has a specific meaning for each root operation. For example, the qualifier can be used to identify the destination site of a *Bypass*. The first through fifth characters are always assigned a specific value, but the device (sixth character) and the qualifier (seventh character) are not applicable to all procedures. The value *Z* is used for the sixth and seventh characters to indicate that a specific device or qualifier does not apply to the procedure.

Section (Character 1)

Medical and Surgical procedure codes all have a first character value of Ø.

Body Systems (Character 2)

Body systems for Medical and Surgical section codes are specified in the second character.

Body Systems
Ø   Central Nervous System and Cranial Nerves
1   Peripheral Nervous System
2   Heart and Great Vessels
3   Upper Arteries
4   Lower Arteries
5   Upper Veins
6   Lower Veins
7   Lymphatic and Hemic Systems
8   Eye
9   Ear, Nose, Sinus
B   Respiratory System
C   Mouth and Throat
D   Gastrointestinal System
F   Hepatobiliary System and Pancreas
G   Endocrine System
H   Skin and Breast
J   Subcutaneous Tissue and Fascia
K   Muscles
L   Tendons
M   Bursae and Ligaments
N   Head and Facial Bones
P   Upper Bones
Q   Lower Bones
R   Upper Joints
S   Lower Joints
T   Urinary System
U   Female Reproductive System
V   Male Reproductive System
W   Anatomical Regions, General
X   Anatomical Regions, Upper Extremities
Y   Anatomical Regions, Lower Extremities

Root Operations (Character 3)

The root operation is specified in the third character. In the Medical and Surgical section there are 31 different root operations. The root operation identifies the objective of the procedure. Each root operation has a precise definition.

- *Alteration:* Modifying the natural anatomic structure of a body part without affecting the function of the body part

- *Bypass:* Altering the route of passage of the contents of a tubular body part

- *Change:* Taking out or off a device from a body part and putting back an identical or similar device in or on the same body part without cutting or puncturing the skin or a mucous membrane

- *Control:* Stopping, or attempting to stop, postprocedural or other acute bleeding

- *Creation:* Putting in or on biological or synthetic material to form a new body part that to the extent possible replicates the anatomic structure or function of an absent body part

- *Destruction:* Physical eradication of all or a portion of a body part by the direct use of energy, force, or a destructive agent

- *Detachment:* Cutting off all or a portion of the upper or lower extremities

- *Dilation:* Expanding an orifice or the lumen of a tubular body part

- *Division:* Cutting into a body part without draining fluids and/or gases from the body part in order to separate or transect a body part

- *Drainage:* Taking or letting out fluids and/or gases from a body part

- *Excision:* Cutting out or off, without replacement, a portion of a body part

- *Extirpation:* Taking or cutting out solid matter from a body part

- *Extraction:* Pulling or stripping out or off all or a portion of a body part by the use of force

- *Fragmentation:* Breaking solid matter in a body part into pieces

- *Fusion:* Joining together portions of an articular body part rendering the articular body part immobile

- *Insertion:* Putting in a nonbiological appliance that monitors, assists, performs, or prevents a physiological function but does not physically take the place of a body part

- *Inspection:* Visually and/or manually exploring a body part

- *Map:* Locating the route of passage of electrical impulses and/or locating functional areas in a body part

- *Occlusion:* Completely closing an orifice or lumen of a tubular body part

- *Reattachment:* Putting back in or on all or a portion of a separated body part to its normal location or other suitable location

- *Release:* Freeing a body part from an abnormal physical constraint by cutting or by use of force

- *Removal:* Taking out or off a device from a body part

- *Repair:* Restoring, to the extent possible, a body part to its normal anatomic structure and function

- *Replacement:* Putting in or on biological or synthetic material that physically takes the place and/or function of all or a portion of a body part

- *Reposition:* Moving to its normal location or other suitable location all or a portion of a body part

- *Resection:* Cutting out or off, without replacement, all of a body part

- *Restriction:* Partially closing an orifice or lumen of a tubular body part

- *Revision:* Correcting, to the extent possible, a portion of a malfunctioning device or the position of a displaced device

- *Supplement:* Putting in or on biological or synthetic material that physically reinforces and/or augments the function of a portion of a body part

- *Transfer:* Moving, without taking out, all or a portion of a body part to another location to take over the function of all or a portion of a body part

- *Transplantation:* Putting in or on all or a portion of a living body part taken from another individual or animal to physically take the place and/or function of all or a portion of a similar body part

The above definitions of root operations illustrate the precision of code values defined in the system. There is a clear distinction between each root operation.

A root operation specifies the objective of the procedure. The term *anastomosis* is not a root operation, because it is a means of joining and is always an integral part of another procedure (e.g., Bypass, Resection) with a specific objective. Similarly, *incision* is not a root operation, since it is always part of the objective of another procedure (e.g., Division, Drainage). The root operation *Repair* in the Medical and Surgical section functions as a "not elsewhere classified" option. *Repair* is used when the procedure performed is not one of the other specific root operations.

Appendix B provides additional explanation and representative examples of the Medical and Surgical root operations. Appendix C groups all root operations in the Medical and Surgical section into subcategories and provides an example of each root operation.

Body Part (Character 4)
The body part is specified in the fourth character. The body part indicates the specific anatomical site of the body system on which the procedure was performed (e.g., Duodenum). Tubular body parts are defined in ICD-10-PCS as those hollow body parts that provide a route of passage for solids, liquids, or gases. They include the cardiovascular system and body parts such as those contained in the gastrointestinal tract, genitourinary tract, biliary tract, and respiratory tract.

Approach (Character 5)
The technique used to reach the site of the procedure is specified in the fifth character. There are seven different approaches:

- *Open*: Cutting through the skin or mucous membrane and any other body layers necessary to expose the site of the procedure

- *Percutaneous*: Entry, by puncture or minor incision, of instrumentation through the skin or mucous membrane and any other body layers necessary to reach the site of the procedure

- *Percutaneous Endoscopic*: Entry, by puncture or minor incision, of instrumentation through the skin or mucous membrane and any other body layers necessary to reach and visualize the site of the procedure

- *Via Natural or Artificial Opening*: Entry of instrumentation through a natural or artificial external opening to reach the site of the procedure

- *Via Natural or Artificial Opening Endoscopic*: Entry of instrumentation through a natural or artificial external opening to reach and visualize the site of the procedure

- *Via Natural or Artificial Opening with Percutaneous Endoscopic Assistance:* Entry of instrumentation through a natural or artificial external opening and entry, by puncture or minor incision, of instrumentation through the skin or mucous membrane and any other body layers necessary to aid in the performance of the procedure

- *External*: Procedures performed directly on the skin or mucous membrane and procedures performed indirectly by the application of external force through the skin or mucous membrane

The approach comprises three components: the access location, method, and type of instrumentation.

Access location: For procedures performed on an internal body part, the access location specifies the external site through which the site of the procedure is reached. There are two general types of access locations: skin or mucous membranes, and external orifices. Every approach value except external includes one of these two access locations. The skin or mucous membrane can be cut or punctured to reach the procedure site. All open and percutaneous approach values use this access location. The site of a procedure can also be reached through an external opening. External openings can be natural (e.g., mouth) or artificial (e.g., colostomy stoma).

Method: For procedures performed on an internal body part, the method specifies how the external access location is entered. An open method specifies cutting through the skin or mucous membrane and any other intervening body layers necessary to expose the site of the procedure. An instrumentation method specifies the entry of instrumentation through the access location to the internal procedure site. Instrumentation can be introduced by puncture or minor incision, or through an external opening. The puncture or minor incision does not constitute an open approach because it does not expose the site of the procedure. An approach can define multiple methods. For example, *Via Natural or Artificial Opening with Percutaneous Endoscopic Assistance* includes both the initial entry of instrumentation to reach the site of the procedure, and the placement of additional percutaneous instrumentation into the body part to visualize and assist in the performance of the procedure.

Type of instrumentation: For procedures performed on an internal body part, instrumentation means that specialized equipment is used to perform the procedure. Instrumentation is used in all internal approaches other than the basic open approach. Instrumentation may or may not include the capacity to visualize the procedure site. For example, the instrumentation used to perform a sigmoidoscopy permits the internal site of the procedure to be visualized, while the instrumentation used to perform a needle biopsy of the liver does not. The term "endoscopic" as used in approach values refers to instrumentation that permits a site to be visualized.

Procedures performed directly on the skin or mucous membrane are identified by the external approach (e.g., skin excision). Procedures performed indirectly by the application of external force are also identified by the external approach (e.g., closed reduction of fracture).

Appendix A compares the components (access location, method, and type of instrumentation) of each approach and provides an example and illustration of each approach.

Device (Character 6)

The device is specified in the sixth character. There are four general types of devices:

- Biological or synthetic material that takes the place of all or a portion of a body part (e.g, skin graft, joint prosthesis).

- Biological or synthetic material that assists or prevents a physiological function (e.g., IUD).

- Therapeutic material that is not absorbed by, eliminated by, or incorporated into a body part (e.g., radioactive implant).

- Mechanical or electronic appliances used to assist, monitor, take the place of or prevent a physiological function (e.g., cardiac pacemaker, orthopedic pin).

Appendix F compares the general device types and provides examples of each.

While all devices can be removed, some cannot be removed without putting in another nonbiological appliance or body-part substitute.

When a specific device value is used to identify the device for a root operation, such as *Insertion* and that same device value is not an option for a more broad range root operation such as *Removal*, select the general device value. For example, in the body system Heart and Great Vessels, the specific device character for Cardiac Lead, Pacemaker in root operation *Insertion* is J. For the root operation *Removal*, the general device character M Cardiac Lead would be selected for the pacemaker lead.

ICD-10-PCS contains a PCS Device Aggregation Table (see appendix G) that crosswalks the *specific* device character values that have been created for specific root operations and specific body part character values to the *general* device character value that would be used for root operations that represent a broad range of procedures and general body part character values, such as Removal and Revision.

Instruments used to visualize the procedure site are specified in the approach, not the device, value.

If the objective of the procedure is to put in the device, then the root operation is *Insertion*. If the device is put in to meet an objective other than *Insertion*, then the root operation defining the underlying objective of the procedure is used, with the device specified in the device character. For example, if a procedure to replace the hip joint is performed, the root operation *Replacement* is coded, and the prosthetic device is specified in the device character. Materials that are incidental to a procedure such as clips, ligatures, and sutures are not specified in the device character. Because new devices can be developed, the value *Other Device* is provided as a temporary option for use until a specific device value is added to the system.

Qualifier (Character 7)

The qualifier is specified in the seventh character. The qualifier contains unique values for individual procedures. For example, the qualifier can be used to identify the destination site in a *Bypass*.

Medical and Surgical Section Principles

In developing the Medical and Surgical procedure codes, several specific principles were followed.

Composite Terms Are Not Root Operations

Composite terms such as colonoscopy, sigmoidectomy, or appendectomy do not describe root operations, but they do specify multiple components of a specific root operation. In ICD-10-PCS, the components of a procedure are defined separately by the characters making up the complete code. The only component of a procedure specified in the root operation is the objective of the procedure. With each complete code the underlying objective of the procedure is specified by the root operation (third character), the precise part is specified by the body part (fourth character), and the method used to reach and visualize the procedure site is specified by the approach (fifth character). While colonoscopy, sigmoidectomy, and appendectomy are included in the Index, they do not constitute root operations in the Tables section. The objective of colonoscopy is the visualization of the colon and the root operation (character 3) is *Inspection*. Character 4 specifies the body part, which in this case is part of the colon. These composite terms, like colonoscopy or appendectomy, are included as cross-reference only. The index provides the correct root operation reference. Examples of other types of composite terms not representative of root operations are *partial* sigmoidectomy, *total* hysterectomy, and *partial* hip replacement. Always refer to the correct root operation in the Index and Tables section.

Root Operation Based on Objective of Procedure

The root operation is based on the objective of the procedure, such as *Resection* of transverse colon or *Dilation* of an artery. The assignment of the root operation is based on the procedure actually performed, which may or may not have been the intended procedure. If the intended procedure is modified or discontinued (e.g., excision instead of resection is performed), the root operation is determined by the procedure actually performed. If the desired result is not attained after completing the procedure (i.e., the artery does not remain expanded after the dilation procedure), the root operation is still determined by the procedure actually performed.

Examples:

- Dilating the urethra is coded as *Dilation* since the objective of the procedure is to dilate the urethra. If dilation of the urethra includes putting in an intraluminal stent, the root operation remains *Dilation* and not *Insertion* of the intraluminal device because the underlying objective of the procedure is dilation of the urethra. The stent is identified by the intraluminal device value in the sixth character of the dilation procedure code.

- If the objective is solely to put a radioactive element in the urethra, then the procedure is coded to the root operation *Insertion*, with the radioactive element identified in the sixth character of the code.

- If the objective of the procedure is to correct a malfunctioning or displaced device, then the procedure is coded to the root operation *Revision*. In the root operation *Revision*, the original device being revised is identified in the device character. *Revision* is typically performed on mechanical appliances (e.g., pacemaker) or materials used in replacement procedures (e.g., synthetic substitute). Typical revision procedures include adjustment of pacemaker position and correction of malfunctioning knee prosthesis.

Combination Procedures Are Coded Separately

If multiple procedures as defined by distinct objectives are performed during an operative episode, then multiple codes are used. For example, obtaining the vein graft used for coronary bypass surgery is coded as a separate procedure from the bypass itself.

Redo of Procedures

The complete or partial redo of the original procedure is coded to the root operation that identifies the procedure performed rather than *Revision*.

Example:

> A complete redo of a hip replacement procedure that requires putting in a new prosthesis is coded to the root operation *Replacement* rather than *Revision*.

The correction of complications arising from the original procedure, other than device complications, is coded to the procedure performed. Correction of a malfunctioning or displaced device would be coded to the root operation *Revision*.

Example:

> A procedure to control hemorrhage arising from the original procedure is coded to *Control* rather than *Revision*.

Examples of Procedures Coded in the Medical Surgical Section

The following are examples of procedures from the Medical and Surgical section, coded in ICD-10-PCS.

- Suture of skin laceration, left lower arm: ØHQEXZZ

  Medical and Surgical section (Ø), body system *Skin and Breast* (H), root operation *Repair* (Q), body part *Skin, Left Lower Arm* (E), *External* Approach (X) *No device* (Z), and *No qualifier* (Z).

- Laparoscopic appendectomy: ØDTJ4ZZ

  Medical and Surgical section (Ø), body system *Gastrointestinal* (D), root operation *Resection* (T), body part *Appendix* (J), *Percutaneous Endoscopic* approach (4), No Device (Z), and No qualifier (Z).

- Sigmoidoscopy with biopsy: ØDBN8ZX

  Medical and Surgical section (Ø), body system *Gastrointestinal* (D), root operation *Excision* (B), body part *Sigmoid Colon* (N), *Via Natural or Artificial Opening Endoscopic* approach (8), *No Device* (Z), and with qualifier *Diagnostic* (X).

- Tracheostomy with tracheostomy tube: ØB11ØF4

  Medical and Surgical section (Ø), body system *Respiratory* (B), root operation *Bypass* (1), body part *Trachea* (1), *Open* approach (Ø), with *Tracheostomy Device* (F), and qualifier *Cutaneous* (4).

Obstetrics Section (1)

Character Meanings

The seven characters in the Obstetrics section have the same meaning as in the Medical and Surgical section.

Character	Meaning
1	Section
2	Body System
3	Root Operation
4	Body Part
5	Approach
6	Device
7	Qualifier

The Obstetrics section includes procedures performed on the products of conception only. Procedures on the pregnant female are coded in the Medical and Surgical section (e.g., episiotomy). The term "products of conception" refers to all physical components of a pregnancy, including the fetus, amnion, umbilical cord, and placenta. There is no differentiation of the products of conception based on gestational age.

Thus, the specification of the products of conception as a zygote, embryo or fetus, or the trimester of the pregnancy is not part of the procedure code but can be found in the diagnosis code.

Section (Character 1)
Obstetrics procedure codes have a first character value of *1*.

Body System (Character 2)
The second character value for body system is *Pregnancy*.

Root Operation (Character 3)
The root operations *Change, Drainage, Extraction, Insertion, Inspection, Removal, Repair, Reposition, Resection,* and *Transplantation* are used in the obstetrics section and have the same meaning as in the Medical and Surgical section.

The Obstetrics section also includes two additional root operations, *Abortion* and *Delivery*, defined below:

- *Abortion*: Artificially terminating a pregnancy

- *Delivery*: Assisting the passage of the products of conception from the genital canal

A cesarean section is not a separate root operation because the underlying objective is *Extraction* (i.e., pulling out all or a portion of a body part).

Body Part (Character 4)
The body part values in the obstetrics section are:

- *Products of conception*

- *Products of conception, retained*

- *Products of conception, ectopic*

Approach (Character 5)
The fifth character specifies approaches and is defined as are those in the Medical and Surgical section. In the case of an abortion procedure that uses a laminaria or an abortifacient, the approach is *Via Natural or Artificial Opening*.

Device (Character 6)
The sixth character is used for devices such as fetal monitoring electrodes.

Qualifier (Character 7)
Qualifier values are specific to the root operation and are used to capture details of the procedure, such as whether forceps or a vacuum were used during an Extraction, the type of fluid taken out during a Drainage procedure, or the products of conception body system that was repaired.

Placement Section (2)

Character Meanings
The seven characters in the Placement section have the following meaning:

Character	Meaning
1	Section
2	Body System
3	Root Operation
4	Body Region
5	Approach
6	Device
7	Qualifier

Placement section codes represent procedures for putting a device in or on a body region for the purpose of protection, immobilization, stretching, compression, or packing.

Section (Character 1)
Placement procedure codes have a first character value of *2*.

Body System (Character 2)
The second character contains two values specifying either *Anatomical Regions* or *Anatomical Orifices*.

Root Operation (Character 3)
The root operations in the Placement section include only those procedures that are performed without making an incision or a puncture. The root operations *Change* and *Removal* are in the Placement section and have the same meaning as in the Medical and Surgical section.

The Placement section also includes five additional root operations, defined as follows:

- *Compression*: Putting pressure on a body region

- *Dressing*: Putting material on a body region for protection

- *Immobilization*: Limiting or preventing motion of an external body region

- *Packing*: Putting material in a body region or orifice

- *Traction*: Exerting a pulling force on a body region in a distal direction

Body Region (Character 4)
The fourth character values are either body regions (e.g., *Upper Leg*) or natural orifices (e.g., *Ear*).

Approach (Character 5)
Since all placement procedures are performed directly on the skin or mucous membrane, or performed indirectly by applying external force through the skin or mucous membrane, the approach value is always *External*.

Device (Character 6)
The device character is always specified (except in the case of manual traction) and indicates the device placed during the procedure (e.g., cast, splint, bandage, etc.). Except for casts for fractures and dislocations, devices in the Placement section are off the shelf and do not require any extensive design, fabrication, or fitting. Placement of devices that require extensive design, fabrication, or fitting are coded in the Rehabilitation section.

Qualifier (Character 7)

The qualifier character is not specified in the Placement section; the qualifier value is always *No Qualifier*.

Administration Section (3)

Character Meanings

The seven characters in the Administration section have the following meaning:

Character	Meaning
1	Section
2	Body System
3	Root Operation
4	Body System/Region
5	Approach
6	Substance
7	Qualifier

Administration section codes represent procedures for putting in or on a therapeutic, prophylactic, protective, diagnostic, nutritional, or physiological substance. The section includes transfusions, infusions, and injections, along with other similar services such as irrigation and tattooing.

Section (Character 1)

Administration procedure codes have a first character value of *3*.

Body System (Character 2)

The body system character contains only three values: *Indwelling Device, Physiological Systems and Anatomical Regions,* or *Circulatory System*. The *Circulatory System* is used for transfusion procedures.

Root Operation (Character 3)

There are three root operations in the Administration section.

* *Introduction*: Putting in or on a therapeutic, diagnostic, nutritional, physiological, or prophylactic substance except blood or blood products

* *Irrigation*: Putting in or on a cleansing substance

* *Transfusion*: Putting in blood or blood products

Body/System Region (Character 4)

The fourth character specifies the body system/region. The fourth character identifies the site where the substance is administered, not the site where the substance administered takes effect. Sites include *Skin and Mucous Membranes, Subcutaneous Tissue,* and *Muscle*. These differentiate intradermal, subcutaneous, and intramuscular injections, respectively. Other sites include *Eye, Respiratory Tract, Peritoneal Cavity,* and *Epidural Space*.

The body systems/regions for arteries and veins are *Peripheral Artery, Central Artery, Peripheral Vein,* and *Central Vein*. The *Peripheral Artery* or *Vein* is typically used when a substance is introduced locally into an artery or vein. For example, chemotherapy is the introduction of an antineoplastic substance into a peripheral artery or vein by a percutaneous approach. In general, the substance introduced into a peripheral artery or vein has a systemic effect.

The *Central Artery* or *Vein* is typically used when the site where the substance is introduced is distant from the point of entry into the artery or vein. For example, the introduction of a substance directly at the site of a clot within an artery or vein using a catheter is coded as an introduction of a thrombolytic substance into a central artery or vein by a percutaneous approach. In general, the substance introduced into a central artery or vein has a local effect.

Approach (Character 5)

The fifth character specifies approaches as defined in the Medical and Surgical section. The approach for intradermal, subcutaneous, and intramuscular introductions (i.e., injections) is *Percutaneous*. If a catheter is placed to introduce a substance into an internal site within the circulatory system, then the approach is also *Percutaneous*. For example, if a catheter is used to introduce contrast directly into the heart for angiography, then the procedure would be coded as a percutaneous introduction of contrast into the heart.

Substance (Character 6)

The sixth character specifies the substance being introduced. Broad categories of substances are defined, such as anesthetic, contrast, dialysate, and blood products such as platelets.

Qualifier (Character 7)

The seventh character is a qualifier and is used to indicate whether the substance is *Autologous* or *Nonautologous*, or to further specify the substance.

Measurement and Monitoring Section (4)

Character Meanings

The seven characters in the Measurement and Monitoring section have the following meaning:

Character	Meaning
1	Section
2	Body System
3	Root Operation
4	Body System
5	Approach
6	Function/Device
7	Qualifier

Measurement and Monitoring section codes represent procedures for determining the level of a physiological or physical function.

Section (Character 1)

Measurement and Monitoring procedure codes have a first character value of *4*.

Body System (Character 2)

The second character values for body system are A, *Physiological Systems* or B, *Physiological Devices*.

Root Operation (Character 3)

There are two root operations in the Measurement and Monitoring section, as defined below:

* *Measurement*: Determining the level of a physiological or physical function at a point in time

* *Monitoring*: Determining the level of a physiological or physical function repetitively over a period of time

Body System (Character 4)

The fourth character specifies the specific body system measured or monitored.

Approach (Character 5)

The fifth character specifies approaches as defined in the Medical and Surgical section.

Function/Device (Character 6)

The sixth character specifies the physiological or physical function being measured or monitored. Examples of physiological or physical functions are *Conductivity, Metabolism, Pulse, Temperature,* and *Volume.* If a device used to perform the measurement or monitoring is inserted and left in, then insertion of the device is coded as a separate Medical and Surgical procedure.

Qualifier (Character 7)

The seventh character qualifier contains specific values as needed to further specify the body part (e.g., central, portal, pulmonary) or a variation of the procedure performed (e.g., ambulatory, stress). Examples of typical procedures coded in this section are EKG, EEG, and cardiac catheterization. An EKG is the measurement of cardiac electrical activity, while an EEG is the measurement of electrical activity of the central nervous system. A cardiac catheterization performed to measure the pressure in the heart is coded as the measurement of cardiac pressure by percutaneous approach.

Extracorporeal or Systemic Assistance and Performance Section (5)

Character Meanings

The seven characters in the Extracorporeal or Systemic Assistance and Performance section have the following meaning:

Character	Meaning
1	Section
2	Body System
3	Root Operation
4	Body System
5	Duration
6	Function
7	Qualifier

In Extracorporeal or Systemic Assistance and Performance procedures, equipment outside the body is used to assist or perform a physiological function. The section includes procedures performed in a critical care setting, such as mechanical ventilation and cardioversion; it also includes other services such as hyperbaric oxygen treatment and hemodialysis.

Section (Character 1)

Extracorporeal or Systemic Assistance and Performance procedure codes have a first character value of *5*.

Body System (Character 2)

The second character value for body system is A, *Physiological Systems.*

Root Operation (Character 3)

There are three root operations in the Extracorporeal or Systemic Assistance and Performance section, as defined below.

- *Assistance*: Taking over a portion of a physiological function by extracorporeal means
- *Performance*: Completely taking over a physiological function by extracorporeal means
- *Restoration*: Returning, or attempting to return, a physiological function to its natural state by extracorporeal means

The root operation *Restoration* contains a single procedure code that identifies extracorporeal cardioversion.

Body System (Character 4)

The fourth character specifies the body system (e.g., cardiac, respiratory) to which extracorporeal or systemic assistance or performance is applied.

Duration (Character 5)

The fifth character specifies the duration of the procedure.

Function (Character 6)

The sixth character specifies the physiological function assisted or performed (e.g., oxygenation, ventilation) during the procedure.

Qualifier (Character 7)

The seventh character qualifier specifies the type of equipment used, if any.

Extracorporeal or Systemic Therapies Section (6)

Character Meanings

The seven characters in the Extracorporeal or Systemic Therapies section have the following meaning:

Character	Meaning
1	Section
2	Body System
3	Root Operation
4	Body System
5	Duration
6	Qualifier
7	Qualifier

In extracorporeal or systemic therapy, equipment outside the body is used for a therapeutic purpose that does not involve the assistance or performance of a physiological function.

Section (Character 1)

Extracorporeal or Systemic Therapy procedure codes have a first character value of 6.

Body System (Character 2)

The second character value for body system is *Physiological Systems.*

Root Operation (Character 3)

There are 11 root operations in the Extracorporeal or Systemic Therapy section, as defined below.

- *Atmospheric Control*: Extracorporeal control of atmospheric pressure and composition

- *Decompression*: Extracorporeal elimination of undissolved gas from body fluids

  Coding note: The root operation *Decompression* involves only one type of procedure: treatment for decompression sickness (the bends) in a hyperbaric chamber.

- *Electromagnetic Therapy*: Extracorporeal treatment by electromagnetic rays

- *Hyperthermia*: Extracorporeal raising of body temperature

  Coding note: The term hyperthermia is used to describe both a temperature imbalance treatment and also as an adjunct radiation treatment for cancer. When treating the temperature imbalance, it is coded to this section; for the cancer treatment, it is coded in section *D Radiation Therapy*.

- *Hypothermia*: Extracorporeal lowering of body temperature

- *Perfusion*: Extracorporeal treatment by diffusion of therapeutic fluid

- *Pheresis*: Extracorporeal separation of blood products

  Coding note: Pheresis may be used for two main purposes: to treat diseases when too much of a blood component is produced (e.g., leukemia) and to remove a blood product such as platelets from a donor, for transfusion into another patient.

- *Phototherapy*: Extracorporeal treatment by light rays

  Coding note: Phototherapy involves using a machine that exposes the blood to light rays outside the body, recirculates it, and then returns it to the body.

- *Shock Wave Therapy*: Extracorporeal treatment by shock waves

- *Ultrasound Therapy*: Extracorporeal treatment by ultrasound

- *Ultraviolet Light Therapy*: Extracorporeal treatment by ultraviolet light

Body System (Character 4)

The fourth character specifies the body system on which the extracorporeal or systemic therapy is performed (e.g., skin, circulatory).

Duration (Character 5)

The fifth character specifies whether the procedure was performed once (single) or multiple times.

Qualifier (Character 6)

The sixth character for Extracorporeal or Systemic Therapies is *No Qualifier*, except for root operation Perfusion which has a sixth character qualifier of *Donor Organ*.

Qualifier (Character 7)

The seventh character qualifier is used in the root operation *Pheresis* to specify the blood component on which pheresis is performed and in the root operation *Ultrasound Therapy* to specify site of treatment.

Osteopathic Section (7)

Character Meanings

The seven characters in the Osteopathic section have the following meaning:

Character	Meaning
1	Section
2	Body System
3	Root Operation
4	Body Region
5	Approach
6	Method
7	Qualifier

Section (Character 1)

Osteopathic procedure codes have a first character value of *7*.

Body System (Character 2)

The body system character contains the value *Anatomical Regions*.

Root Operation (Character 3)

There is only one root operation in the Osteopathic section.

- *Treatment*: Manual treatment to eliminate or alleviate somatic dysfunction and related disorders

Body Region (Character 4)

The fourth character specifies the body region on which the osteopathic treatment is performed.

Approach (Character 5)

The approach for osteopathic treatment is always *External*.

Method (Character 6)

The sixth character specifies the method by which the treatment is accomplished.

Qualifier (Character 7)

The seventh character is not specified in the Osteopathic section and always has the value *None*.

Other Procedures Section (8)

Character Meanings

The seven characters in the Other Procedures section have the following meaning:

Character	Meaning
1	Section
2	Body System
3	Root Operation
4	Body Region
5	Approach
6	Method
7	Qualifier

The Other Procedures section includes acupuncture, suture removal, and in vitro fertilization.

Section (Character 1)

Other Procedure section codes have a first character value of *8*.

Body System (Character 2)

The second character values for body systems are *Physiological Systems and Anatomical Regions* and *Indwelling Device*.

Root Operation (Character 3)

The Other Procedures section has only one root operation, defined as follows:

*   *Other Procedures*: Methodologies that attempt to remediate or cure a disorder or disease.

Body Region (Character 4)

The fourth character contains specified body-region values, and also the body-region value *None*.

Approach (Character 5)

The fifth character specifies approaches as defined in the Medical and Surgical section.

Method (Character 6)

The sixth character specifies the method (e.g., *Acupuncture, Therapeutic Massage*).

Qualifier (Character 7)

The seventh character is a qualifier and contains specific values as needed.

Chiropractic Section (9)

Character Meanings

The seven characters in the Chiropractic section have the following meaning:

Character	Meaning
1	Section
2	Body System
3	Root Operation
4	Body Region
5	Approach
6	Method
7	Qualifier

Section (Character 1)

Chiropractic section procedure codes have a first character value of 9.

Body System (Character 2)

The second character value for body system is *Anatomical Regions*.

Root Operation (Character 3)

There is only one root operation in the *Chiropractic* section.

*   *Manipulation:* Manual procedure that involves a directed thrust to move a joint past the physiological range of motion, without exceeding the anatomical limit.

Body Region (Character 4)

The fourth character specifies the body region on which the chiropractic manipulation is performed.

Approach (Character 5)

The approach for chiropractic manipulation is always *External*.

Method (Character 6)

The sixth character is the method by which the manipulation is accomplished.

Qualifier (Character 7)

The seventh character is not specified in the Chiropractic section and always has the value *None*.

Imaging Section (B)

Character Meanings

The seven characters in Imaging procedures have the following meaning:

Character	Meaning
1	Section
2	Body System
3	Type
4	Body Part
5	Contrast
6	Qualifier
7	Qualifier

Imaging procedures include plain radiography, fluoroscopy, CT, MRI, and ultrasound. Nuclear medicine procedures, including PET, uptakes, and scans, are in the nuclear medicine section. Therapeutic radiation procedure codes are in a separate radiation therapy section.

Section (Character 1)

Imaging procedure codes have a first character value of *B*.

Body System (Character 2)

In the Imaging section, the second character defines the body system, such as *Heart* or *Gastrointestinal System*.

Type (Character 3)

The third character defines the type of imaging procedure (e.g., MRI, ultrasound). The following list includes all types in the *Imaging* section with a definition of each type:

*   *Computerized Tomography (CT Scan)*: Computer reformatted digital display of multiplanar images developed from the capture of multiple exposures of external ionizing radiation

*   *Fluoroscopy*: Single plane or bi-plane real time display of an image developed from the capture of external ionizing radiation on a fluorescent screen. The image may also be stored by either digital or analog means

*   *Magnetic Resonance Imaging (MRI)*: Computer reformatted digital display of multiplanar images developed from the capture of radiofrequency signals emitted by nuclei in a body site excited within a magnetic field

*   *Other Imaging:* Other specified modality for visualizing a body part

- *Plain Radiography*: Planar display of an image developed from the capture of external ionizing radiation on photographic or photoconductive plate
- *Ultrasonography*: Real time display of images of anatomy or flow information developed from the capture of reflected and attenuated high frequency sound waves

Body Part (Character 4)

The fourth character defines the body part with different values for each body system (character 2) value.

Contrast (Character 5)

The fifth character specifies whether the contrast material used in the imaging procedure is *High Osmolar, Low Osmolar,* or *Other Contrast* when applicable.

Qualifier (Character 6)

The sixth character qualifier provides further detail regarding the nature of the substance or technologies used, such as *Unenhanced and Enhanced (contrast), Laser,* or *Intravascular Optical Coherence*.

Qualifier (Character 7)

The seventh character is a qualifier that may be used to specify certain procedural circumstances, the method by which the procedure was performed, or technologies utilized, such as *Intraoperative, Intravascular, or Transesophageal*.

Nuclear Medicine Section (C)

Character Meanings

The seven characters in the Nuclear Medicine section have the following meaning:

Character	Meaning
1	Section
2	Body System
3	Type
4	Body Part
5	Radionuclide
6	Qualifier
7	Qualifier

Nuclear Medicine is the introduction of radioactive material into the body to create an image, to diagnose and treat pathologic conditions, or to assess metabolic functions. The Nuclear Medicine section does not include the introduction of encapsulated radioactive material for the treatment of cancer. These procedures are included in the Radiation Therapy section.

Section (Character 1)

Nuclear Medicine procedure codes have a first character value of *C*.

Body System (Character 2)

The second character specifies the body system on which the nuclear medicine procedure is performed.

Type (Character 3)

The third character indicates the type of nuclear medicine procedure (e.g., planar imaging or nonimaging uptake). The following list includes the types of nuclear medicine procedures with a definition of each type.

- *Nonimaging Nuclear Medicine Assay:* Introduction of radioactive materials into the body for the study of body fluids and blood elements, by the detection of radioactive emissions
- *Nonimaging Nuclear Medicine Probe:* Introduction of radioactive materials into the body for the study of distribution and fate of certain substances by the detection of radioactive emissions; or alternatively, measurement of absorption of radioactive emissions from an external source
- *Nonimaging Nuclear Medicine Uptake:* Introduction of radioactive materials into the body for measurements of organ function, from the detection of radioactive emissions
- *Planar Nuclear Medicine Imaging*: Introduction of radioactive materials into the body for single-plane display of images developed from the capture of radioactive emissions
- *Positron Emission Tomography (PET) Imaging:* Introduction of radioactive materials into the body for three dimensional display of images developed from the simultaneous capture, 180 degrees apart, of radioactive emissions
- *Systemic Nuclear Medicine Therapy:* Introduction of unsealed radioactive materials into the body for treatment
- *Tomographic (Tomo) Nuclear Medicine Imaging*: Introduction of radioactive materials into the body for three dimensional display of images developed from the capture of radioactive emissions

Body Part (Character 4)

The fourth character indicates the body part or body region studied; with regional (e.g., *lower extremity veins*) and combination (e.g., *liver and spleen*) body parts commonly used.

Radionuclide (Character 5)

The fifth character specifies the radionuclide, the radiation source. The option *Other Radionuclide* is provided in the nuclear medicine section for newly approved radionuclides until they can be added to the coding system. If more than one radiopharmaceutical is given to perform the procedure, then more than one code is used.

Qualifier (Character 6 and 7)

The sixth and seventh characters are qualifiers but are not specified in the *Nuclear Medicine* section; the value is always *None*.

Radiation Therapy Section (D)

Character Meanings

The seven characters in the Radiation Therapy section have the following meaning:

Character	Meaning
1	Section
2	Body System
3	Modality
4	Treatment Site
5	Modality Qualifier
6	Isotope
7	Qualifier

Section (Character 1)

Radiation therapy procedure codes have a first character value of *D*.

Body System (Character 2)

The second character specifies the body system (e.g., central nervous system, musculoskeletal) irradiated.

Modality (Character 3)

The third character specifies the general modality used (e.g., beam radiation).

Treatment Site (Character 4)

The fourth character specifies the body part that is the focus of the radiation therapy.

Modality Qualifier (Character 5)

The fifth character further specifies the radiation modality used (e.g., photons, electrons).

Isotope (Character 6)

The sixth character specifies the isotopes introduced into the body, if applicable.

Qualifier (Character 7)

The seventh character may specify whether the procedure was performed intraoperatively.

Physical Rehabilitation and Diagnostic Audiology Section (F)

Character Meanings

The seven characters in the Physical Rehabilitation and Diagnostic Audiology section have the following meaning:

Character	Meaning
1	Section
2	Section Qualifier
3	Type
4	Body System/Region
5	Type Qualifier
6	Equipment
7	Qualifier

Physical rehabilitation procedures include physical therapy, occupational therapy, and speech-language pathology. Osteopathic procedures and chiropractic procedures are in separate sections.

Section (Character 1)

Physical Rehabilitation and Diagnostic Audiology procedure codes have a first character value of *F*.

Section Qualifier (Character 2)

The section qualifier *Rehabilitation* or *Diagnostic Audiology* is specified in the second character.

Type (Character 3)

The third character specifies the type. There are 14 different values, which can be classified into four basic types of rehabilitation and diagnostic audiology procedures, defined as follows:

Assessment: Includes a determination of the patient's diagnosis when appropriate, need for treatment, planning for treatment, periodic assessment, and documentation related to these activities

Assessments are further classified into more than 100 different tests or methods. The majority of these focus on the faculties of hearing and speech, but others focus on various aspects of body function, and on the patient's quality of life, such as muscle performance, neuromotor development, and reintegration skills.

- *Speech Assessment*: Measurement of speech and related functions

- *Motor and/or Nerve Function Assessment*: Measurement of motor, nerve, and related functions

- *Activities of Daily Living Assessment*: Measurement of functional level for activities of daily living

- *Hearing Assessment*: Measurement of hearing and related functions

- *Hearing Aid Assessment*: Measurement of the appropriateness and/or effectiveness of a hearing device

- *Vestibular Assessment*: Measurement of the vestibular system and related functions

Caregiver Training: Educating caregiver with the skills and knowledge used to interact with and assist the patient

Caregiver Training is divided into 18 different broad subjects taught to help a caregiver provide proper patient care.

- *Caregiver Training*: Training in activities to support patient's optimal level of function

Fitting(s): Design, fabrication, modification, selection, and/or application of splint, orthosis, prosthesis, hearing aids, and/or other rehabilitation device

The fifth character used in *Device Fitting* procedures describes the device being fitted rather than the method used to fit the device. Definitions of devices, when provided, are located in the definitions portion of the ICD-10-PCS tables and index, under section F, character 5.

- *Device Fitting*: Fitting of a device designed to facilitate or support achievement of a higher level of function

Treatment: Use of specific activities or methods to develop, improve, and/or restore the performance of necessary functions, compensate for dysfunction and/or minimize debilitation

Treatment procedures include swallowing dysfunction exercises, bathing and showering techniques, wound management, gait training, and a host of activities typically associated with rehabilitation.

- *Speech Treatment*: Application of techniques to improve, augment, or compensate for speech and related functional impairment

- *Motor Treatment*: Exercise or activities to increase or facilitate motor function

- *Activities of Daily Living Treatment*: Exercise or activities to facilitate functional competence for activities of daily living

- *Hearing Treatment*: Application of techniques to improve, augment, or compensate for hearing and related functional impairment

- *Cochlear Implant Treatment*: Application of techniques to improve the communication abilities of individuals with cochlear implant
- *Vestibular Treatment*: Application of techniques to improve, augment, or compensate for vestibular and related functional impairment

The type of treatment includes training as well as activities that restore function.

Body System/Region (Character 4)
The fourth character specifies the body region and/or system on which the procedure is performed.

Type Qualifier (Character 5)
The fifth character is a type qualifier that further specifies the procedure performed. Examples include therapy to improve the range of motion and training for bathing techniques. Refer to appendix J for definitions of these types of procedures.

Equipment (Character 6)
The sixth character specifies the equipment used. Specific equipment is not defined in the equipment value. Instead, broad categories of equipment are specified (e.g., aerobic endurance and conditioning, assistive/adaptive/supportive, etc.)

Qualifier (Character 7)
The seventh character is not specified in the Physical Rehabilitation and Diagnostic Audiology section and always has the value *None*.

Mental Health Section (G)

Character Meanings
The seven characters in the Mental Health section have the following meaning:

Character	Meaning
1	Section
2	Body System
3	Type
4	Qualifier
5	Qualifier
6	Qualifier
7	Qualifier

Section (Character 1)
Mental health procedure codes have a first character value of *G*.

Body System (Character 2)
The second character is used to identify the body system elsewhere in ICD-10-PCS. In this section it always has the value *None*.

Type (Character 3)
The third character specifies the procedure type, such as crisis intervention or counseling. There are 12 types of mental health procedures.

- *Psychological Tests:* The administration and interpretation of standardized psychological tests and measurement instruments for the assessment of psychological function

- *Crisis Intervention:* Treatment of a traumatized, acutely disturbed, or distressed individual for the purpose of short-term stabilization
- *Medication Management:* Monitoring and adjusting the use of medications for the treatment of a mental health disorder
- *Individual Psychotherapy:* Treatment of an individual with a mental health disorder by behavioral, cognitive, psychoanalytic, psychodynamic, or psychophysiological means to improve functioning or well-being
- *Counseling:* The application of psychological methods to treat an individual with normal developmental issues and psychological problems in order to increase function, improve well-being, alleviate distress, maladjustment, or resolve crises
- *Family Psychotherapy:* Treatment that includes one or more family members of an individual with a mental health disorder by behavioral, cognitive, psychoanalytic, psychodynamic, or psychophysiological means to improve functioning or well-being
- *Electroconvulsive Therapy:* The application of controlled electrical voltages to treat a mental health disorder
- *Biofeedback:* Provision of information from the monitoring and regulating of physiological processes in conjunction with cognitive-behavioral techniques to improve patient functioning or well-being
- *Hypnosis:* Induction of a state of heightened suggestibility by auditory, visual, and tactile techniques to elicit an emotional or behavioral response
- *Narcosynthesis:* Administration of intravenous barbiturates in order to release suppressed or repressed thoughts
- *Group Psychotherapy:* Treatment of two or more individuals with a mental health disorder by behavioral, cognitive, psychoanalytic, psychodynamic, or psychophysiological means to improve functioning or well-being
- *Light Therapy:* Application of specialized light treatments to improve functioning or well-being

Qualifier (Character 4)
The fourth character is a qualifier to indicate that counseling was educational or vocational or to indicate type of test or method of therapy.

Qualifier (Character 5, 6 and 7)
The fifth, sixth, and seventh characters are not specified and always have the value *None*.

Substance Abuse Treatment Section (H)

Character Meanings
The seven characters in the Substance Abuse Treatment section have the following meaning:

Character	Meaning
1	Section
2	Body System
3	Type
4	Qualifier
5	Qualifier
6	Qualifier
7	Qualifier

Section (Character 1)
Substance Abuse Treatment codes have a first character value of *H*.

Body System (Character 2)
The second character is used to identify the body system elsewhere in ICD-10-PCS. In this section, it always has the value *None*.

Type (Character 3)
The third character specifies the type of procedure. There are seven values classified in this section, as listed below:

- *Detoxification Services:* Detoxification from alcohol and/or drugs
- *Individual Counseling:* The application of psychological methods to treat an individual with addictive behavior
- *Group Counseling:* The application of psychological methods to treat two or more individuals with addictive behavior
- *Individual Psychotherapy:* Treatment of an individual with addictive behavior by behavioral, cognitive, psychoanalytic, psychodynamic, or psychophysiological means
- *Family Counseling:* The application of psychological methods that includes one or more family members to treat an individual with addictive behavior
- *Medication Management:* Monitoring and adjusting the use of replacement medications for the treatment of addiction
- *Pharmacotherapy:* The use of replacement medications for the treatment of addiction

Qualifier (Character 4)
The fourth character further specifies the procedure type. These qualifier values vary dependent upon the Root Type procedure (Character 3). Root type 2, *Detoxification Services* contains only the value Z, *None* and Root type 6, *Family Counseling* contains only the value 3, *Other Family Counseling*, whereas the remainder Root Type procedures include multiple possible values.

Qualifier (Character 5, 6 and 7)
The fifth through seventh characters are designated as qualifiers but are never specified, so they always have the value *None*.

New Technology Section (X)

General Information
Section X New Technology is a section added to ICD-10-PCS beginning October 1, 2015. The new section provides a place for codes that uniquely identify procedures requested via the New Technology Application Process or that capture other new technologies not currently classified in ICD-10-PCS.

Section X does not introduce any new coding concepts or unusual guidelines for correct coding. In fact, Section X codes maintain continuity with the other sections in ICD-10-PCS by using the same root operation and body part values as their closest counterparts in other sections of ICD-10-PCS. For example, the codes for the infusion of ceftazidime-avibactam, use the same root operation (Introduction) and body part values (Central Vein and Peripheral Vein) in section X as the infusion codes in section 3 Administration, which are their closest counterparts in the other sections of ICD-10-PCS.

Character Meanings
The seven characters in the new technology section have the following meaning:

Character	Meaning
1	Section
2	Body System
3	Root Operation
4	Body Part
5	Approach
6	Device/Substance/Technology
7	Qualifier

Section (Character 1)
New technology procedure codes have a first character value of *X*.

Body System (Character 2)
The second character values for body system combine the uses of body system, body region, and physiological system as specified in other sections in ICD-10-PCS.

Root Operation (Character 3)
The third character utilizes the same root operation values as their counterparts in other sections of ICD-10-PCS.

Body Part (Character 4)
The fourth character specifies the same body part values as their closest counterparts in other sections of ICD-10-PCS.

Approach (Character 5)
The fifth character specifies approaches as defined in the Medical and Surgical section.

Device/Substance/Technology (Character 6)
The sixth character specifies the key feature of the new technology procedure. It may be specified as a new device, a new substance, or other new technology. Examples of sixth character values are *blinatumomab antineoplastic immunotherapy*, *orbital atherectomy technology*, and *intraoperative knee replacement sensor*.

Qualifier (Character 7)
The seventh character qualifier is used exclusively to specify the new technology group, a number or letter that changes each year that new technology codes are added to the system. For example, Section X codes added for the first year have the seventh character value 1, *New Technology Group 1*, and the next year that Section X codes are added have the seventh character value 2, *New Technology Group 2*, and so on. Changing the seventh character value to a unique letter or number every year that there are new codes in the new technology section allows the ICD-10-PCS to "recycle" the values in the third, fourth, and sixth characters as needed.

New Technology Coding Instruction
Section X codes are standalone codes. They are not supplemental codes. Section X codes fully represent the specific procedure described in the code title, and do not require any additional codes from other sections of ICD-10-PCS. When section X contains a code title which describes a specific new technology procedure, only that X code is reported for the procedure. There is no need to report a broader, non-specific code in another section of ICD-10-PCS.

For example, code XWØ4321 Introduction of Ceftazidime-Avibactam Anti-infective into Central Vein, Percutaneous Approach, New Technology Group 1, would be reported to indicate that Ceftazidime-Avibactam Anti-infective was administered via central vein. A separate code from table 3EØ in the Administration section of ICD-10-PCS would not be reported in addition to this code. The X section code fully identifies the administration of the ceftazidime-avibactam antibiotic, and no additional code is needed.

The New Technology section codes are easily found by looking in the ICD-10-PCS Index or the Tables. In the Index, the name of the new technology device, substance or technology for a section X code is included as a main term. In addition, all codes in section X are listed under the main term New Technology. The new technology code index entry for ceftazidime-avibactam is shown below.

Ceftazidime-Avibactam Anti-infective XWØ

New Technology
    Ceftazidime-Avibactam Anti-infective XWØ

ICD-10-PCS Index and Tabular Format

The *ICD-10-PCS: The Complete Official Code Set* is based on the official version of the International Classification of Diseases, 10th Revision, Procedure Classification System, issued by the U.S. Department of Health and Human Services, Centers for Medicare and Medicaid Services. This book is consistent with the content of the government's version of ICD-10-PCS and follows their official format.

Index

The Alphabetic Index can be used to locate the appropriate table containing all the information necessary to construct a procedure code, however, the PCS tables should always be consulted to find the most appropriate valid code. Users may choose a valid code directly from the tables—he or she need not consult the index before proceeding to the tables to complete the code.

Main Terms

The Alphabetic Index reflects the structure of the tables. Therefore, the index is organized as an alphabetic listing. The index:

- Is based on the value of the third character
- Contains common procedure terms
- Lists anatomic sites
- Uses device terms

The main terms in the Alphabetic Index are root operations, root procedure types, or common procedure names. In addition, anatomic sites from the Body Part Key and device terms from the Device Key have been added for ease of use.

Examples:

> *Resection* (root operation)
>
> *Fluoroscopy* (root type)
>
> *Prostatectomy* (common procedure name)
>
> *Brachiocephalic artery* (body part)
>
> *Bard® Dulex™ mesh* (device)

The index provides at least the first three or four values of the code, and some entries may provide complete valid codes. However, the user should always consult the appropriate table to verify that the most appropriate valid code has been selected.

Root Operation and Procedure Type Main Terms

For the *Medical and Surgical* and related sections, the root operation values are used as main terms in the index. The subterms under the root operation main terms are body parts. For the Ancillary section of the tables, the main terms in the index are the general type of procedure performed.

Examples:

> **Biofeedback** GZC9ZZZ
> **Destruction**
>   Acetabulum
>   Left ØQ55
>   Right ØQ54
>   Adenoids ØC5Q
>   Ampulla of Vater ØF5C
> **Planar Nuclear Medicine Imaging**
>   Abdomen CW1Ø

See Reference

The second type of term in the index uses common procedure names, such as "appendectomy" or "fundoplication." These common terms are listed as main terms with a "see" reference noting the PCS root operations that are possible valid code tables based on the objective of the procedure.

Examples:

> **Tendonectomy**
>   *see* Excision, Tendons ØLB
>   *see* Resection, Tendons ØLT

Use Reference

The index also lists anatomic sites from the Body Part Key and device terms from the Device Key. These terms are listed with a "use" reference. The purpose of these references is to act as an additional reference to the terms located in the Appendix Keys. The term provided is the Body Part value or Device value to be selected when constructing a procedure code using the code tables. This type of index reference is not intended to direct the user to another term in the index, but to provide guidance regarding character value selection. Therefore, "use" references generally do not refer to specific valid code tables.

Examples:

> **CoAxia NeuroFlo catheter**
>   *use* Intraluminal Device
> **Epitrochlear lymph node**
>   *use* Lymphatic, Left Upper Extremity
>   *use* Lymphatic, Right Upper Extremity
> **SynCardia Total Artificial Heart**
>   *use* Synthetic Substitute

Code Tables

ICD-10-PCS contains 17 sections of Code Tables organized by general type of procedure. The first three characters of a procedure code define each table. The tables consist of columns providing the possible last four characters of codes and rows providing valid values for each character. Within a PCS table, valid codes include all combinations of choices in characters 4 through 7 contained in the same row of the table. All seven characters must be specified to form a valid code.

There are three main sections of tables:

- Medical and Surgical section:
  - *Medical and Surgical* (Ø)
- Medical and Surgical-related sections:
  - *Obstetrics* (1)
  - *Placement* (2)
  - *Administration* (3)
  - *Measurement and Monitoring* (4)
  - *Extracorporeal or Systemic Assistance and Performance* (5)
  - *Extracorporeal or Systemic Therapies* (6)
  - *Osteopathic* (7)
  - *Other Procedures* (8)
  - *Chiropractic* (9)

- Ancillary sections:
  - — *Imaging* (B)
  - — *Nuclear Medicine* (C)
  - — *Radiation Therapy* (D)
  - — *Physical Rehabilitation and Diagnostic Audiology* (F)
  - — *Mental Health* (G)
  - — *Substance Abuse Treatment* (H)
- New Technology section:
  - — *New Technology* (X)

The first three character values define each table. The root operation or root type designated for each table is accompanied by its official definition.

Example:

Table ØØF provides codes for procedures on the central nervous system that involve breaking up of solid matter into pieces:

Character 1, Section	Ø: Medical and Surgical
Character 2, Body System	Ø: Central Nervous System and Cranial Nerves
Character 3, Root Operation	F: Fragmentation: Breaking solid matter in a body part into pieces

Tables are arranged numerically, then alphabetically.

When reviewing tables, the user should keep in mind that:

- Some tables may cover multiple pages in the code book—to ensure maximum clarity about character choices, valid entries do not split rows between pages. For instance, the entire table of valid characters completing a code beginning with 4A1 is split between two pages, but the split is between, not within, rows. This means that all the valid sixth and seventh characters for, say, body system *Arterial* (3) and approach *External* (X) are contained on one page.
- Individual entries may be listed in several horizontal "selection" lines.
- When a table is continued onto another page, a note to this effect has been added in red.

Body Part Definitions:

An exclusive Optum360 feature in the tables is the incorporation of the body part definitions provided in appendix E into the Medical and Surgical section (Ø) tables under their appropriate body part characters in the first column (character 4). This provides the user a direct reference to all anatomical descriptions, terms, and sites that could be coded to that particular body part value.

Paired body parts typically have values for the right and left side and in some cases a value for bilateral. These paired body parts often have the same list of inclusive body part definitions. When there are paired body parts with the same body part definitions, the first listed body part (usually the right side) contains the list of body part definitions while the second listed body part (usually the left side) contains a **See** instruction. This **See** instruction references the body part value that contains the body part definitions. In the table below, body part value P – Upper Eyelid, Left is followed by a **See** instruction that states **See** *N Upper Eyelid, Right*. All body part descriptions under value N also apply to body part value P.

Example:

Ø   Medical and Surgical
8   Eye
M   Reattachment   Definition: Putting back in or on all or a portion of a separated body part to its normal location or other suitable location
    Explanation: Vascular circulation and nervous pathways may or may not be reestablished

Body Part Character 4	Approach Character 5	Device Character 6	Qualifier Character 7
N Upper Eyelid, Right Lateral canthus Levator palpebrae superioris muscle Orbicularis oculi muscle Superior tarsal plate **P Upper Eyelid, Left** *See N Upper Eyelid, Right* **Q Lower Eyelid, Right** Inferior tarsal plate Medial canthus **R Lower Eyelid, Left** *See Q Lower Eyelid, Right*	**X External**	**Z No Device**	**Z No Qualifier**

ICD-10-PCS Additional Features

Use of Official Sources

Color-coding, symbol, and other annotations in this manual that identify coding and reimbursement issues are derived from various official federal government sources, including the *Federal Register*, volume 85, number 104, May 29, 2020 ("Hospital Inpatient Prospective Payment Systems for Acute Care Hospitals and the Long Term Care Hospital Prospective Payment System and Proposed Policy Changes and Fiscal Year 2021 Rates; Proposed Rule") and the proposed, version 38, MS-DRG Grouper software, Definitions Manual files and Medicare Code Editor (MCE) files published with the fiscal 2021 IPPS proposed rule. For the most current files related to IPPS, please refer to the following:

- FY2021 IPPS Final Rule
  https://www.cms.gov/Medicare/Medicare-Fee-for-Service-Payment/AcuteInpatientPPS/IPPS-Regulations-and-Notices

- FY2021 Final Version 38, MS-DRG Grouper software
  https://www.cms.gov/Medicare/Medicare-Fee-for-Service-Payment/AcuteInpatientPPS/MS-DRG-Classifications-and-Software

Table Notations

Many tables in ICD-10-PCS contain color or symbol annotations that may aid in code selection, provide clinical or coding information, or alert the coder to reimbursement issues affected by the PCS code assignment. These annotations are most often displayed on or next to a character 4 value. Some character 4 values may have more than one annotation.

Refer to the color/symbol legend at the bottom of each page in the tables section for an abridged description of each color and symbol.

Annotation Box

An annotation box has been appended to all tables that contain color-coding or symbol annotations. The color bar or symbol attached to a character 4 value is provided in the box, as well as a list of the valid PCS code(s) to which that edit applies. The box may also list conditional criteria that must be met to satisfy the edit.

For example, see Table 00F. Four character 4 body part values have a gray color bar. In the annotation box below the table, the gray color bar is defined as "Non-OR," or a nonoperating room procedure edit. Following the Non-OR annotation are the PCS codes that are considered nonoperating room procedures from that row of Table 00F.

Bracketed Code Notation

The use of bracketed codes is an efficient convention to provide all valid character value alternatives for a specific set of circumstances. The character values in the brackets correspond to the valid values for the character in the position the bracket appears.

Examples:

In the annotation box for Table 00F the Noncovered Procedure edit (NC) applies to codes represented in the bracketed code 00F[3,4,5,6]XZZ.

00F[3,4,5,6]XZZ   Fragmentation in (Central Nervous System and Cranial Nerves), External Approach

The valid fourth character values (Body Part) that may be selected for this specific circumstance are as follows:

3	Epidural Space, Intracranial
4	Subdural Space, Intracranial
5	Subarachnoid Space, Intracranial
6	Cerebral Ventricle

The fragmentation of matter in the spinal canal, Body Part value U, is not included in the noncovered procedure code edits.

Color-Coding/Symbols

New and Revised Text

To highlight changes to the PCS tables for the current year, the new and revised text is provided in green font.

Medicare Code Edits

Medicare administrative contractors (MACs) and many payers use Medicare code edits to check the coding accuracy on claims. The coding edits provided in this manual include only those directly related to ICD-10-PCS codes used for acute care hospital inpatient admissions. These edits are based on the proposed, version 38, Medicare Code Editor (MCE) files published with the fiscal 2021 IPPS proposed rule.

The PCS related Medicare code edits are listed below:

- Invalid procedure code
- *Sex conflict
- *Questionable obstetric admission
- *Noncovered procedure
- *Limited coverage procedure

Starred edits above that are related to PCS issues are identified in this manual by symbols as described below.

Sex Edit Symbols
The sex edit symbols below are used to detect inconsistencies between the patient's sex and the procedure. The symbols below most often appear to the right of the body part (character 4) value but may also be found to the right of the qualifier (character 7) value:

♂   Male procedure only

♀   Female procedure only

QA Questionable Obstetric Admission
An inpatient admission is considered questionable when a vaginal or cesarean delivery code is assigned without a corresponding secondary diagnosis code describing the outcome of delivery. Both a delivery (ICD-10-PCS) code and an outcome-of-delivery (ICD-10-CM) code must be present to avoid errors in MS-DRG assignment. This symbol is found only in the Obstetrics Section, appearing to the right of the body part (character 4) value.

NC Noncovered Procedure
Medicare does not cover all procedures. However, some noncovered procedures, due to the presence of certain diagnoses, are reimbursed.

LC **Limited Coverage**

For certain procedures whose medical complexity and serious nature incur extraordinary associated costs, Medicare limits coverage to a portion of the cost. The limited coverage edit indicates the type of limited coverage.

ICD-10 MS-DRG Definitions Manual Edits

An MS-DRG is assigned based on specific patient attributes, such as principal diagnosis, secondary diagnoses, procedures, and discharge status. The attributes (edits) provided in this manual include only those directly related to ICD-10-PCS codes used for acute care hospital inpatient admissions. These edits are based on the proposed, version 38, MS-DRG Grouper software and Definitions Manual published with the fiscal 2021 IPPS proposed rule.

Non-Operating Room Procedures Not Affecting MS-DRG Assignment

In the Medical and Surgical section (ØØ1–ØYW) and the Obstetric section (1Ø2–1ØY) tables **only,** ICD-10-PCS procedures codes that DO NOT affect MS-DRG assignment are identified by a gray color bar over the body part (character 4) value and are considered non-operating room (non-OR) procedures.

NOTE: The majority of the ICD-10-PCS codes in the Medical and Surgical-Related, Ancillary and New Technology section tables are non-operating room procedures that do not typically affect MS-DRG assignment. Only the Valid Operating Room and DRG Non-Operating Room procedures are highlighted in these sections, *see* Non-Operating Room Procedures Affecting MS-DRG Assignment and Valid OR Procedure description below.

Non-Operating Room Procedures Affecting MS-DRG Assignment

Some ICD-10-PCS procedure codes, although considered non-operating room procedures, may still affect MS-DRG assignment. In all sections of the ICD-10-PCS book, these procedures are identified by a **purple color bar** over the body part (character 4) value.

Valid OR Procedure

In the Medical and Surgical-Related (2WØ–9WB), Ancillary (BØØ–HZ9) and New Technology (X2A–XYØ) section tables **only**, any codes that are considered a valid operating room procedure are identified with a **blue color bar** over the body part (character 4) value and will affect MS-DRG assignment. All codes without a color bar (blue or purple) are considered non-operating room procedures.

Hospital-Acquired Condition Related Procedures

Procedures associated with hospital-acquired conditions (HAC) are identified with the **yellow color bar** over the body part (character 4) value. Appendix K provides each specific HAC category and its associated ICD-10-CM and ICD-10-PCS codes.

Combination Only

Some ICD-10-PCS procedure codes that describe non-operating room procedures can group to a specific MS-DRG but only when used in combination with certain other ICD-10-PCS procedure codes. Such codes are designated by a **red color bar** over the body part (character 4) value.

⊞ **Combination Member**

A combination member, which can be either a valid operating room procedure or a non-operating room procedure, is an ICD-10-PCS procedure code that can influence MS-DRG assignment either on its own or in combination with other specific ICD-10-PCS procedure codes. Combination member codes are designated by a plus sign (⊞) to the right of the body part (character 4) value.

Note: In the few instances when a code is both a combination member and a non-operating room procedure affecting the MS-DRG assignment, the body part (character 4) value will have a purple color bar and the combination member icon.

See Appendix L for Procedure Combinations

Under certain circumstances, more than one procedure code is needed in order to group to a specific MS-DRG. When codes within a table have been identified as a Combination Only (**red color bar**) or Combination Member (⊞) code, there is also a footnote instructing the coder to *see Appendix L*. Appendix L contains tables that identify the other procedure codes needed in the combination and the title and number of the MS-DRG to which the combination will group.

Other Table Notations

AHA Coding Clinic:

Official citations from AHA's *Coding Clinic for ICD-10-CM/PCS* have been provided at the beginning of each section, when applicable. Each specific citation is listed below a header identifying the table to which that particular *Coding Clinic* citation applies. The citations appear in purple type with the year, quarter, and page of the reference as well as the title of the question as it appears in that *Coding Clinic's* table of contents. *Coding Clinic* citations included in this edition have been updated through second quarter 2020.

Appendixes

The resources described below have been included as appendixes for *ICD-10-PCS The Complete Official Code Set*. These resources further instruct the coder on the appropriate application of the ICD-10-PCS code set.

Appendix A: Components of the Medical and Surgical Approach Definitions

This resource further defines the approach characters used in the Medical and Surgical (Ø) section. Complementing the detailed definition of the approach, additional information includes whether or not instrumentation is a part of the approach, the typical access location, the method used to initiate the approach, related procedural examples, and illustrations all of which will help the user determine the appropriate approach value.

Appendix B: Root Operation Definitions

This resource is a compilation of all root operations found in the Medical and Surgical-related sections (Ø-9) of this PCS manual. It provides a definition and in some cases a more detailed explanation of the root operation, to better reflect the purpose or objective. Examples of related procedure(s) may also be provided.

Appendix C: Comparison of Medical and Surgical Root Operations

The Medical and Surgical root operations are divided into groups that share similar attributes. These groups, and the root operations in each group, are listed in this resource along with information identifying the target of the root operation, the action used to perform the root operation, any clarification or further explanation on the objective of the root operation, and procedure examples.

Appendix D: Body Part Key

When an anatomical term or description is provided in the documentation but does not have a specific body part character within a table, the user can reference this resource to search for the anatomical description or site noted in the documentation to determine if there is a specific PCS body part character (character 4) to which the anatomical description or site could be coded.

Appendix E: Body Part Definitions

This resource is the reverse look-up of the Body Part Key. Each table in the Medical and Surgical section (Ø) of the PCS manual contains anatomical terms linked to a body part character or value, for example, in Table ØBB the Body Part (character 4) of 1 is Trachea. The body part Trachea may have anatomical structures or descriptions that may be used in procedure documentation instead of the term trachea. The Body Part Definitions list other anatomical structures or synonyms that are included in specific ICD-10-PCS body part values. According to the body part definitions, in the example above, cricoid cartilage is included in the Trachea (character 1) body part.

Appendix F: Device Classification

This resource provides an explanation of how a device is defined in the ICD-10-PCS classification along with two tables. The first table groups devices used in the ICD-10-PCS tables into general categories, including a definition of each device type and related examples. The second table provides definitions of transplant and grafting tissue types and associated terminology that may be found in the documentation.

Appendix G: Device Key and Aggregation Table

The Device Key helps users code the appropriate PCS sixth character for device. Devices are listed alphabetically by brand name or commonly used medical terminology and are translated to the appropriate PCS language or value. The key also reflects the body system where the device is located. For example, a SAPIEN valve used for transaortic valve replacement translates to Zooplastic Tissue in Heart and Great Vessels.

The Aggregation Table crosswalks specific device character value definitions for specific root operations in a specific body system to the more general device character value to be used when the root operation covers a wide range of body parts and the device character represents an entire family of devices.

Appendix H: Device Definitions

This resource is a reverse look-up to the Device Key. The user may reference this resource to see all the specific devices that may be grouped to a particular device character (character 6).

Example:
The operative report states, "An internal fixation device was used to repair a fractured femur. Kirschner wire, bone screws and neutralization plate all used and left in the bone at the end of the procedure. "

Although PCS requires all devices left in the body to be coded and the operative report lists three different devices, a check in the device definitions shows that all of these devices are included in the PCS value "Internal Fixation Device" and require only one code.

Appendix I: Substance Key/Substance Definitions

The Substance Key lists substances by trade name or synonym and relates them to a PCS character in the Administration (3) or New Technology (X) section in the Substance (sixth character) or Qualifier (seventh character) column.

The Substance Definitions table is the reverse look-up of the substance key, relating all substance categories, the sixth- or seventh character values, to all trade name or synonyms that may be classified to that particular character.

Appendix J: Sections B-H Character Definitions

In each ancillary section (B-H) the characters in a particular column may have different meanings depending on which section the user is working from. This resource provides the values for the characters in these sections as well as a definition of the character value.

Appendix K: Hospital Acquired Conditions

Hospital acquired conditions (HACs) are conditions that are considered reasonably preventable when occurring during the hospital admission and may prevent a case from grouping to a higher-paying MS-DRG. In certain instances the HACs are conditional, requiring a specific ICD-10-CM diagnosis code in combination with a specific ICD-10-PCS procedure code. This resource identifies these conditional HACs, listing the diagnosis and procedure codes that, in combination, may trigger a HAC edit. All codes, ICD-10-CM and ICD-10-PCS, are listed with their full descriptions.

Appendix L: Procedure Combination Tables

The procedure combination tables provided in this resource illustrate certain procedure combinations that must occur in order to assign a specific MS-DRG.

Appendix M: Coding Exercises and Answers

This resource provides the coding exercises with answers, and in some cases a brief explanation as to the reason that particular code was used.

ICD-10-PCS Official Guidelines for Coding and Reporting 2021

Narrative changes appear in **bold** text.

The Centers for Medicare and Medicaid Services (CMS) and the National Center for Health Statistics (NCHS), two departments within the U.S. Federal Government's Department of Health and Human Services (DHHS) provide the following guidelines for coding and reporting using the International Classification of Diseases, 10th Revision, Procedure Coding System (ICD-10-PCS). These guidelines should be used as a companion document to the official version of the ICD-10-PCS as published on the CMS website. The ICD-10-PCS is a procedure classification published by the United States for classifying procedures performed in hospital inpatient health care settings.

These guidelines have been approved by the four organizations that make up the Cooperating Parties for the ICD-10-PCS: the American Hospital Association (AHA), the American Health Information Management Association (AHIMA), CMS, and NCHS.

These guidelines are a set of rules that have been developed to accompany and complement the official conventions and instructions provided within the ICD-10-PCS itself. They are intended to provide direction that is applicable in most circumstances. However, there may be unique circumstances where exceptions are applied. The instructions and conventions of the classification take precedence over guidelines. These guidelines are based on the coding and sequencing instructions in the Tables, Index and Definitions of ICD-10-PCS, but provide additional instruction. Adherence to these guidelines when assigning ICD-10-PCS procedure codes is required under the Health Insurance Portability and Accountability Act (HIPAA). The procedure codes have been adopted under HIPAA for hospital inpatient healthcare settings. A joint effort between the healthcare provider and the coder is essential to achieve complete and accurate documentation, code assignment, and reporting of diagnoses and procedures. These guidelines have been developed to assist both the healthcare provider and the coder in identifying those procedures that are to be reported. The importance of consistent, complete documentation in the medical record cannot be overemphasized. Without such documentation accurate coding cannot be achieved.

Conventions

A1. ICD-10-PCS codes are composed of seven characters. Each character is an axis of classification that specifies information about the procedure performed. Within a defined code range, a character specifies the same type of information in that axis of classification.

Example:
The fifth axis of classification specifies the approach in sections Ø through 4 and 7 through 9 of the system.

A2. One of 34 possible values can be assigned to each axis of classification in the seven-character code: they are the numbers Ø through 9 and the alphabet (except I and O because they are easily confused with the numbers 1 and Ø). The number of unique values used in an axis of classification differs as needed.

Example:
Where the fifth axis of classification specifies the approach, seven different approach values are currently used to specify the approach.

A3. The valid values for an axis of classification can be added to as needed.

Example:
If a significantly distinct type of device is used in a new procedure, a new device value can be added to the system.

A4. As with words in their context, the meaning of any single value is a combination of its axis of classification and any preceding values on which it may be dependent.

Example:
The meaning of a body part value in the Medical and Surgical section is always dependent on the body system value. The body part value Ø in the Central Nervous body system specifies Brain and the body part value Ø in the Peripheral Nervous body system specifies Cervical Plexus.

A5. As the system is expanded to become increasingly detailed, over time more values will depend on preceding values for their meaning.

Example:
In the Lower Joints body system, the device value 3 in the root operation Insertion specifies Infusion Device and the device value 3 in the root operation Replacement specifies Ceramic Synthetic Substitute.

A6. The purpose of the alphabetic index is to locate the appropriate table that contains all information necessary to construct a procedure code. The PCS Tables should always be consulted to find the most appropriate valid code.

A7. It is not required to consult the index first before proceeding to the tables to complete the code. A valid code may be chosen directly from the tables.

A8. All seven characters must be specified to be a valid code. If the documentation is incomplete for coding purposes, the physician should be queried for the necessary information.

A9. Within a PCS table, valid codes include all combinations of choices in characters 4 through 7 contained in the same row of the table. In the example below, ØJHT3VZ is a valid code, and ØJHW3VZ is *not* a valid code.

Section:	Ø	**Medical and Surgical**
Body System:	J	**Subcutaneous Tissue and Fascia**
Operation:	H	**Insertion** Putting in a nonbiological appliance that monitors, assists, performs, or prevents a physiological function but does not physically take the place of a body part

Body Part		Approach		Device		Qualifier	
S Subcutaneous Tissue and Fascia, Head and Neck **V** Subcutaneous Tissue and Fascia, Upper Extremity **W** Subcutaneous Tissue and Fascia, Lower Extremity		**Ø** Open **3** Percutaneous		**1** Radioactive Element **3** Infusion Device **Y** Other Device		**Z** No Qualifier	
T Subcutaneous Tissue and Fascia, Trunk		**Ø** Open **3** Percutaneous		**1** Radioactive Element **3** Infusion Device **V** Infusion Pump **Y** Other Device		**Z** No Qualifier	

A10. "And," when used in a code description, means "and/or," except when used to describe a combination of multiple body parts for which separate values exist for each body part (e.g., Skin and Subcutaneous Tissue used as a qualifier, where there are separate body part values for "Skin" and "Subcutaneous Tissue").

Example:

Lower Arm and Wrist Muscle means lower arm and/or wrist muscle.

A11. Many of the terms used to construct PCS codes are defined within the system. It is the coder's responsibility to determine what the documentation in the medical record equates to in the PCS definitions. The physician is not expected to use the terms used in PCS code descriptions, nor is the coder required to query the physician when the correlation between the documentation and the defined PCS terms is clear.

Example:

When the physician documents "partial resection" the coder can independently correlate "partial resection" to the root operation Excision without querying the physician for clarification.

Medical and Surgical Section Guidelines (section Ø)

B2. Body System

General guidelines

B2.1a. The procedure codes in Anatomical Regions, General, Anatomical Regions, Upper Extremities and Anatomical Regions, Lower Extremities can be used when the procedure is performed on an anatomical region rather than a specific body part, or on the rare occasion when no information is available to support assignment of a code to a specific body part.

Examples:

Chest tube drainage of the pleural cavity is coded to the root operation Drainage found in the body system Anatomical Regions, General.

Suture repair of the abdominal wall is coded to the root operation Repair in the body system Anatomical Regions, General.

Amputation of the foot is coded to the root operation Detachment in the body system Anatomical Regions, Lower Extremities.

B2.1b. Where the general body part values "upper" and "lower" are provided as an option in the Upper Arteries, Lower Arteries, Upper Veins, Lower Veins, Muscles and Tendons body systems, "upper" or "lower" specifies body parts located above or below the diaphragm respectively.

Example:

Vein body parts above the diaphragm are found in the Upper Veins body system; vein body parts below the diaphragm are found in the Lower Veins body system.

B3. Root Operation

General guidelines

B3.1a. In order to determine the appropriate root operation, the full definition of the root operation as contained in the PCS Tables must be applied.

B3.1b. Components of a procedure specified in the root operation definition or explanation as integral to that root operation are not coded separately. Procedural steps necessary to reach the operative site

and close the operative site, including anastomosis of a tubular body part, are also not coded separately.

Examples:

Resection of a joint as part of a joint replacement procedure is included in the root operation definition of Replacement and is not coded separately.

Laparotomy performed to reach the site of an open liver biopsy is not coded separately.

In a resection of sigmoid colon with anastomosis of descending colon to rectum, the anastomosis is not coded separately.

Multiple procedures

B3.2. During the same operative episode, multiple procedures are coded if:

a. The same root operation is performed on different body parts as defined by distinct values of the body part character.

   Examples:

   Diagnostic excision of liver and pancreas are coded separately.

   Excision of lesion in the ascending colon and excision of lesion in the transverse colon are coded separately.

b. The same root operation is repeated in multiple body parts, and those body parts are separate and distinct body parts classified to a single ICD-10-PCS body part value.

   Examples:

   Excision of the sartorius muscle and excision of the gracilis muscle are both included in the upper leg muscle body part value, and multiple procedures are coded.

   Extraction of multiple toenails are coded separately.

c. Multiple root operations with distinct objectives are performed on the same body part.

   Example:

   Destruction of sigmoid lesion and bypass of sigmoid colon are coded separately.

d. The intended root operation is attempted using one approach but is converted to a different approach.

   Example:

   Laparoscopic cholecystectomy converted to an open cholecystectomy is coded as percutaneous endoscopic Inspection and open Resection.

Discontinued or incomplete procedures

B3.3. If the intended procedure is discontinued or otherwise not completed, code the procedure to the root operation performed. If a procedure is discontinued before any other root operation is performed, code the root operation Inspection of the body part or anatomical region inspected.

Example:

A planned aortic valve replacement procedure is discontinued after the initial thoracotomy and before any incision is made in the heart muscle, when the patient becomes hemodynamically unstable. This procedure is coded as an open Inspection of the mediastinum.

Biopsy procedures

B3.4a. Biopsy procedures are coded using the root operations Excision, Extraction, or Drainage and the qualifier Diagnostic.

Examples:

Fine needle aspiration biopsy of fluid in the lung is coded to the root operation Drainage with the qualifier Diagnostic.

Biopsy of bone marrow is coded to the root operation Extraction with the qualifier Diagnostic.

Lymph node sampling for biopsy is coded to the root operation Excision with the qualifier Diagnostic.

Biopsy followed by more definitive treatment

B3.4b. If a diagnostic Excision, Extraction, or Drainage procedure (biopsy) is followed by a more definitive procedure, such as Destruction, Excision or Resection at the same procedure site, both the biopsy and the more definitive treatment are coded.

Example:
Biopsy of breast followed by partial mastectomy at the same procedure site, both the biopsy and the partial mastectomy procedure are coded.

Overlapping body layers

B3.5. If root operations such as Excision, Extraction, Repair or Inspection are performed on overlapping layers of the musculoskeletal system, the body part specifying the deepest layer is coded.

Example:
Excisional debridement that includes skin and subcutaneous tissue and muscle is coded to the muscle body part.

Bypass procedures

B3.6a. Bypass procedures are coded by identifying the body part bypassed "from" and the body part bypassed "to." The fourth character body part specifies the body part bypassed from, and the qualifier specifies the body part bypassed to.

Example:
Bypass from stomach to jejunum, stomach is the body part and jejunum is the qualifier.

B3.6b. Coronary artery bypass procedures are coded differently than other bypass procedures as described in the previous guideline. Rather than identifying the body part bypassed from, the body part identifies the number of coronary arteries bypassed to, and the qualifier specifies the vessel bypassed from.

Example:
Aortocoronary artery bypass of the left anterior descending coronary artery and the obtuse marginal coronary artery is classified in the body part axis of classification as two coronary arteries, and the qualifier specifies the aorta as the body part bypassed from.

B3.6c. If multiple coronary arteries are bypassed, a separate procedure is coded for each coronary artery that uses a different device and/or qualifier.

Example:
Aortocoronary artery bypass and internal mammary coronary artery bypass are coded separately.

Control vs. more definitive root operations

B3.7. The root operation Control is defined as, "Stopping, or attempting to stop, postprocedural or other acute bleeding." If an attempt to stop postprocedural or other acute bleeding is unsuccessful, and to stop the bleeding requires performing a more definitive root operation, such as Bypass, Detachment, Excision, Extraction, Reposition, Replacement, or Resection, then the more definitive root operation is coded instead of Control.

Example:
Resection of spleen to stop bleeding is coded to Resection instead of Control.

Excision vs. Resection

B3.8. PCS contains specific body parts for anatomical subdivisions of a body part, such as lobes of the lungs or liver and regions of the intestine. Resection of the specific body part is coded whenever all of the body part is cut out or off, rather than coding Excision of a less specific body part.

Example:
Left upper lung lobectomy is coded to Resection of Upper Lung Lobe, Left rather than Excision of Lung, Left.

Excision for graft

B3.9. If an autograft is obtained from a different procedure site in order to complete the objective of the procedure, a separate procedure is coded, except when the seventh character qualifier value in the ICD-10-PCS table fully specifies the site from which the autograft was obtained.

Examples:
Coronary bypass with excision of saphenous vein graft, excision of saphenous vein is coded separately.

Replacement of breast with autologous deep inferior epigastric artery perforator (DIEP) flap, excision of the DIEP flap is not coded separately. The seventh character qualifier value Deep Inferior Epigastric Artery Perforator Flap in the Replacement table fully specifies the site of the autograft harvest.

Fusion procedures of the spine

B3.10a. The body part coded for a spinal vertebral joint(s) rendered immobile by a spinal fusion procedure is classified by the level of the spine (e.g. thoracic). There are distinct body part values for a single vertebral joint and for multiple vertebral joints at each spinal level.

Example:
Body part values specify Lumbar Vertebral Joint, Lumbar Vertebral Joints, 2 or More and Lumbosacral Vertebral Joint.

B3.10b. If multiple vertebral joints are fused, a separate procedure is coded for each vertebral joint that uses a different device and/or qualifier.

Example:
Fusion of lumbar vertebral joint, posterior approach, anterior column and fusion of lumbar vertebral joint, posterior approach, posterior column are coded separately.

B3.10c. Combinations of devices and materials are often used on a vertebral joint to render the joint immobile. When combinations of devices are used on the same vertebral joint, the device value coded for the procedure is as follows:

- If an interbody fusion device is used to render the joint immobile **(containing bone graft or bone graft substitute)**, the procedure is coded with the device value Interbody Fusion Device
- If bone graft is the *only* device used to render the joint immobile, the procedure is coded with the device value Nonautologous Tissue Substitute or Autologous Tissue Substitute
- If a mixture of autologous and nonautologous bone graft (with or without biological or synthetic extenders or binders) is used to render the joint immobile, code the procedure with the device value Autologous Tissue Substitute

Examples:
Fusion of a vertebral joint using a cage style interbody fusion device containing morsellized bone graft is coded to the device Interbody Fusion Device.

Fusion of a vertebral joint using a bone dowel interbody fusion device made of cadaver bone and packed with a mixture of local morsellized bone and demineralized bone matrix is coded to the device Interbody Fusion Device.

Fusion of a vertebral joint using both autologous bone graft and bone bank bone graft is coded to the device Autologous Tissue Substitute.

Inspection procedures

B3.11a. Inspection of a body part(s) performed in order to achieve the objective of a procedure is not coded separately.

Example:
Fiberoptic bronchoscopy performed for irrigation of bronchus, only the irrigation procedure is coded.

B3.11b. If multiple tubular body parts are inspected, the most distal body part (the body part furthest from the starting point of the inspection) is coded. If multiple non-tubular body parts in a region are inspected, the body part that specifies the entire area inspected is coded.

Examples:
Cystoureteroscopy with inspection of bladder and ureters is coded to the ureter body part value.

Exploratory laparotomy with general inspection of abdominal contents is coded to the peritoneal cavity body part value.

B3.11c. When both an Inspection procedure and another procedure are performed on the same body part during the same episode, if the Inspection procedure is performed using a different approach than the other procedure, the Inspection procedure is coded separately.

Example:
Endoscopic Inspection of the duodenum is coded separately when open Excision of the duodenum is performed during the same procedural episode.

Occlusion vs. Restriction for vessel embolization procedures

B3.12. If the objective of an embolization procedure is to completely close a vessel, the root operation Occlusion is coded. If the objective of an embolization procedure is to narrow the lumen of a vessel, the root operation Restriction is coded.

Examples:
Tumor embolization is coded to the root operation Occlusion, because the objective of the procedure is to cut off the blood supply to the vessel.

Embolization of a cerebral aneurysm is coded to the root operation Restriction, because the objective of the procedure is not to close off the vessel entirely, but to narrow the lumen of the vessel at the site of the aneurysm where it is abnormally wide.

Release procedures

B3.13. In the root operation Release, the body part value coded is the body part being freed and not the tissue being manipulated or cut to free the body part.

Example:
Lysis of intestinal adhesions is coded to the specific intestine body part value.

Release vs. Division

B3.14. If the sole objective of the procedure is freeing a body part without cutting the body part, the root operation is Release. If the sole objective of the procedure is separating or transecting a body part, the root operation is Division.

Examples:
Freeing a nerve root from surrounding scar tissue to relieve pain is coded to the root operation Release.

Severing a nerve root to relieve pain is coded to the root operation Division.

Reposition for fracture treatment

B3.15. Reduction of a displaced fracture is coded to the root operation Reposition and the application of a cast or splint in conjunction with the Reposition procedure is not coded separately. Treatment of a nondisplaced fracture is coded to the procedure performed.

Examples:
Casting of a nondisplaced fracture is coded to the root operation Immobilization in the Placement section.

Putting a pin in a nondisplaced fracture is coded to the root operation Insertion.

Transplantation vs. Administration

B3.16. Putting in a mature and functioning living body part taken from another individual or animal is coded to the root operation Transplantation. Putting in autologous or nonautologous cells is coded to the Administration section.

Example:
Putting in autologous or nonautologous bone marrow, pancreatic islet cells or stem cells is coded to the Administration section.

Transfer procedures using multiple tissue layers

B3.17. The root operation Transfer contains qualifiers that can be used to specify when a transfer flap is composed of more than one tissue layer, such as a musculocutaneous flap. For procedures involving transfer of multiple tissue layers including skin, subcutaneous tissue, fascia or muscle, the procedure is coded to the body part value that describes the deepest tissue layer in the flap, and the qualifier can be used to describe the other tissue layer(s) in the transfer flap.

Example:
A musculocutaneous flap transfer is coded to the appropriate body part value in the body system Muscles, and the qualifier is used to describe the additional tissue layer(s) in the transfer flap.

Excision/Resection followed by replacement

B3.18. If an excision or resection of a body part is followed by a replacement procedure, code both procedures to identify each distinct objective, except when the excision or resection is considered integral and preparatory for the replacement procedure.

Examples:
Mastectomy followed by reconstruction, both resection and replacement of the breast are coded to fully capture the distinct objectives of the procedures performed.

Maxillectomy with obturator reconstruction, both excision and replacement of the maxilla are coded to fully capture the distinct objectives of the procedures performed.

Excisional debridement of tendon with skin graft, both the excision of the tendon and the replacement of the skin with a graft are coded to fully capture the distinct objectives of the procedures performed.

Esophagectomy followed by reconstruction with colonic interposition, both the resection and the transfer of the large intestine to function as the esophagus are coded to fully capture the distinct objectives of the procedures performed.

Examples:
Resection of a joint as part of a joint replacement procedure is considered integral and preparatory for the replacement of the joint and the resection is not coded separately.

Resection of a valve as part of a valve replacement procedure is considered integral and preparatory for the valve replacement and the resection is not coded separately.

B4. Body Part

General guidelines

B4.1a. If a procedure is performed on a portion of a body part that does not have a separate body part value, code the body part value corresponding to the whole body part.

> *Example:*
> A procedure performed on the alveolar process of the mandible is coded to the mandible body part.

B4.1b. If the prefix "peri" is combined with a body part to identify the site of the procedure, and the site of the procedure is not further specified, then the procedure is coded to the body part named. This guideline applies only when a more specific body part value is not available.

> *Examples:*
> A procedure site identified as perirenal is coded to the kidney body part when the site of the procedure is not further specified.
>
> A procedure site described in the documentation as peri-urethral, and the documentation also indicates that it is the vulvar tissue and not the urethral tissue that is the site of the procedure, then the procedure is coded to the vulva body part.
>
> A procedure site documented as involving the periosteum is coded to the corresponding bone body part.

B4.1c. If a procedure is performed on a continuous section of a tubular body part, code the body part value corresponding to the furthest anatomical site from the point of entry.

> *Example:*
> A procedure performed on a continuous section of artery from the femoral artery to the external iliac artery with the point of entry at the femoral artery is coded to the external iliac body part.

Branches of body parts

B4.2. Where a specific branch of a body part does not have its own body part value in PCS, the body part is typically coded to the closest proximal branch that has a specific body part value. In the cardiovascular body systems, if a general body part is available in the correct root operation table, and coding to a proximal branch would require assigning a code in a different body system, the procedure is coded using the general body part value.

> *Examples:*
> A procedure performed on the mandibular branch of the trigeminal nerve is coded to the trigeminal nerve body part value.
>
> Occlusion of the bronchial artery is coded to the body part value Upper Artery in the body system Upper Arteries, and not to the body part value Thoracic Aorta, Descending in the body system Heart and Great Vessels.

Bilateral body part values

B4.3. Bilateral body part values are available for a limited number of body parts. If the identical procedure is performed on contralateral body parts, and a bilateral body part value exists for that body part, a single procedure is coded using the bilateral body part value. If no bilateral body part value exists, each procedure is coded separately using the appropriate body part value.

> *Examples:*
> The identical procedure performed on both fallopian tubes is coded once using the body part value Fallopian Tube, Bilateral.

The identical procedure performed on both knee joints is coded twice using the body part values Knee Joint, Right and Knee Joint, Left.

Coronary arteries

B4.4. The coronary arteries are classified as a single body part that is further specified by number of arteries treated. One procedure code specifying multiple arteries is used when the same procedure is performed, including the same device and qualifier values.

> *Examples:*
> Angioplasty of two distinct coronary arteries with placement of two stents is coded as Dilation of Coronary Artery, Two Arteries with Two Intraluminal Devices.
>
> Angioplasty of two distinct coronary arteries, one with stent placed and one without, is coded separately as Dilation of Coronary Artery, One Artery with Intraluminal Device, and Dilation of Coronary Artery, One Artery with no device.

Tendons, ligaments, bursae and fascia near a joint

B4.5. Procedures performed on tendons, ligaments, bursae and fascia supporting a joint are coded to the body part in the respective body system that is the focus of the procedure. Procedures performed on joint structures themselves are coded to the body part in the joint body systems.

> *Examples:*
> Repair of the anterior cruciate ligament of the knee is coded to the knee bursa and ligament body part in the bursae and ligaments body system.
>
> Knee arthroscopy with shaving of articular cartilage is coded to the knee joint body part in the Lower Joints body system.

Skin, subcutaneous tissue and fascia overlying a joint

B4.6. If a procedure is performed on the skin, subcutaneous tissue or fascia overlying a joint, the procedure is coded to the following body part:

- Shoulder is coded to Upper Arm
- Elbow is coded to Lower Arm
- Wrist is coded to Lower Arm
- Hip is coded to Upper Leg
- Knee is coded to Lower Leg
- Ankle is coded to Foot

Fingers and toes

B4.7. If a body system does not contain a separate body part value for fingers, procedures performed on the fingers are coded to the body part value for the hand. If a body system does not contain a separate body part value for toes, procedures performed on the toes are coded to the body part value for the foot.

> *Example:*
> Excision of finger muscle is coded to one of the hand muscle body part values in the Muscles body system.

Upper and lower intestinal tract

B4.8. In the Gastrointestinal body system, the general body part values Upper Intestinal Tract and Lower Intestinal Tract are provided as an option for the root operations Change, Inspection, Removal and Revision. Upper Intestinal Tract includes the portion of the gastrointestinal tract from the esophagus down to and including the duodenum, and Lower Intestinal Tract includes the portion of the gastrointestinal tract from the jejunum down to and including the rectum and anus.

Example:
In the root operation Change table, change of a device in the jejunum is coded using the body part Lower Intestinal Tract.

B5. Approach

Open approach with percutaneous endoscopic assistance

B5.2a. Procedures performed using the open approach with percutaneous endoscopic assistance are coded to the approach Open.

Example:
Laparoscopic-assisted sigmoidectomy is coded to the approach Open.

Percutaneous endoscopic approach with extension of incision

B5.2b. Procedures performed using the percutaneous endoscopic approach, with incision or extension of an incision to assist in the removal of all or a portion of a body part or to anastomose a tubular body part to complete the procedure, are coded to the approach value Percutaneous Endoscopic.

Examples:

Laparoscopic sigmoid colectomy with extension of stapling port for removal of specimen and direct anastomosis is coded to the approach value percutaneous endoscopic.

Laparoscopic nephrectomy with midline incision for removing the resected kidney is coded to the approach value percutaneous endoscopic.

Robotic-assisted laparoscopic prostatectomy with extension of incision for removal of the resected prostate is coded to the approach value percutaneous endoscopic.

External approach

B5.3a. Procedures performed within an orifice on structures that are visible without the aid of any instrumentation are coded to the approach External.

Example:
Resection of tonsils is coded to the approach External.

B5.3b. Procedures performed indirectly by the application of external force through the intervening body layers are coded to the approach External.

Example:
Closed reduction of fracture is coded to the approach External.

Percutaneous procedure via device

B5.4. Procedures performed percutaneously via a device placed for the procedure are coded to the approach Percutaneous.

Example:
Fragmentation of kidney stone performed via percutaneous nephrostomy is coded to the approach Percutaneous.

B6. Device

General guidelines

B6.1a. A device is coded only if a device remains after the procedure is completed. If no device remains, the device value No Device is coded. In limited root operations, the classification provides the qualifier values Temporary and Intraoperative, for specific procedures involving clinically significant devices, where the purpose of the device is to be utilized for a brief duration during the procedure or current inpatient stay. If a device that is intended to remain after the procedure is completed requires removal before the end of the operative episode in which it was inserted (for example, the device size is inadequate or a

complication occurs), both the insertion and removal of the device should be coded.

B6.1b. Materials such as sutures, ligatures, radiological markers and temporary post-operative wound drains are considered integral to the performance of a procedure and are not coded as devices.

B6.1c. Procedures performed on a device only and not on a body part are specified in the root operations Change, Irrigation, Removal and Revision, and are coded to the procedure performed.

Example:
Irrigation of percutaneous nephrostomy tube is coded to the root operation Irrigation of indwelling device in the Administration section.

Drainage device

B6.2. A separate procedure to put in a drainage device is coded to the root operation Drainage with the device value Drainage Device.

Obstetric Section Guidelines (section 1)

C. Obstetrics Section

Products of conception

C1. Procedures performed on the products of conception are coded to the Obstetrics section. Procedures performed on the pregnant female other than the products of conception are coded to the appropriate root operation in the Medical and Surgical section.

Examples:
Amniocentesis is coded to the products of conception body part in the Obstetrics section.

Repair of obstetric urethral laceration is coded to the urethra body part in the Medical and Surgical section.

Procedures following delivery or abortion

C2. Procedures performed following a delivery or abortion for curettage of the endometrium or evacuation of retained products of conception are all coded in the Obstetrics section, to the root operation Extraction and the body part Products of Conception, Retained.

Diagnostic or therapeutic dilation and curettage performed during times other than the postpartum or post-abortion period are all coded in the Medical and Surgical section, to the root operation Extraction and the body part Endometrium.

Radiation Therapy Section Guidelines (section D)

D. Radiation Therapy Section

Brachytherapy

D1.a. Brachytherapy is coded to the modality Brachytherapy in the Radiation Therapy section. When a radioactive brachytherapy source is left in the body at the end of the procedure, it is coded separately to the root operation Insertion with the device value Radioactive Element.

Example:
Brachytherapy with implantation of a low dose rate brachytherapy source left in the body at the end of the procedure is coded to the applicable treatment site in section D, Radiation Therapy, with the modality Brachytherapy, the modality qualifier value Low Dose Rate, and the applicable isotope value and qualifier value. The implantation of the brachytherapy source is coded separately to the device value Radioactive Element in the appropriate Insertion

table of the Medical and Surgical section. The Radiation Therapy section code identifies the specific modality and isotope of the brachytherapy, and the root operation Insertion code identifies the implantation of the brachytherapy source that remains in the body at the end of the procedure.

Exception:

Implantation of Cesium-131 brachytherapy seeds embedded in a collagen matrix to the treatment site after resection of brain tumor is coded to the root operation Insertion with the device value Radioactive Element, Cesium-131 Collagen Implant. The procedure is coded to the root operation Insertion only, because the device value identifies both the implantation of the radioactive element and a specific brachytherapy isotope that is not included in the Radiation Therapy section tables.

D1.b. A separate procedure to place a temporary applicator for delivering the brachytherapy is coded to the root operation Insertion and the device value Other Device.

Examples:

Intrauterine brachytherapy applicator placed as a separate procedure from the brachytherapy procedure is coded to Insertion of Other Device, and the brachytherapy is coded separately using the modality Brachytherapy in the Radiation Therapy section.

Intrauterine brachytherapy applicator placed concomitantly with delivery of the brachytherapy dose is coded with a single code using the modality Brachytherapy in the Radiation Therapy section.

New Technology Section Guidelines (section X)

E. New Technology Section

General guidelines

E1.a. Section X codes fully represent the specific procedure described in the code title, and do not require additional codes from other sections of ICD-10-PCS. When section X contains a code title which fully describes a specific new technology procedure, and it is the only procedure performed, only the section X code is reported for the procedure. There is no need to report an additional code in another section of ICD-10-PCS.

Example:

XW04321 Introduction of Ceftazidime-Avibactam Anti-infective into Central Vein, Percutaneous Approach, New Technology Group 1, can be coded to indicate that Ceftazidime-Avibactam Anti-infective was administered via a central vein. A separate code from

table 3E0 in the Administration section of ICD-10-PCS is not coded in addition to this code.

E1.b. When multiple procedures are performed, New Technology section X codes are coded following the multiple procedures guideline.

Examples:

Dual filter cerebral embolic filtration used during transcatheter aortic valve replacement (TAVR), X2A5312 Cerebral Embolic Filtration, Dual Filter in Innominate Artery and Left Common Carotid Artery, Percutaneous Approach, New Technology Group 2, is coded for the cerebral embolic filtration, along with an ICD-10-PCS code for the TAVR procedure.

Magnetically controlled growth rod (MCGR) placed during a spinal fusion procedure, a code from table XNS, Reposition of the Bones is coded for the MCGR, along with an ICD-10-PCS code for the spinal fusion procedure.

F. Selection of Principal Procedure

The following instructions should be applied in the selection of principal procedure and clarification on the importance of the relation to the principal diagnosis when more than one procedure is performed:

1. Procedure performed for definitive treatment of both principal diagnosis and secondary diagnosis

   a. Sequence procedure performed for definitive treatment most related to principal diagnosis as principal procedure.

2. Procedure performed for definitive treatment and diagnostic procedures performed for both principal diagnosis and secondary diagnosis.

   a. Sequence procedure performed for definitive treatment most related to principal diagnosis as principal procedure

3. A diagnostic procedure was performed for the principal diagnosis and a procedure is performed for definitive treatment of a secondary diagnosis.

   a. Sequence diagnostic procedure as principal procedure, since the procedure most related to the principal diagnosis takes precedence.

4. No procedures performed that are related to principal diagnosis; procedures performed for definitive treatment and diagnostic procedures were performed for secondary diagnosis

   a. Sequence procedure performed for definitive treatment of secondary diagnosis as principal procedure, since there are no procedures (definitive or nondefinitive treatment) related to principal diagnosis.

# #

3f (Aortic) Bioprosthesis valve *use* Zooplastic Tissue in Heart and Great Vessels

A

Abdominal aortic plexus *use* Abdominal Sympathetic Nerve
Abdominal esophagus *use* Esophagus, Lower
Abdominohysterectomy *see* Resection, Uterus ØUT9
Abdominoplasty
  see Alteration, Abdominal Wall ØWØF
  see Repair, Abdominal Wall ØWQF
  see Supplement, Abdominal Wall ØWUF
Abductor hallucis muscle
  use Foot Muscle, Left
  use Foot Muscle, Right
AbioCor® Total Replacement Heart *use* Synthetic Substitute
Ablation
  see Control bleeding in
  see Destruction
Abortion
  Abortifacient 10A07ZX
  Laminaria 10A07ZW
  Products of Conception 10A0
  Vacuum 10A07Z6
Abrasion *see* Extraction
Absolute Pro Vascular (OTW) Self-Expanding Stent System *use* Intraluminal Device
Accelerate PhenoTest™ BC XXE5XN6
Accessory cephalic vein
  use Cephalic Vein, Left
  use Cephalic Vein, Right
Accessory obturator nerve *use* Lumbar Plexus
Accessory phrenic nerve *use* Phrenic Nerve
Accessory spleen *use* Spleen
Acculink (RX) Carotid Stent System *use* Intraluminal Device
Acellular Hydrated Dermis *use* Nonautologous Tissue Substitute
Acetabular cup *use* Liner in Lower Joints
Acetabulectomy
  see Excision, Lower Bones ØQB
  see Resection, Lower Bones ØQT
Acetabulofemoral joint
  use Hip Joint, Left
  use Hip Joint, Right
Acetabuloplasty
  see Repair, Lower Bones ØQQ
  see Replacement, Lower Bones ØQR
  see Supplement, Lower Bones ØQU
Achilles tendon
  use Lower Leg Tendon, Left
  use Lower Leg Tendon, Right
Achillorrhaphy *see* Repair, Tendons ØLQ
Achillotenotomy, achillotomy
  see Division, Tendons ØL8
  see Drainage, Tendons ØL9
Acoustic Pulse Thrombolysis *see* Fragmentation, Artery
Acromioclavicular ligament
  use Shoulder Bursa and Ligament, Left
  use Shoulder Bursa and Ligament, Right
Acromion (process)
  use Scapula, Left
  use Scapula, Right
Acromionectomy
  see Excision, Upper Joints ØRB
  see Resection, Upper Joints ØRT
Acromioplasty
  see Repair, Upper Joints ØRQ
  see Replacement, Upper Joints ØRR
  see Supplement, Upper Joints ØRU
Activa PC neurostimulator *use* Stimulator Generator, Multiple Array in ØJH
Activa RC neurostimulator *use* Stimulator Generator, Multiple Array Rechargeable in ØJH
Activa SC neurostimulator *use* Stimulator Generator, Single Array in ØJH
Activities of Daily Living Assessment F02
Activities of Daily Living Treatment F08
ACUITY™ Steerable Lead
  use Cardiac Lead, Defibrillator in Ø2H

ACUITY™ Steerable Lead — *continued*
  use Cardiac Lead, Pacemaker in Ø2H
Acupuncture
  Breast
    Anesthesia 8E0H300
    No Qualifier 8E0H30Z
  Integumentary System
    Anesthesia 8E0H300
    No Qualifier 8E0H30Z
Adductor brevis muscle
  use Upper Leg Muscle, Left
  use Upper Leg Muscle, Right
Adductor hallucis muscle
  use Foot Muscle, Left
  use Foot Muscle, Right
Adductor longus muscle
  use Upper Leg Muscle, Left
  use Upper Leg Muscle, Right
Adductor magnus muscle
  use Upper Leg Muscle, Left
  use Upper Leg Muscle, Right
Adenohypophysis *use* Pituitary Gland
Adenoidectomy
  see Excision, Adenoids ØCBQ
  see Resection, Adenoids ØCTQ
Adenoidotomy *see* Drainage, Adenoids ØC9Q
Adhesiolysis *see* Release
Administration
  Blood products *see* Transfusion
  Other substance *see* Introduction of substance in or on
Adrenalectomy
  see Excision, Endocrine System ØGB
  see Resection, Endocrine System ØGT
Adrenalorrhaphy *see* Repair, Endocrine System ØGQ
Adrenalotomy *see* Drainage, Endocrine System ØG9
Advancement
  see Reposition
  see Transfer
Advisa (MRI) *use* Pacemaker, Dual Chamber in ØJH
AFX® Endovascular AAA System *use* Intraluminal Device
AIGISRx Antibacterial Envelope *use* Anti-Infective Envelope
Alar ligament of axis *use* Head and Neck Bursa and Ligament
Alfieri Stitch Valvuloplasty *see* Restriction, Valve, Mitral Ø2VG
Alimentation *see* Introduction of substance in or on
Alteration
  Abdominal Wall ØWØF
  Ankle Region
    Left ØYØL
    Right ØYØK
  Arm
    Lower
      Left ØXØF
      Right ØXØD
    Upper
      Left ØXØ9
      Right ØXØ8
  Axilla
    Left ØXØ5
    Right ØXØ4
  Back
    Lower ØWØL
    Upper ØWØK
  Breast
    Bilateral ØHØV
    Left ØHØU
    Right ØHØT
  Buttock
    Left ØYØ1
    Right ØYØØ
  Chest Wall ØWØ8
  Ear
    Bilateral Ø9Ø2
    Left Ø9Ø1
    Right Ø9ØØ
  Elbow Region
    Left ØXØC
    Right ØXØB
  Extremity
    Lower
      Left ØYØB
      Right ØYØ9
    Upper
      Left ØXØ7

Alteration — *continued*
  Extremity — *continued*
    Upper — *continued*
      Right ØXØ6
  Eyelid
    Lower
      Left Ø8ØR
      Right Ø8ØQ
    Upper
      Left Ø8ØP
      Right Ø8ØN
  Face ØWØ2
  Head ØWØØ
  Jaw
    Lower ØWØ5
    Upper ØWØ4
  Knee Region
    Left ØYØG
    Right ØYØF
  Leg
    Lower
      Left ØYØJ
      Right ØYØH
    Upper
      Left ØYØD
      Right ØYØC
  Lip
    Lower ØCØ1X
    Upper ØCØØX
  Nasal Mucosa and Soft Tissue Ø9ØK
  Neck ØWØ6
  Perineum
    Female ØWØN
    Male ØWØM
  Shoulder Region
    Left ØXØ3
    Right ØXØ2
  Subcutaneous Tissue and Fascia
    Abdomen ØJØ8
    Back ØJØ7
    Buttock ØJØ9
    Chest ØJØ6
    Face ØJØ1
    Lower Arm
      Left ØJØH
      Right ØJØG
    Lower Leg
      Left ØJØP
      Right ØJØN
    Neck
      Left ØJØ5
      Right ØJØ4
    Upper Arm
      Left ØJØF
      Right ØJØD
    Upper Leg
      Left ØJØM
      Right ØJØL
  Wrist Region
    Left ØXØH
    Right ØXØG
Alveolar process of mandible
  use Mandible, Left
  use Mandible, Right
Alveolar process of maxilla *use* Maxilla
Alveolectomy
  see Excision, Head and Facial Bones ØNB
  see Resection, Head and Facial Bones ØNT
Alveoloplasty
  see Repair, Head and Facial Bones ØNQ
  see Replacement, Head and Facial Bones ØNR
  see Supplement, Head and Facial Bones ØNU
Alveolotomy
  see Division, Head and Facial Bones ØN8
  see Drainage, Head and Facial Bones ØN9
Ambulatory cardiac monitoring 4A12X45
Amniocentesis *see* Drainage, Products of Conception 1090
Amnioinfusion *see* Introduction of substance in or on, Products of Conception 3E0E
Amnioscopy 10J08ZZ
Amniotomy *see* Drainage, Products of Conception 1090
AMPLATZER® Muscular VSD Occluder *use* Synthetic Substitute
Amputation *see* Detachment
AMS 800® Urinary Control System *use* Artificial Sphincter in Urinary System
Anal orifice *use* Anus

Analog radiography see Plain Radiography
Analog radiology see Plain Radiography
Anastomosis see Bypass
Anatomical snuffbox
 use Lower Arm and Wrist Muscle, Left
 use Lower Arm and Wrist Muscle, Right
Andexanet Alfa, Factor Xa Inhibitor Reversal Agent
 use Coagulation Factor Xa, Inactivated
Andexxa use Coagulation Factor Xa, Inactivated
AneuRx® AAA Advantage® use Intraluminal Device
Angiectomy
 see Excision, Heart and Great Vessels 02B
 see Excision, Lower Arteries 04B
 see Excision, Lower Veins 06B
 see Excision, Upper Arteries 03B
 see Excision, Upper Veins 05B
Angiocardiography
 Combined right and left heart see Fluoroscopy, Heart, Right and Left B216
 Left Heart see Fluoroscopy, Heart, Left B215
 Right Heart see Fluoroscopy, Heart, Right B214
 SPY system intravascular fluorescence see Monitoring, Physiological Systems 4A1
Angiography
 see Fluoroscopy, Heart B21
 see Plain Radiography, Heart B20
Angioplasty
 see Dilation, Heart and Great Vessels 027
 see Dilation, Lower Arteries 047
 see Dilation, Upper Arteries 037
 see Repair, Heart and Great Vessels 02Q
 see Repair, Lower Arteries 04Q
 see Repair, Upper Arteries 03Q
 see Replacement, Heart and Great Vessels 02R
 see Replacement, Lower Arteries 04R
 see Replacement, Upper Arteries 03R
 see Supplement, Heart and Great Vessels 02U
 see Supplement, Lower Arteries 04U
 see Supplement, Upper Arteries 03U
Angiorrhaphy
 see Repair, Heart and Great Vessels 02Q
 see Repair, Lower Arteries 04Q
 see Repair, Upper Arteries 03Q
Angioscopy 02JY4ZZ, 03JY4ZZ, 04JY4ZZ
Angiotensin II use Synthetic Human Angiotensin II
Angiotripsy
 see Occlusion, Lower Arteries 04L
 see Occlusion, Upper Arteries 03L
Angular artery use Face Artery
Angular vein
 use Face Vein, Left
 use Face Vein, Right
Annular ligament
 use Elbow Bursa and Ligament, Left
 use Elbow Bursa and Ligament, Right
Annuloplasty
 see Repair, Heart and Great Vessels 02Q
 see Supplement, Heart and Great Vessels 02U
Annuloplasty ring use Synthetic Substitute
Anoplasty
 see Repair, Anus 0DQQ
 see Supplement, Anus 0DUQ
Anorectal junction use Rectum
Anoscopy 0DJD8ZZ
Ansa cervicalis use Cervical Plexus
Antabuse therapy HZ93ZZZ
Antebrachial fascia
 use Subcutaneous Tissue and Fascia, Left Lower Arm
 use Subcutaneous Tissue and Fascia, Right Lower Arm
Anterior cerebral artery use Intracranial Artery
Anterior cerebral vein use Intracranial Vein
Anterior choroidal artery use Intracranial Artery
Anterior circumflex humeral artery
 use Axillary Artery, Left
 use Axillary Artery, Right
Anterior communicating artery use Intracranial Artery
Anterior cruciate ligament (ACL)
 use Knee Bursa and Ligament, Left
 use Knee Bursa and Ligament, Right
Anterior crural nerve use Femoral Nerve
Anterior facial vein
 use Face Vein, Left
 use Face Vein, Right

Anterior intercostal artery
 use Internal Mammary Artery, Left
 use Internal Mammary Artery, Right
Anterior interosseous nerve use Median Nerve
Anterior lateral malleolar artery
 use Anterior Tibial Artery, Left
 use Anterior Tibial Artery, Right
Anterior lingual gland use Minor Salivary Gland
Anterior (pectoral) lymph node
 use Lymphatic, Left Axillary
 use Lymphatic, Right Axillary
Anterior medial malleolar artery
 use Anterior Tibial Artery, Left
 use Anterior Tibial Artery, Right
Anterior spinal artery
 use Vertebral Artery, Left
 use Vertebral Artery, Right
Anterior tibial recurrent artery
 use Anterior Tibial Artery, Left
 use Anterior Tibial Artery, Right
Anterior ulnar recurrent artery
 use Ulnar Artery, Left
 use Ulnar Artery, Right
Anterior vagal trunk use Vagus Nerve
Anterior vertebral muscle
 use Neck Muscle, Left
 use Neck Muscle, Right
Antibacterial Envelope (TYRX) (AIGISRx) use Anti-Infective Envelope
Antigen-free air conditioning see Atmospheric Control, Physiological Systems 6A0
Antihelix
 use External Ear, Bilateral
 use External Ear, Left
 use External Ear, Right
Antimicrobial envelope use Anti-Infective Envelope
Antitragus
 use External Ear, Bilateral
 use External Ear, Left
 use External Ear, Right
Antrostomy see Drainage, Ear, Nose, Sinus 099
Antrotomy see Drainage, Ear, Nose, Sinus 099
Antrum of Highmore
 use Maxillary Sinus, Left
 use Maxillary Sinus, Right
Aortic annulus use Aortic Valve
Aortic arch use Thoracic Aorta, Ascending/Arch
Aortic intercostal artery use Upper Artery
Aortography
 see Fluoroscopy, Lower Arteries B41
 see Fluoroscopy, Upper Arteries B31
 see Plain Radiography, Lower Arteries B40
 see Plain Radiography, Upper Arteries B30
Aortoplasty
 see Repair, Aorta, Abdominal 04Q0
 see Repair, Aorta, Thoracic, Ascending/Arch 02QX
 see Repair, Aorta, Thoracic, Descending 02QW
 see Replacement, Aorta, Abdominal 04R0
 see Replacement, Aorta, Thoracic, Ascending/Arch 02RX
 see Replacement, Aorta, Thoracic, Descending 02RW
 see Supplement, Aorta, Abdominal 04U0
 see Supplement, Aorta, Thoracic, Ascending/Arch 02UX
 see Supplement, Aorta, Thoracic, Descending 02UW
Apalutamide Antineoplastic XW0DXJ5
Apical (subclavicular) lymph node
 use Lymphatic, Left Axillary
 use Lymphatic, Right Axillary
Apneustic center use Pons
Appendectomy
 see Excision, Appendix 0DBJ
 see Resection, Appendix 0DTJ
Appendicolysis see Release, Appendix 0DNJ
Appendicotomy see Drainage, Appendix 0D9J
Application see Introduction of substance in or on
Aquablation therapy, prostate XV508A4
Aquapheresis 6A550Z3
Aqueduct of Sylvius use Cerebral Ventricle
Aqueous humour
 use Anterior Chamber, Left
 use Anterior Chamber, Right
Arachnoid mater, intracranial use Cerebral Meninges
Arachnoid mater, spinal use Spinal Meninges

Arcuate artery
 use Foot Artery, Left
 use Foot Artery, Right
Areola
 use Nipple, Left
 use Nipple, Right
AROM (artificial rupture of membranes) 10907ZC
Arterial canal (duct) use Pulmonary Artery, Left
Arterial pulse tracing see Measurement, Arterial 4A03
Arteriectomy
 see Excision, Heart and Great Vessels 02B
 see Excision, Lower Arteries 04B
 see Excision, Upper Arteries 03B
Arteriography
 see Fluoroscopy, Heart B21
 see Fluoroscopy, Lower Arteries B41
 see Fluoroscopy, Upper Arteries B31
 see Plain Radiography, Heart B20
 see Plain Radiography, Lower Arteries B40
 see Plain Radiography, Upper Arteries B30
Arterioplasty
 see Repair, Heart and Great Vessels 02Q
 see Repair, Lower Arteries 04Q
 see Repair, Upper Arteries 03Q
 see Replacement, Heart and Great Vessels 02R
 see Replacement, Lower Arteries 04R
 see Replacement, Upper Arteries 03R
 see Supplement, Heart and Great Vessels 02U
 see Supplement, Lower Arteries 04U
 see Supplement, Upper Arteries 03U
Arteriorrhaphy
 see Repair, Heart and Great Vessels 02Q
 see Repair, Lower Arteries 04Q
 see Repair, Upper Arteries 03Q
Arterioscopy
 see Inspection, Artery, Lower 04JY
 see Inspection, Artery, Upper 03JY
 see Inspection, Great Vessel 02JY
Arthrectomy
 see Excision, Lower Joints 0SB
 see Excision, Upper Joints 0RB
 see Resection, Lower Joints 0ST
 see Resection, Upper Joints 0RT
Arthrocentesis
 see Drainage, Lower Joints 0S9
 see Drainage, Upper Joints 0R9
Arthrodesis
 see Fusion, Lower Joints 0SG
 see Fusion, Upper Joints 0RG
Arthrography
 see Plain Radiography, Non-Axial Lower Bones BQ0
 see Plain Radiography, Non-Axial Upper Bones BP0
 see Plain Radiography, Skull and Facial Bones BN0
Arthrolysis
 see Release, Lower Joints 0SN
 see Release, Upper Joints 0RN
Arthropexy
 see Repair, Lower Joints 0SQ
 see Repair, Upper Joints 0RQ
 see Reposition, Lower Joints 0SS
 see Reposition, Upper Joints 0RS
Arthroplasty
 see Repair, Lower Joints 0SQ
 see Repair, Upper Joints 0RQ
 see Replacement, Lower Joints 0SR
 see Replacement, Upper Joints 0RR
 see Supplement, Lower Joints 0SU
 see Supplement, Upper Joints 0RU
Arthroplasty, radial head
 see Replacement, Radius, Left 0PRJ
 see Replacement, Radius, Right 0PRH
Arthroscopy
 see Inspection, Lower Joints 0SJ
 see Inspection, Upper Joints 0RJ
Arthrotomy
 see Drainage, Lower Joints 0S9
 see Drainage, Upper Joints 0R9
Articulating Spacer (Antibiotic) use Articulating Spacer in Lower Joints
Artificial anal sphincter (AAS) use Artificial Sphincter in Gastrointestinal System
Artificial bowel sphincter (neosphincter) use Artificial Sphincter in Gastrointestinal System
Artificial Sphincter
 Insertion of device in
  Anus 0DHQ

▽ Subterms under main terms may continue to next column or page

Artificial Sphincter — *continued*
  Insertion of device in — *continued*
    Bladder ØTHB
    Bladder Neck ØTHC
    Urethra ØTHD
  Removal of device from
    Anus ØDPQ
    Bladder ØTPB
    Urethra ØTPD
  Revision of device in
    Anus ØDWQ
    Bladder ØTWB
    Urethra ØTWD
Artificial urinary sphincter (AUS) *use* Artificial Sphincter in Urinary System
Aryepiglottic fold *use* Larynx
Arytenoid cartilage *use* Larynx
Arytenoid muscle
  use Neck Muscle, Left
  use Neck Muscle, Right
Arytenoidectomy *see* Excision, Larynx ØCBS
Arytenoidopexy *see* Repair, Larynx ØCQS
Ascenda Intrathecal Catheter *use* Infusion Device
Ascending aorta *use* Thoracic Aorta, Ascending/Arch
Ascending palatine artery *use* Face Artery
Ascending pharyngeal artery
  use External Carotid Artery, Left
  use External Carotid Artery, Right
Aspiration, fine needle
  Fluid or gas *see* Drainage
  Tissue biopsy
    see Excision
    see Extraction
Assessment
  Activities of daily living *see* Activities of Daily Living Assessment, Rehabilitation FØ2
  Hearing *see* Hearing Assessment, Diagnostic Audiology F13
  Hearing aid *see* Hearing Aid Assessment, Diagnostic Audiology F14
  Intravascular perfusion, using indocyanine green (ICG) dye *see* Monitoring, Physiological Systems 4A1
  Motor function *see* Motor Function Assessment, Rehabilitation FØ1
  Nerve function *see* Motor Function Assessment, Rehabilitation FØ1
  Speech *see* Speech Assessment, Rehabilitation FØØ
  Vestibular *see* Vestibular Assessment, Diagnostic Audiology F15
  Vocational *see* Activities of Daily Living Treatment, Rehabilitation FØ8
Assistance
  Cardiac
    Continuous
      Balloon Pump 5AØ221Ø
      Impeller Pump 5AØ221D
      Other Pump 5AØ2216
      Pulsatile Compression 5AØ2215
    Intermittent
      Balloon Pump 5AØ211Ø
      Impeller Pump 5AØ211D
      Other Pump 5AØ2116
      Pulsatile Compression 5AØ2115
  Circulatory
    Continuous
      Hyperbaric 5AØ5221
      Supersaturated 5AØ522C
    Intermittent
      Hyperbaric 5AØ5121
      Supersaturated 5AØ512C
  Respiratory
    24-96 Consecutive Hours
      Continuous Negative Airway Pressure 5AØ9459
      Continuous Positive Airway Pressure 5AØ9457
      High Nasal Flow/Velocity 5AØ945A
      Intermittent Negative Airway Pressure 5AØ945B
      Intermittent Positive Airway Pressure 5AØ9458
      No Qualifier 5AØ945Z
    Continuous, Filtration 5AØ92ØZ
    Greater than 96 Consecutive Hours
      Continuous Negative Airway Pressure 5AØ9559

Assistance — *continued*
  Respiratory — *continued*
    Greater than 96 Consecutive Hours — *continued*
      Continuous Positive Airway Pressure 5AØ9557
      High Nasal Flow/Velocity 5AØ955A
      Intermittent Negative Airway Pressure 5AØ955B
      Intermittent Positive Airway Pressure 5AØ9558
      No Qualifier 5AØ955Z
    Less than 24 Consecutive Hours
      Continuous Negative Airway Pressure 5AØ9359
      Continuous Positive Airway Pressure 5AØ9357
      High Nasal Flow/Velocity 5AØ935A
      Intermittent Negative Airway Pressure 5AØ935B
      Intermittent Positive Airway Pressure 5AØ9358
      No Qualifier 5AØ935Z
Assurant (Cobalt) stent *use* Intraluminal Device
Atezolizumab Antineoplastic XWØ
Atherectomy
  see Extirpation, Heart and Great Vessels Ø2C
  see Extirpation, Lower Arteries Ø4C
  see Extirpation, Upper Arteries Ø3C
Atlantoaxial joint *use* Cervical Vertebral Joint
Atmospheric Control 6AØZ
AtriClip LAA Exclusion System *use* Extraluminal Device
Atrioseptoplasty
  see Repair, Heart and Great Vessels Ø2Q
  see Replacement, Heart and Great Vessels Ø2R
  see Supplement, Heart and Great Vessels Ø2U
Atrioventricular node *use* Conduction Mechanism
Atrium dextrum cordis *use* Atrium, Right
Atrium pulmonale *use* Atrium, Left
Attain Ability® lead Ø2H
  use Cardiac Lead, Defibrillator in Ø2H
  use Cardiac Lead, Pacemaker in Ø2H
Attain Starfix® (OTW) lead
  use Cardiac Lead, Defibrillator in Ø2H
  use Cardiac Lead, Pacemaker in Ø2H
Audiology, diagnostic
  see Hearing Aid Assessment, Diagnostic Audiology F14
  see Hearing Assessment, Diagnostic Audiology F13
  see Vestibular Assessment, Diagnostic Audiology F15
Audiometry *see* Hearing Assessment, Diagnostic Audiology F13
Auditory tube
  use Eustachian Tube, Left
  use Eustachian Tube, Right
Auerbach's (myenteric) plexus *use* Abdominal Sympathetic Nerve
Auricle
  use External Ear, Bilateral
  use External Ear, Left
  use External Ear, Right
Auricularis muscle *use* Head Muscle
Autograft *use* Autologous Tissue Substitute
Autologous artery graft
  use Autologous Arterial Tissue in Heart and Great Vessels
  use Autologous Arterial Tissue in Lower Arteries
  use Autologous Arterial Tissue in Lower Veins
  use Autologous Arterial Tissue in Upper Arteries
  use Autologous Arterial Tissue in Upper Veins
Autologous vein graft
  use Autologous Venous Tissue in Heart and Great Vessels
  use Autologous Venous Tissue in Lower Arteries
  use Autologous Venous Tissue in Lower Veins
  use Autologous Venous Tissue in Upper Arteries
  use Autologous Venous Tissue in Upper Veins
Autotransfusion *see* Transfusion
Autotransplant
  Adrenal tissue *see* Reposition, Endocrine System ØGS
  Kidney *see* Reposition, Urinary System ØTS
  Pancreatic tissue *see* Reposition, Pancreas ØFSG

Autotransplant — *continued*
  Parathyroid tissue *see* Reposition, Endocrine System ØGS
  Thyroid tissue *see* Reposition, Endocrine System ØGS
  Tooth *see* Reattachment, Mouth and Throat ØCM
Avulsion *see* Extraction
Axial Lumbar Interbody Fusion System *use* Interbody Fusion Device in Lower Joints
AxiaLIF® System *use* Interbody Fusion Device in Lower Joints
Axicabtagene Ciloeucel *use* Engineered Autologous Chimeric Antigen Receptor T-cell Immunotherapy
Axillary fascia
  use Subcutaneous Tissue and Fascia, Left Upper Arm
  use Subcutaneous Tissue and Fascia, Right Upper Arm
Axillary nerve *use* Brachial Plexus
AZEDRA® *use* Iobenguane I-131 Antineoplastic

B

BAK/C® Interbody Cervical Fusion System *use* Interbody Fusion Device in Upper Joints
BAL (bronchial alveolar lavage), diagnostic *see* Drainage, Respiratory System ØB9
Balanoplasty
  see Repair, Penis ØVQS
  see Supplement, Penis ØVUS
Balloon atrial septostomy (BAS) Ø2163Z7
Balloon Pump
  Continuous, Output 5AØ221Ø
  Intermittent, Output 5AØ211Ø
Bandage, Elastic *see* Compression
Banding
  see Occlusion
  see Restriction
Banding, esophageal varices *see* Occlusion, Vein, Esophageal Ø6L3
Banding, laparoscopic (adjustable) gastric
  Initial procedure ØDV64CZ
  Surgical correction *see* Revision of device in, Stomach ØDW6
Bard® Composix® Kugel® patch *use* Synthetic Substitute
Bard® Composix® (E/X) (LP) mesh *use* Synthetic Substitute
Bard® Dulex™ mesh *use* Synthetic Substitute
Bard® Ventralex™ Hernia Patch *use* Synthetic Substitute
Barium swallow *see* Fluoroscopy, Gastrointestinal System BD1
Baroreflex Activation Therapy® (BAT®)
  use Stimulator Generator in Subcutaneous Tissue and Fascia
  use Stimulator Lead in Upper Arteries
Barricaid® Annular Closure Device (ACD) *use* Synthetic Substitute
Bartholin's (greater vestibular) gland *use* Vestibular Gland
Basal (internal) cerebral vein *use* Intracranial Vein
Basal metabolic rate (BMR) *see* Measurement, Physiological Systems 4AØZ
Basal nuclei *use* Basal Ganglia
Base of Tongue *use* Pharynx
Basilar artery *use* Intracranial Artery
Basis pontis *use* Pons
Beam Radiation
  Abdomen DWØ3
    Intraoperative DWØ33ZØ
  Adrenal Gland DGØ2
    Intraoperative DGØ23ZØ
  Bile Ducts DFØ2
    Intraoperative DFØ23ZØ
  Bladder DTØ2
    Intraoperative DTØ23ZØ
  Bone
    Intraoperative DPØC3ZØ
    Other DPØC
  Bone Marrow D7ØØ
    Intraoperative D7ØØ3ZØ
  Brain DØØØ
    Intraoperative DØØØ3ZØ
  Brain Stem DØØ1
    Intraoperative DØØ13ZØ

Beam Radiation — *continued*
  Breast
    Left DM00
      Intraoperative DM003Z0
    Right DM01
      Intraoperative DM013Z0
  Bronchus DB01
    Intraoperative DB013Z0
  Cervix DU01
    Intraoperative DU013Z0
  Chest DW02
    Intraoperative DW023Z0
  Chest Wall DB07
    Intraoperative DB073Z0
  Colon DD05
    Intraoperative DD053Z0
  Diaphragm DB08
    Intraoperative DB083Z0
  Duodenum DD02
    Intraoperative DD023Z0
  Ear D900
    Intraoperative D9003Z0
  Esophagus DD00
    Intraoperative DD003Z0
  Eye D800
    Intraoperative D8003Z0
  Femur DP09
    Intraoperative DP093Z0
  Fibula DP0B
    Intraoperative DP0B3Z0
  Gallbladder DF01
    Intraoperative DF013Z0
  Gland
    Adrenal DG02
      Intraoperative DG023Z0
    Parathyroid DG04
      Intraoperative DG043Z0
    Pituitary DG00
      Intraoperative DG003Z0
    Thyroid DG05
      Intraoperative DG053Z0
  Glands
    Intraoperative D9063Z0
    Salivary D906
  Head and Neck DW01
    Intraoperative DW013Z0
  Hemibody DW04
    Intraoperative DW043Z0
  Humerus DP06
    Intraoperative DP063Z0
  Hypopharynx D903
    Intraoperative D9033Z0
  Ileum DD04
    Intraoperative DD043Z0
  Jejunum DD03
    Intraoperative DD033Z0
  Kidney DT00
    Intraoperative DT003Z0
  Larynx D90B
    Intraoperative D90B3Z0
  Liver DF00
    Intraoperative DF003Z0
  Lung DB02
    Intraoperative DB023Z0
  Lymphatics
    Abdomen D706
      Intraoperative D7063Z0
    Axillary D704
      Intraoperative D7043Z0
    Inguinal D708
      Intraoperative D7083Z0
    Neck D703
      Intraoperative D7033Z0
    Pelvis D707
      Intraoperative D7073Z0
    Thorax D705
      Intraoperative D7053Z0
  Mandible DP03
    Intraoperative DP033Z0
  Maxilla DP02
    Intraoperative DP023Z0
  Mediastinum DB06
    Intraoperative DB063Z0
  Mouth D904
    Intraoperative D9043Z0
  Nasopharynx D90D
    Intraoperative D90D3Z0
  Neck and Head DW01
    Intraoperative DW013Z0

Beam Radiation — *continued*
  Nerve
    Intraoperative D0073Z0
    Peripheral D007
  Nose D901
    Intraoperative D9013Z0
  Oropharynx D90F
    Intraoperative D90F3Z0
  Ovary DU00
    Intraoperative DU003Z0
  Palate
    Hard D908
      Intraoperative D9083Z0
    Soft D909
      Intraoperative D9093Z0
  Pancreas DF03
    Intraoperative DF033Z0
  Parathyroid Gland DG04
    Intraoperative DG043Z0
  Pelvic Bones DP08
    Intraoperative DP083Z0
  Pelvic Region DW06
    Intraoperative DW063Z0
  Pineal Body DG01
    Intraoperative DG013Z0
  Pituitary Gland DG00
    Intraoperative DG003Z0
  Pleura DB05
    Intraoperative DB053Z0
  Prostate DV00
    Intraoperative DV003Z0
  Radius DP07
    Intraoperative DP073Z0
  Rectum DD07
    Intraoperative DD073Z0
  Rib DP05
    Intraoperative DP053Z0
  Sinuses D907
    Intraoperative D9073Z0
  Skin
    Abdomen DH08
      Intraoperative DH083Z0
    Arm DH04
      Intraoperative DH043Z0
    Back DH07
      Intraoperative DH073Z0
    Buttock DH09
      Intraoperative DH093Z0
    Chest DH06
      Intraoperative DH063Z0
    Face DH02
      Intraopérative DH023Z0
    Leg DH0B
      Intraoperative DH0B3Z0
    Neck DH03
      Intraoperative DH033Z0
  Skull DP00
    Intraoperative DP003Z0
  Spinal Cord D006
    Intraoperative D0063Z0
  Spleen D702
    Intraoperative D7023Z0
  Sternum DP04
    Intraoperative DP043Z0
  Stomach DD01
    Intraoperative DD013Z0
  Testis DV01
    Intraoperative DV013Z0
  Thymus D701
    Intraoperative D7013Z0
  Thyroid Gland DG05
    Intraoperative DG053Z0
  Tibia DP0B
    Intraoperative DP0B3Z0
  Tongue D905
    Intraoperative D9053Z0
  Trachea DB00
    Intraoperative DB003Z0
  Ulna DP07
    Intraoperative DP073Z0
  Ureter DT01
    Intraoperative DT013Z0
  Urethra DT03
    Intraoperative DT033Z0
  Uterus DU02
    Intraoperative DU023Z0
  Whole Body DW05
    Intraoperative DW053Z0
Bedside swallow F00ZJWZ

Berlin Heart Ventricular Assist Device *use* Implantable Heart Assist System in Heart and Great Vessels
Bezlotoxumab Monoclonal Antibody XW0
Biceps brachii muscle
  use Upper Arm Muscle, Left
  use Upper Arm Muscle, Right
Biceps femoris muscle
  use Upper Leg Muscle, Left
  use Upper Leg Muscle, Right
Bicipital aponeurosis
  use Subcutaneous Tissue and Fascia, Left Lower Arm
  use Subcutaneous Tissue and Fascia, Right Lower Arm
Bicuspid valve *use* Mitral Valve
Bili light therapy *see* Phototherapy, Skin 6A60
Bioactive embolization coil(s) *use* Intraluminal Device, Bioactive in Upper Arteries
Biofeedback GZC9ZZZ
BioFire® FilmArray® Pneumonia Panel XXEBXQ6
Biopsy
  see Drainage with qualifier Diagnostic
  see Excision with qualifier Diagnostic
  see Extraction with qualifier Diagnostic
BiPAP *see* Assistance, Respiratory 5A09
Bisection *see* Division
Biventricular external heart assist system *use* Short-term External Heart Assist System in Heart and Great Vessels
Blepharectomy
  see Excision, Eye 08B
  see Resection, Eye 08T
Blepharoplasty
  see Repair, Eye 08Q
  see Replacement, Eye 08R
  see Reposition, Eye 08S
  see Supplement, Eye 08U
Blepharorrhaphy *see* Repair, Eye 08Q
Blepharotomy *see* Drainage, Eye 089
Blinatumomab Antineoplastic Immunotherapy XW0
Block, Nerve, anesthetic injection 3E0T3BZ
Blood glucose monitoring system *use* Monitoring Device
Blood pressure *see* Measurement, Arterial 4A03
BMR (basal metabolic rate) *see* Measurement, Physiological Systems 4A0Z
Body of femur
  use Femoral Shaft, Left
  use Femoral Shaft, Right
Body of fibula
  use Fibula, Left
  use Fibula, Right
Bone anchored hearing device
  use Hearing Device, Bone Conduction in 09H
  use Hearing Device in Head and Facial Bones
Bone bank bone graft *use* Nonautologous Tissue Substitute
Bone Growth Stimulator
  Insertion of device in
    Bone
      Facial 0NHW
      Lower 0QHY
      Nasal 0NHB
      Upper 0PHY
    Skull 0NH0
  Removal of device from
    Bone
      Facial 0NPW
      Lower 0QPY
      Nasal 0NPB
      Upper 0PPY
    Skull 0NP0
  Revision of device in
    Bone
      Facial 0NWW
      Lower 0QWY
      Nasal 0NWB
      Upper 0PWY
    Skull 0NW0
Bone marrow transplant *see* Transfusion, Circulatory 302
Bone morphogenetic protein 2 (BMP 2) *use* Recombinant Bone Morphogenetic Protein

Bone screw (interlocking) (lag) (pedicle) (recessed)
  use Internal Fixation Device in Head and Facial
    Bones
  use Internal Fixation Device in Lower Bones
  use Internal Fixation Device in Upper Bones
Bony labyrinth
  use Inner Ear, Left
  use Inner Ear, Right
Bony orbit
  use Orbit, Left
  use Orbit, Right
Bony vestibule
  use Inner Ear, Left
  use Inner Ear, Right
Botallo's duct use Pulmonary Artery, Left
Bovine pericardial valve use Zooplastic Tissue in Heart
    and Great Vessels
Bovine pericardium graft use Zooplastic Tissue in
    Heart and Great Vessels
BP (blood pressure) see Measurement, Arterial 4A03
Brachial (lateral) lymph node
  use Lymphatic, Left Axillary
  use Lymphatic, Right Axillary
Brachialis muscle
  use Upper Arm Muscle, Left
  use Upper Arm Muscle, Right
Brachiocephalic artery use Innominate Artery
Brachiocephalic trunk use Innominate Artery
Brachiocephalic vein
  use Innominate Vein, Left
  use Innominate Vein, Right
Brachioradialis muscle
  use Lower Arm and Wrist Muscle, Left
  use Lower Arm and Wrist Muscle, Right
Brachytherapy
  Abdomen DW13
  Adrenal Gland DG12
  Back
    Lower DW1LBB
    Upper DW1KBB
  Bile Ducts DF12
  Bladder DT12
  Bone Marrow D710
  Brain D010
  Brain Stem D011
  Breast
    Left DM10
    Right DM11
  Bronchus DB11
  Cervix DU11
  Chest DW12
  Chest Wall DB17
  Colon DD15
  Cranial Cavity DW10BB
  Diaphragm DB18
  Duodenum DD12
  Ear D910
  Esophagus DD10
  Extremity
    Lower DW1YBB
    Upper DW1XBB
  Eye D810
  Gallbladder DF11
  Gastrointestinal Tract DW1PBB
  Genitourinary Tract DW1RBB
  Gland
    Adrenal DG12
    Parathyroid DG14
    Pituitary DG10
    Thyroid DG15
  Glands, Salivary D916
  Head and Neck DW11
  Hypopharynx D913
  Ileum DD14
  Jejunum DD13
  Kidney DT10
  Larynx D91B
  Liver DF10
  Lung DB12
  Lymphatics
    Abdomen D716
    Axillary D714
    Inguinal D718
    Neck D713
    Pelvis D717
    Thorax D715
  Mediastinum DB16
  Mouth D914

Brachytherapy — continued
  Nasopharynx D91D
  Neck and Head DW11
  Nerve, Peripheral D017
  Nose D911
  Oropharynx D91F
  Ovary DU10
  Palate
    Hard D918
    Soft D919
  Pancreas DF13
  Parathyroid Gland DG14
  Pelvic Region DW16
  Pineal Body DG11
  Pituitary Gland DG10
  Pleura DB15
  Prostate DV10
  Rectum DD17
  Respiratory Tract DW1QBB
  Sinuses D917
  Spinal Cord D016
  Spleen D712
  Stomach DD11
  Testis DV11
  Thymus D711
  Thyroid Gland DG15
  Tongue D915
  Trachea DB10
  Ureter DT11
  Urethra DT13
  Uterus DU12
Brachytherapy, CivaSheet®
  see Brachytherapy with qualifier Unidirectional
    Source
  see Insertion with device Radioactive Element
Brachytherapy seeds use Radioactive Element
Breast procedures, skin only use Skin, Chest
Brexanolone XW0
Brexucabtagene Autoleucel use Brexucabtagene
    Autoleucel Immunotherapy
Brexucabtagene Autoleucel Immunotherapy XW2
Broad ligament use Uterine Supporting Structure
Bronchial artery use Upper Artery
Bronchography
  see Fluoroscopy, Respiratory System BB1
  see Plain Radiography, Respiratory System BB0
Bronchoplasty
  see Repair, Respiratory System 0BQ
  see Supplement, Respiratory System 0BU
Bronchorrhaphy see Repair, Respiratory System 0BQ
Bronchoscopy 0BJ08ZZ
Bronchotomy see Drainage, Respiratory System 0B9
Bronchus Intermedius use Main Bronchus, Right
BRYAN® Cervical Disc System use Synthetic Substitute
Buccal gland use Buccal Mucosa
Buccinator lymph node use Lymphatic, Head
Buccinator muscle use Facial Muscle
Buckling, scleral with implant see Supplement, Eye
    08U
Bulbospongiosus muscle use Perineum Muscle
Bulbourethral (Cowper's) gland use Urethra
Bundle of His use Conduction Mechanism
Bundle of Kent use Conduction Mechanism
Bunionectomy see Excision, Lower Bones 0QB
Bursectomy
  see Excision, Bursae and Ligaments 0MB
  see Resection, Bursae and Ligaments 0MT
Bursocentesis see Drainage, Bursae and Ligaments
    0M9
Bursography
  see Plain Radiography, Non-Axial Lower Bones BQ0
  see Plain Radiography, Non-Axial Upper Bones BP0
Bursotomy
  see Division, Bursae and Ligaments 0M8
  see Drainage, Bursae and Ligaments 0M9
BVS 5000 Ventricular Assist Device use Short-term
    External Heart Assist System in Heart and Great
    Vessels
Bypass
  Anterior Chamber
    Left 08133
    Right 08123
  Aorta
    Abdominal 0410
    Thoracic
      Ascending/Arch 021X
      Descending 021W

Bypass — continued
  Artery
    Anterior Tibial
      Left 041Q
      Right 041P
    Axillary
      Left 03160
      Right 03150
    Brachial
      Left 03180
      Right 03170
    Common Carotid
      Left 031J0
      Right 031H0
    Common Iliac
      Left 041D
      Right 041C
    Coronary
      Four or More Arteries 0213
      One Artery 0210
      Three Arteries 0212
      Two Arteries 0211
    External Carotid
      Left 031N0
      Right 031M0
    External Iliac
      Left 041J
      Right 041H
    Femoral
      Left 041L
      Right 041K
    Foot
      Left 041W
      Right 041V
    Hepatic 0413
    Innominate 03120
    Internal Carotid
      Left 031L0
      Right 031K0
    Internal Iliac
      Left 041F
      Right 041E
    Intracranial 031G0
    Peroneal
      Left 041U
      Right 041T
    Popliteal
      Left 041N
      Right 041M
    Posterior Tibial
      Left 041S
      Right 041R
    Pulmonary
      Left 021R
      Right 021Q
    Pulmonary Trunk 021P
    Radial
      Left 031C
      Right 031B
    Splenic 0414
    Subclavian
      Left 03140
      Right 03130
    Temporal
      Left 031T0
      Right 031S0
    Ulnar
      Left 031A
      Right 0319
  Atrium
    Left 0217
    Right 0216
  Bladder 0T1B
  Cavity, Cranial 0W110J
  Cecum 0D1H
  Cerebral Ventricle 0016
  Colon
    Ascending 0D1K
    Descending 0D1M
    Sigmoid 0D1N
    Transverse 0D1L
  Duct
    Common Bile 0F19
    Cystic 0F18
    Hepatic
      Common 0F17
      Left 0F16
      Right 0F15

Bypass — *continued*
Duct — *continued*
Lacrimal
Left Ø81Y
Right Ø81X
Pancreatic ØF1D
Accessory ØF1F
Duodenum ØD19
Ear
Left Ø91EØ
Right Ø91DØ
Esophagus ØD15
Lower ØD13
Middle ØD12
Upper ØD11
Fallopian Tube
Left ØU16
Right ØU15
Gallbladder ØF14
Ileum ØD1B
Intestine
Large ØD1E
Small ØD18
Jejunum ØD1A
Kidney Pelvis
Left ØT14
Right ØT13
Pancreas ØF1G
Pelvic Cavity ØW1J
Peritoneal Cavity ØW1G
Pleural Cavity
Left ØW1B
Right ØW19
Spinal Canal ØØ1U
Stomach ØD16
Trachea ØB11
Ureter
Left ØT17
Right ØT16
Ureters, Bilateral ØT18
Vas Deferens
Bilateral ØV1Q
Left ØV1P
Right ØV1N
Vein
Axillary
Left Ø518
Right Ø517
Azygos Ø51Ø
Basilic
Left Ø51C
Right Ø51B
Brachial
Left Ø51A
Right Ø519
Cephalic
Left Ø51F
Right Ø51D
Colic Ø617
Common Iliac
Left Ø61D
Right Ø61C
Esophageal Ø613
External Iliac
Left Ø61G
Right Ø61F
External Jugular
Left Ø51Q
Right Ø51P
Face
Left Ø51V
Right Ø51T
Femoral
Left Ø61N
Right Ø61M
Foot
Left Ø61V
Right Ø61T
Gastric Ø612
Hand
Left Ø51H
Right Ø51G
Hemiazygos Ø511
Hepatic Ø614
Hypogastric
Left Ø61J
Right Ø61H
Inferior Mesenteric Ø616

Bypass — *continued*
Vein — *continued*
Innominate
Left Ø514
Right Ø513
Internal Jugular
Left Ø51N
Right Ø51M
Intracranial Ø51L
Portal Ø618
Renal
Left Ø61B
Right Ø619
Saphenous
Left Ø61Q
Right Ø61P
Splenic Ø611
Subclavian
Left Ø516
Right Ø515
Superior Mesenteric Ø615
Vertebral
Left Ø51S
Right Ø51R
Vena Cava
Inferior Ø61Ø
Superior Ø21V
Ventricle
Left Ø21L
Right Ø21K
Bypass, cardiopulmonary 5A1221Z

C

Caesarean section *see* Extraction, Products of Conception 10DØ
Calcaneocuboid joint
use Tarsal Joint, Left
use Tarsal Joint, Right
Calcaneocuboid ligament
use Foot Bursa and Ligament, Left
use Foot Bursa and Ligament, Right
Calcaneofibular ligament
use Ankle Bursa and Ligament, Left
use Ankle Bursa and Ligament, Right
Calcaneus
use Tarsal, Left
use Tarsal, Right
Cannulation
see Bypass
see Dilation
see Drainage
see Irrigation
Canthorrhaphy *see* Repair, Eye Ø8Q
Canthotomy *see* Release, Eye Ø8N
Capitate bone
use Carpal, Left
use Carpal, Right
Caplacizumab XWØ
Capsulectomy, lens *see* Excision, Eye Ø8B
Capsulorrhaphy, joint
see Repair, Lower Joints ØSQ
see Repair, Upper Joints ØRQ
Cardia *use* Esophagogastric Junction
Cardiac contractility modulation lead *use* Cardiac Lead in Heart and Great Vessels
Cardiac event recorder *use* Monitoring Device
Cardiac Lead
Defibrillator
Atrium
Left Ø2H7
Right Ø2H6
Pericardium Ø2HN
Vein, Coronary Ø2H4
Ventricle
Left Ø2HL
Right Ø2HK
Insertion of device in
Atrium
Left Ø2H7
Right Ø2H6
Pericardium Ø2HN
Vein, Coronary Ø2H4
Ventricle
Left Ø2HL
Right Ø2HK

Cardiac Lead — *continued*
Pacemaker
Atrium
Left Ø2H7
Right Ø2H6
Pericardium Ø2HN
Vein, Coronary Ø2H4
Ventricle
Left Ø2HL
Right Ø2HK
Removal of device from, Heart Ø2PA
Revision of device in, Heart Ø2WA
Cardiac plexus *use* Thoracic Sympathetic Nerve
Cardiac Resynchronization Defibrillator Pulse Generator
Abdomen ØJH8
Chest ØJH6
Cardiac Resynchronization Pacemaker Pulse Generator
Abdomen ØJH8
Chest ØJH6
Cardiac resynchronization therapy (CRT) lead
use Cardiac Lead, Defibrillator in Ø2H
use Cardiac Lead, Pacemaker in Ø2H
Cardiac Rhythm Related Device
Insertion of device in
Abdomen ØJH8
Chest ØJH6
Removal of device from, Subcutaneous Tissue and Fascia, Trunk ØJPT
Revision of device in, Subcutaneous Tissue and Fascia, Trunk ØJWT
Cardiocentesis *see* Drainage, Pericardial Cavity ØW9D
Cardioesophageal junction *use* Esophagogastric Junction
Cardiolysis *see* Release, Heart and Great Vessels Ø2N
CardioMEMS® pressure sensor *use* Monitoring Device, Pressure Sensor in Ø2H
Cardiomyotomy *see* Division, Esophagogastric Junction ØD84
Cardioplegia *see* Introduction of substance in or on, Heart 3EØ8
Cardiorrhaphy *see* Repair, Heart and Great Vessels Ø2Q
Cardioversion 5A22Ø4Z
Caregiver Training FØFZ
Caroticotympanic artery
use Internal Carotid Artery, Left
use Internal Carotid Artery, Right
Carotid glomus
use Carotid Bodies, Bilateral
use Carotid Body, Left
use Carotid Body, Right
Carotid sinus
use Internal Carotid Artery, Left
use Internal Carotid Artery, Right
Carotid (artery) sinus (baroreceptor) lead *use* Stimulator Lead in Upper Arteries
Carotid sinus nerve *use* Glossopharyngeal Nerve
Carotid WALLSTENT® Monorail® Endoprosthesis *use* Intraluminal Device
Carpectomy
see Excision, Upper Bones ØPB
see Resection, Upper Bones ØPT
Carpometacarpal ligament
use Hand Bursa and Ligament, Left
use Hand Bursa and Ligament, Right
Casting *see* Immobilization
CAT scan *see* Computerized Tomography (CT Scan)
Catheterization
see Dilation
see Drainage
see Insertion of device in
see Irrigation
Heart *see* Measurement, Cardiac 4AØ2
Umbilical vein, for infusion Ø6HØ33T
Cauda equina *use* Lumbar Spinal Cord
Cauterization
see Destruction
see Repair
Cavernous plexus *use* Head and Neck Sympathetic Nerve
CBMA (Concentrated Bone Marrow Aspirate) *use* Concentrated Bone Marrow Aspirate
CBMA (Concentrated Bone Marrow Aspirate) injection, intramuscular XKØ23Ø3
Cecectomy
see Excision, Cecum ØDBH

Cecectomy — *continued*
 see Resection, Cecum ØDTH
Cecocolostomy
 see Bypass, Gastrointestinal System ØD1
 see Drainage, Gastrointestinal System ØD9
Cecopexy
 see Repair, Cecum ØDQH
 see Reposition, Cecum ØDSH
Cecoplication *see* Restriction, Cecum ØDVH
Cecorrhaphy *see* Repair, Cecum ØDQH
Cecostomy
 see Bypass, Cecum ØD1H
 see Drainage, Cecum ØD9H
Cecotomy *see* Drainage, Cecum ØD9H
Cefiderocol Anti-infective XWØ
Ceftazidime-Avibactam Anti-infective XWØ
Ceftolozane/Tazobactam Anti-infective XWØ
Celiac ganglion *use* Abdominal Sympathetic Nerve
Celiac lymph node *use* Lymphatic, Aortic
Celiac (solar) plexus *use* Abdominal Sympathetic Nerve
Celiac trunk *use* Celiac Artery
Central axillary lymph node
 use Lymphatic, Left Axillary
 use Lymphatic, Right Axillary
Central venous pressure *see* Measurement, Venous 4AØ4
Centrimag® Blood Pump *use* Short-term External Heart Assist System in Heart and Great Vessels
Cephalogram BNØØZZZ
Ceramic on ceramic bearing surface *use* Synthetic Substitute, Ceramic in ØSR
Cerclage *see* Restriction
Cerebral aqueduct (Sylvius) *use* Cerebral Ventricle
Cerebral Embolic Filtration
 Dual Filter X2A5312
 Extracorporeal Flow Reversal Circuit X2A
 Single Deflection Filter X2A6325
Cerebrum *use* Brain
Cervical esophagus *use* Esophagus, Upper
Cervical facet joint
 use Cervical Vertebral Joint
 use Cervical Vertebral Joint, 2 or more
Cervical ganglion *use* Head and Neck Sympathetic Nerve
Cervical interspinous ligament *use* Head and Neck Bursa and Ligament
Cervical intertransverse ligament *use* Head and Neck Bursa and Ligament
Cervical Ligamentum Flavum *use* Head and Neck Bursa and Ligament
Cervical Lymph Node
 use Lymphatic, Left Neck
 use Lymphatic, Right Neck
Cervicectomy
 see Excision, Cervix ØUBC
 see Resection, Cervix ØUTC
Cervicothoracic facet joint *use* Cervicothoracic Vertebral Joint
Cesarean section *see* Extraction, Products of Conception 10DØ
Cesium-131 Collagen Implant *use* Radioactive Element, Cesium-131 Collagen Implant in ØØH
Change Device in
 Abdominal Wall ØW2FX
 Back
  Lower ØW2LX
  Upper ØW2KX
 Bladder ØT2BX
 Bone
  Facial ØN2WX
  Lower ØQ2YX
  Nasal ØN2BX
  Upper ØP2YX
 Bone Marrow Ø72TX
 Brain ØØ2ØX
 Breast
  Left ØH2UX
  Right ØH2TX
 Bursa and Ligament
  Lower ØM2YX
  Upper ØM2XX
 Cavity, Cranial ØW21X
 Chest Wall ØW28X
 Cisterna Chyli Ø72LX
 Diaphragm ØB2TX

Change Device in — *continued*
 Duct
  Hepatobiliary ØF2BX
  Pancreatic ØF2DX
 Ear
  Left Ø92JX
  Right Ø92HX
 Epididymis and Spermatic Cord ØV2MX
 Extremity
  Lower
   Left ØY2BX
   Right ØY29X
  Upper
   Left ØX27X
   Right ØX26X
 Eye
  Left Ø821X
  Right Ø82ØX
 Face ØW22X
 Fallopian Tube ØU28X
 Gallbladder ØF24X
 Gland
  Adrenal ØG25X
  Endocrine ØG2SX
  Pituitary ØG2ØX
  Salivary ØC2AX
 Head ØW2ØX
 Intestinal Tract
  Lower ØD2DXUZ
  Upper ØD2ØXUZ
 Jaw
  Lower ØW25X
  Upper ØW24X
 Joint
  Lower ØS2YX
  Upper ØR2YX
 Kidney ØT25X
 Larynx ØC2SX
 Liver ØF2ØX
 Lung
  Left ØB2LX
  Right ØB2KX
 Lymphatic Ø72NX
  Thoracic Duct Ø72KX
 Mediastinum ØW2CX
 Mesentery ØD2VX
 Mouth and Throat ØC2YX
 Muscle
  Lower ØK2YX
  Upper ØK2XX
 Nasal Mucosa and Soft Tissue Ø92KX
 Neck ØW26X
 Nerve
  Cranial ØØ2EX
  Peripheral Ø12YX
 Omentum ØD2UX
 Ovary ØU23X
 Pancreas ØF2GX
 Parathyroid Gland ØG2RX
 Pelvic Cavity ØW2JX
 Penis ØV2SX
 Pericardial Cavity ØW2DX
 Perineum
  Female ØW2NX
  Male ØW2MX
 Peritoneal Cavity ØW2GX
 Peritoneum ØD2WX
 Pineal Body ØG21X
 Pleura ØB2QX
 Pleural Cavity
  Left ØW2BX
  Right ØW29X
 Products of Conception 10207
 Prostate and Seminal Vesicles ØV24X
 Retroperitoneum ØW2HX
 Scrotum and Tunica Vaginalis ØV28X
 Sinus Ø92YX
 Skin ØH2PX
 Skull ØN2ØX
 Spinal Canal ØØ2UX
 Spleen Ø72PX
 Subcutaneous Tissue and Fascia
  Head and Neck ØJ2SX
  Lower Extremity ØJ2WX
  Trunk ØJ2TX
  Upper Extremity ØJ2VX
 Tendon
  Lower ØL2YX
  Upper ØL2XX

Change Device in — *continued*
 Testis ØV2DX
 Thymus Ø72MX
 Thyroid Gland ØG2KX
 Trachea ØB21X
 Tracheobronchial Tree ØB2ØX
 Ureter ØT29X
 Urethra ØT2DX
 Uterus and Cervix ØU2DXHZ
 Vagina and Cul-de-sac ØU2HXGZ
 Vas Deferens ØV2RX
 Vulva ØU2MX
Change Device in or on
 Abdominal Wall 2WØ3X
 Anorectal 2YØ3X5Z
 Arm
  Lower
   Left 2WØDX
   Right 2WØCX
  Upper
   Left 2WØBX
   Right 2WØAX
 Back 2WØ5X
 Chest Wall 2WØ4X
 Ear 2YØ2X5Z
 Extremity
  Lower
   Left 2WØMX
   Right 2WØLX
  Upper
   Left 2WØ9X
   Right 2WØ8X
 Face 2WØ1X
 Finger
  Left 2WØKX
  Right 2WØJX
 Foot
  Left 2WØTX
  Right 2WØSX
 Genital Tract, Female 2YØ4X5Z
 Hand
  Left 2WØFX
  Right 2WØEX
 Head 2WØØX
 Inguinal Region
  Left 2WØ7X
  Right 2WØ6X
 Leg
  Lower
   Left 2WØRX
   Right 2WØQX
  Upper
   Left 2WØPX
   Right 2WØNX
 Mouth and Pharynx 2YØØX5Z
 Nasal 2YØ1X5Z
 Neck 2WØ2X
 Thumb
  Left 2WØHX
  Right 2WØGX
 Toe
  Left 2WØVX
  Right 2WØUX
 Urethra 2YØ5X5Z
Chemoembolization *see* Introduction of substance in or on
Chemosurgery, Skin 3EØØXTZ
Chemothalamectomy *see* Destruction, Thalamus ØØ59
Chemotherapy, Infusion for Cancer *see* Introduction of substance in or on
Chest x-ray *see* Plain Radiography, Chest BWØ3
Chiropractic Manipulation
 Abdomen 9WB9X
 Cervical 9WB1X
 Extremities
  Lower 9WB6X
  Upper 9WB7X
 Head 9WBØX
 Lumbar 9WB3X
 Pelvis 9WB5X
 Rib Cage 9WB8X
 Sacrum 9WB4X
 Thoracic 9WB2X
Choana *use* Nasopharynx
Cholangiogram
 see Fluoroscopy, Hepatobiliary System and Pancreas BF1

Cholangiogram — *continued*
  see Plain Radiography, Hepatobiliary System and Pancreas BF0
Cholecystectomy
  see Excision, Gallbladder 0FB4
  see Resection, Gallbladder 0FT4
Cholecystojejunostomy
  see Bypass, Hepatobiliary System and Pancreas 0F1
  see Drainage, Hepatobiliary System and Pancreas 0F9
Cholecystopexy
  see Repair, Gallbladder 0FQ4
  see Reposition, Gallbladder 0FS4
Cholecystoscopy 0FJ44ZZ
Cholecystostomy
  see Bypass, Gallbladder 0F14
  see Drainage, Gallbladder 0F94
Cholecystotomy *see* Drainage, Gallbladder 0F94
Choledochectomy
  see Excision, Hepatobiliary System and Pancreas 0FB
  see Resection, Hepatobiliary System and Pancreas 0FT
Choledocholithotomy *see* Extirpation, Duct, Common Bile 0FC9
Choledochoplasty
  see Repair, Hepatobiliary System and Pancreas 0FQ
  see Replacement, Hepatobiliary System and Pancreas 0FR
  see Supplement, Hepatobiliary System and Pancreas 0FU
Choledochoscopy 0FJB8ZZ
Choledochotomy *see* Drainage, Hepatobiliary System and Pancreas 0F9
Cholelithotomy *see* Extirpation, Hepatobiliary System and Pancreas 0FC
Chondrectomy
  see Excision, Lower Joints 0SB
  see Excision, Upper Joints 0RB
  Knee *see* Excision, Lower Joints 0SB
  Semilunar cartilage *see* Excision, Lower Joints 0SB
Chondroglossus muscle *use* Tongue, Palate, Pharynx Muscle
Chorda tympani *use* Facial Nerve
Chordotomy *see* Division, Central Nervous System and Cranial Nerves 008
Choroid plexus *use* Cerebral Ventricle
Choroidectomy
  see Excision, Eye 08B
  see Resection, Eye 08T
Ciliary body
  use Eye, Left
  use Eye, Right
Ciliary ganglion *use* Head and Neck Sympathetic Nerve
Circle of Willis *use* Intracranial Artery
Circumcision 0VTTXZZ
Circumflex iliac artery
  use Femoral Artery, Left
  use Femoral Artery, Right
CivaSheet® *use* Radioactive Element
CivaSheet® Brachytherapy
  see Brachytherapy with qualifier Unidirectional Source
  see Insertion with device Radioactive Element
Clamp and rod internal fixation system (CRIF)
  use Internal Fixation Device in Lower Bones
  use Internal Fixation Device in Upper Bones
Clamping *see* Occlusion
Claustrum *use* Basal Ganglia
Claviculectomy
  see Excision, Upper Bones 0PB
  see Resection, Upper Bones 0PT
Claviculotomy
  see Division, Upper Bones 0P8
  see Drainage, Upper Bones 0P9
Clipping, aneurysm
  see Occlusion using Extraluminal Device
  see Restriction using Extraluminal Device
Clitorectomy, clitoridectomy
  see Excision, Clitoris 0UBJ
  see Resection, Clitoris 0UTJ
Clolar *use* Clofarabine
Closure
  see Occlusion
  see Repair

Clysis *see* Introduction of substance in or on
Coagulation *see* Destruction
Coagulation Factor Xa, Inactivated XW0
Coagulation Factor Xa, (Recombinant) Inactivated
  use Coagulation Factor Xa, Inactivated
COALESCE® radiolucent interbody fusion device
  use Interbody Fusion Device, Radiolucent Porous in New Technology
CoAxia NeuroFlo catheter *use* Intraluminal Device
Cobalt/chromium head and polyethylene socket
  use Synthetic Substitute, Metal on Polyethylene in 0SR
Cobalt/chromium head and socket *use* Synthetic Substitute, Metal in 0SR
Coccygeal body *use* Coccygeal Glomus
Coccygeus muscle
  use Trunk Muscle, Left
  use Trunk Muscle, Right
Cochlea
  use Inner Ear, Left
  use Inner Ear, Right
Cochlear implant (CI), multiple channel (electrode)
  use Hearing Device, Multiple Channel Cochlear Prosthesis in 09H
Cochlear implant (CI), single channel (electrode)
  use Hearing Device, Single Channel Cochlear Prosthesis in 09H
Cochlear Implant Treatment F0BZ0
Cochlear nerve *use* Acoustic Nerve
COGNIS® CRT-D *use* Cardiac Resynchronization Defibrillator Pulse Generator in 0JH
COHERE® radiolucent interbody fusion device *use* Interbody Fusion Device, Radiolucent Porous in New Technology
Colectomy
  see Excision, Gastrointestinal System 0DB
  see Resection, Gastrointestinal System 0DT
Collapse *see* Occlusion
Collection from
  Breast, Breast Milk 8E0HX62
  Indwelling Device
    Circulatory System
      Blood 8C02X6K
      Other Fluid 8C02X6L
    Nervous System
      Cerebrospinal Fluid 8C01X6J
      Other Fluid 8C01X6L
  Integumentary System, Breast Milk 8E0HX62
  Reproductive System, Male, Sperm 8E0VX63
Colocentesis *see* Drainage, Gastrointestinal System 0D9
Colofixation
  see Repair, Gastrointestinal System 0DQ
  see Reposition, Gastrointestinal System 0DS
Cololysis *see* Release, Gastrointestinal System 0DN
Colonic Z-Stent® *use* Intraluminal Device
Colonoscopy 0DJD8ZZ
Colopexy
  see Repair, Gastrointestinal System 0DQ
  see Reposition, Gastrointestinal System 0DS
Coloplication *see* Restriction, Gastrointestinal System 0DV
Coloproctectomy
  see Excision, Gastrointestinal System 0DB
  see Resection, Gastrointestinal System 0DT
Coloproctostomy
  see Bypass, Gastrointestinal System 0D1
  see Drainage, Gastrointestinal System 0D9
Colopuncture *see* Drainage, Gastrointestinal System 0D9
Colorrhaphy *see* Repair, Gastrointestinal System 0DQ
Colostomy
  see Bypass, Gastrointestinal System 0D1
  see Drainage, Gastrointestinal System 0D9
Colpectomy
  see Excision, Vagina 0UBG
  see Resection, Vagina 0UTG
Colpocentesis *see* Drainage, Vagina 0U9G
Colpopexy
  see Repair, Vagina 0UQG
  see Reposition, Vagina 0USG
Colpoplasty
  see Repair, Vagina 0UQG
  see Supplement, Vagina 0UUG
Colporrhaphy *see* Repair, Vagina 0UQG
Colposcopy 0UJH8ZZ
Columella *use* Nasal Mucosa and Soft Tissue

Common digital vein
  use Foot Vein, Left
  use Foot Vein, Right
Common facial vein
  use Face Vein, Left
  use Face Vein, Right
Common fibular nerve *use* Peroneal Nerve
Common hepatic artery *use* Hepatic Artery
Common iliac (subaortic) lymph node *use* Lymphatic, Pelvis
Common interosseous artery
  use Ulnar Artery, Left
  use Ulnar Artery, Right
Common peroneal nerve *use* Peroneal Nerve
Complete (SE) stent *use* Intraluminal Device
Compression
  see Restriction
  Abdominal Wall 2W13X
  Arm
    Lower
      Left 2W1DX
      Right 2W1CX
    Upper
      Left 2W1BX
      Right 2W1AX
  Back 2W15X
  Chest Wall 2W14X
  Extremity
    Lower
      Left 2W1MX
      Right 2W1LX
    Upper
      Left 2W19X
      Right 2W18X
  Face 2W11X
  Finger
    Left 2W1KX
    Right 2W1JX
  Foot
    Left 2W1TX
    Right 2W1SX
  Hand
    Left 2W1FX
    Right 2W1EX
  Head 2W10X
  Inguinal Region
    Left 2W17X
    Right 2W16X
  Leg
    Lower
      Left 2W1RX
      Right 2W1QX
    Upper
      Left 2W1PX
      Right 2W1NX
  Neck 2W12X
  Thumb
    Left 2W1HX
    Right 2W1GX
  Toe
    Left 2W1VX
    Right 2W1UX
Computer Assisted Procedure
  Extremity
    Lower
      No Qualifier 8E0YXBZ
      With Computerized Tomography 8E0YXBG
      With Fluoroscopy 8E0YXBF
      With Magnetic Resonance Imaging 8E0YXBH
    Upper
      No Qualifier 8E0XXBZ
      With Computerized Tomography 8E0XXBG
      With Fluoroscopy 8E0XXBF
      With Magnetic Resonance Imaging 8E0XXBH
  Head and Neck Region
    No Qualifier 8E09XBZ
    With Computerized Tomography 8E09XBG
    With Fluoroscopy 8E09XBF
    With Magnetic Resonance Imaging 8E09XBH
  Trunk Region
    No Qualifier 8E0WXBZ
    With Computerized Tomography 8E0WXBG
    With Fluoroscopy 8E0WXBF
    With Magnetic Resonance Imaging 8E0WXBH

Index

Computerized Tomography (CT Scan) — Computerized Tomography (CT Scan)

Computerized Tomography (CT Scan) — *continued*
  Vein — *continued*
    Renal — *continued*
      Left B52K
        Intravascular Optical Coherence
          B52KZ2Z
      Right B52J
        Intravascular Optical Coherence
          B52JZ2Z
    Spanchnic B52T
      Intravascular Optical Coherence
        B52TZ2Z
  Vena Cava
    Inferior B529
      Intravascular Optical Coherence
        B529Z2Z
    Superior B528
      Intravascular Optical Coherence
        B528Z2Z
  Ventricle, Cerebral B028
  Wrist
    Left BP2M
    Right BP2L
Concentrated Bone Marrow Aspirate (CBMA) injection, intramuscular XK02303
Concerto II CRT-D *use* Cardiac Resynchronization Defibrillator Pulse Generator in 0JH
Condylectomy
  see Excision, Head and Facial Bones 0NB
  see Excision, Lower Bones 0QB
  see Excision, Upper Bones 0PB
Condyloid process
  use Mandible, Left
  use Mandible, Right
Condylotomy
  see Division, Head and Facial Bones 0N8
  see Division, Lower Bones 0Q8
  see Division, Upper Bones 0P8
  see Drainage, Head and Facial Bones 0N9
  see Drainage, Lower Bones 0Q9
  see Drainage, Upper Bones 0P9
Condylysis
  see Release, Head and Facial Bones 0NN
  see Release, Lower Bones 0QN
  see Release, Upper Bones 0PN
Conization, cervix *see* Excision, Cervix 0UBC
Conjunctivoplasty
  see Repair, Eye 08Q
  see Replacement, Eye 08R
CONSERVE® PLUS Total Resurfacing Hip System *use* Resurfacing Device in Lower Joints
Construction
  Auricle, ear *see* Replacement, Ear, Nose, Sinus 09R
  Ileal conduit *see* Bypass, Urinary System 0T1
Consulta CRT-D *use* Cardiac Resynchronization Defibrillator Pulse Generator in 0JH
Consulta CRT-P *use* Cardiac Resynchronization Pacemaker Pulse Generator in 0JH
Contact Radiation
  Abdomen DWY37ZZ
  Adrenal Gland DGY27ZZ
  Bile Ducts DFY27ZZ
  Bladder DTY27ZZ
  Bone, Other DPYC7ZZ
  Brain D0Y07ZZ
  Brain Stem D0Y17ZZ
  Breast
    Left DMY07ZZ
    Right DMY17ZZ
  Bronchus DBY17ZZ
  Cervix DUY17ZZ
  Chest DWY27ZZ
  Chest Wall DBY77ZZ
  Colon DDY57ZZ
  Diaphragm DBY87ZZ
  Duodenum DDY27ZZ
  Ear D9Y07ZZ
  Esophagus DDY07ZZ
  Eye D8Y07ZZ
  Femur DPY97ZZ
  Fibula DPYB7ZZ
  Gallbladder DFY17ZZ
  Gland
    Adrenal DGY27ZZ
    Parathyroid DGY47ZZ
    Pituitary DGY07ZZ
    Thyroid DGY57ZZ
  Glands, Salivary D9Y67ZZ

Contact Radiation — *continued*
  Head and Neck DWY17ZZ
  Hemibody DWY47ZZ
  Humerus DPY67ZZ
  Hypopharynx D9Y37ZZ
  Ileum DDY47ZZ
  Jejunum DDY37ZZ
  Kidney DTY07ZZ
  Larynx D9YB7ZZ
  Liver DFY07ZZ
  Lung DBY27ZZ
  Mandible DPY37ZZ
  Maxilla DPY27ZZ
  Mediastinum DBY67ZZ
  Mouth D9Y47ZZ
  Nasopharynx D9YD7ZZ
  Neck and Head DWY17ZZ
  Nerve, Peripheral D0Y77ZZ
  Nose D9Y17ZZ
  Oropharynx D9YF7ZZ
  Ovary DUY07ZZ
  Palate
    Hard D9Y87ZZ
    Soft D9Y97ZZ
  Pancreas DFY37ZZ
  Parathyroid Gland DGY47ZZ
  Pelvic Bones DPY87ZZ
  Pelvic Region DWY67ZZ
  Pineal Body DGY17ZZ
  Pituitary Gland DGY07ZZ
  Pleura DBY57ZZ
  Prostate DVY07ZZ
  Radius DPY77ZZ
  Rectum DDY77ZZ
  Rib DPY57ZZ
  Sinuses D9Y77ZZ
  Skin
    Abdomen DHY87ZZ
    Arm DHY47ZZ
    Back DHY77ZZ
    Buttock DHY97ZZ
    Chest DHY67ZZ
    Face DHY27ZZ
    Leg DHYB7ZZ
    Neck DHY37ZZ
  Skull DPY07ZZ
  Spinal Cord D0Y67ZZ
  Sternum DPY47ZZ
  Stomach DDY17ZZ
  Testis DVY17ZZ
  Thyroid Gland DGY57ZZ
  Tibia DPYB7ZZ
  Tongue D9Y57ZZ
  Trachea DBY07ZZ
  Ulna DPY77ZZ
  Ureter DTY17ZZ
  Urethra DTY37ZZ
  Uterus DUY27ZZ
  Whole Body DWY57ZZ
ContaCT software (Measurement of intracranial arterial flow) 4A03X5D
CONTAK RENEWAL® 3 RF (HE) CRT-D *use* Cardiac Resynchronization Defibrillator Pulse Generator in 0JH
Contegra Pulmonary Valved Conduit *use* Zooplastic Tissue in Heart and Great Vessels
CONTEPO™ *use* Fosfomycin Anti-Infective
Continuous Glucose Monitoring (CGM) device *use* Monitoring Device
Continuous Negative Airway Pressure
  24-96 Consecutive Hours, Ventilation 5A09459
  Greater than 96 Consecutive Hours, Ventilation 5A09559
  Less than 24 Consecutive Hours, Ventilation 5A09359
Continuous Positive Airway Pressure
  24-96 Consecutive Hours, Ventilation 5A09457
  Greater than 96 Consecutive Hours, Ventilation 5A09557
  Less than 24 Consecutive Hours, Ventilation 5A09357
Continuous renal replacement therapy (CRRT) 5A1D90Z
Contraceptive Device
  Change device in, Uterus and Cervix 0U2DXHZ
  Insertion of device in
    Cervix 0UHC

Contraceptive Device — *continued*
  Insertion of device in — *continued*
    Subcutaneous Tissue and Fascia
      Abdomen 0JH8
      Chest 0JH6
      Lower Arm
        Left 0JHH
        Right 0JHG
      Lower Leg
        Left 0JHP
        Right 0JHN
      Upper Arm
        Left 0JHF
        Right 0JHD
      Upper Leg
        Left 0JHM
        Right 0JHL
    Uterus 0UH9
  Removal of device from
    Subcutaneous Tissue and Fascia
      Lower Extremity 0JPW
      Trunk 0JPT
      Upper Extremity 0JPV
    Uterus and Cervix 0UPD
  Revision of device in
    Subcutaneous Tissue and Fascia
      Lower Extremity 0JWW
      Trunk 0JWT
      Upper Extremity 0JWV
    Uterus and Cervix 0UWD
Contractility Modulation Device
  Abdomen 0JH8
  Chest 0JH6
Control bleeding in
  Abdominal Wall 0W3F
  Ankle Region
    Left 0Y3L
    Right 0Y3K
  Arm
    Lower
      Left 0X3F
      Right 0X3D
    Upper
      Left 0X39
      Right 0X38
  Axilla
    Left 0X35
    Right 0X34
  Back
    Lower 0W3L
    Upper 0W3K
  Buttock
    Left 0Y31
    Right 0Y30
  Cavity, Cranial 0W31
  Chest Wall 0W38
  Elbow Region
    Left 0X3C
    Right 0X3B
  Extremity
    Lower
      Left 0Y3B
      Right 0Y39
    Upper
      Left 0X37
      Right 0X36
  Face 0W32
  Femoral Region
    Left 0Y38
    Right 0Y37
  Foot
    Left 0Y3N
    Right 0Y3M
  Gastrointestinal Tract 0W3P
  Genitourinary Tract 0W3R
  Hand
    Left 0X3K
    Right 0X3J
  Head 0W30
  Inguinal Region
    Left 0Y36
    Right 0Y35
  Jaw
    Lower 0W35
    Upper 0W34
  Knee Region
    Left 0Y3G
    Right 0Y3F

Control bleeding in — *continued*
  Leg
    Lower
      Left 0Y3J
      Right 0Y3H
    Upper
      Left 0Y3D
      Right 0Y3C
  Mediastinum 0W3C
  Nasal Mucosa and Soft Tissue 093K
  Neck 0W36
  Oral Cavity and Throat 0W33
  Pelvic Cavity 0W3J
  Pericardial Cavity 0W3D
  Perineum
    Female 0W3N
    Male 0W3M
  Peritoneal Cavity 0W3G
  Pleural Cavity
    Left 0W3B
    Right 0W39
  Respiratory Tract 0W3Q
  Retroperitoneum 0W3H
  Shoulder Region
    Left 0X33
    Right 0X32
  Wrist Region
    Left 0X3H
    Right 0X3G
Control, Epistaxis *see* Control bleeding in, Nasal Mucosa and Soft Tissue 093K
Conus arteriosus *use* Ventricle, Right
Conus medullaris *use* Lumbar Spinal Cord
Conversion
  Cardiac rhythm 5A2204Z
  Gastrostomy to jejunostomy feeding device *see* Insertion of device in, Jejunum 0DHA
Cook Biodesign® Fistula Plug(s) *use* Nonautologous Tissue Substitute
Cook Biodesign® Hernia Graft(s) *use* Nonautologous Tissue Substitute
Cook Biodesign® Layered Graft(s) *use* Nonautologous Tissue Substitute
Cook Zenaprom™ Layered Graft(s) *use* Nonautologous Tissue Substitute
Cook Zenith AAA Endovascular Graft *use* Intraluminal Device
Cook Zenith® Fenestrated AAA Endovascular Graft
  use Intraluminal Device, Branched or Fenestrated, One or Two Arteries in 04V
  use Intraluminal Device, Branched or Fenestrated, Three or More Arteries in 04V
Coracoacromial ligament
  use Shoulder Bursa and Ligament, Left
  use Shoulder Bursa and Ligament, Right
Coracobrachialis muscle
  use Upper Arm Muscle, Left
  use Upper Arm Muscle, Right
Coracoclavicular ligament
  use Shoulder Bursa and Ligament, Left
  use Shoulder Bursa and Ligament, Right
Coracohumeral ligament
  use Shoulder Bursa and Ligament, Left
  use Shoulder Bursa and Ligament, Right
Coracoid process
  use Scapula, Left
  use Scapula, Right
Cordotomy *see* Division, Central Nervous System and Cranial Nerves 008
Core needle biopsy *see* Excision with qualifier Diagnostic
CoreValve transcatheter aortic valve *use* Zooplastic Tissue in Heart and Great Vessels
Cormet Hip Resurfacing System *use* Resurfacing Device in Lower Joints
Corniculate cartilage *use* Larynx
CoRoent® XL *use* Interbody Fusion Device in Lower Joints
Coronary arteriography
  see Fluoroscopy, Heart B21
  see Plain Radiography, Heart B20
Corox (OTW) Bipolar Lead
  use Cardiac Lead, Defibrillator in 02H
  use Cardiac Lead, Pacemaker in 02H
Corpus callosum *use* Brain
Corpus cavernosum *use* Penis
Corpus spongiosum *use* Penis

Corpus striatum *use* Basal Ganglia
Corrugator supercilii muscle *use* Facial Muscle
Cortical strip neurostimulator lead *use* Neurostimulator Lead in Central Nervous System and Cranial Nerves
Corvia IASD® *use* Synthetic Substitute
Costatectomy
  see Excision, Upper Bones 0PB
  see Resection, Upper Bones 0PT
Costectomy
  see Excision, Upper Bones 0PB
  see Resection, Upper Bones 0PT
Costocervical trunk
  use Subclavian Artery, Left
  use Subclavian Artery, Right
Costochondrectomy
  see Excision, Upper Bones 0PB
  see Resection, Upper Bones 0PT
Costoclavicular ligament
  use Shoulder Bursa and Ligament, Left
  use Shoulder Bursa and Ligament, Right
Costosternoplasty
  see Repair, Upper Bones 0PQ
  see Replacement, Upper Bones 0PR
  see Supplement, Upper Bones 0PU
Costotomy
  see Division, Upper Bones 0P8
  see Drainage, Upper Bones 0P9
Costotransverse joint *use* Thoracic Vertebral Joint
Costotransverse ligament *use* Rib(s) Bursa and Ligament
Costovertebral joint *use* Thoracic Vertebral Joint
Costoxiphoid ligament *use* Sternum Bursa and Ligament
Counseling
  Family, for substance abuse, Other Family Counseling HZ63ZZZ
  Group
    12-Step HZ43ZZZ
    Behavioral HZ41ZZZ
    Cognitive HZ40ZZZ
    Cognitive-Behavioral HZ42ZZZ
    Confrontational HZ48ZZZ
    Continuing Care HZ49ZZZ
    Infectious Disease
      Post-Test HZ4CZZZ
      Pre-Test HZ4CZZZ
    Interpersonal HZ44ZZZ
    Motivational Enhancement HZ47ZZZ
    Psychoeducation HZ46ZZZ
    Spiritual HZ4BZZZ
    Vocational HZ45ZZZ
  Individual
    12-Step HZ33ZZZ
    Behavioral HZ31ZZZ
    Cognitive HZ30ZZZ
    Cognitive-Behavioral HZ32ZZZ
    Confrontational HZ38ZZZ
    Continuing Care HZ39ZZZ
    Infectious Disease
      Post-Test HZ3CZZZ
      Pre-Test HZ3CZZZ
    Interpersonal HZ34ZZZ
    Motivational Enhancement HZ37ZZZ
    Psychoeducation HZ36ZZZ
    Spiritual HZ3BZZZ
    Vocational HZ35ZZZ
  Mental Health Services
    Educational GZ60ZZZ
    Other Counseling GZ63ZZZ
    Vocational GZ61ZZZ
Countershock, cardiac 5A2204Z
Cowper's (bulbourethral) gland *use* Urethra
CPAP (continuous positive airway pressure) *see* Assistance, Respiratory 5A09
Craniectomy
  see Excision, Head and Facial Bones 0NB
  see Resection, Head and Facial Bones 0NT
Cranioplasty
  see Repair, Head and Facial Bones 0NQ
  see Replacement, Head and Facial Bones 0NR
  see Supplement, Head and Facial Bones 0NU
Craniotomy
  see Division, Head and Facial Bones 0N8
  see Drainage, Central Nervous System and Cranial Nerves 009
  see Drainage, Head and Facial Bones 0N9

Creation
  Perineum
    Female 0W4N0
    Male 0W4M0
  Valve
    Aortic 024F0
    Mitral 024G0
    Tricuspid 024J0
Cremaster muscle *use* Perineum Muscle
Cribriform plate
  use Ethmoid Bone, Left
  use Ethmoid Bone, Right
Cricoid cartilage *use* Trachea
Cricoidectomy *see* Excision, Larynx 0CBS
Cricothyroid artery
  use Thyroid Artery, Left
  use Thyroid Artery, Right
Cricothyroid muscle
  use Neck Muscle, Left
  use Neck Muscle, Right
Crisis Intervention GZ2ZZZZ
CRRT (Continuous renal replacement therapy) 5A1D90Z
Crural fascia
  use Subcutaneous Tissue and Fascia, Left Upper Leg
  use Subcutaneous Tissue and Fascia, Right Upper Leg
Crushing, nerve
  Cranial *see* Destruction, Central Nervous System and Cranial Nerves 005
  Peripheral *see* Destruction, Peripheral Nervous System 015
Cryoablation *see* Destruction
Cryotherapy *see* Destruction
Cryptorchidectomy
  see Excision, Male Reproductive System 0VB
  see Resection, Male Reproductive System 0VT
Cryptorchiectomy
  see Excision, Male Reproductive System 0VB
  see Resection, Male Reproductive System 0VT
Cryptotomy
  see Division, Gastrointestinal System 0D8
  see Drainage, Gastrointestinal System 0D9
CT scan *see* Computerized Tomography (CT Scan)
CT sialogram *see* Computerized Tomography (CT Scan), Ear, Nose, Mouth and Throat B92
Cubital lymph node
  use Lymphatic, Left Upper Extremity
  use Lymphatic, Right Upper Extremity
Cubital nerve *use* Ulnar Nerve
Cuboid bone
  use Tarsal, Left
  use Tarsal, Right
Cuboideonavicular joint
  use Tarsal Joint, Left
  use Tarsal Joint, Right
Culdocentesis *see* Drainage, Cul-de-sac 0U9F
Culdoplasty
  see Repair, Cul-de-sac 0UQF
  see Supplement, Cul-de-sac 0UUF
Culdoscopy 0UJH8ZZ
Culdotomy *see* Drainage, Cul-de-sac 0U9F
Culmen *use* Cerebellum
Cultured epidermal cell autograft *use* Autologous Tissue Substitute
Cuneiform cartilage *use* Larynx
Cuneonavicular joint
  use Joint, Tarsal, Left
  use Joint, Tarsal, Right
Cuneonavicular ligament
  use Foot Bursa and Ligament, Left
  use Foot Bursa and Ligament, Right
Curettage
  see Excision
  see Extraction
Cutaneous (transverse) cervical nerve *use* Cervical Plexus
CVP (central venous pressure) *see* Measurement, Venous 4A04
Cyclodiathermy *see* Destruction, Eye 085
Cyclophotocoagulation *see* Destruction, Eye 085
CYPHER® Stent *use* Intraluminal Device, Drug-eluting in Heart and Great Vessels
Cystectomy
  see Excision, Bladder 0TBB
  see Resection, Bladder 0TTB

Cystocele repair *see* Repair, Subcutaneous Tissue and Fascia, Pelvic Region ØJQC

Cystography
  see Fluoroscopy, Urinary System BT1
  see Plain Radiography, Urinary System BTØ

Cystolithotomy *see* Extirpation, Bladder ØTCB

Cystopexy
  see Repair, Bladder ØTQB
  see Reposition, Bladder ØTSB

Cystoplasty
  see Repair, Bladder ØTQB
  see Replacement, Bladder ØTRB
  see Supplement, Bladder ØTUB

Cystorrhaphy *see* Repair, Bladder ØTQB

Cystoscopy ØTJB8ZZ

Cystostomy *see* Bypass, Bladder ØT1B

Cystostomy tube *use* Drainage Device

Cystotomy *see* Drainage, Bladder ØT9B

Cystourethrography
  see Fluoroscopy, Urinary System BT1
  see Plain Radiography, Urinary System BTØ

Cystourethroplasty
  see Repair, Urinary System ØTQ
  see Replacement, Urinary System ØTR
  see Supplement, Urinary System ØTU

Cytarabine and Daunorubicin Liposome Antineoplastic XWØ

D

DBS lead *use* Neurostimulator Lead in Central Nervous System and Cranial Nerves

DeBakey Left Ventricular Assist Device *use* Implantable Heart Assist System in Heart and Great Vessels

Debridement
  Excisional *see* Excision
  Non-excisional *see* Extraction

Decompression, Circulatory 6A15

Decortication, lung
  see Extirpation, Respiratory System ØBC
  see Release, Respiratory System ØBN

Deep brain neurostimulator lead *use* Neurostimulator Lead in Central Nervous and Cranial Nerves

Deep cervical fascia
  use Subcutaneous Tissue and Fascia, Left Neck
  use Subcutaneous Tissue and Fascia, Right Neck

Deep cervical vein
  use Vertebral Vein, Left
  use Vertebral Vein, Right

Deep circumflex iliac artery
  use External Iliac Artery, Left
  use External Iliac Artery, Right

Deep facial vein
  use Face Vein, Left
  use Face Vein, Right

Deep femoral artery
  use Femoral Artery, Left
  use Femoral Artery, Right

Deep femoral (profunda femoris) vein
  use Femoral Vein, Left
  use Femoral Vein, Right

Deep Inferior Epigastric Artery Perforator Flap
  Replacement
    Bilateral ØHRVØ77
    Left ØHRUØ77
    Right ØHRTØ77
  Transfer
    Left ØKXG
    Right ØKXF

Deep palmar arch
  use Hand Artery, Left
  use Hand Artery, Right

Deep transverse perineal muscle *use* Perineum Muscle

Deferential artery
  use Internal Iliac Artery, Left
  use Internal Iliac Artery, Right

Defibrillator Generator
  Abdomen ØJH8
  Chest ØJH6

Defibrotide Sodium Anticoagulant XWØ

Defitelio *use* Defibrotide Sodium Anticoagulant

Delivery
  Cesarean *see* Extraction, Products of Conception 1ØDØ
  Forceps *see* Extraction, Products of Conception 1ØDØ
  Manually assisted 1ØEØXZZ
  Products of Conception 1ØEØXZZ
  Vacuum assisted *see* Extraction, Products of Conception 1ØDØ

Delta frame external fixator
  use External Fixation Device, Hybrid in ØPH
  use External Fixation Device, Hybrid in ØPS
  use External Fixation Device, Hybrid in ØQH
  use External Fixation Device, Hybrid in ØQS

Delta III Reverse shoulder prosthesis *use* Synthetic Substitute, Reverse Ball and Socket in ØRR

Deltoid fascia
  use Subcutaneous Tissue and Fascia, Left Upper Arm
  use Subcutaneous Tissue and Fascia, Right Upper Arm

Deltoid ligament
  use Ankle Bursa and Ligament, Left
  use Ankle Bursa and Ligament, Right

Deltoid muscle
  use Shoulder Muscle, Left
  use Shoulder Muscle, Right

Deltopectoral (infraclavicular) lymph node
  use Lymphatic, Left Upper Extremity
  use Lymphatic, Right Upper Extremity

Denervation
  Cranial nerve *see* Destruction, Central Nervous System and Cranial Nerves ØØ5
  Peripheral nerve *see* Destruction, Peripheral Nervous System Ø15

Dens *use* Cervical Vertebra

Densitometry
  Plain Radiography
    Femur
      Left BQØ4ZZ1
      Right BQØ3ZZ1
    Hip
      Left BQØ1ZZ1
      Right BQØØZZ1
    Spine
      Cervical BRØØZZ1
      Lumbar BRØ9ZZ1
      Thoracic BRØ7ZZ1
      Whole BRØGZZ1
  Ultrasonography
    Elbow
      Left BP4HZZ1
      Right BP4GZZ1
    Hand
      Left BP4PZZ1
      Right BP4NZZ1
    Shoulder
      Left BP49ZZ1
      Right BP48ZZ1
    Wrist
      Left BP4MZZ1
      Right BP4LZZ1

Denticulate (dentate) ligament *use* Spinal Meninges

Depressor anguli oris muscle *use* Facial Muscle

Depressor labii inferioris muscle *use* Facial Muscle

Depressor septi nasi muscle *use* Facial Muscle

Depressor supercilii muscle *use* Facial Muscle

Dermabrasion *see* Extraction, Skin and Breast ØHD

Dermis *use* Skin

Descending genicular artery
  use Femoral Artery, Left
  use Femoral Artery, Right

Destruction
  Acetabulum
    Left ØQ55
    Right ØQ54
  Adenoids ØC5Q
  Ampulla of Vater ØF5C
  Anal Sphincter ØD5R
  Anterior Chamber
    Left Ø8533ZZ
    Right Ø8523ZZ
  Anus ØD5Q
  Aorta
    Abdominal
    Thoracic
      Ascending/Arch Ø25X
      Descending Ø25W

Destruction — *continued*
  Aortic Body ØG5D
  Appendix ØD5J
  Artery
    Anterior Tibial
      Left Ø45Q
      Right Ø45P
    Axillary
      Left Ø356
      Right Ø355
    Brachial
      Left Ø358
      Right Ø357
    Celiac Ø451
    Colic
      Left Ø457
      Middle Ø458
      Right Ø456
    Common Carotid
      Left Ø35J
      Right Ø35H
    Common Iliac
      Left Ø45D
      Right Ø45C
    External Carotid
      Left Ø35N
      Right Ø35M
    External Iliac
      Left Ø45J
      Right Ø45H
    Face Ø35R
    Femoral
      Left Ø45L
      Right Ø45K
    Foot
      Left Ø45W
      Right Ø45V
    Gastric Ø452
    Hand
      Left Ø35F
      Right Ø35D
    Hepatic Ø453
    Inferior Mesenteric Ø45B
    Innominate Ø352
    Internal Carotid
      Left Ø35L
      Right Ø35K
    Internal Iliac
      Left Ø45F
      Right Ø45E
    Internal Mammary
      Left Ø351
      Right Ø35Ø
    Intracranial Ø35G
    Lower Ø45Y
    Peroneal
      Left Ø45U
      Right Ø45T
    Popliteal
      Left Ø45N
      Right Ø45M
    Posterior Tibial
      Left Ø45S
      Right Ø45R
    Pulmonary
      Left Ø25R
      Right Ø25Q
    Pulmonary Trunk Ø25P
    Radial
      Left Ø35C
      Right Ø35B
    Renal
      Left Ø45A
      Right Ø459
    Splenic Ø454
    Subclavian
      Left Ø354
      Right Ø353
    Superior Mesenteric Ø455
    Temporal
      Left Ø35T
      Right Ø35S
    Thyroid
      Left Ø35V
      Right Ø35U
    Ulnar
      Left Ø35A
      Right Ø359
    Upper Ø35Y

Subterms under main terms may continue to next column or page

Destruction — *continued*
Artery — *continued*
Vertebral
Left Ø35Q
Right Ø35P
Atrium
Left Ø257
Right Ø256
Auditory Ossicle
Left Ø95A
Right Ø959
Basal Ganglia ØØ58
Bladder ØT5B
Bladder Neck ØT5C
Bone
Ethmoid
Left ØN5G
Right ØN5F
Frontal ØN51
Hyoid ØN5X
Lacrimal
Left ØN5J
Right ØN5H
Nasal ØN5B
Occipital ØN57
Palatine
Left ØN5L
Right ØN5K
Parietal
Left ØN54
Right ØN53
Pelvic
Left ØQ53
Right ØQ52
Sphenoid ØN5C
Temporal
Left ØN56
Right ØN55
Zygomatic
Left ØN5N
Right ØN5M
Brain ØØ5Ø
Breast
Bilateral ØH5V
Left ØH5U
Right ØH5T
Bronchus
Lingula ØB59
Lower Lobe
Left ØB5B
Right ØB56
Main
Left ØB57
Right ØB53
Middle Lobe, Right ØB55
Upper Lobe
Left ØB58
Right ØB54
Buccal Mucosa ØC54
Bursa and Ligament
Abdomen
Left ØM5J
Right ØM5H
Ankle
Left ØM5R
Right ØM5Q
Elbow
Left ØM54
Right ØM53
Foot
Left ØM5T
Right ØM5S
Hand
Left ØM58
Right ØM57
Head and Neck ØM5Ø
Hip
Left ØM5M
Right ØM5L
Knee
Left ØM5P
Right ØM5N
Lower Extremity
Left ØM5W
Right ØM5V
Perineum ØM5K
Rib(s) ØM5G
Shoulder
Left ØM52

Destruction — *continued*
Bursa and Ligament — *continued*
Shoulder — *continued*
Right ØM51
Spine
Lower ØM5D
Upper ØM5C
Sternum ØM5F
Upper Extremity
Left ØM5B
Right ØM59
Wrist
Left ØM56
Right ØM55
Carina ØB52
Carotid Bodies, Bilateral ØG58
Carotid Body
Left ØG56
Right ØG57
Carpal
Left ØP5N
Right ØP5M
Cecum ØD5H
Cerebellum ØØ5C
Cerebral Hemisphere ØØ57
Cerebral Meninges ØØ51
Cerebral Ventricle ØØ56
Cervix ØU5C
Chordae Tendineae Ø259
Choroid
Left Ø85B
Right Ø85A
Cisterna Chyli Ø75L
Clavicle
Left ØP5B
Right ØP59
Clitoris ØU5J
Coccygeal Glomus ØG5B
Coccyx ØQ5S
Colon
Ascending ØD5K
Descending ØD5M
Sigmoid ØD5N
Transverse ØD5L
Conduction Mechanism Ø258
Conjunctiva
Left Ø85TXZZ
Right Ø85SXZZ
Cord
Bilateral ØV5H
Left ØV5G
Right ØV5F
Cornea
Left Ø859XZZ
Right Ø858XZZ
Cul-de-sac ØU5F
Diaphragm ØB5T
Disc
Cervical Vertebral ØR53
Cervicothoracic Vertebral ØR55
Lumbar Vertebral ØS52
Lumbosacral ØS54
Thoracic Vertebral ØR59
Thoracolumbar Vertebral ØR5B
Duct
Common Bile ØF59
Cystic ØF58
Hepatic
Common ØF57
Left ØF56
Right ØF55
Lacrimal
Left Ø85Y
Right Ø85X
Pancreatic ØF5D
Accessory ØF5F
Parotid
Left ØC5C
Right ØC5B
Duodenum ØD59
Dura Mater ØØ52
Ear
External
Left Ø951
Right Ø95Ø
External Auditory Canal
Left Ø954
Right Ø953

Destruction — *continued*
Ear — *continued*
Inner
Left Ø95E
Right Ø95D
Middle
Left Ø956
Right Ø955
Endometrium ØU5B
Epididymis
Bilateral ØV5L
Left ØV5K
Right ØV5J
Epiglottis ØC5R
Esophagogastric Junction ØD54
Esophagus ØD55
Lower ØD53
Middle ØD52
Upper ØD51
Eustachian Tube
Left Ø95G
Right Ø95F
Eye
Left Ø851XZZ
Right Ø850XZZ
Eyelid
Lower
Left Ø85R
Right Ø85Q
Upper
Left Ø85P
Right Ø85N
Fallopian Tube
Left ØU56
Right ØU55
Fallopian Tubes, Bilateral ØU57
Femoral Shaft
Left ØQ59
Right ØQ58
Femur
Lower
Left ØQ5C
Right ØQ5B
Upper
Left ØQ57
Right ØQ56
Fibula
Left ØQ5K
Right ØQ5J
Finger Nail ØH5QXZZ
Gallbladder ØF54
Gingiva
Lower ØC56
Upper ØC55
Gland
Adrenal
Bilateral ØG54
Left ØG52
Right ØG53
Lacrimal
Left Ø85W
Right Ø85V
Minor Salivary ØC5J
Parotid
Left ØC59
Right ØC58
Pituitary ØG5Ø
Sublingual
Left ØC5F
Right ØC5D
Submaxillary
Left ØC5H
Right ØC5G
Vestibular ØU5L
Glenoid Cavity
Left ØP58
Right ØP57
Glomus Jugulare ØG5C
Humeral Head
Left ØP5D
Right ØP5C
Humeral Shaft
Left ØP5G
Right ØP5F
Hymen ØU5K
Hypothalamus ØØ5A
Ileocecal Valve ØD5C
Ileum ØD5B

Destruction — continued
- Intestine
  - Large ØD5E
    - Left ØD5G
    - Right ØD5F
  - Small ØD58
- Iris
  - Left Ø85D3ZZ
  - Right Ø85C3ZZ
- Jejunum ØD5A
- Joint
  - Acromioclavicular
    - Left ØR5H
    - Right ØR5G
  - Ankle
    - Left ØS5G
    - Right ØS5F
  - Carpal
    - Left ØR5R
    - Right ØR5Q
  - Carpometacarpal
    - Left ØR5T
    - Right ØR5S
  - Cervical Vertebral ØR51
  - Cervicothoracic Vertebral ØR54
  - Coccygeal ØS56
  - Elbow
    - Left ØR5M
    - Right ØR5L
  - Finger Phalangeal
    - Left ØR5X
    - Right ØR5W
  - Hip
    - Left ØS5B
    - Right ØS59
  - Knee
    - Left ØS5D
    - Right ØS5C
  - Lumbar Vertebral ØS5Ø
  - Lumbosacral ØS53
  - Metacarpophalangeal
    - Left ØR5V
    - Right ØR5U
  - Metatarsal-Phalangeal
    - Left ØS5N
    - Right ØS5M
  - Occipital-cervical ØR5Ø
  - Sacrococcygeal ØS55
  - Sacroiliac
    - Left ØS58
    - Right ØS57
  - Shoulder
    - Left ØR5K
    - Right ØR5J
  - Sternoclavicular
    - Left ØR5F
    - Right ØR5E
  - Tarsal
    - Left ØS5J
    - Right ØS5H
  - Tarsometatarsal
    - Left ØS5L
    - Right ØS5K
  - Temporomandibular
    - Left ØR5D
    - Right ØR5C
  - Thoracic Vertebral ØR56
  - Thoracolumbar Vertebral ØR5A
  - Toe Phalangeal
    - Left ØS5Q
    - Right ØS5P
  - Wrist
    - Left ØR5P
    - Right ØR5N
- Kidney
  - Left ØT51
  - Right ØT5Ø
- Kidney Pelvis
  - Left ØT54
  - Right ØT53
- Larynx ØC5S
- Lens
  - Left Ø85K3ZZ
  - Right Ø85J3ZZ
- Lip
  - Lower ØC51
  - Upper ØC5Ø
- Liver ØF5Ø
  - Left Lobe ØF52

Destruction — continued
- Liver — continued
  - Right Lobe ØF51
- Lung
  - Bilateral ØB5M
  - Left ØB5L
  - Lower Lobe
    - Left ØB5J
    - Right ØB5F
  - Middle Lobe, Right ØB5D
  - Right ØB5K
  - Upper Lobe
    - Left ØB5G
    - Right ØB5C
- Lung Lingula ØB5H
- Lymphatic
  - Aortic Ø75D
  - Axillary
    - Left Ø756
    - Right Ø755
  - Head Ø75Ø
  - Inguinal
    - Left Ø75J
    - Right Ø75H
  - Internal Mammary
    - Left Ø759
    - Right Ø758
  - Lower Extremity
    - Left Ø75G
    - Right Ø75F
  - Mesenteric Ø75B
  - Neck
    - Left Ø752
    - Right Ø751
  - Pelvis Ø75C
  - Thoracic Duct Ø75K
  - Thorax Ø757
  - Upper Extremity
    - Left Ø754
    - Right Ø753
- Mandible
  - Left ØN5V
  - Right ØN5T
- Maxilla ØN5R
- Medulla Oblongata ØØ5D
- Mesentery ØD5V
- Metacarpal
  - Left ØP5Q
  - Right ØP5P
- Metatarsal
  - Left ØQ5P
  - Right ØQ5N
- Muscle
  - Abdomen
    - Left ØK5L
    - Right ØK5K
  - Extraocular
    - Left Ø85M
    - Right Ø85L
  - Facial ØK51
  - Foot
    - Left ØK5W
    - Right ØK5V
  - Hand
    - Left ØK5D
    - Right ØK5C
  - Head ØK5Ø
  - Hip
    - Left ØK5P
    - Right ØK5N
  - Lower Arm and Wrist
    - Left ØK5B
    - Right ØK59
  - Lower Leg
    - Left ØK5T
    - Right ØK5S
  - Neck
    - Left ØK53
    - Right ØK52
  - Papillary Ø25D
  - Perineum ØK5M
  - Shoulder
    - Left ØK56
    - Right ØK55
  - Thorax
    - Left ØK5J
    - Right ØK5H
  - Tongue, Palate, Pharynx ØK54

Destruction — continued
- Muscle — continued
  - Trunk
    - Left ØK5G
    - Right ØK5F
  - Upper Arm
    - Left ØK58
    - Right ØK57
  - Upper Leg
    - Left ØK5R
    - Right ØK5Q
- Nasal Mucosa and Soft Tissue Ø95K
- Nasopharynx Ø95N
- Nerve
  - Abdominal Sympathetic Ø15M
  - Abducens ØØ5L
  - Accessory ØØ5R
  - Acoustic ØØ5N
  - Brachial Plexus Ø153
  - Cervical Ø151
  - Cervical Plexus Ø15Ø
  - Facial ØØ5M
  - Femoral Ø15D
  - Glossopharyngeal ØØ5P
  - Head and Neck Sympathetic Ø15K
  - Hypoglossal ØØ5S
  - Lumbar Ø15B
  - Lumbar Plexus Ø159
  - Lumbar Sympathetic Ø15N
  - Lumbosacral Plexus Ø15A
  - Median Ø155
  - Oculomotor ØØ5H
  - Olfactory ØØ5F
  - Optic ØØ5G
  - Peroneal Ø15H
  - Phrenic Ø152
  - Pudendal Ø15C
  - Radial Ø156
  - Sacral Ø15R
  - Sacral Plexus Ø15Q
  - Sacral Sympathetic Ø15P
  - Sciatic Ø15F
  - Thoracic Ø158
  - Thoracic Sympathetic Ø15L
  - Tibial Ø15G
  - Trigeminal ØØ5K
  - Trochlear ØØ5J
  - Ulnar Ø154
  - Vagus ØØ5Q
- Nipple
  - Left ØH5X
  - Right ØH5W
- Omentum ØD5U
- Orbit
  - Left ØN5Q
  - Right ØN5P
- Ovary
  - Bilateral ØU52
  - Left ØU51
  - Right ØU5Ø
- Palate
  - Hard ØC52
  - Soft ØC53
- Pancreas ØF5G
- Para-aortic Body ØG59
- Paraganglion Extremity ØG5F
- Parathyroid Gland ØG5R
  - Inferior
    - Left ØG5P
    - Right ØG5N
  - Multiple ØG5Q
  - Superior
    - Left ØG5M
    - Right ØG5L
- Patella
  - Left ØQ5F
  - Right ØQ5D
- Penis ØV5S
- Pericardium Ø25N
- Peritoneum ØD5W
- Phalanx
  - Finger
    - Left ØP5V
    - Right ØP5T
  - Thumb
    - Left ØP5S
    - Right ØP5R
  - Toe
    - Left ØQ5R

◁ **Subterms under main terms may continue to next column or page**

Destruction — *continued*
  Phalanx — *continued*
    Toe — *continued*
      Right 0Q5Q
  Pharynx 0C5M
  Pineal Body 0G51
  Pleura
    Left 0B5P
    Right 0B5N
  Pons 005B
  Prepuce 0V5T
  Prostate 0V50
    Robotic Waterjet Ablation XV508A4
  Radius
    Left 0P5J
    Right 0P5H
  Rectum 0D5P
  Retina
    Left 085F3ZZ
    Right 085E3ZZ
  Retinal Vessel
    Left 085H3ZZ
    Right 085G3ZZ
  Ribs
    1 to 2 0P51
    3 or More 0P52
  Sacrum 0Q51
  Scapula
    Left 0P56
    Right 0P55
  Sclera
    Left 0857XZZ
    Right 0856XZZ
  Scrotum 0V55
  Septum
    Atrial 0255
    Nasal 095M
    Ventricular 025M
  Sinus
    Accessory 095P
    Ethmoid
      Left 095V
      Right 095U
    Frontal
      Left 095T
      Right 095S
    Mastoid
      Left 095C
      Right 095B
    Maxillary
      Left 095R
      Right 095Q
    Sphenoid
      Left 095X
      Right 095W
  Skin
    Abdomen 0H57XZ
    Back 0H56XZ
    Buttock 0H58XZ
    Chest 0H55XZ
    Ear
      Left 0H53XZ
      Right 0H52XZ
    Face 0H51XZ
    Foot
      Left 0H5NXZ
      Right 0H5MXZ
    Hand
      Left 0H5GXZ
      Right 0H5FXZ
    Inguinal 0H5AXZ
    Lower Arm
      Left 0H5EXZ
      Right 0H5DXZ
    Lower Leg
      Left 0H5LXZ
      Right 0H5KXZ
    Neck 0H54XZ
    Perineum 0H59XZ
    Scalp 0H50XZ
    Upper Arm
      Left 0H5CXZ
      Right 0H5BXZ
    Upper Leg
      Left 0H5JXZ
      Right 0H5HXZ
  Skull 0N50
  Spinal Cord
    Cervical 005W

Destruction — *continued*
  Spinal Cord — *continued*
    Lumbar 005Y
    Thoracic 005X
  Spinal Meninges 005T
  Spleen 075P
  Sternum 0P50
  Stomach 0D56
    Pylorus 0D57
  Subcutaneous Tissue and Fascia
    Abdomen 0J58
    Back 0J57
    Buttock 0J59
    Chest 0J56
    Face 0J51
    Foot
      Left 0J5R
      Right 0J5Q
    Hand
      Left 0J5K
      Right 0J5J
    Lower Arm
      Left 0J5H
      Right 0J5G
    Lower Leg
      Left 0J5P
      Right 0J5N
    Neck
      Left 0J55
      Right 0J54
    Pelvic Region 0J5C
    Perineum 0J5B
    Scalp 0J50
    Upper Arm
      Left 0J5F
      Right 0J5D
    Upper Leg
      Left 0J5M
      Right 0J5L
  Tarsal
    Left 0Q5M
    Right 0Q5L
  Tendon
    Abdomen
      Left 0L5G
      Right 0L5F
    Ankle
      Left 0L5T
      Right 0L5S
    Foot
      Left 0L5W
      Right 0L5V
    Hand
      Left 0L58
      Right 0L57
    Head and Neck 0L50
    Hip
      Left 0L5K
      Right 0L5J
    Knee
      Left 0L5R
      Right 0L5Q
    Lower Arm and Wrist
      Left 0L56
      Right 0L55
    Lower Leg
      Left 0L5P
      Right 0L5N
    Perineum 0L5H
    Shoulder
      Left 0L52
      Right 0L51
    Thorax
      Left 0L5D
      Right 0L5C
    Trunk
      Left 0L5B
      Right 0L59
    Upper Arm
      Left 0L54
      Right 0L53
    Upper Leg
      Left 0L5M
      Right 0L5L
  Testis
    Bilateral 0V5C
    Left 0V5B
    Right 0V59
  Thalamus 0059

Destruction — *continued*
  Thymus 075M
  Thyroid Gland 0G5K
    Left Lobe 0G5G
    Right Lobe 0G5H
  Tibia
    Left 0Q5H
    Right 0Q5G
  Toe Nail 0H5RXZZ
  Tongue 0C57
  Tonsils 0C5P
  Tooth
    Lower 0C5X
    Upper 0C5W
  Trachea 0B51
  Tunica Vaginalis
    Left 0V57
    Right 0V56
  Turbinate, Nasal 095L
  Tympanic Membrane
    Left 0958
    Right 0957
  Ulna
    Left 0P5L
    Right 0P5K
  Ureter
    Left 0T57
    Right 0T56
  Urethra 0T5D
  Uterine Supporting Structure 0U54
  Uterus 0U59
  Uvula 0C5N
  Vagina 0U5G
  Valve
    Aortic 025F
    Mitral 025G
    Pulmonary 025H
    Tricuspid 025J
  Vas Deferens
    Bilateral 0V5Q
    Left 0V5P
    Right 0V5N
  Vein
    Axillary
      Left 0558
      Right 0557
    Azygos 0550
    Basilic
      Left 055C
      Right 055B
    Brachial
      Left 055A
      Right 0559
    Cephalic
      Left 055F
      Right 055D
    Colic 0657
    Common Iliac
      Left 065D
      Right 065C
    Coronary 0254
    Esophageal 0653
    External Iliac
      Left 065G
      Right 065F
    External Jugular
      Left 055Q
      Right 055P
    Face
      Left 055V
      Right 055T
    Femoral
      Left 065N
      Right 065M
    Foot
      Left 065V
      Right 065T
    Gastric 0652
    Hand
      Left 055H
      Right 055G
    Hemiazygos 0551
    Hepatic 0654
    Hypogastric
      Left 065J
      Right 065H
    Inferior Mesenteric 0656
    Innominate
      Left 0554

Destruction — *continued*
  Vein — *continued*
    Innominate — *continued*
      Right Ø553
    Internal Jugular
      Left Ø55N
      Right Ø55M
    Intracranial Ø55L
    Lower Ø65Y
    Portal Ø658
    Pulmonary
      Left Ø25T
      Right Ø25S
    Renal
      Left Ø65B
      Right Ø659
    Saphenous
      Left Ø65Q
      Right Ø65P
    Splenic Ø651
    Subclavian
      Left Ø556
      Right Ø555
    Superior Mesenteric Ø655
    Upper Ø55Y
    Vertebral
      Left Ø55S
      Right Ø55R
  Vena Cava
    Inferior Ø65Ø
    Superior Ø25V
  Ventricle
    Left Ø25L
    Right Ø25K
  Vertebra
    Cervical ØP53
    Lumbar ØQ5Ø
    Thoracic ØP54
  Vesicle
    Bilateral ØV53
    Left ØV52
    Right ØV51
  Vitreous
    Left Ø8553ZZ
    Right Ø8543ZZ
  Vocal Cord
    Left ØC5V
    Right ØC5T
  Vulva ØU5M
Detachment
  Arm
    Lower
      Left ØX6FØZ
      Right ØX6DØZ
    Upper
      Left ØX69ØZ
      Right ØX68ØZ
  Elbow Region
    Left ØX6CØZZ
    Right ØX6BØZZ
  Femoral Region
    Left ØY68ØZZ
    Right ØY67ØZZ
  Finger
    Index
      Left ØX6PØZ
      Right ØX6NØZ
    Little
      Left ØX6WØZ
      Right ØX6VØZ
    Middle
      Left ØX6RØZ
      Right ØX6QØZ
    Ring
      Left ØX6TØZ
      Right ØX6SØZ
  Foot
    Left ØY6NØZ
    Right ØY6MØZ
  Forequarter
    Left ØX61ØZZ
    Right ØX6ØØZZ
  Hand
    Left ØX6KØZ
    Right ØX6JØZ
  Hindquarter
    Bilateral ØY64ØZZ
    Left ØY63ØZZ
    Right ØY62ØZZ

Detachment — *continued*
  Knee Region
    Left ØY6GØZZ
    Right ØY6FØZZ
  Leg
    Lower
      Left ØY6JØZ
      Right ØY6HØZ
    Upper
      Left ØY6DØZ
      Right ØY6CØZ
  Shoulder Region
    Left ØX63ØZZ
    Right ØX62ØZZ
  Thumb
    Left ØX6MØZ
    Right ØX6LØZ
  Toe
    1st
      Left ØY6QØZ
      Right ØY6PØZ
    2nd
      Left ØY6SØZ
      Right ØY6RØZ
    3rd
      Left ØY6UØZ
      Right ØY6TØZ
    4th
      Left ØY6WØZ
      Right ØY6VØZ
    5th
      Left ØY6YØZ
      Right ØY6XØZ
Determination, Mental status GZ14ZZZ
Detorsion
  see Release
  see Reposition
Detoxification Services, for substance abuse
  HZ2ZZZZ
Device Fitting FØDZ
Diagnostic Audiology *see* Audiology, Diagnostic
Diagnostic imaging *see* Imaging, Diagnostic
Diagnostic radiology *see* Imaging, Diagnostic
Dialysis
  Hemodialysis *see* Performance, Urinary 5A1D
  Peritoneal 3E1M39Z
Diaphragma sellae *use* Dura Mater
Diaphragmatic pacemaker generator *use* Stimulator
  Generator in Subcutaneous Tissue and Fascia
Diaphragmatic Pacemaker Lead
  Insertion of device in, Diaphragm ØBHT
  Removal of device from, Diaphragm ØBPT
  Revision of device in, Diaphragm ØBWT
Digital radiography, plain *see* Plain Radiography
Dilation
  Ampulla of Vater ØF7C
  Anus ØD7Q
  Aorta
    Abdominal
    Thoracic
      Ascending/Arch Ø27X
      Descending Ø27W
  Artery
    Anterior Tibial
      Left Ø47Q
        Sustained Release Drug-eluting
          Intraluminal Device
            X27Q385
          Four or More X27Q3C5
          Three X27Q3B5
          Two X27Q395
      Right Ø47P
        Sustained Release Drug-eluting
          Intraluminal Device
            X27P385
          Four or More X27P3C5
          Three X27P3B5
          Two X27P395
    Axillary
      Left Ø376
      Right Ø375
    Brachial
      Left Ø378
      Right Ø377
    Celiac Ø471
    Colic
      Left Ø477
      Middle Ø478

Dilation — *continued*
  Artery — *continued*
    Colic — *continued*
      Right Ø476
    Common Carotid
      Left Ø37J
      Right Ø37H
    Common Iliac
      Left Ø47D
      Right Ø47C
    Coronary
      Four or More Arteries Ø273
      One Artery Ø27Ø
      Three Arteries Ø272
      Two Arteries Ø271
    External Carotid
      Left Ø37N
      Right Ø37M
    External Iliac
      Left Ø47J
      Right Ø47H
    Face Ø37R
    Femoral
      Left Ø47L
        Sustained Release Drug-eluting
          Intraluminal Device
            X27J385
          Four or More X27J3C5
          Three X27J3B5
          Two X27J395
      Right Ø47K
        Sustained Release Drug-eluting
          Intraluminal Device
            X27H385
          Four or More X27H3C5
          Three X27H3B5
          Two X27H395
    Foot
      Left Ø47W
      Right Ø47V
    Gastric Ø472
    Hand
      Left Ø37F
      Right Ø37D
    Hepatic Ø473
    Inferior Mesenteric Ø47B
    Innominate Ø372
    Internal Carotid
      Left Ø37L
      Right Ø37K
    Internal Iliac
      Left Ø47F
      Right Ø47E
    Internal Mammary
      Left Ø371
      Right Ø37Ø
    Intracranial Ø37G
    Lower Ø47Y
    Peroneal
      Left Ø47U
        Sustained Release Drug-eluting
          Intraluminal Device
            X27U385
          Four or More X27U3C5
          Three X27U3B5
          Two X27U395
      Right Ø47T
        Sustained Release Drug-eluting
          Intraluminal Device
            X27T385
          Four or More X27T3C5
          Three X27T3B5
          Two X27T395
    Popliteal
      Left Ø47N
      Left Distal
        Sustained Release Drug-eluting
          Intraluminal Device
            X27N385
          Four or More X27N3C5
          Three X27N3B5
          Two X27N395
      Left Proximal
        Sustained Release Drug-eluting
          Intraluminal Device
            X27L385
          Four or More X27L3C5
          Three X27L3B5
          Two X27L395

▽ **Subterms under main terms may continue to next column or page**

Dilation — *continued*
  Artery — *continued*
    Popliteal — *continued*
      Right Ø47M
      Right Distal
        Sustained Release Drug-eluting
          Intraluminal Device
            X27M385
          Four or More X27M3C5
          Three X27M3B5
          Two X27M395
      Right Proximal
        Sustained Release Drug-eluting
          Intraluminal Device
            X27K385
          Four or More X27K3C5
          Three X27K3B5
          Two X27K395
    Posterior Tibial
      Left Ø47S
        Sustained Release Drug-eluting
          Intraluminal Device
            X27S385
          Four or More X27S3C5
          Three X27S3B5
          Two X27S395
      Right Ø47R
        Sustained Release Drug-eluting
          Intraluminal Device
            X27R385
          Four or More X27R3C5
          Three X27R3B5
          Two X27R395
    Pulmonary
      Left Ø27R
      Right Ø27Q
    Pulmonary Trunk Ø27P
    Radial
      Left Ø37C
      Right Ø37B
    Renal
      Left Ø47A
      Right Ø479
    Splenic Ø474
    Subclavian
      Left Ø374
      Right Ø373
    Superior Mesenteric Ø475
    Temporal
      Left Ø37T
      Right Ø37S
    Thyroid
      Left Ø37V
      Right Ø37U
    Ulnar
      Left Ø37A
      Right Ø379
    Upper Ø37Y
    Vertebral
      Left Ø37Q
      Right Ø37P
  Bladder ØT7B
  Bladder Neck ØT7C
  Bronchus
    Lingula ØB79
    Lower Lobe
      Left ØB7B
      Right ØB76
    Main
      Left ØB77
      Right ØB73
    Middle Lobe, Right ØB75
    Upper Lobe
      Left ØB78
      Right ØB74
  Carina ØB72
  Cecum ØD7H
  Cerebral Ventricle ØØ76
  Cervix ØU7C
  Colon
    Ascending ØD7K
    Descending ØD7M
    Sigmoid ØD7N
    Transverse ØD7L
  Duct
    Common Bile ØF79
    Cystic ØF78
    Hepatic
      Common ØF77

Dilation — *continued*
  Duct — *continued*
    Hepatic — *continued*
      Left ØF76
      Right ØF75
    Lacrimal
      Left Ø87Y
      Right Ø87X
    Pancreatic ØF7D
      Accessory ØF7F
    Parotid
      Left ØC7C
      Right ØC7B
  Duodenum ØD79
  Esophagogastric Junction ØD74
  Esophagus ØD75
    Lower ØD73
    Middle ØD72
    Upper ØD71
  Eustachian Tube
    Left Ø97G
    Right Ø97F
  Fallopian Tube
    Left ØU76
    Right ØU75
  Fallopian Tubes, Bilateral ØU77
  Hymen ØU7K
  Ileocecal Valve ØD7C
  Ileum ØD7B
  Intestine
    Large ØD7E
      Left ØD7G
      Right ØD7F
    Small ØD78
  Jejunum ØD7A
  Kidney Pelvis
    Left ØT74
    Right ØT73
  Larynx ØC7S
  Pharynx ØC7M
  Rectum ØD7P
  Stomach ØD76
    Pylorus ØD77
  Trachea ØB71
  Ureter
    Left ØT77
    Right ØT76
  Ureters, Bilateral ØT78
  Urethra ØT7D
  Uterus ØU79
  Vagina ØU7G
  Valve
    Aortic Ø27F
    Mitral Ø27G
    Pulmonary Ø27H
    Tricuspid Ø27J
  Vas Deferens
    Bilateral ØV7Q
    Left ØV7P
    Right ØV7N
  Vein
    Axillary
      Left Ø578
      Right Ø577
    Azygos Ø57Ø
    Basilic
      Left Ø57C
      Right Ø57B
    Brachial
      Left Ø57A
      Right Ø579
    Cephalic
      Left Ø57F
      Right Ø57D
    Colic Ø677
    Common Iliac
      Left Ø67D
      Right Ø67C
    Esophageal Ø673
    External Iliac
      Left Ø67G
      Right Ø67F
    External Jugular
      Left Ø57Q
      Right Ø57P
    Face
      Left Ø57V
      Right Ø57T

Dilation — *continued*
  Vein — *continued*
    Femoral
      Left Ø67N
      Right Ø67M
    Foot
      Left Ø67V
      Right Ø67T
    Gastric Ø672
    Hand
      Left Ø57H
      Right Ø57G
    Hemiazygos Ø571
    Hepatic Ø674
    Hypogastric
      Left Ø67J
      Right Ø67H
    Inferior Mesenteric Ø676
    Innominate
      Left Ø574
      Right Ø573
    Internal Jugular
      Left Ø57N
      Right Ø57M
    Intracranial Ø57L
    Lower Ø67Y
    Portal Ø678
    Pulmonary
      Left Ø27T
      Right Ø27S
    Renal
      Left Ø67B
      Right Ø679
    Saphenous
      Left Ø67Q
      Right Ø67P
    Splenic Ø671
    Subclavian
      Left Ø576
      Right Ø575
    Superior Mesenteric Ø675
    Upper Ø57Y
    Vertebral
      Left Ø57S
      Right Ø57R
  Vena Cava
    Inferior Ø67Ø
    Superior Ø27V
  Ventricle
    Left Ø27L
    Right Ø27K
Direct Lateral Interbody Fusion (DLIF) device *use*
    Interbody Fusion Device in Lower Joints
Disarticulation *see* Detachment
Discectomy, diskectomy
    see Excision, Lower Joints ØSB
    see Excision, Upper Joints ØRB
    see Resection, Lower Joints ØST
    see Resection, Upper Joints ØRT
Discography
    see Fluoroscopy, Axial Skeleton, Except Skull and
      Facial Bones BR1
    see Plain Radiography, Axial Skeleton, Except Skull
      and Facial Bones BRØ
Dismembered pyeloplasty *see* Repair, Kidney Pelvis
Distal humerus
    use Humeral Shaft, Left
    use Humeral Shaft, Right
Distal humerus, involving joint
    use Elbow Joint, Left
    use Elbow Joint, Right
Distal radioulnar joint
    use Wrist Joint, Left
    use Wrist Joint, Right
Diversion *see* Bypass
Diverticulectomy *see* Excision, Gastrointestinal System
    ØDB
Division
  Acetabulum
    Left ØQ85
    Right ØQ84
  Anal Sphincter ØD8R
  Basal Ganglia ØØ88
  Bladder Neck ØT8C
  Bone
    Ethmoid
      Left ØN8G
      Right ØN8F

▽ **Subterms under main terms may continue to next column or page**

Division — *continued*
  Subcutaneous Tissue and Fascia — *continued*
    Back 0J87
    Buttock 0J89
    Chest 0J86
    Face 0J81
    Foot
      Left 0J8R
      Right 0J8Q
    Hand
      Left 0J8K
      Right 0J8J
    Head and Neck 0J8S
    Lower Arm
      Left 0J8H
      Right 0J8G
    Lower Extremity 0J8W
    Lower Leg
      Left 0J8P
      Right 0J8N
    Neck
      Left 0J85
      Right 0J84
    Pelvic Region 0J8C
    Perineum 0J8B
    Scalp 0J80
    Trunk 0J8T
    Upper Arm
      Left 0J8F
      Right 0J8D
    Upper Extremity 0J8V
    Upper Leg
      Left 0J8M
      Right 0J8L
  Tarsal
    Left 0Q8M
    Right 0Q8L
  Tendon
    Abdomen
      Left 0L8G
      Right 0L8F
    Ankle
      Left 0L8T
      Right 0L8S
    Foot
      Left 0L8W
      Right 0L8V
    Hand
      Left 0L88
      Right 0L87
    Head and Neck 0L80
    Hip
      Left 0L8K
      Right 0L8J
    Knee
      Left 0L8R
      Right 0L8Q
    Lower Arm and Wrist
      Left 0L86
      Right 0L85
    Lower Leg
      Left 0L8P
      Right 0L8N
    Perineum 0L8H
    Shoulder
      Left 0L82
      Right 0L81
    Thorax
      Left 0L8D
      Right 0L8C
    Trunk
      Left 0L8B
      Right 0L89
    Upper Arm
      Left 0L84
      Right 0L83
    Upper Leg
      Left 0L8M
      Right 0L8L
  Thyroid Gland Isthmus 0G8J
  Tibia
    Left 0Q8H
    Right 0Q8G
  Turbinate, Nasal 098L
  Ulna
    Left 0P8L
    Right 0P8K
  Uterine Supporting Structure 0U84

Division — *continued*
  Vertebra
    Cervical 0P83
    Lumbar 0Q80
    Thoracic 0P84
Doppler study *see* Ultrasonography
Dorsal digital nerve *use* Radial Nerve
Dorsal metacarpal vein
  use Hand Vein, Left
  use Hand Vein, Right
Dorsal metatarsal artery
  use Foot Artery, Left
  use Foot Artery, Right
Dorsal metatarsal vein
  use Foot Vein, Left
  use Foot Vein, Right
Dorsal scapular artery
  use Subclavian Artery, Left
  use Subclavian Artery, Right
Dorsal scapular nerve *use* Brachial Plexus
Dorsal venous arch
  use Foot Vein, Left
  use Foot Vein, Right
Dorsalis pedis artery
  use Anterior Tibial Artery, Left
  use Anterior Tibial Artery, Right
DownStream® System 5A0512C, 5A0522C
Drainage
  Abdominal Wall 0W9F
  Acetabulum
    Left 0Q95
    Right 0Q94
  Adenoids 0C9Q
  Ampulla of Vater 0F9C
  Anal Sphincter 0D9R
  Ankle Region
    Left 0Y9L
    Right 0Y9K
  Anterior Chamber
    Left 0893
    Right 0892
  Anus 0D9Q
  Aorta, Abdominal 0490
  Aortic Body 0G9D
  Appendix 0D9J
  Arm
    Lower
      Left 0X9F
      Right 0X9D
    Upper
      Left 0X99
      Right 0X98
  Artery
    Anterior Tibial
      Left 049Q
      Right 049P
    Axillary
      Left 0396
      Right 0395
    Brachial
      Left 0398
      Right 0397
    Celiac 0491
    Colic
      Left 0497
      Middle 0498
      Right 0496
    Common Carotid
      Left 039J
      Right 039H
    Common Iliac
      Left 049D
      Right 049C
    External Carotid
      Left 039N
      Right 039M
    External Iliac
      Left 049J
      Right 049H
    Face 039R
    Femoral
      Left 049L
      Right 049K
    Foot
      Left 049W
      Right 049V
    Gastric 0492

Drainage — *continued*
  Artery — *continued*
    Hand
      Left 039F
      Right 039D
    Hepatic 0493
    Inferior Mesenteric 049B
    Innominate 0392
    Internal Carotid
      Left 039L
      Right 039K
    Internal Iliac
      Left 049F
      Right 049E
    Internal Mammary
      Left 0391
      Right 0390
    Intracranial 039G
    Lower 049Y
    Peroneal
      Left 049U
      Right 049T
    Popliteal
      Left 049N
      Right 049M
    Posterior Tibial
      Left 049S
      Right 049R
    Radial
      Left 039C
      Right 039B
    Renal
      Left 049A
      Right 0499
    Splenic 0494
    Subclavian
      Left 0394
      Right 0393
    Superior Mesenteric 0495
    Temporal
      Left 039T
      Right 039S
    Thyroid
      Left 039V
      Right 039U
    Ulnar
      Left 039A
      Right 0399
    Upper 039Y
    Vertebral
      Left 039Q
      Right 039P
  Auditory Ossicle
    Left 099A
    Right 0999
  Axilla
    Left 0X95
    Right 0X94
  Back
    Lower 0W9L
    Upper 0W9K
  Basal Ganglia 0098
  Bladder 0T9B
  Bladder Neck 0T9C
  Bone
    Ethmoid
      Left 0N9G
      Right 0N9F
    Frontal 0N91
    Hyoid 0N9X
    Lacrimal
      Left 0N9J
      Right 0N9H
    Nasal 0N9B
    Occipital 0N97
    Palatine
      Left 0N9L
      Right 0N9K
    Parietal
      Left 0N94
      Right 0N93
    Pelvic
      Left 0Q93
      Right 0Q92
    Sphenoid 0N9C
    Temporal
      Left 0N96
      Right 0N95

Drainage — *continued*
Bone — *continued*
  Zygomatic
    Left ØN9N
    Right ØN9M
Bone Marrow Ø79T
Brain ØØ9Ø
Breast
  Bilateral ØH9V
  Left ØH9U
  Right ØH9T
Bronchus
  Lingula ØB99
  Lower Lobe
    Left ØB9B
    Right ØB96
  Main
    Left ØB97
    Right ØB93
  Middle Lobe, Right ØB95
  Upper Lobe
    Left ØB98
    Right ØB94
Buccal Mucosa ØC94
Bursa and Ligament
  Abdomen
    Left ØM9J
    Right ØM9H
  Ankle
    Left ØM9R
    Right ØM9Q
  Elbow
    Left ØM94
    Right ØM93
  Foot
    Left ØM9T
    Right ØM9S
  Hand
    Left ØM98
    Right ØM97
  Head and Neck ØM9Ø
  Hip
    Left ØM9M
    Right ØM9L
  Knee
    Left ØM9P
    Right ØM9N
  Lower Extremity
    Left ØM9W
    Right ØM9V
  Perineum ØM9K
  Rib(s) ØM9G
  Shoulder
    Left ØM92
    Right ØM91
  Spine
    Lower ØM9D
    Upper ØM9C
  Sternum ØM9F
  Upper Extremity
    Left ØM9B
    Right ØM99
  Wrist
    Left ØM96
    Right ØM95
Buttock
  Left ØY91
  Right ØY9Ø
Carina ØB92
Carotid Bodies, Bilateral ØG98
Carotid Body
  Left ØG96
  Right ØG97
Carpal
  Left ØP9N
  Right ØP9M
Cavity, Cranial ØW91
Cecum ØD9H
Cerebellum ØØ9C
Cerebral Hemisphere ØØ97
Cerebral Meninges ØØ91
Cerebral Ventricle ØØ96
Cervix ØU9C
Chest Wall ØW98
Choroid
  Left Ø89B
  Right Ø89A
Cisterna Chyli Ø79L

Drainage — *continued*
Clavicle
  Left ØP9B
  Right ØP99
Clitoris ØU9J
Coccygeal Glomus ØG9B
Coccyx ØQ9S
Colon
  Ascending ØD9K
  Descending ØD9M
  Sigmoid ØD9N
  Transverse ØD9L
Conjunctiva
  Left Ø89T
  Right Ø89S
Cord
  Bilateral ØV9H
  Left ØV9G
  Right ØV9F
Cornea
  Left Ø899
  Right Ø898
Cul-de-sac ØU9F
Diaphragm ØB9T
Disc
  Cervical Vertebral ØR93
  Cervicothoracic Vertebral ØR95
  Lumbar Vertebral ØS92
  Lumbosacral ØS94
  Thoracic Vertebral ØR99
  Thoracolumbar Vertebral ØR9B
Duct
  Common Bile ØF99
  Cystic ØF98
  Hepatic
    Common ØF97
    Left ØF96
    Right ØF95
  Lacrimal
    Left Ø89Y
    Right Ø89X
  Pancreatic ØF9D
    Accessory ØF9F
  Parotid
    Left ØC9C
    Right ØC9B
Duodenum ØD99
Dura Mater ØØ92
Ear
  External
    Left Ø991
    Right Ø99Ø
  External Auditory Canal
    Left Ø994
    Right Ø993
  Inner
    Left Ø99E
    Right Ø99D
  Middle
    Left Ø996
    Right Ø995
Elbow Region
  Left ØX9C
  Right ØX9B
Epididymis
  Bilateral ØV9L
  Left ØV9K
  Right ØV9J
Epidural Space, Intracranial ØØ93
Epiglottis ØC9R
Esophagogastric Junction ØD94
Esophagus ØD95
  Lower ØD93
  Middle ØD92
  Upper ØD91
Eustachian Tube
  Left Ø99G
  Right Ø99F
Extremity
  Lower
    Left ØY9B
    Right ØY99
  Upper
    Left ØX97
    Right ØX96
Eye
  Left Ø891
  Right Ø89Ø

Drainage — *continued*
Eyelid
  Lower
    Left Ø89R
    Right Ø89Q
  Upper
    Left Ø89P
    Right Ø89N
Face ØW92
Fallopian Tube
  Left ØU96
  Right ØU95
Fallopian Tubes, Bilateral ØU97
Femoral Region
  Left ØY98
  Right ØY97
Femoral Shaft
  Left ØQ99
  Right ØQ98
Femur
  Lower
    Left ØQ9C
    Right ØQ9B
  Upper
    Left ØQ97
    Right ØQ96
Fibula
  Left ØQ9K
  Right ØQ9J
Finger Nail ØH9Q
Foot
  Left ØY9N
  Right ØY9M
Gallbladder ØF94
Gingiva
  Lower ØC96
  Upper ØC95
Gland
  Adrenal
    Bilateral ØG94
    Left ØG92
    Right ØG93
  Lacrimal
    Left Ø89W
    Right Ø89V
  Minor Salivary ØC9J
  Parotid
    Left ØC99
    Right ØC98
  Pituitary ØG9Ø
  Sublingual
    Left ØC9F
    Right ØC9D
  Submaxillary
    Left ØC9H
    Right ØC9G
  Vestibular ØU9L
Glenoid Cavity
  Left ØP98
  Right ØP97
Glomus Jugulare ØG9C
Hand
  Left ØX9K
  Right ØX9J
Head ØW9Ø
Humeral Head
  Left ØP9D
  Right ØP9C
Humeral Shaft
  Left ØP9G
  Right ØP9F
Hymen ØU9K
Hypothalamus ØØ9A
Ileocecal Valve ØD9C
Ileum ØD9B
Inguinal Region
  Left ØY96
  Right ØY95
Intestine
  Large ØD9E
    Left ØD9G
    Right ØD9F
  Small ØD98
Iris
  Left Ø89D
  Right Ø89C
Jaw
  Lower ØW95
  Upper ØW94

Subterms under main terms may continue to next column or page

Drainage — *continued*
Jejunum Ø D9A
Joint
  Acromioclavicular
    Left ØR9H
    Right ØR9G
  Ankle
    Left ØS9G
    Right ØS9F
  Carpal
    Left ØR9R
    Right ØR9Q
  Carpometacarpal
    Left ØR9T
    Right ØR9S
  Cervical Vertebral ØR91
  Cervicothoracic Vertebral ØR94
  Coccygeal ØS96
  Elbow
    Left ØR9M
    Right ØR9L
  Finger Phalangeal
    Left ØR9X
    Right ØR9W
  Hip
    Left ØS9B
    Right ØS99
  Knee
    Left ØS9D
    Right ØS9C
  Lumbar Vertebral ØS9Ø
  Lumbosacral ØS93
  Metacarpophalangeal
    Left ØR9V
    Right ØR9U
  Metatarsal-Phalangeal
    Left ØS9N
    Right ØS9M
  Occipital-cervical ØR9Ø
  Sacrococcygeal ØS95
  Sacroiliac
    Left ØS98
    Right ØS97
  Shoulder
    Left ØR9K
    Right ØR9J
  Sternoclavicular
    Left ØR9F
    Right ØR9E
  Tarsal
    Left ØS9J
    Right ØS9H
  Tarsometatarsal
    Left ØS9L
    Right ØS9K
  Temporomandibular
    Left ØR9D
    Right ØR9C
  Thoracic Vertebral ØR96
  Thoracolumbar Vertebral ØR9A
  Toe Phalangeal
    Left ØS9Q
    Right ØS9P
  Wrist
    Left ØR9P
    Right ØR9N
Kidney
  Left ØT91
  Right ØT9Ø
Kidney Pelvis
  Left ØT94
  Right ØT93
Knee Region
  Left ØY9G
  Right ØY9F
Larynx ØC9S
Leg
  Lower
    Left ØY9J
    Right ØY9H
  Upper
    Left ØY9D
    Right ØY9C
Lens
  Left Ø89K
  Right Ø89J
Lip
  Lower ØC91
  Upper ØC9Ø

Drainage — *continued*
Liver ØF9Ø
  Left Lobe ØF92
  Right Lobe ØF91
Lung
  Bilateral ØB9M
  Left ØB9L
  Lower Lobe
    Left ØB9J
    Right ØB9F
  Middle Lobe, Right ØB9D
  Right ØB9K
  Upper Lobe
    Left ØB9G
    Right ØB9C
Lung Lingula ØB9H
Lymphatic
  Aortic Ø79D
  Axillary
    Left Ø796
    Right Ø795
  Head Ø79Ø
  Inguinal
    Left Ø79J
    Right Ø79H
  Internal Mammary
    Left Ø799
    Right Ø798
  Lower Extremity
    Left Ø79G
    Right Ø79F
  Mesenteric Ø79B
  Neck
    Left Ø792
    Right Ø791
  Pelvis Ø79C
  Thoracic Duct Ø79K
  Thorax Ø797
  Upper Extremity
    Left Ø794
    Right Ø793
Mandible
  Left ØN9V
  Right ØN9T
Maxilla ØN9R
Mediastinum ØW9C
Medulla Oblongata ØØ9D
Mesentery ØD9V
Metacarpal
  Left ØP9Q
  Right ØP9P
Metatarsal
  Left ØQ9P
  Right ØQ9N
Muscle
  Abdomen
    Left ØK9L
    Right ØK9K
  Extraocular
    Left Ø89M
    Right Ø89L
  Facial ØK91
  Foot
    Left ØK9W
    Right ØK9V
  Hand
    Left ØK9D
    Right ØK9C
  Head ØK9Ø
  Hip
    Left ØK9P
    Right ØK9N
  Lower Arm and Wrist
    Left ØK9B
    Right ØK99
  Lower Leg
    Left ØK9T
    Right ØK9S
  Neck
    Left ØK93
    Right ØK92
  Perineum ØK9M
  Shoulder
    Left ØK96
    Right ØK95
  Thorax
    Left ØK9J
    Right ØK9H
  Tongue, Palate, Pharynx ØK94

Drainage — *continued*
Muscle — *continued*
  Trunk
    Left ØK9G
    Right ØK9F
  Upper Arm
    Left ØK98
    Right ØK97
  Upper Leg
    Left ØK9R
    Right ØK9Q
Nasal Mucosa and Soft Tissue Ø99K
Nasopharynx Ø99N
Neck ØW96
Nerve
  Abdominal Sympathetic Ø19M
  Abducens ØØ9L
  Accessory ØØ9R
  Acoustic ØØ9N
  Brachial Plexus Ø193
  Cervical Ø191
  Cervical Plexus Ø19Ø
  Facial ØØ9M
  Femoral Ø19D
  Glossopharyngeal ØØ9P
  Head and Neck Sympathetic Ø19K
  Hypoglossal ØØ9S
  Lumbar Ø19B
  Lumbar Plexus Ø199
  Lumbar Sympathetic Ø19N
  Lumbosacral Plexus Ø19A
  Median Ø195
  Oculomotor ØØ9H
  Olfactory ØØ9F
  Optic ØØ9G
  Peroneal Ø19H
  Phrenic Ø192
  Pudendal Ø19C
  Radial Ø196
  Sacral Ø19R
  Sacral Plexus Ø19Q
  Sacral Sympathetic Ø19P
  Sciatic Ø19F
  Thoracic Ø198
  Thoracic Sympathetic Ø19L
  Tibial Ø19G
  Trigeminal ØØ9K
  Trochlear ØØ9J
  Ulnar Ø194
  Vagus ØØ9Q
Nipple
  Left ØH9X
  Right ØH9W
Omentum ØD9U
Oral Cavity and Throat ØW93
Orbit
  Left ØN9Q
  Right ØN9P
Ovary
  Bilateral ØU92
  Left ØU91
  Right ØU9Ø
Palate
  Hard ØC92
  Soft ØC93
Pancreas ØF9G
Para-aortic Body ØG99
Paraganglion Extremity ØG9F
Parathyroid Gland ØG9R
  Inferior
    Left ØG9P
    Right ØG9N
  Multiple ØG9Q
  Superior
    Left ØG9M
    Right ØG9L
Patella
  Left ØQ9F
  Right ØQ9D
Pelvic Cavity ØW9J
Penis ØV9S
Pericardial Cavity ØW9D
Perineum
  Female ØW9N
  Male ØW9M
Peritoneal Cavity ØW9G
Peritoneum ØD9W

Subterms under main terms may continue to next column or page

Drainage — *continued*
- Vein — *continued*
  - Femoral
    - Left Ø69N
    - Right Ø69M
  - Foot
    - Left Ø69V
    - Right Ø69T
  - Gastric Ø692
  - Hand
    - Left Ø59H
    - Right Ø59G
  - Hemiazygos Ø591
  - Hepatic Ø694
  - Hypogastric
    - Left Ø69J
    - Right Ø69H
  - Inferior Mesenteric Ø696
  - Innominate
    - Left Ø594
    - Right Ø593
  - Internal Jugular
    - Left Ø59N
    - Right Ø59M
  - Intracranial Ø59L
  - Lower Ø69Y
  - Portal Ø698
  - Renal
    - Left Ø69B
    - Right Ø699
  - Saphenous
    - Left Ø69Q
    - Right Ø69P
  - Splenic Ø691
  - Subclavian
    - Left Ø596
    - Right Ø595
  - Superior Mesenteric Ø695
  - Upper Ø59Y
  - Vertebral
    - Left Ø59S
    - Right Ø59R
- Vena Cava, Inferior Ø69Ø
- Vertebra
  - Cervical ØP93
  - Lumbar ØQ9Ø
  - Thoracic ØP94
- Vesicle
  - Bilateral ØV93
  - Left ØV92
  - Right ØV91
- Vitreous
  - Left Ø895
  - Right Ø894
- Vocal Cord
  - Left ØC9V
  - Right ØC9T
- Vulva ØU9M
- Wrist Region
  - Left ØX9H
  - Right ØX9G

Dressing
- Abdominal Wall 2W23X4Z
- Arm
  - Lower
    - Left 2W2DX4Z
    - Right 2W2CX4Z
  - Upper
    - Left 2W2BX4Z
    - Right 2W2AX4Z
- Back 2W25X4Z
- Chest Wall 2W24X4Z
- Extremity
  - Lower
    - Left 2W2MX4Z
    - Right 2W2LX4Z
  - Upper
    - Left 2W29X4Z
    - Right 2W28X4Z
- Face 2W21X4Z
- Finger
  - Left 2W2KX4Z
  - Right 2W2JX4Z
- Foot
  - Left 2W2TX4Z
  - Right 2W2SX4Z
- Hand
  - Left 2W2FX4Z
  - Right 2W2EX4Z

Dressing — *continued*
- Head 2W2ØX4Z
- Inguinal Region
  - Left 2W27X4Z
  - Right 2W26X4Z
- Leg
  - Lower
    - Left 2W2RX4Z
    - Right 2W2QX4Z
  - Upper
    - Left 2W2PX4Z
    - Right 2W2NX4Z
- Neck 2W22X4Z
- Thumb
  - Left 2W2HX4Z
  - Right 2W2GX4Z
- Toe
  - Left 2W2VX4Z
  - Right 2W2UX4Z

Driver stent (RX) (OTW) *use* Intraluminal Device
Drotrecogin alfa, infusion *see* Introduction of Recombinant Human-activated Protein C
Duct of Santorini *use* Pancreatic Duct, Accessory
Duct of Wirsung *use* Pancreatic Duct
Ductogram, mammary *see* Plain Radiography, Skin, Subcutaneous Tissue and Breast BHØ
Ductography, mammary *see* Plain Radiography, Skin, Subcutaneous Tissue and Breast BHØ
Ductus deferens
- *use* Vas Deferens
- *use* Vas Deferens, Bilateral
- *use* Vas Deferens, Left
- *use* Vas Deferens, Right

Duodenal ampulla *use* Ampulla of Vater
Duodenectomy
- *see* Excision, Duodenum ØDB9
- *see* Resection, Duodenum ØDT9

Duodenocholedochotomy *see* Drainage, Gallbladder ØF94
Duodenocystostomy
- *see* Bypass, Gallbladder ØF14
- *see* Drainage, Gallbladder ØF94

Duodenoenterostomy
- *see* Bypass, Gastrointestinal System ØD1
- *see* Drainage, Gastrointestinal System ØD9

Duodenojejunal flexure *use* Jejunum
Duodenolysis *see* Release, Duodenum ØDN9
Duodenorrhaphy *see* Repair, Duodenum ØDQ9
Duodenostomy
- *see* Bypass, Duodenum ØD19
- *see* Drainage, Duodenum ØD99

Duodenotomy *see* Drainage, Duodenum ØD99
Dura mater, intracranial *use* Dura Mater
Dura mater, spinal *use* Spinal Meninges
DuraGraft® Endothelial Damage Inhibitor *use* Endothelial Damage Inhibitor
DuraHeart Left Ventricular Assist System *use* Implantable Heart Assist System in Heart and Great Vessels
Dural venous sinus *use* Intracranial Vein
Durata® Defibrillation Lead *use* Cardiac Lead, Defibrillator in Ø2H
Durvalumab Antineoplastic XWØ
DynaNail Mini®
- *use* Internal Fixation Device, Sustained Compression in ØRG
- *use* Internal Fixation Device, Sustained Compression in ØSG

DynaNail®
- *use* Internal Fixation Device, Sustained Compression in ØRG
- *use* Internal Fixation Device, Sustained Compression in ØSG

Dynesys® Dynamic Stabilization System
- *use* Spinal Stabilization Device, Pedicle-Based in ØRH
- *use* Spinal Stabilization Device, Pedicle-Based in ØSH

E

Earlobe
- *use* Ear, External, Bilateral
- *use* Ear, External, Left
- *use* Ear, External, Right

ECCO2R (Extracorporeal Carbon Dioxide Removal) 5AØ92ØZ
Echocardiogram *see* Ultrasonography, Heart B24
Echography *see* Ultrasonography
EchoTip® Insight™ Portosystemic Pressure Gradient Measurement System 4AØ44B2
ECMO *see* Performance, Circulatory 5A15
ECMO, intraoperative *see* Performance, Circulatory 5A15A
Eculizumab XWØ
EDWARDS INTUITY Elite valve system *use* Zooplastic Tissue, Rapid Deployment Technique in New Technology
EEG (electroencephalogram) *see* Measurement, Central Nervous 4AØØ
EGD (esophagogastroduodenoscopy) ØDJØ8ZZ
Eighth cranial nerve *use* Acoustic Nerve
Ejaculatory duct
- *use* Vas Deferens
- *use* Vas Deferens, Bilateral
- *use* Vas Deferens, Left
- *use* Vas Deferens, Right

EKG (electrocardiogram) *see* Measurement, Cardiac 4AØ2
EKOS™ EkoSonic® Endovascular System *see* Fragmentation, Artery
Eladocagene exuparvovec XWØQ316
Electrical bone growth stimulator (EBGS)
- *use* Bone Growth Stimulator in Head and Facial Bones
- *use* Bone Growth Stimulator in Lower Bones
- *use* Bone Growth Stimulator in Upper Bones

Electrical muscle stimulation (EMS) lead *use* Stimulator Lead in Muscles
Electrocautery
- Destruction *see* Destruction
- Repair *see* Repair

Electroconvulsive Therapy
- Bilateral-Multiple Seizure GZB3ZZZ
- Bilateral-Single Seizure GZB2ZZZ
- Electroconvulsive Therapy, Other GZB4ZZZ
- Unilateral-Multiple Seizure GZB1ZZZ
- Unilateral-Single Seizure GZBØZZZ

Electroencephalogram (EEG) *see* Measurement, Central Nervous 4AØØ
Electromagnetic Therapy
- Central Nervous 6A22
- Urinary 6A21

Electronic muscle stimulator lead *use* Stimulator Lead in Muscles
Electrophysiologic stimulation (EPS) *see* Measurement, Cardiac 4AØ2
Electroshock therapy *see* Electroconvulsive Therapy
Elevation, bone fragments, skull *see* Reposition, Head and Facial Bones ØNS
Eleventh cranial nerve *use* Accessory Nerve
Ellipsys® vascular access system
- Radial Artery, Left Ø31C3ZF
- Radial Artery, Right Ø31B3ZF
- Ulnar Artery, Left Ø31A3ZF
- Ulnar Artery, Right Ø3193ZF

E-Luminexx™ (Biliary) (Vascular) Stent *use* Intraluminal Device
Eluvia™ Drug-Eluting Vascular Stent System
- *use* Intraluminal Device, Sustained Release Drug-eluting in New Technology
- *use* Intraluminal Device, Sustained Release Drug-eluting, Two in New Technology
- *use* Intraluminal Device, Sustained Release Drug-eluting, Three in New Technology
- *use* Intraluminal Device, Sustained Release Drug-eluting, Four or More in New Technology

ELZONRIS™ *use* Tagraxofusp-erzs Antineoplastic
Embolectomy *see* Extirpation
Embolization
- *see* Occlusion
- *see* Restriction

Embolization coil(s) *use* Intraluminal Device
EMG (electromyogram) *see* Measurement, Musculoskeletal 4AØF
Encephalon *use* Brain
Endarterectomy
- *see* Extirpation, Lower Arteries Ø4C
- *see* Extirpation, Upper Arteries Ø3C

Endeavor® (III) (IV) (Sprint) Zotarolimus-eluting Coronary Stent System *use* Intraluminal Device, Drug-eluting in Heart and Great Vessels

EndoAVF procedure
  Radial Artery, Left Ø31C3ZF
  Radial Artery, Right Ø31B3ZF
  Ulnar Artery, Left Ø31A3ZF
  Ulnar Artery, Right Ø3193ZF
Endologix® AFX Endovascular AAA System *use* Intraluminal Device
EndoSure® sensor *use* Monitoring Device, Pressure Sensor in Ø2H
ENDOTAK RELIANCE® (G) Defibrillation Lead *use* Cardiac Lead, Defibrillator in Ø2H
Endothelial damage inhibitor, applied to vein graft XYØVX83
Endotracheal tube (cuffed) (double-lumen) *use* Intraluminal Device, Endotracheal Airway in Respiratory System
Endovascular fistula creation
  Radial Artery, Left Ø31C3ZF
  Radial Artery, Right Ø31B3ZF
  Ulnar Artery, Left Ø31A3ZF
  Ulnar Artery, Right Ø3193ZF
Endurant® Endovascular Stent Graft *use* Intraluminal Device
Endurant® II AAA stent graft system *use* Intraluminal Device
Engineered Autologous Chimeric Antigen Receptor T-cell Immunotherapy XWØ
Enlargement
  see Dilation
  see Repair
EnRhythm *use* Pacemaker, Dual Chamber in ØJH
ENROUTE® Transcarotid Neuroprotection System *see* New Technology, Cardiovascular System X2A
Enterorrhaphy *see* Repair, Gastrointestinal System ØDQ
Enterra gastric neurostimulator *use* Stimulator Generator, Multiple Array in ØJH
Enucleation
  Eyeball *see* Resection, Eye Ø8T
  Eyeball with prosthetic implant *see* Replacement, Eye Ø8R
Ependyma *use* Cerebral Ventricle
Epicel® cultured epidermal autograft *use* Autologous Tissue Substitute
Epic™ Stented Tissue Valve (aortic) *use* Zooplastic Tissue in Heart and Great Vessels
Epidermis *use* Skin
Epididymectomy
  see Excision, Male Reproductive System ØVB
  see Resection, Male Reproductive System ØVT
Epididymoplasty
  see Repair, Male Reproductive System ØVQ
  see Supplement, Male Reproductive System ØVU
Epididymorrhaphy *see* Repair, Male Reproductive System ØVQ
Epididymotomy *see* Drainage, Male Reproductive System ØV9
Epidural space, spinal *use* Spinal Canal
Epiphysiodesis
  see Insertion of device in, Lower Bones ØQH
  see Insertion of device in, Upper Bones ØPH
  see Repair, Lower Bones ØQQ
  see Repair, Upper Bones ØPQ
Epiploic foramen *use* Peritoneum
Epiretinal Visual Prosthesis
  Left Ø8H1Ø5Z
  Right Ø8HØØ5Z
Episiorrhaphy *see* Repair, Perineum, Female ØWQN
Episiotomy *see* Division, Perineum, Female ØW8N
Epithalamus *use* Thalamus
Epitrochlear lymph node
  use Lymphatic, Left Upper Extremity
  use Lymphatic, Right Upper Extremity
EPS (electrophysiologic stimulation) *see* Measurement, Cardiac 4AØ2
Eptifibatide, infusion *see* Introduction of Platelet Inhibitor
ERCP (endoscopic retrograde cholangiopancreatography) *see* Fluoroscopy, Hepatobiliary System and Pancreas BF1
Erdafitinib Antineoplastic XWØDXL5
ERLEADA™ *use* Apalutamide Antineoplastic
Erector spinae muscle
  use Trunk Muscle, Left
  use Trunk Muscle, Right
ERLEADA™ *use* Apalutamide Antineoplastic
Esketamine Hydrochloride XWØ97M5
Esophageal artery *use* Upper Artery

Esophageal obturator airway (EOA) *use* Intraluminal Device, Airway in Gastrointestinal System
Esophageal plexus *use* Thoracic Sympathetic Nerve
Esophagectomy
  see Excision, Gastrointestinal System ØDB
  see Resection, Gastrointestinal System ØDT
Esophagocoloplasty
  see Repair, Gastrointestinal System ØDQ
  see Supplement, Gastrointestinal System ØDU
Esophagoenterostomy
  see Bypass, Gastrointestinal System ØD1
  see Drainage, Gastrointestinal System ØD9
Esophagoesophagostomy
  see Bypass, Gastrointestinal System ØD1
  see Drainage, Gastrointestinal System ØD9
Esophagogastrectomy
  see Excision, Gastrointestinal System ØDB
  see Resection, Gastrointestinal System ØDT
Esophagogastroduodenoscopy (EGD) ØDJØ8ZZ
Esophagogastroplasty
  see Repair, Gastrointestinal System ØDQ
  see Supplement, Gastrointestinal System ØDU
Esophagogastroscopy ØDJ68ZZ
Esophagogastrostomy
  see Bypass, Gastrointestinal System ØD1
  see Drainage, Gastrointestinal System ØD9
Esophagojejunoplasty *see* Supplement, Gastrointestinal System ØDU
Esophagojejunostomy
  see Bypass, Gastrointestinal System ØD1
  see Drainage, Gastrointestinal System ØD9
Esophagomyotomy *see* Division, Esophagogastric Junction ØD84
Esophagoplasty
  see Repair, Gastrointestinal System ØDQ
  see Replacement, Esophagus ØDR5
  see Supplement, Gastrointestinal System ØDU
Esophagoplication *see* Restriction, Gastrointestinal System ØDV
Esophagorrhaphy *see* Repair, Gastrointestinal System ØDQ
Esophagoscopy ØDJØ8ZZ
Esophagotomy *see* Drainage, Gastrointestinal System ØD9
Esteem® implantable hearing system *use* Hearing Device in Ear, Nose, Sinus
ESWL (extracorporeal shock wave lithotripsy) *see* Fragmentation
Ethmoidal air cell
  use Ethmoid Sinus, Left
  use Ethmoid Sinus, Right
Ethmoidectomy
  see Excision, Ear, Nose, Sinus Ø9B
  see Excision, Head and Facial Bones ØNB
  see Resection, Ear, Nose, Sinus Ø9T
  see Resection, Head and Facial Bones ØNT
Ethmoidotomy *see* Drainage, Ear, Nose, Sinus Ø99
Evacuation
  Hematoma *see* Extirpation
  Other Fluid *see* Drainage
Evera (XT) (S) (DR/VR) *use* Defibrillator Generator in ØJH
Everolimus-eluting coronary stent *use* Intraluminal Device, Drug-eluting in Heart and Great Vessels
Evisceration
  Eyeball *see* Resection, Eye Ø8T
  Eyeball with prosthetic implant *see* Replacement, Eye Ø8R
Examination *see* Inspection
Exchange *see* Change device in
Excision
  Abdominal Wall ØWBF
  Acetabulum
    Left ØQB5
    Right ØQB4
  Adenoids ØCBQ
  Ampulla of Vater ØFBC
  Anal Sphincter ØDBR
  Ankle Region
    Left ØYBL
    Right ØYBK
  Anus ØDBQ
  Aorta
    Abdominal
    Thoracic
      Ascending/Arch Ø2BX
      Descending Ø2BW

Excision — *continued*
Aortic Body ØGBD
Appendix ØDBJ
Arm
  Lower
    Left ØXBF
    Right ØXBD
  Upper
    Left ØXB9
    Right ØXB8
Artery
  Anterior Tibial
    Left Ø4BQ
    Right Ø4BP
  Axillary
    Left Ø3B6
    Right Ø3B5
  Brachial
    Left Ø3B8
    Right Ø3B7
  Celiac Ø4B1
  Colic
    Left Ø4B7
    Middle Ø4B8
    Right Ø4B6
  Common Carotid
    Left Ø3BJ
    Right Ø3BH
  Common Iliac
    Left Ø4BD
    Right Ø4BC
  External Carotid
    Left Ø3BN
    Right Ø3BM
  External Iliac
    Left Ø4BJ
    Right Ø4BH
  Face Ø3BR
  Femoral
    Left Ø4BL
    Right Ø4BK
  Foot
    Left Ø4BW
    Right Ø4BV
  Gastric Ø4B2
  Hand
    Left Ø3BF
    Right Ø3BD
  Hepatic Ø4B3
  Inferior Mesenteric Ø4BB
  Innominate Ø3B2
  Internal Carotid
    Left Ø3BL
    Right Ø3BK
  Internal Iliac
    Left Ø4BF
    Right Ø4BE
  Internal Mammary
    Left Ø3B1
    Right Ø3BØ
  Intracranial Ø3BG
  Lower Ø4BY
  Peroneal
    Left Ø4BU
    Right Ø4BT
  Popliteal
    Left Ø4BN
    Right Ø4BM
  Posterior Tibial
    Left Ø4BS
    Right Ø4BR
  Pulmonary
    Left Ø2BR
    Right Ø2BQ
  Pulmonary Trunk Ø2BP
  Radial
    Left Ø3BC
    Right Ø3BB`
  Renal
    Left Ø4BA
    Right Ø4B9
  Splenic Ø4B4
  Subclavian
    Left Ø3B4
    Right Ø3B3
  Superior Mesenteric Ø4B5
  Temporal
    Left Ø3BT
    Right Ø3BS

Excision — *continued*
  Artery — *continued*
    Thyroid
      Left Ø3BV
      Right Ø3BU
    Ulnar
      Left Ø3BA
      Right Ø3B9
    Upper Ø3BY
    Vertebral
      Left Ø3BQ
      Right Ø3BP
  Atrium
    Left Ø2B7
    Right Ø2B6
  Auditory Ossicle
    Left Ø9BA
    Right Ø9B9
  Axilla
    Left ØXB5
    Right ØXB4
  Back
    Lower ØWBL
    Upper ØWBK
  Basal Ganglia ØØB8
  Bladder ØTBB
  Bladder Neck ØTBC
  Bone
    Ethmoid
      Left ØNBG
      Right ØNBF
    Frontal ØNB1
    Hyoid ØNBX
    Lacrimal
      Left ØNBJ
      Right ØNBH
    Nasal ØNBB
    Occipital ØNB7
    Palatine
      Left ØNBL
      Right ØNBK
    Parietal
      Left ØNB4
      Right ØNB3
    Pelvic
      Left ØQB3
      Right ØQB2
    Sphenoid ØNBC
    Temporal
      Left ØNB6
      Right ØNB5
    Zygomatic
      Left ØNBN
      Right ØNBM
  Brain ØØBØ
  Breast
    Bilateral ØHBV
    Left ØHBU
    Right ØHBT
    Supernumerary ØHBY
  Bronchus
    Lingula ØBB9
    Lower Lobe
      Left ØBBB
      Right ØBB6
    Main
      Left ØBB7
      Right ØBB3
    Middle Lobe, Right ØBB5
    Upper Lobe
      Left ØBB8
      Right ØBB4
  Buccal Mucosa ØCB4
  Bursa and Ligament
    Abdomen
      Left ØMBJ
      Right ØMBH
    Ankle
      Left ØMBR
      Right ØMBQ
    Elbow
      Left ØMB4
      Right ØMB3
    Foot
      Left ØMBT
      Right ØMBS
    Hand
      Left ØMB8
      Right ØMB7

Excision — *continued*
  Bursa and Ligament — *continued*
    Head and Neck ØMBØ
    Hip
      Left ØMBM
      Right ØMBL
    Knee
      Left ØMBP
      Right ØMBN
    Lower Extremity
      Left ØMBW
      Right ØMBV
    Perineum ØMBK
    Rib(s) ØMBG
    Shoulder
      Left ØMB2
      Right ØMB1
    Spine
      Lower ØMBD
      Upper ØMBC
    Sternum ØMBF
    Upper Extremity
      Left ØMBB
      Right ØMB9
    Wrist
      Left ØMB6
      Right ØMB5
  Buttock
    Left ØYB1
    Right ØYBØ
  Carina ØBB2
  Carotid Bodies, Bilateral ØGB8
  Carotid Body
    Left ØGB6
    Right ØGB7
  Carpal
    Left ØPBN
    Right ØPBM
  Cecum ØDBH
  Cerebellum ØØBC
  Cerebral Hemisphere ØØB7
  Cerebral Meninges ØØB1
  Cerebral Ventricle ØØB6
  Cervix ØUBC
  Chest Wall ØWB8
  Chordae Tendineae Ø2B9
  Choroid
    Left Ø8BB
    Right Ø8BA
  Cisterna Chyli Ø7BL
  Clavicle
    Left ØPBB
    Right ØPB9
  Clitoris ØUBJ
  Coccygeal Glomus ØGBB
  Coccyx ØQBS
  Colon
    Ascending ØDBK
    Descending ØDBM
    Sigmoid ØDBN
    Transverse ØDBL
  Conduction Mechanism Ø2B8
  Conjunctiva
    Left Ø8BTXZ
    Right Ø8BSXZ
  Cord
    Bilateral ØVBH
    Left ØVBG
    Right ØVBF
  Cornea
    Left Ø8B9XZ
    Right Ø8B8XZ
  Cul-de-sac ØUBF
  Diaphragm ØBBT
  Disc
    Cervical Vertebral ØRB3
    Cervicothoracic Vertebral ØRB5
    Lumbar Vertebral ØSB2
    Lumbosacral ØSB4
    Thoracic Vertebral ØRB9
    Thoracolumbar Vertebral ØRBB
  Duct
    Common Bile ØFB9
    Cystic ØFB8
    Hepatic
      Common ØFB7
      Left ØFB6
      Right ØFB5

Excision — *continued*
  Duct — *continued*
    Lacrimal
      Left Ø8BY
      Right Ø8BX
    Pancreatic ØFBD
      Accessory ØFBF
    Parotid
      Left ØCBC
      Right ØCBB
  Duodenum ØDB9
  Dura Mater ØØB2
  Ear
    External
      Left Ø9B1
      Right Ø9BØ
    External Auditory Canal
      Left Ø9B4
      Right Ø9B3
    Inner
      Left Ø9BE
      Right Ø9BD
    Middle
      Left Ø9B6
      Right Ø9B5
  Elbow Region
    Left ØXBC
    Right ØXBB
  Epididymis
    Bilateral ØVBL
    Left ØVBK
    Right ØVBJ
  Epiglottis ØCBR
  Esophagogastric Junction ØDB4
  Esophagus ØDB5
    Lower ØDB3
    Middle ØDB2
    Upper ØDB1
  Eustachian Tube
    Left Ø9BG
    Right Ø9BF
  Extremity
    Lower
      Left ØYBB
      Right ØYB9
    Upper
      Left ØXB7
      Right ØXB6
  Eye
    Left Ø8B1
    Right Ø8BØ
  Eyelid
    Lower
      Left Ø8BR
      Right Ø8BQ
    Upper
      Left Ø8BP
      Right Ø8BN
  Face ØWB2
  Fallopian Tube
    Left ØUB6
    Right ØUB5
  Fallopian Tubes, Bilateral ØUB7
  Femoral Region
    Left ØYB8
    Right ØYB7
  Femoral Shaft
    Left ØQB9
    Right ØQB8
  Femur
    Lower
      Left ØQBC
      Right ØQBB
    Upper
      Left ØQB7
      Right ØQB6
  Fibula
    Left ØQBK
    Right ØQBJ
  Finger Nail ØHBQXZ
  Floor of mouth *see* Excision, Oral Cavity and Throat ØWB3
  Foot
    Left ØYBN
    Right ØYBM
  Gallbladder ØFB4
  Gingiva
    Lower ØCB6
    Upper ØCB5

Excision — continued
- Gland
  - Adrenal
    - Bilateral 0GB4
    - Left 0GB2
    - Right 0GB3
  - Lacrimal
    - Left 08BW
    - Right 08BV
  - Minor Salivary 0CBJ
  - Parotid
    - Left 0CB9
    - Right 0CB8
  - Pituitary 0GB0
  - Sublingual
    - Left 0CBF
    - Right 0CBD
  - Submaxillary
    - Left 0CBH
    - Right 0CBG
  - Vestibular 0UBL
- Glenoid Cavity
  - Left 0PB8
  - Right 0PB7
- Glomus Jugulare 0GBC
- Hand
  - Left 0XBK
  - Right 0XBJ
- Head 0WB0
- Humeral Head
  - Left 0PBD
  - Right 0PBC
- Humeral Shaft
  - Left 0PBG
  - Right 0PBF
- Hymen 0UBK
- Hypothalamus 00BA
- Ileocecal Valve 0DBC
- Ileum 0DBB
- Inguinal Region
  - Left 0YB6
  - Right 0YB5
- Intestine
  - Large 0DBE
    - Left 0DBG
    - Right 0DBF
  - Small 0DB8
- Iris
  - Left 08BD3Z
  - Right 08BC3Z
- Jaw
  - Lower 0WB5
  - Upper 0WB4
- Jejunum 0DBA
- Joint
  - Acromioclavicular
    - Left 0RBH
    - Right 0RBG
  - Ankle
    - Left 0SBG
    - Right 0SBF
  - Carpal
    - Left 0RBR
    - Right 0RBQ
  - Carpometacarpal
    - Left 0RBT
    - Right 0RBS
  - Cervical Vertebral 0RB1
  - Cervicothoracic Vertebral 0RB4
  - Coccygeal 0SB6
  - Elbow
    - Left 0RBM
    - Right 0RBL
  - Finger Phalangeal
    - Left 0RBX
    - Right 0RBW
  - Hip
    - Left 0SBB
    - Right 0SB9
  - Knee
    - Left 0SBD
    - Right 0SBC
  - Lumbar Vertebral 0SB0
  - Lumbosacral 0SB3
  - Metacarpophalangeal
    - Left 0RBV
    - Right 0RBU
  - Metatarsal-Phalangeal
    - Left 0SBN

Excision — continued
- Joint — continued
  - Metatarsal-Phalangeal — continued
    - Right 0SBM
  - Occipital-cervical 0RB0
  - Sacrococcygeal 0SB5
  - Sacroiliac
    - Left 0SB8
    - Right 0SB7
  - Shoulder
    - Left 0RBK
    - Right 0RBJ
  - Sternoclavicular
    - Left 0RBF
    - Right 0RBE
  - Tarsal
    - Left 0SBJ
    - Right 0SBH
  - Tarsometatarsal
    - Left 0SBL
    - Right 0SBK
  - Temporomandibular
    - Left 0RBD
    - Right 0RBC
  - Thoracic Vertebral 0RB6
  - Thoracolumbar Vertebral 0RBA
  - Toe Phalangeal
    - Left 0SBQ
    - Right 0SBP
  - Wrist
    - Left 0RBP
    - Right 0RBN
- Kidney
  - Left 0TB1
  - Right 0TB0
- Kidney Pelvis
  - Left 0TB4
  - Right 0TB3
- Knee Region
  - Left 0YBG
  - Right 0YBF
- Larynx 0CBS
- Leg
  - Lower
    - Left 0YBJ
    - Right 0YBH
  - Upper
    - Left 0YBD
    - Right 0YBC
- Lens
  - Left 08BK3Z
  - Right 08BJ3Z
- Lip
  - Lower 0CB1
  - Upper 0CB0
- Liver 0FB0
  - Left Lobe 0FB2
  - Right Lobe 0FB1
- Lung
  - Bilateral 0BBM
  - Left 0BBL
  - Lower Lobe
    - Left 0BBJ
    - Right 0BBF
  - Middle Lobe, Right 0BBD
  - Right 0BBK
  - Upper Lobe
    - Left 0BBG
    - Right 0BBC
- Lung Lingula 0BBH
- Lymphatic
  - Aortic 07BD
  - Axillary
    - Left 07B6
    - Right 07B5
  - Head 07B0
  - Inguinal
    - Left 07BJ
    - Right 07BH
  - Internal Mammary
    - Left 07B9
    - Right 07B8
  - Lower Extremity
    - Left 07BG
    - Right 07BF
  - Mesenteric 07BB
  - Neck
    - Left 07B2
    - Right 07B1

Excision — continued
- Lymphatic — continued
  - Pelvis 07BC
  - Thoracic Duct 07BK
  - Thorax 07B7
  - Upper Extremity
    - Left 07B4
    - Right 07B3
- Mandible
  - Left 0NBV
  - Right 0NBT
- Maxilla 0NBR
- Mediastinum 0WBC
- Medulla Oblongata 00BD
- Mesentery 0DBV
- Metacarpal
  - Left 0PBQ
  - Right 0PBP
- Metatarsal
  - Left 0QBP
  - Right 0QBN
- Muscle
  - Abdomen
    - Left 0KBL
    - Right 0KBK
  - Extraocular
    - Left 08BM
    - Right 08BL
  - Facial 0KB1
  - Foot
    - Left 0KBW
    - Right 0KBV
  - Hand
    - Left 0KBD
    - Right 0KBC
  - Head 0KB0
  - Hip
    - Left 0KBP
    - Right 0KBN
  - Lower Arm and Wrist
    - Left 0KBB
    - Right 0KB9
  - Lower Leg
    - Left 0KBT
    - Right 0KBS
  - Neck
    - Left 0KB3
    - Right 0KB2
  - Papillary 02BD
  - Perineum 0KBM
  - Shoulder
    - Left 0KB6
    - Right 0KB5
  - Thorax
    - Left 0KBJ
    - Right 0KBH
  - Tongue, Palate, Pharynx 0KB4
  - Trunk
    - Left 0KBG
    - Right 0KBF
  - Upper Arm
    - Left 0KB8
    - Right 0KB7
  - Upper Leg
    - Left 0KBR
    - Right 0KBQ
- Nasal Mucosa and Soft Tissue 09BK
- Nasopharynx 09BN
- Neck 0WB6
- Nerve
  - Abdominal Sympathetic 01BM
  - Abducens 00BL
  - Accessory 00BR
  - Acoustic 00BN
  - Brachial Plexus 01B3
  - Cervical 01B1
  - Cervical Plexus 01B0
  - Facial 00BM
  - Femoral 01BD
  - Glossopharyngeal 00BP
  - Head and Neck Sympathetic 01BK
  - Hypoglossal 00BS
  - Lumbar 01BB
  - Lumbar Plexus 01B9
  - Lumbar Sympathetic 01BN
  - Lumbosacral Plexus 01BA
  - Median 01B5
  - Oculomotor 00BH
  - Olfactory 00BF

Subterms under main terms may continue to next column or page

Excision — *continued*
  Uterine Supporting Structure ØUB4
  Uterus ØUB9
  Uvula ØCBN
  Vagina ØUBG
  Valve
    Aortic Ø2BF
    Mitral Ø2BG
    Pulmonary Ø2BH
    Tricuspid Ø2BJ
  Vas Deferens
    Bilateral ØVBQ
    Left ØVBP
    Right ØVBN
  Vein
    Axillary
      Left Ø5B8
      Right Ø5B7
    Azygos Ø5BØ
    Basilic
      Left Ø5BC
      Right Ø5BB
    Brachial
      Left Ø5BA
      Right Ø5B9
    Cephalic
      Left Ø5BF
      Right Ø5BD
    Colic Ø6B7
    Common Iliac
      Left Ø6BD
      Right Ø6BC
    Coronary Ø2B4
    Esophageal Ø6B3
    External Iliac
      Left Ø6BG
      Right Ø6BF
    External Jugular
      Left Ø5BQ
      Right Ø5BP
    Face
      Left Ø5BV
      Right Ø5BT
    Femoral
      Left Ø6BN
      Right Ø6BM
    Foot
      Left Ø6BV
      Right Ø6BT
    Gastric Ø6B2
    Hand
      Left Ø5BH
      Right Ø5BG
    Hemiazygos Ø5B1
    Hepatic Ø6B4
    Hypogastric
      Left Ø6BJ
      Right Ø6BH
    Inferior Mesenteric Ø6B6
    Innominate
      Left Ø5B4
      Right Ø5B3
    Internal Jugular
      Left Ø5BN
      Right Ø5BM
    Intracranial Ø5BL
    Lower Ø6BY
    Portal Ø6B8
    Pulmonary
      Left Ø2BT
      Right Ø2BS
    Renal
      Left Ø6BB
      Right Ø6B9
    Saphenous
      Left Ø6BQ
      Right Ø6BP
    Splenic Ø6B1
    Subclavian
      Left Ø5B6
      Right Ø5B5
    Superior Mesenteric Ø6B5
    Upper Ø5BY
    Vertebral
      Left Ø5BS
      Right Ø5BR
  Vena Cava
    Inferior Ø6BØ
    Superior Ø2BV

Excision — *continued*
  Ventricle
    Left Ø2BL
    Right Ø2BK
  Vertebra
    Cervical ØPB3
    Lumbar ØQBØ
    Thoracic ØPB4
  Vesicle
    Bilateral ØVB3
    Left ØVB2
    Right ØVB1
  Vitreous
    Left Ø8B53Z
    Right Ø8B43Z
  Vocal Cord
    Left ØCBV
    Right ØCBT
  Vulva ØUBM
  Wrist Region
    Left ØXBH
    Right ØXBG
EXCLUDER® AAA Endoprosthesis
  use Intraluminal Device
  use Intraluminal Device, Branched or Fenestrated, One or Two Arteries in Ø4V
  use Intraluminal Device, Branched or Fenestrated, Three or More Arteries in Ø4V
EXCLUDER® IBE Endoprosthesis *use* Intraluminal Device, Branched or Fenestrated, One or Two Arteries in Ø4V
Exclusion, Left atrial appendage (LAA) *see* Occlusion, Atrium, Left Ø2L7
Exercise, rehabilitation *see* Motor Treatment, Rehabilitation FØ7
Exploration *see* Inspection
Express® Biliary SD Monorail® Premounted Stent System *use* Intraluminal Device
Express® (LD) Premounted Stent System *use* Intraluminal Device
Express® SD Renal Monorail® Premounted Stent System *use* Intraluminal Device
Ex-PRESS™ mini glaucoma shunt *use* Synthetic Substitute
Extensor carpi radialis muscle
  use Lower Arm and Wrist Muscle, Left
  use Lower Arm and Wrist Muscle, Right
Extensor carpi ulnaris muscle
  use Lower Arm and Wrist Muscle, Left
  use Lower Arm and Wrist Muscle, Right
Extensor digitorum brevis muscle
  use Foot Muscle, Left
  use Foot Muscle, Right
Extensor digitorum longus muscle
  use Lower Leg Muscle, Left
  use Lower Leg Muscle, Right
Extensor hallucis brevis muscle
  use Foot Muscle, Left
  use Foot Muscle, Right
Extensor hallucis longus muscle
  use Lower Leg Muscle, Left
  use Lower Leg Muscle, Right
External anal sphincter *use* Anal Sphincter
External auditory meatus
  use External Auditory Canal, Left
  use External Auditory Canal, Right
External fixator
  use External Fixation Device in Head and Facial Bones
  use External Fixation Device in Lower Bones
  use External Fixation Device in Lower Joints
  use External Fixation Device in Upper Bones
  use External Fixation Device in Upper Joints
External maxillary artery *use* Face Artery
External naris *use* Nasal Mucosa and Soft Tissue
External oblique aponeurosis *use* Subcutaneous Tissue and Fascia, Trunk
External oblique muscle
  use Abdomen Muscle, Left
  use Abdomen Muscle, Right
External popliteal nerve *use* Peroneal Nerve
External pudendal artery
  use Femoral Artery, Left
  use Femoral Artery, Right
External pudendal vein
  use Saphenous Vein, Left
  use Saphenous Vein, Right

External urethral sphincter *use* Urethra
Extirpation
  Acetabulum
    Left ØQC5
    Right ØQC4
  Adenoids ØCCQ
  Ampulla of Vater ØFCC
  Anal Sphincter ØDCR
  Anterior Chamber
    Left Ø8C3
    Right Ø8C2
  Anus ØDCQ
  Aorta
    Abdominal Ø4CØ
    Thoracic
      Ascending/Arch Ø2CX
      Descending Ø2CW
  Aortic Body ØGCD
  Appendix ØDCJ
  Artery
    Anterior Tibial
      Left Ø4CQ
      Right Ø4CP
    Axillary
      Left Ø3C6
      Right Ø3C5
    Brachial
      Left Ø3C8
      Right Ø3C7
    Celiac Ø4C1
    Colic
      Left Ø4C7
      Middle Ø4C8
      Right Ø4C6
    Common Carotid
      Left Ø3CJ
      Right Ø3CH
    Common Iliac
      Left Ø4CD
      Right Ø4CC
    Coronary
      Four or More Arteries Ø2C3
      One Artery Ø2CØ
      Three Arteries Ø2C2
      Two Arteries Ø2C1
    External Carotid
      Left Ø3CN
      Right Ø3CM
    External Iliac
      Left Ø4CJ
      Right Ø4CH
    Face Ø3CR
    Femoral
      Left Ø4CL
      Right Ø4CK
    Foot
      Left Ø4CW
      Right Ø4CV
    Gastric Ø4C2
    Hand
      Left Ø3CF
      Right Ø3CD
    Hepatic Ø4C3
    Inferior Mesenteric Ø4CB
    Innominate Ø3C2
    Internal Carotid
      Left Ø3CL
      Right Ø3CK
    Internal Iliac
      Left Ø4CF
      Right Ø4CE
    Internal Mammary
      Left Ø3C1
      Right Ø3CØ
    Intracranial Ø3CG
    Lower Ø4CY
    Peroneal
      Left Ø4CU
      Right Ø4CT
    Popliteal
      Left Ø4CN
      Right Ø4CM
    Posterior Tibial
      Left Ø4CS
      Right Ø4CR
    Pulmonary
      Left Ø2CR
      Right Ø2CQ
    Pulmonary Trunk Ø2CP

Extirpation — continued
Artery — continued
Radial
Left 03CC
Right 03CB
Renal
Left 04CA
Right 04C9
Splenic 04C4
Subclavian
Left 03C4
Right 03C3
Superior Mesenteric 04C5
Temporal
Left 03CT
Right 03CS
Thyroid
Left 03CV
Right 03CU
Ulnar
Left 03CA
Right 03C9
Upper 03CY
Vertebral
Left 03CQ
Right 03CP
Atrium
Left 02C7
Right 02C6
Auditory Ossicle
Left 09CA
Right 09C9
Basal Ganglia 00C8
Bladder 0TCB
Bladder Neck 0TCC
Bone
Ethmoid
Left 0NCG
Right 0NCF
Frontal 0NC1
Hyoid 0NCX
Lacrimal
Left 0NCJ
Right 0NCH
Nasal 0NCB
Occipital 0NC7
Palatine
Left 0NCL
Right 0NCK
Parietal
Left 0NC4
Right 0NC3
Pelvic
Left 0QC3
Right 0QC2
Sphenoid 0NCC
Temporal
Left 0NC6
Right 0NC5
Zygomatic
Left 0NCN
Right 0NCM
Brain 00C0
Breast
Bilateral 0HCV
Left 0HCU
Right 0HCT
Bronchus
Lingula 0BC9
Lower Lobe
Left 0BCB
Right 0BC6
Main
Left 0BC7
Right 0BC3
Middle Lobe, Right 0BC5
Upper Lobe
Left 0BC8
Right 0BC4
Buccal Mucosa 0CC4
Bursa and Ligament
Abdomen
Left 0MCJ
Right 0MCH
Ankle
Left 0MCR
Right 0MCQ
Elbow
Left 0MC4

Extirpation — continued
Bursa and Ligament — continued
Elbow — continued
Right 0MC3
Foot
Left 0MCT
Right 0MCS
Hand
Left 0MC8
Right 0MC7
Head and Neck 0MC0
Hip
Left 0MCM
Right 0MCL
Knee
Left 0MCP
Right 0MCN
Lower Extremity
Left 0MCW
Right 0MCV
Perineum 0MCK
Rib(s) 0MCG
Shoulder
Left 0MC2
Right 0MC1
Spine
Lower 0MCD
Upper 0MCC
Sternum 0MCF
Upper Extremity
Left 0MCB
Right 0MC9
Wrist
Left 0MC6
Right 0MC5
Carina 0BC2
Carotid Bodies, Bilateral 0GC8
Carotid Body
Left 0GC6
Right 0GC7
Carpal
Left 0PCN
Right 0PCM
Cavity, Cranial 0WC1
Cecum 0DCH
Cerebellum 00CC
Cerebral Hemisphere 00C7
Cerebral Meninges 00C1
Cerebral Ventricle 00C6
Cervix 0UCC
Chordae Tendineae 02C9
Choroid
Left 08CB
Right 08CA
Cisterna Chyli 07CL
Clavicle
Left 0PCB
Right 0PC9
Clitoris 0UCJ
Coccygeal Glomus 0GCB
Coccyx 0QCS
Colon
Ascending 0DCK
Descending 0DCM
Sigmoid 0DCN
Transverse 0DCL
Conduction Mechanism 02C8
Conjunctiva
Left 08CTXZZ
Right 08CSXZZ
Cord
Bilateral 0VCH
Left 0VCG
Right 0VCF
Cornea
Left 08C9XZZ
Right 08C8XZZ
Cul-de-sac 0UCF
Diaphragm 0BCT
Disc
Cervical Vertebral 0RC3
Cervicothoracic Vertebral 0RC5
Lumbar Vertebral 0SC2
Lumbosacral 0SC4
Thoracic Vertebral 0RC9
Thoracolumbar Vertebral 0RCB
Duct
Common Bile 0FC9
Cystic 0FC8

Extirpation — continued
Duct — continued
Hepatic
Common 0FC7
Left 0FC6
Right 0FC5
Lacrimal
Left 08CY
Right 08CX
Pancreatic 0FCD
Accessory 0FCF
Parotid
Left 0CCC
Right 0CCB
Duodenum 0DC9
Dura Mater 00C2
Ear
External
Left 09C1
Right 09C0
External Auditory Canal
Left 09C4
Right 09C3
Inner
Left 09CE
Right 09CD
Middle
Left 09C6
Right 09C5
Endometrium 0UCB
Epididymis
Bilateral 0VCL
Left 0VCK
Right 0VCJ
Epidural Space, Intracranial 00C3
Epiglottis 0CCR
Esophagogastric Junction 0DC4
Esophagus 0DC5
Lower 0DC3
Middle 0DC2
Upper 0DC1
Eustachian Tube
Left 09CG
Right 09CF
Eye
Left 08C1XZZ
Right 08C0XZZ
Eyelid
Lower
Left 08CR
Right 08CQ
Upper
Left 08CP
Right 08CN
Fallopian Tube
Left 0UC6
Right 0UC5
Fallopian Tubes, Bilateral 0UC7
Femoral Shaft
Left 0QC9
Right 0QC8
Femur
Lower
Left 0QCC
Right 0QCB
Upper
Left 0QC7
Right 0QC6
Fibula
Left 0QCK
Right 0QCJ
Finger Nail 0HCQXZZ
Gallbladder 0FC4
Gastrointestinal Tract 0WCP
Genitourinary Tract 0WCR
Gingiva
Lower 0CC6
Upper 0CC5
Gland
Adrenal
Bilateral 0GC4
Left 0GC2
Right 0GC3
Lacrimal
Left 08CW
Right 08CV
Minor Salivary 0CCJ
Parotid
Left 0CC9

▽ **Subterms under main terms may continue to next column or page**

Extirpation — continued

Gland — continued
Parotid — continued
Right 0CC8
Pituitary 0GC0
Sublingual
Left 0CCF
Right 0CCD
Submaxillary
Left 0CCH
Right 0CCG
Vestibular 0UCL
Glenoid Cavity
Left 0PC8
Right 0PC7
Glomus Jugulare 0GCC
Humeral Head
Left 0PCD
Right 0PCC
Humeral Shaft
Left 0PCG
Right 0PCF
Hymen 0UCK
Hypothalamus 00CA
Ileocecal Valve 0DCC
Ileum 0DCB
Intestine
Large 0DCE
Left 0DCG
Right 0DCF
Small 0DC8
Iris
Left 08CD
Right 08CC
Jaw
Lower 0WC5
Upper 0WC4
Jejunum 0DCA
Joint
Acromioclavicular
Left 0RCH
Right 0RCG
Ankle
Left 0SCG
Right 0SCF
Carpal
Left 0RCR
Right 0RCQ
Carpometacarpal
Left 0RCT
Right 0RCS
Cervical Vertebral 0RC1
Cervicothoracic Vertebral 0RC4
Coccygeal 0SC6
Elbow
Left 0RCM
Right 0RCL
Finger Phalangeal
Left 0RCX
Right 0RCW
Hip
Left 0SCB
Right 0SC9
Knee
Left 0SCD
Right 0SCC
Lumbar Vertebral 0SC0
Lumbosacral 0SC3
Metacarpophalangeal
Left 0RCV
Right 0RCU
Metatarsal-Phalangeal
Left 0SCN
Right 0SCM
Occipital-cervical 0RC0
Sacrococcygeal 0SC5
Sacroiliac
Left 0SC8
Right 0SC7
Shoulder
Left 0RCK
Right 0RCJ
Sternoclavicular
Left 0RCF
Right 0RCE
Tarsal
Left 0SCJ
Right 0SCH

Extirpation — continued

Joint — continued
Tarsometatarsal
Left 0SCL
Right 0SCK
Temporomandibular
Left 0RCD
Right 0RCC
Thoracic Vertebral 0RC6
Thoracolumbar Vertebral 0RCA
Toe Phalangeal
Left 0SCQ
Right 0SCP
Wrist
Left 0RCP
Right 0RCN
Kidney
Left 0TC1
Right 0TC0
Kidney Pelvis
Left 0TC4
Right 0TC3
Larynx 0CCS
Lens
Left 08CK
Right 08CJ
Lip
Lower 0CC1
Upper 0CC0
Liver 0FC0
Left Lobe 0FC2
Right Lobe 0FC1
Lung
Bilateral 0BCM
Left 0BCL
Lower Lobe
Left 0BCJ
Right 0BCF
Middle Lobe, Right 0BCD
Right 0BCK
Upper Lobe
Left 0BCG
Right 0BCC
Lung Lingula 0BCH
Lymphatic
Aortic 07CD
Axillary
Left 07C6
Right 07C5
Head 07C0
Inguinal
Left 07CJ
Right 07CH
Internal Mammary
Left 07C9
Right 07C8
Lower Extremity
Left 07CG
Right 07CF
Mesenteric 07CB
Neck
Left 07C2
Right 07C1
Pelvis 07CC
Thoracic Duct 07CK
Thorax 07C7
Upper Extremity
Left 07C4
Right 07C3
Mandible
Left 0NCV
Right 0NCT
Maxilla 0NCR
Mediastinum 0WCC
Medulla Oblongata 00CD
Mesentery 0DCV
Metacarpal
Left 0PCQ
Right 0PCP
Metatarsal
Left 0QCP
Right 0QCN
Muscle
Abdomen
Left 0KCL
Right 0KCK
Extraocular
Left 08CM
Right 08CL

Extirpation — continued

Muscle — continued
Facial 0KC1
Foot
Left 0KCW
Right 0KCV
Hand
Left 0KCD
Right 0KCC
Head 0KC0
Hip
Left 0KCP
Right 0KCN
Lower Arm and Wrist
Left 0KCB
Right 0KC9
Lower Leg
Left 0KCT
Right 0KCS
Neck
Left 0KC3
Right 0KC2
Papillary 02CD
Perineum 0KCM
Shoulder
Left 0KC6
Right 0KC5
Thorax
Left 0KCJ
Right 0KCH
Tongue, Palate, Pharynx 0KC4
Trunk
Left 0KCG
Right 0KCF
Upper Arm
Left 0KC8
Right 0KC7
Upper Leg
Left 0KCR
Right 0KCQ
Nasal Mucosa and Soft Tissue 09CK
Nasopharynx 09CN
Nerve
Abdominal Sympathetic 01CM
Abducens 00CL
Accessory 00CR
Acoustic 00CN
Brachial Plexus 01C3
Cervical 01C1
Cervical Plexus 01C0
Facial 00CM
Femoral 01CD
Glossopharyngeal 00CP
Head and Neck Sympathetic 01CK
Hypoglossal 00CS
Lumbar 01CB
Lumbar Plexus 01C9
Lumbar Sympathetic 01CN
Lumbosacral Plexus 01CA
Median 01C5
Oculomotor 00CH
Olfactory 00CF
Optic 00CG
Peroneal 01CH
Phrenic 01C2
Pudendal 01CC
Radial 01C6
Sacral 01CR
Sacral Plexus 01CQ
Sacral Sympathetic 01CP
Sciatic 01CF
Thoracic 01C8
Thoracic Sympathetic 01CL
Tibial 01CG
Trigeminal 00CK
Trochlear 00CJ
Ulnar 01C4
Vagus 00CQ
Nipple
Left 0HCX
Right 0HCW
Omentum 0DCU
Oral Cavity and Throat 0WC3
Orbit
Left 0NCQ
Right 0NCP
Orbital Atherectomy Technology X2C
Ovary
Bilateral 0UC2

Subterms under main terms may continue to next column or page

Extirpation — *continued*
Ovary — *continued*
Left ØUC1
Right ØUCØ
Palate
Hard ØCC2
Soft ØCC3
Pancreas ØFCG
Para-aortic Body ØGC9
Paraganglion Extremity ØGCF
Parathyroid Gland ØGCR
Inferior
Left ØGCP
Right ØGCN
Multiple ØGCQ
Superior
Left ØGCM
Right ØGCL
Patella
Left ØQCF
Right ØQCD
Pelvic Cavity ØWCJ
Penis ØVCS
Pericardial Cavity ØWCD
Pericardium Ø2CN
Peritoneal Cavity ØWCG
Peritoneum ØDCW
Phalanx
Finger
Left ØPCV
Right ØPCT
Thumb
Left ØPCS
Right ØPCR
Toe
Left ØQCR
Right ØQCQ
Pharynx ØCCM
Pineal Body ØGC1
Pleura
Left ØBCP
Right ØBCN
Pleural Cavity
Left ØWCB
Right ØWC9
Pons ØØCB
Prepuce ØVCT
Prostate ØVCØ
Radius
Left ØPCJ
Right ØPCH
Rectum ØDCP
Respiratory Tract ØWCQ
Retina
Left Ø8CF
Right Ø8CE
Retinal Vessel
Left Ø8CH
Right Ø8CG
Retroperitoneum ØWCH
Ribs
1 to 2 ØPC1
3 or More ØPC2
Sacrum ØQC1
Scapula
Left ØPC6
Right ØPC5
Sclera
Left Ø8C7XZZ
Right Ø8C6XZZ
Scrotum ØVC5
Septum
Atrial Ø2C5
Nasal Ø9CM
Ventricular Ø2CM
Sinus
Accessory Ø9CP
Ethmoid
Left Ø9CV
Right Ø9CU
Frontal
Left Ø9CT
Right Ø9CS
Mastoid
Left Ø9CC
Right Ø9CB
Maxillary
Left Ø9CR
Right Ø9CQ

Extirpation — *continued*
Sinus — *continued*
Sphenoid
Left Ø9CX
Right Ø9CW
Skin
Abdomen ØHC7XZZ
Back ØHC6XZZ
Buttock ØHC8XZZ
Chest ØHC5XZZ
Ear
Left ØHC3XZZ
Right ØHC2XZZ
Face ØHC1XZZ
Foot
Left ØHCNXZZ
Right ØHCMXZZ
Hand
Left ØHCGXZZ
Right ØHCFXZZ
Inguinal ØHCAXZZ
Lower Arm
Left ØHCEXZZ
Right ØHCDXZZ
Lower Leg
Left ØHCLXZZ
Right ØHCKXZZ
Neck ØHC4XZZ
Perineum ØHC9XZZ
Scalp ØHCØXZZ
Upper Arm
Left ØHCCXZZ
Right ØHCBXZZ
Upper Leg
Left ØHCJXZZ
Right ØHCHXZZ
Spinal Canal ØØCU
Spinal Cord
Cervical ØØCW
Lumbar ØØCY
Thoracic ØØCX
Spinal Meninges ØØCT
Spleen Ø7CP
Sternum ØPCØ
Stomach ØDC6
Pylorus ØDC7
Subarachnoid Space, Intracranial ØØC5
Subcutaneous Tissue and Fascia
Abdomen ØJC8
Back ØJC7
Buttock ØJC9
Chest ØJC6
Face ØJC1
Foot
Left ØJCR
Right ØJCQ
Hand
Left ØJCK
Right ØJCJ
Lower Arm
Left ØJCH
Right ØJCG
Lower Leg
Left ØJCP
Right ØJCN
Neck
Left ØJC5
Right ØJC4
Pelvic Region ØJCC
Perineum ØJCB
Scalp ØJCØ
Upper Arm
Left ØJCF
Right ØJCD
Upper Leg
Left ØJCM
Right ØJCL
Subdural Space, Intracranial ØØC4
Tarsal
Left ØQCM
Right ØQCL
Tendon
Abdomen
Left ØLCG
Right ØLCF
Ankle
Left ØLCT
Right ØLCS

Extirpation — *continued*
Tendon — *continued*
Foot
Left ØLCW
Right ØLCV
Hand
Left ØLC8
Right ØLC7
Head and Neck ØLCØ
Hip
Left ØLCK
Right ØLCJ
Knee
Left ØLCR
Right ØLCQ
Lower Arm and Wrist
Left ØLC6
Right ØLC5
Lower Leg
Left ØLCP
Right ØLCN
Perineum ØLCH
Shoulder
Left ØLC2
Right ØLC1
Thorax
Left ØLCD
Right ØLCC
Trunk
Left ØLCB
Right ØLC9
Upper Arm
Left ØLC4
Right ØLC3
Upper Leg
Left ØLCM
Right ØLCL
Testis
Bilateral ØVCC
Left ØVCB
Right ØVC9
Thalamus ØØC9
Thymus Ø7CM
Thyroid Gland ØGCK
Left Lobe ØGCG
Right Lobe ØGCH
Tibia
Left ØQCH
Right ØQCG
Toe Nail ØHCRXZZ
Tongue ØCC7
Tonsils ØCCP
Tooth
Lower ØCCX
Upper ØCCW
Trachea ØBC1
Tunica Vaginalis
Left ØVC7
Right ØVC6
Turbinate, Nasal Ø9CL
Tympanic Membrane
Left Ø9C8
Right Ø9C7
Ulna
Left ØPCL
Right ØPCK
Ureter
Left ØTC7
Right ØTC6
Urethra ØTCD
Uterine Supporting Structure ØUC4
Uterus ØUC9
Uvula ØCCN
Vagina ØUCG
Valve
Aortic Ø2CF
Mitral Ø2CG
Pulmonary Ø2CH
Tricuspid Ø2CJ
Vas Deferens
Bilateral ØVCQ
Left ØVCP
Right ØVCN
Vein
Axillary
Left Ø5C8
Right Ø5C7
Azygos Ø5CØ

Index

Extirpation — Extraction

Extirpation — *continued*
- Vein — *continued*
  - Basilic
    - Left 05CC
    - Right 05CB
  - Brachial
    - Left 05CA
    - Right 05C9
  - Cephalic
    - Left 05CF
    - Right 05CD
  - Colic 06C7
  - Common Iliac
    - Left 06CD
    - Right 06CC
  - Coronary 02C4
  - Esophageal 06C3
  - External Iliac
    - Left 06CG
    - Right 06CF
  - External Jugular
    - Left 05CQ
    - Right 05CP
  - Face
    - Left 05CV
    - Right 05CT
  - Femoral
    - Left 06CN
    - Right 06CM
  - Foot
    - Left 06CV
    - Right 06CT
  - Gastric 06C2
  - Hand
    - Left 05CH
    - Right 05CG
  - Hemiazygos 05C1
  - Hepatic 06C4
  - Hypogastric
    - Left 06CJ
    - Right 06CH
  - Inferior Mesenteric 06C6
  - Innominate
    - Left 05C4
    - Right 05C3
  - Internal Jugular
    - Left 05CN
    - Right 05CM
  - Intracranial 05CL
  - Lower 06CY
  - Portal 06C8
  - Pulmonary
    - Left 02CT
    - Right 02CS
  - Renal
    - Left 06CB
    - Right 06C9
  - Saphenous
    - Left 06CQ
    - Right 06CP
  - Splenic 06C1
  - Subclavian
    - Left 05C6
    - Right 05C5
  - Superior Mesenteric 06C5
  - Upper 05CY
  - Vertebral
    - Left 05CS
    - Right 05CR
- Vena Cava
  - Inferior 06C0
  - Superior 02CV
- Ventricle
  - Left 02CL
  - Right 02CK
- Vertebra
  - Cervical 0PC3
  - Lumbar 0QC0
  - Thoracic 0PC4
- Vesicle
  - Bilateral 0VC3
  - Left 0VC2
  - Right 0VC1
- Vitreous
  - Left 08C5
  - Right 08C4
- Vocal Cord
  - Left 0CCV
  - Right 0CCT

Extirpation — *continued*
- Vulva 0UCM

Extracorporeal Carbon Dioxide Removal (ECCO2R)
- 5A0920Z

Extracorporeal shock wave lithotripsy *see* Fragmentation

Extracranial-intracranial bypass (EC-IC) *see* Bypass, Upper Arteries 031

Extraction
- Acetabulum
  - Left 0QD50ZZ
  - Right 0QD40ZZ
- Ampulla of Vater 0FDC
- Anus 0DDQ
- Appendix 0DDJ
- Auditory Ossicle
  - Left 09DA0ZZ
  - Right 09D90ZZ
- Bone
  - Ethmoid
    - Left 0NDG0ZZ
    - Right 0NDF0ZZ
  - Frontal 0ND10ZZ
  - Hyoid 0NDX0ZZ
  - Lacrimal
    - Left 0NDJ0ZZ
    - Right 0NDH0ZZ
  - Nasal 0NDB0ZZ
  - Occipital 0ND70ZZ
  - Palatine
    - Left 0NDL0ZZ
    - Right 0NDK0ZZ
  - Parietal
    - Left 0ND40ZZ
    - Right 0ND30ZZ
  - Pelvic
    - Left 0QD30ZZ
    - Right 0QD20ZZ
  - Sphenoid 0NDC0ZZ
  - Temporal
    - Left 0ND60ZZ
    - Right 0ND50ZZ
  - Zygomatic
    - Left 0NDN0ZZ
    - Right 0NDM0ZZ
- Bone Marrow
  - Iliac 07DR
  - Sternum 07DQ
  - Vertebral 07DS
- Breast
  - Bilateral 0HDV0ZZ
  - Left 0HDU0ZZ
  - Right 0HDT0ZZ
  - Supernumerary 0HDY0ZZ
- Bronchus
  - Lingula 0BD9
  - Lower Lobe
    - Left 0BDB
    - Right 0BD6
  - Main
    - Left 0BD7
    - Right 0BD3
  - Middle Lobe, Right 0BD5
  - Upper Lobe
    - Left 0BD8
    - Right 0BD4
- Bursa and Ligament
  - Abdomen
    - Left 0MDJ
    - Right 0MDH
  - Ankle
    - Left 0MDR
    - Right 0MDQ
  - Elbow
    - Left 0MD4
    - Right 0MD3
  - Foot
    - Left 0MDT
    - Right 0MDS
  - Hand
    - Left 0MD8
    - Right 0MD7
  - Head and Neck 0MD0
  - Hip
    - Left 0MDM
    - Right 0MDL
  - Knee
    - Left 0MDP
    - Right 0MDN

Extraction — *continued*
- Bursa and Ligament — *continued*
  - Lower Extremity
    - Left 0MDW
    - Right 0MDV
  - Perineum 0MDK
  - Rib(s) 0MDG
  - Shoulder
    - Left 0MD2
    - Right 0MD1
  - Spine
    - Lower 0MDD
    - Upper 0MDC
  - Sternum 0MDF
  - Upper Extremity
    - Left 0MDB
    - Right 0MD9
  - Wrist
    - Left 0MD6
    - Right 0MD5
- Carina 0BD2
- Carpal
  - Left 0PDN0ZZ
  - Right 0PDM0ZZ
- Cecum 0DDH
- Cerebral Meninges 00D1
- Cisterna Chyli 07DL
- Clavicle
  - Left 0PDB0ZZ
  - Right 0PD90ZZ
- Coccyx 0QDS0ZZ
- Colon
  - Ascending 0DDK
  - Descending 0DDM
  - Sigmoid 0DDN
  - Transverse 0DDL
- Cornea
  - Left 08D9XZ
  - Right 08D8XZ
- Duct
  - Common Bile 0FD9
  - Cystic 0FD8
  - Hepatic
    - Common 0FD7
    - Left 0FD6
    - Right 0FD5
  - Pancreatic 0FDD
    - Accessory 0FDF
- Duodenum 0DD9
- Dura Mater 00D2
- Endometrium 0UDB
- Esophagogastric Junction 0DD4
- Esophagus 0DD5
  - Lower 0DD3
  - Middle 0DD2
  - Upper 0DD1
- Femoral Shaft
  - Left 0QD90ZZ
  - Right 0QD80ZZ
- Femur
  - Lower
    - Left 0QDC0ZZ
    - Right 0QDB0ZZ
  - Upper
    - Left 0QD70ZZ
    - Right 0QD60ZZ
- Fibula
  - Left 0QDK0ZZ
  - Right 0QDJ0ZZ
- Finger Nail 0HDQXZZ
- Gallbladder 0FD4
- Glenoid Cavity
  - Left 0PD80ZZ
  - Right 0PD70ZZ
- Hair 0HDSXZZ
- Humeral Head
  - Left 0PDD0ZZ
  - Right 0PDC0ZZ
- Humeral Shaft
  - Left 0PDG0ZZ
  - Right 0PDF0ZZ
- Ileocecal Valve 0DDC
- Ileum 0DDB
- Intestine
  - Large 0DDE
    - Left 0DDG
    - Right 0DDF
  - Small 0DD8
- Jejunum 0DDA

Extraction — *continued*

Kidney
- Left 0TD1
- Right 0TD0

Lens
- Left 08DK3ZZ
- Right 08DJ3ZZ

Liver 0FD0
- Left Lobe 0FD2
- Right Lobe 0FD1

Lung
- Bilateral 0BDM
- Left 0BDL
- Lower Lobe
  - Left 0BDJ
  - Right 0BDF
- Middle Lobe, Right 0BDD
- Right 0BDK
- Upper Lobe
  - Left 0BDG
  - Right 0BDC

Lung Lingula 0BDH

Lymphatic
- Aortic 07DD
- Axillary
  - Left 07D6
  - Right 07D5
- Head 07D0
- Inguinal
  - Left 07DJ
  - Right 07DH
- Internal Mammary
  - Left 07D9
  - Right 07D8
- Lower Extremity
  - Left 07DG
  - Right 07DF
- Mesenteric 07DB
- Neck
  - Left 07D2
  - Right 07D1
- Pelvis 07DC
- Thoracic Duct 07DK
- Thorax 07D7
- Upper Extremity
  - Left 07D4
  - Right 07D3

Mandible
- Left 0NDVZZ
- Right 0NDT0ZZ

Maxilla 0NDR0ZZ

Metacarpal
- Left 0PDQ0ZZ
- Right 0PDP0ZZ

Metatarsal
- Left 0QDP0ZZ
- Right 0QDN0ZZ

Muscle
- Abdomen
  - Left 0KDL0ZZ
  - Right 0KDK0ZZ
- Facial 0KD10ZZ
- Foot
  - Left 0KDW0ZZ
  - Right 0KDV0ZZ
- Hand
  - Left 0KDD0ZZ
  - Right 0KDC0ZZ
- Head 0KD00ZZ
- Hip
  - Left 0KDP0ZZ
  - Right 0KDN0ZZ
- Lower Arm and Wrist
  - Left 0KDB0ZZ
  - Right 0KD90ZZ
- Lower Leg
  - Left 0KDT0ZZ
  - Right 0KDS0ZZ
- Neck
  - Left 0KD30ZZ
  - Right 0KD20ZZ
- Perineum 0KDM0ZZ
- Shoulder
  - Left 0KD60ZZ
  - Right 0KD50ZZ
- Thorax
  - Left 0KDJ0ZZ
  - Right 0KDH0ZZ
- Tongue, Palate, Pharynx 0KD40ZZ

Extraction — *continued*

Muscle — *continued*
- Trunk
  - Left 0KDG0ZZ
  - Right 0KDF0ZZ
- Upper Arm
  - Left 0KD80ZZ
  - Right 0KD70ZZ
- Upper Leg
  - Left 0KDR0ZZ
  - Right 0KDQ0ZZ

Nerve
- Abdominal Sympathetic 01DM
- Abducens 00DL
- Accessory 00DR
- Acoustic 00DN
- Brachial Plexus 01D3
- Cervical 01D1
- Cervical Plexus 01D0
- Facial 00DM
- Femoral 01DD
- Glossopharyngeal 00DP
- Head and Neck Sympathetic 01DK
- Hypoglossal 00DS
- Lumbar 01DB
- Lumbar Plexus 01D9
- Lumbar Sympathetic 01DN
- Lumbosacral Plexus 01DA
- Median 01D5
- Oculomotor 00DH
- Olfactory 00DF
- Optic 00DG
- Peroneal 01DH
- Phrenic 01D2
- Pudendal 01DC
- Radial 01D6
- Sacral 01DR
- Sacral Plexus 01DQ
- Sacral Sympathetic 01DP
- Sciatic 01DF
- Thoracic 01D8
- Thoracic Sympathetic 01DL
- Tibial 01DG
- Trigeminal 00DK
- Trochlear 00DJ
- Ulnar 01D4
- Vagus 00DQ

Orbit
- Left 0NDQ0ZZ
- Right 0NDP0ZZ

Ova 0UDN

Pancreas 0FDG

Patella
- Left 0QDF0ZZ
- Right 0QDD0ZZ

Phalanx
- Finger
  - Left 0PDV0ZZ
  - Right 0PDT0ZZ
- Thumb
  - Left 0PDS0ZZ
  - Right 0PDR0ZZ
- Toe
  - Left 0QDR0ZZ
  - Right 0QDQ0ZZ

Pleura
- Left 0BDP
- Right 0BDN

Products of Conception
- Ectopic 10D2
- Extraperitoneal 10D00Z2
- High 10D00Z0
- High Forceps 10D07Z5
- Internal Version 10D07Z7
- Low 10D00Z1
- Low Forceps 10D07Z3
- Mid Forceps 10D07Z4
- Other 10D07Z8
- Retained 10D1
- Vacuum 10D07Z6

Radius
- Left 0PDJ0ZZ
- Right 0PDH0ZZ

Rectum 0DDP

Ribs
- 1 to 2 0PD10ZZ
- 3 or More 0PD20ZZ

Sacrum 0QD10ZZ

Extraction — *continued*

Scapula
- Left 0PD60ZZ
- Right 0PD50ZZ

Septum, Nasal 09DM

Sinus
- Accessory 09DP
- Ethmoid
  - Left 09DV
  - Right 09DU
- Frontal
  - Left 09DT
  - Right 09DS
- Mastoid
  - Left 09DC
  - Right 09DB
- Maxillary
  - Left 09DR
  - Right 09DQ
- Sphenoid
  - Left 09DX
  - Right 09DW

Skin
- Abdomen 0HD7XZZ
- Back 0HD6XZZ
- Buttock 0HD8XZZ
- Chest 0HD5XZZ
- Ear
  - Left 0HD3XZZ
  - Right 0HD2XZZ
- Face 0HD1XZZ
- Foot
  - Left 0HDNXZZ
  - Right 0HDMXZZ
- Hand
  - Left 0HDGXZZ
  - Right 0HDFXZZ
- Inguinal 0HDAXZZ
- Lower Arm
  - Left 0HDEXZZ
  - Right 0HDDXZZ
- Lower Leg
  - Left 0HDLXZZ
  - Right 0HDKXZZ
- Neck 0HD4XZZ
- Perineum 0HD9XZZ
- Scalp 0HD0XZZ
- Upper Arm
  - Left 0HDCXZZ
  - Right 0HDBXZZ
- Upper Leg
  - Left 0HDJXZZ
  - Right 0HDHXZZ

Skull 0ND00ZZ

Spinal Meninges 00DT

Spleen 07DP

Sternum 0PD00ZZ

Stomach 0DD6
- Pylorus 0DD7

Subcutaneous Tissue and Fascia
- Abdomen 0JD8
- Back 0JD7
- Buttock 0JD9
- Chest 0JD6
- Face 0JD1
- Foot
  - Left 0JDR
  - Right 0JDQ
- Hand
  - Left 0JDK
  - Right 0JDJ
- Lower Arm
  - Left 0JDH
  - Right 0JDG
- Lower Leg
  - Left 0JDP
  - Right 0JDN
- Neck
  - Left 0JD5
  - Right 0JD4
- Pelvic Region 0JDC
- Perineum 0JDB
- Scalp 0JD0
- Upper Arm
  - Left 0JDF
  - Right 0JDD
- Upper Leg
  - Left 0JDM
  - Right 0JDL

Extraction — *continued*
Tarsal
Left 0QDM0ZZ
Right 0QDL0ZZ
Tendon
Abdomen
Left 0LDG0ZZ
Right 0LDF0ZZ
Ankle
Left 0LDT0ZZ
Right 0LDS0ZZ
Foot
Left 0LDW0ZZ
Right 0LDV0ZZ
Hand
Left 0LD80ZZ
Right 0LD70ZZ
Head and Neck 0LD00ZZ
Hip
Left 0LDK0ZZ
Right 0LDJ0ZZ
Knee
Left 0LDR0ZZ
Right 0LDQ0ZZ
Lower Arm and Wrist
Left 0LD60ZZ
Right 0LD50ZZ
Lower Leg
Left 0LDP0ZZ
Right 0LDN0ZZ
Perineum 0LDH0ZZ
Shoulder
Left 0LD20ZZ
Right 0LD10ZZ
Thorax
Left 0LDD0ZZ
Right 0LDC0ZZ
Trunk
Left 0LDB0ZZ
Right 0LD90ZZ
Upper Arm
Left 0LD40ZZ
Right 0LD30ZZ
Upper Leg
Left 0LDM0ZZ
Right 0DLL0ZZ
Thymus 07DM
Tibia
Left 0QDH0ZZ
Right 0QDG0ZZ
Toe Nail 0HDRXZZ
Tooth
Lower 0CDXXZ
Upper 0CDWXZ
Trachea 0BD1
Turbinate, Nasal 09DL
Tympanic Membrane
Left 09D8
Right 09D7
Ulna
Left 0PDL0ZZ
Right 0PDK0ZZ
Vein
Basilic
Left 05DC
Right 05DB
Brachial
Left 05DA
Right 05D9
Cephalic
Left 05DF
Right 05DD
Femoral
Left 06DN
Right 06DM
Foot
Left 06DV
Right 06DT
Hand
Left 05DH
Right 05DG
Lower 06DY
Saphenous
Left 06DQ
Right 06DP
Upper 05DY
Vertebra
Cervical 0PD30ZZ
Lumbar 0QD00ZZ

Extraction — *continued*
Vertebra — *continued*
Thoracic 0PD40ZZ
Vocal Cord
Left 0CDV
Right 0CDT
Extradural space, intracranial *use* Epidural Space, Intracranial
Extradural space, spinal *use* Spinal Canal
EXtreme Lateral Interbody Fusion (XLIF) device *use* Interbody Fusion Device in Lower Joints

F

Face lift *see* Alteration, Face 0W02
Facet replacement spinal stabilization device
use Spinal Stabilization Device, Facet Replacement in 0RH
use Spinal Stabilization Device, Facet Replacement in 0SH
Facial artery *use* Face Artery
Factor Xa Inhibitor Reversal Agent, Andexanet Alfa *use* Coagulation Factor Xa, Inactivated
False vocal cord *use* Larynx
Falx cerebri *use* Dura Mater
Fascia lata
use Subcutaneous Tissue and Fascia, Left Upper Leg
use Subcutaneous Tissue and Fascia, Right Upper Leg
Fasciaplasty, fascioplasty
see Repair, Subcutaneous Tissue and Fascia 0JQ
see Replacement, Subcutaneous Tissue and Fascia 0JR
Fasciectomy *see* Excision, Subcutaneous Tissue and Fascia 0JB
Fasciorrhaphy *see* Repair, Subcutaneous Tissue and Fascia 0JQ
Fasciotomy
see Division, Subcutaneous Tissue and Fascia 0J8
see Drainage, Subcutaneous Tissue and Fascia 0J9
see Release
Feeding Device
Change device in
Lower 0D2DXUZ
Upper 0D20XUZ
Insertion of device in
Duodenum 0DH9
Esophagus 0DH5
Ileum 0DHB
Intestine, Small 0DH8
Jejunum 0DHA
Stomach 0DH6
Removal of device from
Esophagus 0DP5
Intestinal Tract
Lower 0DPD
Upper 0DP0
Stomach 0DP6
Revision of device in
Intestinal Tract
Lower 0DWD
Upper 0DW0
Stomach 0DW6
Femoral head
use Upper Femur, Left
use Upper Femur, Right
Femoral lymph node
use Lymphatic, Left Lower Extremity
use Lymphatic, Right Lower Extremity
Femoropatellar joint
use Knee Joint, Left
use Knee Joint, Left, Tibial Surface
use Knee Joint, Right
use Knee Joint, Right, Femoral Surface
Femorotibial joint
use Knee Joint, Left
use Knee Joint, Left, Tibial Surface
use Knee Joint, Right
use Knee Joint, Right, Tibial Surface
FETROJA® *use* Cefiderocol Anti-infective
FGS (fluorescence-guided surgery) *see* Fluorescence Guided Procedure
Fibular artery
use Peroneal Artery, Left
use Peroneal Artery, Right

Fibularis brevis muscle
use Lower Leg Muscle, Left
use Lower Leg Muscle, Right
Fibularis longus muscle
use Lower Leg Muscle, Left
use Lower Leg Muscle, Right
Fifth cranial nerve *use* Trigeminal Nerve
Filum terminale *use* Spinal Meninges
Fimbriectomy
see Excision, Female Reproductive System 0UB
see Resection, Female Reproductive System 0UT
Fine needle aspiration
Fluid or gas *see* Drainage
Tissue biopsy
see Excision
see Extraction
First cranial nerve *use* Olfactory Nerve
First intercostal nerve *use* Brachial Plexus
Fistulization
see Bypass
see Drainage
see Repair
Fitting
Arch bars, for fracture reduction *see* Reposition, Mouth and Throat 0CS
Arch bars, for immobilization *see* Immobilization, Face 2W31
Artificial limb *see* Device Fitting, Rehabilitation F0D
Hearing aid *see* Device Fitting, Rehabilitation F0D
Ocular prosthesis F0DZ8UZ
Prosthesis, limb *see* Device Fitting, Rehabilitation F0D
Prosthesis, ocular F0DZ8UZ
Fixation, bone
External, with fracture reduction *see* Reposition
External, without fracture reduction *see* Insertion
Internal, with fracture reduction *see* Reposition
Internal, without fracture reduction *see* Insertion
FLAIR® Endovascular Stent Graft *use* Intraluminal Device
Flexible Composite Mesh *use* Synthetic Substitute
Flexor carpi radialis muscle
use Lower Arm and Wrist Muscle, Left
use Lower Arm and Wrist Muscle, Right
Flexor carpi ulnaris muscle
use Lower Arm and Wrist Muscle, Left
use Lower Arm and Wrist Muscle, Right
Flexor digitorum brevis muscle
use Foot Muscle, Left
use Foot Muscle, Right
Flexor digitorum longus muscle
use Lower Leg Muscle, Left
use Lower Leg Muscle, Right
Flexor hallucis brevis muscle
use Foot Muscle, Left
use Foot Muscle, Right
Flexor hallucis longus muscle
use Lower Leg Muscle, Left
use Lower Leg Muscle, Right
Flexor pollicis longus muscle
use Lower Arm and Wrist Muscle, Left
use Lower Arm and Wrist Muscle, Right
Flow Diverter embolization device *use* Intraluminal Device, Flow Diverter in 03V
Fluorescence Guided Procedure
Extremity
Lower 8E0Y
Upper 8E0X
Head and Neck Region 8E09
Aminolevulinic Acid 8E090EM
No Qualifier 8E090EZ
Trunk Region 8E0W
Fluorescent Pyrazine, Kidney XT25XE5
Fluoroscopy
Abdomen and Pelvis BW11
Airway, Upper BB1DZZZ
Ankle
Left BQ1H
Right BQ1G
Aorta
Abdominal B410
Laser, Intraoperative B410
Thoracic B310
Laser, Intraoperative B310
Thoraco-Abdominal B31P
Laser, Intraoperative B31P

Subterms under main terms may continue to next column or page

Fluoroscopy — *continued*
Aorta and Bilateral Lower Extremity Arteries B41D
  Laser, Intraoperative B41D
Arm
  Left BP1FZZZ
  Right BP1EZZZ
Artery
  Brachiocephalic-Subclavian
    Laser, Intraoperative B311
    Right B311
  Bronchial B31L
    Laser, Intraoperative B31L
  Bypass Graft, Other B21F
  Cervico-Cerebral Arch B31Q
    Laser, Intraoperative B31Q
  Common Carotid
    Bilateral B315
      Laser, Intraoperative B315
    Left B314
      Laser, Intraoperative B314
    Right B313
      Laser, Intraoperative B313
  Coronary
    Bypass Graft
      Multiple B213
        Laser, Intraoperative B213
      Single B212
        Laser, Intraoperative B212
    Multiple B211
      Laser, Intraoperative B211
    Single B210
      Laser, Intraoperative B210
  External Carotid
    Bilateral B31C
      Laser, Intraoperative B31C
    Left B31B
      Laser, Intraoperative B31B
    Right B319
      Laser, Intraoperative B319
  Hepatic B412
    Laser, Intraoperative B412
  Inferior Mesenteric B415
    Laser, Intraoperative B415
  Intercostal B31L
    Laser, Intraoperative B31L
  Internal Carotid
    Bilateral B318
      Laser, Intraoperative B318
    Left B317
      Laser, Intraoperative B317
    Right B316
      Laser, Intraoperative B316
  Internal Mammary Bypass Graft
    Left B218
    Right B217
  Intra-Abdominal
    Laser, Intraoperative B41B
    Other B41B
  Intracranial B31R
    Laser, Intraoperative B31R
  Lower
    Laser, Intraoperative B41J
    Other B41J
  Lower Extremity
    Bilateral and Aorta B41D
      Laser, Intraoperative B41D
    Left B41G
      Laser, Intraoperative B41G
    Right B41F
      Laser, Intraoperative B41F
  Lumbar B419
    Laser, Intraoperative B419
  Pelvic B41C
    Laser, Intraoperative B41C
  Pulmonary
    Left B31T
      Laser, Intraoperative B31T
    Right B31S
      Laser, Intraoperative B31S
  Pulmonary Trunk B31U
    Laser, Intraoperative B31U
  Renal
    Bilateral B418
      Laser, Intraoperative B418
    Left B417
      Laser, Intraoperative B417
    Right B416
      Laser, Intraoperative B416
  Spinal B31M

Fluoroscopy — *continued*
Artery — *continued*
  Spinal — *continued*
    Laser, Intraoperative B31M
  Splenic B413
    Laser, Intraoperative B413
  Subclavian
    Laser, Intraoperative B312
    Left B312
  Superior Mesenteric B414
    Laser, Intraoperative B414
  Upper
    Laser, Intraoperative B31N
    Other B31N
  Upper Extremity
    Bilateral B31K
      Laser, Intraoperative B31K
    Left B31J
      Laser, Intraoperative B31J
    Right B31H
      Laser, Intraoperative B31H
  Vertebral
    Bilateral B31G
      Laser, Intraoperative B31G
    Left B31F
      Laser, Intraoperative B31F
    Right B31D
      Laser, Intraoperative B31D
Bile Duct BF10
  Pancreatic Duct and Gallbladder BF14
Bile Duct and Gallbladder BF13
Biliary Duct BF11
Bladder BT10
  Kidney and Ureter BT14
    Left BT1F
    Right BT1D
Bladder and Urethra BT1B
Bowel, Small BD1
Calcaneus
  Left BQ1KZZZ
  Right BQ1JZZZ
Clavicle
  Left BP15ZZZ
  Right BP14ZZZ
Coccyx BR1F
Colon BD14
Corpora Cavernosa BV10
Dialysis Fistula B51W
Dialysis Shunt B51W
Diaphragm BB16ZZZ
Disc
  Cervical BR11
  Lumbar BR13
  Thoracic BR12
Duodenum BD19
Elbow
  Left BP1H
  Right BP1G
Epiglottis B91G
Esophagus BD11
Extremity
  Lower BW1C
  Upper BW1J
Facet Joint
  Cervical BR14
  Lumbar BR16
  Thoracic BR15
Fallopian Tube
  Bilateral BU12
  Left BU11
  Right BU10
Fallopian Tube and Uterus BU18
Femur
  Left BQ14ZZZ
  Right BQ13ZZZ
Finger
  Left BP1SZZZ
  Right BP1RZZZ
Foot
  Left BQ1MZZZ
  Right BQ1LZZZ
Forearm
  Left BP1KZZZ
  Right BP1JZZZ
Gallbladder BF12
  Bile Duct and Pancreatic Duct BF14
Gallbladder and Bile Duct BF13
Gastrointestinal, Upper BD1

Fluoroscopy — *continued*
Hand
  Left BP1PZZZ
  Right BP1NZZZ
Head and Neck BW19
Heart
  Left B215
  Right B214
  Right and Left B216
Hip
  Left BQ11
  Right BQ10
Humerus
  Left BP1BZZZ
  Right BP1AZZZ
Ileal Diversion Loop BT1C
Ileal Loop, Ureters and Kidney BT1G
Intracranial Sinus B512
Joint
  Acromioclavicular, Bilateral BP13ZZZ
  Finger
    Left BP1D
    Right BP1C
  Foot
    Left BQ1Y
    Right BQ1X
  Hand
    Left BP1D
    Right BP1C
  Lumbosacral BR1B
  Sacroiliac BR1D
  Sternoclavicular
    Bilateral BP12ZZZ
    Left BP11ZZZ
    Right BP10ZZZ
  Temporomandibular
    Bilateral BN19
    Left BN18
    Right BN17
  Thoracolumbar BR18
  Toe
    Left BQ1Y
    Right BQ1X
Kidney
  Bilateral BT13
  Ileal Loop and Ureter BT1G
  Left BT12
  Right BT11
  Ureter and Bladder BT14
    Left BT1F
    Right BT1D
Knee
  Left BQ18
  Right BQ17
Larynx B91J
Leg
  Left BQ1FZZZ
  Right BQ1DZZZ
Lung
  Bilateral BB14ZZZ
  Left BB13ZZZ
  Right BB12ZZZ
Mediastinum BB1CZZZ
Mouth BD1B
Neck and Head BW19
Oropharynx BD1B
Pancreatic Duct BF1
  Gallbladder and Bile Buct BF14
Patella
  Left BQ1WZZZ
  Right BQ1VZZZ
Pelvis BR1C
Pelvis and Abdomen BW11
Pharynix B91G
Ribs
  Left BP1YZZZ
  Right BP1XZZZ
Sacrum BR1F
Scapula
  Left BP17ZZZ
  Right BP16ZZZ
Shoulder
  Left BP19
  Right BP18
Sinus, Intracranial B512
Spinal Cord B01B
Spine
  Cervical BR10
  Lumbar BR19

Fluoroscopy — *continued*
  Spine — *continued*
    Thoracic BR17
    Whole BR1G
  Sternum BR1H
  Stomach BD12
  Toe
    Left BQ1QZZZ
    Right BQ1PZZZ
  Tracheobronchial Tree
    Bilateral BB19YZZ
    Left BB18YZZ
    Right BB17YZZ
  Ureter
    Ileal Loop and Kidney BT1G
    Kidney and Bladder BT14
      Left BT1F
      Right BT1D
    Left BT17
    Right BT16
  Urethra BT15
  Urethra and Bladder BT1B
  Uterus BU16
  Uterus and Fallopian Tube BU18
  Vagina BU19
  Vasa Vasorum BV18
  Vein
    Cerebellar B511
    Cerebral B511
    Epidural B510
    Jugular
      Bilateral B515
      Left B514
      Right B513
    Lower Extremity
      Bilateral B51D
      Left B51C
      Right B51B
    Other B51V
    Pelvic (Iliac)
      Left B51G
      Right B51F
    Pelvic (Iliac) Bilateral B51H
    Portal B51T
    Pulmonary
      Bilateral B51S
      Left B51R
      Right B51Q
    Renal
      Bilateral B51L
      Left B51K
      Right B51J
    Spanchnic B51T
    Subclavian
      Left B517
      Right B516
    Upper Extremity
      Bilateral B51P
      Left B51N
      Right B51M
  Vena Cava
    Inferior B519
    Superior B518
  Wrist
    Left BP1M
    Right BP1L
Fluoroscopy, laser intraoperative
  see Fluoroscopy, Heart B21
  see Fluoroscopy, Lower Arteries B41
  see Fluoroscopy, Upper Arteries B31
Flushing *see* Irrigation
Foley catheter *use* Drainage Device
Fontan completion procedure Stage II *see* Bypass, Vena Cava, Inferior 0610
Foramen magnum *use* Occipital Bone
Foramen of Monro (intraventricular) *use* Cerebral Ventricle
Foreskin *use* Prepuce
Formula™ Balloon-Expandable Renal Stent System *use* Intraluminal Device
Fosfomycin Anti-infective XW0
Fosfomycin injection *use* Fosfomycin Anti-infective
Fossa of Rosenmuller *use* Nasopharynx
Fourth cranial nerve *use* Trochlear Nerve
Fourth ventricle *use* Cerebral Ventricle
Fovea
  use Retina, Left
  use Retina, Right

Fragmentation
  Ampulla of Vater 0FFC
  Anus 0DFQ
  Appendix 0DFJ
  Artery
    Anterior Tibial
      Left 04FQ3Z
      Right 04FP3Z
    Axillary
      Left 03F63Z
      Right 03F53Z
    Brachial
      Left 03F83Z
      Right 03F73Z
    Common Iliac
      Left 04FD3Z
      Right 04FC3Z
    External Iliac
      Left 04FJ3Z
      Right 04FH3Z
    Femoral
      Left 04FL3Z
      Right 04FK3Z
    Innominate 03F23Z
    Internal Iliac
      Left 04FF3Z
      Right 04FE3Z
    Lower 04FY3Z
    Peroneal
      Left 04FU3Z
      Right 04FT3Z
    Popliteal
      Left 04FN3Z
      Right 04FM3Z
    Posterior Tibial
      Left 04FS3Z
      Right 04FR3Z
    Pulmonary
      Left 02FR3Z
      Right 02FQ3Z
    Pulmonary Trunk 02FP3Z
    Radial
      Left 03FC3Z
      Right 03FB3Z
    Subclavian
      Left 03F43Z
      Right 03F33Z
    Ulnar
      Left 03FA3Z
      Right 03F93Z
    Upper 03FY3Z
  Bladder 0TFB
  Bladder Neck 0TFC
  Bronchus
    Lingula 0BF9
    Lower Lobe
      Left 0BFB
      Right 0BF6
    Main
      Left 0BF7
      Right 0BF3
    Middle Lobe, Right 0BF5
    Upper Lobe
      Left 0BF8
      Right 0BF4
  Carina 0BF2
  Cavity, Cranial 0WF1
  Cecum 0DFH
  Cerebral Ventricle 00F6
  Colon
    Ascending 0DFK
    Descending 0DFM
    Sigmoid 0DFN
    Transverse 0DFL
  Duct
    Common Bile 0FF9
    Cystic 0FF8
    Hepatic
      Common 0FF7
      Left 0FF6
      Right 0FF5
    Pancreatic 0FFD
      Accessory 0FFF
    Parotid
      Left 0CFC
      Right 0CFB
  Duodenum 0DF9
  Epidural Space, Intracranial 00F3
  Esophagus 0DF5

Fragmentation — *continued*
  Fallopian Tube
    Left 0UF6
    Right 0UF5
  Fallopian Tubes, Bilateral 0UF7
  Gallbladder 0FF4
  Gastrointestinal Tract 0WFP
  Genitourinary Tract 0WFR
  Ileum 0DFB
  Intestine
    Large 0DFE
      Left 0DFG
      Right 0DFF
    Small 0DF8
  Jejunum 0DFA
  Kidney Pelvis
    Left 0TF4
    Right 0TF3
  Mediastinum 0WFC
  Oral Cavity and Throat 0WF3
  Pelvic Cavity 0WFJ
  Pericardial Cavity 0WFD
  Pericardium 02FN
  Peritoneal Cavity 0WFG
  Pleural Cavity
    Left 0WFB
    Right 0WF9
  Rectum 0DFP
  Respiratory Tract 0WFQ
  Spinal Canal 00FU
  Stomach 0DF6
  Subarachnoid Space, Intracranial 00F5
  Subdural Space, Intracranial 00F4
  Trachea 0BF1
  Ureter
    Left 0TF7
    Right 0TF6
  Urethra 0TFD
  Uterus 0UF9
  Vein
    Axillary
      Left 05F83Z
      Right 05F73Z
    Basilic
      Left 05FC3Z
      Right 05FB3Z
    Brachial
      Left 05FA3Z
      Right 05F93Z
    Cephalic
      Left 05FF3Z
      Right 05FD3Z
    Common Iliac
      Left 06FD3Z
      Right 06FC3Z
    External Iliac
      Left 06FG3Z
      Right 06FF3Z
    Femoral
      Left 06FN3Z
      Right 06FM3Z
    Hypogastric
      Left 06FJ3Z
      Right 06FH3Z
    Innominate
      Left 05F43Z
      Right 05F33Z
    Lower 06FY3Z
    Pulmonary
      Left 02FT3Z
      Right 02FS3Z
    Saphenous
      Left 06FQ3Z
      Right 06FP3Z
    Subclavian
      Left 05F63Z
      Right 05F53Z
    Upper 05FY3Z
  Vitreous
    Left 08F5
    Right 08F4
Fragmentation, Ultrasonic *see* Fragmentation, Artery
Freestyle (Stentless) Aortic Root Bioprosthesis *use* Zooplastic Tissue in Heart and Great Vessels
Frenectomy
  see Excision, Mouth and Throat 0CB
  see Resection, Mouth and Throat 0CT

Frenoplasty, frenuloplasty
   see Repair, Mouth and Throat 0CQ
   see Replacement, Mouth and Throat 0CR
   see Supplement, Mouth and Throat 0CU
Frenotomy
   see Drainage, Mouth and Throat 0C9
   see Release, Mouth and Throat 0CN
Frenulotomy
   see Drainage, Mouth and Throat 0C9
   see Release, Mouth and Throat 0CN
Frenulum labii inferioris *use* Lower Lip
Frenulum labii superioris *use* Upper Lip
Frenulum linguae *use* Tongue
Frenulumectomy
   see Excision, Mouth and Throat 0CB
   see Resection, Mouth and Throat 0CT
Frontal lobe *use* Cerebral Hemisphere
Frontal vein
   use Face Vein, Left
   use Face Vein, Right
Fulguration *see* Destruction
Fundoplication, gastroesophageal *see* Restriction,
   Esophagogastric Junction 0DV4
Fundus uteri *use* Uterus
Fusion
   Acromioclavicular
      Left 0RGH
      Right 0RGG
   Ankle
      Left 0SGG
      Right 0SGF
   Carpal
      Left 0RGR
      Right 0RGQ
   Carpometacarpal
      Left 0RGT
      Right 0RGS
   Cervical Vertebral 0RG1
      2 or more 0RG2
         Interbody Fusion Device
            Nanotextured Surface XRG2092
            Radiolucent Porous XRG20F3
      Interbody Fusion Device
         Nanotextured Surface XRG1092
         Radiolucent Porous XRG10F3
   Cervicothoracic Vertebral 0RG4
      Interbody Fusion Device
         Nanotextured Surface XRG4092
         Radiolucent Porous XRG40F3
   Coccygeal 0SG6
   Elbow
      Left 0RGM
      Right 0RGL
   Finger Phalangeal
      Left 0RGX
      Right 0RGW
   Hip
      Left 0SGB
      Right 0SG9
   Knee
      Left 0SGD
      Right 0SGC
   Lumbar Vertebral 0SG0
      2 or more 0SG1
         Interbody Fusion Device
            Nanotextured Surface XRGC092
            Radiolucent Porous XRGC0F3
      Interbody Fusion Device
         Nanotextured Surface XRGB092
         Radiolucent Porous XRGB0F3
   Lumbosacral 0SG3
      Interbody Fusion Device
         Nanotextured Surface XRGD092
         Radiolucent Porous XRGD0F3
   Metacarpophalangeal
      Left 0RGV
      Right 0RGU
   Metatarsal-Phalangeal
      Left 0SGN
      Right 0SGM
   Occipital-cervical 0RG0
      Interbody Fusion Device
         Nanotextured Surface XRG0092
         Radiolucent Porous XRG00F3
   Sacrococcygeal 0SG5
   Sacroiliac
      Left 0SG8
      Right 0SG7

Fusion — *continued*
   Shoulder
      Left 0RGK
      Right 0RGJ
   Sternoclavicular
      Left 0RGF
      Right 0RGE
   Tarsal
      Left 0SGJ
      Right 0SGH
   Tarsometatarsal
      Left 0SGL
      Right 0SGK
   Temporomandibular
      Left 0RGD
      Right 0RGC
   Thoracic Vertebral 0RG6
      2 to 7 0RG7
         Interbody Fusion Device
            Nanotextured Surface XRG7092
            Radiolucent Porous XRG70F3
      8 or more 0RG8
         Interbody Fusion Device
            Nanotextured Surface XRG8092
            Radiolucent Porous XRG80F3
      Interbody Fusion Device
         Nanotextured Surface XRG6092
         Radiolucent Porous XRG60F3
   Thoracolumbar Vertebral 0RGA
      Interbody Fusion Device
         Nanotextured Surface XRGA092
         Radiolucent Porous XRGA0F3
   Toe Phalangeal
      Left 0SGQ
      Right 0SGP
   Wrist
      Left 0RGP
      Right 0RGN
Fusion screw (compression) (lag) (locking)
   use Internal Fixation Device in Lower Joints
   use Internal Fixation Device in Upper Joints

G

Gait training *see* Motor Treatment, Rehabilitation F07
Galea aponeurotica *use* Subcutaneous Tissue and
   Fascia, Scalp
GammaTile™ *use* Radioactive Element, Cesium-131
   Collagen Implant in 00H
Ganglion impar (ganglion of Walther) *use* Sacral
   Sympathetic Nerve
Ganglionectomy
   Destruction of lesion *see* Destruction
   Excision of lesion *see* Excision
Gasserian ganglion *use* Trigeminal Nerve
Gastrectomy
   Partial *see* Excision, Stomach 0DB6
   Total *see* Resection, Stomach 0DT6
   Vertical (sleeve) *see* Excision, Stomach 0DB6
Gastric electrical stimulation (GES) lead *use* Stimu-
   lator Lead in Gastrointestinal System
Gastric lymph node *use* Lymphatic, Aortic
Gastric pacemaker lead *use* Stimulator Lead in Gas-
   trointestinal System
Gastric plexus *use* Abdominal Sympathetic Nerve
Gastrocnemius muscle
   use Lower Leg Muscle, Left
   use Lower Leg Muscle, Right
Gastrocolic ligament *use* Omentum
Gastrocolic omentum *use* Omentum
Gastrocolostomy
   see Bypass, Gastrointestinal System 0D1
   see Drainage, Gastrointestinal System 0D9
Gastroduodenal artery *use* Hepatic Artery
Gastroduodenectomy
   see Excision, Gastrointestinal System 0DB
   see Resection, Gastrointestinal System 0DT
Gastroduodenoscopy 0DJ08ZZ
Gastroenteroplasty
   see Repair, Gastrointestinal System 0DQ
   see Supplement, Gastrointestinal System 0DU
Gastroenterostomy
   see Bypass, Gastrointestinal System 0D1
   see Drainage, Gastrointestinal System 0D9
Gastroesophageal (GE) junction *use* Esophagogastric
   Junction

Gastrogastrostomy
   see Bypass, Stomach 0D16
   see Drainage, Stomach 0D96
Gastrohepatic omentum *use* Omentum
Gastrojejunostomy
   see Bypass, Stomach 0D16
   see Drainage, Stomach 0D96
Gastrolysis *see* Release, Stomach 0DN6
Gastropexy
   see Repair, Stomach 0DQ6
   see Reposition, Stomach 0DS6
Gastrophrenic ligament *use* Omentum
Gastroplasty
   see Repair, Stomach 0DQ6
   see Supplement, Stomach 0DU6
Gastroplication *see* Restriction, Stomach 0DV6
Gastropylorectomy *see* Excision, Gastrointestinal
   System 0DB
Gastrorrhaphy *see* Repair, Stomach 0DQ6
Gastroscopy 0DJ68ZZ
Gastrosplenic ligament *use* Omentum
Gastrostomy
   see Bypass, Stomach 0D16
   see Drainage, Stomach 0D96
Gastrotomy *see* Drainage, Stomach 0D96
Gemellus muscle
   use Hip Muscle, Left
   use Hip Muscle, Right
Geniculate ganglion *use* Facial Nerve
Geniculate nucleus *use* Thalamus
Genioglossus muscle *use* Tongue, Palate, Pharynx
   Muscle
Genioplasty *see* Alteration, Jaw, Lower 0W05
Genitofemoral nerve *use* Lumbar Plexus
GIAPREZA™ *use* Synthetic Human Angiotensin II
Gilteritinib Antineoplastic XW0DXV5
Gingivectomy *see* Excision, Mouth and Throat 0CB
Gingivoplasty
   see Repair, Mouth and Throat 0CQ
   see Replacement, Mouth and Throat 0CR
   see Supplement, Mouth and Throat 0CU
Glans penis *use* Prepuce
Glenohumeral joint
   use Shoulder Joint, Left
   use Shoulder Joint, Right
Glenohumeral ligament
   use Shoulder Bursa and Ligament, Left
   use Shoulder Bursa and Ligament, Right
Glenoid fossa (of scapula)
   use Glenoid Cavity, Left
   use Glenoid Cavity, Right
Glenoid ligament (labrum)
   use Shoulder Joint, Left
   use Shoulder Joint, Right
Globus pallidus *use* Basal Ganglia
Glomectomy
   see Excision, Endocrine System 0GB
   see Resection, Endocrine System 0GT
Glossectomy
   see Excision, Tongue 0CB7
   see Resection, Tongue 0CT7
Glossoepiglottic fold *use* Epiglottis
Glossopexy
   see Repair, Tongue 0CQ7
   see Reposition, Tongue 0CS7
Glossoplasty
   see Repair, Tongue 0CQ7
   see Replacement, Tongue 0CR7
   see Supplement, Tongue 0CU7
Glossorrhaphy *see* Repair, Tongue 0CQ7
Glossotomy *see* Drainage, Tongue 0C97
Glottis *use* Larynx
Gluteal Artery Perforator Flap
   Replacement
      Bilateral 0HRV079
      Left 0HRU079
      Right 0HRT079
   Transfer
      Left 0KXG
      Right 0KXF
Gluteal lymph node *use* Lymphatic, Pelvis
Gluteal vein
   use Hypogastric Vein, Left
   use Hypogastric Vein, Right
Gluteus maximus muscle
   use Hip Muscle, Left

Gluteus maximus muscle — *continued*
   use Hip Muscle, Right
Gluteus medius muscle
   use Hip Muscle, Left
   use Hip Muscle, Right
Gluteus minimus muscle
   use Hip Muscle, Left
   use Hip Muscle, Right
GORE EXCLUDER® AAA Endoprosthesis
   use Intraluminal Device
   use Intraluminal Device, Branched or Fenestrated,
     One or Two Arteries in 04V
   use Intraluminal Device, Branched or Fenestrated,
     Three or More Arteries in 04V
GORE EXCLUDER® IBE Endoprosthesis *use* Intraluminal Device, Branched or Fenestrated, One or Two
   Arteries in 04V
GORE TAG® Thoracic Endoprosthesis *use* Intraluminal Device
GORE® DUALMESH® *use* Synthetic Substitute
Gracilis muscle
   use Upper Leg Muscle, Left
   use Upper Leg Muscle, Right
Graft
   see Replacement
   see Supplement
Great auricular nerve *use* Cervical Plexus
Great cerebral vein *use* Intracranial Vein
Great(er) saphenous vein
   use Saphenous Vein, Left
   use Saphenous Vein, Right
Greater alar cartilage *use* Nasal Mucosa and Soft Tis-
   sue
Greater occipital nerve *use* Cervical Nerve
Greater Omentum *use* Omentum
Greater splanchnic nerve *use* Thoracic Sympathetic
   Nerve
Greater superficial petrosal nerve *use* Facial Nerve
Greater trochanter
   use Upper Femur, Left
   use Upper Femur, Right
Greater tuberosity
   use Humeral Head, Left
   use Humeral Head, Right
Greater vestibular (Bartholin's) gland *use* Vestibular
   Gland
Greater wing *use* Sphenoid Bone
Guedel airway *use* Intraluminal Device, Airway in
   Mouth and Throat
Guidance, catheter placement
   EKG *see* Measurement, Physiological Systems 4A0
   Fluoroscopy *see* Fluoroscopy, Veins B51
   Ultrasound *see* Ultrasonography, Veins B54

H

Hallux
   use 1st Toe, Left
   use 1st Toe, Right
Hamate bone
   use Carpal, Left
   use Carpal, Right
Hancock Bioprosthesis (aortic) (mitral) valve *use*
   Zooplastic Tissue in Heart and Great Vessels
Hancock Bioprosthetic Valved Conduit *use*
   Zooplastic Tissue in Heart and Great Vessels
Harvesting, stem cells *see* Pheresis, Circulatory 6A55
Head of fibula
   use Fibula, Left
   use Fibula, Right
Hearing Aid Assessment F14Z
Hearing Assessment F13Z
Hearing Device
   Bone Conduction
     Left 09HE
     Right 09HD
   Insertion of device in
     Left 0NH6
     Right 0NH5
   Multiple Channel Cochlear Prosthesis
     Left 09HE
     Right 09HD
   Removal of device from, Skull 0NP0
   Revision of device in, Skull 0NW0
   Single Channel Cochlear Prosthesis
     Left 09HE

Hearing Device — *continued*
   Single Channel Cochlear Prosthesis — *continued*
     Right 09HD
Hearing Treatment F09Z
Heart Assist System
   Implantable
     Insertion of device in, Heart 02HA
     Removal of device from, Heart 02PA
     Revision of device in, Heart 02WA
   Short-term External
     Insertion of device in, Heart 02HA
     Removal of device from, Heart 02PA
     Revision of device in, Heart 02WA
HeartMate 3™ LVAS *use* Implantable Heart Assist
   System in Heart and Great Vessels
HeartMate II® Left Ventricular Assist Device (LVAD)
   use Implantable Heart Assist System in Heart and
   Great Vessels
HeartMate XVE® Left Ventricular Assist Device
   (LVAD) *use* Implantable Heart Assist System in
   Heart and Great Vessels
HeartMate® implantable heart assist system *see*
   Insertion of device in, Heart 02HA
Helix
   use Ear, External, Bilateral
   use Ear, External, Left
   use Ear, External, Right
Hematopoietic cell transplant (HCT) *see* Transfusion,
   Circulatory 302
Hemicolectomy *see* Resection, Gastrointestinal System
   0DT
Hemicystectomy *see* Excision, Urinary System 0TB
Hemigastrectomy *see* Excision, Gastrointestinal System 0DB
Hemiglossectomy *see* Excision, Mouth and Throat 0CB
Hemilaminectomy
   see Excision, Lower Bones 0QB
   see Excision, Upper Bones 0PB
Hemilaminotomy
   see Drainage, Lower Bones 0Q9
   see Drainage, Upper Bones 0P9
   see Excision, Lower Bones 0QB
   see Excision, Upper Bones 0PB
   see Release, Central Nervous System and Cranial
     Nerves 00N
   see Release, Lower Bones 0QN
   see Release, Peripheral Nervous System 01N
   see Release, Upper Bones 0PN
Hemilaryngectomy *see* Excision, Larynx 0CBS
Hemimandibulectomy *see* Excision, Head and Facial
   Bones 0NB
Hemimaxillectomy *see* Excision, Head and Facial Bones
   0NB
Hemipylorectomy *see* Excision, Gastrointestinal System 0DB
Hemispherectomy
   see Excision, Central Nervous System and Cranial
     Nerves 00B
   see Resection, Central Nervous System and Cranial
     Nerves 00T
Hemithyroidectomy
   see Excision, Endocrine System 0GB
   see Resection, Endocrine System 0GT
Hemodialysis *see* Performance, Urinary 5A1D
Hemolung® Respiratory Assist System (RAS)
   5A0920Z
Hemospray® Endoscopic Hemostat *use* Mineral-
   based Topical Hemostatic Agent
Hepatectomy
   see Excision, Hepatobiliary System and Pancreas
     0FB
   see Resection, Hepatobiliary System and Pancreas
     0FT
Hepatic artery proper *use* Hepatic Artery
Hepatic flexure *use* Transverse Colon
Hepatic lymph node *use* Lymphatic, Aortic
Hepatic plexus *use* Abdominal Sympathetic Nerve
Hepatic portal vein *use* Portal Vein
Hepaticoduodenostomy
   see Bypass, Hepatobiliary System and Pancreas
     0F1
   see Drainage, Hepatobiliary System and Pancreas
     0F9
Hepaticotomy *see* Drainage, Hepatobiliary System and
   Pancreas 0F9
Hepatocholedochostomy *see* Drainage, Duct, Com-
   mon Bile 0F99

Hepatogastric ligament *use* Omentum
Hepatopancreatic ampulla *use* Ampulla of Vater
Hepatopexy
   see Repair, Hepatobiliary System and Pancreas 0FQ
   see Reposition, Hepatobiliary System and Pancreas
     0FS
Hepatorrhaphy *see* Repair, Hepatobiliary System and
   Pancreas 0FQ
Hepatotomy *see* Drainage, Hepatobiliary System and
   Pancreas 0F9
Herculink (RX) Elite Renal Stent System *use* Intralu-
   minal Device
Herniorrhaphy
   see Repair, Anatomical Regions, General 0WQ
   see Repair, Anatomical Regions, Lower Extremities
     0YQ
   With synthetic substitute
     see Supplement, Anatomical Regions, Gener-
       al 0WU
     see Supplement, Anatomical Regions, Lower
       Extremities 0YU
Hip (joint) liner *use* Liner in Lower Joints
HIPEC (hyperthermic intraperitoneal chemother-
   apy) 3E0M30Y
Holter monitoring 4A12X45
Holter valve ventricular shunt *use* Synthetic Substi-
   tute
Human angiotensin II, synthetic *use* Synthetic Hu-
   man Angiotensin II
Humeroradial joint
   use Elbow Joint, Left
   use Elbow Joint, Right
Humeroulnar joint
   use Elbow Joint, Left
   use Elbow Joint, Right
Humerus, distal
   use Humeral Shaft, Left
   use Humeral Shaft, Right
Hydrocelectomy *see* Excision, Male Reproductive System 0VB
Hydrotherapy
   Assisted exercise in pool *see* Motor Treatment,
     Rehabilitation F07
   Whirlpool *see* Activities of Daily Living Treatment,
     Rehabilitation F08
Hymenectomy
   see Excision, Hymen 0UBK
   see Resection, Hymen 0UTK
Hymenoplasty
   see Repair, Hymen 0UQK
   see Supplement, Hymen 0UUK
Hymenorrhaphy *see* Repair, Hymen 0UQK
Hymenotomy
   see Division, Hymen 0U8K
   see Drainage, Hymen 0U9K
Hyoglossus muscle *use* Tongue, Palate, Pharynx
   Muscle
Hyoid artery
   use Thyroid Artery, Left
   use Thyroid Artery, Right
Hyperalimentation *see* Introduction of substance in
   or on
Hyperbaric oxygenation
   Decompression sickness treatment *see* Decompres-
     sion, Circulatory 6A15
   Wound treatment *see* Assistance, Circulatory 5A05
Hyperthermia
   Radiation Therapy
     Abdomen DWY38ZZ
     Adrenal Gland DGY28ZZ
     Bile Ducts DFY28ZZ
     Bladder DTY28ZZ
     Bone Marrow D7Y08ZZ
     Bone, Other DPYC8ZZ
     Brain D0Y08ZZ
     Brain Stem D0Y18ZZ
     Breast
       Left DMY08ZZ
       Right DMY18ZZ
     Bronchus DBY18ZZ
     Cervix DUY18ZZ
     Chest DWY28ZZ
     Chest Wall DBY78ZZ
     Colon DDY58ZZ
     Diaphragm DBY88ZZ
     Duodenum DDY28ZZ
     Ear D9Y08ZZ

Hyperthermia — continued
Radiation Therapy — continued
   Esophagus DDY08ZZ
   Eye D8Y08ZZ
   Femur DPY98ZZ
   Fibula DPYB8ZZ
   Gallbladder DFY18ZZ
   Gland
      Adrenal DGY28ZZ
      Parathyroid DGY48ZZ
      Pituitary DGY08ZZ
      Thyroid DGY58ZZ
   Glands, Salivary D9Y68ZZ
   Head and Neck DWY18ZZ
   Hemibody DWY48ZZ
   Humerus DPY68ZZ
   Hypopharynx D9Y38ZZ
   Ileum DDY48ZZ
   Jejunum DDY38ZZ
   Kidney DTY08ZZ
   Larynx D9YB8ZZ
   Liver DFY08ZZ
   Lung DBY28ZZ
   Lymphatics
      Abdomen D7Y68ZZ
      Axillary D7Y48ZZ
      Inguinal D7Y88ZZ
      Neck D7Y38ZZ
      Pelvis D7Y78ZZ
      Thorax D7Y58ZZ
   Mandible DPY38ZZ
   Maxilla DPY28ZZ
   Mediastinum DBY68ZZ
   Mouth D9Y48ZZ
   Nasopharynx D9YD8ZZ
   Neck and Head DWY18ZZ
   Nerve, Peripheral D0Y78ZZ
   Nose D9Y18ZZ
   Oropharynx D9YF8ZZ
   Ovary DUY08ZZ
   Palate
      Hard D9Y88ZZ
      Soft D9Y98ZZ
   Pancreas DFY38ZZ
   Parathyroid Gland DGY48ZZ
   Pelvic Bones DPY88ZZ
   Pelvic Region DWY68ZZ
   Pineal Body DGY18ZZ
   Pituitary Gland DGY08ZZ
   Pleura DBY58ZZ
   Prostate DVY08ZZ
   Radius DPY78ZZ
   Rectum DDY78ZZ
   Rib DPY58ZZ
   Sinuses D9Y78ZZ
   Skin
      Abdomen DHY88ZZ
      Arm DHY48ZZ
      Back DHY78ZZ
      Buttock DHY98ZZ
      Chest DHY68ZZ
      Face DHY28ZZ
      Leg DHYB8ZZ
      Neck DHY38ZZ
   Skull DPY08ZZ
   Spinal Cord D0Y68ZZ
   Spleen D7Y28ZZ
   Sternum DPY48ZZ
   Stomach DDY18ZZ
   Testis DVY18ZZ
   Thymus D7Y18ZZ
   Thyroid Gland DGY58ZZ
   Tibia DPYB8ZZ
   Tongue D9Y58ZZ
   Trachea DBY08ZZ
   Ulna DPY78ZZ
   Ureter DTY18ZZ
   Urethra DTY38ZZ
   Uterus DUY28ZZ
   Whole Body DWY58ZZ
  Whole Body 6A3Z
Hyperthermic intraperitoneal chemotherapy (HIPEC) 3E0M30Y
Hypnosis GZFZZZZ
Hypogastric artery
  use Internal Iliac Artery, Left
  use Internal Iliac Artery, Right
Hypopharynx *use* Pharynx

Hypophysectomy
  see Excision, Gland, Pituitary 0GB0
  see Resection, Gland, Pituitary 0GT0
Hypophysis *use* Pituitary Gland
Hypothalamotomy *see* Destruction, Thalamus 0059
Hypothenar muscle
  use Hand Muscle, Left
  use Hand Muscle, Right
Hypothermia, Whole Body 6A4Z
Hysterectomy
  Supracervical *see* Resection, Uterus 0UT9
  Total *see* Resection, Uterus 0UT9
Hysterolysis *see* Release, Uterus 0UN9
Hysteropexy
  see Repair, Uterus 0UQ9
  see Reposition, Uterus 0US9
Hysteroplasty *see* Repair, Uterus 0UQ9
Hysterorrhaphy *see* Repair, Uterus 0UQ9
Hysteroscopy 0UJD8ZZ
Hysterotomy *see* Drainage, Uterus 0U99
Hysterotrachelectomy
  see Resection, Cervix 0UTC
  see Resection, Uterus 0UT9
Hysterotracheloplasty *see* Repair, Uterus 0UQ9
Hysterotrachelorrhaphy *see* Repair, Uterus 0UQ9

I

IABP (Intra-aortic balloon pump) *see* Assistance, Cardiac 5A02
IAEMT (Intraoperative anesthetic effect monitoring and titration) *see* Monitoring, Central Nervous 4A10
IASD® (InterAtrial Shunt Device), Corvia *use* Synthetic Substitute
Idarucizumab, Dabigatran Reversal Agent XW0
IHD (Intermittent hemodialysis) 5A1D70Z
Ileal artery *use* Superior Mesenteric Artery
Ileectomy
  see Excision, Ileum 0DBB
  see Resection, Ileum 0DTB
Ileocolic artery *use* Superior Mesenteric Artery
Ileocolic vein *use* Colic Vein
Ileopexy
  see Repair, Ileum 0DQB
  see Reposition, Ileum 0DSB
Ileorrhaphy *see* Repair, Ileum 0DQB
Ileoscopy 0DJD8ZZ
Ileostomy
  see Bypass, Ileum 0D1B
  see Drainage, Ileum 0D9B
Ileotomy *see* Drainage, Ileum 0D9B
Ileoureterostomy *see* Bypass, Urinary System 0T1
Iliac crest
  use Pelvic Bone, Left
  use Pelvic Bone, Right
Iliac fascia
  use Subcutaneous Tissue and Fascia, Left Upper Leg
  use Subcutaneous Tissue and Fascia, Right Upper Leg
Iliac lymph node *use* Lymphatic, Pelvis
Iliacus muscle
  use Hip Muscle, Left
  use Hip Muscle, Right
Iliofemoral ligament
  use Hip Bursa and Ligament, Left
  use Hip Bursa and Ligament, Right
Iliohypogastric nerve *use* Lumbar Plexus
Ilioinguinal nerve *use* Lumbar Plexus
Iliolumbar artery
  use Internal Iliac Artery, Left
  use Internal Iliac Artery, Right
Iliolumbar ligament *use* Lower Spine Bursa and Ligament
Iliotibial tract (band)
  use Subcutaneous Tissue and Fascia, Left Upper Leg
  use Subcutaneous Tissue and Fascia, Right Upper Leg
Ilium
  use Pelvic Bone, Left
  use Pelvic Bone, Right
Ilizarov external fixator
  use External Fixation Device, Ring in 0PH
  use External Fixation Device, Ring in 0PS

Ilizarov external fixator — continued
  use External Fixation Device, Ring in 0QH
  use External Fixation Device, Ring in 0QS
Ilizarov-Vecklich device
  use External Fixation Device, Limb Lengthening in 0PH
  use External Fixation Device, Limb Lengthening in 0QH
Imaging, diagnostic
  see Computerized Tomography (CT Scan)
  see Fluoroscopy
  see Magnetic Resonance Imaging (MRI)
  see Plain Radiography
  see Ultrasonography
IMFINZI® *use* Durvalumab Antineoplastic
Imipenem-cilastatin-relebactam Anti-infective XW0
IMI/REL *use* Imipenem-cilastatin-relebactam Anti-infective
Immobilization
  Abdominal Wall 2W33X
  Arm
    Lower
      Left 2W3DX
      Right 2W3CX
    Upper
      Left 2W3BX
      Right 2W3AX
  Back 2W35X
  Chest Wall 2W34X
  Extremity
    Lower
      Left 2W3MX
      Right 2W3LX
    Upper
      Left 2W39X
      Right 2W38X
  Face 2W31X
  Finger
    Left 2W3KX
    Right 2W3JX
  Foot
    Left 2W3TX
    Right 2W3SX
  Hand
    Left 2W3FX
    Right 2W3EX
  Head 2W30X
  Inguinal Region
    Left 2W37X
    Right 2W36X
  Leg
    Lower
      Left 2W3RX
      Right 2W3QX
    Upper
      Left 2W3PX
      Right 2W3NX
  Neck 2W32X
  Thumb
    Left 2W3HX
    Right 2W3GX
  Toe
    Left 2W3VX
    Right 2W3UX
Immunization *see* Introduction of Serum, Toxoid, and Vaccine
Immunotherapy *see* Introduction of Immunotherapeutic Substance
Immunotherapy, antineoplastic
  Interferon *see* Introduction of Low-dose Interleukin-2
  Interleukin-2, high-dose *see* Introduction of High-dose Interleukin-2
  Interleukin-2, low-dose *see* Introduction of Low-dose Interleukin-2
  Monoclonal antibody *see* Introduction of Monoclonal Antibody
  Proleukin, high-dose *see* Introduction of High-dose Interleukin-2
  Proleukin, low-dose *see* Introduction of Low-dose Interleukin-2
Impella® heart pump *use* Short-term External Heart Assist System in Heart and Great Vessels
Impeller Pump
  Continuous, Output 5A0221D
  Intermittent, Output 5A0211D

Implantable cardioverter-defibrillator (ICD) *use* Defibrillator Generator in 0JH
Implantable drug infusion pump (anti-spasmodic) (chemotherapy) (pain) *use* Infusion Device, Pump in Subcutaneous Tissue and Fascia
Implantable glucose monitoring device *use* Monitoring Device
Implantable hemodynamic monitor (IHM) *use* Monitoring Device, Hemodynamic in 0JH
Implantable hemodynamic monitoring system (IHMS) *use* Monitoring Device, Hemodynamic in 0JH
Implantable Miniature Telescope™ (IMT) *use* Synthetic Substitute, Intraocular Telescope in 08R
Implantation
　see Insertion
　see Replacement
Implanted (venous)(access) port *use* Vascular Access Device, Totally Implantable in Subcutaneous Tissue and Fascia
IMV (intermittent mandatory ventilation) *see* Assistance, Respiratory 5A09
In Vitro Fertilization 8E0ZXY1
Incision, abscess *see* Drainage
Incudectomy
　see Excision, Ear, Nose, Sinus 09B
　see Resection, Ear, Nose, Sinus 09T
Incudopexy
　see Repair, Ear, Nose, Sinus 09Q
　see Reposition, Ear, Nose, Sinus 09S
Incus
　use Auditory Ossicle, Left
　use Auditory Ossicle, Right
Induction of labor
　Artificial rupture of membranes *see* Drainage, Pregnancy 109
　Oxytocin *see* Introduction of Hormone
InDura, intrathecal catheter (1P) (spinal) *use* Infusion Device
Inferior cardiac nerve *use* Thoracic Sympathetic Nerve
Inferior cerebellar vein *use* Intracranial Vein
Inferior cerebral vein *use* Intracranial Vein
Inferior epigastric artery
　use External Iliac Artery, Left
　use External Iliac Artery, Right
Inferior epigastric lymph node *use* Lymphatic, Pelvis
Inferior genicular artery
　use Popliteal Artery, Left
　use Popliteal Artery, Right
Inferior gluteal artery
　use Internal Iliac Artery, Left
　use Internal Iliac Artery, Right
Inferior gluteal nerve *use* Sacral Plexus
Inferior hypogastric plexus *use* Abdominal Sympathetic Nerve
Inferior labial artery *use* Face Artery
Inferior longitudinal muscle *use* Tongue, Palate, Pharynx Muscle
Inferior mesenteric ganglion *use* Abdominal Sympathetic Nerve
Inferior mesenteric lymph node *use* Lymphatic, Mesenteric
Inferior mesenteric plexus *use* Abdominal Sympathetic Nerve
Inferior oblique muscle
　use Extraocular Muscle, Left
　use Extraocular Muscle, Right
Inferior pancreaticoduodenal artery *use* Superior Mesenteric Artery
Inferior phrenic artery *use* Abdominal Aorta
Inferior rectus muscle
　use Extraocular Muscle, Left
　use Extraocular Muscle, Right
Inferior suprarenal artery
　use Renal Artery, Left
　use Renal Artery, Right
Inferior tarsal plate
　use Lower Eyelid, Left
　use Lower Eyelid, Right
Inferior thyroid vein
　use Innominate Vein, Left
　use Innominate Vein, Right
Inferior tibiofibular joint
　use Ankle Joint, Left
　use Ankle Joint, Right
Inferior turbinate *use* Nasal Turbinate

Inferior ulnar collateral artery
　use Brachial Artery, Left
　use Brachial Artery, Right
Inferior vesical artery
　use Internal Iliac Artery, Left
　use Internal Iliac Artery, Right
Infraauricular lymph node *use* Lymphatic, Head
Infraclavicular (deltopectoral) lymph node
　use Lymphatic, Left Upper Extremity
　use Lymphatic, Right Upper Extremity
Infrahyoid muscle
　use Neck Muscle, Left
　use Neck Muscle, Right
Infraparotid lymph node *use* Lymphatic, Head
Infraspinatus fascia
　use Subcutaneous Tissue and Fascia, Left Upper Arm
　use Subcutaneous Tissue and Fascia, Right Upper Arm
Infraspinatus muscle
　use Shoulder Muscle, Left
　use Shoulder Muscle, Right
Infundibulopelvic ligament *use* Uterine Supporting Structure
Infusion *see* Introduction of substance in or on
Infusion Device, Pump
　Insertion of device in
　　Abdomen 0JH8
　　Back 0JH7
　　Chest 0JH6
　　Lower Arm
　　　Left 0JHH
　　　Right 0JHG
　　Lower Leg
　　　Left 0JHP
　　　Right 0JHN
　　Trunk 0JHT
　　Upper Arm
　　　Left 0JHF
　　　Right 0JHD
　　Upper Leg
　　　Left 0JHM
　　　Right 0JHL
　Removal of device from
　　Lower Extremity 0JPW
　　Trunk 0JPT
　　Upper Extremity 0JPV
　Revision of device in
　　Lower Extremity 0JWW
　　Trunk 0JWT
　　Upper Extremity 0JWV
Infusion, glucarpidase
　Central Vein 3E043GQ
　Peripheral Vein 3E033GQ
Inguinal canal
　use Inguinal Region, Bilateral
　use Inguinal Region, Left
　use Inguinal Region, Right
Inguinal triangle
　use Inguinal Region, Bilateral
　use Inguinal Region, Left
　use Inguinal Region, Right
Injection *see* Introduction of substance in or on
Injection, Concentrated Bone Marrow Aspirate (CBMA), intramuscular XK02303
Injection reservoir, port *use* Vascular Access Device, Totally Implantable in Subcutaneous Tissue and Fascia
Injection reservoir, pump *use* Infusion Device, Pump in Subcutaneous Tissue and Fascia
Insemination, artificial 3E0P7LZ
Insertion
　Antimicrobial envelope *see* Introduction of Anti-infective
　Aqueous drainage shunt
　　see Bypass, Eye 081
　　see Drainage, Eye 089
　Products of Conception 10H0
　Spinal Stabilization Device
　　see Insertion of device in, Lower Joints 0SH
　　see Insertion of device in, Upper Joints 0RH
Insertion of device in
　Abdominal Wall 0WHF
　Acetabulum
　　Left 0QH5
　　Right 0QH4
　Anal Sphincter 0DHR

Insertion of device in — *continued*
　Ankle Region
　　Left 0YHL
　　Right 0YHK
　Anus 0DHQ
　Aorta
　　Abdominal 04H0
　　Thoracic
　　　Ascending/Arch 02HX
　　　Descending 02HW
　Arm
　　Lower
　　　Left 0XHF
　　　Right 0XHD
　　Upper
　　　Left 0XH9
　　　Right 0XH8
　Artery
　　Anterior Tibial
　　　Left 04HQ
　　　Right 04HP
　　Axillary
　　　Left 03H6
　　　Right 03H5
　　Brachial
　　　Left 03H8
　　　Right 03H7
　　Celiac 04H1
　　Colic
　　　Left 04H7
　　　Middle 04H8
　　　Right 04H6
　　Common Carotid
　　　Left 03HJ
　　　Right 03HH
　　Common Iliac
　　　Left 04HD
　　　Right 04HC
　　Coronary
　　　Four or More Arteries 02H3
　　　One Artery 02H0
　　　Three Arteries 02H2
　　　Two Arteries 02H1
　　External Carotid
　　　Left 03HN
　　　Right 03HM
　　External Iliac
　　　Left 04HJ
　　　Right 04HH
　　Face 03HR
　　Femoral
　　　Left 04HL
　　　Right 04HK
　　Foot
　　　Left 04HW
　　　Right 04HV
　　Gastric 04H2
　　Hand
　　　Left 03HF
　　　Right 03HD
　　Hepatic 04H3
　　Inferior Mesenteric 04HB
　　Innominate 03H2
　　Internal Carotid
　　　Left 03HL
　　　Right 03HK
　　Internal Iliac
　　　Left 04HF
　　　Right 04HE
　　Internal Mammary
　　　Left 03H1
　　　Right 03H0
　　Intracranial 03HG
　　Lower 04HY
　　Peroneal
　　　Left 04HU
　　　Right 04HT
　　Popliteal
　　　Left 04HN
　　　Right 04HM
　　Posterior Tibial
　　　Left 04HS
　　　Right 04HR
　　Pulmonary
　　　Left 02HR
　　　Right 02HQ
　　Pulmonary Trunk 02HP
　　Radial
　　　Left 03HC

Insertion of device in — continued
  Artery — continued
    Radial — continued
      Right 03HB
    Renal
      Left 04HA
      Right 04H9
    Splenic 04H4
    Subclavian
      Left 03H4
      Right 03H3
    Superior Mesenteric 04H5
    Temporal
      Left 03HT
      Right 03HS
    Thyroid
      Left 03HV
      Right 03HU
    Ulnar
      Left 03HA
      Right 03H9
    Upper 03HY
    Vertebral
      Left 03HQ
      Right 03HP
  Atrium
    Left 02H7
    Right 02H6
  Axilla
    Left 0XH5
    Right 0XH4
  Back
    Lower 0WHL
    Upper 0WHK
  Bladder 0THB
  Bladder Neck 0THC
  Bone
    Ethmoid
      Left 0NHG
      Right 0NHF
    Facial 0NHW
    Frontal 0NH1
    Hyoid 0NHX
    Lacrimal
      Left 0NHJ
      Right 0NHH
    Lower 0QHY
    Nasal 0NHB
    Occipital 0NH7
    Palatine
      Left 0NHL
      Right 0NHK
    Parietal
      Left 0NH4
      Right 0NH3
    Pelvic
      Left 0QH3
      Right 0QH2
    Sphenoid 0NHC
    Temporal
      Left 0NH6
      Right 0NH5
    Upper 0PHY
    Zygomatic
      Left 0NHN
      Right 0NHM
  Bone Marrow 07HT
  Brain 00H0
  Breast
    Bilateral 0HHV
    Left 0HHU
    Right 0HHT
  Bronchus
    Lingula 0BH9
    Lower Lobe
      Left 0BHB
      Right 0BH6
    Main
      Left 0BH7
      Right 0BH3
    Middle Lobe, Right 0BH5
    Upper Lobe
      Left 0BH8
      Right 0BH4
  Bursa and Ligament
    Lower 0MHY
    Upper 0MHX
  Buttock
    Left 0YH1

Insertion of device in — continued
  Buttock — continued
    Right 0YH0
  Carpal
    Left 0PHN
    Right 0PHM
  Cavity, Cranial 0WH1
  Cerebral Ventricle 00H6
  Cervix 0UHC
  Chest Wall 0WH8
  Cisterna Chyli 07HL
  Clavicle
    Left 0PHB
    Right 0PH9
  Coccyx 0QHS
  Cul-de-sac 0UHF
  Diaphragm 0BHT
  Disc
    Cervical Vertebral 0RH3
    Cervicothoracic Vertebral 0RH5
    Lumbar Vertebral 0SH2
    Lumbosacral 0SH4
    Thoracic Vertebral 0RH9
    Thoracolumbar Vertebral 0RHB
  Duct
    Hepatobiliary 0FHB
    Pancreatic 0FHD
  Duodenum 0DH9
  Ear
    Inner
      Left 09HE
      Right 09HD
    Left 09HJ
    Right 09HH
  Elbow Region
    Left 0XHC
    Right 0XHB
  Epididymis and Spermatic Cord 0VHM
  Esophagus 0DH5
  Extremity
    Lower
      Left 0YHB
      Right 0YH9
    Upper
      Left 0XH7
      Right 0XH6
  Eye
    Left 08H1
    Right 08H0
  Face 0WH2
  Fallopian Tube 0UH8
  Femoral Region
    Left 0YH8
    Right 0YH7
  Femoral Shaft
    Left 0QH9
    Right 0QH8
  Femur
    Lower
      Left 0QHC
      Right 0QHB
    Upper
      Left 0QH7
      Right 0QH6
  Fibula
    Left 0QHK
    Right 0QHJ
  Foot
    Left 0YHN
    Right 0YHM
  Gallbladder 0FH4
  Gastrointestinal Tract 0WHP
  Genitourinary Tract 0WHR
  Gland
    Endocrine 0GHS
    Salivary 0CHA
  Glenoid Cavity
    Left 0PH8
    Right 0PH7
  Hand
    Left 0XHK
    Right 0XHJ
  Head 0WH0
  Heart 02HA
  Humeral Head
    Left 0PHD
    Right 0PHC
  Humeral Shaft
    Left 0PHG

Insertion of device in — continued
  Humeral Shaft — continued
    Right 0PHF
  Ileum 0DHB
  Inguinal Region
    Left 0YH6
    Right 0YH5
  Intestinal Tract
    Lower 0DHD
    Upper 0DH0
  Intestine
    Large 0DHE
    Small 0DH8
  Jaw
    Lower 0WH5
    Upper 0WH4
  Jejunum 0DHA
  Joint
    Acromioclavicular
      Left 0RHH
      Right 0RHG
    Ankle
      Left 0SHG
      Right 0SHF
    Carpal
      Left 0RHR
      Right 0RHQ
    Carpometacarpal
      Left 0RHT
      Right 0RHS
    Cervical Vertebral 0RH1
    Cervicothoracic Vertebral 0RH4
    Coccygeal 0SH6
    Elbow
      Left 0RHM
      Right 0RHL
    Finger Phalangeal
      Left 0RHX
      Right 0RHW
    Hip
      Left 0SHB
      Right 0SH9
    Knee
      Left 0SHD
      Right 0SHC
    Lumbar Vertebral 0SH0
    Lumbosacral 0SH3
    Metacarpophalangeal
      Left 0RHV
      Right 0RHU
    Metatarsal-Phalangeal
      Left 0SHN
      Right 0SHM
    Occipital-cervical 0RH0
    Sacrococcygeal 0SH5
    Sacroiliac
      Left 0SH8
      Right 0SH7
    Shoulder
      Left 0RHK
      Right 0RHJ
    Sternoclavicular
      Left 0RHF
      Right 0RHE
    Tarsal
      Left 0SHJ
      Right 0SHH
    Tarsometatarsal
      Left 0SHL
      Right 0SHK
    Temporomandibular
      Left 0RHD
      Right 0RHC
    Thoracic Vertebral 0RH6
    Thoracolumbar Vertebral 0RHA
    Toe Phalangeal
      Left 0SHQ
      Right 0SHP
    Wrist
      Left 0RHP
      Right 0RHN
  Kidney 0TH5
  Knee Region
    Left 0YHG
    Right 0YHF
  Larynx 0CHS
  Leg
    Lower
      Left 0YHJ

Insertion of device in — *continued*
Leg — *continued*
 Lower — *continued*
  Right ØYHH
 Upper
  Left ØYHD
  Right ØYHC
Liver ØFHØ
 Left Lobe ØFH2
 Right Lobe ØFH1
Lung
 Left ØBHL
 Right ØBHK
Lymphatic Ø7HN
 Thoracic Duct Ø7HK
Mandible
 Left ØNHV
 Right ØNHT
Maxilla ØNHR
Mediastinum ØWHC
Metacarpal
 Left ØPHQ
 Right ØPHP
Metatarsal
 Left ØQHP
 Right ØQHN
Mouth and Throat ØCHY
Muscle
 Lower ØKHY
 Upper ØKHX
Nasal Mucosa and Soft Tissue Ø9HK
Nasopharynx Ø9HN
Neck ØWH6
Nerve
 Cranial ØØHE
 Peripheral Ø1HY
Nipple
 Left ØHHX
 Right ØHHW
Oral Cavity and Throat ØWH3
Orbit
 Left ØNHQ
 Right ØNHP
Ovary ØUH3
Pancreas ØFHG
Patella
 Left ØQHF
 Right ØQHD
Pelvic Cavity ØWHJ
Penis ØVHS
Pericardial Cavity ØWHD
Pericardium Ø2HN
Perineum
 Female ØWHN
 Male ØWHM
Peritoneal Cavity ØWHG
Phalanx
 Finger
  Left ØPHV
  Right ØPHT
 Thumb
  Left ØPHS
  Right ØPHR
 Toe
  Left ØQHR
  Right ØQHQ
Pleura ØBHQ
Pleural Cavity
 Left ØWHB
 Right ØWH9
Prostate ØVHØ
Prostate and Seminal Vesicles ØVH4
Radius
 Left ØPHJ
 Right ØPHH
Rectum ØDHP
Respiratory Tract ØWHQ
Retroperitoneum ØWHH
Ribs
 1 to 2 ØPH1
 3 or More ØPH2
Sacrum ØQH1
Scapula
 Left ØPH6
 Right ØPH5
Scrotum and Tunica Vaginalis ØVH8
Shoulder Region
 Left ØXH3
 Right ØXH2

Insertion of device in — *continued*
Sinus Ø9HY
Skin ØHHPXYZ
Skull ØNHØ
Spinal Canal ØØHU
Spinal Cord ØØHV
Spleen Ø7HP
Sternum ØPHØ
Stomach ØDH6
Subcutaneous Tissue and Fascia
 Abdomen ØJH8
 Back ØJH7
 Buttock ØJH9
 Chest ØJH6
 Face ØJH1
 Foot
  Left ØJHR
  Right ØJHQ
 Hand
  Left ØJHK
  Right ØJHJ
 Head and Neck ØJHS
 Lower Arm
  Left ØJHH
  Right ØJHG
 Lower Extremity ØJHW
 Lower Leg
  Left ØJHP
  Right ØJHN
 Neck
  Left ØJH5
  Right ØJH4
 Pelvic Region ØJHC
 Perineum ØJHB
 Scalp ØJHØ
 Trunk ØJHT
 Upper Arm
  Left ØJHF
  Right ØJHD
 Upper Extremity ØJHV
 Upper Leg
  Left ØJHM
  Right ØJHL
Tarsal
 Left ØQHM
 Right ØQHL
Tendon
 Lower ØLHY
 Upper ØLHX
Testis ØVHD
Thymus Ø7HM
Tibia
 Left ØQHH
 Right ØQHG
Tongue ØCH7
Trachea ØBH1
Tracheobronchial Tree ØBHØ
Ulna
 Left ØPHL
 Right ØPHK
Ureter ØTH9
Urethra ØTHD
Uterus ØUH9
Uterus and Cervix ØUHD
Vagina ØUHG
Vagina and Cul-de-sac ØUHH
Vas Deferens ØVHR
Vein
 Axillary
  Left Ø5H8
  Right Ø5H7
 Azygos Ø5HØ
 Basilic
  Left Ø5HC
  Right Ø5HB
 Brachial
  Left Ø5HA
  Right Ø5H9
 Cephalic
  Left Ø5HF
  Right Ø5HD
 Colic Ø6H7
 Common Iliac
  Left Ø6HD
  Right Ø6HC
 Coronary Ø2H4
 Esophageal Ø6H3
 External Iliac
  Left Ø6HG

Insertion of device in — *continued*
Vein — *continued*
 External Iliac — *continued*
  Right Ø6HF
 External Jugular
  Left Ø5HQ
  Right Ø5HP
 Face
  Left Ø5HV
  Right Ø5HT
 Femoral
  Left Ø6HN
  Right Ø6HM
 Foot
  Left Ø6HV
  Right Ø6HT
 Gastric Ø6H2
 Hand
  Left Ø5HH
  Right Ø5HG
 Hemiazygos Ø5H1
 Hepatic Ø6H4
 Hypogastric
  Left Ø6HJ
  Right Ø6HH
 Inferior Mesenteric Ø6H6
 Innominate
  Left Ø5H4
  Right Ø5H3
 Internal Jugular
  Left Ø5HN
  Right Ø5HM
 Intracranial Ø5HL
 Lower Ø6HY
 Portal Ø6H8
 Pulmonary
  Left Ø2HT
  Right Ø2HS
 Renal
  Left Ø6HB
  Right Ø6H9
 Saphenous
  Left Ø6HQ
  Right Ø6HP
 Splenic Ø6H1
 Subclavian
  Left Ø5H6
  Right Ø5H5
 Superior Mesenteric Ø6H5
 Upper Ø5HY
 Vertebral
  Left Ø5HS
  Right Ø5HR
Vena Cava
 Inferior Ø6HØ
 Superior Ø2HV
Ventricle
 Left Ø2HL
 Right Ø2HK
Vertebra
 Cervical ØPH3
 Lumbar ØQHØ
 Thoracic ØPH4
Wrist Region
 Left ØXHH
 Right ØXHG
Inspection
Abdominal Wall ØWJF
Ankle Region
 Left ØYJL
 Right ØYJK
Arm
 Lower
  Left ØXJF
  Right ØXJD
 Upper
  Left ØXJ9
  Right ØXJ8
Artery
 Lower Ø4JY
 Upper Ø3JY
Axilla
 Left ØXJ5
 Right ØXJ4
Back
 Lower ØWJL
 Upper ØWJK
Bladder ØTJB

Inspection — *continued*
- Bone
  - Facial ØNJW
  - Lower ØQJY
  - Nasal ØNJB
  - Upper ØPJY
- Bone Marrow Ø7JT
- Brain ØØJØ
- Breast
  - Left ØHJU
  - Right ØHJT
- Bursa and Ligament
  - Lower ØMJY
  - Upper ØMJX
- Buttock
  - Left ØYJ1
  - Right ØYJØ
- Cavity, Cranial ØWJ1
- Chest Wall ØWJ8
- Cisterna Chyli Ø7JL
- Diaphragm ØBJT
- Disc
  - Cervical Vertebral ØRJ3
  - Cervicothoracic Vertebral ØRJ5
  - Lumbar Vertebral ØSJ2
  - Lumbosacral ØSJ4
  - Thoracic Vertebral ØRJ9
  - Thoracolumbar Vertebral ØRJB
- Duct
  - Hepatobiliary ØFJB
  - Pancreatic ØFJD
- Ear
  - Inner
    - Left Ø9JE
    - Right Ø9JD
  - Left Ø9JJ
  - Right Ø9JH
- Elbow Region
  - Left ØXJC
  - Right ØXJB
- Epididymis and Spermatic Cord ØVJM
- Extremity
  - Lower
    - Left ØYJB
    - Right ØYJ9
  - Upper
    - Left ØXJ7
    - Right ØXJ6
- Eye
  - Left Ø8J1XZZ
  - Right Ø8JØXZZ
- Face ØWJ2
- Fallopian Tube ØUJ8
- Femoral Region
  - Bilateral ØYJE
  - Left ØYJ8
  - Right ØYJ7
- Finger Nail ØHJQXZZ
- Foot
  - Left ØYJN
  - Right ØYJM
- Gallbladder ØFJ4
- Gastrointestinal Tract ØWJP
- Genitourinary Tract ØWJR
- Gland
  - Adrenal ØGJ5
  - Endocrine ØGJS
  - Pituitary ØGJØ
  - Salivary ØCJA
- Great Vessel Ø2JY
- Hand
  - Left ØXJK
  - Right ØXJJ
- Head ØWJØ
- Heart Ø2JA
- Inguinal Region
  - Bilateral ØYJA
  - Left ØYJ6
  - Right ØYJ5
- Intestinal Tract
  - Lower ØDJD
  - Upper ØDJØ
- Jaw
  - Lower ØWJ5
  - Upper ØWJ4
- Joint
  - Acromioclavicular
    - Left ØRJH
    - Right ØRJG

Inspection — *continued*
- Joint — *continued*
  - Ankle
    - Left ØSJG
    - Right ØSJF
  - Carpal
    - Left ØRJR
    - Right ØRJQ
  - Carpometacarpal
    - Left ØRJT
    - Right ØRJS
  - Cervical Vertebral ØRJ1
  - Cervicothoracic Vertebral ØRJ4
  - Coccygeal ØSJ6
  - Elbow
    - Left ØRJM
    - Right ØRJL
  - Finger Phalangeal
    - Left ØRJX
    - Right ØRJW
  - Hip
    - Left ØSJB
    - Right ØSJ9
  - Knee
    - Left ØSJD
    - Right ØSJC
  - Lumbar Vertebral ØSJØ
  - Lumbosacral ØSJ3
  - Metacarpophalangeal
    - Left ØRJV
    - Right ØRJU
  - Metatarsal-Phalangeal
    - Left ØSJN
    - Right ØSJM
  - Occipital-cervical ØRJØ
  - Sacrococcygeal ØSJ5
  - Sacroiliac
    - Left ØSJ8
    - Right ØSJ7
  - Shoulder
    - Left ØRJK
    - Right ØRJJ
  - Sternoclavicular
    - Left ØRJF
    - Right ØRJE
  - Tarsal
    - Left ØSJJ
    - Right ØSJH
  - Tarsometatarsal
    - Left ØSJL
    - Right ØSJK
  - Temporomandibular
    - Left ØRJD
    - Right ØRJC
  - Thoracic Vertebral ØRJ6
  - Thoracolumbar Vertebral ØRJA
  - Toe Phalangeal
    - Left ØSJQ
    - Right ØSJP
  - Wrist
    - Left ØRJP
    - Right ØRJN
- Kidney ØTJ5
- Knee Region
  - Left ØYJG
  - Right ØYJF
- Larynx ØCJS
- Leg
  - Lower
    - Left ØYJJ
    - Right ØYJH
  - Upper
    - Left ØYJD
    - Right ØYJC
- Lens
  - Left Ø8JKXZZ
  - Right Ø8JJXZZ
- Liver ØFJØ
- Lung
  - Left ØBJL
  - Right ØBJK
- Lymphatic Ø7JN
  - Thoracic Duct Ø7JK
- Mediastinum ØWJC
- Mesentery ØDJV
- Mouth and Throat ØCJY
- Muscle
  - Extraocular
    - Left Ø8JM

Inspection — *continued*
- Muscle — *continued*
  - Extraocular — *continued*
    - Right Ø8JL
  - Lower ØKJY
  - Upper ØKJX
- Nasal Mucosa and Soft Tissue Ø9JK
- Neck ØWJ6
- Nerve
  - Cranial ØØJE
  - Peripheral Ø1JY
- Omentum ØDJU
- Oral Cavity and Throat ØWJ3
- Ovary ØUJ3
- Pancreas ØFJG
- Parathyroid Gland ØGJR
- Pelvic Cavity ØWJJ
- Penis ØVJS
- Pericardial Cavity ØWJD
- Perineum
  - Female ØWJN
  - Male ØWJM
- Peritoneal Cavity ØWJG
- Peritoneum ØDJW
- Pineal Body ØGJ1
- Pleura ØBJQ
- Pleural Cavity
  - Left ØWJB
  - Right ØWJ9
- Products of Conception 1ØJØ
  - Ectopic 1ØJ2
  - Retained 1ØJ1
- Prostate and Seminal Vesicles ØVJ4
- Respiratory Tract ØWJQ
- Retroperitoneum ØWJH
- Scrotum and Tunica Vaginalis ØVJ8
- Shoulder Region
  - Left ØXJ3
  - Right ØXJ2
- Sinus Ø9JY
- Skin ØHJPXZZ
- Skull ØNJØ
- Spinal Canal ØØJU
- Spinal Cord ØØJV
- Spleen Ø7JP
- Stomach ØDJ6
- Subcutaneous Tissue and Fascia
  - Head and Neck ØJJS
  - Lower Extremity ØJJW
  - Trunk ØJJT
  - Upper Extremity ØJJV
- Tendon
  - Lower ØLJY
  - Upper ØLJX
- Testis ØVJD
- Thymus Ø7JM
- Thyroid Gland ØGJK
- Toe Nail ØHJRXZZ
- Trachea ØBJ1
- Tracheobronchial Tree ØBJØ
- Tympanic Membrane
  - Left Ø9J8
  - Right Ø9J7
- Ureter ØTJ9
- Urethra ØTJD
- Uterus and Cervix ØUJD
- Vagina and Cul-de-sac ØUJH
- Vas Deferens ØVJR
- Vein
  - Lower Ø6JY
  - Upper Ø5JY
- Vulva ØUJM
- Wrist Region
  - Left ØXJH
  - Right ØXJG

Instillation *see* Introduction of substance in or on
Insufflation *see* Introduction of substance in or on
Interatrial septum *use* Atrial Septum
InterAtrial Shunt Device IASD®, Corvia *use* Synthetic Substitute
Interbody fusion (spine) cage
  use Interbody Fusion Device in Lower Joints
  use Interbody Fusion Device in Upper Joints
Interbody Fusion Device
  Nanotextured Surface
    Cervical Vertebral XRG1Ø92
      2 or more XRG2Ø92
    Cervicothoracic Vertebral XRG4Ø92

Interbody Fusion Device — *continued*
  Nanotextured Surface — *continued*
    Lumbar Vertebral XRGB092
      2 or more XRGC092
    Lumbosacral XRGD092
    Occipital-cervical XRGC092
    Thoracic Vertebral XRG6092
      2 to 7 XRG7092
      8 or more XRG8092
    Thoracolumbar Vertebral XRGA092
  Radiolucent Porous
    Cervical Vertebral XRG10F3
      2 or more XRG20F3
    Cervicothoracic Vertebral XRG40F3
    Lumbar Vertebral XRGB0F3
      2 or more XRGC0F3
    Lumbosacral XRGD0F3
    Occipital-cervical XRG00F3
    Thoracic Vertebral XRG60F3
      2 to 7 XRG70F3
      8 or more XRG80F3
    Thoracolumbar Vertebral XRGA0F3
Intercarpal joint
  use Carpal Joint, Left
  use Carpal Joint, Right
Intercarpal ligament
  use Hand Bursa and Ligament, Left
  use Hand Bursa and Ligament, Right
Interclavicular ligament
  use Shoulder Bursa and Ligament, Left
  use Shoulder Bursa and Ligament, Right
Intercostal lymph node *use* Lymphatic, Thorax
Intercostal muscle
  use Thorax Muscle, Left
  use Thorax Muscle, Right
Intercostal nerve *use* Thoracic Nerve
Intercostobrachial nerve *use* Thoracic Nerve
Intercuneiform joint
  use Tarsal Joint, Left
  use Tarsal Joint, Right
Intercuneiform ligament
  use Foot Bursa and Ligament, Left
  use Foot Bursa and Ligament, Right
Intermediate bronchus *use* Main Bronchus, Right
Intermediate cuneiform bone
  use Tarsal, Left
  use Tarsal, Right
Intermittent hemodialysis (IHD) 5A1D70Z
Intermittent mandatory ventilation *see* Assistance, Respiratory 5A09
Intermittent Negative Airway Pressure
  24-96 Consecutive Hours, Ventilation 5A0945B
  Greater than 96 Consecutive Hours, Ventilation 5A0955B
  Less than 24 Consecutive Hours, Ventilation 5A0935B
Intermittent Positive Airway Pressure
  24-96 Consecutive Hours, Ventilation 5A09458
  Greater than 96 Consecutive Hours, Ventilation 5A09558
  Less than 24 Consecutive Hours, Ventilation 5A09358
Intermittent positive pressure breathing *see* Assistance, Respiratory 5A09
Internal anal sphincter *use* Anal Sphincter
Internal carotid artery, intracranial portion *use* Intracranial Artery
Internal carotid plexus *use* Head and Neck Sympathetic Nerve
Internal (basal) cerebral vein *use* Intracranial Vein
Internal iliac vein
  use Hypogastric Vein, Left
  use Hypogastric Vein, Right
Internal maxillary artery
  use External Carotid Artery, Left
  use External Carotid Artery, Right
Internal naris *use* Nasal Mucosa and Soft Tissue
Internal oblique muscle
  use Abdomen Muscle, Left
  use Abdomen Muscle, Right
Internal pudendal artery
  use Internal Iliac Artery, Left
  use Internal Iliac Artery, Right
Internal pudendal vein
  use Hypogastric Vein, Left
  use Hypogastric Vein, Right

Internal thoracic artery
  use Internal Mammary Artery, Left
  use Internal Mammary Artery, Right
  use Subclavian Artery, Left
  use Subclavian Artery, Right
Internal urethral sphincter *use* Urethra
Interphalangeal (IP) joint
  use Finger Phalangeal Joint, Left
  use Finger Phalangeal Joint, Right
  use Toe Phalangeal Joint, Left
  use Toe Phalangeal Joint, Right
Interphalangeal ligament
  use Foot Bursa and Ligament, Left
  use Foot Bursa and Ligament, Right
  use Hand Bursa and Ligament, Left
  use Hand Bursa and Ligament, Right
Interrogation, cardiac rhythm related device
  Interrogation only *see* Measurement, Cardiac 4B02
  With cardiac function testing *see* Measurement, Cardiac 4A02
Interruption *see* Occlusion
Interspinalis muscle
  use Trunk Muscle, Left
  use Trunk Muscle, Right
Interspinous ligament, cervical *use* Head and Neck Bursa and Ligament
Interspinous ligament, lumbar *use* Lower Spine Bursa and Ligament
Interspinous ligament, thoracic *use* Upper Spine Bursa and Ligament
Interspinous process spinal stabilization device
  use Spinal Stabilization Device, Interspinous Process in 0RH
  use Spinal Stabilization Device, Interspinous Process in 0SH
InterStim® Therapy lead *use* Neurostimulator Lead in Peripheral Nervous System
InterStim® Therapy neurostimulator *use* Stimulator Generator, Single Array in 0JH
Intertransversarius muscle
  use Trunk Muscle, Left
  use Trunk Muscle, Right
Intertransverse ligament, cervical *use* Head and Neck Bursa and Ligament
Intertransverse ligament, lumbar *use* Lower Spine Bursa and Ligament
Intertransverse ligament, thoracic *use* Upper Spine Bursa and Ligament
Interventricular foramen (Monro) *use* Cerebral Ventricle
Interventricular septum *use* Ventricular Septum
Intestinal lymphatic trunk *use* Cisterna Chyli
Intraluminal Device
  Airway
    Esophagus 0DH5
    Mouth and Throat 0CHY
    Nasopharynx 09HN
  Bioactive
    Occlusion
      Common Carotid
        Left 03LJ
        Right 03LH
      External Carotid
        Left 03LN
        Right 03LM
      Internal Carotid
        Left 03LL
        Right 03LK
      Intracranial 03LG
      Vertebral
        Left 03LQ
        Right 03LP
    Restriction
      Common Carotid
        Left 03VJ
        Right 03VH
      External Carotid
        Left 03VN
        Right 03VM
      Internal Carotid
        Left 03VL
        Right 03VK
      Intracranial 03VG
      Vertebral
        Left 03VQ
        Right 03VP

Intraluminal Device — *continued*
  Endobronchial Valve
    Lingula 0BH9
    Lower Lobe
      Left 0BHB
      Right 0BH6
    Main
      Left 0BH7
      Right 0BH3
    Middle Lobe, Right 0BH5
    Upper Lobe
      Left 0BH8
      Right 0BH4
  Endotracheal Airway
    Change device in, Trachea 0B21XEZ
    Insertion of device in, Trachea 0BH1
  Pessary
    Change device in, Vagina and Cul-de-sac 0U2HXGZ
    Insertion of device in
      Cul-de-sac 0UHF
      Vagina 0UHG
Intramedullary (IM) rod (nail)
  use Internal Fixation Device, Intramedullary in Lower Bones
  use Internal Fixation Device, Intramedullary in Upper Bones
Intramedullary skeletal kinetic distractor (ISKD)
  use Internal Fixation Device, Intramedullary in Lower Bones
  use Internal Fixation Device, Intramedullary in Upper Bones
Intraocular Telescope
  Left 08RK30Z
  Right 08RJ30Z
Intraoperative Knee Replacement Sensor XR2
Intraoperative Radiation Therapy (IORT)
  Anus DDY8CZZ
  Bile Ducts DFY2CZZ
  Bladder DTY2CZZ
  Brain D0Y0CZZ
  Brain Stem D0Y1CZZ
  Cervix DUY1CZZ
  Colon DDY5CZZ
  Duodenum DDY2CZZ
  Gallbladder DFY1CZZ
  Ileum DDY4CZZ
  Jejunum DDY3CZZ
  Kidney DTY0CZZ
  Larynx D9YBCZZ
  Liver DFY0CZZ
  Mouth D9Y4CZZ
  Nasopharynx D9YDCZZ
  Nerve, Peripheral D0Y7CZZ
  Ovary DUY0CZZ
  Pancreas DFY3CZZ
  Pharynx D9YCCZZ
  Prostate DVY0CZZ
  Rectum DDY7CZZ
  Spinal Cord D0Y6CZZ
  Stomach DDY1CZZ
  Ureter DTY1CZZ
  Urethra DTY3CZZ
  Uterus DUY2CZZ
Intra.OX 8E02XDZ
Intrauterine Device (IUD) *use* Contraceptive Device in Female Reproductive System
Intravascular fluorescence angiography (IFA) *see* Monitoring, Physiological Systems 4A1
Intravascular Lithotripsy (IVL) *see* Fragmentation
Intravascular ultrasound assisted thrombolysis *see* Fragmentation, Artery
Introduction of substance in or on
  Artery
    Central 3E06
      Analgesics 3E06
      Anesthetic, Intracirculatory 3E06
      Antiarrhythmic 3E06
      Anti-infective 3E06
      Anti-inflammatory 3E06
      Antineoplastic 3E06
      Destructive Agent 3E06
      Diagnostic Substance, Other 3E06
      Electrolytic Substance 3E06
      Hormone 3E06
      Hypnotics 3E06
      Immunotherapeutic 3E06
      Nutritional Substance 3E06

Introduction of substance in or on — *continued*
- Artery — *continued*
  - Central — *continued*
    - Platelet Inhibitor 3E06
    - Radioactive Substance 3E06
    - Sedatives 3E06
    - Serum 3E06
    - Thrombolytic 3E06
    - Toxoid 3E06
    - Vaccine 3E06
    - Vasopressor 3E06
    - Water Balance Substance 3E06
  - Coronary 3E07
    - Diagnostic Substance, Other 3E07
    - Platelet Inhibitor 3E07
    - Thrombolytic 3E07
  - Peripheral 3E05
    - Analgesics 3E05
    - Anesthetic, Intracirculatory 3E05
    - Antiarrhythmic 3E05
    - Anti-infective 3E05
    - Anti-inflammatory 3E05
    - Antineoplastic 3E05
    - Destructive Agent 3E05
    - Diagnostic Substance, Other 3E05
    - Electrolytic Substance 3E05
    - Hormone 3E05
    - Hypnotics 3E05
    - Immunotherapeutic 3E05
    - Nutritional Substance 3E05
    - Platelet Inhibitor 3E05
    - Radioactive Substance 3E05
    - Sedatives 3E05
    - Serum 3E05
    - Thrombolytic 3E05
    - Toxoid 3E05
    - Vaccine 3E05
    - Vasopressor 3E05
    - Water Balance Substance 3E05
- Biliary Tract 3E0J
  - Analgesics 3E0J
  - Anesthetic Agent 3E0J
  - Anti-infective 3E0J
  - Anti-inflammatory 3E0J
  - Antineoplastic 3E0J
  - Destructive Agent 3E0J
  - Diagnostic Substance, Other 3E0J
  - Electrolytic Substance 3E0J
  - Gas 3E0J
  - Hypnotics 3E0J
  - Islet Cells, Pancreatic 3E0J
  - Nutritional Substance 3E0J
  - Radioactive Substance 3E0J
  - Sedatives 3E0J
  - Water Balance Substance 3E0J
- Bone 3E0V
  - Analgesics 3E0V3NZ
  - Anesthetic Agent 3E0V3BZ
  - Anti-infective 3E0V32
  - Anti-inflammatory 3E0V33Z
  - Antineoplastic 3E0V30
  - Destructive Agent 3E0V3TZ
  - Diagnostic Substance, Other 3E0V3KZ
  - Electrolytic Substance 3E0V37Z
  - Hypnotics 3E0V3NZ
  - Nutritional Substance 3E0V36Z
  - Radioactive Substance 3E0V3HZ
  - Sedatives 3E0V3NZ
  - Water Balance Substance 3E0V37Z
- Bone Marrow 3E0A3GC
  - Antineoplastic 3E0A30
- Brain 3E0Q
  - Analgesics 3E0Q
  - Anesthetic Agent 3E0Q
  - Anti-infective 3E0Q
  - Anti-inflammatory 3E0Q
  - Antineoplastic 3E0Q
  - Destructive Agent 3E0Q
  - Diagnostic Substance, Other 3E0Q
  - Electrolytic Substance 3E0Q
  - Gas 3E0Q
  - Hypnotics 3E0Q
  - Nutritional Substance 3E0Q
  - Radioactive Substance 3E0Q
  - Sedatives 3E0Q
  - Stem Cells
    - Embryonic 3E0Q
    - Somatic 3E0Q
  - Water Balance Substance 3E0Q

Introduction of substance in or on — *continued*
- Cranial Cavity 3E0Q
  - Analgesics 3E0Q
  - Anesthetic Agent 3E0Q
  - Anti-infective 3E0Q
  - Anti-inflammatory 3E0Q
  - Antineoplastic 3E0Q
  - Destructive Agent 3E0Q
  - Diagnostic Substance, Other 3E0Q
  - Electrolytic Substance 3E0Q
  - Gas 3E0Q
  - Hypnotics 3E0Q
  - Nutritional Substance 3E0Q
  - Radioactive Substance 3E0Q
  - Sedatives 3E0Q
  - Stem Cells
    - Embryonic 3E0Q
    - Somatic 3E0Q
  - Water Balance Substance 3E0Q
- Ear 3E0B
  - Analgesics 3E0B
  - Anesthetic Agent 3E0B
  - Anti-infective 3E0B
  - Anti-inflammatory 3E0B
  - Antineoplastic 3E0B
  - Destructive Agent 3E0B
  - Diagnostic Substance, Other 3E0B
  - Hypnotics 3E0B
  - Radioactive Substance 3E0B
  - Sedatives 3E0B
- Epidural Space 3E0S3GC
  - Analgesics 3E0S3NZ
  - Anesthetic Agent 3E0S3BZ
  - Anti-infective 3E0S32
  - Anti-inflammatory 3E0S33Z
  - Antineoplastic 3E0S30
  - Destructive Agent 3E0S3TZ
  - Diagnostic Substance, Other 3E0S3KZ
  - Electrolytic Substance 3E0S37Z
  - Gas 3E0S
  - Hypnotics 3E0S3NZ
  - Nutritional Substance 3E0S36Z
  - Radioactive Substance 3E0S3HZ
  - Sedatives 3E0S3NZ
  - Water Balance Substance 3E0S37Z
- Eye 3E0C
  - Analgesics 3E0C
  - Anesthetic Agent 3E0C
  - Anti-infective 3E0C
  - Anti-inflammatory 3E0C
  - Antineoplastic 3E0C
  - Destructive Agent 3E0C
  - Diagnostic Substance, Other 3E0C
  - Gas 3E0C
  - Hypnotics 3E0C
  - Pigment 3E0C
  - Radioactive Substance 3E0C
  - Sedatives 3E0C
- Gastrointestinal Tract
  - Lower 3E0H
    - Analgesics 3E0H
    - Anesthetic Agent 3E0H
    - Anti-infective 3E0H
    - Anti-inflammatory 3E0H
    - Antineoplastic 3E0H
    - Destructive Agent 3E0H
    - Diagnostic Substance, Other 3E0H
    - Electrolytic Substance 3E0H
    - Gas 3E0H
    - Hypnotics 3E0H
    - Nutritional Substance 3E0H
    - Radioactive Substance 3E0H
    - Sedatives 3E0H
    - Water Balance Substance 3E0H
  - Upper 3E0G
    - Analgesics 3E0G
    - Anesthetic Agent 3E0G
    - Anti-infective 3E0G
    - Anti-inflammatory 3E0G
    - Antineoplastic 3E0G
    - Destructive Agent 3E0G
    - Diagnostic Substance, Other 3E0G
    - Electrolytic Substance 3E0G
    - Gas 3E0G
    - Hypnotics 3E0G
    - Nutritional Substance 3E0G
    - Radioactive Substance 3E0G
    - Sedatives 3E0G
    - Water Balance Substance 3E0G

Introduction of substance in or on — *continued*
- Genitourinary Tract 3E0K
  - Analgesics 3E0K
  - Anesthetic Agent 3E0K
  - Anti-infective 3E0K
  - Anti-inflammatory 3E0K
  - Antineoplastic 3E0K
  - Destructive Agent 3E0K
  - Diagnostic Substance, Other 3E0K
  - Electrolytic Substance 3E0K
  - Gas 3E0K
  - Hypnotics 3E0K
  - Nutritional Substance 3E0K
  - Radioactive Substance 3E0K
  - Sedatives 3E0K
  - Water Balance Substance 3E0K
- Heart 3E08
  - Diagnostic Substance, Other 3E08
  - Platelet Inhibitor 3E08
  - Thrombolytic 3E08
- Joint 3E0U
  - Analgesics 3E0U3NZ
  - Anesthetic Agent 3E0U3BZ
  - Anti-infective 3E0U
  - Anti-inflammatory 3E0U33Z
  - Antineoplastic 3E0U30
  - Destructive Agent 3E0U3TZ
  - Diagnostic Substance, Other 3E0U3KZ
  - Electrolytic Substance 3E0U37Z
  - Gas 3E0U3SF
  - Hypnotics 3E0U3NZ
  - Nutritional Substance 3E0U36Z
  - Radioactive Substance 3E0U3HZ
  - Sedatives 3E0U3NZ
  - Water Balance Substance 3E0U37Z
- Lymphatic 3E0W3GC
  - Analgesics 3E0W3NZ
  - Anesthetic Agent 3E0W3BZ
  - Anti-infective 3E0W32
  - Anti-inflammatory 3E0W33Z
  - Antineoplastic 3E0W30
  - Destructive Agent 3E0W3TZ
  - Diagnostic Substance, Other 3E0W3KZ
  - Electrolytic Substance 3E0W37Z
  - Hypnotics 3E0W3NZ
  - Nutritional Substance 3E0W36Z
  - Radioactive Substance 3E0W3HZ
  - Sedatives 3E0W3NZ
  - Water Balance Substance 3E0W37Z
- Mouth 3E0D
  - Analgesics 3E0D
  - Anesthetic Agent 3E0D
  - Antiarrhythmic 3E0D
  - Anti-infective 3E0D
  - Anti-inflammatory 3E0D
  - Antineoplastic 3E0D
  - Destructive Agent 3E0D
  - Diagnostic Substance, Other 3E0D
  - Electrolytic Substance 3E0D
  - Hypnotics 3E0D
  - Nutritional Substance 3E0D
  - Radioactive Substance 3E0D
  - Sedatives 3E0D
  - Serum 3E0D
  - Toxoid 3E0D
  - Vaccine 3E0D
  - Water Balance Substance 3E0D
- Mucous Membrane 3E00XGC
  - Analgesics 3E00XNZ
  - Anesthetic Agent 3E00XBZ
  - Anti-infective 3E00X2
  - Anti-inflammatory 3E00X3Z
  - Antineoplastic 3E00X0
  - Destructive Agent 3E00XTZ
  - Diagnostic Substance, Other 3E00XKZ
  - Hypnotics 3E00XNZ
  - Pigment 3E00XMZ
  - Sedatives 3E00XNZ
  - Serum 3E00X4Z
  - Toxoid 3E00X4Z
  - Vaccine 3E00X4Z
- Muscle 3E023GC
  - Analgesics 3E023NZ
  - Anesthetic Agent 3E023BZ
  - Anti-infective 3E0232
  - Anti-inflammatory 3E0233Z
  - Antineoplastic 3E0230
  - Destructive Agent 3E023TZ
  - Diagnostic Substance, Other 3E023KZ

Introduction of substance in or on — *continued*
- Muscle — *continued*
  - Electrolytic Substance 3E0237Z
  - Hypnotics 3E023NZ
  - Nutritional Substance 3E0236Z
  - Radioactive Substance 3E023HZ
  - Sedatives 3E023NZ
  - Serum 3E0234Z
  - Toxoid 3E0234Z
  - Vaccine 3E0234Z
  - Water Balance Substance 3E0237Z
- Nerve
  - Cranial 3E0X3GC
    - Anesthetic Agent 3E0X3BZ
    - Anti-inflammatory 3E0X33Z
    - Destructive Agent 3E0X3TZ
  - Peripheral 3E0T3GC
    - Anesthetic Agent 3E0T3BZ
    - Anti-inflammatory 3E0T33Z
    - Destructive Agent 3E0T3TZ
  - Plexus 3E0T3GC
    - Anesthetic Agent 3E0T3BZ
    - Anti-inflammatory 3E0T33Z
    - Destructive Agent 3E0T3TZ
- Nose 3E09
  - Analgesics 3E09
  - Anesthetic Agent 3E09
  - Anti-infective 3E09
  - Anti-inflammatory 3E09
  - Antineoplastic 3E09
  - Destructive Agent 3E09
  - Diagnostic Substance, Other 3E09
  - Hypnotics 3E09
  - Radioactive Substance 3E09
  - Sedatives 3E09
  - Serum 3E09
  - Toxoid 3E09
  - Vaccine 3E09
- Pancreatic Tract 3E0J
  - Analgesics 3E0J
  - Anesthetic Agent 3E0J
  - Anti-infective 3E0J
  - Anti-inflammatory 3E0J
  - Antineoplastic 3E0J
  - Destructive Agent 3E0J
  - Diagnostic Substance, Other 3E0J
  - Electrolytic Substance 3E0J
  - Gas 3E0J
  - Hypnotics 3E0J
  - Islet Cells, Pancreatic 3E0J
  - Nutritional Substance 3E0J
  - Radioactive Substance 3E0J
  - Sedatives 3E0J
  - Water Balance Substance 3E0J
- Pericardial Cavity 3E0Y
  - Analgesics 3E0Y3NZ
  - Anesthetic Agent 3E0Y3BZ
  - Anti-infective 3E0Y32
  - Anti-inflammatory 3E0Y33Z
  - Antineoplastic 3E0Y
  - Destructive Agent 3E0Y3TZ
  - Diagnostic Substance, Other 3E0Y3KZ
  - Electrolytic Substance 3E0Y37Z
  - Gas 3E0Y
  - Hypnotics 3E0Y3NZ
  - Nutritional Substance 3E0Y36Z
  - Radioactive Substance 3E0Y3HZ
  - Sedatives 3E0Y3NZ
  - Water Balance Substance 3E0Y37Z
- Peritoneal Cavity 3E0M
  - Adhesion Barrier 3E0M
  - Analgesics 3E0M3NZ
  - Anesthetic Agent 3E0M3BZ
  - Anti-infective 3E0M32
  - Anti-inflammatory 3E0M33Z
  - Antineoplastic 3E0M
  - Destructive Agent 3E0M3TZ
  - Diagnostic Substance, Other 3E0M3KZ
  - Electrolytic Substance 3E0M37Z
  - Gas 3E0M
  - Hypnotics 3E0M3NZ
  - Nutritional Substance 3E0M36Z
  - Radioactive Substance 3E0M3HZ
  - Sedatives 3E0M3NZ
  - Water Balance Substance 3E0M37Z
- Pharynx 3E0D
  - Analgesics 3E0D
  - Anesthetic Agent 3E0D
  - Antiarrhythmic 3E0D

Introduction of substance in or on — *continued*
- Pharynx — *continued*
  - Anti-infective 3E0D
  - Anti-inflammatory 3E0D
  - Antineoplastic 3E0D
  - Destructive Agent 3E0D
  - Diagnostic Substance, Other 3E0D
  - Electrolytic Substance 3E0D
  - Hypnotics 3E0D
  - Nutritional Substance 3E0D
  - Radioactive Substance 3E0D
  - Sedatives 3E0D
  - Serum 3E0D
  - Toxoid 3E0D
  - Vaccine 3E0D
  - Water Balance Substance 3E0D
- Pleural Cavity 3E0L
  - Adhesion Barrier 3E0L
  - Analgesics 3E0L3NZ
  - Anesthetic Agent 3E0L3BZ
  - Anti-infective 3E0L32
  - Anti-inflammatory 3E0L33Z
  - Antineoplastic 3E0L
  - Destructive Agent 3E0L3TZ
  - Diagnostic Substance, Other 3E0L3KZ
  - Electrolytic Substance 3E0L37Z
  - Gas 3E0L
  - Hypnotics 3E0L3NZ
  - Nutritional Substance 3E0L36Z
  - Radioactive Substance 3E0L3HZ
  - Sedatives 3E0L3NZ
  - Water Balance Substance 3E0L37Z
- Products of Conception 3E0E
  - Analgesics 3E0E
  - Anesthetic Agent 3E0E
  - Anti-infective 3E0E
  - Anti-inflammatory 3E0E
  - Antineoplastic 3E0E
  - Destructive Agent 3E0E
  - Diagnostic Substance, Other 3E0E
  - Electrolytic Substance 3E0E
  - Gas 3E0E
  - Hypnotics 3E0E
  - Nutritional Substance 3E0E
  - Radioactive Substance 3E0E
  - Sedatives 3E0E
  - Water Balance Substance 3E0E
- Reproductive
  - Female 3E0P
    - Adhesion Barrier 3E0P
    - Analgesics 3E0P
    - Anesthetic Agent 3E0P
    - Anti-infective 3E0P
    - Anti-inflammatory 3E0P
    - Antineoplastic 3E0P
    - Destructive Agent 3E0P
    - Diagnostic Substance, Other 3E0P
    - Electrolytic Substance 3E0P
    - Gas 3E0P
    - Hormone 3E0P
    - Hypnotics 3E0P
    - Nutritional Substance 3E0P
    - Ovum, Fertilized 3E0P
    - Radioactive Substance 3E0P
    - Sedatives 3E0P
    - Sperm 3E0P
    - Water Balance Substance 3E0P
  - Male 3E0N
    - Analgesics 3E0N
    - Anesthetic Agent 3E0N
    - Anti-infective 3E0N
    - Anti-inflammatory 3E0N
    - Antineoplastic 3E0N
    - Destructive Agent 3E0N
    - Diagnostic Substance, Other 3E0N
    - Electrolytic Substance 3E0N
    - Gas 3E0N
    - Hypnotics 3E0N
    - Nutritional Substance 3E0N
    - Radioactive Substance 3E0N
    - Sedatives 3E0N
    - Water Balance Substance 3E0N
- Respiratory Tract 3E0F
  - Analgesics 3E0F
  - Anesthetic Agent 3E0F
  - Anti-infective 3E0F
  - Anti-inflammatory 3E0F
  - Antineoplastic 3E0F
  - Destructive Agent 3E0F

Introduction of substance in or on — *continued*
- Respiratory Tract — *continued*
  - Diagnostic Substance, Other 3E0F
  - Electrolytic Substance 3E0F
  - Gas 3E0F
  - Hypnotics 3E0F
  - Nutritional Substance 3E0F
  - Radioactive Substance 3E0F
  - Sedatives 3E0F
  - Water Balance Substance 3E0F
- Skin 3E00XGC
  - Analgesics 3E00XNZ
  - Anesthetic Agent 3E00XBZ
  - Anti-infective 3E00X2
  - Anti-inflammatory 3E00X3Z
  - Antineoplastic 3E00X0
  - Destructive Agent 3E00XTZ
  - Diagnostic Substance, Other 3E00XKZ
  - Hypnotics 3E00XNZ
  - Pigment 3E00XMZ
  - Sedatives 3E00XNZ
  - Serum 3E00X4Z
  - Toxoid 3E00X4Z
  - Vaccine 3E00X4Z
- Spinal Canal 3E0R3GC
  - Analgesics 3E0R3NZ
  - Anesthetic Agent 3E0R3BZ
  - Anti-infective 3E0R32
  - Anti-inflammatory 3E0R33Z
  - Antineoplastic 3E0R30
  - Destructive Agent 3E0R3TZ
  - Diagnostic Substance, Other 3E0R3KZ
  - Electrolytic Substance 3E0R37Z
  - Gas 3E0R
  - Hypnotics 3E0R3NZ
  - Nutritional Substance 3E0R36Z
  - Radioactive Substance 3E0R3HZ
  - Sedatives 3E0R3NZ
  - Stem Cells
    - Embryonic 3E0R
    - Somatic 3E0R
  - Water Balance Substance 3E0R37Z
- Subcutaneous Tissue 3E013GC
  - Analgesics 3E013NZ
  - Anesthetic Agent 3E013BZ
  - Anti-infective 3E01
  - Anti-inflammatory 3E0133Z
  - Antineoplastic 3E0130
  - Destructive Agent 3E013TZ
  - Diagnostic Substance, Other 3E013KZ
  - Electrolytic Substance 3E0137Z
  - Hormone 3E013V
  - Hypnotics 3E013NZ
  - Nutritional Substance 3E0136Z
  - Radioactive Substance 3E013HZ
  - Sedatives 3E013NZ
  - Serum 3E0134Z
  - Toxoid 3E0134Z
  - Vaccine 3E0134Z
  - Water Balance Substance 3E0137Z
- Vein
  - Central 3E04
    - Analgesics 3E04
    - Anesthetic, Intracirculatory 3E04
    - Antiarrhythmic 3E04
    - Anti-infective 3E04
    - Anti-inflammatory 3E04
    - Antineoplastic 3E04
    - Destructive Agent 3E04
    - Diagnostic Substance, Other 3E04
    - Electrolytic Substance 3E04
    - Hormone 3E04
    - Hypnotics 3E04
    - Immunotherapeutic 3E04
    - Nutritional Substance 3E04
    - Platelet Inhibitor 3E04
    - Radioactive Substance 3E04
    - Sedatives 3E04
    - Serum 3E04
    - Thrombolytic 3E04
    - Toxoid 3E04
    - Vaccine 3E04
    - Vasopressor 3E04
    - Water Balance Substance 3E04
  - Peripheral 3E03
    - Analgesics 3E03
    - Anesthetic, Intracirculatory 3E03
    - Antiarrhythmic 3E03
    - Anti-infective 3E03

Subterms under main terms may continue to next column or page

Introduction of substance in or on — *continued*
    Vein — *continued*
        Peripheral — *continued*
            Anti-inflammatory 3E03
            Antineoplastic 3E03
            Destructive Agent 3E03
            Diagnostic Substance, Other 3E03
            Electrolytic Substance 3E03
            Hormone 3E03
            Hypnotics 3E03
            Immunotherapeutic 3E03
            Islet Cells, Pancreatic 3E03
            Nutritional Substance 3E03
            Platelet Inhibitor 3E03
            Radioactive Substance 3E03
            Sedatives 3E03
            Serum 3E03
            Thrombolytic 3E03
            Toxoid 3E03
            Vaccine 3E03
            Vasopressor 3E03
            Water Balance Substance 3E03
Intubation
    Airway
        see Insertion of device in, Esophagus ØDH5
        see Insertion of device in, Mouth and Throat
            ØCHY
        see Insertion of device in, Trachea ØBH1
    Drainage device *see* Drainage
    Feeding Device *see* Insertion of device in, Gastroin-
        testinal System ØDH
INTUITY Elite valve system, EDWARDS *use*
    Zooplastic Tissue, Rapid Deployment Technique
    in New Technology
Iobenguane I-131 Antineoplastic XWØ
Iobenguane I-131, High Specific Activity (HSA) *use*
    Iobenguane I-131 Antineoplastic
IPPB (intermittent positive pressure breathing)
    see Assistance, Respiratory 5A09
IRE (Irreversible Electroporation) *see* Destruction,
    Hepatobiliary System and Pancreas ØF5
Iridectomy
    see Excision, Eye Ø8B
    see Resection, Eye Ø8T
Iridoplasty
    see Repair, Eye Ø8Q
    see Replacement, Eye Ø8R
    see Supplement, Eye Ø8U
Iridotomy *see* Drainage, Eye Ø89
Irreversible Electroporation (IRE) *see* Destruction,
    Hepatobiliary System and Pancreas ØF5
Irrigation
    Biliary Tract, Irrigating Substance 3E1J
    Brain, Irrigating Substance 3E1Q38Z
    Cranial Cavity, Irrigating Substance 3E1Q38Z
    Ear, Irrigating Substance 3E1B
    Epidural Space, Irrigating Substance 3E1S38Z
    Eye, Irrigating Substance 3E1C
    Gastrointestinal Tract
        Lower, Irrigating Substance 3E1H
        Upper, Irrigating Substance 3E1G
    Genitourinary Tract, Irrigating Substance 3E1K
    Irrigating Substance 3C1ZX8Z
    Joint, Irrigating Substance 3E1U
    Mucous Membrane, Irrigating Substance 3E10
    Nose, Irrigating Substance 3E19
    Pancreatic Tract, Irrigating Substance 3E1J
    Pericardial Cavity, Irrigating Substance 3E1Y38Z
    Peritoneal Cavity
        Dialysate 3E1M39Z
        Irrigating Substance 3E1M38Z
    Pleural Cavity, Irrigating Substance 3E1L38Z
    Reproductive
        Female, Irrigating Substance 3E1P
        Male, Irrigating Substance 3E1N
    Respiratory Tract, Irrigating Substance 3E1F
    Skin, Irrigating Substance 3E10
    Spinal Canal, Irrigating Substance 3E1R38Z
Isavuconazole Anti-infective XWØ
Ischiatic nerve *use* Sciatic Nerve
Ischiocavernosus muscle *use* Perineum Muscle
Ischiofemoral ligament
    use Hip Bursa and Ligament, Left
    use Hip Bursa and Ligament, Right
Ischium
    use Pelvic Bone, Left
    use Pelvic Bone, Right
Isolation 8E0ZXY6

Isotope Administration, Whole Body DWY5G
Itrel (3) (4) neurostimulator *use* Stimulator Generator,
    Single Array in ØJH

J

Jakafi® *use* Ruxolitinib
Jejunal artery *use* Superior Mesenteric Artery
Jejunectomy
    see Excision, Jejunum ØDBA
    see Resection, Jejunum ØDTA
Jejunocolostomy
    see Bypass, Gastrointestinal System ØD1
    see Drainage, Gastrointestinal System ØD9
Jejunopexy
    see Repair, Jejunum ØDQA
    see Reposition, Jejunum ØDSA
Jejunostomy
    see Bypass, Jejunum ØD1A
    see Drainage, Jejunum ØD9A
Jejunotomy *see* Drainage, Jejunum ØD9A
Joint fixation plate
    use Internal Fixation Device in Lower Joints
    use Internal Fixation Device in Upper Joints
Joint liner (insert) *use* Liner in Lower Joints
Joint spacer (antibiotic)
    use Spacer in Lower Joints
    use Spacer in Upper Joints
Jugular body *use* Glomus Jugulare
Jugular lymph node
    use Lymphatic, Left Neck
    use Lymphatic, Right Neck

K

Kappa *use* Pacemaker, Dual Chamber in ØJH
Kcentra *use* 4-Factor Prothrombin Complex Concen-
    trate
Keratectomy, kerectomy
    see Excision, Eye Ø8B
    see Resection, Eye Ø8T
Keratocentesis *see* Drainage, Eye Ø89
Keratoplasty
    see Repair, Eye Ø8Q
    see Replacement, Eye Ø8R
    see Supplement, Eye Ø8U
Keratotomy
    see Drainage, Eye Ø89
    see Repair, Eye Ø8Q
**Keystone Heart TriGuard 3™ CEPD (cerebral embol-
    ic protection device)** X2A6325
Kirschner wire (K-wire)
    use Internal Fixation Device in Head and Facial
        Bones
    use Internal Fixation Device in Lower Bones
    use Internal Fixation Device in Lower Joints
    use Internal Fixation Device in Upper Bones
    use Internal Fixation Device in Upper Joints
Knee (implant) insert *use* Liner in Lower Joints
KUB x-ray *see* Plain Radiography, Kidney, Ureter and
    Bladder BTØ4
Kuntscher nail
    use Internal Fixation Device, Intramedullary in
        Lower Bones
    use Internal Fixation Device, Intramedullary in
        Upper Bones
KYMRIAH *use* Engineered Autologous Chimeric Antigen
    Receptor T-cell Immunotherapy

L

Labia majora *use* Vulva
Labia minora *use* Vulva
Labial gland
    use Lower Lip
    use Upper Lip
Labiectomy
    see Excision, Female Reproductive System ØUB
    see Resection, Female Reproductive System ØUT
Lacrimal canaliculus
    use Lacrimal Duct, Left
    use Lacrimal Duct, Right
Lacrimal punctum
    use Lacrimal Duct, Left

Lacrimal punctum — *continued*
    use Lacrimal Duct, Right
Lacrimal sac
    use Lacrimal Duct, Left
    use Lacrimal Duct, Right
LAGB (laparoscopic adjustable gastric banding)
    Initial procedure ØDV64CZ
    Surgical correction *see* Revision of device in,
        Stomach ØDW6
Laminectomy
    see Excision, Lower Bones ØQB
    see Excision, Upper Bones ØPB
    see Release, Central Nervous System and Cranial
        Nerves ØØN
    see Release, Peripheral Nervous System Ø1N
Laminotomy
    see Drainage, Lower Bones ØQ9
    see Drainage, Upper Bones ØP9
    see Excision, Lower Bones ØQB
    see Excision, Upper Bones ØPB
    see Release, Central Nervous System and Cranial
        Nerves ØØN
    see Release, Lower Bones ØQN
    see Release, Peripheral Nervous System Ø1N
    see Release, Upper Bones ØPN
Laparoscopic-assisted transanal pull-through
    see Excision, Gastrointestinal System ØDB
    see Resection, Gastrointestinal System ØDT
Laparoscopy *see* Inspection
Laparotomy
    Drainage *see* Drainage, Peritoneal Cavity ØW9G
    Exploratory *see* Inspection, Peritoneal Cavity ØWJG
LAP-BAND® Adjustable Gastric Banding System
    use Extraluminal Device
Laryngectomy
    see Excision, Larynx ØCBS
    see Resection, Larynx ØCTS
Laryngocentesis *see* Drainage, Larynx ØC9S
Laryngogram *see* Fluoroscopy, Larynx B91J
Laryngopexy *see* Repair, Larynx ØCQS
Laryngopharynx *use* Pharynx
Laryngoplasty
    see Repair, Larynx ØCQS
    see Replacement, Larynx ØCRS
    see Supplement, Larynx ØCUS
Laryngorrhaphy *see* Repair, Larynx ØCQS
Laryngoscopy ØCJS8ZZ
Laryngotomy *see* Drainage, Larynx ØC9S
Laser Interstitial Thermal Therapy
    Adrenal Gland DGY2KZZ
    Anus DDY8KZZ
    Bile Ducts DFY2KZZ
    Brain DØYØKZZ
    Brain Stem DØY1KZZ
    Breast
        Left DMYØKZZ
        Right DMY1KZZ
    Bronchus DBY1KZZ
    Chest Wall DBY7KZZ
    Colon DDY5KZZ
    Diaphragm DBY8KZZ
    Duodenum DDY2KZZ
    Esophagus DDYØKZZ
    Gallbladder DFY1KZZ
    Gland
        Adrenal DGY2KZZ
        Parathyroid DGY4KZZ
        Pituitary DGYØKZZ
        Thyroid DGY5KZZ
    Ileum DDY4KZZ
    Jejunum DDY3KZZ
    Liver DFYØKZZ
    Lung DBY2KZZ
    Mediastinum DBY6KZZ
    Nerve, Peripheral DØY7KZZ
    Pancreas DFY3KZZ
    Parathyroid Gland DGY4KZZ
    Pineal Body DGY1KZZ
    Pituitary Gland DGYØKZZ
    Pleura DBY5KZZ
    Prostate DVYØKZZ
    Rectum DDY7KZZ
    Spinal Cord DØY6KZZ
    Stomach DDY1KZZ
    Thyroid Gland DGY5KZZ
    Trachea DBYØKZZ

Lateral canthus
  use Upper Eyelid, Left
  use Upper Eyelid, Right
Lateral collateral ligament (LCL)
  use Knee Bursa and Ligament, Left
  use Knee Bursa and Ligament, Right
Lateral condyle of femur
  use Lower Femur, Left
  use Lower Femur, Right
Lateral condyle of tibia
  use Tibia, Left
  use Tibia, Right
Lateral cuneiform bone
  use Tarsal, Left
  use Tarsal, Right
Lateral epicondyle of femur
  use Lower Femur, Left
  use Lower Femur, Right
Lateral epicondyle of humerus
  use Humeral Shaft, Left
  use Humeral Shaft, Right
Lateral femoral cutaneous nerve *use* Lumbar Plexus
Lateral (brachial) lymph node
  use Lymphatic, Left Axillary
  use Lymphatic, Right Axillary
Lateral malleolus
  use Fibula, Left
  use Fibula, Right
Lateral meniscus
  use Knee Joint, Left
  use Knee Joint, Right
Lateral nasal cartilage *use* Nasal Mucosa and Soft
  Tissue
Lateral plantar artery
  use Foot Artery, Left
  use Foot Artery, Right
Lateral plantar nerve *use* Tibial Nerve
Lateral rectus muscle
  use Extraocular Muscle, Left
  use Extraocular Muscle, Right
Lateral sacral artery
  use Internal Iliac Artery, Left
  use Internal Iliac Artery, Right
Lateral sacral vein
  use Hypogastric Vein, Left
  use Hypogastric Vein, Right
Lateral sural cutaneous nerve *use* Peroneal Nerve
Lateral tarsal artery
  use Foot Artery, Left
  use Foot Artery, Right
Lateral temporomandibular ligament *use* Head and
  Neck Bursa and Ligament
Lateral thoracic artery
  use Axillary Artery, Left
  use Axillary Artery, Right
Latissimus dorsi muscle
  use Trunk Muscle, Left
  use Trunk Muscle, Right
Latissimus Dorsi Myocutaneous Flap
  Replacement
    Bilateral ØHRVØ75
    Left ØHRUØ75
    Right ØHRTØ75
  Transfer
    Left ØKXG
    Right ØKXF
Lavage
  see Irrigation
  Bronchial alveolar, diagnostic *see* Drainage, Respiratory System ØB9
Least splanchnic nerve *use* Thoracic Sympathetic
  Nerve
Lefamulin Anti-infective XWØ
Left ascending lumbar vein *use* Hemiazygos Vein
Left atrioventricular valve *use* Mitral Valve
Left auricular appendix *use* Atrium, Left
Left colic vein *use* Colic Vein
Left coronary sulcus *use* Heart, Left
Left gastric artery *use* Gastric Artery
Left gastroepiploic artery *use* Splenic Artery
Left gastroepiploic vein *use* Splenic Vein
Left inferior phrenic vein *use* Renal Vein, Left
Left inferior pulmonary vein *use* Pulmonary Vein,
  Left
Left jugular trunk *use* Thoracic Duct
Left lateral ventricle *use* Cerebral Ventricle

Left ovarian vein *use* Renal Vein, Left
Left second lumbar vein *use* Renal Vein, Left
Left subclavian trunk *use* Thoracic Duct
Left subcostal vein *use* Hemiazygos Vein
Left superior pulmonary vein *use* Pulmonary Vein,
  Left
Left suprarenal vein *use* Renal Vein, Left
Left testicular vein *use* Renal Vein, Left
Lengthening
  Bone, with device *see* Insertion of Limb Lengthening Device
  Muscle, by incision *see* Division, Muscles ØK8
  Tendon, by incision *see* Division, Tendons ØL8
Leptomeninges, intracranial *use* Cerebral Meninges
Leptomeninges, spinal *use* Spinal Meninges
Lesser alar cartilage *use* Nasal Mucosa and Soft Tissue
Lesser occipital nerve *use* Cervical Plexus
Lesser Omentum *use* Omentum
Lesser saphenous vein
  use Saphenous Vein, Left
  use Saphenous Vein, Right
Lesser splanchnic nerve *use* Thoracic Sympathetic
  Nerve
Lesser trochanter
  use Upper Femur, Left
  use Upper Femur, Right
Lesser tuberosity
  use Humeral Head, Left
  use Humeral Head, Right
Lesser wing *use* Sphenoid Bone
Leukopheresis, therapeutic *see* Pheresis, Circulatory
  6A55
Levator anguli oris muscle *use* Facial Muscle
Levator ani muscle *use* Perineum Muscle
Levator labii superioris alaeque nasi muscle *use*
  Facial Muscle
Levator labii superioris muscle *use* Facial Muscle
Levator palpebrae superioris muscle
  use Upper Eyelid, Left
  use Upper Eyelid, Right
Levator scapulae muscle
  use Neck Muscle, Left
  use Neck Muscle, Right
Levator veli palatini muscle *use* Tongue, Palate,
  Pharynx Muscle
Levatores costarum muscle
  use Thorax Muscle, Left
  use Thorax Muscle, Right
LifeStent® (Flexstar) (XL) Vascular Stent System
  use Intraluminal Device
Ligament of head of fibula
  use Knee Bursa and Ligament, Left
  use Knee Bursa and Ligament, Right
Ligament of the lateral malleolus
  use Ankle Bursa and Ligament, Left
  use Ankle Bursa and Ligament, Right
Ligamentum flavum, cervical *use* Head and Neck
  Bursa and Ligament
Ligamentum flavum, lumbar *use* Lower Spine Bursa
  and Ligament
Ligamentum flavum, thoracic *use* Upper Spine Bursa
  and Ligament
Ligation *see* Occlusion
Ligation, hemorrhoid *see* Occlusion, Lower Veins,
  Hemorrhoidal Plexus
Light Therapy GZJZZZZ
Liner
  Removal of device from
    Hip
      Left ØSPBØ9Z
      Right ØSP9Ø9Z
    Knee
      Left ØSPDØ9Z
      Right ØSPCØ9Z
  Revision of device in
    Hip
      Left ØSWBØ9Z
      Right ØSW9Ø9Z
    Knee
      Left ØSWDØ9Z
      Right ØSWCØ9Z
  Supplement
    Hip
      Left ØSUBØ9Z
        Acetabular Surface ØSUEØ9Z
        Femoral Surface ØSUSØ9Z
      Right ØSU9Ø9Z

Liner — *continued*
  Supplement — *continued*
    Hip — *continued*
      Right — *continued*
        Acetabular Surface ØSUAØ9Z
        Femoral Surface ØSURØ9Z
    Knee
      Left ØSUDØ9
        Femoral Surface ØSUUØ9Z
        Tibial Surface ØSUWØ9Z
      Right ØSUCØ9
        Femoral Surface ØSUTØ9Z
        Tibial Surface ØSUVØ9Z
Lingual artery
  use External Carotid Artery, Left
  use External Carotid Artery, Right
Lingual tonsil *use* Pharynx
Lingulectomy, lung
  see Excision, Lung Lingula ØBBH
  see Resection, Lung Lingula ØBTH
Lisocabtagene Maraleucel *use* Lisocabtagene Maraleucel Immunotherapy
Lisocabtagene Maraleucel Immunotherapy XW2
Lithoplasty *see* Fragmentation
Lithotripsy
  see Fragmentation
  With removal of fragments *see* Extirpation
LITT (laser interstitial thermal therapy) *see* Laser
  Interstitial Thermal Therapy
LIVIAN™ CRT-D *use* Cardiac Resynchronization Defibrillator Pulse Generator in ØJH
Lobectomy
  see Excision, Central Nervous System and Cranial
    Nerves ØØB
  see Excision, Endocrine System ØGB
  see Excision, Hepatobiliary System and Pancreas
    ØFB
  see Excision, Respiratory System ØBB
  see Resection, Endocrine System ØGT
  see Resection, Hepatobiliary System and Pancreas
    ØFT
  see Resection, Respiratory System ØBT
Lobotomy *see* Division, Brain ØØ8Ø
Localization
  see Imaging
  see Map
Locus ceruleus *use* Pons
Long thoracic nerve *use* Brachial Plexus
Loop ileostomy *see* Bypass, Ileum ØD1B
Loop recorder, implantable *use* Monitoring Device
Lower GI series *see* Fluoroscopy, Colon BD14
Lower Respiratory Fluid Nucleic Acid-base Microbial Detection XXEBXQ6
Lumbar artery *use* Abdominal Aorta
Lumbar facet joint *use* Lumbar Vertebral Joint
Lumbar ganglion *use* Lumbar Sympathetic Nerve
Lumbar lymph node *use* Lymphatic, Aortic
Lumbar lymphatic trunk *use* Cisterna Chyli
Lumbar splanchnic nerve *use* Lumbar Sympathetic
  Nerve
Lumbosacral facet joint *use* Lumbosacral Joint
Lumbosacral trunk *use* Lumbar Nerve
Lumpectomy *see* Excision
Lunate bone
  use Carpal, Left
  use Carpal, Right
Lunotriquetral ligament
  use Hand Bursa and Ligament, Left
  use Hand Bursa and Ligament, Right
Lymphadenectomy
  see Excision, Lymphatic and Hemic Systems Ø7B
  see Resection, Lymphatic and Hemic Systems Ø7T
Lymphadenotomy *see* Drainage, Lymphatic and Hemic
  Systems Ø79
Lymphangiectomy
  see Excision, Lymphatic and Hemic Systems Ø7B
  see Resection, Lymphatic and Hemic Systems Ø7T
Lymphangiogram *see* Plain Radiography, Lymphatic
  System B7Ø
Lymphangioplasty
  see Repair, Lymphatic and Hemic Systems Ø7Q
  see Supplement, Lymphatic and Hemic Systems
    Ø7U
Lymphangiorrhaphy *see* Repair, Lymphatic and Hemic
  Systems Ø7Q
Lymphangiotomy *see* Drainage, Lymphatic and Hemic
  Systems Ø79

Lysis *see* Release

M

Macula
  use Retina, Left
  use Retina, Right
MAGEC® Spinal Bracing and Distraction System
  use Magnetically Controlled Growth Rod(s) in New Technology
Magnet extraction, ocular foreign body *see* Extirpation, Eye Ø8C
Magnetic Resonance Imaging (MRI)
  Abdomen BW3Ø
  Ankle
    Left BQ3H
    Right BQ3G
  Aorta
    Abdominal B43Ø
    Thoracic B33Ø
  Arm
    Left BP3F
    Right BP3E
  Artery
    Celiac B431
    Cervico-Cerebral Arch B33Q
    Common Carotid, Bilateral B335
    Coronary
      Bypass Graft, Multiple B233
      Multiple B231
    Internal Carotid, Bilateral B338
    Intracranial B33R
    Lower Extremity
      Bilateral B43H
      Left B43G
      Right B43F
    Pelvic B43C
    Renal, Bilateral B438
    Spinal B33M
    Superior Mesenteric B434
    Upper Extremity
      Bilateral B33K
      Left B33J
      Right B33H
    Vertebral, Bilateral B33G
  Bladder BT3Ø
  Brachial Plexus BW3P
  Brain BØ3Ø
  Breast
    Bilateral BH32
    Left BH31
    Right BH3Ø
  Calcaneus
    Left BQ3K
    Right BQ3J
  Chest BW33Y
  Coccyx BR3F
  Connective Tissue
    Lower Extremity BL31
    Upper Extremity BL3Ø
  Corpora Cavernosa BV3Ø
  Disc
    Cervical BR31
    Lumbar BR33
    Thoracic BR32
  Ear B93Ø
  Elbow
    Left BP3H
    Right BP3G
  Eye
    Bilateral B837
    Left B836
    Right B835
  Femur
    Left BQ34
    Right BQ33
  Fetal Abdomen BY33
  Fetal Extremity BY35
  Fetal Head BY3Ø
  Fetal Heart BY31
  Fetal Spine BY34
  Fetal Thorax BY32
  Fetus, Whole BY36
  Foot
    Left BQ3M
    Right BQ3L
  Forearm
    Left BP3K

Magnetic Resonance Imaging (MRI) — *continued*
  Forearm — *continued*
    Right BP3J
  Gland
    Adrenal, Bilateral BG32
    Parathyroid BG33
    Parotid, Bilateral B936
    Salivary, Bilateral B93D
    Submandibular, Bilateral B939
    Thyroid BG34
  Head BW38
  Heart, Right and Left B236
  Hip
    Left BQ31
    Right BQ3Ø
  Intracranial Sinus B532
  Joint
    Finger
      Left BP3D
      Right BP3C
    Hand
      Left BP3D
      Right BP3C
    Temporomandibular, Bilateral BN39
  Kidney
    Bilateral BT33
    Left BT32
    Right BT31
    Transplant BT39
  Knee
    Left BQ38
    Right BQ37
  Larynx B93J
  Leg
    Left BQ3F
    Right BQ3D
  Liver BF35
  Liver and Spleen BF36
  Lung Apices BB3G
  Nasopharynx B93F
  Neck BW3F
  Nerve
    Acoustic BØ3C
    Brachial Plexus BW3P
  Oropharynx B93F
  Ovary
    Bilateral BU35
    Left BU34
    Right BU33
  Ovary and Uterus BU3C
  Pancreas BF37
  Patella
    Left BQ3W
    Right BQ3V
  Pelvic Region BW3G
  Pelvis BR3C
  Pituitary Gland BØ39
  Plexus, Brachial BW3P
  Prostate BV33
  Retroperitoneum BW3H
  Sacrum BR3F
  Scrotum BV34
  Sella Turcica BØ39
  Shoulder
    Left BP39
    Right BP38
  Sinus
    Intracranial B532
    Paranasal B932
  Spinal Cord BØ3B
  Spine
    Cervical BR3Ø
    Lumbar BR39
    Thoracic BR37
  Spleen and Liver BF36
  Subcutaneous Tissue
    Abdomen BH3H
    Extremity
      Lower BH3J
      Upper BH3F
    Head BH3D
    Neck BH3D
    Pelvis BH3H
    Thorax BH3G
  Tendon
    Lower Extremity BL33
    Upper Extremity BL32
  Testicle
    Bilateral BV37

Magnetic Resonance Imaging (MRI) — *continued*
  Testicle — *continued*
    Left BV36
    Right BV35
  Toe
    Left BQ3Q
    Right BQ3P
  Uterus BU36
    Pregnant BU3B
  Uterus and Ovary BU3C
  Vagina BU39
  Vein
    Cerebellar B531
    Cerebral B531
    Jugular, Bilateral B535
    Lower Extremity
      Bilateral B53D
      Left B53C
      Right B53B
    Other B53V
    Pelvic (Iliac) Bilateral B53H
    Portal B53T
    Pulmonary, Bilateral B53S
    Renal, Bilateral B53L
    Spanchnic B53T
    Upper Extremity
      Bilateral B53P
      Left B53N
      Right B53M
  Vena Cava
    Inferior B539
    Superior B538
  Wrist
    Left BP3M
    Right BP3L
Magnetically Controlled Growth Rod(s)
  Cervical XNS3
  Lumbar XNSØ
  Thoracic XNS4
Magnetic-guided radiofrequency endovascular fistula
  Radial Artery, Left Ø31C3ZF
  Radial Artery, Right Ø31B3ZF
  Ulnar Artery, Left Ø31A3ZF
  Ulnar Artery, Right Ø3193ZF
Malleotomy *see* Drainage, Ear, Nose, Sinus Ø99
Malleus
  use Auditory Ossicle, Left
  use Auditory Ossicle, Right
Mammaplasty, mammoplasty
  see Alteration, Skin and Breast ØHØ
  see Repair, Skin and Breast ØHQ
  see Replacement, Skin and Breast ØHR
  see Supplement, Skin and Breast ØHU
Mammary duct
  use Breast, Bilateral
  use Breast, Left
  use Breast, Right
Mammary gland
  use Breast, Bilateral
  use Breast, Left
  use Breast, Right
Mammectomy
  see Excision, Skin and Breast ØHB
  see Resection, Skin and Breast ØHT
Mammillary body *use* Hypothalamus
Mammography *see* Plain Radiography, Skin, Subcutaneous Tissue and Breast BHØ
Mammotomy *see* Drainage, Skin and Breast ØH9
Mandibular nerve *use* Trigeminal Nerve
Mandibular notch
  use Mandible, Left
  use Mandible, Right
Mandibulectomy
  see Excision, Head and Facial Bones ØNB
  see Resection, Head and Facial Bones ØNT
Manipulation
  Adhesions *see* Release
  Chiropractic *see* Chiropractic Manipulation
Manual removal, retained placenta *see* Extraction, Products of Conception, Retained 1ØD1
Manubrium *use* Sternum
Map
  Basal Ganglia ØØK8
  Brain ØØKØ
  Cerebellum ØØKC
  Cerebral Hemisphere ØØK7

Subterms under main terms may continue to next column or page

Index

Map — Metacarpal ligament

Metacarpophalangeal ligament
  use Hand Bursa and Ligament, Left
  use Hand Bursa and Ligament, Right
Metal on metal bearing surface *use* Synthetic Substitute, Metal in ØSR
Metatarsal ligament
  use Foot Bursa and Ligament, Left
  use Foot Bursa and Ligament, Right
Metatarsectomy
  see Excision, Lower Bones ØQB
  see Resection, Lower Bones ØQT
Metatarsophalangeal (MTP) joint
  use Metatarsal-Phalangeal Joint, Left
  use Metatarsal-Phalangeal Joint, Right
Metatarsophalangeal ligament
  use Foot Bursa and Ligament, Left
  use Foot Bursa and Ligament, Right
Metathalamus *use* Thalamus
Micro-Driver stent (RX) (OTW) *use* Intraluminal Device
MicroMed HeartAssist *use* Implantable Heart Assist System in Heart and Great Vessels
Micrus CERECYTE Microcoil *use* Intraluminal Device, Bioactive in Upper Arteries
Midcarpal joint
  use Carpal Joint, Left
  use Carpal Joint, Right
Middle cardiac nerve *use* Thoracic Sympathetic Nerve
Middle cerebral artery *use* Intracranial Artery
Middle cerebral vein *use* Intracranial Vein
Middle colic vein *use* Colic Vein
Middle genicular artery
  use Popliteal Artery, Left
  use Popliteal Artery, Right
Middle hemorrhoidal vein
  use Hypogastric Vein, Left
  use Hypogastric Vein, Right
Middle rectal artery
  use Internal Iliac Artery, Left
  use Internal Iliac Artery, Right
Middle suprarenal artery *use* Abdominal Aorta
Middle temporal artery
  use Temporal Artery, Left
  use Temporal Artery, Right
Middle turbinate *use* Nasal Turbinate
Mineral-based Topical Hemostatic Agent XWØ
MIRODERM™ Biologic Wound Matrix *use* Skin Substitute, Porcine Liver Derived in New Technology
MitraClip valve repair system *use* Synthetic Substitute
Mitral annulus *use* Mitral Valve
Mitroflow® Aortic Pericardial Heart Valve *use* Zooplastic Tissue in Heart and Great Vessels
Mobilization, adhesions *see* Release
Molar gland *use* Buccal Mucosa
MolecuLight i:X® wound imaging *see* Other Imaging, Anatomical Regions BW5
Monitoring
  Arterial
    Flow
      Coronary 4A13
      Peripheral 4A13
      Pulmonary 4A13
    Pressure
      Coronary 4A13
      Peripheral 4A13
      Pulmonary 4A13
    Pulse
      Coronary 4A13
      Peripheral 4A13
      Pulmonary 4A13
    Saturation, Peripheral 4A13
    Sound, Peripheral 4A13
  Cardiac
    Electrical Activity 4A12
      Ambulatory 4A12X45
      No Qualifier 4A12X4Z
    Output 4A12
    Rate 4A12
    Rhythm 4A12
    Sound 4A12
    Total Activity, Stress 4A12XM4
    Vascular Perfusion, Indocyanine Green Dye 4A12XSH
  Central Nervous
    Conductivity 4A1Ø
    Electrical Activity
      Intraoperative 4A1Ø

Monitoring — *continued*
  Central Nervous — *continued*
    Electrical Activity — *continued*
      No Qualifier 4A1Ø
    Pressure 4A1ØØBZ
      Intracranial 4A1Ø
    Saturation, Intracranial 4A1Ø
    Temperature, Intracranial 4A1Ø
  Gastrointestinal
    Motility 4A1B
    Pressure 4A1B
    Secretion 4A1B
    Vascular Perfusion, Indocyanine Green Dye 4A1BXSH
  Intraoperative Knee Replacement Sensor XR2
  Kidney, Fluorescent Pyrazine XT25XE5
  Lymphatic
    Flow
      Indocyanine Green Dye 4A16
      No Qualifier 4A16
    Pressure 4A16
  Peripheral Nervous
    Conductivity
      Motor 4A11
      Sensory 4A11
    Electrical Activity
      Intraoperative 4A11
      No Qualifier 4A11
  Products of Conception
    Cardiac
      Electrical Activity 4A1H
      Rate 4A1H
      Rhythm 4A1H
      Sound 4A1H
    Nervous
      Conductivity 4A1J
      Electrical Activity 4A1J
      Pressure 4A1J
  Respiratory
    Capacity 4A19
    Flow 4A19
    Rate 4A19
    Resistance 4A19
    Volume 4A19
  Skin and Breast, Vascular Perfusion, Indocyanine Green Dye 4A1GXSH
  Sleep 4A1ZXQZ
  Temperature 4A1Z
  Urinary
    Contractility 4A1D
    Flow 4A1D
    Pressure 4A1D
    Resistance 4A1D
    Volume 4A1D
  Venous
    Flow
      Central 4A14
      Peripheral 4A14
      Portal 4A14
      Pulmonary 4A14
    Pressure
      Central 4A14
      Peripheral 4A14
      Portal 4A14
      Pulmonary 4A14
    Pulse
      Central 4A14
      Peripheral 4A14
      Portal 4A14
      Pulmonary 4A14
    Saturation
      Central 4A14
      Portal 4A14
      Pulmonary 4A14
Monitoring Device, Hemodynamic
  Abdomen ØJH8
  Chest ØJH6
Mosaic Bioprosthesis (aortic) (mitral) valve *use* Zooplastic Tissue in Heart and Great Vessels
Motor Function Assessment FØ1
Motor Treatment FØ7
MR Angiography
  see Magnetic Resonance Imaging (MRI), Heart B23
  see Magnetic Resonance Imaging (MRI), Lower Arteries B43
  see Magnetic Resonance Imaging (MRI), Upper Arteries B33

MULTI-LINK (VISION) (MINI-VISION) (ULTRA) Coronary Stent System *use* Intraluminal Device
Multiple sleep latency test 4AØZXQZ
Musculocutaneous nerve *use* Brachial Plexus
Musculopexy
  see Repair, Muscles ØKQ
  see Reposition, Muscles ØKS
Musculophrenic artery
  use Internal Mammary Artery, Left
  use Internal Mammary Artery, Right
Musculoplasty
  see Repair, Muscles ØKQ
  see Supplement, Muscles ØKU
Musculorrhaphy *see* Repair, Muscles ØKQ
Musculospiral nerve *use* Radial Nerve
Myectomy
  see Excision, Muscles ØKB
  see Resection, Muscles ØKT
Myelencephalon *use* Medulla Oblongata
Myelogram
  CT *see* Computerized Tomography (CT Scan), Central Nervous System BØ2
  MRI *see* Magnetic Resonance Imaging (MRI), Central Nervous System BØ3
Myenteric (Auerbach's) plexus *use* Abdominal Sympathetic Nerve
Myocardial Bridge Release *see* Release, Artery, Coronary
Myomectomy *see* Excision, Female Reproductive System ØUB
Myometrium *use* Uterus
Myopexy
  see Repair, Muscles ØKQ
  see Reposition, Muscles ØKS
Myoplasty
  see Repair, Muscles ØKQ
  see Supplement, Muscles ØKU
Myorrhaphy *see* Repair, Muscles ØKQ
Myoscopy *see* Inspection, Muscles ØKJ
Myotomy
  see Division, Muscles ØK8
  see Drainage, Muscles ØK9
Myringectomy
  see Excision, Ear, Nose, Sinus Ø9B
  see Resection, Ear, Nose, Sinus Ø9T
Myringoplasty
  see Repair, Ear, Nose, Sinus Ø9Q
  see Replacement, Ear, Nose, Sinus Ø9R
  see Supplement, Ear, Nose, Sinus Ø9U
Myringostomy *see* Drainage, Ear, Nose, Sinus Ø99
Myringotomy *see* Drainage, Ear, Nose, Sinus Ø99

N

NA-1 (Nerinitide) *use* Nerinitide
Nail bed
  use Finger Nail
  use Toe Nail
Nail plate
  use Finger Nail
  use Toe Nail
nanoLOCK™ interbody fusion device *use* Interbody Fusion Device, Nanotextured Surface in New Technology
Narcosynthesis GZGZZZZ
Nasal cavity *use* Nasal Mucosa and Soft Tissue
Nasal concha *use* Nasal Turbinate
Nasalis muscle *use* Facial Muscle
Nasolacrimal duct
  use Lacrimal Duct, Left
  use Lacrimal Duct, Right
Nasopharyngeal airway (NPA) *use* Intraluminal Device, Airway in Ear, Nose, Sinus
Navicular bone
  use Tarsal, Left
  use Tarsal, Right
Near Infrared Spectroscopy, Circulatory System 8EØ2
Neck of femur
  use Upper Femur, Left
  use Upper Femur, Right
Neck of humerus (anatomical) (surgical)
  use Humeral Head, Left
  use Humeral Head, Right
Nephrectomy
  see Excision, Urinary System ØTB

Nephrectomy — continued
see Resection, Urinary System 0TT
Nephrolithotomy see Extirpation, Urinary System 0TC
Nephrolysis see Release, Urinary System 0TN
Nephropexy
see Repair, Urinary System 0TQ
see Reposition, Urinary System 0TS
Nephroplasty
see Repair, Urinary System 0TQ
see Supplement, Urinary System 0TU
Nephropyeloureterostomy
see Bypass, Urinary System 0T1
see Drainage, Urinary System 0T9
Nephrorrhaphy see Repair, Urinary System 0TQ
Nephroscopy, transurethral 0TJ58ZZ
Nephrostomy
see Bypass, Urinary System 0T1
see Drainage, Urinary System 0T9
Nephrotomography
see Fluoroscopy, Urinary System BT1
see Plain Radiography, Urinary System BT0
Nephrotomy
see Division, Urinary System 0T8
see Drainage, Urinary System 0T9
Nerinitide XW0
Nerve conduction study
see Measurement, Central Nervous 4A00
see Measurement, Peripheral Nervous 4A01
Nerve Function Assessment F01
Nerve to the stapedius use Facial Nerve
Nesiritide use Human B-Type Natriuretic Peptide
Neurectomy
see Excision, Central Nervous System and Cranial Nerves 00B
see Excision, Peripheral Nervous System 01B
Neurexeresis
see Extraction, Central Nervous System and Cranial Nerves 00D
see Extraction, Peripheral Nervous System 01D
Neurohypophysis use Pituitary Gland
Neurolysis
see Release, Central Nervous System and Cranial Nerves 00N
see Release, Peripheral Nervous System 01N
Neuromuscular electrical stimulation (NEMS) lead
use Stimulator Lead in Muscles
Neurophysiologic monitoring see Monitoring, Central Nervous 4A10
Neuroplasty
see Repair, Central Nervous System and Cranial Nerves 00Q
see Repair, Peripheral Nervous System 01Q
see Supplement, Central Nervous System and Cranial Nerves 00U
see Supplement, Peripheral Nervous System 01U
Neurorrhaphy
see Repair, Central Nervous System and Cranial Nerves 00Q
see Repair, Peripheral Nervous System 01Q
Neurostimulator Generator
Insertion of device in, Skull 0NH00NZ
Removal of device from, Skull 0NP00NZ
Revision of device in, Skull 0NW00NZ
Neurostimulator generator, multiple channel use Stimulator Generator, Multiple Array in 0JH
Neurostimulator generator, multiple channel rechargeable use Stimulator Generator, Multiple Array Rechargeable in 0JH
Neurostimulator generator, single channel use Stimulator Generator, Single Array in 0JH
Neurostimulator generator, single channel rechargeable use Stimulator Generator, Single Array Rechargeable in 0JH
Neurostimulator Lead
Insertion of device in
Brain 00H0
Cerebral Ventricle 00H6
Nerve
Cranial 00HE
Peripheral 01HY
Spinal Canal 00HU
Spinal Cord 00HV
Vein
Azygos 05H0
Innominate
Left 05H4
Right 05H3

Neurostimulator Lead — continued
Removal of device from
Brain 00P0
Cerebral Ventricle 00P6
Nerve
Cranial 00PE
Peripheral 01PY
Spinal Canal 00PU
Spinal Cord 00PV
Vein
Azygos 05P0
Innominate
Left 05P4
Right 05P3
Revision of device in
Brain 00W0
Cerebral Ventricle 00W6
Nerve
Cranial 00WE
Peripheral 01WY
Spinal Canal 00WU
Spinal Cord 00WV
Vein
Azygos 05W0
Innominate
Left 05W4
Right 05W3
Neurotomy
see Division, Central Nervous System and Cranial Nerves 008
see Division, Peripheral Nervous System 018
Neurotripsy
see Destruction, Central Nervous System and Cranial Nerves 005
see Destruction, Peripheral Nervous System 015
Neutralization plate
use Internal Fixation Device in Head and Facial Bones
use Internal Fixation Device in Lower Bones
use Internal Fixation Device in Upper Bones
New Technology
Apalutamide Antineoplastic XW0DXJ5
Atezolizumab Antineoplastic XW0
Bezlotoxumab Monoclonal Antibody XW0
Blinatumomab Antineoplastic Immunotherapy XW0
Brexanolone XW0
Brexucabtagene Autoleucel Immunotherapy XW2
Caplacizumab XW0
Cefiderocol Anti-infective XW0
Ceftazidime-Avibactam Anti-infective XW0
Ceftolozane/Tazobactam Anti-infective XW0
Cerebral Embolic Filtration
Dual Filter X2A5312
Extracorporeal Flow Reversal Circuit X2A
Single Deflection Filter X2A6325
Coagulation Factor Xa, Inactivated XW0
Concentrated Bone Marrow Aspirate XK02303
Cytarabine and Daunorubicin Liposome Antineoplastic XW0
Defibrotide Sodium Anticoagulant XW0
Destruction, Prostate, Robotic Waterjet Ablation XV508A4
Dilation
Anterior Tibial
Left
Sustained Release Drug-eluting Intraluminal Device X27Q385
Four or More X27Q3C5
Three X27Q3B5
Two X27Q395
Right
Sustained Release Drug-eluting Intraluminal Device X27P385
Four or More X27P3C5
Three X27P3B5
Two X27P395
Femoral
Left
Sustained Release Drug-eluting Intraluminal Device X27J385
Four or More X27J3C5
Three X27J3B5
Two X27J395

New Technology — continued
Dilation — continued
Femoral — continued
Right
Sustained Release Drug-eluting Intraluminal Device X27H385
Four or More X27H3C5
Three X27H3B5
Two X27H395
Peroneal
Left
Sustained Release Drug-eluting Intraluminal Device X27U385
Four or More X27U3C5
Three X27U3B5
Two X27U395
Right
Sustained Release Drug-eluting Intraluminal Device X27T385
Four or More X27T3C5
Three X27T3B5
Two X27T395
Popliteal
Left Distal
Sustained Release Drug-eluting Intraluminal Device X27N385
Four or More X27N3C5
Three X27N3B5
Two X27N395
Left Proximal
Sustained Release Drug-eluting Intraluminal Device X27L385
Four or More X27L3C5
Three X27L3B5
Two X27L395
Right Distal
Sustained Release Drug-eluting Intraluminal Device X27M385
Four or More X27M3C5
Three X27M3B5
Two X27M395
Right Proximal
Sustained Release Drug-eluting Intraluminal Device X27K385
Four or More X27K3C5
Three X27K3B5
Two X27K395
Posterior Tibial
Left
Sustained Release Drug-eluting Intraluminal Device X27S385
Four or More X27S3C5
Three X27S3B5
Two X27S395
Right
Sustained Release Drug-eluting Intraluminal Device X27R385
Four or More X27R3C5
Three X27R3B5
Two X27R395
Durvalumab Antineoplastic XW0
Eculizumab XW0
Eladocagene exuparvovec XW0Q316
Endothelial Damage Inhibitor XY0VX83
Engineered Autologous Chimeric Antigen Receptor T-cell Immunotherapy XW0
Erdafitinib Antineoplastic XW0DXL5
Esketamine Hydrochloride XW097M5
Fosfomycin Anti-infective XW0
Fusion
Cervical Vertebral
2 or more
Nanotextured Surface XRG2092
Radiolucent Porous XRG20F3
Interbody Fusion Device
Nanotextured Surface XRG1092
Radiolucent Porous XRG10F3
Cervicothoracic Vertebral
Nanotextured Surface XRG4092
Radiolucent Porous XRG40F3

Subterms under main terms may continue to next column or page

New Technology — *continued*
  Fusion — *continued*
    Lumbar Vertebral
      2 or more
        Nanotextured Surface XRGC092
        Radiolucent Porous XRGC0F3
      Interbody Fusion Device
        Nanotextured Surface XRGB092
        Radiolucent Porous XRGB0F3
    Lumbosacral
      Nanotextured Surface XRGD092
      Radiolucent Porous XRGD0F3
    Occipital-cervical
      Nanotextured Surface XRG0092
      Radiolucent Porous XRG00F3
    Thoracic Vertebral
      2 to 7
        Nanotextured Surface XRG7092
        Radiolucent Porous XRG70F3
      8 or more
        Nanotextured Surface XRG8092
        Radiolucent Porous XRG80F3
      Interbody Fusion Device
        Nanotextured Surface XRG6092
        Radiolucent Porous XRG60F3
    Thoracolumbar Vertebral
      Nanotextured Surface XRGA092
      Radiolucent Porous XRGA0F3
  Gilteritinib Antineoplastic XW0DXV5
  Idarucizumab, Dabigatran Reversal Agent XW0
  Imipenem-cilastatin-relebactam Anti-infective XW0
  Intraoperative Knee Replacement Sensor XR2
  Iobenguane I-131 Antineoplastic XW0
  Isavuconazole Anti-infective XW0
  Kidney, Fluorescent Pyrazine XT25XE5
  Lefamulin Anti-infective XW0
  Lisocabtagene Maraleucel Immunotherapy XW2
  Lower Respiratory Fluid Nucleic Acid-base Micro-bial Detection XXEBXQ6
  Meropenem-vaborbactam Anti-infective XW0
  Mineral-based Topical Hemostatic Agent XW0
  Nerinitide XW0
  Omadacycline Anti-infective XW0
  Orbital Atherectomy Technology X2C
  Other New Technology Therapeutic Substance XW0
  Plazomicin Anti-infective XW0
  Positive Blood Culture Fluorescence Hybridization for Organism Identification, Concentration and Susceptibility XXE5XN6
  Replacement
    Skin Substitute, Porcine Liver Derived XHRPXL2
    Zooplastic Tissue, Rapid Deployment Tech-nique X2RF
  Reposition
    Cervical, Magnetically Controlled Growth Rod(s) XNS3
    Lumbar, Magnetically Controlled Growth Rod(s) XNS0
    Thoracic, Magnetically Controlled Growth Rod(s) XNS4
  Ruxolitinib XW0DXT5
  Supplement
    Lumbar, Mechanically Expandable (Paired) Synthetic Substitute XNU0356
    Thoracic, Mechanically Expandable (Paired) Synthetic Substitute XNU4356
  Synthetic Human Angiotensin II XW0
  Tagraxofusp-erzs Antineoplastic XW0
  Uridine Triacetate XW0DX82
  Venetoclax Antineoplastic XW0DXR5
  Whole Blood Nucleic Acid-base Microbial Detection XXE5XM5
Ninth cranial nerve *use* Glossopharyngeal Nerve
NIRS (Near Infrared Spectroscopy) *see* Physiological Systems and Anatomical Regions 8E0
Nitinol framed polymer mesh *use* Synthetic Substi-tute
Nonimaging Nuclear Medicine Assay
  Bladder, Kidneys and Ureters CT63
  Blood C763
  Kidneys, Ureters and Bladder CT63
  Lymphatics and Hematologic System C76YYZZ
  Ureters, Kidneys and Bladder CT63
  Urinary System CT6YYZZ
Nonimaging Nuclear Medicine Probe
  Abdomen CW50

Nonimaging Nuclear Medicine Probe — *continued*
  Abdomen and Chest CW54
  Abdomen and Pelvis CW51
  Brain C050
  Central Nervous System C05YYZZ
  Chest CW53
  Chest and Abdomen CW54
  Chest and Neck CW56
  Extremity
    Lower CP5PZZZ
    Upper CP5NZZZ
  Head and Neck CW5B
  Heart C25YYZZ
    Right and Left C256
  Lymphatics
    Head C75J
    Head and Neck C755
    Lower Extremity C75P
    Neck C75K
    Pelvic C75D
    Trunk C75M
    Upper Chest C75L
    Upper Extremity C75N
  Lymphatics and Hematologic System C75YYZZ
  Musculoskeletal System, Other CP5YYZZ
  Neck and Chest CW56
  Neck and Head CW5B
  Pelvic Region CW5J
  Pelvis and Abdomen CW51
  Spine CP55ZZZ
Nonimaging Nuclear Medicine Uptake
  Endocrine System CG4YYZZ
  Gland, Thyroid CG42
Non-tunneled central venous catheter *use* Infusion Device
Nostril *use* Nasal Mucosa and Soft Tissue
Novacor Left Ventricular Assist Device *use* Im-plantable Heart Assist System in Heart and Great Vessels
Novation® Ceramic AHS® (Articulation Hip System) *use* Synthetic Substitute, Ceramic in 0SR
Nuclear medicine
  see Nonimaging Nuclear Medicine Assay
  see Nonimaging Nuclear Medicine Probe
  see Nonimaging Nuclear Medicine Uptake
  see Planar Nuclear Medicine Imaging
  see Positron Emission Tomographic (PET) Imaging
  see Systemic Nuclear Medicine Therapy
  see Tomographic (Tomo) Nuclear Medicine Imag-ing
Nuclear scintigraphy *see* Nuclear Medicine
Nutrition, concentrated substances
  Enteral infusion 3E0G36Z
  Parenteral (peripheral) infusion *see* Introduction of Nutritional Substance
NUZYRA™ *use* Omadacycline Anti-infective

O

Obliteration *see* Destruction
Obturator artery
  use Internal Iliac Artery, Left
  use Internal Iliac Artery, Right
Obturator lymph node *use* Lymphatic, Pelvis
Obturator muscle
  use Hip Muscle, Left
  use Hip Muscle, Right
Obturator nerve *use* Lumbar Plexus
Obturator vein
  use Hypogastric Vein, Left
  use Hypogastric Vein, Right
Obtuse margin *use* Heart, Left
Occipital artery
  use External Carotid Artery, Left
  use External Carotid Artery, Right
Occipital lobe *use* Cerebral Hemisphere
Occipital lymph node
  use Lymphatic, Left Neck
  use Lymphatic, Right Neck
Occipitofrontalis muscle *use* Facial Muscle
Occlusion
  Ampulla of Vater 0FLC
  Anus 0DLQ
  Aorta
    Abdominal 04L0
    Thoracic, Descending 02LW3DJ

Occlusion — *continued*
  Artery
    Anterior Tibial
      Left 04LQ
      Right 04LP
    Axillary
      Left 03L6
      Right 03L5
    Brachial
      Left 03L8
      Right 03L7
    Celiac 04L1
    Colic
      Left 04L7
      Middle 04L8
      Right 04L6
    Common Carotid
      Left 03LJ
      Right 03LH
    Common Iliac
      Left 04LD
      Right 04LC
    External Carotid
      Left 03LN
      Right 03LM
    External Iliac
      Left 04LJ
      Right 04LH
    Face 03LR
    Femoral
      Left 04LL
      Right 04LK
    Foot
      Left 04LW
      Right 04LV
    Gastric 04L2
    Hand
      Left 03LF
      Right 03LD
    Hepatic 04L3
    Inferior Mesenteric 04LB
    Innominate 03L2
    Internal Carotid
      Left 03LL
      Right 03LK
    Internal Iliac
      Left 04LF
      Right 04LE
    Internal Mammary
      Left 03L1
      Right 03L0
    Intracranial 03LG
    Lower 04LY
    Peroneal
      Left 04LU
      Right 04LT
    Popliteal
      Left 04LN
      Right 04LM
    Posterior Tibial
      Left 04LS
      Right 04LR
    Pulmonary
      Left 02LR
      Right 02LQ
    Pulmonary Trunk 02LP
    Radial
      Left 03LC
      Right 03LB
    Renal
      Left 04LA
      Right 04L9
    Splenic 04L4
    Subclavian
      Left 03L4
      Right 03L3
    Superior Mesenteric 04L5
    Temporal
      Left 03LT
      Right 03LS
    Thyroid
      Left 03LV
      Right 03LU
    Ulnar
      Left 03LA
      Right 03L9
    Upper 03LY
    Vertebral
      Left 03LQ

Orbicularis oculi muscle
  use Upper Eyelid, Left
  use Upper Eyelid, Right
Orbicularis oris muscle *use* Facial Muscle
Orbital Atherectomy Technology X2C
Orbital fascia *use* Subcutaneous Tissue and Fascia,
  Face
Orbital portion of ethmoid bone
  use Orbit, Left
  use Orbit, Right
Orbital portion of frontal bone
  use Orbit, Left
  use Orbit, Right
Orbital portion of lacrimal bone
  use Orbit, Left
  use Orbit, Right
Orbital portion of maxilla
  use Orbit, Left
  use Orbit, Right
Orbital portion of palatine bone
  use Orbit, Left
  use Orbit, Right
Orbital portion of sphenoid bone
  use Orbit, Left
  use Orbit, Right
Orbital portion of zygomatic bone
  use Orbit, Left
  use Orbit, Right
Orchectomy, orchidectomy, orchiectomy
  see Excision, Male Reproductive System ØVB
  see Resection, Male Reproductive System ØVT
Orchidoplasty, orchioplasty
  see Repair, Male Reproductive System ØVQ
  see Replacement, Male Reproductive System ØVR
  see Supplement, Male Reproductive System ØVU
Orchidorrhaphy, orchiorrhaphy *see* Repair, Male
  Reproductive System ØVQ
Orchidotomy, orchiotomy, orchotomy *see* Drainage,
  Male Reproductive System ØV9
Orchiopexy
  see Repair, Male Reproductive System ØVQ
  see Reposition, Male Reproductive System ØVS
Oropharyngeal airway (OPA) *use* Intraluminal Device,
  Airway in Mouth and Throat
Oropharynx *use* Pharynx
Ossiculectomy
  see Excision, Ear, Nose, Sinus Ø9B
  see Resection, Ear, Nose, Sinus Ø9T
Ossiculotomy *see* Drainage, Ear, Nose, Sinus Ø99
Ostectomy
  see Excision, Head and Facial Bones ØNB
  see Excision, Lower Bones ØQB
  see Excision, Upper Bones ØPB
  see Resection, Head and Facial Bones ØNT
  see Resection, Lower Bones ØQT
  see Resection, Upper Bones ØPT
Osteoclasis
  see Division, Head and Facial Bones ØN8
  see Division, Lower Bones ØQ8
  see Division, Upper Bones ØP8
Osteolysis
  see Release, Head and Facial Bones ØNN
  see Release, Lower Bones ØQN
  see Release, Upper Bones ØPN
Osteopathic Treatment
  Abdomen 7WØ9X
  Cervical 7WØ1X
  Extremity
    Lower 7WØ6X
    Upper 7WØ7X
  Head 7WØØX
  Lumbar 7WØ3X
  Pelvis 7WØ5X
  Rib Cage 7WØ8X
  Sacrum 7WØ4X
  Thoracic 7WØ2X
Osteopexy
  see Repair, Head and Facial Bones ØNQ
  see Repair, Lower Bones ØQQ
  see Repair, Upper Bones ØPQ
  see Reposition, Head and Facial Bones ØNS
  see Reposition, Lower Bones ØQS
  see Reposition, Upper Bones ØPS
Osteoplasty
  see Repair, Head and Facial Bones ØNQ
  see Repair, Lower Bones ØQQ

Osteoplasty — *continued*
  see Repair, Upper Bones ØPQ
  see Replacement, Head and Facial Bones ØNR
  see Replacement, Lower Bones ØQR
  see Replacement, Upper Bones ØPR
  see Supplement, Head and Facial Bones ØNU
  see Supplement, Lower Bones ØQU
  see Supplement, Upper Bones ØPU
Osteorrhaphy
  see Repair, Head and Facial Bones ØNQ
  see Repair, Lower Bones ØQQ
  see Repair, Upper Bones ØPQ
Osteotomy, ostotomy
  see Division, Head and Facial Bones ØN8
  see Division, Lower Bones ØQ8
  see Division, Upper Bones ØP8
  see Drainage, Head and Facial Bones ØN9
  see Drainage, Lower Bones ØQ9
  see Drainage, Upper Bones ØP9
Other Imaging
  Bile Duct and Gallbladder, Indocyanine Green Dye,
    Intraoperative BF53200
  Bile Duct, Indocyanine Green Dye, Intraoperative
    BF50200
  Extremity
    Lower BW5CZ1Z
    Upper BW5JZ1Z
  Gallbladder and Bile Duct, Indocyanine Green Dye,
    Intraoperative BF53200
  Gallbladder, Indocyanine Green Dye, Intraoperative
    BF52200
  Head and Neck BW59Z1Z
  Hepatobiliary System, All, Indocyanine Green Dye,
    Intraoperative BF5C200
  Liver and Spleen, Indocyanine Green Dye, Intraop-
    erative BF56200
  Liver, Indocyanine Green Dye, Intraoperative
    BF55200
  Neck and Head BW59Z1Z
  Pancreas, Indocyanine Green Dye, Intraoperative
    BF57200
  Spleen and Liver, Indocyanine Green Dye, Intraop-
    erative BF56200
  Trunk BW52Z1Z
Other New Technology Therapeutic Substance
  XWØ
Otic ganglion *use* Head and Neck Sympathetic Nerve
OTL-101 *use* Hematopoietic Stem/Progenitor Cells,
  Genetically Modified
Otoplasty
  see Repair, Ear, Nose, Sinus Ø9Q
  see Replacement, Ear, Nose, Sinus Ø9R
  see Supplement, Ear, Nose, Sinus Ø9U
Otoscopy *see* Inspection, Ear, Nose, Sinus Ø9J
Oval window
  use Middle Ear, Left
  use Middle Ear, Right
Ovarian artery *use* Abdominal Aorta
Ovarian ligament *use* Uterine Supporting Structure
Ovariectomy
  see Excision, Female Reproductive System ØUB
  see Resection, Female Reproductive System ØUT
Ovariocentesis *see* Drainage, Female Reproductive
  System ØU9
Ovariopexy
  see Repair, Female Reproductive System ØUQ
  see Reposition, Female Reproductive System ØUS
Ovariotomy
  see Division, Female Reproductive System ØU8
  see Drainage, Female Reproductive System ØU9
Ovatio™ CRT-D *use* Cardiac Resynchronization Defibril-
  lator Pulse Generator in ØJH
Oversewing
  Gastrointestinal ulcer *see* Repair, Gastrointestinal
    System ØDQ
  Pleural bleb *see* Repair, Respiratory System ØBQ
Oviduct
  use Fallopian Tube, Left
  use Fallopian Tube, Right
Oximetry, Fetal pulse 10H073Z
OXINIUM *use* Synthetic Substitute, Oxidized Zirconium
  on Polyethylene in ØSR
Oxygenation
  Extracorporeal membrane (ECMO) *see* Perfor-
    mance, Circulatory 5A15
  Hyperbaric *see* Assistance, Circulatory 5AØ5
  Supersaturated *see* Assistance, Circulatory 5AØ5

P

Pacemaker
  Dual Chamber
    Abdomen ØJH8
    Chest ØJH6
  Intracardiac
    Insertion of device in
      Atrium
        Left Ø2H7
        Right Ø2H6
      Vein, Coronary Ø2H4
      Ventricle
        Left Ø2HL
        Right Ø2HK
    Removal of device from, Heart Ø2PA
    Revision of device in, Heart Ø2WA
  Single Chamber
    Abdomen ØJH8
    Chest ØJH6
  Single Chamber Rate Responsive
    Abdomen ØJH8
    Chest ØJH6
Packing
  Abdominal Wall 2W43X5Z
  Anorectal 2Y43X5Z
  Arm
    Lower
      Left 2W4DX5Z
      Right 2W4CX5Z
    Upper
      Left 2W4BX5Z
      Right 2W4AX5Z
  Back 2W45X5Z
  Chest Wall 2W44X5Z
  Ear 2Y42X5Z
  Extremity
    Lower
      Left 2W4MX5Z
      Right 2W4LX5Z
    Upper
      Left 2W49X5Z
      Right 2W48X5Z
  Face 2W41X5Z
  Finger
    Left 2W4KX5Z
    Right 2W4JX5Z
  Foot
    Left 2W4TX5Z
    Right 2W4SX5Z
  Genital Tract, Female 2Y44X5Z
  Hand
    Left 2W4FX5Z
    Right 2W4EX5Z
  Head 2W40X5Z
  Inguinal Region
    Left 2W47X5Z
    Right 2W46X5Z
  Leg
    Lower
      Left 2W4RX5Z
      Right 2W4QX5Z
    Upper
      Left 2W4PX5Z
      Right 2W4NX5Z
  Mouth and Pharynx 2Y40X5Z
  Nasal 2Y41X5Z
  Neck 2W42X5Z
  Thumb
    Left 2W4HX5Z
    Right 2W4GX5Z
  Toe
    Left 2W4VX5Z
    Right 2W4UX5Z
  Urethra 2Y45X5Z
Paclitaxel-eluting coronary stent *use* Intraluminal
  Device, Drug-eluting in Heart and Great Vessels
Paclitaxel-eluting peripheral stent
  use Intraluminal Device, Drug-eluting in Lower
    Arteries
  use Intraluminal Device, Drug-eluting in Upper
    Arteries
Palatine gland *use* Buccal Mucosa
Palatine tonsil *use* Tonsils
Palatine uvula *use* Uvula
Palatoglossal muscle *use* Tongue, Palate, Pharynx
  Muscle

Palatopharyngeal muscle *use* Tongue, Palate, Pharynx Muscle
Palatoplasty
  see Repair, Mouth and Throat ØCQ
  see Replacement, Mouth and Throat ØCR
  see Supplement, Mouth and Throat ØCU
Palatorrhaphy *see* Repair, Mouth and Throat ØCQ
Palmar cutaneous nerve
  use Median Nerve
  use Radial Nerve
Palmar (volar) digital vein
  use Hand Vein, Left
  use Hand Vein, Right
Palmar fascia (aponeurosis)
  use Subcutaneous Tissue and Fascia, Left Hand
  use Subcutaneous Tissue and Fascia, Right Hand
Palmar interosseous muscle
  use Hand Muscle, Left
  use Hand Muscle, Right
Palmar (volar) metacarpal vein
  use Hand Vein, Left
  use Hand Vein, Right
Palmar ulnocarpal ligament
  use Wrist Bursa and Ligament, Left
  use Wrist Bursa and Ligament, Right
Palmaris longus muscle
  use Lower Arm and Wrist Muscle, Left
  use Lower Arm and Wrist Muscle, Right
Pancreatectomy
  see Excision, Pancreas ØFBG
  see Resection, Pancreas ØFTG
Pancreatic artery *use* Splenic Artery
Pancreatic plexus *use* Abdominal Sympathetic Nerve
Pancreatic vein *use* Splenic Vein
Pancreaticoduodenostomy *see* Bypass, Hepatobiliary System and Pancreas ØF1
Pancreaticosplenic lymph node *use* Lymphatic, Aortic
Pancreatogram, endoscopic retrograde *see* Fluoroscopy, Pancreatic Duct BF18
Pancreatolithotomy *see* Extirpation, Pancreas ØFCG
Pancreatotomy
  see Division, Pancreas ØF8G
  see Drainage, Pancreas ØF9G
Panniculectomy
  see Excision, Skin, Abdomen ØHB7
  see Excision, Subcutaneous Tissue and Fascia, Abdomen ØJB8
Paraaortic lymph node *use* Lymphatic, Aortic
Paracentesis
  Eye *see* Drainage, Eye Ø89
  Peritoneal Cavity *see* Drainage, Peritoneal Cavity ØW9G
  Tympanum *see* Drainage, Ear, Nose, Sinus Ø99
Pararectal lymph node *use* Lymphatic, Mesenteric
Parasternal lymph node *use* Lymphatic, Thorax
Parathyroidectomy
  see Excision, Endocrine System ØGB
  see Resection, Endocrine System ØGT
Paratracheal lymph node *use* Lymphatic, Thorax
Paraurethral (Skene's) gland *use* Vestibular Gland
Parenteral nutrition, total *see* Introduction of Nutritional Substance
Parietal lobe *use* Cerebral Hemisphere
Parotid lymph node *use* Lymphatic, Head
Parotid plexus *use* Facial Nerve
Parotidectomy
  see Excision, Mouth and Throat ØCB
  see Resection, Mouth and Throat ØCT
Pars flaccida
  use Tympanic Membrane, Left
  use Tympanic Membrane, Right
Partial joint replacement
  Hip *see* Replacement, Lower Joints ØSR
  Knee *see* Replacement, Lower Joints ØSR
  Shoulder *see* Replacement, Upper Joints ØRR
Partially absorbable mesh *use* Synthetic Substitute
Patch, blood, spinal 3EØR3GC
Patellapexy
  see Repair, Lower Bones ØQQ
  see Reposition, Lower Bones ØQS
Patellaplasty
  see Repair, Lower Bones ØQQ
  see Replacement, Lower Bones ØQR
  see Supplement, Lower Bones ØQU

Patellar ligament
  use Knee Bursa and Ligament, Left
  use Knee Bursa and Ligament, Right
Patellar tendon
  use Knee Tendon, Left
  use Knee Tendon, Right
Patellectomy
  see Excision, Lower Bones ØQB
  see Resection, Lower Bones ØQT
Patellofemoral joint
  use Knee Joint, Left
  use Knee Joint, Left, Femoral Surface
  use Knee Joint, Right
  use Knee Joint, Right, Femoral Surface
Pectineus muscle
  use Upper Leg Muscle, Left
  use Upper Leg Muscle, Right
Pectoral fascia *use* Subcutaneous Tissue and Fascia, Chest
Pectoral (anterior) lymph node
  use Lymphatic Left, Axillary
  use Lymphatic Right, Axillary
Pectoralis major muscle
  use Thorax Muscle, Left
  use Thorax Muscle, Right
Pectoralis minor muscle
  use Thorax Muscle, Left
  use Thorax Muscle, Right
Pedicle-based dynamic stabilization device
  use Spinal Stabilization Device, Pedicle-Based in ØSH
  use Spinal Stabilization Device, Pedicle-Based in ØRH
PEEP (positive end expiratory pressure) *see* Assistance, Respiratory 5AØ9
PEG (percutaneous endoscopic gastrostomy) ØDH63UZ
PEJ (percutaneous endoscopic jejunostomy) ØDHA3UZ
Pelvic splanchnic nerve
  use Abdominal Sympathetic Nerve
  use Sacral Sympathetic Nerve
Penectomy
  see Excision, Male Reproductive System ØVB
  see Resection, Male Reproductive System ØVT
Penile urethra *use* Urethra
Perceval sutureless valve *use* Zooplastic Tissue, Rapid Deployment Technique in New Technology
Percutaneous endoscopic gastrojejunostomy (PEG/J) tube *use* Feeding Device in Gastrointestinal System
Percutaneous endoscopic gastrostomy (PEG) tube *use* Feeding Device in Gastrointestinal System
Percutaneous nephrostomy catheter *use* Drainage Device
Percutaneous transluminal coronary angioplasty (PTCA) *see* Dilation, Heart and Great Vessels Ø27
Performance
  Biliary
    Multiple, Filtration 5A1C6ØZ
    Single, Filtration 5A1CØØZ
  Cardiac
    Continuous
      Output 5A1221Z
      Pacing 5A1223Z
    Intermittent, Pacing 5A1213Z
    Single, Output, Manual 5A12Ø12
  Circulatory
    Continuous
      Central Membrane 5A1522F
      Peripheral Veno-arterial Membrane 5A1522G
      Peripheral Veno-venous Membrane 5A1522H
    Intraoperative
      Central Membrane 5A15A2F
      Peripheral Veno-arterial Membrane 5A15A2G
      Peripheral Veno-venous Membrane 5A15A2H
  Respiratory
    24-96 Consecutive Hours, Ventilation 5A1945Z
    Greater than 96 Consecutive Hours, Ventilation 5A1955Z
    Less than 24 Consecutive Hours, Ventilation 5A1935Z

Performance — *continued*
  Respiratory — *continued*
    Single, Ventilation, Nonmechanical 5A19Ø54
  Urinary
    Continuous, Greater than 18 hours per day, Filtration 5A1D9ØZ
    Intermittent, Less than 6 Hours Per Day, Filtration 5A1D7ØZ
    Prolonged Intermittent, 6-18 hours per day, Filtration 5A1D8ØZ
Perfusion *see* Introduction of substance in or on
Perfusion, donor organ
  Heart 6AB5ØBZ
  Kidney(s) 6ABTØBZ
  Liver 6ABFØBZ
  Lung(s) 6ABBØBZ
Pericardiectomy
  see Excision, Pericardium Ø2BN
  see Resection, Pericardium Ø2TN
Pericardiocentesis *see* Drainage, Pericardial Cavity ØW9D
Pericardiolysis *see* Release, Pericardium Ø2NN
Pericardiophrenic artery
  use Internal Mammary Artery, Left
  use Internal Mammary Artery, Right
Pericardioplasty
  see Repair, Pericardium Ø2QN
  see Replacement, Pericardium Ø2RN
  see Supplement, Pericardium Ø2UN
Pericardiorrhaphy *see* Repair, Pericardium Ø2QN
Pericardiostomy *see* Drainage, Pericardial Cavity ØW9D
Pericardiotomy *see* Drainage, Pericardial Cavity ØW9D
Perimetrium *use* Uterus
Peripheral Intravascular Lithotripsy (Peripheral IVL) *see* Fragmentation
Peripheral parenteral nutrition *see* Introduction of Nutritional Substance
Peripherally inserted central catheter (PICC) *use* Infusion Device
Peritoneal dialysis 3E1M39Z
Peritoneocentesis
  see Drainage, Peritoneal Cavity ØW9G
  see Drainage, Peritoneum ØD9W
Peritoneoplasty
  see Repair, Peritoneum ØDQW
  see Replacement, Peritoneum ØDRW
  see Supplement, Peritoneum ØDUW
Peritoneoscopy ØDJW4ZZ
Peritoneotomy *see* Drainage, Peritoneum ØD9W
Peritoneumectomy *see* Excision, Peritoneum ØDBW
Peroneus brevis muscle
  use Lower Leg Muscle, Left
  use Lower Leg Muscle, Right
Peroneus longus muscle
  use Lower Leg Muscle, Left
  use Lower Leg Muscle, Right
Pessary ring *use* Intraluminal Device, Pessary in Female Reproductive System
PET scan *see* Positron Emission Tomographic (PET) Imaging
Petrous part of temoporal bone
  use Temporal Bone, Left
  use Temporal Bone, Right
Phacoemulsification, lens
  With IOL implant *see* Replacement, Eye Ø8R
  Without IOL implant *see* Extraction, Eye Ø8D
Phalangectomy
  see Excision, Lower Bones ØQB
  see Excision, Upper Bones ØPB
  see Resection, Lower Bones ØQT
  see Resection, Upper Bones ØPT
Phallectomy
  see Excision, Penis ØVBS
  see Resection, Penis ØVTS
Phalloplasty
  see Repair, Penis ØVQS
  see Supplement, Penis ØVUS
Phallotomy *see* Drainage, Penis ØV9S
Pharmacotherapy, for substance abuse
  Antabuse HZ93ZZZ
  Bupropion HZ97ZZZ
  Clonidine HZ96ZZZ
  Levo-alpha-acetyl-methadol (LAAM) HZ92ZZZ
  Methadone Maintenance HZ91ZZZ
  Naloxone HZ95ZZZ
  Naltrexone HZ94ZZZ
  Nicotine Replacement HZ9ØZZZ

Pharmacotherapy, for substance abuse —
   continued
   Psychiatric Medication HZ98ZZZ
   Replacement Medication, Other HZ99ZZZ
Pharyngeal constrictor muscle *use* Tongue, Palate,
   Pharynx Muscle
Pharyngeal plexus *use* Vagus Nerve
Pharyngeal recess *use* Nasopharynx
Pharyngeal tonsil *use* Adenoids
Pharyngogram *see* Fluoroscopy, Pharynix B91G
Pharyngoplasty
   see Repair, Mouth and Throat 0CQ
   see Replacement, Mouth and Throat 0CR
   see Supplement, Mouth and Throat 0CU
Pharyngorrhaphy *see* Repair, Mouth and Throat 0CQ
Pharyngotomy *see* Drainage, Mouth and Throat 0C9
Pharyngotympanic tube
   use Eustachian Tube, Left
   use Eustachian Tube, Right
Pheresis
   Erythrocytes 6A55
   Leukocytes 6A55
   Plasma 6A55
   Platelets 6A55
   Stem Cells
      Cord Blood 6A55
      Hematopoietic 6A55
Phlebectomy
   see Excision, Lower Veins 06B
   see Excision, Upper Veins 05B
   see Extraction, Lower Veins 06D
   see Extraction, Upper Veins 05D
Phlebography
   see Plain Radiography, Veins B50
   Impedance 4A04X51
Phleborrhaphy
   see Repair, Lower Veins 06Q
   see Repair, Upper Veins 05Q
Phlebotomy
   see Drainage, Lower Veins 069
   see Drainage, Upper Veins 059
Photocoagulation
   For Destruction *see* Destruction
   For Repair *see* Repair
Photopheresis, therapeutic *see* Phototherapy, Circu-
   latory 6A65
Phototherapy
   Circulatory 6A65
   Skin 6A60
   Ultraviolet light *see* Ultraviolet Light Therapy,
      Physiological Systems 6A8
Phrenectomy, phrenoneurectomy *see* Excision,
   Nerve, Phrenic 01B2
Phrenemphraxis *see* Destruction, Nerve, Phrenic 0152
Phrenic nerve stimulator generator *use* Stimulator
   Generator in Subcutaneous Tissue and Fascia
Phrenic nerve stimulator lead *use* Diaphragmatic
   Pacemaker Lead in Respiratory System
Phreniclasis *see* Destruction, Nerve, Phrenic 0152
Phrenicoexeresis *see* Extraction, Nerve, Phrenic 01D2
Phrenicotomy *see* Division, Nerve, Phrenic 0182
Phrenicotripsy *see* Destruction, Nerve, Phrenic 0152
Phrenoplasty
   see Repair, Respiratory System 0BQ
   see Supplement, Respiratory System 0BU
Phrenotomy *see* Drainage, Respiratory System 0B9
Physiatry *see* Motor Treatment, Rehabilitation F07
Physical medicine *see* Motor Treatment, Rehabilitation
   F07
Physical therapy *see* Motor Treatment, Rehabilitation
   F07
PHYSIOMESH™ Flexible Composite Mesh *use* Syn-
   thetic Substitute
Pia mater, intracranial *use* Cerebral Meninges
Pia mater, spinal *use* Spinal Meninges
Pinealectomy
   see Excision, Pineal Body 0GB1
   see Resection, Pineal Body 0GT1
Pinealoscopy 0GJ14ZZ
Pinealotomy *see* Drainage, Pineal Body 0G91
Pinna
   use External Ear, Bilateral
   use External Ear, Left
   use External Ear, Right
Pipeline™ (Flex) embolization device *use* Intralumi-
   nal Device, Flow Diverter in 03V
Piriform recess (sinus) *use* Pharynx

Piriformis muscle
   use Hip Muscle, Left
   use Hip Muscle, Right
**PIRRT (Prolonged intermittent renal replacement
   therapy)** 5A1D80Z
Pisiform bone
   use Carpal, Left
   use Carpal, Right
Pisohamate ligament
   use Hand Bursa and Ligament, Left
   use Hand Bursa and Ligament, Right
Pisometacarpal ligament
   use Hand Bursa and Ligament, Left
   use Hand Bursa and Ligament, Right
Pituitectomy
   see Excision, Gland, Pituitary 0GB0
   see Resection, Gland, Pituitary 0GT0
Plain film radiology *see* Plain Radiography
Plain Radiography
   Abdomen BW00ZZZ
   Abdomen and Pelvis BW01ZZZ
   Abdominal Lymphatic
      Bilateral B701
      Unilateral B700
   Airway, Upper BB0DZZZ
   Ankle
      Left BQ0H
      Right BQ0G
   Aorta
      Abdominal B400
      Thoracic B300
      Thoraco-Abdominal B30P
   Aorta and Bilateral Lower Extremity Arteries B40D
   Arch
      Bilateral BN0DZZZ
      Left BN0CZZZ
      Right BN0BZZZ
   Arm
      Left BP0FZZZ
      Right BP0EZZZ
   Artery
      Brachiocephalic-Subclavian, Right B301
      Bronchial B30L
      Bypass Graft, Other B20F
      Cervico-Cerebral Arch B30Q
      Common Carotid
         Bilateral B305
         Left B304
         Right B303
      Coronary
         Bypass Graft
            Multiple B203
            Single B202
         Multiple B201
         Single B200
      External Carotid
         Bilateral B30C
         Left B30B
         Right B309
      Hepatic B402
      Inferior Mesenteric B405
      Intercostal B30L
      Internal Carotid
         Bilateral B308
         Left B307
         Right B306
      Internal Mammary Bypass Graft
         Left B208
         Right B207
      Intra-Abdominal, Other B40B
      Intracranial B30R
      Lower Extremity
         Bilateral and Aorta B40D
         Left B40G
         Right B40F
      Lower, Other B40J
      Lumbar B409
      Pelvic B40C
      Pulmonary
         Left B30T
         Right B30S
      Renal
         Bilateral B408
         Left B407
         Right B406
         Transplant B40M
      Spinal B30M
      Splenic B403

Plain Radiography — *continued*
   Artery — *continued*
      Subclavian, Left B302
      Superior Mesenteric B404
      Upper Extremity
         Bilateral B30K
         Left B30J
         Right B30H
      Upper, Other B30N
      Vertebral
         Bilateral B30G
         Left B30F
         Right B30D
   Bile Duct BF00
   Bile Duct and Gallbladder BF03
   Bladder BT00
      Kidney and Ureter BT04
   Bladder and Urethra BT0B
   Bone
      Facial BN05ZZZ
      Nasal BN04ZZZ
   Bones, Long, All BW0BZZZ
   Breast
      Bilateral BH02ZZZ
      Left BH01ZZZ
      Right BH00ZZZ
   Calcaneus
      Left BQ0KZZZ
      Right BQ0JZZZ
   Chest BW03ZZZ
   Clavicle
      Left BP05ZZZ
      Right BP04ZZZ
   Coccyx BR0FZZZ
   Corpora Cavernosa BV00
   Dialysis Fistula B50W
   Dialysis Shunt B50W
   Disc
      Cervical BR01
      Lumbar BR03
      Thoracic BR02
   Duct
      Lacrimal
         Bilateral B802
         Left B801
         Right B800
      Mammary
         Multiple
            Left BH06
            Right BH05
         Single
            Left BH04
            Right BH03
   Elbow
      Left BP0H
      Right BP0G
   Epididymis
      Left BV02
      Right BV01
   Extremity
      Lower BW0CZZZ
      Upper BW0JZZZ
   Eye
      Bilateral B807ZZZ
      Left B806ZZZ
      Right B805ZZZ
   Facet Joint
      Cervical BR04
      Lumbar BR06
      Thoracic BR05
   Fallopian Tube
      Bilateral BU02
      Left BU01
      Right BU00
   Fallopian Tube and Uterus BU08
   Femur
      Left, Densitometry BQ04ZZ1
      Right, Densitometry BQ03ZZ1
   Finger
      Left BP0SZZZ
      Right BP0RZZZ
   Foot
      Left BQ0MZZZ
      Right BQ0LZZZ
   Forearm
      Left BP0KZZZ
      Right BP0JZZZ
   Gallbladder and Bile Duct BF03

Plain Radiography — *continued*
Gland
  Parotid
    Bilateral B906
    Left B905
    Right B904
  Salivary
    Bilateral B90D
    Left B90C
    Right B90B
  Submandibular
    Bilateral B909
    Left B908
    Right B907
Hand
  Left BP0PZZZ
  Right BP0NZZZ
Heart
  Left B205
  Right B204
  Right and Left B206
Hepatobiliary System, All BF0C
Hip
  Left BQ01
    Densitometry BQ01ZZ1
  Right BQ00
    Densitometry BQ00ZZ1
Humerus
  Left BP0BZZZ
  Right BP0AZZZ
Ileal Diversion Loop BT0C
Intracranial Sinus B502
Joint
  Acromioclavicular, Bilateral BP03ZZZ
  Finger
    Left BP0D
    Right BP0C
  Foot
    Left BQ0Y
    Right BQ0X
  Hand
    Left BP0D
    Right BP0C
  Lumbosacral BR0BZZZ
  Sacroiliac BR0D
  Sternoclavicular
    Bilateral BP02ZZZ
    Left BP01ZZZ
    Right BP00ZZZ
  Temporomandibular
    Bilateral BN09
    Left BN08
    Right BN07
  Thoracolumbar BR08ZZZ
  Toe
    Left BQ0Y
    Right BQ0X
Kidney
  Bilateral BT03
  Left BT02
  Right BT01
  Ureter and Bladder BT04
Knee
  Left BQ08
  Right BQ07
Leg
  Left BQ0FZZZ
  Right BQ0DZZZ
Lymphatic
  Head B704
  Lower Extremity
    Bilateral B70B
    Left B709
    Right B708
  Neck B704
  Pelvic B70C
  Upper Extremity
    Bilateral B707
    Left B706
    Right B705
Mandible BN06ZZZ
Mastoid B90HZZZ
Nasopharynx B90FZZZ
Optic Foramina
  Left B804ZZZ
  Right B803ZZZ
Orbit
  Bilateral BN03ZZZ
  Left BN02ZZZ

Plain Radiography — *continued*
Orbit — *continued*
  Right BN01ZZZ
Oropharynx B90FZZZ
Patella
  Left BQ0WZZZ
  Right BQ0VZZZ
Pelvis BR0CZZZ
Pelvis and Abdomen BW01ZZZ
Prostate BV03
Retroperitoneal Lymphatic
  Bilateral B701
  Unilateral B700
Ribs
  Left BP0YZZZ
  Right BP0XZZZ
Sacrum BR0FZZZ
Scapula
  Left BP07ZZZ
  Right BP06ZZZ
Shoulder
  Left BP09
  Right BP08
Sinus
  Intracranial B502
  Paranasal B902ZZZ
Skull BN00ZZZ
Spinal Cord B00B
Spine
  Cervical, Densitometry BR00ZZ1
  Lumbar, Densitometry BR09ZZ1
  Thoracic, Densitometry BR07ZZ1
  Whole, Densitometry BR0GZZ1
Sternum BR0HZZZ
Teeth
  All BN0JZZZ
  Multiple BN0HZZZ
Testicle
  Left BV06
  Right BV05
Toe
  Left BQ0QZZZ
  Right BQ0PZZZ
Tooth, Single BN0GZZZ
Tracheobronchial Tree
  Bilateral BB09YZZ
  Left BB08YZZ
  Right BB07YZZ
Ureter
  Bilateral BT08
  Kidney and Bladder BT04
  Left BT07
  Right BT06
Urethra BT05
Urethra and Bladder BT0B
Uterus BU06
Uterus and Fallopian Tube BU08
Vagina BU09
Vasa Vasorum BV08
Vein
  Cerebellar B501
  Cerebral B501
  Epidural B500
  Jugular
    Bilateral B505
    Left B504
    Right B503
  Lower Extremity
    Bilateral B50D
    Left B50C
    Right B50B
  Other B50V
  Pelvic (Iliac)
    Left B50G
    Right B50F
  Pelvic (Iliac) Bilateral B50H
  Portal B50T
  Pulmonary
    Bilateral B50S
    Left B50R
    Right B50Q
  Renal
    Bilateral B50L
    Left B50K
    Right B50J
  Spanchnic B50T
  Subclavian
    Left B507
    Right B506

Plain Radiography — *continued*
Vein — *continued*
  Upper Extremity
    Bilateral B50P
    Left B50N
    Right B50M
Vena Cava
  Inferior B509
  Superior B508
Whole Body BW0KZZZ
  Infant BW0MZZZ
Whole Skeleton BW0LZZZ
Wrist
  Left BP0M
  Right BP0L

Planar Nuclear Medicine Imaging
Abdomen CW10
Abdomen and Chest CW14
Abdomen and Pelvis CW11
Anatomical Region, Other CW1ZZZZ
Anatomical Regions, Multiple CW1YYZZ
Bladder and Ureters CT1H
Bladder, Kidneys and Ureters CT13
Blood C713
Bone Marrow C710
Brain C010
Breast CH1YYZZ
  Bilateral CH12
  Left CH11
  Right CH10
Bronchi and Lungs CB12
Central Nervous System C01YYZZ
Cerebrospinal Fluid C015
Chest CW13
Chest and Abdomen CW14
Chest and Neck CW16
Digestive System CD1YYZZ
Ducts, Lacrimal, Bilateral C819
Ear, Nose, Mouth and Throat C91YYZZ
Endocrine System CG1YYZZ
Extremity
  Lower CW1D
    Bilateral CP1F
    Left CP1D
    Right CP1C
  Upper CW1M
    Bilateral CP1B
    Left CP19
    Right CP18
Eye C81YYZZ
Gallbladder CF14
Gastrointestinal Tract CD17
  Upper CD15
Gland
  Adrenal, Bilateral CG14
  Parathyroid CG11
  Thyroid CG12
Glands, Salivary, Bilateral C91B
Head and Neck CW1B
Heart C21YYZZ
  Right and Left C216
Hepatobiliary System, All CF1C
Hepatobiliary System and Pancreas CF1YYZZ
Kidneys, Ureters and Bladder CT13
Liver CF15
Liver and Spleen CF16
Lungs and Bronchi CB12
Lymphatics
  Head C71J
  Head and Neck C715
  Lower Extremity C71P
  Neck C71K
  Pelvic C71D
  Trunk C71M
  Upper Chest C71L
  Upper Extremity C71N
Lymphatics and Hematologic System C71YYZZ
Musculoskeletal System
  All CP1Z
  Other CP1YYZZ
Myocardium C21G
Neck and Chest CW16
Neck and Head CW1B
Pancreas and Hepatobiliary System CF1YYZZ
Pelvic Region CW1J
Pelvis CP16
Pelvis and Abdomen CW11
Pelvis and Spine CP17
Reproductive System, Male CV1YYZZ

Subterms under main terms may continue to next column or page

Posterior ulnar recurrent artery
  use Ulnar Artery, Left
  use Ulnar Artery, Right
Posterior vagal trunk *use* Vagus Nerve
PPN (peripheral parenteral nutrition) *see* Introduction of Nutritional Substance
Preauricular lymph node *use* Lymphatic, Head
Precava *use* Superior Vena Cava
PRECICE intramedullary limb lengthening system
  use Internal Fixation Device, Intramedullary Limb Lengthening in ØPH
  use Internal Fixation Device, Intramedullary Limb Lengthening in ØQH
Prepatellar bursa
  use Knee Bursa and Ligament, Left
  use Knee Bursa and Ligament, Right
Preputiotomy *see* Drainage, Male Reproductive System ØV9
Pressure support ventilation *see* Performance, Respiratory 5A19
PRESTIGE® Cervical Disc *use* Synthetic Substitute
Pretracheal fascia
  use Subcutaneous Tissue and Fascia, Left Neck
  use Subcutaneous Tissue and Fascia, Right Neck
Prevertebral fascia
  use Subcutaneous Tissue and Fascia, Left Neck
  use Subcutaneous Tissue and Fascia, Right Neck
PrimeAdvanced neurostimulator (SureScan) (MRI Safe) *use* Stimulator Generator, Multiple Array in ØJH
Princeps pollicis artery
  use Hand Artery, Left
  use Hand Artery, Right
Probing, duct
  Diagnostic *see* Inspection
  Dilation *see* Dilation
PROCEED™ Ventral Patch *use* Synthetic Substitute
Procerus muscle *use* Facial Muscle
Proctectomy
  see Excision, Rectum ØDBP
  see Resection, Rectum ØDTP
Proctoclysis *see* Introduction of substance in or on, Gastrointestinal Tract, Lower 3EØH
Proctocolectomy
  see Excision, Gastrointestinal System ØDB
  see Resection, Gastrointestinal System ØDT
Proctocolpoplasty
  see Repair, Gastrointestinal System ØDQ
  see Supplement, Gastrointestinal System ØDU
Proctoperineoplasty
  see Repair, Gastrointestinal System ØDQ
  see Supplement, Gastrointestinal System ØDU
Proctoperineorrhaphy *see* Repair, Gastrointestinal System ØDQ
Proctopexy
  see Repair, Rectum ØDQP
  see Reposition, Rectum ØDSP
Proctoplasty
  see Repair, Rectum ØDQP
  see Supplement, Rectum ØDUP
Proctorrhaphy *see* Repair, Rectum ØDQP
Proctoscopy ØDJD8ZZ
Proctosigmoidectomy
  see Excision, Gastrointestinal System ØDB
  see Resection, Gastrointestinal System ØDT
Proctosigmoidoscopy ØDJD8ZZ
Proctostomy *see* Drainage, Rectum ØD9P
Proctotomy *see* Drainage, Rectum ØD9P
Prodisc-C *use* Synthetic Substitute
Prodisc-L *use* Synthetic Substitute
Production, atrial septal defect *see* Excision, Septum, Atrial Ø2B5
Profunda brachii
  use Brachial Artery, Left
  use Brachial Artery, Right
Profunda femoris (deep femoral) vein
  use Femoral Vein, Left
  use Femoral Vein, Right
PROLENE Polypropylene Hernia System (PHS) *use* Synthetic Substitute
Prolonged intermittent renal replacement therapy (PIRRT) 5A1D80Z
Pronator quadratus muscle
  use Lower Arm and Wrist Muscle, Left
  use Lower Arm and Wrist Muscle, Right

Pronator teres muscle
  use Lower Arm and Wrist Muscle, Left
  use Lower Arm and Wrist Muscle, Right
Prostatectomy
  see Excision, Prostate ØVBØ
  see Resection, Prostate ØVTØ
Prostatic urethra *use* Urethra
Prostatomy, prostatotomy *see* Drainage, Prostate ØV9Ø
Protecta XT CRT-D *use* Cardiac Resynchronization Defibrillator Pulse Generator in ØJH
Protecta XT DR (XT VR) *use* Defibrillator Generator in ØJH
Protégé® RX Carotid Stent System *use* Intraluminal Device
Proximal radioulnar joint
  use Elbow Joint, Left
  use Elbow Joint, Right
Psoas muscle
  use Hip Muscle, Left
  use Hip Muscle, Right
PSV (pressure support ventilation) *see* Performance, Respiratory 5A19
Psychoanalysis GZ54ZZZ
Psychological Tests
  Cognitive Status GZ14ZZZ
  Developmental GZ1ØZZZ
  Intellectual and Psychoeducational GZ12ZZZ
  Neurobehavioral Status GZ14ZZZ
  Neuropsychological GZ13ZZZ
  Personality and Behavioral GZ11ZZZ
Psychotherapy
  Family, Mental Health Services GZ72ZZZ
  Group GZHZZZZ
    Mental Health Services GZHZZZZ
  Individual
    see Psychotherapy, Individual, Mental Health Services
    for substance abuse
      12-Step HZ53ZZZ
      Behavioral HZ51ZZZ
      Cognitive HZ5ØZZZ
      Cognitive-Behavioral HZ52ZZZ
      Confrontational HZ58ZZZ
      Interactive HZ55ZZZ
      Interpersonal HZ54ZZZ
      Motivational Enhancement HZ57ZZZ
      Psychoanalysis HZ5BZZZ
      Psychodynamic HZ5CZZZ
      Psychoeducation HZ56ZZZ
      Psychophysiological HZ5DZZZ
      Supportive HZ59ZZZ
  Mental Health Services
    Behavioral GZ51ZZZ
    Cognitive GZ52ZZZ
    Cognitive-Behavioral GZ58ZZZ
    Interactive GZ5ØZZZ
    Interpersonal GZ53ZZZ
    Psychoanalysis GZ54ZZZ
    Psychodynamic GZ55ZZZ
    Psychophysiological GZ59ZZZ
    Supportive GZ56ZZZ
PTCA (percutaneous transluminal coronary angioplasty) *see* Dilation, Heart and Great Vessels Ø27
Pterygoid muscle *use* Head Muscle
Pterygoid process *use* Sphenoid Bone
Pterygopalatine (sphenopalatine) ganglion *use* Head and Neck Sympathetic Nerve
Pubis
  use Pelvic Bone, Left
  use Pelvic Bone, Right
Pubofemoral ligament
  use Hip Bursa and Ligament, Left
  use Hip Bursa and Ligament, Right
Pudendal nerve *use* Sacral Plexus
Pull-through, laparoscopic-assisted transanal
  see Excision, Gastrointestinal System ØDB
  see Resection, Gastrointestinal System ØDT
Pull-through, rectal *see* Resection, Rectum ØDTP
Pulmoaortic canal *use* Pulmonary Artery, Left
Pulmonary annulus *use* Pulmonary Valve
Pulmonary artery wedge monitoring *see* Monitoring, Arterial 4A13
Pulmonary plexus
  use Thoracic Sympathetic Nerve
  use Vagus Nerve
Pulmonic valve *use* Pulmonary Valve

Pulpectomy *see* Excision, Mouth and Throat ØCB
Pulverization *see* Fragmentation
Pulvinar *use* Thalamus
Pump reservoir *use* Infusion Device, Pump in Subcutaneous Tissue and Fascia
Punch biopsy *see* Excision with qualifier Diagnostic
Puncture *see* Drainage
Puncture, lumbar *see* Drainage, Spinal Canal ØØ9U
Pyelography
  see Fluoroscopy, Urinary System BT1
  see Plain Radiography, Urinary System BTØ
Pyeloileostomy, urinary diversion *see* Bypass, Urinary System ØT1
Pyeloplasty
  see Repair, Urinary System ØTQ
  see Replacement, Urinary System ØTR
  see Supplement, Urinary System ØTU
Pyeloplasty, dismembered *see* Repair, Kidney Pelvis
Pyelorrhaphy *see* Repair, Urinary System ØTQ
Pyeloscopy ØTJ58ZZ
Pyelostomy
  see Bypass, Urinary System ØT1
  see Drainage, Urinary System ØT9
Pyelotomy *see* Drainage, Urinary System ØT9
Pylorectomy
  see Excision, Stomach, Pylorus ØDB7
  see Resection, Stomach, Pylorus ØDT7
Pyloric antrum *use* Stomach, Pylorus
Pyloric canal *use* Stomach, Pylorus
Pyloric sphincter *use* Stomach, Pylorus
Pylorodiosis *see* Dilation, Stomach, Pylorus ØD77
Pylorogastrectomy
  see Excision, Gastrointestinal System ØDB
  see Resection, Gastrointestinal System ØDT
Pyloroplasty
  see Repair, Stomach, Pylorus ØDQ7
  see Supplement, Stomach, Pylorus ØDU7
Pyloroscopy ØDJ68ZZ
Pylorotomy *see* Drainage, Stomach, Pylorus ØD97
Pyramidalis muscle
  use Abdomen Muscle, Left
  use Abdomen Muscle, Right

Q

Quadrangular cartilage *use* Nasal Septum
Quadrant resection of breast *see* Excision, Skin and Breast ØHB
Quadrate lobe *use* Liver
Quadratus femoris muscle
  use Hip Muscle, Left
  use Hip Muscle, Right
Quadratus lumborum muscle
  use Trunk Muscle, Left
  use Trunk Muscle, Right
Quadratus plantae muscle
  use Foot Muscle, Left
  use Foot Muscle, Right
Quadriceps (femoris)
  use Upper Leg Muscle, Left
  use Upper Leg Muscle, Right
Quarantine 8EØZXY6

R

Radial collateral carpal ligament
  use Wrist Bursa and Ligament, Left
  use Wrist Bursa and Ligament, Right
Radial collateral ligament
  use Elbow Bursa and Ligament, Left
  use Elbow Bursa and Ligament, Right
Radial notch
  use Ulna, Left
  use Ulna, Right
Radial recurrent artery
  use Radial Artery, Left
  use Radial Artery, Right
Radial vein
  use Brachial Vein, Left
  use Brachial Vein, Right
Radialis indicis
  use Hand Artery, Left
  use Hand Artery, Right
Radiation Therapy
  see Beam Radiation

Radiation Therapy — continued
see Brachytherapy
see Stereotactic Radiosurgery
Radiation treatment see Radiation Therapy
Radiocarpal joint
use Wrist Joint, Left
use Wrist Joint, Right
Radiocarpal ligament
use Wrist Bursa and Ligament, Left
use Wrist Bursa and Ligament, Right
Radiography see Plain Radiography
Radiology, analog see Plain Radiography
Radiology, diagnostic see Imaging, Diagnostic
Radioulnar ligament
use Wrist Bursa and Ligament, Left
use Wrist Bursa and Ligament, Right
Range of motion testing see Motor Function Assessment, Rehabilitation F01
REALIZE® Adjustable Gastric Band use Extraluminal Device
Reattachment
Abdominal Wall ØWMFØZZ
Ampulla of Vater ØFMC
Ankle Region
  Left ØYMLØZZ
  Right ØYMKØZZ
Arm
  Lower
    Left ØXMFØZZ
    Right ØXMDØZZ
  Upper
    Left ØXM9ØZZ
    Right ØXM8ØZZ
Axilla
  Left ØXM5ØZZ
  Right ØXM4ØZZ
Back
  Lower ØWMLØZZ
  Upper ØWMKØZZ
Bladder ØTMB
Bladder Neck ØTMC
Breast
  Bilateral ØHMVXZZ
  Left ØHMUXZZ
  Right ØHMTXZZ
Bronchus
  Lingula ØBM9ØZZ
  Lower Lobe
    Left ØBMBØZZ
    Right ØBM6ØZZ
  Main
    Left ØBM7ØZZ
    Right ØBM3ØZZ
  Middle Lobe, Right ØBM5ØZZ
  Upper Lobe
    Left ØBM8ØZZ
    Right ØBM4ØZZ
Bursa and Ligament
  Abdomen
    Left ØMMJ
    Right ØMMH
  Ankle
    Left ØMMR
    Right ØMMQ
  Elbow
    Left ØMM4
    Right ØMM3
  Foot
    Left ØMMT
    Right ØMMS
  Hand
    Left ØMM8
    Right ØMM7
  Head and Neck ØMMØ
  Hip
    Left ØMMM
    Right ØMML
  Knee
    Left ØMMP
    Right ØMMN
  Lower Extremity
    Left ØMMW
    Right ØMMV
  Perineum ØMMK
  Rib(s) ØMMG
  Shoulder
    Left ØMM2
    Right ØMM1

Reattachment — continued
Bursa and Ligament — continued
  Spine
    Lower ØMMD
    Upper ØMMC
  Sternum ØMMF
  Upper Extremity
    Left ØMMB
    Right ØMM9
  Wrist
    Left ØMM6
    Right ØMM5
Buttock
  Left ØYM1ØZZ
  Right ØYMØØZZ
Carina ØBM2ØZZ
Cecum ØDMH
Cervix ØUMC
Chest Wall ØWM8ØZZ
Clitoris ØUMJXZZ
Colon
  Ascending ØDMK
  Descending ØDMM
  Sigmoid ØDMN
  Transverse ØDML
Cord
  Bilateral ØVMH
  Left ØVMG
  Right ØVMF
Cul-de-sac ØUMF
Diaphragm ØBMTØZZ
Duct
  Common Bile ØFM9
  Cystic ØFM8
  Hepatic
    Common ØFM7
    Left ØFM6
    Right ØFM5
  Pancreatic ØFMD
    Accessory ØFMF
Duodenum ØDM9
Ear
  Left Ø9M1XZZ
  Right Ø9MØXZZ
Elbow Region
  Left ØXMCØZZ
  Right ØXMBØZZ
Esophagus ØDM5
Extremity
  Lower
    Left ØYMBØZZ
    Right ØYM9ØZZ
  Upper
    Left ØXM7ØZZ
    Right ØXM6ØZZ
Eyelid
  Lower
    Left Ø8MRXZZ
    Right Ø8MQXZZ
  Upper
    Left Ø8MPXZZ
    Right Ø8MNXZZ
Face ØWM2ØZZ
Fallopian Tube
  Left ØUM6
  Right ØUM5
Fallopian Tubes, Bilateral ØUM7
Femoral Region
  Left ØYM8ØZZ
  Right ØYM7ØZZ
Finger
  Index
    Left ØXMPØZZ
    Right ØXMNØZZ
  Little
    Left ØXMWØZZ
    Right ØXMVØZZ
  Middle
    Left ØXMRØZZ
    Right ØXMQØZZ
  Ring
    Left ØXMTØZZ
    Right ØXMSØZZ
Foot
  Left ØYMNØZZ
  Right ØYMMØZZ
Forequarter
  Left ØXM1ØZZ
  Right ØXMØØZZ

Reattachment — continued
Gallbladder ØFM4
Gland
  Left ØGM2
  Right ØGM3
Hand
  Left ØXMKØZZ
  Right ØXMJØZZ
Hindquarter
  Bilateral ØYM4ØZZ
  Left ØYM3ØZZ
  Right ØYM2ØZZ
Hymen ØUMK
Ileum ØDMB
Inguinal Region
  Left ØYM6ØZZ
  Right ØYM5ØZZ
Intestine
  Large ØDME
    Left ØDMG
    Right ØDMF
  Small ØDM8
Jaw
  Lower ØWM5ØZZ
  Upper ØWM4ØZZ
Jejunum ØDMA
Kidney
  Left ØTM1
  Right ØTMØ
Kidney Pelvis
  Left ØTM4
  Right ØTM3
Kidneys, Bilateral ØTM2
Knee Region
  Left ØYMGØZZ
  Right ØYMFØZZ
Leg
  Lower
    Left ØYMJØZZ
    Right ØYMHØZZ
  Upper
    Left ØYMDØZZ
    Right ØYMCØZZ
Lip
  Lower ØCM1ØZZ
  Upper ØCMØØZZ
Liver ØFMØ
  Left Lobe ØFM2
  Right Lobe ØFM1
Lung
  Left ØBMLØZZ
  Lower Lobe
    Left ØBMJØZZ
    Right ØBMFØZZ
  Middle Lobe, Right ØBMDØZZ
  Right ØBMKØZZ
  Upper Lobe
    Left ØBMGØZZ
    Right ØBMCØZZ
Lung Lingula ØBMHØZZ
Muscle
  Abdomen
    Left ØKML
    Right ØKMK
  Facial ØKM1
  Foot
    Left ØKMW
    Right ØKMV
  Hand
    Left ØKMD
    Right ØKMC
  Head ØKMØ
  Hip
    Left ØKMP
    Right ØKMN
  Lower Arm and Wrist
    Left ØKMB
    Right ØKM9
  Lower Leg
    Left ØKMT
    Right ØKMS
  Neck
    Left ØKM3
    Right ØKM2
  Perineum ØKMM
  Shoulder
    Left ØKM6
    Right ØKM5

Reattachment — *continued*
Muscle — *continued*
Thorax
Left ØKMJ
Right ØKMH
Tongue, Palate, Pharynx ØKM4
Trunk
Left ØKMG
Right ØKMF
Upper Arm
Left ØKM8
Right ØKM7
Upper Leg
Left ØKMR
Right ØKMQ
Nasal Mucosa and Soft Tissue Ø9MKXZZ
Neck ØWM6ØZZ
Nipple
Left ØHMXXZZ
Right ØHMWXZZ
Ovary
Bilateral ØUM2
Left ØUM1
Right ØUMØ
Palate, Soft ØCM3ØZZ
Pancreas ØFMG
Parathyroid Gland ØGMR
Inferior
Left ØGMP
Right ØGMN
Multiple ØGMQ
Superior
Left ØGMM
Right ØGML
Penis ØVMSXZZ
Perineum
Female ØWMNØZZ
Male ØWMMØZZ
Rectum ØDMP
Scrotum ØVM5XZZ
Shoulder Region
Left ØXM3ØZZ
Right ØXM2ØZZ
Skin
Abdomen ØHM7XZZ
Back ØHM6XZZ
Buttock ØHM8XZZ
Chest ØHM5XZZ
Ear
Left ØHM3XZZ
Right ØHM2XZZ
Face ØHM1XZZ
Foot
Left ØHMNXZZ
Right ØHMMXZZ
Hand
Left ØHMGXZZ
Right ØHMFXZZ
Inguinal ØHMAXZZ
Lower Arm
Left ØHMEXZZ
Right ØHMDXZZ
Lower Leg
Left ØHMLXZZ
Right ØHMKXZZ
Neck ØHM4XZZ
Perineum ØHM9XZZ
Scalp ØHMØXZZ
Upper Arm
Left ØHMCXZZ
Right ØHMBXZZ
Upper Leg
Left ØHMJXZZ
Right ØHMHXZZ
Stomach ØDM6
Tendon
Abdomen
Left ØLMG
Right ØLMF
Ankle
Left ØLMT
Right ØLMS
Foot
Left ØLMW
Right ØLMV
Hand
Left ØLM8
Right ØLM7
Head and Neck ØLMØ

Reattachment — *continued*
Tendon — *continued*
Hip
Left ØLMK
Right ØLMJ
Knee
Left ØLMR
Right ØLMQ
Lower Arm and Wrist
Left ØLM6
Right ØLM5
Lower Leg
Left ØLMP
Right ØLMN
Perineum ØLMH
Shoulder
Left ØLM2
Right ØLM1
Thorax
Left ØLMD
Right ØLMC
Trunk
Left ØLMB
Right ØLM9
Upper Arm
Left ØLM4
Right ØLM3
Upper Leg
Left ØLMM
Right ØLML
Testis
Bilateral ØVMC
Left ØVMB
Right ØVM9
Thumb
Left ØXMMØZZ
Right ØXMLØZZ
Thyroid Gland
Left Lobe ØGMG
Right Lobe ØGMH
Toe
1st
Left ØYMQØZZ
Right ØYMPØZZ
2nd
Left ØYMSØZZ
Right ØYMRØZZ
3rd
Left ØYMUØZZ
Right ØYMTØZZ
4th
Left ØYMWØZZ
Right ØYMVØZZ
5th
Left ØYMYØZZ
Right ØYMXØZZ
Tongue ØCM7ØZZ
Tooth
Lower ØCMX
Upper ØCMW
Trachea ØBM1ØZZ
Tunica Vaginalis
Left ØVM7
Right ØVM6
Ureter
Left ØTM7
Right ØTM6
Ureters, Bilateral ØTM8
Urethra ØTMD
Uterine Supporting Structure ØUM4
Uterus ØUM9
Uvula ØCMNØZZ
Vagina ØUMG
Vulva ØUMMXZZ
Wrist Region
Left ØXMHØZZ
Right ØXMGØZZ
REBOA (resuscitative endovascular balloon occlusion of the aorta)
Ø2LW3DJ
Ø4LØ3DJ
Rebound HRD® (Hernia Repair Device) *use* Synthetic Substitute
RECELL® cell suspension autograft *see* Replacement, Skin and Breast ØHR
Recession
see Repair
see Reposition

Reclosure, disrupted abdominal wall ØWQFXZZ
Reconstruction
see Repair
see Replacement
see Supplement
Rectectomy
see Excision, Rectum ØDBP
see Resection, Rectum ØDTP
Rectocele repair *see* Repair, Subcutaneous Tissue and Fascia, Pelvic Region ØJQC
Rectopexy
see Repair, Gastrointestinal System ØDQ
see Reposition, Gastrointestinal System ØDS
Rectoplasty
see Repair, Gastrointestinal System ØDQ
see Supplement, Gastrointestinal System ØDU
Rectorrhaphy *see* Repair, Gastrointestinal System ØDQ
Rectoscopy ØDJD8ZZ
Rectosigmoid junction *use* Sigmoid Colon
Rectosigmoidectomy
see Excision, Gastrointestinal System ØDB
see Resection, Gastrointestinal System ØDT
Rectostomy *see* Drainage, Rectum ØD9P
Rectotomy *see* Drainage, Rectum ØD9P
Rectus abdominis muscle
use Abdomen Muscle, Left
use Abdomen Muscle, Right
Rectus femoris muscle
use Upper Leg Muscle, Left
use Upper Leg Muscle, Right
Recurrent laryngeal nerve *use* Vagus Nerve
Reduction
Dislocation *see* Reposition
Fracture *see* Reposition
Intussusception, intestinal *see* Reposition, Gastrointestinal System ØDS
Mammoplasty *see* Excision, Skin and Breast ØHB
Prolapse *see* Reposition
Torsion *see* Reposition
Volvulus, gastrointestinal *see* Reposition, Gastrointestinal System ØDS
Refusion *see* Fusion
Rehabilitation
see Activities of Daily Living Assessment, Rehabilitation FØ2
see Activities of Daily Living Treatment, Rehabilitation FØ8
see Caregiver Training, Rehabilitation FØF
see Cochlear Implant Treatment, Rehabilitation FØB
see Device Fitting, Rehabilitation FØD
see Hearing Treatment, Rehabilitation FØ9
see Motor Function Assessment, Rehabilitation FØ1
see Motor Treatment, Rehabilitation FØ7
see Speech Assessment, Rehabilitation FØØ
see Speech Treatment, Rehabilitation FØ6
see Vestibular Treatment, Rehabilitation FØC
Reimplantation
see Reattachment
see Reposition
see Transfer
Reinforcement
see Repair
see Supplement
Relaxation, scar tissue *see* Release
Release
Acetabulum
Left ØQN5
Right ØQN4
Adenoids ØCNQ
Ampulla of Vater ØFNC
Anal Sphincter ØDNR
Anterior Chamber
Left Ø8N33ZZ
Right Ø8N23ZZ
Anus ØDNQ
Aorta
Abdominal Ø4NØ
Thoracic
Ascending/Arch Ø2NX
Descending Ø2NW
Aortic Body ØGND
Appendix ØDNJ
Artery
Anterior Tibial
Left Ø4NQ

Subterms under main terms may continue to next column or page

Release — continued
  Artery — continued
    Anterior Tibial — continued
      Right 04NP
    Axillary
      Left 03N6
      Right 03N5
    Brachial
      Left 03N8
      Right 03N7
    Celiac 04N1
    Colic
      Left 04N7
      Middle 04N8
      Right 04N6
    Common Carotid
      Left 03NJ
      Right 03NH
    Common Iliac
      Left 04ND
      Right 04NC
    Coronary
      Four or More Arteries 02N3
      One Artery 02N0
      Three Arteries 02N2
      Two Arteries 02N1
    External Carotid
      Left 03NN
      Right 03NM
    External Iliac
      Left 04NJ
      Right 04NH
    Face 03NR
    Femoral
      Left 04NL
      Right 04NK
    Foot
      Left 04NW
      Right 04NV
    Gastric 04N2
    Hand
      Left 03NF
      Right 03ND
    Hepatic 04N3
    Inferior Mesenteric 04NB
    Innominate 03N2
    Internal Carotid
      Left 03NL
      Right 03NK
    Internal Iliac
      Left 04NF
      Right 04NE
    Internal Mammary
      Left 03N1
      Right 03N0
    Intracranial 03NG
    Lower 04NY
    Peroneal
      Left 04NU
      Right 04NT
    Popliteal
      Left 04NN
      Right 04NM
    Posterior Tibial
      Left 04NS
      Right 04NR
    Pulmonary
      Left 02NR
      Right 02NQ
    Pulmonary Trunk 02NP
    Radial
      Left 03NC
      Right 03NB
    Renal
      Left 04NA
      Right 04N9
    Splenic 04N4
    Subclavian
      Left 03N4
      Right 03N3
    Superior Mesenteric 04N5
    Temporal
      Left 03NT
      Right 03NS
    Thyroid
      Left 03NV
      Right 03NU
    Ulnar
      Left 03NA

Release — continued
  Artery — continued
    Ulnar — continued
      Right 03N9
    Upper 03NY
    Vertebral
      Left 03NQ
      Right 03NP
  Atrium
    Left 02N7
    Right 02N6
  Auditory Ossicle
    Left 09NA
    Right 09N9
  Basal Ganglia 00N8
  Bladder 0TNB
  Bladder Neck 0TNC
  Bone
    Ethmoid
      Left 0NNG
      Right 0NNF
    Frontal 0NN1
    Hyoid 0NNX
    Lacrimal
      Left 0NNJ
      Right 0NNH
    Nasal 0NNB
    Occipital 0NN7
    Palatine
      Left 0NNL
      Right 0NNK
    Parietal
      Left 0NN4
      Right 0NN3
    Pelvic
      Left 0QN3
      Right 0QN2
    Sphenoid 0NNC
    Temporal
      Left 0NN6
      Right 0NN5
    Zygomatic
      Left 0NNN
      Right 0NNM
  Brain 00N0
  Breast
    Bilateral 0HNV
    Left 0HNU
    Right 0HNT
  Bronchus
    Lingula 0BN9
    Lower Lobe
      Left 0BNB
      Right 0BN6
    Main
      Left 0BN7
      Right 0BN3
    Middle Lobe, Right 0BN5
    Upper Lobe
      Left 0BN8
      Right 0BN4
  Buccal Mucosa 0CN4
  Bursa and Ligament
    Abdomen
      Left 0MNJ
      Right 0MNH
    Ankle
      Left 0MNR
      Right 0MNQ
    Elbow
      Left 0MN4
      Right 0MN3
    Foot
      Left 0MNT
      Right 0MNS
    Hand
      Left 0MN8
      Right 0MN7
    Head and Neck 0MN0
    Hip
      Left 0MNM
      Right 0MNL
    Knee
      Left 0MNP
      Right 0MNN
    Lower Extremity
      Left 0MNW
      Right 0MNV
    Perineum 0MNK

Release — continued
  Bursa and Ligament — continued
    Rib(s) 0MNG
    Shoulder
      Left 0MN2
      Right 0MN1
    Spine
      Lower 0MND
      Upper 0MNC
    Sternum 0MNF
    Upper Extremity
      Left 0MNB
      Right 0MN9
    Wrist
      Left 0MN6
      Right 0MN5
  Carina 0BN2
  Carotid Bodies, Bilateral 0GN8
  Carotid Body
    Left 0GN6
    Right 0GN7
  Carpal
    Left 0PNN
    Right 0PNM
  Cecum 0DNH
  Cerebellum 00NC
  Cerebral Hemisphere 00N7
  Cerebral Meninges 00N1
  Cerebral Ventricle 00N6
  Cervix 0UNC
  Chordae Tendineae 02N9
  Choroid
    Left 08NB
    Right 08NA
  Cisterna Chyli 07NL
  Clavicle
    Left 0PNB
    Right 0PN9
  Clitoris 0UNJ
  Coccygeal Glomus 0GNB
  Coccyx 0QNS
  Colon
    Ascending 0DNK
    Descending 0DNM
    Sigmoid 0DNN
    Transverse 0DNL
  Conduction Mechanism 02N8
  Conjunctiva
    Left 08NTXZZ
    Right 08NSXZZ
  Cord
    Bilateral 0VNH
    Left 0VNG
    Right 0VNF
  Cornea
    Left 08N9XZZ
    Right 08N8XZZ
  Cul-de-sac 0UNF
  Diaphragm 0BNT
  Disc
    Cervical Vertebral 0RN3
    Cervicothoracic Vertebral 0RN5
    Lumbar Vertebral 0SN2
    Lumbosacral 0SN4
    Thoracic Vertebral 0RN9
    Thoracolumbar Vertebral 0RNB
  Duct
    Common Bile 0FN9
    Cystic 0FN8
    Hepatic
      Common 0FN7
      Left 0FN6
      Right 0FN5
    Lacrimal
      Left 08NY
      Right 08NX
    Pancreatic 0FND
      Accessory 0FNF
    Parotid
      Left 0CNC
      Right 0CNB
  Duodenum 0DN9
  Dura Mater 00N2
  Ear
    External
      Left 09N1
      Right 09N0
    External Auditory Canal
      Left 09N4

Release — *continued*
  Ear — *continued*
    External Auditory Canal — *continued*
      Right Ø9N3
    Inner
      Left Ø9NE
      Right Ø9ND
    Middle
      Left Ø9N6
      Right Ø9N5
  Epididymis
    Bilateral ØVNL
    Left ØVNK
    Right ØVNJ
  Epiglottis ØCNR
  Esophagogastric Junction ØDN4
  Esophagus ØDN5
    Lower ØDN3
    Middle ØDN2
    Upper ØDN1
  Eustachian Tube
    Left Ø9NG
    Right Ø9NF
  Eye
    Left Ø8N1XZZ
    Right Ø8NØXZZ
  Eyelid
    Lower
      Left Ø8NR
      Right Ø8NQ
    Upper
      Left Ø8NP
      Right Ø8NN
  Fallopian Tube
    Left ØUN6
    Right ØUN5
  Fallopian Tubes, Bilateral ØUN7
  Femoral Shaft
    Left ØQN9
    Right ØQN8
  Femur
    Lower
      Left ØQNC
      Right ØQNB
    Upper
      Left ØQN7
      Right ØQN6
  Fibula
    Left ØQNK
    Right ØQNJ
  Finger Nail ØHNQXZZ
  Gallbladder ØFN4
  Gingiva
    Lower ØCN6
    Upper ØCN5
  Gland
    Adrenal
      Bilateral ØGN4
      Left ØGN2
      Right ØGN3
    Lacrimal
      Left Ø8NW
      Right Ø8NV
    Minor Salivary ØCNJ
    Parotid
      Left ØCN9
      Right ØCN8
    Pituitary ØGNØ
    Sublingual
      Left ØCNF
      Right ØCND
    Submaxillary
      Left ØCNH
      Right ØCNG
    Vestibular ØUNL
  Glenoid Cavity
    Left ØPN8
    Right ØPN7
  Glomus Jugulare ØGNC
  Humeral Head
    Left ØPND
    Right ØPNC
  Humeral Shaft
    Left ØPNG
    Right ØPNF
  Hymen ØUNK
  Hypothalamus ØØNA
  Ileocecal Valve ØDNC
  Ileum ØDNB

Release — *continued*
  Intestine
    Large ØDNE
      Left ØDNG
      Right ØDNF
    Small ØDN8
  Iris
    Left Ø8ND3ZZ
    Right Ø8NC3ZZ
  Jejunum ØDNA
  Joint
    Acromioclavicular
      Left ØRNH
      Right ØRNG
    Ankle
      Left ØSNG
      Right ØSNF
    Carpal
      Left ØRNR
      Right ØRNQ
    Carpometacarpal
      Left ØRNT
      Right ØRNS
    Cervical Vertebral ØRN1
    Cervicothoracic Vertebral ØRN4
    Coccygeal ØSN6
    Elbow
      Left ØRNM
      Right ØRNL
    Finger Phalangeal
      Left ØRNX
      Right ØRNW
    Hip
      Left ØSNB
      Right ØSN9
    Knee
      Left ØSND
      Right ØSNC
    Lumbar Vertebral ØSNØ
    Lumbosacral ØSN3
    Metacarpophalangeal
      Left ØRNV
      Right ØRNU
    Metatarsal-Phalangeal
      Left ØSNN
      Right ØSNM
    Occipital-cervical ØRNØ
    Sacrococcygeal ØSN5
    Sacroiliac
      Left ØSN8
      Right ØSN7
    Shoulder
      Left ØRNK
      Right ØRNJ
    Sternoclavicular
      Left ØRNF
      Right ØRNE
    Tarsal
      Left ØSNJ
      Right ØSNH
    Tarsometatarsal
      Left ØSNL
      Right ØSNK
    Temporomandibular
      Left ØRND
      Right ØRNC
    Thoracic Vertebral ØRN6
    Thoracolumbar Vertebral ØRNA
    Toe Phalangeal
      Left ØSNQ
      Right ØSNP
    Wrist
      Left ØRNP
      Right ØRNN
  Kidney
    Left ØTN1
    Right ØTNØ
  Kidney Pelvis
    Left ØTN4
    Right ØTN3
  Larynx ØCNS
  Lens
    Left Ø8NK3ZZ
    Right Ø8NJ3ZZ
  Lip
    Lower ØCN1
    Upper ØCNØ
  Liver ØFNØ
    Left Lobe ØFN2

Release — *continued*
  Liver — *continued*
    Right Lobe ØFN1
  Lung
    Bilateral ØBNM
    Left ØBNL
    Lower Lobe
      Left ØBNJ
      Right ØBNF
    Middle Lobe, Right ØBND
    Right ØBNK
    Upper Lobe
      Left ØBNG
      Right ØBNC
  Lung Lingula ØBNH
  Lymphatic
    Aortic Ø7ND
    Axillary
      Left Ø7N6
      Right Ø7N5
    Head Ø7NØ
    Inguinal
      Left Ø7NJ
      Right Ø7NH
    Internal Mammary
      Left Ø7N9
      Right Ø7N8
    Lower Extremity
      Left Ø7NG
      Right Ø7NF
    Mesenteric Ø7NB
    Neck
      Left Ø7N2
      Right Ø7N1
    Pelvis Ø7NC
    Thoracic Duct Ø7NK
    Thorax Ø7N7
    Upper Extremity
      Left Ø7N4
      Right Ø7N3
  Mandible
    Left ØNNV
    Right ØNNT
  Maxilla ØNNR
  Medulla Oblongata ØØND
  Mesentery ØDNV
  Metacarpal
    Left ØPNQ
    Right ØPNP
  Metatarsal
    Left ØQNP
    Right ØQNN
  Muscle
    Abdomen
      Left ØKNL
      Right ØKNK
    Extraocular
      Left Ø8NM
      Right Ø8NL
    Facial ØKN1
    Foot
      Left ØKNW
      Right ØKNV
    Hand
      Left ØKND
      Right ØKNC
    Head ØKNØ
    Hip
      Left ØKNP
      Right ØKNN
    Lower Arm and Wrist
      Left ØKNB
      Right ØKN9
    Lower Leg
      Left ØKNT
      Right ØKNS
    Neck
      Left ØKN3
      Right ØKN2
    Papillary Ø2ND
    Perineum ØKNM
    Shoulder
      Left ØKN6
      Right ØKN5
    Thorax
      Left ØKNJ
      Right ØKNH
    Tongue, Palate, Pharynx ØKN4

▽ Subterms under main terms may continue to next column or page

Release — continued
  Muscle — continued
    Trunk
      Left ØKNG
      Right ØKNF
    Upper Arm
      Left ØKN8
      Right ØKN7
    Upper Leg
      Left ØKNR
      Right ØKNQ
  Myocardial Bridge *see* Release, Artery, Coronary
  Nasal Mucosa and Soft Tissue 09NK
  Nasopharynx 09NN
  Nerve
    Abdominal Sympathetic 01NM
    Abducens 00NL
    Accessory 00NR
    Acoustic 00NN
    Brachial Plexus 01N3
    Cervical 01N1
    Cervical Plexus 01N0
    Facial 00NM
    Femoral 01ND
    Glossopharyngeal 00NP
    Head and Neck Sympathetic 01NK
    Hypoglossal 00NS
    Lumbar 01NB
    Lumbar Plexus 01N9
    Lumbar Sympathetic 01NN
    Lumbosacral Plexus 01NA
    Median 01N5
    Oculomotor 00NH
    Olfactory 00NF
    Optic 00NG
    Peroneal 01NH
    Phrenic 01N2
    Pudendal 01NC
    Radial 01N6
    Sacral 01NR
    Sacral Plexus 01NQ
    Sacral Sympathetic 01NP
    Sciatic 01NF
    Thoracic 01N8
    Thoracic Sympathetic 01NL
    Tibial 01NG
    Trigeminal 00NK
    Trochlear 00NJ
    Ulnar 01N4
    Vagus 00NQ
  Nipple
    Left ØHNX
    Right ØHNW
  Omentum ØDNU
  Orbit
    Left ØNNQ
    Right ØNNP
  Ovary
    Bilateral ØUN2
    Left ØUN1
    Right ØUN0
  Palate
    Hard ØCN2
    Soft ØCN3
  Pancreas ØFNG
  Para-aortic Body ØGN9
  Paraganglion Extremity ØGNF
  Parathyroid Gland ØGNR
    Inferior
      Left ØGNP
      Right ØGNN
    Multiple ØGNQ
    Superior
      Left ØGNM
      Right ØGNL
  Patella
    Left ØQNF
    Right ØQND
  Penis ØVNS
  Pericardium 02NN
  Peritoneum ØDNW
  Phalanx
    Finger
      Left ØPNV
      Right ØPNT
    Thumb
      Left ØPNS
      Right ØPNR

Release — continued
  Phalanx — continued
    Toe
      Left ØQNR
      Right ØQNQ
  Pharynx ØCNM
  Pineal Body ØGN1
  Pleura
    Left ØBNP
    Right ØBNN
  Pons 00NB
  Prepuce ØVNT
  Prostate ØVN0
  Radius
    Left ØPNJ
    Right ØPNH
  Rectum ØDNP
  Retina
    Left 08NF3ZZ
    Right 08NE3ZZ
  Retinal Vessel
    Left 08NH3ZZ
    Right 08NG3ZZ
  Ribs
    1 to 2 ØPN1
    3 or More ØPN2
  Sacrum ØQN1
  Scapula
    Left ØPN6
    Right ØPN5
  Sclera
    Left 08N7XZZ
    Right 08N6XZZ
  Scrotum ØVN5
  Septum
    Atrial 02N5
    Nasal 09NM
    Ventricular 02NM
  Sinus
    Accessory 09NP
    Ethmoid
      Left 09NV
      Right 09NU
    Frontal
      Left 09NT
      Right 09NS
    Mastoid
      Left 09NC
      Right 09NB
    Maxillary
      Left 09NR
      Right 09NQ
    Sphenoid
      Left 09NX
      Right 09NW
  Skin
    Abdomen ØHN7XZZ
    Back ØHN6XZZ
    Buttock ØHN8XZZ
    Chest ØHN5XZZ
    Ear
      Left ØHN3XZZ
      Right ØHN2XZZ
    Face ØHN1XZZ
    Foot
      Left ØHNNXZZ
      Right ØHNMXZZ
    Hand
      Left ØHNGXZZ
      Right ØHNFXZZ
    Inguinal ØHNAXZZ
    Lower Arm
      Left ØHNEXZZ
      Right ØHNDXZZ
    Lower Leg
      Left ØHNLXZZ
      Right ØHNKXZZ
    Neck ØHN4XZZ
    Perineum ØHN9XZZ
    Scalp ØHN0XZZ
    Upper Arm
      Left ØHNCXZZ
      Right ØHNBXZZ
    Upper Leg
      Left ØHNJXZZ
      Right ØHNHXZZ
  Spinal Cord
    Cervical 00NW
    Lumbar 00NY

Release — continued
  Spinal Cord — continued
    Thoracic 00NX
  Spinal Meninges 00NT
  Spleen 07NP
  Sternum ØPN0
  Stomach ØDN6
    Pylorus ØDN7
  Subcutaneous Tissue and Fascia
    Abdomen ØJN8
    Back ØJN7
    Buttock ØJN9
    Chest ØJN6
    Face ØJN1
    Foot
      Left ØJNR
      Right ØJNQ
    Hand
      Left ØJNK
      Right ØJNJ
    Lower Arm
      Left ØJNH
      Right ØJNG
    Lower Leg
      Left ØJNP
      Right ØJNN
    Neck
      Left ØJN5
      Right ØJN4
    Pelvic Region ØJNC
    Perineum ØJNB
    Scalp ØJN0
    Upper Arm
      Left ØJNF
      Right ØJND
    Upper Leg
      Left ØJNM
      Right ØJNL
  Tarsal
    Left ØQNM
    Right ØQNL
  Tendon
    Abdomen
      Left ØLNG
      Right ØLNF
    Ankle
      Left ØLNT
      Right ØLNS
    Foot
      Left ØLNW
      Right ØLNV
    Hand
      Left ØLN8
      Right ØLN7
    Head and Neck ØLN0
    Hip
      Left ØLNK
      Right ØLNJ
    Knee
      Left ØLNR
      Right ØLNQ
    Lower Arm and Wrist
      Left ØLN6
      Right ØLN5
    Lower Leg
      Left ØLNP
      Right ØLNN
    Perineum ØLNH
    Shoulder
      Left ØLN2
      Right ØLN1
    Thorax
      Left ØLND
      Right ØLNC
    Trunk
      Left ØLNB
      Right ØLN9
    Upper Arm
      Left ØLN4
      Right ØLN3
    Upper Leg
      Left ØLNM
      Right ØLNL
  Testis
    Bilateral ØVNC
    Left ØVNB
    Right ØVN9
  Thalamus 00N9
  Thymus 07NM

Release — continued
  Thyroid Gland ØGNK
    Left Lobe ØGNG
    Right Lobe ØGNH
  Tibia
    Left ØQNH
    Right ØQNG
  Toe Nail ØHNRXZZ
  Tongue ØCN7
  Tonsils ØCNP
  Tooth
    Lower ØCNX
    Upper ØCNW
  Trachea ØBN1
  Tunica Vaginalis
    Left ØVN7
    Right ØVN6
  Turbinate, Nasal Ø9NL
  Tympanic Membrane
    Left Ø9N8
    Right Ø9N7
  Ulna
    Left ØPNL
    Right ØPNK
  Ureter
    Left ØTN7
    Right ØTN6
  Urethra ØTND
  Uterine Supporting Structure ØUN4
  Uterus ØUN9
  Uvula ØCNN
  Vagina ØUNG
  Valve
    Aortic Ø2NF
    Mitral Ø2NG
    Pulmonary Ø2NH
    Tricuspid Ø2NJ
  Vas Deferens
    Bilateral ØVNQ
    Left ØVNP
    Right ØVNN
  Vein
    Axillary
      Left Ø5N8
      Right Ø5N7
    Azygos Ø5NØ
    Basilic
      Left Ø5NC
      Right Ø5NB
    Brachial
      Left Ø5NA
      Right Ø5N9
    Cephalic
      Left Ø5NF
      Right Ø5ND
    Colic Ø6N7
    Common Iliac
      Left Ø6ND
      Right Ø6NC
    Coronary Ø2N4
    Esophageal Ø6N3
    External Iliac
      Left Ø6NG
      Right Ø6NF
    External Jugular
      Left Ø5NQ
      Right Ø5NP
    Face
      Left Ø5NV
      Right Ø5NT
    Femoral
      Left Ø6NN
      Right Ø6NM
    Foot
      Left Ø6NV
      Right Ø6NT
    Gastric Ø6N2
    Hand
      Left Ø5NH
      Right Ø5NG
    Hemiazygos Ø5N1
    Hepatic Ø6N4
    Hypogastric
      Left Ø6NJ
      Right Ø6NH
    Inferior Mesenteric Ø6N6
    Innominate
      Left Ø5N4
      Right Ø5N3

Release — continued
  Vein — continued
    Internal Jugular
      Left Ø5NN
      Right Ø5NM
    Intracranial Ø5NL
    Lower Ø6NY
    Portal Ø6N8
    Pulmonary
      Left Ø2NT
      Right Ø2NS
    Renal
      Left Ø6NB
      Right Ø6N9
    Saphenous
      Left Ø6NQ
      Right Ø6NP
    Splenic Ø6N1
    Subclavian
      Left Ø5N6
      Right Ø5N5
    Superior Mesenteric Ø6N5
    Upper Ø5NY
    Vertebral
      Left Ø5NS
      Right Ø5NR
  Vena Cava
    Inferior Ø6NØ
    Superior Ø2NV
  Ventricle
    Left Ø2NL
    Right Ø2NK
  Vertebra
    Cervical ØPN3
    Lumbar ØQNØ
    Thoracic ØPN4
  Vesicle
    Bilateral ØVN3
    Left ØVN2
    Right ØVN1
  Vitreous
    Left Ø8N53ZZ
    Right Ø8N43ZZ
  Vocal Cord
    Left ØCNV
    Right ØCNT
  Vulva ØUNM
Relocation see Reposition
Removal
  Abdominal Wall 2W53X
  Anorectal 2Y53X5Z
  Arm
    Lower
      Left 2W5DX
      Right 2W5CX
    Upper
      Left 2W5BX
      Right 2W5AX
  Back 2W55X
  Chest Wall 2W54X
  Ear 2Y52X5Z
  Extremity
    Lower
      Left 2W5MX
      Right 2W5LX
    Upper
      Left 2W59X
      Right 2W58X
  Face 2W51X
  Finger
    Left 2W5KX
    Right 2W5JX
  Foot
    Left 2W5TX
    Right 2W5SX
  Genital Tract, Female 2Y54X5Z
  Hand
    Left 2W5FX
    Right 2W5EX
  Head 2W50X
  Inguinal Region
    Left 2W57X
    Right 2W56X
  Leg
    Lower
      Left 2W5RX
      Right 2W5QX
    Upper
      Left 2W5PX

Removal — continued
  Leg — continued
    Upper — continued
      Right 2W5NX
  Mouth and Pharynx 2Y5ØX5Z
  Nasal 2Y51X5Z
  Neck 2W52X
  Thumb
    Left 2W5HX
    Right 2W5GX
  Toe
    Left 2W5VX
    Right 2W5UX
  Urethra 2Y55X5Z
Removal of device from
  Abdominal Wall ØWPF
  Acetabulum
    Left ØQP5
    Right ØQP4
  Anal Sphincter ØDPR
  Anus ØDPQ
  Artery
    Lower Ø4PY
    Upper Ø3PY
  Back
    Lower ØWPL
    Upper ØWPK
  Bladder ØTPB
  Bone
    Facial ØNPW
    Lower ØQPY
    Nasal ØNPB
    Pelvic
      Left ØQP3
      Right ØQP2
    Upper ØPPY
  Bone Marrow Ø7PT
  Brain ØØPØ
  Breast
    Left ØHPU
    Right ØHPT
  Bursa and Ligament
    Lower ØMPY
    Upper ØMPX
  Carpal
    Left ØPPN
    Right ØPPM
  Cavity, Cranial ØWP1
  Cerebral Ventricle ØØP6
  Chest Wall ØWP8
  Cisterna Chyli Ø7PL
  Clavicle
    Left ØPPB
    Right ØPP9
  Coccyx ØQPS
  Diaphragm ØBPT
  Disc
    Cervical Vertebral ØRP3
    Cervicothoracic Vertebral ØRP5
    Lumbar Vertebral ØSP2
    Lumbosacral ØSP4
    Thoracic Vertebral ØRP9
    Thoracolumbar Vertebral ØRPB
  Duct
    Hepatobiliary ØFPB
    Pancreatic ØFPD
  Ear
    Inner
      Left Ø9PJ
      Right Ø9PD
    Left Ø9PJ
    Right Ø9PH
  Epididymis and Spermatic Cord ØVPM
  Esophagus ØDP5
  Extremity
    Lower
      Left ØYPB
      Right ØYP9
    Upper
      Left ØXP7
      Right ØXP6
  Eye
    Left Ø8P1
    Right Ø8PØ
  Face ØWP2
  Fallopian Tube ØUP8
  Femoral Shaft
    Left ØQP9
    Right ØQP8

Removal of device from — *continued*
Femur
  Lower
    Left ØQPC
    Right ØQPB
  Upper
    Left ØQP7
    Right ØQP6
Fibula
  Left ØQPK
  Right ØQPJ
Finger Nail ØHPQX
Gallbladder ØFP4
Gastrointestinal Tract ØWPP
Genitourinary Tract ØWPR
Gland
  Adrenal ØGP5
  Endocrine ØGPS
  Pituitary ØGPØ
  Salivary ØCPA
Glenoid Cavity
  Left ØPP8
  Right ØPP7
Great Vessel Ø2PY
Hair ØHPSX
Head ØWPØ
Heart Ø2PA
Humeral Head
  Left ØPPD
  Right ØPPC
Humeral Shaft
  Left ØPPG
  Right ØPPF
Intestinal Tract
  Lower ØDPD
  Upper ØDPØ
Jaw
  Lower ØWP5
  Upper ØWP4
Joint
  Acromioclavicular
    Left ØRPH
    Right ØRPG
  Ankle
    Left ØSPG
    Right ØSPF
  Carpal
    Left ØRPR
    Right ØRPQ
  Carpometacarpal
    Left ØRPT
    Right ØRPS
  Cervical Vertebral ØRP1
  Cervicothoracic Vertebral ØRP4
  Coccygeal ØSP6
  Elbow
    Left ØRPM
    Right ØRPL
  Finger Phalangeal
    Left ØRPX
    Right ØRPW
  Hip
    Left ØSPB
      Acetabular Surface ØSPE
      Femoral Surface ØSPS
    Right ØSP9
      Acetabular Surface ØSPA
      Femoral Surface ØSPR
  Knee
    Left ØSPD
      Femoral Surface ØSPU
      Tibial Surface ØSPW
    Right ØSPC
      Femoral Surface ØSPT
      Tibial Surface ØSPV
  Lumbar Vertebral ØSPØ
  Lumbosacral ØSP3
  Metacarpophalangeal
    Left ØRPV
    Right ØRPU
  Metatarsal-Phalangeal
    Left ØSPN
    Right ØSPM
  Occipital-cervical ØRPØ
  Sacrococcygeal ØSP5
  Sacroiliac
    Left ØSP8
    Right ØSP7

Removal of device from — *continued*
Joint — *continued*
  Shoulder
    Left ØRPK
    Right ØRPJ
  Sternoclavicular
    Left ØRPF
    Right ØRPE
  Tarsal
    Left ØSPJ
    Right ØSPH
  Tarsometatarsal
    Left ØSPL
    Right ØSPK
  Temporomandibular
    Left ØRPD
    Right ØRPC
  Thoracic Vertebral ØRP6
  Thoracolumbar Vertebral ØRPA
  Toe Phalangeal
    Left ØSPQ
    Right ØSPP
  Wrist
    Left ØRPP
    Right ØRPN
Kidney ØTP5
Larynx ØCPS
Lens
  Left Ø8PK3
  Right Ø8PJ3
Liver ØFPØ
Lung
  Left ØBPL
  Right ØBPK
Lymphatic Ø7PN
  Thoracic Duct Ø7PK
Mediastinum ØWPC
Mesentery ØDPV
Metacarpal
  Left ØPPQ
  Right ØPPP
Metatarsal
  Left ØQPP
  Right ØQPN
Mouth and Throat ØCPY
Muscle
  Extraocular
    Left Ø8PM
    Right Ø8PL
  Lower ØKPY
  Upper ØKPX
Nasal Mucosa and Soft Tissue Ø9PK
Neck ØWP6
Nerve
  Cranial ØØPE
  Peripheral Ø1PY
Omentum ØDPU
Ovary ØUP3
Pancreas ØFPG
Parathyroid Gland ØGPR
Patella
  Left ØQPF
  Right ØQPD
Pelvic Cavity ØWPJ
Penis ØVPS
Pericardial Cavity ØWPD
Perineum
  Female ØWPN
  Male ØWPM
Peritoneal Cavity ØWPG
Peritoneum ØDPW
Phalanx
  Finger
    Left ØPPV
    Right ØPPT
  Thumb
    Left ØPPS
    Right ØPPR
  Toe
    Left ØQPR
    Right ØQPQ
Pineal Body ØGP1
Pleura ØBPQ
Pleural Cavity
  Left ØWPB
  Right ØWP9
Products of Conception 10PØ
Prostate and Seminal Vesicles ØVP4

Removal of device from — *continued*
Radius
  Left ØPPJ
  Right ØPPH
Rectum ØDPP
Respiratory Tract ØWPQ
Retroperitoneum ØWPH
Ribs
  1 to 2 ØPP1
  3 or More ØPP2
Sacrum ØQP1
Scapula
  Left ØPP6
  Right ØPP5
Scrotum and Tunica Vaginalis ØVP8
Sinus Ø9PY
Skin ØHPPX
Skull ØNPØ
Spinal Canal ØØPU
Spinal Cord ØØPV
Spleen Ø7PP
Sternum ØPPØ
Stomach ØDP6
Subcutaneous Tissue and Fascia
  Head and Neck ØJPS
  Lower Extremity ØJPW
  Trunk ØJPT
  Upper Extremity ØJPV
Tarsal
  Left ØQPM
  Right ØQPL
Tendon
  Lower ØLPY
  Upper ØLPX
Testis ØVPD
Thymus Ø7PM
Thyroid Gland ØGPK
Tibia
  Left ØQPH
  Right ØQPG
Toe Nail ØHPRX
Trachea ØBP1
Tracheobronchial Tree ØBPØ
Tympanic Membrane
  Left Ø9P8
  Right Ø9P7
Ulna
  Left ØPPL
  Right ØPPK
Ureter ØTP9
Urethra ØTPD
Uterus and Cervix ØUPD
Vagina and Cul-de-sac ØUPH
Vas Deferens ØVPR
Vein
  Azygos Ø5PØ
  Innominate
    Left Ø5P4
    Right Ø5P3
  Lower Ø6PY
  Upper Ø5PY
Vertebra
  Cervical ØPP3
  Lumbar ØQPØ
  Thoracic ØPP4
Vulva ØUPM
Renal calyx
  use Kidney
  use Kidney, Left
  use Kidney, Right
  use Kidneys, Bilateral
Renal capsule
  use Kidney
  use Kidney, Left
  use Kidney, Right
  use Kidneys, Bilateral
Renal cortex
  use Kidney
  use Kidney, Left
  use Kidney, Right
  use Kidneys, Bilateral
Renal dialysis *see* Performance, Urinary 5A1D
Renal nerve *use* Abdominal Sympathetic Nerve
Renal plexus *use* Abdominal Sympathetic Nerve
Renal segment
  use Kidney
  use Kidney, Left
  use Kidney, Right

Renal segment — *continued*
  use Kidneys, Bilateral
Renal segmental artery
  use Renal Artery, Left
  use Renal Artery, Right
Reopening, operative site
  Control of bleeding *see* Control bleeding in
  Inspection only *see* Inspection
Repair
  Abdominal Wall 0WQF
  Acetabulum
    Left 0QQ5
    Right 0QQ4
  Adenoids 0CQQ
  Ampulla of Vater 0FQC
  Anal Sphincter 0DQR
  Ankle Region
    Left 0YQL
    Right 0YQK
  Anterior Chamber
    Left 08Q33ZZ
    Right 08Q23ZZ
  Anus 0DQQ
  Aorta
    Abdominal 04Q0
    Thoracic
      Ascending/Arch 02QX
      Descending 02QW
  Aortic Body 0GQD
  Appendix 0DQJ
  Arm
    Lower
      Left 0XQF
      Right 0XQD
    Upper
      Left 0XQ9
      Right 0XQ8
  Artery
    Anterior Tibial
      Left 04QQ
      Right 04QP
    Axillary
      Left 03Q6
      Right 03Q5
    Brachial
      Left 03Q8
      Right 03Q7
    Celiac 04Q1
    Colic
      Left 04Q7
      Middle 04Q8
      Right 04Q6
    Common Carotid
      Left 03QJ
      Right 03QH
    Common Iliac
      Left 04QD
      Right 04QC
    Coronary
      Four or More Arteries 02Q3
      One Artery 02Q0
      Three Arteries 02Q2
      Two Arteries 02Q1
    External Carotid
      Left 03QN
      Right 03QM
    External Iliac
      Left 04QJ
      Right 04QH
    Face 03QR
    Femoral
      Left 04QL
      Right 04QK
    Foot
      Left 04QW
      Right 04QV
    Gastric 04Q2
    Hand
      Left 03QF
      Right 03QD
    Hepatic 04Q3
    Inferior Mesenteric 04QB
    Innominate 03Q2
    Internal Carotid
      Left 03QL
      Right 03QK
    Internal Iliac
      Left 04QF

Repair — *continued*
  Artery — *continued*
    Internal Iliac — *continued*
      Right 04QE
    Internal Mammary
      Left 03Q1
      Right 03Q0
    Intracranial 03QG
    Lower 04QY
    Peroneal
      Left 04QU
      Right 04QT
    Popliteal
      Left 04QN
      Right 04QM
    Posterior Tibial
      Left 04QS
      Right 04QR
    Pulmonary
      Left 02QR
      Right 02QQ
    Pulmonary Trunk 02QP
    Radial
      Left 03QC
      Right 03QB
    Renal
      Left 04QA
      Right 04Q9
    Splenic 04Q4
    Subclavian
      Left 03Q4
      Right 03Q3
    Superior Mesenteric 04Q5
    Temporal
      Left 03QT
      Right 03QS
    Thyroid
      Left 03QV
      Right 03QU
    Ulnar
      Left 03QA
      Right 03Q9
    Upper 03QY
    Vertebral
      Left 03QQ
      Right 03QP
  Atrium
    Left 02Q7
    Right 02Q6
  Auditory Ossicle
    Left 09QA
    Right 09Q9
  Axilla
    Left 0XQ5
    Right 0XQ4
  Back
    Lower 0WQL
    Upper 0WQK
  Basal Ganglia 00Q8
  Bladder 0TQB
  Bladder Neck 0TQC
  Bone
    Ethmoid
      Left 0NQG
      Right 0NQF
    Frontal 0NQ1
    Hyoid 0NQX
    Lacrimal
      Left 0NQJ
      Right 0NQH
    Nasal 0NQB
    Occipital 0NQ7
    Palatine
      Left 0NQL
      Right 0NQK
    Parietal
      Left 0NQ4
      Right 0NQ3
    Pelvic
      Left 0QQ3
      Right 0QQ2
    Sphenoid 0NQC
    Temporal
      Left 0NQ6
      Right 0NQ5
    Zygomatic
      Left 0NQN
      Right 0NQM
  Brain 00Q0

Repair — *continued*
  Breast
    Bilateral 0HQV
    Left 0HQU
    Right 0HQT
    Supernumerary 0HQY
  Bronchus
    Lingula 0BQ9
    Lower Lobe
      Left 0BQB
      Right 0BQ6
    Main
      Left 0BQ7
      Right 0BQ3
    Middle Lobe, Right 0BQ5
    Upper Lobe
      Left 0BQ8
      Right 0BQ4
  Buccal Mucosa 0CQ4
  Bursa and Ligament
    Abdomen
      Left 0MQJ
      Right 0MQH
    Ankle
      Left 0MQR
      Right 0MQQ
    Elbow
      Left 0MQ4
      Right 0MQ3
    Foot
      Left 0MQT
      Right 0MQS
    Hand
      Left 0MQ8
      Right 0MQ7
    Head and Neck 0MQ0
    Hip
      Left 0MQM
      Right 0MQL
    Knee
      Left 0MQP
      Right 0MQN
    Lower Extremity
      Left 0MQW
      Right 0MQV
    Perineum 0MQK
    Rib(s) 0MQG
    Shoulder
      Left 0MQ2
      Right 0MQ1
    Spine
      Lower 0MQD
      Upper 0MQC
    Sternum 0MQF
    Upper Extremity
      Left 0MQB
      Right 0MQ9
    Wrist
      Left 0MQ6
      Right 0MQ5
  Buttock
    Left 0YQ1
    Right 0YQ0
  Carina 0BQ2
  Carotid Bodies, Bilateral 0GQ8
  Carotid Body
    Left 0GQ6
    Right 0GQ7
  Carpal
    Left 0PQN
    Right 0PQM
  Cecum 0DQH
  Cerebellum 00QC
  Cerebral Hemisphere 00Q7
  Cerebral Meninges 00Q1
  Cerebral Ventricle 00Q6
  Cervix 0UQC
  Chest Wall 0WQ8
  Chordae Tendineae 02Q9
  Choroid
    Left 08QB
    Right 08QA
  Cisterna Chyli 07QL
  Clavicle
    Left 0PQB
    Right 0PQ9
  Clitoris 0UQJ
  Coccygeal Glomus 0GQB
  Coccyx 0QQS

▽ Subterms under main terms may continue to next column or page

Repair — *continued*
- Colon
  - Ascending ØDQK
  - Descending ØDQM
  - Sigmoid ØDQN
  - Transverse ØDQL
- Conduction Mechanism Ø2Q8
- Conjunctiva
  - Left Ø8QTXZZ
  - Right Ø8QSXZZ
- Cord
  - Bilateral ØVQH
  - Left ØVQG
  - Right ØVQF
- Cornea
  - Left Ø8Q9XZZ
  - Right Ø8Q8XZZ
- Cul-de-sac ØUQF
- Diaphragm ØBQT
- Disc
  - Cervical Vertebral ØRQ3
  - Cervicothoracic Vertebral ØRQ5
  - Lumbar Vertebral ØSQ2
  - Lumbosacral ØSQ4
  - Thoracic Vertebral ØRQ9
  - Thoracolumbar Vertebral ØRQB
- Duct
  - Common Bile ØFQ9
  - Cystic ØFQ8
  - Hepatic
    - Common ØFQ7
    - Left ØFQ6
    - Right ØFQ5
  - Lacrimal
    - Left Ø8QY
    - Right Ø8QX
  - Pancreatic ØFQD
    - Accessory ØFQF
  - Parotid
    - Left ØCQC
    - Right ØCQB
- Duodenum ØDQ9
- Dura Mater ØØQ2
- Ear
  - External
    - Bilateral Ø9Q2
    - Left Ø9Q1
    - Right Ø9QØ
  - External Auditory Canal
    - Left Ø9Q4
    - Right Ø9Q3
  - Inner
    - Left Ø9QE
    - Right Ø9QD
  - Middle
    - Left Ø9Q6
    - Right Ø9Q5
- Elbow Region
  - Left ØXQC
  - Right ØXQB
- Epididymis
  - Bilateral ØVQL
  - Left ØVQK
  - Right ØVQJ
- Epiglottis ØCQR
- Esophagogastric Junction ØDQ4
- Esophagus ØDQ5
  - Lower ØDQ3
  - Middle ØDQ2
  - Upper ØDQ1
- Eustachian Tube
  - Left Ø9QG
  - Right Ø9QF
- Extremity
  - Lower
    - Left ØYQB
    - Right ØYQ9
  - Upper
    - Left ØXQ7
    - Right ØXQ6
- Eye
  - Left Ø8Q1XZZ
  - Right Ø8QØXZZ
- Eyelid
  - Lower
    - Left Ø8QR
    - Right Ø8QQ
  - Upper
    - Left Ø8QP

Repair — *continued*
- Eyelid — *continued*
  - Upper — *continued*
    - Right Ø8QN
- Face ØWQ2
- Fallopian Tube
  - Left ØUQ6
  - Right ØUQ5
- Fallopian Tubes, Bilateral ØUQ7
- Femoral Region
  - Bilateral ØYQE
  - Left ØYQ8
  - Right ØYQ7
- Femoral Shaft
  - Left ØQQ9
  - Right ØQQ8
- Femur
  - Lower
    - Left ØQQC
    - Right ØQQB
  - Upper
    - Left ØQQ7
    - Right ØQQ6
- Fibula
  - Left ØQQK
  - Right ØQQJ
- Finger
  - Index
    - Left ØXQP
    - Right ØXQN
  - Little
    - Left ØXQW
    - Right ØXQV
  - Middle
    - Left ØXQR
    - Right ØXQQ
  - Ring
    - Left ØXQT
    - Right ØXQS
- Finger Nail ØHQQXZZ
- Floor of mouth *see* Repair, Oral Cavity and Throat ØWQ3
- Foot
  - Left ØYQN
  - Right ØYQM
- Gallbladder ØFQ4
- Gingiva
  - Lower ØCQ6
  - Upper ØCQ5
- Gland
  - Adrenal
    - Bilateral ØGQ4
    - Left ØGQ2
    - Right ØGQ3
  - Lacrimal
    - Left Ø8QW
    - Right Ø8QV
  - Minor Salivary ØCQJ
  - Parotid
    - Left ØCQ9
    - Right ØCQ8
  - Pituitary ØGQØ
  - Sublingual
    - Left ØCQF
    - Right ØCQD
  - Submaxillary
    - Left ØCQH
    - Right ØCQG
  - Vestibular ØUQL
- Glenoid Cavity
  - Left ØPQ8
  - Right ØPQ7
- Glomus Jugulare ØGQC
- Hand
  - Left ØXQK
  - Right ØXQJ
- Head ØWQØ
- Heart Ø2QA
  - Left Ø2QC
  - Right Ø2QB
- Humeral Head
  - Left ØPQD
  - Right ØPQC
- Humeral Shaft
  - Left ØPQG
  - Right ØPQF
- Hymen ØUQK
- Hypothalamus ØØQA
- Ileocecal Valve ØDQC

Repair — *continued*
- Ileum ØDQB
- Inguinal Region
  - Bilateral ØYQA
  - Left ØYQ6
  - Right ØYQ5
- Intestine
  - Large ØDQE
    - Left ØDQG
    - Right ØDQF
  - Small ØDQ8
- Iris
  - Left Ø8QD3ZZ
  - Right Ø8QC3ZZ
- Jaw
  - Lower ØWQ5
  - Upper ØWQ4
- Jejunum ØDQA
- Joint
  - Acromioclavicular
    - Left ØRQH
    - Right ØRQG
  - Ankle
    - Left ØSQG
    - Right ØSQF
  - Carpal
    - Left ØRQR
    - Right ØRQQ
  - Carpometacarpal
    - Left ØRQT
    - Right ØRQS
  - Cervical Vertebral ØRQ1
  - Cervicothoracic Vertebral ØRQ4
  - Coccygeal ØSQ6
  - Elbow
    - Left ØRQM
    - Right ØRQL
  - Finger Phalangeal
    - Left ØRQX
    - Right ØRQW
  - Hip
    - Left ØSQB
    - Right ØSQ9
  - Knee
    - Left ØSQD
    - Right ØSQC
  - Lumbar Vertebral ØSQØ
  - Lumbosacral ØSQ3
  - Metacarpophalangeal
    - Left ØRQV
    - Right ØRQU
  - Metatarsal-Phalangeal
    - Left ØSQN
    - Right ØSQM
  - Occipital-cervical ØRQØ
  - Sacrococcygeal ØSQ5
  - Sacroiliac
    - Left ØSQ8
    - Right ØSQ7
  - Shoulder
    - Left ØRQK
    - Right ØRQJ
  - Sternoclavicular
    - Left ØRQF
    - Right ØRQE
  - Tarsal
    - Left ØSQJ
    - Right ØSQH
  - Tarsometatarsal
    - Left ØSQL
    - Right ØSQK
  - Temporomandibular
    - Left ØRQD
    - Right ØRQC
  - Thoracic Vertebral ØRQ6
  - Thoracolumbar Vertebral ØRQA
  - Toe Phalangeal
    - Left ØSQQ
    - Right ØSQP
  - Wrist
    - Left ØRQP
    - Right ØRQN
- Kidney
  - Left ØTQ1
  - Right ØTQØ
- Kidney Pelvis
  - Left ØTQ4
  - Right ØTQ3

Repair — *continued*
- Knee Region
  - Left ØYQG
  - Right ØYQF
- Larynx ØCQS
- Leg
  - Lower
    - Left ØYQJ
    - Right ØYQH
  - Upper
    - Left ØYQD
    - Right ØYQC
- Lens
  - Left Ø8QK3ZZ
  - Right Ø8QJ3ZZ
- Lip
  - Lower ØCQ1
  - Upper ØCQØ
- Liver ØFQØ
  - Left Lobe ØFQ2
  - Right Lobe ØFQ1
- Lung
  - Bilateral ØBQM
  - Left ØBQL
  - Lower Lobe
    - Left ØBQJ
    - Right ØBQF
  - Middle Lobe, Right ØBQD
  - Right ØBQK
  - Upper Lobe
    - Left ØBQG
    - Right ØBQC
- Lung Lingula ØBQH
- Lymphatic
  - Aortic Ø7QD
  - Axillary
    - Left Ø7Q6
    - Right Ø7Q5
  - Head Ø7QØ
  - Inguinal
    - Left Ø7QJ
    - Right Ø7QH
  - Internal Mammary
    - Left Ø7Q9
    - Right Ø7Q8
  - Lower Extremity
    - Left Ø7QG
    - Right Ø7QF
  - Mesenteric Ø7QB
  - Neck
    - Left Ø7Q2
    - Right Ø7Q1
  - Pelvis Ø7QC
  - Thoracic Duct Ø7QK
  - Thorax Ø7Q7
  - Upper Extremity
    - Left Ø7Q4
    - Right Ø7Q3
- Mandible
  - Left ØNQV
  - Right ØNQT
- Maxilla ØNQR
- Mediastinum ØWQC
- Medulla Oblongata ØØQD
- Mesentery ØDQV
- Metacarpal
  - Left ØPQQ
  - Right ØPQP
- Metatarsal
  - Left ØQQP
  - Right ØQQN
- Muscle
  - Abdomen
    - Left ØKQL
    - Right ØKQK
  - Extraocular
    - Left Ø8QM
    - Right Ø8QL
  - Facial ØKQ1
  - Foot
    - Left ØKQW
    - Right ØKQV
  - Hand
    - Left ØKQD
    - Right ØKQC
  - Head ØKQØ
  - Hip
    - Left ØKQP
    - Right ØKQN

Repair — *continued*
- Muscle — *continued*
  - Lower Arm and Wrist
    - Left ØKQB
    - Right ØKQ9
  - Lower Leg
    - Left ØKQT
    - Right ØKQS
  - Neck
    - Left ØKQ3
    - Right ØKQ2
  - Papillary Ø2QD
  - Perineum ØKQM
  - Shoulder
    - Left ØKQ6
    - Right ØKQ5
  - Thorax
    - Left ØKQJ
    - Right ØKQH
  - Tongue, Palate, Pharynx ØKQ4
  - Trunk
    - Left ØKQG
    - Right ØKQF
  - Upper Arm
    - Left ØKQ8
    - Right ØKQ7
  - Upper Leg
    - Left ØKQR
    - Right ØKQQ
- Nasal Mucosa and Soft Tissue Ø9QK
- Nasopharynx Ø9QN
- Neck ØWQ6
- Nerve
  - Abdominal Sympathetic Ø1QM
  - Abducens ØØQL
  - Accessory ØØQR
  - Acoustic ØØQN
  - Brachial Plexus Ø1Q3
  - Cervical Ø1Q1
  - Cervical Plexus Ø1QØ
  - Facial ØØQM
  - Femoral Ø1QD
  - Glossopharyngeal ØØQP
  - Head and Neck Sympathetic Ø1QK
  - Hypoglossal ØØQS
  - Lumbar Ø1QB
  - Lumbar Plexus Ø1Q9
  - Lumbar Sympathetic Ø1QN
  - Lumbosacral Plexus Ø1QA
  - Median Ø1Q5
  - Oculomotor ØØQH
  - Olfactory ØØQF
  - Optic ØØQG
  - Peroneal Ø1QH
  - Phrenic Ø1Q2
  - Pudendal Ø1QC
  - Radial Ø1Q6
  - Sacral Ø1QR
  - Sacral Plexus Ø1QQ
  - Sacral Sympathetic Ø1QP
  - Sciatic Ø1QF
  - Thoracic Ø1Q8
  - Thoracic Sympathetic Ø1QL
  - Tibial Ø1QG
  - Trigeminal ØØQK
  - Trochlear ØØQJ
  - Ulnar Ø1Q4
  - Vagus ØØQQ
- Nipple
  - Left ØHQX
  - Right ØHQW
- Omentum ØDQU
- Oral Cavity and Throat ØWQ3
- Orbit
  - Left ØNQQ
  - Right ØNQP
- Ovary
  - Bilateral ØUQ2
  - Left ØUQ1
  - Right ØUQØ
- Palate
  - Hard ØCQ2
  - Soft ØCQ3
- Pancreas ØFQG
- Para-aortic Body ØGQ9
- Paraganglion Extremity ØGQF
- Parathyroid Gland ØGQR
  - Inferior
    - Left ØGQP

Repair — *continued*
- Parathyroid Gland — *continued*
  - Inferior — *continued*
    - Right ØGQN
  - Multiple ØGQQ
  - Superior
    - Left ØGQM
    - Right ØGQL
- Patella
  - Left ØQQF
  - Right ØQQD
- Penis ØVQS
- Pericardium Ø2QN
- Perineum
  - Female ØWQN
  - Male ØWQM
- Peritoneum ØDQW
- Phalanx
  - Finger
    - Left ØPQV
    - Right ØPQT
  - Thumb
    - Left ØPQS
    - Right ØPQR
  - Toe
    - Left ØQQR
    - Right ØQQQ
- Pharynx ØCQM
- Pineal Body ØGQ1
- Pleura
  - Left ØBQP
  - Right ØBQN
- Pons ØØQB
- Prepuce ØVQT
- Products of Conception 1ØQØ
- Prostate ØVQØ
- Radius
  - Left ØPQJ
  - Right ØPQH
- Rectum ØDQP
- Retina
  - Left Ø8QF3ZZ
  - Right Ø8QE3ZZ
- Retinal Vessel
  - Left Ø8QH3ZZ
  - Right Ø8QG3ZZ
- Ribs
  - 1 to 2 ØPQ1
  - 3 or More ØPQ2
- Sacrum ØQQ1
- Scapula
  - Left ØPQ6
  - Right ØPQ5
- Sclera
  - Left Ø8Q7XZZ
  - Right Ø8Q6XZZ
- Scrotum ØVQ5
- Septum
  - Atrial Ø2Q5
  - Nasal Ø9QM
  - Ventricular Ø2QM
- Shoulder Region
  - Left ØXQ3
  - Right ØXQ2
- Sinus
  - Accessory Ø9QP
  - Ethmoid
    - Left Ø9QV
    - Right Ø9QU
  - Frontal
    - Left Ø9QT
    - Right Ø9QS
  - Mastoid
    - Left Ø9QC
    - Right Ø9QB
  - Maxillary
    - Left Ø9QR
    - Right Ø9QQ
  - Sphenoid
    - Left Ø9QX
    - Right Ø9QW
- Skin
  - Abdomen ØHQ7XZZ
  - Back ØHQ6XZZ
  - Buttock ØHQ8XZZ
  - Chest ØHQ5XZZ
  - Ear
    - Left ØHQ3XZZ
    - Right ØHQ2XZZ

Subterms under main terms may continue to next column or page

Repair — *continued*
  Skin — *continued*
    Face ØHQ1XZZ
    Foot
      Left ØHQNXZZ
      Right ØHQMXZZ
    Hand
      Left ØHQGXZZ
      Right ØHQFXZZ
    Inguinal ØHQAXZZ
    Lower Arm
      Left ØHQEXZZ
      Right ØHQDXZZ
    Lower Leg
      Left ØHQLXZZ
      Right ØHQKXZZ
    Neck ØHQ4XZZ
    Perineum ØHQ9XZZ
    Scalp ØHQ0XZZ
    Upper Arm
      Left ØHQCXZZ
      Right ØHQBXZZ
    Upper Leg
      Left ØHQJXZZ
      Right ØHQHXZZ
  Skull ØNQ0
  Spinal Cord
    Cervical 00QW
    Lumbar 00QY
    Thoracic 00QX
  Spinal Meninges 00QT
  Spleen 07QP
  Sternum ØPQ0
  Stomach ØDQ6
    Pylorus ØDQ7
  Subcutaneous Tissue and Fascia
    Abdomen ØJQ8
    Back ØJQ7
    Buttock ØJQ9
    Chest ØJQ6
    Face ØJQ1
    Foot
      Left ØJQR
      Right ØJQQ
    Hand
      Left ØJQK
      Right ØJQJ
    Lower Arm
      Left ØJQH
      Right ØJQG
    Lower Leg
      Left ØJQP
      Right ØJQN
    Neck
      Left ØJQ5
      Right ØJQ4
    Pelvic Region ØJQC
    Perineum ØJQB
    Scalp ØJQ0
    Upper Arm
      Left ØJQF
      Right ØJQD
    Upper Leg
      Left ØJQM
      Right ØJQL
  Tarsal
    Left ØQQM
    Right ØQQL
  Tendon
    Abdomen
      Left ØLQG
      Right ØLQF
    Ankle
      Left ØLQT
      Right ØLQS
    Foot
      Left ØLQW
      Right ØLQV
    Hand
      Left ØLQ8
      Right ØLQ7
    Head and Neck ØLQ0
    Hip
      Left ØLQK
      Right ØLQJ
    Knee
      Left ØLQR
      Right ØLQQ

Repair — *continued*
  Tendon — *continued*
    Lower Arm and Wrist
      Left ØLQ6
      Right ØLQ5
    Lower Leg
      Left ØLQP
      Right ØLQN
    Perineum ØLQH
    Shoulder
      Left ØLQ2
      Right ØLQ1
    Thorax
      Left ØLQD
      Right ØLQC
    Trunk
      Left ØLQB
      Right ØLQ9
    Upper Arm
      Left ØLQ4
      Right ØLQ3
    Upper Leg
      Left ØLQM
      Right ØLQL
  Testis
    Bilateral ØVQC
    Left ØVQB
    Right ØVQ9
  Thalamus 00Q9
  Thumb
    Left ØXQM
    Right ØXQL
  Thymus 07QM
  Thyroid Gland ØGQK
    Left Lobe ØGQG
    Right Lobe ØGQH
  Thyroid Gland Isthmus ØGQJ
  Tibia
    Left ØQQH
    Right ØQQG
  Toe
    1st
      Left ØYQQ
      Right ØYQP
    2nd
      Left ØYQS
      Right ØYQR
    3rd
      Left ØYQU
      Right ØYQT
    4th
      Left ØYQW
      Right ØYQV
    5th
      Left ØYQY
      Right ØYQX
  Toe Nail ØHQRXZZ
  Tongue ØCQ7
  Tonsils ØCQP
  Tooth
    Lower ØCQX
    Upper ØCQW
  Trachea ØBQ1
  Tunica Vaginalis
    Left ØVQ7
    Right ØVQ6
  Turbinate, Nasal 09QL
  Tympanic Membrane
    Left 09Q8
    Right 09Q7
  Ulna
    Left ØPQL
    Right ØPQK
  Ureter
    Left ØTQ7
    Right ØTQ6
  Urethra ØTQD
  Uterine Supporting Structure ØUQ4
  Uterus ØUQ9
  Uvula ØCQN
  Vagina ØUQG
  Valve
    Aortic 02QF
    Mitral 02QG
    Pulmonary 02QH
    Tricuspid 02QJ
  Vas Deferens
    Bilateral ØVQQ
    Left ØVQP

Repair — *continued*
  Vas Deferens — *continued*
    Right ØVQN
  Vein
    Axillary
      Left 05Q8
      Right 05Q7
    Azygos 05Q0
    Basilic
      Left 05QC
      Right 05QB
    Brachial
      Left 05QA
      Right 05Q9
    Cephalic
      Left 05QF
      Right 05QD
    Colic 06Q7
    Common Iliac
      Left 06QD
      Right 06QC
    Coronary 02Q4
    Esophageal 06Q3
    External Iliac
      Left 06QG
      Right 06QF
    External Jugular
      Left 05QQ
      Right 05QP
    Face
      Left 05QV
      Right 05QT
    Femoral
      Left 06QN
      Right 06QM
    Foot
      Left 06QV
      Right 06QT
    Gastric 06Q2
    Hand
      Left 05QH
      Right 05QG
    Hemiazygos 05Q1
    Hepatic 06Q4
    Hypogastric
      Left 06QJ
      Right 06QH
    Inferior Mesenteric 06Q6
    Innominate
      Left 05Q4
      Right 05Q3
    Internal Jugular
      Left 05QN
      Right 05QM
    Intracranial 05QL
    Lower 06QY
    Portal 06Q8
    Pulmonary
      Left 02QT
      Right 02QS
    Renal
      Left 06QB
      Right 06Q9
    Saphenous
      Left 06QQ
      Right 06QP
    Splenic 06Q1
    Subclavian
      Left 05Q6
      Right 05Q5
    Superior Mesenteric 06Q5
    Upper 05QY
    Vertebral
      Left 05QS
      Right 05QR
  Vena Cava
    Inferior 06Q0
    Superior 02QV
  Ventricle
    Left 02QL
    Right 02QK
  Vertebra
    Cervical ØPQ3
    Lumbar ØQQ0
    Thoracic ØPQ4
  Vesicle
    Bilateral ØVQ3
    Left ØVQ2
    Right ØVQ1

Subterms under main terms may continue to next column or page

Replacement — *continued*
  Esophagus ØDR5
  Eye
    Left Ø8R1
    Right Ø8RØ
  Eyelid
    Lower
      Left Ø8RR
      Right Ø8RQ
    Upper
      Left Ø8RP
      Right Ø8RN
  Femoral Shaft
    Left ØQR9
    Right ØQR8
  Femur
    Lower
      Left ØQRC
      Right ØQRB
    Upper
      Left ØQR7
      Right ØQR6
  Fibula
    Left ØQRK
    Right ØQRJ
  Finger Nail ØHRQX
  Gingiva
    Lower ØCR6
    Upper ØCR5
  Glenoid Cavity
    Left ØPR8
    Right ØPR7
  Hair ØHRSX
  Humeral Head
    Left ØPRD
    Right ØPRC
  Humeral Shaft
    Left ØPRG
    Right ØPRF
  Iris
    Left Ø8RD3
    Right Ø8RC3
  Joint
    Acromioclavicular
      Left ØRRHØ
      Right ØRRGØ
    Ankle
      Left ØSRG
      Right ØSRF
    Carpal
      Left ØRRRØ
      Right ØRRQØ
    Carpometacarpal
      Left ØRRTØ
      Right ØRRSØ
    Cervical Vertebral ØRR1Ø
    Cervicothoracic Vertebral ØRR4Ø
    Coccygeal ØSR6Ø
    Elbow
      Left ØRRMØ
      Right ØRRLØ
    Finger Phalangeal
      Left ØRRXØ
      Right ØRRWØ
    Hip
      Left ØSRB
        Acetabular Surface ØSRE
        Femoral Surface ØSRS
      Right ØSR9
        Acetabular Surface ØSRA
        Femoral Surface ØSRR
    Knee
      Left ØSRD
        Femoral Surface ØSRU
        Tibial Surface ØSRW
      Right ØSRC
        Femoral Surface ØSRT
        Tibial Surface ØSRV
    Lumbar Vertebral ØSRØØ
    Lumbosacral ØSR3Ø
    Metacarpophalangeal
      Left ØRRVØ
      Right ØRRUØ
    Metatarsal-Phalangeal
      Left ØSRNØ
      Right ØSRMØ
    Occipital-cervical ØRRØØ
    Sacrococcygeal ØSR5Ø

Replacement — *continued*
  Joint — *continued*
    Sacroiliac
      Left ØSR8Ø
      Right ØSR7Ø
    Shoulder
      Left ØRRK
      Right ØRRJ
    Sternoclavicular
      Left ØRRFØ
      Right ØRREØ
    Tarsal
      Left ØSRJØ
      Right ØSRHØ
    Tarsometatarsal
      Left ØSRLØ
      Right ØSRKØ
    Temporomandibular
      Left ØRRDØ
      Right ØRRCØ
    Thoracic Vertebral ØRR6Ø
    Thoracolumbar Vertebral ØRRAØ
    Toe Phalangeal
      Left ØSRQØ
      Right ØSRPØ
    Wrist
      Left ØRRPØ
      Right ØRRNØ
  Kidney Pelvis
    Left ØTR4
    Right ØTR3
  Larynx ØCRS
  Lens
    Left Ø8RK3ØZ
    Right Ø8RJ3ØZ
  Lip
    Lower ØCR1
    Upper ØCRØ
  Mandible
    Left ØNRV
    Right ØNRT
  Maxilla ØNRR
  Mesentery ØDRV
  Metacarpal
    Left ØPRQ
    Right ØPRP
  Metatarsal
    Left ØQRP
    Right ØQRN
  Muscle
    Abdomen
      Left ØKRL
      Right ØKRK
    Facial ØKR1
    Foot
      Left ØKRW
      Right ØKRV
    Hand
      Left ØKRD
      Right ØKRC
    Head ØKRØ
    Hip
      Left ØKRP
      Right ØKRN
    Lower Arm and Wrist
      Left ØKRB
      Right ØKR9
    Lower Leg
      Left ØKRT
      Right ØKRS
    Neck
      Left ØKR3
      Right ØKR2
    Papillary Ø2RD
    Perineum ØKRM
    Shoulder
      Left ØKR6
      Right ØKR5
    Thorax
      Left ØKRJ
      Right ØKRH
    Tongue, Palate, Pharynx ØKR4
    Trunk
      Left ØKRG
      Right ØKRF
    Upper Arm
      Left ØKR8
      Right ØKR7

Replacement — *continued*
  Muscle — *continued*
    Upper Leg
      Left ØKRR
      Right ØKRQ
  Nasal Mucosa and Soft Tissue Ø9RK
  Nasopharynx Ø9RN
  Nerve
    Abducens ØØRL
    Accessory ØØRR
    Acoustic ØØRN
    Cervical Ø1R1
    Facial ØØRM
    Femoral Ø1RD
    Glossopharyngeal ØØRP
    Hypoglossal ØØRS
    Lumbar Ø1RB
    Median Ø1R5
    Oculomotor ØØRH
    Olfactory ØØRF
    Optic ØØRG
    Peroneal Ø1RH
    Phrenic Ø1R2
    Pudendal Ø1RC
    Radial Ø1R6
    Sacral Ø1RR
    Sciatic Ø1RF
    Thoracic Ø1R8
    Tibial Ø1RG
    Trigeminal ØØRK
    Trochlear ØØRJ
    Ulnar Ø1R4
    Vagus ØØRQ
  Nipple
    Left ØHRX
    Right ØHRW
  Omentum ØDRU
  Orbit
    Left ØNRQ
    Right ØNRP
  Palate
    Hard ØCR2
    Soft ØCR3
  Patella
    Left ØQRF
    Right ØQRD
  Pericardium Ø2RN
  Peritoneum ØDRW
  Phalanx
    Finger
      Left ØPRV
      Right ØPRT
    Thumb
      Left ØPRS
      Right ØPRR
    Toe
      Left ØQRR
      Right ØQRQ
  Pharynx ØCRM
  Radius
    Left ØPRJ
    Right ØPRH
  Retinal Vessel
    Left Ø8RH3
    Right Ø8RG3
  Ribs
    1 to 2 ØPR1
    3 or More ØPR2
  Sacrum ØQR1
  Scapula
    Left ØPR6
    Right ØPR5
  Sclera
    Left Ø8R7X
    Right Ø8R6X
  Septum
    Atrial Ø2R5
    Nasal Ø9RM
    Ventricular Ø2RM
  Skin
    Abdomen ØHR7
    Back ØHR6
    Buttock ØHR8
    Chest ØHR5
    Ear
      Left ØHR3
      Right ØHR2
    Face ØHR1

Replacement — *continued*
Skin — *continued*
Foot
Left ØHRN
Right ØHRM
Hand
Left ØHRG
Right ØHRF
Inguinal ØHRA
Lower Arm
Left ØHRE
Right ØHRD
Lower Leg
Left ØHRL
Right ØHRK
Neck ØHR4
Perineum ØHR9
Scalp ØHRØ
Upper Arm
Left ØHRC
Right ØHRB
Upper Leg
Left ØHRJ
Right ØHRH
Skin Substitute, Porcine Liver Derived XHRPXL2
Skull ØNRØ
Spinal Meninges ØØRT
Sternum ØPRØ
Subcutaneous Tissue and Fascia
Abdomen ØJR8
Back ØJR7
Buttock ØJR9
Chest ØJR6
Face ØJR1
Foot
Left ØJRR
Right ØJRQ
Hand
Left ØJRK
Right ØJRJ
Lower Arm
Left ØJRH
Right ØJRG
Lower Leg
Left ØJRP
Right ØJRN
Neck
Left ØJR5
Right ØJR4
Pelvic Region ØJRC
Perineum ØJRB
Scalp ØJRØ
Upper Arm
Left ØJRF
Right ØJRD
Upper Leg
Left ØJRM
Right ØJRL
Tarsal
Left ØQRM
Right ØQRL
Tendon
Abdomen
Left ØLRG
Right ØLRF
Ankle
Left ØLRT
Right ØLRS
Foot
Left ØLRW
Right ØLRV
Hand
Left ØLR8
Right ØLR7
Head and Neck ØLRØ
Hip
Left ØLRK
Right ØLRJ
Knee
Left ØLRR
Right ØLRQ
Lower Arm and Wrist
Left ØLR6
Right ØLR5
Lower Leg
Left ØLRP
Right ØLRN
Perineum ØLRH

Replacement — *continued*
Tendon — *continued*
Shoulder
Left ØLR2
Right ØLR1
Thorax
Left ØLRD
Right ØLRC
Trunk
Left ØLRB
Right ØLR9
Upper Arm
Left ØLR4
Right ØLR3
Upper Leg
Left ØLRM
Right ØLRL
Testis
Bilateral ØVRCØJZ
Left ØVRBØJZ
Right ØVR9ØJZ
Thumb
Left ØXRM
Right ØXRL
Tibia
Left ØQRH
Right ØQRG
Toe Nail ØHRRX
Tongue ØCR7
Tooth
Lower ØCRX
Upper ØCRW
Trachea ØBR1
Turbinate, Nasal Ø9RL
Tympanic Membrane
Left Ø9R8
Right Ø9R7
Ulna
Left ØPRL
Right ØPRK
Ureter
Left ØTR7
Right ØTR6
Urethra ØTRD
Uvula ØCRN
Valve
Aortic Ø2RF
Mitral Ø2RG
Pulmonary Ø2RH
Tricuspid Ø2RJ
Vein
Axillary
Left Ø5R8
Right Ø5R7
Azygos Ø5RØ
Basilic
Left Ø5RC
Right Ø5RB
Brachial
Left Ø5RA
Right Ø5R9
Cephalic
Left Ø5RF
Right Ø5RD
Colic Ø6R7
Common Iliac
Left Ø6RD
Right Ø6RC
Esophageal Ø6R3
External Iliac
Left Ø6RG
Right Ø6RF
External Jugular
Left Ø5RQ
Right Ø5RP
Face
Left Ø5RV
Right Ø5RT
Femoral
Left Ø6RN
Right Ø6RM
Foot
Left Ø6RV
Right Ø6RT
Gastric Ø6R2
Hand
Left Ø5RH
Right Ø5RG
Hemiazygos Ø5R1

Replacement — *continued*
Vein — *continued*
Hepatic Ø6R4
Hypogastric
Left Ø6RJ
Right Ø6RH
Inferior Mesenteric Ø6R6
Innominate
Left Ø5R4
Right Ø5R3
Internal Jugular
Left Ø5RN
Right Ø5RM
Intracranial Ø5RL
Lower Ø6RY
Portal Ø6R8
Pulmonary
Left Ø2RT
Right Ø2RS
Renal
Left Ø6RB
Right Ø6R9
Saphenous
Left Ø6RQ
Right Ø6RP
Splenic Ø6R1
Subclavian
Left Ø5R6
Right Ø5R5
Superior Mesenteric Ø6R5
Upper Ø5RY
Vertebral
Left Ø5RS
Right Ø5RR
Vena Cava
Inferior Ø6RØ
Superior Ø2RV
Ventricle
Left Ø2RL
Right Ø2RK
Vertebra
Cervical ØPR3
Lumbar ØQRØ
Thoracic ØPR4
Vitreous
Left Ø8R53
Right Ø8R43
Vocal Cord
Left ØCRV
Right ØCRT
Zooplastic Tissue, Rapid Deployment Technique X2RF
Replacement, hip
Partial or total *see* Replacement, Lower Joints ØSR
Resurfacing only *see* Supplement, Lower Joints ØSU
Replantation *see* Reposition
Replantation, scalp *see* Reattachment, Skin, Scalp ØHMØ
Reposition
Acetabulum
Left ØQS5
Right ØQS4
Ampulla of Vater ØFSC
Anus ØDSQ
Aorta
Abdominal Ø4SØ
Thoracic
Ascending/Arch Ø2SXØZZ
Descending Ø2SWØZZ
Artery
Anterior Tibial
Left Ø4SQ
Right Ø4SP
Axillary
Left Ø3S6
Right Ø3S5
Brachial
Left Ø3S8
Right Ø3S7
Celiac Ø4S1
Colic
Left Ø4S7
Middle Ø4S8
Right Ø4S6
Common Carotid
Left Ø3SJ
Right Ø3SH

▽ **Subterms under main terms may continue to next column or page**

Reposition — *continued*
  Artery — *continued*
    Common Iliac
      Left 04SD
      Right 04SC
    Coronary
      One Artery 02S00ZZ
      Two Arteries 02S10ZZ
    External Carotid
      Left 03SN
      Right 03SM
    External Iliac
      Left 04SJ
      Right 04SH
    Face 03SR
    Femoral
      Left 04SL
      Right 04SK
    Foot
      Left 04SW
      Right 04SV
    Gastric 04S2
    Hand
      Left 03SF
      Right 03SD
    Hepatic 04S3
    Inferior Mesenteric 04SB
    Innominate 03S2
    Internal Carotid
      Left 03SL
      Right 03SK
    Internal Iliac
      Left 04SF
      Right 04SE
    Internal Mammary
      Left 03S1
      Right 03S0
    Intracranial 03SG
    Lower 04SY
    Peroneal
      Left 04SU
      Right 04ST
    Popliteal
      Left 04SN
      Right 04SM
    Posterior Tibial
      Left 04SS
      Right 04SR
    Pulmonary
      Left 02SR0ZZ
      Right 02SQ0ZZ
    Pulmonary Trunk 02SP0ZZ
    Radial
      Left 03SC
      Right 03SB
    Renal
      Left 04SA
      Right 04S9
    Splenic 04S4
    Subclavian
      Left 03S4
      Right 03S3
    Superior Mesenteric 04S5
    Temporal
      Left 03ST
      Right 03SS
    Thyroid
      Left 03SV
      Right 03SU
    Ulnar
      Left 03SA
      Right 03S9
    Upper 03SY
    Vertebral
      Left 03SQ
      Right 03SP
  Auditory Ossicle
    Left 09SA
    Right 09S9
  Bladder 0TSB
  Bladder Neck 0TSC
  Bone
    Ethmoid
      Left 0NSG
      Right 0NSF
    Frontal 0NS1
    Hyoid 0NSX
    Lacrimal
      Left 0NSJ

Reposition — *continued*
  Bone — *continued*
    Lacrimal — *continued*
      Right 0NSH
    Nasal 0NSB
    Occipital 0NS7
    Palatine
      Left 0NSL
      Right 0NSK
    Parietal
      Left 0NS4
      Right 0NS3
    Pelvic
      Left 0QS3
      Right 0QS2
    Sphenoid 0NSC
    Temporal
      Left 0NS6
      Right 0NS5
    Zygomatic
      Left 0NSN
      Right 0NSM
  Breast
    Bilateral 0HSV0ZZ
    Left 0HSU0ZZ
    Right 0HST0ZZ
  Bronchus
    Lingula 0BS90ZZ
    Lower Lobe
      Left 0BSB0ZZ
      Right 0BS60ZZ
    Main
      Left 0BS70ZZ
      Right 0BS30ZZ
    Middle Lobe, Right 0BS50ZZ
    Upper Lobe
      Left 0BS80ZZ
      Right 0BS40ZZ
  Bursa and Ligament
    Abdomen
      Left 0MSJ
      Right 0MSH
    Ankle
      Left 0MSR
      Right 0MSQ
    Elbow
      Left 0MS4
      Right 0MS3
    Foot
      Left 0MST
      Right 0MSS
    Hand
      Left 0MS8
      Right 0MS7
    Head and Neck 0MS0
    Hip
      Left 0MSM
      Right 0MSL
    Knee
      Left 0MSP
      Right 0MSN
    Lower Extremity
      Left 0MSW
      Right 0MSV
    Perineum 0MSK
    Rib(s) 0MSG
    Shoulder
      Left 0MS2
      Right 0MS1
    Spine
      Lower 0MSD
      Upper 0MSC
    Sternum 0MSF
    Upper Extremity
      Left 0MSB
      Right 0MS9
    Wrist
      Left 0MS6
      Right 0MS5
  Carina 0BS20ZZ
  Carpal
    Left 0PSN
    Right 0PSM
  Cecum 0DSH
  Cervix 0USC
  Clavicle
    Left 0PSB
    Right 0PS9
  Coccyx 0QSS

Reposition — *continued*
  Colon
    Ascending 0DSK
    Descending 0DSM
    Sigmoid 0DSN
    Transverse 0DSL
  Cord
    Bilateral 0VSH
    Left 0VSG
    Right 0VSF
  Cul-de-sac 0USF
  Diaphragm 0BST0ZZ
  Duct
    Common Bile 0FS9
    Cystic 0FS8
    Hepatic
      Common 0FS7
      Left 0FS6
      Right 0FS5
    Lacrimal
      Left 08SY
      Right 08SX
    Pancreatic 0FSD
      Accessory 0FSF
    Parotid
      Left 0CSC
      Right 0CSB
  Duodenum 0DS9
  Ear
    Bilateral 09S2
    Left 09S1
    Right 09S0
  Epiglottis 0CSR
  Esophagus 0DS5
  Eustachian Tube
    Left 09SG
    Right 09SF
  Eyelid
    Lower
      Left 08SR
      Right 08SQ
    Upper
      Left 08SP
      Right 08SN
  Fallopian Tube
    Left 0US6
    Right 0US5
  Fallopian Tubes, Bilateral 0US7
  Femoral Shaft
    Left 0QS9
    Right 0QS8
  Femur
    Lower
      Left 0QSC
      Right 0QSB
    Upper
      Left 0QS7
      Right 0QS6
  Fibula
    Left 0QSK
    Right 0QSJ
  Gallbladder 0FS4
  Gland
    Adrenal
      Left 0GS2
      Right 0GS3
    Lacrimal
      Left 08SW
      Right 08SV
  Glenoid Cavity
    Left 0PS8
    Right 0PS7
  Hair 0HSSXZZ
  Humeral Head
    Left 0PSD
    Right 0PSC
  Humeral Shaft
    Left 0PSG
    Right 0PSF
  Ileum 0DSB
  Intestine
    Large 0DSE
    Small 0DS8
  Iris
    Left 08SD3ZZ
    Right 08SC3ZZ
  Jejunum 0DSA

— *continued*
Joint
  Acromioclavicular
    Left ØRSH
    Right ØRSG
  Ankle
    Left ØSSG
    Right ØSSF
  Carpal
    Left ØRSR
    Right ØRSQ
  Carpometacarpal
    Left ØRST
    Right ØRSS
  Cervical Vertebral ØRS1
  Cervicothoracic Vertebral ØRS4
  Coccygeal ØSS6
  Elbow
    Left ØRSM
    Right ØRSL
  Finger Phalangeal
    Left ØRSX
    Right ØRSW
  Hip
    Left ØSSB
    Right ØSS9
  Knee
    Left ØSSD
    Right ØSSC
  Lumbar Vertebral ØSSØ
  Lumbosacral ØSS3
  Metacarpophalangeal
    Left ØRSV
    Right ØRSU
  Metatarsal-Phalangeal
    Left ØSSN
    Right ØSSM
  Occipital-cervical ØRSØ
  Sacrococcygeal ØSS5
  Sacroiliac
    Left ØSS8
    Right ØSS7
  Shoulder
    Left ØRSK
    Right ØRSJ
  Sternoclavicular
    Left ØRSF
    Right ØRSE
  Tarsal
    Left ØSSJ
    Right ØSSH
  Tarsometatarsal
    Left ØSSL
    Right ØSSK
  Temporomandibular
    Left ØRSD
    Right ØRSC
  Thoracic Vertebral ØRS6
  Thoracolumbar Vertebral ØRSA
  Toe Phalangeal
    Left ØSSQ
    Right ØSSP
  Wrist
    Left ØRSP
    Right ØRSN
Kidney
  Left ØTS1
  Right ØTSØ
Kidney Pelvis
  Left ØTS4
  Right ØTS3
Kidneys, Bilateral ØTS2
Lens
  Left Ø8SK3ZZ
  Right Ø8SJ3ZZ
Lip
  Lower ØCS1
  Upper ØCSØ
Liver ØFSØ
Lung
  Left ØBSLØZZ
  Lower Lobe
    Left ØBSJØZZ
    Right ØBSFØZZ
  Middle Lobe, Right ØBSDØZZ
  Right ØBSKØZZ
  Upper Lobe
    Left ØBSGØZZ
    Right ØBSCØZZ

— *continued*
  Lung Lingula ØBSHØZZ
Mandible
  Left ØNSV
  Right ØNST
Maxilla ØNSR
Metacarpal
  Left ØPSQ
  Right ØPSP
Metatarsal
  Left ØQSP
  Right ØQSN
Muscle
  Abdomen
    Left ØKSL
    Right ØKSK
  Extraocular
    Left Ø8SM
    Right Ø8SL
  Facial ØKS1
  Foot
    Left ØKSW
    Right ØKSV
  Hand
    Left ØKSD
    Right ØKSC
  Head ØKSØ
  Hip
    Left ØKSP
    Right ØKSN
  Lower Arm and Wrist
    Left ØKSB
    Right ØKS9
  Lower Leg
    Left ØKST
    Right ØKSS
  Neck
    Left ØKS3
    Right ØKS2
  Perineum ØKSM
  Shoulder
    Left ØKS6
    Right ØKS5
  Thorax
    Left ØKSJ
    Right ØKSH
  Tongue, Palate, Pharynx ØKS4
  Trunk
    Left ØKSG
    Right ØKSF
  Upper Arm
    Left ØKS8
    Right ØKS7
  Upper Leg
    Left ØKSR
    Right ØKSQ
Nasal Mucosa and Soft Tissue Ø9SK
Nerve
  Abducens ØØSL
  Accessory ØØSR
  Acoustic ØØSN
  Brachial Plexus Ø1S3
  Cervical Ø1S1
  Cervical Plexus Ø1SØ
  Facial ØØSM
  Femoral Ø1SD
  Glossopharyngeal ØØSP
  Hypoglossal ØØSS
  Lumbar Ø1SB
  Lumbar Plexus Ø1S9
  Lumbosacral Plexus Ø1SA
  Median Ø1S5
  Oculomotor ØØSH
  Olfactory ØØSF
  Optic ØØSG
  Peroneal Ø1SH
  Phrenic Ø1S2
  Pudendal Ø1SC
  Radial Ø1S6
  Sacral Ø1SR
  Sacral Plexus Ø1SQ
  Sciatic Ø1SF
  Thoracic Ø1S8
  Tibial Ø1SG
  Trigeminal ØØSK
  Trochlear ØØSJ
  Ulnar Ø1S4
  Vagus ØØSQ

— *continued*
Nipple
  Left ØHSXXZZ
  Right ØHSWXZZ
Orbit
  Left ØNSQ
  Right ØNSP
Ovary
  Bilateral ØUS2
  Left ØUS1
  Right ØUSØ
Palate
  Hard ØCS2
  Soft ØCS3
Pancreas ØFSG
Parathyroid Gland ØGSR
  Inferior
    Left ØGSP
    Right ØGSN
  Multiple ØGSQ
  Superior
    Left ØGSM
    Right ØGSL
Patella
  Left ØQSF
  Right ØQSD
Phalanx
  Finger
    Left ØPSV
    Right ØPST
  Thumb
    Left ØPSS
    Right ØPSR
  Toe
    Left ØQSR
    Right ØQSQ
Products of Conception 10SØ
  Ectopic 10S2
Radius
  Left ØPSJ
  Right ØPSH
Rectum ØDSP
Retinal Vessel
  Left Ø8SH3ZZ
  Right Ø8SG3ZZ
Ribs
  1 to 2 ØPS1
  3 or More ØPS2
Sacrum ØQS1
Scapula
  Left ØPS6
  Right ØPS5
Septum, Nasal Ø9SM
Sesamoid Bone(s) 1st Toe
  see Reposition, Metatarsal, Left ØQSP
  see Reposition, Metatarsal, Right ØQSN
Skull ØNSØ
Spinal Cord
  Cervical ØØSW
  Lumbar ØØSY
  Thoracic ØØSX
Spleen Ø7SPØZZ
Sternum ØPSØ
Stomach ØDS6
Tarsal
  Left ØQSM
  Right ØQSL
Tendon
  Abdomen
    Left ØLSG
    Right ØLSF
  Ankle
    Left ØLST
    Right ØLSS
  Foot
    Left ØLSW
    Right ØLSV
  Hand
    Left ØLS8
    Right ØLS7
  Head and Neck ØLSØ
  Hip
    Left ØLSK
    Right ØLSJ
  Knee
    Left ØLSR
    Right ØLSQ
  Lower Arm and Wrist
    Left ØLS6

Subterms under main terms may continue to next column or page

Reposition — *continued*

Tendon — *continued*

Lower Arm and Wrist — *continued*

Right 0LS5

Lower Leg

Left 0LSP

Right 0LSN

Perineum 0LSH

Shoulder

Left 0LS2

Right 0LS1

Thorax

Left 0LSD

Right 0LSC

Trunk

Left 0LSB

Right 0LS9

Upper Arm

Left 0LS4

Right 0LS3

Upper Leg

Left 0LSM

Right 0LSL

Testis

Bilateral 0VSC

Left 0VSB

Right 0VS9

Thymus 07SM0ZZ

Thyroid Gland

Left Lobe 0GSG

Right Lobe 0GSH

Tibia

Left 0QSH

Right 0QSG

Tongue 0CS7

Tooth

Lower 0CSX

Upper 0CSW

Trachea 0BS10ZZ

Turbinate, Nasal 09SL

Tympanic Membrane

Left 09S8

Right 09S7

Ulna

Left 0PSL

Right 0PSK

Ureter

Left 0TS7

Right 0TS6

Ureters, Bilateral 0TS8

Urethra 0TSD

Uterine Supporting Structure 0US4

Uterus 0US9

Uvula 0CSN

Vagina 0USG

Vein

Axillary

Left 05S8

Right 05S7

Azygos 05S0

Basilic

Left 05SC

Right 05SB

Brachial

Left 05SA

Right 05S9

Cephalic

Left 05SF

Right 05SD

Colic 06S7

Common Iliac

Left 06SD

Right 06SC

Esophageal 06S3

External Iliac

Left 06SG

Right 06SF

External Jugular

Left 05SQ

Right 05SP

Face

Left 05SV

Right 05ST

Femoral

Left 06SN

Right 06SM

Foot

Left 06SV

Right 06ST

Reposition — *continued*

Vein — *continued*

Gastric 06S2

Hand

Left 05SH

Right 05SG

Hemiazygos 05S1

Hepatic 06S4

Hypogastric

Left 06SJ

Right 06SH

Inferior Mesenteric 06S6

Innominate

Left 05S4

Right 05S3

Internal Jugular

Left 05SN

Right 05SM

Intracranial 05SL

Lower 06SY

Portal 06S8

Pulmonary

Left 02ST0ZZ

Right 02SS0ZZ

Renal

Left 06SB

Right 06S9

Saphenous

Left 06SQ

Right 06SP

Splenic 06S1

Subclavian

Left 05S6

Right 05S5

Superior Mesenteric 06S5

Upper 05SY

Vertebral

Left 05SS

Right 05SR

Vena Cava

Inferior 06S0

Superior 02SV0ZZ

Vertebra

Cervical 0PS3

Magnetically Controlled Growth Rod(s) XNS3

Lumbar 0QS0

Magnetically Controlled Growth Rod(s) XNS0

Thoracic 0PS4

Magnetically Controlled Growth Rod(s) XNS4

Vocal Cord

Left 0CSV

Right 0CST

Resection

Acetabulum

Left 0QT50ZZ

Right 0QT40ZZ

Adenoids 0CTQ

Ampulla of Vater 0FTC

Anal Sphincter 0DTR

Anus 0DTQ

Aortic Body 0GTD

Appendix 0DTJ

Auditory Ossicle

Left 09TA

Right 09T9

Bladder 0TTB

Bladder Neck 0TTC

Bone

Ethmoid

Left 0NTG0ZZ

Right 0NTF0ZZ

Frontal 0NT10ZZ

Hyoid 0NTX0ZZ

Lacrimal

Left 0NTJ0ZZ

Right 0NTH0ZZ

Nasal 0NTB0ZZ

Occipital 0NT70ZZ

Palatine

Left 0NTL0ZZ

Right 0NTK0ZZ

Parietal

Left 0NT40ZZ

Right 0NT30ZZ

Pelvic

Left 0QT30ZZ

Resection — *continued*

Bone — *continued*

Pelvic — *continued*

Right 0QT20ZZ

Sphenoid 0NTC0ZZ

Temporal

Left 0NT60ZZ

Right 0NT50ZZ

Zygomatic

Left 0NTN0ZZ

Right 0NTM0ZZ

Breast

Bilateral 0HTV0ZZ

Left 0HTU0ZZ

Right 0HTT0ZZ

Supernumerary 0HTY0ZZ

Bronchus

Lingula 0BT9

Lower Lobe

Left 0BTB

Right 0BT6

Main

Left 0BT7

Right 0BT3

Middle Lobe, Right 0BT5

Upper Lobe

Left 0BT8

Right 0BT4

Bursa and Ligament

Abdomen

Left 0MTJ

Right 0MTH

Ankle

Left 0MTR

Right 0MTQ

Elbow

Left 0MT4

Right 0MT3

Foot

Left 0MTT

Right 0MTS

Hand

Left 0MT8

Right 0MT7

Head and Neck 0MT0

Hip

Left 0MTM

Right 0MTL

Knee

Left 0MTP

Right 0MTN

Lower Extremity

Left 0MTW

Right 0MTV

Perineum 0MTK

Rib(s) 0MTG

Shoulder

Left 0MT2

Right 0MT1

Spine

Lower 0MTD

Upper 0MTC

Sternum 0MTF

Upper Extremity

Left 0MTB

Right 0MT9

Wrist

Left 0MT6

Right 0MT5

Carina 0BT2

Carotid Bodies, Bilateral 0GT8

Carotid Body

Left 0GT6

Right 0GT7

Carpal

Left 0PTN0ZZ

Right 0PTM0ZZ

Cecum 0DTH

Cerebral Hemisphere 00T7

Cervix 0UTC

Chordae Tendineae 02T9

Cisterna Chyli 07TL

Clavicle

Left 0PTB0ZZ

Right 0PT90ZZ

Clitoris 0UTJ

Coccygeal Glomus 0GTB

Coccyx 0QTS0ZZ

Resection — *continued*
Colon
  Ascending ØDTK
  Descending ØDTM
  Sigmoid ØDTN
  Transverse ØDTL
Conduction Mechanism Ø2T8
Cord
  Bilateral ØVTH
  Left ØVTG
  Right ØVTF
Cornea
  Left Ø8T9XZZ
  Right Ø8T8XZZ
Cul-de-sac ØUTF
Diaphragm ØBTT
Disc
  Cervical Vertebral ØRT3ØZZ
  Cervicothoracic Vertebral ØRT5ØZZ
  Lumbar Vertebral ØST2ØZZ
  Lumbosacral ØST4ØZZ
  Thoracic Vertebral ØRT9ØZZ
  Thoracolumbar Vertebral ØRTBØZZ
Duct
  Common Bile ØFT9
  Cystic ØFT8
  Hepatic
    Common ØFT7
    Left ØFT6
    Right ØFT5
  Lacrimal
    Left Ø8TY
    Right Ø8TX
  Pancreatic ØFTD
    Accessory ØFTF
  Parotid
    Left ØCTCØZZ
    Right ØCTBØZZ
Duodenum ØDT9
Ear
  External
    Left Ø9T1
    Right Ø9TØ
  Inner
    Left Ø9TE
    Right Ø9TD
  Middle
    Left Ø9T6
    Right Ø9T5
Epididymis
  Bilateral ØVTL
  Left ØVTK
  Right ØVTJ
Epiglottis ØCTR
Esophagogastric Junction ØDT4
Esophagus ØDT5
  Lower ØDT3
  Middle ØDT2
  Upper ØDT1
Eustachian Tube
  Left Ø9TG
  Right Ø9TF
Eye
  Left Ø8T1XZZ
  Right Ø8TØXZZ
Eyelid
  Lower
    Left Ø8TR
    Right Ø8TQ
  Upper
    Left Ø8TP
    Right Ø8TN
Fallopian Tube
  Left ØUT6
  Right ØUT5
Fallopian Tubes, Bilateral ØUT7
Femoral Shaft
  Left ØQT9ØZZ
  Right ØQT8ØZZ
Femur
  Lower
    Left ØQTCØZZ
    Right ØQTBØZZ
  Upper
    Left ØQT7ØZZ
    Right ØQT6ØZZ
Fibula
  Left ØQTKØZZ
  Right ØQTJØZZ

Resection — *continued*
Finger Nail ØHTQXZZ
Gallbladder ØFT4
Gland
  Adrenal
    Bilateral ØGT4
    Left ØGT2
    Right ØGT3
  Lacrimal
    Left Ø8TW
    Right Ø8TV
  Minor Salivary ØCTJØZZ
  Parotid
    Left ØCT9ØZZ
    Right ØCT8ØZZ
  Pituitary ØGTØ
  Sublingual
    Left ØCTFØZZ
    Right ØCTDØZZ
  Submaxillary
    Left ØCTHØZZ
    Right ØCTGØZZ
  Vestibular ØUTL
Glenoid Cavity
  Left ØPT8ØZZ
  Right ØPT7ØZZ
Glomus Jugulare ØGTC
Humeral Head
  Left ØPTDØZZ
  Right ØPTCØZZ
Humeral Shaft
  Left ØPTGØZZ
  Right ØPTFØZZ
Hymen ØUTK
Ileocecal Valve ØDTC
Ileum ØDTB
Intestine
  Large ØDTE
    Left ØDTG
    Right ØDTF
  Small ØDT8
Iris
  Left Ø8TD3ZZ
  Right Ø8TC3ZZ
Jejunum ØDTA
Joint
  Acromioclavicular
    Left ØRTHØZZ
    Right ØRTGØZZ
  Ankle
    Left ØSTGØZZ
    Right ØSTFØZZ
  Carpal
    Left ØRTRØZZ
    Right ØRTQØZZ
  Carpometacarpal
    Left ØRTTØZZ
    Right ØRTSØZZ
  Cervicothoracic Vertebral ØRT4ØZZ
  Coccygeal ØST6ØZZ
  Elbow
    Left ØRTMØZZ
    Right ØRTLØZZ
  Finger Phalangeal
    Left ØRTXØZZ
    Right ØRTWØZZ
  Hip
    Left ØSTBØZZ
    Right ØST9ØZZ
  Knee
    Left ØSTDØZZ
    Right ØSTCØZZ
  Metacarpophalangeal
    Left ØRTVØZZ
    Right ØRTUØZZ
  Metatarsal-Phalangeal
    Left ØSTNØZZ
    Right ØSTMØZZ
  Sacrococcygeal ØST5ØZZ
  Sacroiliac
    Left ØST8ØZZ
    Right ØST7ØZZ
  Shoulder
    Left ØRTKØZZ
    Right ØRTJØZZ
  Sternoclavicular
    Left ØRTFØZZ
    Right ØRTEØZZ

Resection — *continued*
Joint — *continued*
  Tarsal
    Left ØSTJØZZ
    Right ØSTHØZZ
  Tarsometatarsal
    Left ØSTLØZZ
    Right ØSTKØZZ
  Temporomandibular
    Left ØRTDØZZ
    Right ØRTCØZZ
  Toe Phalangeal
    Left ØSTQØZZ
    Right ØSTPØZZ
  Wrist
    Left ØRTPØZZ
    Right ØRTNØZZ
Kidney
  Left ØTT1
  Right ØTTØ
Kidney Pelvis
  Left ØTT4
  Right ØTT3
Kidneys, Bilateral ØTT2
Larynx ØCTS
Lens
  Left Ø8TK3ZZ
  Right Ø8TJ3ZZ
Lip
  Lower ØCT1
  Upper ØCTØ
Liver ØFTØ
  Left Lobe ØFT2
  Right Lobe ØFT1
Lung
  Bilateral ØBTM
  Left ØBTL
  Lower Lobe
    Left ØBTJ
    Right ØBTF
  Middle Lobe, Right ØBTD
  Right ØBTK
  Upper Lobe
    Left ØBTG
    Right ØBTC
Lung Lingula ØBTH
Lymphatic
  Aortic Ø7TD
  Axillary
    Left Ø7T6
    Right Ø7T5
  Head Ø7TØ
  Inguinal
    Left Ø7TJ
    Right Ø7TH
  Internal Mammary
    Left Ø7T9
    Right Ø7T8
  Lower Extremity
    Left Ø7TG
    Right Ø7TF
  Mesenteric Ø7TB
  Neck
    Left Ø7T2
    Right Ø7T1
  Pelvis Ø7TC
  Thoracic Duct Ø7TK
  Thorax Ø7T7
  Upper Extremity
    Left Ø7T4
    Right Ø7T3
Mandible
  Left ØNTVØZZ
  Right ØNTTØZZ
Maxilla ØNTRØZZ
Metacarpal
  Left ØPTQØZZ
  Right ØPTPØZZ
Metatarsal
  Left ØQTPØZZ
  Right ØQTNØZZ
Muscle
  Abdomen
    Left ØKTL
    Right ØKTK
  Extraocular
    Left Ø8TM
    Right Ø8TL
  Facial ØKT1

Resection — *continued*
  Muscle — *continued*
    Foot
      Left ØKTW
      Right ØKTV
    Hand
      Left ØKTD
      Right ØKTC
    Head ØKTØ
    Hip
      Left ØKTP
      Right ØKTN
    Lower Arm and Wrist
      Left ØKTB
      Right ØKT9
    Lower Leg
      Left ØKTT
      Right ØKTS
    Neck
      Left ØKT3
      Right ØKT2
    Papillary Ø2TD
    Perineum ØKTM
    Shoulder
      Left ØKT6
      Right ØKT5
    Thorax
      Left ØKTJ
      Right ØKTH
    Tongue, Palate, Pharynx ØKT4
    Trunk
      Left ØKTG
      Right ØKTF
    Upper Arm
      Left ØKT8
      Right ØKT7
    Upper Leg
      Left ØKTR
      Right ØKTQ
  Nasal Mucosa and Soft Tissue Ø9TK
  Nasopharynx Ø9TN
  Nipple
    Left ØHTXXZZ
    Right ØHTWXZZ
  Omentum ØDTU
  Orbit
    Left ØNTQØZZ
    Right ØNTPØZZ
  Ovary
    Bilateral ØUT2
    Left ØUT1
    Right ØUTØ
  Palate
    Hard ØCT2
    Soft ØCT3
  Pancreas ØFTG
  Para-aortic Body ØGT9
  Paraganglion Extremity ØGTF
  Parathyroid Gland ØGTR
    Inferior
      Left ØGTP
      Right ØGTN
    Multiple ØGTQ
    Superior
      Left ØGTM
      Right ØGTL
  Patella
    Left ØQTFØZZ
    Right ØQTDØZZ
  Penis ØVTS
  Pericardium Ø2TN
  Phalanx
    Finger
      Left ØPTVØZZ
      Right ØPTTØZZ
    Thumb
      Left ØPTSØZZ
      Right ØPTRØZZ
    Toe
      Left ØQTRØZZ
      Right ØQTQØZZ
  Pharynx ØCTM
  Pineal Body ØGT1
  Prepuce ØVTT
  Products of Conception, Ectopic 10T2
  Prostate ØVTØ
  Radius
    Left ØPTJØZZ
    Right ØPTHØZZ

Resection — *continued*
  Rectum ØDTP
  Ribs
    1 to 2 ØPT1ØZZ
    3 or More ØPT2ØZZ
  Scapula
    Left ØPT6ØZZ
    Right ØPT5ØZZ
  Scrotum ØVT5
  Septum
    Atrial Ø2T5
    Nasal Ø9TM
    Ventricular Ø2TM
  Sinus
    Accessory Ø9TP
    Ethmoid
      Left Ø9TV
      Right Ø9TU
    Frontal
      Left Ø9TT
      Right Ø9TS
    Mastoid
      Left Ø9TC
      Right Ø9TB
    Maxillary
      Left Ø9TR
      Right Ø9TQ
    Sphenoid
      Left Ø9TX
      Right Ø9TW
  Spleen Ø7TP
  Sternum ØPTØØZZ
  Stomach ØDT6
    Pylorus ØDT7
  Tarsal
    Left ØQTMØZZ
    Right ØQTLØZZ
  Tendon
    Abdomen
      Left ØLTG
      Right ØLTF
    Ankle
      Left ØLTT
      Right ØLTS
    Foot
      Left ØLTW
      Right ØLTV
    Hand
      Left ØLT8
      Right ØLT7
    Head and Neck ØLTØ
    Hip
      Left ØLTK
      Right ØLTJ
    Knee
      Left ØLTR
      Right ØLTQ
    Lower Arm and Wrist
      Left ØLT6
      Right ØLT5
    Lower Leg
      Left ØLTP
      Right ØLTN
    Perineum ØLTH
    Shoulder
      Left ØLT2
      Right ØLT1
    Thorax
      Left ØLTD
      Right ØLTC
    Trunk
      Left ØLTB
      Right ØLT9
    Upper Arm
      Left ØLT4
      Right ØLT3
    Upper Leg
      Left ØLTM
      Right ØLTL
  Testis
    Bilateral ØVTC
    Left ØVTB
    Right ØVT9
  Thymus Ø7TM
  Thyroid Gland ØGTK
    Left Lobe ØGTG
    Right Lobe ØGTH
  Thyroid Gland Isthmus ØGTJ

Resection — *continued*
  Tibia
    Left ØQTHØZZ
    Right ØQTGØZZ
  Toe Nail ØHTRXZZ
  Tongue ØCT7
  Tonsils ØCTP
  Tooth
    Lower ØCTXØZ
    Upper ØCTWØZ
  Trachea ØBT1
  Tunica Vaginalis
    Left ØVT7
    Right ØVT6
  Turbinate, Nasal Ø9TL
  Tympanic Membrane
    Left Ø9T8
    Right Ø9T7
  Ulna
    Left ØPTLØZZ
    Right ØPTKØZZ
  Ureter
    Left ØTT7
    Right ØTT6
  Urethra ØTTD
  Uterine Supporting Structure ØUT4
  Uterus ØUT9
  Uvula ØCTN
  Vagina ØUTG
  Valve, Pulmonary Ø2TH
  Vas Deferens
    Bilateral ØVTQ
    Left ØVTP
    Right ØVTN
  Vesicle
    Bilateral ØVT3
    Left ØVT2
    Right ØVT1
  Vitreous
    Left Ø8T53ZZ
    Right Ø8T43ZZ
  Vocal Cord
    Left ØCTV
    Right ØCTT
  Vulva ØUTM
Resection, Left ventricular outflow tract obstruc-
    tion (LVOT) *see* Dilation, Ventricle, Left Ø27L
Resection, Subaortic membrane (Left ventricular
    outflow tract obstruction) *see* Dilation, Ventri-
    cle, Left Ø27L
Restoration, Cardiac, Single, Rhythm 5A22Ø4Z
RestoreAdvanced neurostimulator (SureScan) (MRI
    Safe) *use* Stimulator Generator, Multiple Array
    Rechargeable in ØJH
RestoreSensor neurostimulator (SureScan) (MRI
    Safe) *use* Stimulator Generator, Multiple Array
    Rechargeable in ØJH
RestoreUltra neurostimulator (SureScan) (MRI
    Safe) *use* Stimulator Generator, Multiple Array
    Rechargeable in ØJH
Restriction
  Ampulla of Vater ØFVC
  Anus ØDVQ
  Aorta
    Abdominal Ø4VØ
      Intraluminal Device, Branched or Fenes-
        trated Ø4VØ
    Thoracic
      Ascending/Arch, Intraluminal Device,
        Branched or Fenestrated Ø2VX
      Descending, Intraluminal Device,
        Branched or Fenestrated Ø2VW
  Artery
    Anterior Tibial
      Left Ø4VQ
      Right Ø4VP
    Axillary
      Left Ø3V6
      Right Ø3V5
    Brachial
      Left Ø3V8
      Right Ø3V7
    Celiac Ø4V1
    Colic
      Left Ø4V7
      Middle Ø4V8
      Right Ø4V6

Resuscitation — *continued*
Pulmonary 5A19054
Resuscitative endovascular balloon occlusion of the aorta (REBOA)
Ø2LW3DJ
Ø4LØ3DJ
Resuture, Heart valve prosthesis *see* Revision of device in, Heart and Great Vessels Ø2W
Retained placenta, manual removal *see* Extraction, Products of Conception, Retained 1ØD1
Retraining
Cardiac *see* Motor Treatment, Rehabilitation FØ7
Vocational *see* Activities of Daily Living Treatment, Rehabilitation FØ8
Retrogasserian rhizotomy *see* Division, Nerve, Trigeminal ØØ8K
Retroperitoneal cavity *use* Retroperitoneum
Retroperitoneal lymph node *use* Lymphatic, Aortic
Retroperitoneal space *use* Retroperitoneum
Retropharyngeal lymph node
use Lymphatic, Left Neck
use Lymphatic, Right Neck
Retropubic space *use* Pelvic Cavity
Reveal (LINQ) (DX) (XT) *use* Monitoring Device
Reverse total shoulder replacement *see* Replacement, Upper Joints ØRR
Reverse® Shoulder Prosthesis *use* Synthetic Substitute, Reverse Ball and Socket in ØRR
Revision
Correcting a portion of existing device *see* Revision of device in
Removal of device without replacement *see* Removal of device from
Replacement of existing device
see Removal of device from
see Root operation to place new device, e.g., Insertion, Replacement, Supplement
Revision of device in
Abdominal Wall ØWWF
Acetabulum
Left ØQW5
Right ØQW4
Anal Sphincter ØDWR
Anus ØDWQ
Artery
Lower Ø4WY
Upper Ø3WY
Auditory Ossicle
Left Ø9WA
Right Ø9W9
Back
Lower ØWWL
Upper ØWWK
Bladder ØTWB
Bone
Facial ØNWW
Lower ØQWY
Nasal ØNWB
Pelvic
Left ØQW3
Right ØQW2
Upper ØPWY
Bone Marrow Ø7WT
Brain ØØWØ
Breast
Left ØHWU
Right ØHWT
Bursa and Ligament
Lower ØMWY
Upper ØMWX
Carpal
Left ØPWN
Right ØPWM
Cavity, Cranial ØWW1
Cerebral Ventricle ØØW6
Chest Wall ØWW8
Cisterna Chyli Ø7WL
Clavicle
Left ØPWB
Right ØPW9
Coccyx ØQWS
Diaphragm ØBWT
Disc
Cervical Vertebral ØRW3
Cervicothoracic Vertebral ØRW5
Lumbar Vertebral ØSW2
Lumbosacral ØSW4
Thoracic Vertebral ØRW9

Revision of device in — *continued*
Disc — *continued*
Thoracolumbar Vertebral ØRWB
Duct
Hepatobiliary ØFWB
Pancreatic ØFWD
Ear
Inner
Left Ø9WE
Right Ø9WD
Left Ø9WJ
Right Ø9WH
Epididymis and Spermatic Cord ØVWM
Esophagus ØDW5
Extremity
Lower
Left ØYWB
Right ØYW9
Upper
Left ØXW7
Right ØXW6
Eye
Left Ø8W1
Right Ø8WØ
Face ØWW2
Fallopian Tube ØUW8
Femoral Shaft
Left ØQW9
Right ØQW8
Femur
Lower
Left ØQWC
Right ØQWB
Upper
Left ØQW7
Right ØQW6
Fibula
Left ØQWK
Right ØQWJ
Finger Nail ØHWQX
Gallbladder ØFW4
Gastrointestinal Tract ØWWP
Genitourinary Tract ØWWR
Gland
Adrenal ØGW5
Endocrine ØGWS
Pituitary ØGWØ
Salivary ØCWA
Glenoid Cavity
Left ØPW8
Right ØPW7
Great Vessel Ø2WY
Hair ØHWSX
Head ØWWØ
Heart Ø2WA
Humeral Head
Left ØPWD
Right ØPWC
Humeral Shaft
Left ØPWG
Right ØPWF
Intestinal Tract
Lower ØDWD
Upper ØDWØ
Intestine
Large ØDWE
Small ØDW8
Jaw
Lower ØWW5
Upper ØWW4
Joint
Acromioclavicular
Left ØRWH
Right ØRWG
Ankle
Left ØSWG
Right ØSWF
Carpal
Left ØRWR
Right ØRWQ
Carpometacarpal
Left ØRWT
Right ØRWS
Cervical Vertebral ØRW1
Cervicothoracic Vertebral ØRW4
Coccygeal ØSW6
Elbow
Left ØRWM
Right ØRWL

Revision of device in — *continued*
Joint — *continued*
Finger Phalangeal
Left ØRWX
Right ØRWW
Hip
Left ØSWB
Acetabular Surface ØSWE
Femoral Surface ØSWS
Right ØSW9
Acetabular Surface ØSWA
Femoral Surface ØSWR
Knee
Left ØSWD
Femoral Surface ØSWU
Tibial Surface ØSWW
Right ØSWC
Femoral Surface ØSWT
Tibial Surface ØSWV
Lumbar Vertebral ØSWØ
Lumbosacral ØSW3
Metacarpophalangeal
Left ØRWV
Right ØRWU
Metatarsal-Phalangeal
Left ØSWN
Right ØSWM
Occipital-cervical ØRWØ
Sacrococcygeal ØSW5
Sacroiliac
Left ØSW8
Right ØSW7
Shoulder
Left ØRWK
Right ØRWJ
Sternoclavicular
Left ØRWF
Right ØRWE
Tarsal
Left ØSWJ
Right ØSWH
Tarsometatarsal
Left ØSWL
Right ØSWK
Temporomandibular
Left ØRWD
Right ØRWC
Thoracic Vertebral ØRW6
Thoracolumbar Vertebral ØRWA
Toe Phalangeal
Left ØSWQ
Right ØSWP
Wrist
Left ØRWP
Right ØRWN
Kidney ØTW5
Larynx ØCWS
Lens
Left Ø8WK
Right Ø8WJ
Liver ØFWØ
Lung
Left ØBWL
Right ØBWK
Lymphatic Ø7WN
Thoracic Duct Ø7WK
Mediastinum ØWWC
Mesentery ØDWV
Metacarpal
Left ØPWQ
Right ØPWP
Metatarsal
Left ØQWP
Right ØQWN
Mouth and Throat ØCWY
Muscle
Extraocular
Left Ø8WM
Right Ø8WL
Lower ØKWY
Upper ØKWX
Nasal Mucosa and Soft Tissue Ø9WK
Neck ØWW6
Nerve
Cranial ØØWE
Peripheral Ø1WY
Omentum ØDWU
Ovary ØUW3
Pancreas ØFWG

Revision of device in — *continued*
  Parathyroid Gland ØGWR
  Patella
    Left ØQWF
    Right ØQWD
  Pelvic Cavity ØWWJ
  Penis ØVWS
  Pericardial Cavity ØWWD
  Perineum
    Female ØWWN
    Male ØWWM
  Peritoneal Cavity ØWWG
  Peritoneum ØDWW
  Phalanx
    Finger
      Left ØPWV
      Right ØPWT
    Thumb
      Left ØPWS
      Right ØPWR
    Toe
      Left ØQWR
      Right ØQWQ
  Pineal Body ØGW1
  Pleura ØBWQ
  Pleural Cavity
    Left ØWWB
    Right ØWW9
  Prostate and Seminal Vesicles ØVW4
  Radius
    Left ØPWJ
    Right ØPWH
  Respiratory Tract ØWWQ
  Retroperitoneum ØWWH
  Ribs
    1 to 2 ØPW1
    3 or More ØPW2
  Sacrum ØQW1
  Scapula
    Left ØPW6
    Right ØPW5
  Scrotum and Tunica Vaginalis ØVW8
  Septum
    Atrial Ø2W5
    Ventricular Ø2WM
  Sinus Ø9WY
  Skin ØHWPX
  Skull ØNWØ
  Spinal Canal ØØWU
  Spinal Cord ØØWV
  Spleen Ø7WP
  Sternum ØPWØ
  Stomach ØDW6
  Subcutaneous Tissue and Fascia
    Head and Neck ØJWS
    Lower Extremity ØJWW
    Trunk ØJWT
    Upper Extremity ØJWV
  Tarsal
    Left ØQWM
    Right ØQWL
  Tendon
    Lower ØLWY
    Upper ØLWX
  Testis ØVWD
  Thymus Ø7WM
  Thyroid Gland ØGWK
  Tibia
    Left ØQWH
    Right ØQWG
  Toe Nail ØHWRX
  Trachea ØBW1
  Tracheobronchial Tree ØBWØ
  Tympanic Membrane
    Left Ø9W8
    Right Ø9W7
  Ulna
    Left ØPWL
    Right ØPWK
  Ureter ØTW9
  Urethra ØTWD
  Uterus and Cervix ØUWD
  Vagina and Cul-de-sac ØUWH
  Valve
    Aortic Ø2WF
    Mitral Ø2WG
    Pulmonary Ø2WH
    Tricuspid Ø2WJ
  Vas Deferens ØVWR

Revision of device in — *continued*
  Vein
    Azygos Ø5WØ
    Innominate
      Left Ø5W4
      Right Ø5W3
    Lower Ø6WY
    Upper Ø5WY
  Vertebra
    Cervical ØPW3
    Lumbar ØQWØ
    Thoracic ØPW4
  Vulva ØUWM
Revo MRI™ SureScan® pacemaker *use* Pacemaker, Dual Chamber in ØJH
rhBMP-2 *use* Recombinant Bone Morphogenetic Protein
Rheos® System device *use* Stimulator Generator in Subcutaneous Tissue and Fascia
Rheos® System lead *use* Stimulator Lead in Upper Arteries
Rhinopharynx *use* Nasopharynx
Rhinoplasty
  see Alteration, Nasal Mucosa and Soft Tissue Ø9ØK
  see Repair, Nasal Mucosa and Soft Tissue Ø9QK
  see Replacement, Nasal Mucosa and Soft Tissue Ø9RK
  see Supplement, Nasal Mucosa and Soft Tissue Ø9UK
Rhinorrhaphy *see* Repair, Nasal Mucosa and Soft Tissue Ø9QK
Rhinoscopy Ø9JKXZZ
Rhizotomy
  see Division, Central Nervous System and Cranial Nerves ØØ8
  see Division, Peripheral Nervous System Ø18
Rhomboid major muscle
  use Trunk Muscle, Left
  use Trunk Muscle, Right
Rhomboid minor muscle
  use Trunk Muscle, Left
  use Trunk Muscle, Right
Rhythm electrocardiogram *see* Measurement, Cardiac 4AØ2
Rhytidectomy *see* Alteration, Face ØWØ2
Right ascending lumbar vein *use* Azygos Vein
Right atrioventricular valve *use* Tricuspid Valve
Right auricular appendix *use* Atrium, Right
Right colic vein *use* Colic Vein
Right coronary sulcus *use* Heart, Right
Right gastric artery *use* Gastric Artery
Right gastroepiploic vein *use* Superior Mesenteric Vein
Right inferior phrenic vein *use* Inferior Vena Cava
Right inferior pulmonary vein *use* Pulmonary Vein, Right
Right jugular trunk *use* Lymphatic, Right Neck
Right lateral ventricle *use* Cerebral Ventricle
Right lymphatic duct *use* Lymphatic, Right Neck
Right ovarian vein *use* Inferior Vena Cava
Right second lumbar vein *use* Inferior Vena Cava
Right subclavian trunk *use* Lymphatic, Right Neck
Right subcostal vein *use* Azygos Vein
Right superior pulmonary vein *use* Pulmonary Vein, Right
Right suprarenal vein *use* Inferior Vena Cava
Right testicular vein *use* Inferior Vena Cava
Rima glottidis *use* Larynx
Risorius muscle *use* Facial Muscle
RNS System lead *use* Neurostimulator Lead in Central Nervous System and Cranial Nerves
RNS system neurostimulator generator *use* Neurostimulator Generator in Head and Facial Bones
Robotic Assisted Procedure
  Extremity
    Lower 8EØY
    Upper 8EØX
  Head and Neck Region 8EØ9
  Trunk Region 8EØW
Robotic Waterjet Ablation, Destruction, Prostate XV5Ø8A4
Rotation of fetal head
  Forceps 1ØSØ7ZZ
  Manual 1ØSØXZZ
Round ligament of uterus *use* Uterine Supporting Structure

Round window
  use Inner Ear, Left
  use Inner Ear, Right
Roux-en-Y operation
  see Bypass, Gastrointestinal System ØD1
  see Bypass, Hepatobiliary System and Pancreas ØF1
Rupture
  Adhesions *see* Release
  Fluid collection *see* Drainage
Ruxolitinib XWØDXT5

S

Sacral ganglion *use* Sacral Sympathetic Nerve
Sacral lymph node *use* Lymphatic, Pelvis
Sacral nerve modulation (SNM) lead *use* Stimulator Lead in Urinary System
Sacral neuromodulation lead *use* Stimulator Lead in Urinary System
Sacral splanchnic nerve *use* Sacral Sympathetic Nerve
Sacrectomy *see* Excision, Lower Bones ØQB
Sacrococcygeal ligament *use* Lower Spine Bursa and Ligament
Sacrococcygeal symphysis *use* Sacrococcygeal Joint
Sacroiliac ligament *use* Lower Spine Bursa and Ligament
Sacrospinous ligament *use* Lower Spine Bursa and Ligament
Sacrotuberous ligament *use* Lower Spine Bursa and Ligament
Salpingectomy
  see Excision, Female Reproductive System ØUB
  see Resection, Female Reproductive System ØUT
Salpingolysis *see* Release, Female Reproductive System ØUN
Salpingopexy
  see Repair, Female Reproductive System ØUQ
  see Reposition, Female Reproductive System ØUS
Salpingopharyngeus muscle *use* Tongue, Palate, Pharynx Muscle
Salpingoplasty
  see Repair, Female Reproductive System ØUQ
  see Supplement, Female Reproductive System ØUU
Salpingorrhaphy *see* Repair, Female Reproductive System ØUQ
Salpingoscopy ØUJ88ZZ
Salpingostomy *see* Drainage, Female Reproductive System ØU9
Salpingotomy *see* Drainage, Female Reproductive System ØU9
Salpinx
  use Fallopian Tube, Left
  use Fallopian Tube, Right
Saphenous nerve *use* Femoral Nerve
SAPIEN transcatheter aortic valve *use* Zooplastic Tissue in Heart and Great Vessels
Sartorius muscle
  use Upper Leg Muscle, Left
  use Upper Leg Muscle, Right
SAVAL below-the-knee (BTK) drug-eluting stent system
  use Intraluminal Device, Sustained Release Drug-eluting in New Technology
  use Intraluminal Device, Sustained Release Drug-eluting, Two in New Technology
  use Intraluminal Device, Sustained Release Drug-eluting, Three in New Technology
  use Intraluminal Device, Sustained Release Drug-eluting, Four or More in New Technology
Scalene muscle
  use Neck Muscle, Left
  use Neck Muscle, Right
Scan
  Computerized Tomography (CT) *see* Computerized Tomography (CT Scan)
  Radioisotope *see* Planar Nuclear Medicine Imaging
Scaphoid bone
  use Carpal, Left
  use Carpal, Right
Scapholunate ligament
  use Wrist Bursa and Ligament, Left
  use Wrist Bursa and Ligament, Right
Scaphotrapezium ligament
  use Hand Bursa and Ligament, Left
  use Hand Bursa and Ligament, Right

Scapulectomy
see Excision, Upper Bones ØPB
see Resection, Upper Bones ØPT
Scapulopexy
see Repair, Upper Bones ØPQ
see Reposition, Upper Bones ØPS
Scarpa's (vestibular) ganglion use Acoustic Nerve
Sclerectomy see Excision, Eye Ø8B
Sclerotherapy, mechanical see Destruction
Sclerotherapy, via injection of sclerosing agent
see Introduction, Destructive Agent
Sclerotomy see Drainage, Eye Ø89
Scrotectomy
see Excision, Male Reproductive System ØVB
see Resection, Male Reproductive System ØVT
Scrotoplasty
see Repair, Male Reproductive System ØVQ
see Supplement, Male Reproductive System ØVU
Scrotorrhaphy see Repair, Male Reproductive System ØVQ
Scrototomy see Drainage, Male Reproductive System ØV9
Sebaceous gland use Skin
Second cranial nerve use Optic Nerve
Section, cesarean see Extraction, Pregnancy 1ØD
Secura (DR) (VR) use Defibrillator Generator in ØJH
Sella turcica use Sphenoid Bone
Semicircular canal
use Inner Ear, Left
use Inner Ear, Right
Semimembranosus muscle
use Upper Leg Muscle, Left
use Upper Leg Muscle, Right
Semitendinosus muscle
use Upper Leg Muscle, Left
use Upper Leg Muscle, Right
Sentinel™ Cerebral Protection System (CPS)
X2A5312
Seprafilm use Adhesion Barrier
Septal cartilage use Nasal Septum
Septectomy
see Excision, Ear, Nose, Sinus Ø9B
see Excision, Heart and Great Vessels Ø2B
see Resection, Ear, Nose, Sinus Ø9T
see Resection, Heart and Great Vessels Ø2T
Septoplasty
see Repair, Ear, Nose, Sinus Ø9Q
see Repair, Heart and Great Vessels Ø2Q
see Replacement, Ear, Nose, Sinus Ø9R
see Replacement, Heart and Great Vessels Ø2R
see Reposition, Ear, Nose, Sinus Ø9S
see Supplement, Ear, Nose, Sinus Ø9U
see Supplement, Heart and Great Vessels Ø2U
Septostomy, balloon atrial Ø2163Z7
Septotomy see Drainage, Ear, Nose, Sinus Ø99
Sequestrectomy, bone see Extirpation
Serratus anterior muscle
use Thorax Muscle, Left
use Thorax Muscle, Right
Serratus posterior muscle
use Trunk Muscle, Left
use Trunk Muscle, Right
Seventh cranial nerve use Facial Nerve
Shapshot_NIR 8EØ2XDZ
Sheffield hybrid external fixator
use External Fixation Device, Hybrid in ØPH
use External Fixation Device, Hybrid in ØPS
use External Fixation Device, Hybrid in ØQH
use External Fixation Device, Hybrid in ØQS
Sheffield ring external fixator
use External Fixation Device, Ring in ØPH
use External Fixation Device, Ring in ØPS
use External Fixation Device, Ring in ØQH
use External Fixation Device, Ring in ØQS
Shirodkar cervical cerclage ØUVC7ZZ
Shock Wave Therapy, Musculoskeletal 6A93
Shockwave Intravascular Lithotripsy (Shockwave IVL) see Fragmentation
Short gastric artery use Splenic Artery
Shortening
see Excision
see Repair
see Reposition
Shunt creation see Bypass
Sialoadenectomy
Complete see Resection, Mouth and Throat ØCT

Sialoadenectomy — continued
Partial see Excision, Mouth and Throat ØCB
Sialodochoplasty
see Repair, Mouth and Throat ØCQ
see Replacement, Mouth and Throat ØCR
see Supplement, Mouth and Throat ØCU
Sialoectomy
see Excision, Mouth and Throat ØCB
see Resection, Mouth and Throat ØCT
Sialography see Plain Radiography, Ear, Nose, Mouth and Throat B9Ø
Sialolithotomy see Extirpation, Mouth and Throat ØCC
S-ICD™ lead use Subcutaneous Defibrillator Lead in Subcutaneous Tissue and Fascia
Sigmoid artery use Inferior Mesenteric Artery
Sigmoid flexure use Sigmoid Colon
Sigmoid vein use Inferior Mesenteric Vein
Sigmoidectomy
see Excision, Gastrointestinal System ØDB
see Resection, Gastrointestinal System ØDT
Sigmoidorrhaphy see Repair, Gastrointestinal System ØDQ
Sigmoidoscopy ØDJD8ZZ
Sigmoidotomy see Drainage, Gastrointestinal System ØD9
Single lead pacemaker (atrium) (ventricle) use Pacemaker, Single Chamber in ØJH
Single lead rate responsive pacemaker (atrium) (ventricle) use Pacemaker, Single Chamber Rate Responsive in ØJH
Sinoatrial node use Conduction Mechanism
Sinogram
Abdominal Wall see Fluoroscopy, Abdomen and Pelvis BW11
Chest Wall see Plain Radiography, Chest BWØ3
Retroperitoneum see Fluoroscopy, Abdomen and Pelvis BW11
Sinus venosus use Atrium, Right
Sinusectomy
see Excision, Ear, Nose, Sinus Ø9B
see Resection, Ear, Nose, Sinus Ø9T
Sinusoscopy Ø9JY4ZZ
Sinusotomy see Drainage, Ear, Nose, Sinus Ø99
Sirolimus-eluting coronary stent use Intraluminal Device, Drug-eluting in Heart and Great Vessels
Sixth cranial nerve use Abducens Nerve
Size reduction, breast see Excision, Skin and Breast ØHB
SJM Biocor® Stented Valve System use Zooplastic Tissue in Heart and Great Vessels
Skene's (paraurethral) gland use Vestibular Gland
Skin Substitute, Porcine Liver Derived, Replacement XHRPXL2
Sling
Fascial, orbicularis muscle (mouth) see Supplement, Muscle, Facial ØKU1
Levator muscle, for urethral suspension see Reposition, Bladder Neck ØTSC
Pubococcygeal, for urethral suspension see Reposition, Bladder Neck ØTSC
Rectum see Reposition, Rectum ØDSP
Small bowel series see Fluoroscopy, Bowel, Small BD13
Small saphenous vein
use Saphenous Vein, Left
use Saphenous Vein, Right
Snapshot_NIR 8EØ2XDZ
Snaring, polyp, colon see Excision, Gastrointestinal System ØDB
Solar (celiac) plexus use Abdominal Sympathetic Nerve
Soleus muscle
use Lower Leg Muscle, Left
use Lower Leg Muscle, Right
Soliris® use Eculizumab
Spacer
Insertion of device in
Disc
Lumbar Vertebral ØSH2
Lumbosacral ØSH4
Joint
Acromioclavicular
Left ØRHH
Right ØRHG
Ankle
Left ØSHG
Right ØSHF

Spacer — continued
Insertion of device in — continued
Joint — continued
Carpal
Left ØRHR
Right ØRHQ
Carpometacarpal
Left ØRHT
Right ØRHS
Cervical Vertebral ØRH1
Cervicothoracic Vertebral ØRH4
Coccygeal ØSH6
Elbow
Left ØRHM
Right ØRHL
Finger Phalangeal
Left ØRHX
Right ØRHW
Hip
Left ØSHB
Right ØSH9
Knee
Left ØSHD
Right ØSHC
Lumbar Vertebral ØSHØ
Lumbosacral ØSH3
Metacarpophalangeal
Left ØRHV
Right ØRHU
Metatarsal-Phalangeal
Left ØSHN
Right ØSHM
Occipital-cervical ØRHØ
Sacrococcygeal ØSH5
Sacroiliac
Left ØSH8
Right ØSH7
Shoulder
Left ØRHK
Right ØRHJ
Sternoclavicular
Left ØRHF
Right ØRHE
Tarsal
Left ØSHJ
Right ØSHH
Tarsometatarsal
Left ØSHL
Right ØSHK
Temporomandibular
Left ØRHD
Right ØRHC
Thoracic Vertebral ØRH6
Thoracolumbar Vertebral ØRHA
Toe Phalangeal
Left ØSHQ
Right ØSHP
Wrist
Left ØRHP
Right ØRHN
Removal of device from
Acromioclavicular
Left ØRPH
Right ØRPG
Ankle
Left ØSPG
Right ØSPF
Carpal
Left ØRPR
Right ØRPQ
Carpometacarpal
Left ØRPT
Right ØRPS
Cervical Vertebral ØRP1
Cervicothoracic Vertebral ØRP4
Coccygeal ØSP6
Elbow
Left ØRPM
Right ØRPL
Finger Phalangeal
Left ØRPX
Right ØRPW
Hip
Left ØSPB
Right ØSP9
Knee
Left ØSPD
Right ØSPC
Lumbar Vertebral ØSPØ

Spacer — continued
Removal of device from — continued
Lumbosacral ØSP3
Metacarpophalangeal
Left ØRPV
Right ØRPU
Metatarsal-Phalangeal
Left ØSPN
Right ØSPM
Occipital-cervical ØRPØ
Sacrococcygeal ØSP5
Sacroiliac
Left ØSP8
Right ØSP7
Shoulder
Left ØRPK
Right ØRPJ
Sternoclavicular
Left ØRPF
Right ØRPE
Tarsal
Left ØSPJ
Right ØSPH
Tarsometatarsal
Left ØSPL
Right ØSPK
Temporomandibular
Left ØRPD
Right ØRPC
Thoracic Vertebral ØRP6
Thoracolumbar Vertebral ØRPA
Toe Phalangeal
Left ØSPQ
Right ØSPP
Wrist
Left ØRPP
Right ØRPN
Revision of device in
Acromioclavicular
Left ØRWH
Right ØRWG
Ankle
Left ØSWG
Right ØSWF
Carpal
Left ØRWR
Right ØRWQ
Carpometacarpal
Left ØRWT
Right ØRWS
Cervical Vertebral ØRW1
Cervicothoracic Vertebral ØRW4
Coccygeal ØSW6
Elbow
Left ØRWM
Right ØRWL
Finger Phalangeal
Left ØRWX
Right ØRWW
Hip
Left ØSWB
Right ØSW9
Knee
Left ØSWD
Right ØSWC
Lumbar Vertebral ØSWØ
Lumbosacral ØSW3
Metacarpophalangeal
Left ØRWV
Right ØRWU
Metatarsal-Phalangeal
Left ØSWN
Right ØSWM
Occipital-cervical ØRWØ
Sacrococcygeal ØSW5
Sacroiliac
Left ØSW8
Right ØSW7
Shoulder
Left ØRWK
Right ØRWJ
Sternoclavicular
Left ØRWF
Right ØRWE
Tarsal
Left ØSWJ
Right ØSWH
Tarsometatarsal
Left ØSWL

Spacer — continued
Revision of device in — continued
Tarsometatarsal — continued
Right ØSWK
Temporomandibular
Left ØRWD
Right ØRWC
Thoracic Vertebral ØRW6
Thoracolumbar Vertebral ØRWA
Toe Phalangeal
Left ØSWQ
Right ØSWP
Wrist
Left ØRWP
Right ØRWN
Spacer, Articulating (Antibiotic) use Articulating Spacer in Lower Joints
Spacer, Static (Antibiotic) use Spacer in Lower Joints
Spectroscopy
Intravascular Near Infrared 8E023DZ
Near Infrared see Physiological Systems and Anatomical Regions 8E0
Speech Assessment FØØ
Speech therapy see Speech Treatment, Rehabilitation FØ6
Speech Treatment FØ6
Sphenoidectomy
see Excision, Ear, Nose, Sinus Ø9B
see Excision, Head and Facial Bones ØNB
see Resection, Ear, Nose, Sinus Ø9T
see Resection, Head and Facial Bones ØNT
Sphenoidotomy see Drainage, Ear, Nose, Sinus Ø99
Sphenomandibular ligament use Head and Neck Bursa and Ligament
Sphenopalatine (pterygopalatine) ganglion use Head and Neck Sympathetic Nerve
Sphincterorrhaphy, anal see Repair, Anal Sphincter ØDQR
Sphincterotomy, anal
see Division, Anal Sphincter ØD8R
see Drainage, Anal Sphincter ØD9R
Spinal cord neurostimulator lead use Neurostimulator Lead in Central Nervous System and Cranial Nerves
Spinal growth rods, magnetically controlled use Magnetically Controlled Growth Rod(s) in New Technology
Spinal nerve, cervical use Cervical Nerve
Spinal nerve, lumbar use Lumbar Nerve
Spinal nerve, sacral use Sacral Nerve
Spinal nerve, thoracic use Thoracic Nerve
Spinal Stabilization Device
Facet Replacement
Cervical Vertebral ØRH1
Cervicothoracic Vertebral ØRH4
Lumbar Vertebral ØSHØ
Lumbosacral ØSH3
Occipital-cervical ØRHØ
Thoracic Vertebral ØRH6
Thoracolumbar Vertebral ØRHA
Interspinous Process
Cervical Vertebral ØRH1
Cervicothoracic Vertebral ØRH4
Lumbar Vertebral ØSHØ
Lumbosacral ØSH3
Occipital-cervical ØRHØ
Thoracic Vertebral ØRH6
Thoracolumbar Vertebral ØRHA
Pedicle-Based
Cervical Vertebral ØRH1
Cervicothoracic Vertebral ØRH4
Lumbar Vertebral ØSHØ
Lumbosacral ØSH3
Occipital-cervical ØRHØ
Thoracic Vertebral ØRH6
Thoracolumbar Vertebral ØRHA
SpineJack® system use Synthetic Substitute, Mechanically Expandable (Paired) in New Technology
Spinous process
use Cervical Vertebra
use Lumbar Vertebra
use Thoracic Vertebra
Spiral ganglion use Acoustic Nerve
Spiration IBV™ Valve System use Intraluminal Device, Endobronchial Valve in Respiratory System
Splenectomy
see Excision, Lymphatic and Hemic Systems Ø7B
see Resection, Lymphatic and Hemic Systems Ø7T

Splenic flexure use Transverse Colon
Splenic plexus use Abdominal Sympathetic Nerve
Splenius capitis muscle use Head Muscle
Splenius cervicis muscle
use Neck Muscle, Left
use Neck Muscle, Right
Splenolysis see Release, Lymphatic and Hemic Systems Ø7N
Splenopexy
see Repair, Lymphatic and Hemic Systems Ø7Q
see Reposition, Lymphatic and Hemic Systems Ø7S
Splenoplasty see Repair, Lymphatic and Hemic Systems Ø7Q
Splenorrhaphy see Repair, Lymphatic and Hemic Systems Ø7Q
Splenotomy see Drainage, Lymphatic and Hemic Systems Ø79
Splinting, musculoskeletal see Immobilization, Anatomical Regions 2W3
SPRAVATO™ use Esketamine Hydrochloride
SPY PINPOINT fluorescence imaging system
see Monitoring, Physiological Systems 4A1
see Other Imaging, Hepatobiliary System and Pancreas BF5
SPY system intraoperative fluorescence cholangiography see Other Imaging, Hepatobiliary System and Pancreas BF5
SPY system intravascular fluorescence angiography see Monitoring, Physiological Systems 4A1
Stapedectomy
see Excision, Ear, Nose, Sinus Ø9B
see Resection, Ear, Nose, Sinus Ø9T
Stapediolysis see Release, Ear, Nose, Sinus Ø9N
Stapedioplasty
see Repair, Ear, Nose, Sinus Ø9Q
see Replacement, Ear, Nose, Sinus Ø9R
see Supplement, Ear, Nose, Sinus Ø9U
Stapedotomy see Drainage, Ear, Nose, Sinus Ø99
Stapes
use Auditory Ossicle, Left
use Auditory Ossicle, Right
Static Spacer (Antibiotic) use Spacer in Lower Joints
STELARA® use Other New Technology Therapeutic Substance
Stellate ganglion use Head and Neck Sympathetic Nerve
Stem cell transplant see Transfusion, Circulatory 3Ø2
Stensen's duct
use Parotid Duct, Left
use Parotid Duct, Right
Stent, intraluminal (cardiovascular) (gastrointestinal) (hepatobiliary) (urinary) use Intraluminal Device
Stent retriever thrombectomy see Extirpation, Upper Arteries Ø3C
Stented tissue valve use Zooplastic Tissue in Heart and Great Vessels
Stereotactic Radiosurgery
Abdomen DW23
Adrenal Gland DG22
Bile Ducts DF22
Bladder DT22
Bone Marrow D72Ø
Brain DØ2Ø
Brain Stem DØ21
Breast
Left DM2Ø
Right DM21
Bronchus DB21
Cervix DU21
Chest DW22
Chest Wall DB27
Colon DD25
Diaphragm DB28
Duodenum DD22
Ear D92Ø
Esophagus DD2Ø
Eye D82Ø
Gallbladder DF21
Gamma Beam
Abdomen DW23JZZ
Adrenal Gland DG22JZZ
Bile Ducts DF22JZZ
Bladder DT22JZZ
Bone Marrow D72ØJZZ
Brain DØ2ØJZZ
Brain Stem DØ21JZZ

Subterms under main terms may continue to next column or page

Stereotactic Radiosurgery — *continued*
  Gamma Beam — *continued*
    Breast
      Left DM20JZZ
      Right DM21JZZ
    Bronchus DB21JZZ
    Cervix DU21JZZ
    Chest DW22JZZ
    Chest Wall DB27JZZ
    Colon DD25JZZ
    Diaphragm DB28JZZ
    Duodenum DD22JZZ
    Ear D920JZZ
    Esophagus DD20JZZ
    Eye D820JZZ
    Gallbladder DF21JZZ
    Gland
      Adrenal DG22JZZ
      Parathyroid DG24JZZ
      Pituitary DG20JZZ
      Thyroid DG25JZZ
    Glands, Salivary D926JZZ
    Head and Neck DW21JZZ
    Ileum DD24JZZ
    Jejunum DD23JZZ
    Kidney DT20JZZ
    Larynx D92BJZZ
    Liver DF20JZZ
    Lung DB22JZZ
    Lymphatics
      Abdomen D726JZZ
      Axillary D724JZZ
      Inguinal D728JZZ
      Neck D723JZZ
      Pelvis D727JZZ
      Thorax D725JZZ
    Mediastinum DB26JZZ
    Mouth D924JZZ
    Nasopharynx D92DJZZ
    Neck and Head DW21JZZ
    Nerve, Peripheral D027JZZ
    Nose D921JZZ
    Ovary DU20JZZ
    Palate
      Hard D928JZZ
      Soft D929JZZ
    Pancreas DF23JZZ
    Parathyroid Gland DG24JZZ
    Pelvic Region DW26JZZ
    Pharynx D92CJZZ
    Pineal Body DG21JZZ
    Pituitary Gland DG20JZZ
    Pleura DB25JZZ
    Prostate DV20JZZ
    Rectum DD27JZZ
    Sinuses D927JZZ
    Spinal Cord D026JZZ
    Spleen D722JZZ
    Stomach DD21JZZ
    Testis DV21JZZ
    Thymus D721JZZ
    Thyroid Gland DG25JZZ
    Tongue D925JZZ
    Trachea DB20JZZ
    Ureter DT21JZZ
    Urethra DT23JZZ
    Uterus DU22JZZ
  Gland
    Adrenal DG22
    Parathyroid DG24
    Pituitary DG20
    Thyroid DG25
  Glands, Salivary D926
  Head and Neck DW21
  Ileum DD24
  Jejunum DD23
  Kidney DT20
  Larynx D92B
  Liver DF20
  Lung DB22
  Lymphatics
    Abdomen D726
    Axillary D724
    Inguinal D728
    Neck D723
    Pelvis D727
    Thorax D725
  Mediastinum DB26
  Mouth D924

Stereotactic Radiosurgery — *continued*
  Nasopharynx D92D
  Neck and Head DW21
  Nerve, Peripheral D027
  Nose D921
  Other Photon
    Abdomen DW23DZZ
    Adrenal Gland DG22DZZ
    Bile Ducts DF22DZZ
    Bladder DT22DZZ
    Bone Marrow D720DZZ
    Brain D020DZZ
    Brain Stem D021DZZ
    Breast
      Left DM20DZZ
      Right DM21DZZ
    Bronchus DB21DZZ
    Cervix DU21DZZ
    Chest DW22DZZ
    Chest Wall DB27DZZ
    Colon DD25DZZ
    Diaphragm DB28DZZ
    Duodenum DD22DZZ
    Ear D920DZZ
    Esophagus DD20DZZ
    Eye D820DZZ
    Gallbladder DF21DZZ
    Gland
      Adrenal DG22DZZ
      Parathyroid DG24DZZ
      Pituitary DG20DZZ
      Thyroid DG25DZZ
    Glands, Salivary D926DZZ
    Head and Neck DW21DZZ
    Ileum DD24DZZ
    Jejunum DD23DZZ
    Kidney DT20DZZ
    Larynx D92BDZZ
    Liver DF20DZZ
    Lung DB22DZZ
    Lymphatics
      Abdomen D726DZZ
      Axillary D724DZZ
      Inguinal D728DZZ
      Neck D723DZZ
      Pelvis D727DZZ
      Thorax D725DZZ
    Mediastinum DB26DZZ
    Mouth D924DZZ
    Nasopharynx D92DDZZ
    Neck and Head DW21DZZ
    Nerve, Peripheral D027DZZ
    Nose D921DZZ
    Ovary DU20DZZ
    Palate
      Hard D928DZZ
      Soft D929DZZ
    Pancreas DF23DZZ
    Parathyroid Gland DG24DZZ
    Pelvic Region DW26DZZ
    Pharynx D92CDZZ
    Pineal Body DG21DZZ
    Pituitary Gland DG20DZZ
    Pleura DB25DZZ
    Prostate DV20DZZ
    Rectum DD27DZZ
    Sinuses D927DZZ
    Spinal Cord D026DZZ
    Spleen D722DZZ
    Stomach DD21DZZ
    Testis DV21DZZ
    Thymus D721DZZ
    Thyroid Gland DG25DZZ
    Tongue D925DZZ
    Trachea DB20DZZ
    Ureter DT21DZZ
    Urethra DT23DZZ
    Uterus DU22DZZ
  Ovary DU20
  Palate
    Hard D928
    Soft D929
  Pancreas DF23
  Parathyroid Gland DG24
  Particulate
    Abdomen DW23HZZ
    Adrenal Gland DG22HZZ
    Bile Ducts DF22HZZ
    Bladder DT22HZZ

Stereotactic Radiosurgery — *continued*
  Particulate — *continued*
    Bone Marrow D720HZZ
    Brain D020HZZ
    Brain Stem D021HZZ
    Breast
      Left DM20HZZ
      Right DM21HZZ
    Bronchus DB21HZZ
    Cervix DU21HZZ
    Chest DW22HZZ
    Chest Wall DB27HZZ
    Colon DD25HZZ
    Diaphragm DB28HZZ
    Duodenum DD22HZZ
    Ear D920HZZ
    Esophagus DD20HZZ
    Eye D820HZZ
    Gallbladder DF21HZZ
    Gland
      Adrenal DG22HZZ
      Parathyroid DG24HZZ
      Pituitary DG20HZZ
      Thyroid DG25HZZ
    Glands, Salivary D926HZZ
    Head and Neck DW21HZZ
    Ileum DD24HZZ
    Jejunum DD23HZZ
    Kidney DT20HZZ
    Larynx D92BHZZ
    Liver DF20HZZ
    Lung DB22HZZ
    Lymphatics
      Abdomen D726HZZ
      Axillary D724HZZ
      Inguinal D728HZZ
      Neck D723HZZ
      Pelvis D727HZZ
      Thorax D725HZZ
    Mediastinum DB26HZZ
    Mouth D924HZZ
    Nasopharynx D92DHZZ
    Neck and Head DW21HZZ
    Nerve, Peripheral D027HZZ
    Nose D921HZZ
    Ovary DU20HZZ
    Palate
      Hard D928HZZ
      Soft D929HZZ
    Pancreas DF23HZZ
    Parathyroid Gland DG24HZZ
    Pelvic Region DW26HZZ
    Pharynx D92CHZZ
    Pineal Body DG21HZZ
    Pituitary Gland DG20HZZ
    Pleura DB25HZZ
    Prostate DV20HZZ
    Rectum DD27HZZ
    Sinuses D927HZZ
    Spinal Cord D026HZZ
    Spleen D722HZZ
    Stomach DD21HZZ
    Testis DV21HZZ
    Thymus D721HZZ
    Thyroid Gland DG25HZZ
    Tongue D925HZZ
    Trachea DB20HZZ
    Ureter DT21HZZ
    Urethra DT23HZZ
    Uterus DU22HZZ
  Pelvic Region DW26
  Pharynx D92C
  Pineal Body DG21
  Pituitary Gland DG20
  Pleura DB25
  Prostate DV20
  Rectum DD27
  Sinuses D927
  Spinal Cord D026
  Spleen D722
  Stomach DD21
  Testis DV21
  Thymus D721
  Thyroid Gland DG25
  Tongue D925
  Trachea DB20
  Ureter DT21
  Urethra DT23
  Uterus DU22

Index

Stereotactic Radiosurgery — Stereotactic Radiosurgery

Sternoclavicular ligament
use Shoulder Bursa and Ligament, Left
use Shoulder Bursa and Ligament, Right
Sternocleidomastoid artery
use Thyroid Artery, Left
use Thyroid Artery, Right
Sternocleidomastoid muscle
use Neck Muscle, Left
use Neck Muscle, Right
Sternocostal ligament use Sternum Bursa and Ligament
Sternotomy
see Division, Sternum 0P80
see Drainage, Sternum 0P90
Stimulation, cardiac
Cardioversion 5A2204Z
Electrophysiologic testing see Measurement, Cardiac 4A02
Stimulator Generator
Insertion of device in
Abdomen 0JH8
Back 0JH7
Chest 0JH6
Multiple Array
Abdomen 0JH8
Back 0JH7
Chest 0JH6
Multiple Array Rechargeable
Abdomen 0JH8
Back 0JH7
Chest 0JH6
Removal of device from, Subcutaneous Tissue and Fascia, Trunk 0JPT
Revision of device in, Subcutaneous Tissue and Fascia, Trunk 0JWT
Single Array
Abdomen 0JH8
Back 0JH7
Chest 0JH6
Single Array Rechargeable
Abdomen 0JH8
Back 0JH7
Chest 0JH6
Stimulator Lead
Insertion of device in
Anal Sphincter 0DHR
Artery
Left 03HL
Right 03HK
Bladder 0THB
Muscle
Lower 0KHY
Upper 0KHX
Stomach 0DH6
Ureter 0TH9
Removal of device from
Anal Sphincter 0DPR
Artery, Upper 03PY
Bladder 0TPB
Muscle
Lower 0KPY
Upper 0KPX
Stomach 0DP6
Ureter 0TP9
Revision of device in
Anal Sphincter 0DWR
Artery, Upper 03WY
Bladder 0TWB
Muscle
Lower 0KWY
Upper 0KWX
Stomach 0DW6
Ureter 0TW9
Stoma
Excision
Abdominal Wall 0WBFXZ2
Neck 0WB6XZ2
Repair
Abdominal Wall 0WQFXZ2
Neck 0WQ6XZ2
Stomatoplasty
see Repair, Mouth and Throat 0CQ
see Replacement, Mouth and Throat 0CR
see Supplement, Mouth and Throat 0CU
Stomatorrhaphy see Repair, Mouth and Throat 0CQ
Stratos LV use Cardiac Resynchronization Pacemaker Pulse Generator in 0JH
Stress test 4A02XM4, 4A12XM4

Stripping see Extraction
Study
Electrophysiologic stimulation, cardiac see Measurement, Cardiac 4A02
Ocular motility 4A07X7Z
Pulmonary airway flow measurement see Measurement, Respiratory 4A09
Visual acuity 4A07X0Z
Styloglossus muscle use Tongue, Palate, Pharynx Muscle
Stylomandibular ligament use Head and Neck Bursa and Ligament
Stylopharyngeus muscle use Tongue, Palate, Pharynx Muscle
Subacromial bursa
use Shoulder Bursa and Ligament, Left
use Shoulder Bursa and Ligament, Right
Subaortic (common iliac) lymph node use Lymphatic, Pelvis
Subarachnoid space, spinal use Spinal Canal
Subclavicular (apical) lymph node
use Lymphatic, Left Axillary
use Lymphatic, Right Axillary
Subclavius muscle
use Thorax Muscle, Left
use Thorax Muscle, Right
Subclavius nerve use Brachial Plexus
Subcostal artery use Upper Artery
Subcostal muscle
use Thorax Muscle, Left
use Thorax Muscle, Right
Subcostal nerve use Thoracic Nerve
Subcutaneous Defibrillator Lead
Insertion of device in, Subcutaneous Tissue and Fascia, Chest 0JH6
Removal of device from, Subcutaneous Tissue and Fascia, Trunk 0JPT
Revision of device in, Subcutaneous Tissue and Fascia, Trunk 0JWT
Subcutaneous injection reservoir, port use Vascular Access Device, Totally Implantable in Subcutaneous Tissue and Fascia
Subcutaneous injection reservoir, pump use Infusion Device, Pump in Subcutaneous Tissue and Fascia
Subdermal progesterone implant use Contraceptive Device in Subcutaneous Tissue and Fascia
Subdural space, spinal use Spinal Canal
Submandibular ganglion
use Facial Nerve
use Head and Neck Sympathetic Nerve
Submandibular gland
use Submaxillary Gland, Left
use Submaxillary Gland, Right
Submandibular lymph node use Lymphatic, Head
Submandibular space use Subcutaneous Tissue and Fascia, Face
Submaxillary ganglion use Head and Neck Sympathetic Nerve
Submaxillary lymph node use Lymphatic, Head
Submental artery use Face Artery
Submental lymph node use Lymphatic, Head
Submucous (Meissner's) plexus use Abdominal Sympathetic Nerve
Suboccipital nerve use Cervical Nerve
Suboccipital venous plexus
use Vertebral Vein, Left
use Vertebral Vein, Right
Subparotid lymph node use Lymphatic, Head
Subscapular aponeurosis
use Subcutaneous Tissue and Fascia, Left Upper Arm
use Subcutaneous Tissue and Fascia, Right Upper Arm
Subscapular artery
use Axillary Artery, Left
use Axillary Artery, Right
Subscapular (posterior) lymph node
use Lymphatic, Axillary, Left
use Lymphatic, Axillary, Right
Subscapularis muscle
use Shoulder Muscle, Left
use Shoulder Muscle, Right
Substance Abuse Treatment
Counseling
Family, for substance abuse, Other Family Counseling HZ63ZZZ

Substance Abuse Treatment — continued
Counseling — continued
Group
12-Step HZ43ZZZ
Behavioral HZ41ZZZ
Cognitive HZ40ZZZ
Cognitive-Behavioral HZ42ZZZ
Confrontational HZ48ZZZ
Continuing Care HZ49ZZZ
Infectious Disease
Post-Test HZ4CZZZ
Pre-Test HZ4CZZZ
Interpersonal HZ44ZZZ
Motivational Enhancement HZ47ZZZ
Psychoeducation HZ46ZZZ
Spiritual HZ4BZZZ
Vocational HZ45ZZZ
Individual
12-Step HZ33ZZZ
Behavioral HZ31ZZZ
Cognitive HZ30ZZZ
Cognitive-Behavioral HZ32ZZZ
Confrontational HZ38ZZZ
Continuing Care HZ39ZZZ
Infectious Disease
Post-Test HZ3CZZZ
Pre-Test HZ3CZZZ
Interpersonal HZ34ZZZ
Motivational Enhancement HZ37ZZZ
Psychoeducation HZ36ZZZ
Spiritual HZ3BZZZ
Vocational HZ35ZZZ
Detoxification Services, for substance abuse HZ2ZZZZ
Medication Management
Antabuse HZ83ZZZ
Bupropion HZ87ZZZ
Clonidine HZ86ZZZ
Levo-alpha-acetyl-methadol (LAAM) HZ82ZZZ
Methadone Maintenance HZ81ZZZ
Naloxone HZ85ZZZ
Naltrexone HZ84ZZZ
Nicotine Replacement HZ80ZZZ
Other Replacement Medication HZ89ZZZ
Psychiatric Medication HZ88ZZZ
Pharmacotherapy
Antabuse HZ93ZZZ
Bupropion HZ97ZZZ
Clonidine HZ96ZZZ
Levo-alpha-acetyl-methadol (LAAM) HZ92ZZZ
Methadone Maintenance HZ91ZZZ
Naloxone HZ95ZZZ
Naltrexone HZ94ZZZ
Nicotine Replacement HZ90ZZZ
Psychiatric Medication HZ98ZZZ
Replacement Medication, Other HZ99ZZZ
Psychotherapy
12-Step HZ53ZZZ
Behavioral HZ51ZZZ
Cognitive HZ50ZZZ
Cognitive-Behavioral HZ52ZZZ
Confrontational HZ58ZZZ
Interactive HZ55ZZZ
Interpersonal HZ54ZZZ
Motivational Enhancement HZ57ZZZ
Psychoanalysis HZ5BZZZ
Psychodynamic HZ5CZZZ
Psychoeducation HZ56ZZZ
Psychophysiological HZ5DZZZ
Supportive HZ59ZZZ
Substantia nigra use Basal Ganglia
Subtalar (talocalcaneal) joint
use Tarsal Joint, Left
use Tarsal Joint, Right
Subtalar ligament
use Foot Bursa and Ligament, Left
use Foot Bursa and Ligament, Right
Subthalamic nucleus use Basal Ganglia
Suction curettage (D&C), nonobstetric see Extraction, Endometrium 0UDB
Suction curettage, obstetric post-delivery see Extraction, Products of Conception, Retained 10D1
Superficial circumflex iliac vein
use Saphenous Vein, Left
use Saphenous Vein, Right

Superficial epigastric artery
 use Femoral Artery, Left
 use Femoral Artery, Right
Superficial epigastric vein
 use Saphenous Vein, Left
 use Saphenous Vein, Right
Superficial Inferior Epigastric Artery Flap
 Replacement
  Bilateral ØHRVØ78
  Left ØHRUØ78
  Right ØHRTØ78
 Transfer
  Left ØKXG
  Right ØKXF
Superficial palmar arch
 use Hand Artery, Left
 use Hand Artery, Right
Superficial palmar venous arch
 use Hand Vein, Left
 use Hand Vein, Right
Superficial temporal artery
 use Temporal Artery, Left
 use Temporal Artery, Right
Superficial transverse perineal muscle *use* Perineum
 Muscle
Superior cardiac nerve *use* Thoracic Sympathetic
 Nerve
Superior cerebellar vein *use* Intracranial Vein
Superior cerebral vein *use* Intracranial Vein
Superior clunic (cluneal) nerve *use* Lumbar Nerve
Superior epigastric artery
 use Internal Mammary Artery, Left
 use Internal Mammary Artery, Right
Superior genicular artery
 use Popliteal Artery, Left
 use Popliteal Artery, Right
Superior gluteal artery
 use Internal Iliac Artery, Left
 use Internal Iliac Artery, Right
Superior gluteal nerve *use* Lumbar Plexus
Superior hypogastric plexus *use* Abdominal Sympa-
 thetic Nerve
Superior labial artery *use* Face Artery
Superior laryngeal artery
 use Thyroid Artery, Left
 use Thyroid Artery, Right
Superior laryngeal nerve *use* Vagus Nerve
Superior longitudinal muscle *use* Tongue, Palate,
 Pharynx Muscle
Superior mesenteric ganglion *use* Abdominal Sym-
 pathetic Nerve
Superior mesenteric lymph node *use* Lymphatic,
 Mesenteric
Superior mesenteric plexus *use* Abdominal Sympa-
 thetic Nerve
Superior oblique muscle
 use Extraocular Muscle, Left
 use Extraocular Muscle, Right
Superior olivary nucleus *use* Pons
Superior rectal artery *use* Inferior Mesenteric Artery
Superior rectal vein *use* Inferior Mesenteric Vein
Superior rectus muscle
 use Extraocular Muscle, Left
 use Extraocular Muscle, Right
Superior tarsal plate
 use Upper Eyelid, Left
 use Upper Eyelid, Right
Superior thoracic artery
 use Axillary Artery, Left
 use Axillary Artery, Right
Superior thyroid artery
 use External Carotid Artery, Left
 use External Carotid Artery, Right
 use Thyroid Artery, Left
 use Thyroid Artery, Right
Superior turbinate *use* Nasal Turbinate
Superior ulnar collateral artery
 use Brachial Artery, Left
 use Brachial Artery, Right
Supersaturated Oxygen therapy 5AØ512C, 5AØ522C
Supplement
 Abdominal Wall ØWUF
 Acetabulum
  Left ØQU5
  Right ØQU4
 Ampulla of Vater ØFUC
 Anal Sphincter ØDUR

Supplement — *continued*
 Ankle Region
  Left ØYUL
  Right ØYUK
 Anus ØDUQ
 Aorta
  Abdominal Ø4UØ
  Thoracic
   Ascending/Arch Ø2UX
   Descending Ø2UW
 Arm
  Lower
   Left ØXUF
   Right ØXUD
  Upper
   Left ØXU9
   Right ØXU8
 Artery
  Anterior Tibial
   Left Ø4UQ
   Right Ø4UP
  Axillary
   Left Ø3U6
   Right Ø3U5
  Brachial
   Left Ø3U8
   Right Ø3U7
  Celiac Ø4U1
  Colic
   Left Ø4U7
   Middle Ø4U8
   Right Ø4U6
  Common Carotid
   Left Ø3UJ
   Right Ø3UH
  Common Iliac
   Left Ø4UD
   Right Ø4UC
  Coronary
   Four or More Arteries Ø2U3
   One Artery Ø2UØ
   Three Arteries Ø2U2
   Two Arteries Ø2U1
  External Carotid
   Left Ø3UN
   Right Ø3UM
  External Iliac
   Left Ø4UJ
   Right Ø4UH
  Face Ø3UR
  Femoral
   Left Ø4UL
   Right Ø4UK
  Foot
   Left Ø4UW
   Right Ø4UV
  Gastric Ø4U2
  Hand
   Left Ø3UF
   Right Ø3UD
  Hepatic Ø4U3
  Inferior Mesenteric Ø4UB
  Innominate Ø3U2
  Internal Carotid
   Left Ø3UL
   Right Ø3UK
  Internal Iliac
   Left Ø4UF
   Right Ø4UE
  Internal Mammary
   Left Ø3U1
   Right Ø3UØ
  Intracranial Ø3UG
  Lower Ø4UY
  Peroneal
   Left Ø4UU
   Right Ø4UT
  Popliteal
   Left Ø4UN
   Right Ø4UM
  Posterior Tibial
   Left Ø4US
   Right Ø4UR
  Pulmonary
   Left Ø2UR
   Right Ø2UQ
  Pulmonary Trunk Ø2UP
  Radial
   Left Ø3UC

Supplement — *continued*
 Artery — *continued*
  Radial — *continued*
   Right Ø3UB
  Renal
   Left Ø4UA
   Right Ø4U9
  Splenic Ø4U4
  Subclavian
   Left Ø3U4
   Right Ø3U3
  Superior Mesenteric Ø4U5
  Temporal
   Left Ø3UT
   Right Ø3US
  Thyroid
   Left Ø3UV
   Right Ø3UU
  Ulnar
   Left Ø3UA
   Right Ø3U9
  Upper Ø3UY
  Vertebral
   Left Ø3UQ
   Right Ø3UP
 Atrium
  Left Ø2U7
  Right Ø2U6
 Auditory Ossicle
  Left Ø9UA
  Right Ø9U9
 Axilla
  Left ØXU5
  Right ØXU4
 Back
  Lower ØWUL
  Upper ØWUK
 Bladder ØTUB
 Bladder Neck ØTUC
 Bone
  Ethmoid
   Left ØNUG
   Right ØNUF
  Frontal ØNU1
  Hyoid ØNUX
  Lacrimal
   Left ØNUJ
   Right ØNUH
  Nasal ØNUB
  Occipital ØNU7
  Palatine
   Left ØNUL
   Right ØNUK
  Parietal
   Left ØNU4
   Right ØNU3
  Pelvic
   Left ØQU3
   Right ØQU2
  Sphenoid ØNUC
  Temporal
   Left ØNU6
   Right ØNU5
  Zygomatic
   Left ØNUN
   Right ØNUM
 Breast
  Bilateral ØHUV
  Left ØHUU
  Right ØHUT
 Bronchus
  Lingula ØBU9
  Lower Lobe
   Left ØBUB
   Right ØBU6
  Main
   Left ØBU7
   Right ØBU3
  Middle Lobe, Right ØBU5
  Upper Lobe
   Left ØBU8
   Right ØBU4
 Buccal Mucosa ØCU4
 Bursa and Ligament
  Abdomen
   Left ØMUJ
   Right ØMUH
  Ankle
   Left ØMUR

Supplement — *continued*
  Bursa and Ligament — *continued*
    Ankle — *continued*
      Right ØMUQ
    Elbow
      Left ØMU4
      Right ØMU3
    Foot
      Left ØMUT
      Right ØMUS
    Hand
      Left ØMU8
      Right ØMU7
    Head and Neck ØMUØ
    Hip
      Left ØMUM
      Right ØMUL
    Knee
      Left ØMUP
      Right ØMUN
    Lower Extremity
      Left ØMUW
      Right ØMUV
    Perineum ØMUK
    Rib(s) ØMUG
    Shoulder
      Left ØMU2
      Right ØMU1
    Spine
      Lower ØMUD
      Upper ØMUC
    Sternum ØMUF
    Upper Extremity
      Left ØMUB
      Right ØMU9
    Wrist
      Left ØMU6
      Right ØMU5
  Buttock
    Left ØYU1
    Right ØYUØ
  Carina ØBU2
  Carpal
    Left ØPUN
    Right ØPUM
  Cecum ØDUH
  Cerebral Meninges ØØU1
  Cerebral Ventricle ØØU6
  Chest Wall ØWU8
  Chordae Tendineae Ø2U9
  Cisterna Chyli Ø7UL
  Clavicle
    Left ØPUB
    Right ØPU9
  Clitoris ØUUJ
  Coccyx ØQUS
  Colon
    Ascending ØDUK
    Descending ØDUM
    Sigmoid ØDUN
    Transverse ØDUL
  Cord
    Bilateral ØVUH
    Left ØVUG
    Right ØVUF
  Cornea
    Left Ø8U9
    Right Ø8U8
  Cul-de-sac ØUUF
  Diaphragm ØBUT
  Disc
    Cervical Vertebral ØRU3
    Cervicothoracic Vertebral ØRU5
    Lumbar Vertebral ØSU2
    Lumbosacral ØSU4
    Thoracic Vertebral ØRU9
    Thoracolumbar Vertebral ØRUB
  Duct
    Common Bile ØFU9
    Cystic ØFU8
    Hepatic
      Common ØFU7
      Left ØFU6
      Right ØFU5
    Lacrimal
      Left Ø8UY
      Right Ø8UX
    Pancreatic ØFUD
      Accessory ØFUF

Supplement — *continued*
  Duodenum ØDU9
  Dura Mater ØØU2
  Ear
    External
      Bilateral Ø9U2
      Left Ø9U1
      Right Ø9UØ
    Inner
      Left Ø9UE
      Right Ø9UD
    Middle
      Left Ø9U6
      Right Ø9U5
  Elbow Region
    Left ØXUC
    Right ØXUB
  Epididymis
    Bilateral ØVUL
    Left ØVUK
    Right ØVUJ
  Epiglottis ØCUR
  Esophagogastric Junction ØDU4
  Esophagus ØDU5
    Lower ØDU3
    Middle ØDU2
    Upper ØDU1
  Extremity
    Lower
      Left ØYUB
      Right ØYU9
    Upper
      Left ØXU7
      Right ØXU6
  Eye
    Left Ø8U1
    Right Ø8UØ
  Eyelid
    Lower
      Left Ø8UR
      Right Ø8UQ
    Upper
      Left Ø8UP
      Right Ø8UN
  Face ØWU2
  Fallopian Tube
    Left ØUU6
    Right ØUU5
  Fallopian Tubes, Bilateral ØUU7
  Femoral Region
    Bilateral ØYUE
    Left ØYU8
    Right ØYU7
  Femoral Shaft
    Left ØQU9
    Right ØQU8
  Femur
    Lower
      Left ØQUC
      Right ØQUB
    Upper
      Left ØQU7
      Right ØQU6
  Fibula
    Left ØQUK
    Right ØQUJ
  Finger
    Index
      Left ØXUP
      Right ØXUN
    Little
      Left ØXUW
      Right ØXUV
    Middle
      Left ØXUR
      Right ØXUQ
    Ring
      Left ØXUT
      Right ØXUS
  Foot
    Left ØYUN
    Right ØYUM
  Gingiva
    Lower ØCU6
    Upper ØCU5
  Glenoid Cavity
    Left ØPU8
    Right ØPU7

Supplement — *continued*
  Hand
    Left ØXUK
    Right ØXUJ
  Head ØWUØ
  Heart Ø2UA
  Humeral Head
    Left ØPUD
    Right ØPUC
  Humeral Shaft
    Left ØPUG
    Right ØPUF
  Hymen ØUUK
  Ileocecal Valve ØDUC
  Ileum ØDUB
  Inguinal Region
    Bilateral ØYUA
    Left ØYU6
    Right ØYU5
  Intestine
    Large ØDUE
      Left ØDUG
      Right ØDUF
    Small ØDU8
  Iris
    Left Ø8UD
    Right Ø8UC
  Jaw
    Lower ØWU5
    Upper ØWU4
  Jejunum ØDUA
  Joint
    Acromioclavicular
      Left ØRUH
      Right ØRUG
    Ankle
      Left ØSUG
      Right ØSUF
    Carpal
      Left ØRUR
      Right ØRUQ
    Carpometacarpal
      Left ØRUT
      Right ØRUS
    Cervical Vertebral ØRU1
    Cervicothoracic Vertebral ØRU4
    Coccygeal ØSU6
    Elbow
      Left ØRUM
      Right ØRUL
    Finger Phalangeal
      Left ØRUX
      Right ØRUW
    Hip
      Left ØSUB
        Acetabular Surface ØSUE
        Femoral Surface ØSUS
      Right ØSU9
        Acetabular Surface ØSUA
        Femoral Surface ØSUR
    Knee
      Left ØSUD
        Femoral Surface ØSUUØ9Z
        Tibial Surface ØSUWØ9Z
      Right ØSUC
        Femoral Surface ØSUTØ9Z
        Tibial Surface ØSUVØ9Z
    Lumbar Vertebral ØSUØ
    Lumbosacral ØSU3
    Metacarpophalangeal
      Left ØRUV
      Right ØRUU
    Metatarsal-Phalangeal
      Left ØSUN
      Right ØSUM
    Occipital-cervical ØRUØ
    Sacrococcygeal ØSU5
    Sacroiliac
      Left ØSU8
      Right ØSU7
    Shoulder
      Left ØRUK
      Right ØRUJ
    Sternoclavicular
      Left ØRUF
      Right ØRUE
    Tarsal
      Left ØSUJ
      Right ØSUH

▽ **Subterms under main terms may continue to next column or page**

Supplement — *continued*
  Tendon — *continued*
    Foot
      Left ØLUW
      Right ØLUV
    Hand
      Left ØLU8
      Right ØLU7
    Head and Neck ØLUØ
    Hip
      Left ØLUK
      Right ØLUJ
    Knee
      Left ØLUR
      Right ØLUQ
    Lower Arm and Wrist
      Left ØLU6
      Right ØLU5
    Lower Leg
      Left ØLUP
      Right ØLUN
    Perineum ØLUH
    Shoulder
      Left ØLU2
      Right ØLU1
    Thorax
      Left ØLUD
      Right ØLUC
    Trunk
      Left ØLUB
      Right ØLU9
    Upper Arm
      Left ØLU4
      Right ØLU3
    Upper Leg
      Left ØLUM
      Right ØLUL
  Testis
    Bilateral ØVUCØ
    Left ØVUBØ
    Right ØVU9Ø
  Thumb
    Left ØXUM
    Right ØXUL
  Tibia
    Left ØQUH
    Right ØQUG
  Toe
    1st
      Left ØYUQ
      Right ØYUP
    2nd
      Left ØYUS
      Right ØYUR
    3rd
      Left ØYUU
      Right ØYUT
    4th
      Left ØYUW
      Right ØYUV
    5th
      Left ØYUY
      Right ØYUX
  Tongue ØCU7
  Trachea ØBU1
  Tunica Vaginalis
    Left ØVU7
    Right ØVU6
  Turbinate, Nasal Ø9UL
  Tympanic Membrane
    Left Ø9U8
    Right Ø9U7
  Ulna
    Left ØPUL
    Right ØPUK
  Ureter
    Left ØTU7
    Right ØTU6
  Urethra ØTUD
  Uterine Supporting Structure ØUU4
  Uvula ØCUN
  Vagina ØUUG
  Valve
    Aortic Ø2UF
    Mitral Ø2UG
    Pulmonary Ø2UH
    Tricuspid Ø2UJ
  Vas Deferens
    Bilateral ØVUQ

Supplement — *continued*
  Vas Deferens — *continued*
    Left ØVUP
    Right ØVUN
  Vein
    Axillary
      Left Ø5U8
      Right Ø5U7
    Azygos Ø5UØ
    Basilic
      Left Ø5UC
      Right Ø5UB
    Brachial
      Left Ø5UA
      Right Ø5U9
    Cephalic
      Left Ø5UF
      Right Ø5UD
    Colic Ø6U7
    Common Iliac
      Left Ø6UD
      Right Ø6UC
    Esophageal Ø6U3
    External Iliac
      Left Ø6UG
      Right Ø6UF
    External Jugular
      Left Ø5UQ
      Right Ø5UP
    Face
      Left Ø5UV
      Right Ø5UT
    Femoral
      Left Ø6UN
      Right Ø6UM
    Foot
      Left Ø6UV
      Right Ø6UT
    Gastric Ø6U2
    Hand
      Left Ø5UH
      Right Ø5UG
    Hemiazygos Ø5U1
    Hepatic Ø6U4
    Hypogastric
      Left Ø6UJ
      Right Ø6UH
    Inferior Mesenteric Ø6U6
    Innominate
      Left Ø5U4
      Right Ø5U3
    Internal Jugular
      Left Ø5UN
      Right Ø5UM
    Intracranial Ø5UL
    Lower Ø6UY
    Portal Ø6U8
    Pulmonary
      Left Ø2UT
      Right Ø2US
    Renal
      Left Ø6UB
      Right Ø6U9
    Saphenous
      Left Ø6UQ
      Right Ø6UP
    Splenic Ø6U1
    Subclavian
      Left Ø5U6
      Right Ø5U5
    Superior Mesenteric Ø6U5
    Upper Ø5UY
    Vertebral
      Left Ø5US
      Right Ø5UR
  Vena Cava
    Inferior Ø6UØ
    Superior Ø2UV
  Ventricle
    Left Ø2UL
    Right Ø2UK
  Vertebra
    Cervical ØPU3
    Lumbar ØQUØ
      Mechanically Expandable (Paired) Synthetic Substitute XNUØ356
    Thoracic ØPU4
      Mechanically Expandable (Paired) Synthetic Substitute XNU4356

Supplement — *continued*
  Vesicle
    Bilateral ØVU3
    Left ØVU2
    Right ØVU1
  Vocal Cord
    Left ØCUV
    Right ØCUT
  Vulva ØUUM
  Wrist Region
    Left ØXUH
    Right ØXUG
Supraclavicular (Virchow's) lymph node
  use Lymphatic, Left Neck
  use Lymphatic, Right Neck
Supraclavicular nerve *use* Cervical Plexus
Suprahyoid lymph node *use* Lymphatic, Head
Suprahyoid muscle
  use Neck Muscle, Left
  use Neck Muscle, Right
Suprainguinal lymph node *use* Lymphatic, Pelvis
Supraorbital vein
  use Face Vein, Left
  use Face Vein, Right
Suprarenal gland
  use Adrenal Gland
  use Adrenal Gland, Bilateral
  use Adrenal Gland, Left
  use Adrenal Gland, Right
Suprarenal plexus *use* Abdominal Sympathetic Nerve
Suprascapular nerve *use* Brachial Plexus
Supraspinatus fascia
  use Subcutaneous Tissue and Fascia, Left Upper Arm
  use Subcutaneous Tissue and Fascia, Right Upper Arm
Supraspinatus muscle
  use Shoulder Muscle, Left
  use Shoulder Muscle, Right
Supraspinous ligament
  use Lower Spine Bursa and Ligament
  use Upper Spine Bursa and Ligament
Suprasternal notch *use* Sternum
Supratrochlear lymph node
  use Lymphatic, Left Upper Extremity
  use Lymphatic, Right Upper Extremity
Sural artery
  use Popliteal Artery, Left
  use Popliteal Artery, Right
Surpass Streamline™ Flow Diverter *use* Intraluminal Device, Flow Diverter in Ø3V
Suspension
  Bladder Neck *see* Reposition, Bladder Neck ØTSC
  Kidney *see* Reposition, Urinary System ØTS
  Urethra *see* Reposition, Urinary System ØTS
  Urethrovesical *see* Reposition, Bladder Neck ØTSC
  Uterus *see* Reposition, Uterus ØUS9
  Vagina *see* Reposition, Vagina ØUSG
Sustained Release Drug-eluting Intraluminal Device
  Dilation
    Anterior Tibial
      Left X27Q385
      Right X27P385
    Femoral
      Left X27J385
      Right X27H385
    Peroneal
      Left X27U385
      Right X27T385
    Popliteal
      Left Distal X27N385
      Left Proximal X27L385
      Right Distal X27M385
      Right Proximal X27K385
    Posterior Tibial
      Left X27S385
      Right X27R385
    Four or More
    Anterior Tibial
      Left X27Q3C5
      Right X27P3C5
    Femoral
      Left X27J3C5
      Right X27H3C5
    Peroneal
      Left X27U3C5

Sustained Release Drug-eluting Intraluminal Device
— *continued*
Four or More — *continued*
Peroneal — *continued*
Right X27T3C5
Popliteal
Left Distal X27N3C5
Left Proximal X27L3C5
Right Distal X27M3C5
Right Proximal X27K3C5
Posterior Tibial
Left X27S3C5
Right X27R3C5
Three
Anterior Tibial
Left X27Q3B5
Right X27P3B5
Femoral
Left X27J3B5
Right X27H3B5
Peroneal
Left X27U3B5
Right X27T3B5
Popliteal
Left Distal X27N3B5
Left Proximal X27L3B5
Right Distal X27M3B5
Right Proximal X27K3B5
Posterior Tibial
Left X27S3B5
Right X27R3B5
Two
Anterior Tibial
Left X27Q395
Right X27P395
Femoral
Left X27J395
Right X27H395
Peroneal
Left X27U395
Right X27T395
Popliteal
Left Distal X27N395
Left Proximal X27L395
Right Distal X27M395
Right Proximal X27K395
Posterior Tibial
Left X27S395
Right X27R395

Suture
Laceration repair *see* Repair
Ligation *see* Occlusion
Suture Removal
Extremity
Lower 8E0YXY8
Upper 8E0XXY8
Head and Neck Region 8E09XY8
Trunk Region 8E0WXY8
Sutureless valve, Perceval *use* Zooplastic Tissue, Rapid Deployment Technique in New Technology
Sweat gland *use* Skin
Sympathectomy *see* Excision, Peripheral Nervous System 01B
SynCardia Total Artificial Heart *use* Synthetic Substitute
Synchra CRT-P *use* Cardiac Resynchronization Pacemaker Pulse Generator in 0JH
SynchroMed pump *use* Infusion Device, Pump in Subcutaneous Tissue and Fascia
Synechiotomy, iris *see* Release, Eye 08N
Synovectomy
Lower joint *see* Excision, Lower Joints 0SB
Upper joint *see* Excision, Upper Joints 0RB
Synthetic Human Angiotensin II XW0
Systemic Nuclear Medicine Therapy
Abdomen CW70
Anatomical Regions, Multiple CW7YYZZ
Chest CW73
Thyroid CW7G
Whole Body CW7N

T

Tagraxofusp-erzs Antineoplastic XW0
Takedown
Arteriovenous shunt *see* Removal of device from, Upper Arteries 03P

Takedown — *continued*
Arteriovenous shunt, with creation of new shunt *see* Bypass, Upper Arteries 031
Stoma
see Excision
see Reposition
Talent® Converter *use* Intraluminal Device
Talent® Occluder *use* Intraluminal Device
Talent® Stent Graft (abdominal) (thoracic) *use* Intraluminal Device
Talocalcaneal (subtalar) joint
use Tarsal Joint, Left
use Tarsal Joint, Right
Talocalcaneal ligament
use Foot Bursa and Ligament, Left
use Foot Bursa and Ligament, Right
Talocalcaneonavicular joint
use Tarsal Joint, Left
use Tarsal Joint, Right
Talocalcaneonavicular ligament
use Foot Bursa and Ligament, Left
use Foot Bursa and Ligament, Right
Talocrural joint
use Ankle Joint, Left
use Joint, Ankle, Right
Talofibular ligament
use Ankle Bursa and Ligament, Left
use Ankle Bursa and Ligament, Right
Talus bone
use Tarsal, Left
use Tarsal, Right
TandemHeart® System *use* Short-term External Heart Assist System in Heart and Great Vessels
Tarsectomy
see Excision, Lower Bones 0QB
see Resection, Lower Bones 0QT
Tarsometatarsal ligament
use Foot Bursa and Ligament, Left
use Foot Bursa and Ligament, Right
Tarsorrhaphy *see* Repair, Eye 08Q
Tattooing
Cornea 3E0CXMZ
Skin *see* Introduction of substance in or on, Skin 3E00
TAXUS® Liberté® Paclitaxel-eluting Coronary Stent System *use* Intraluminal Device, Drug-eluting in Heart and Great Vessels
TBNA (transbronchial needle aspiration)
Fluid or gas *see* Drainage, Respiratory System 0B9
Tissue biopsy *see* Extraction, Respiratory System 0BD
TECENTRIQ® *use* Atezolizumab Antineoplastic
Telemetry 4A12X4Z
Ambulatory 4A12X45
Temperature gradient study 4A0ZXKZ
Temporal lobe *use* Cerebral Hemisphere
Temporalis muscle *use* Head Muscle
Temporoparietalis muscle *use* Head Muscle
Tendolysis *see* Release, Tendons 0LN
Tendonectomy
see Excision, Tendons 0LB
see Resection, Tendons 0LT
Tendonoplasty, tenoplasty
see Repair, Tendons 0LQ
see Replacement, Tendons 0LR
see Supplement, Tendons 0LU
Tendorrhaphy *see* Repair, Tendons 0LQ
Tendototomy
see Division, Tendons 0L8
see Drainage, Tendons 0L9
Tenectomy, tenonectomy
see Excision, Tendons 0LB
see Resection, Tendons 0LT
Tenolysis *see* Release, Tendons 0LN
Tenontorrhaphy *see* Repair, Tendons 0LQ
Tenontotomy
see Division, Tendons 0L8
see Drainage, Tendons 0L9
Tenorrhaphy *see* Repair, Tendons 0LQ
Tenosynovectomy
see Excision, Tendons 0LB
see Resection, Tendons 0LT
Tenotomy
see Division, Tendons 0L8
see Drainage, Tendons 0L9

Tensor fasciae latae muscle
use Hip Muscle, Left
use Hip Muscle, Right
Tensor veli palatini muscle *use* Tongue, Palate, Pharynx Muscle
Tenth cranial nerve *use* Vagus Nerve
Tentorium cerebelli *use* Dura Mater
Teres major muscle
use Shoulder Muscle, Left
use Shoulder Muscle, Right
Teres minor muscle
use Shoulder Muscle, Left
use Shoulder Muscle, Right
Termination of pregnancy
Aspiration curettage 10A07ZZ
Dilation and curettage 10A07ZZ
Hysterotomy 10A00ZZ
Intra-amniotic injection 10A03ZZ
Laminaria 10A07ZW
Vacuum 10A07Z6
Testectomy
see Excision, Male Reproductive System 0VB
see Resection, Male Reproductive System 0VT
Testicular artery *use* Abdominal Aorta
Testing
Glaucoma 4A07XBZ
Hearing *see* Hearing Assessment, Diagnostic Audiology F13
Mental health *see* Psychological Tests
Muscle function, electromyography (EMG) *see* Measurement, Musculoskeletal 4A0F
Muscle function, manual *see* Motor Function Assessment, Rehabilitation F01
Neurophysiologic monitoring, intra-operative *see* Monitoring, Physiological Systems 4A1
Range of motion *see* Motor Function Assessment, Rehabilitation F01
Vestibular function *see* Vestibular Assessment, Diagnostic Audiology F15
Thalamectomy *see* Excision, Thalamus 00B9
Thalamotomy *see* Drainage, Thalamus 0099
Thenar muscle
use Hand Muscle, Left
use Hand Muscle, Right
Therapeutic Massage
Musculoskeletal System 8E0KX1Z
Reproductive System
Prostate 8E0VX1C
Rectum 8E0VX1D
Therapeutic occlusion coil(s) *use* Intraluminal Device
Thermography 4A0ZXKZ
Thermotherapy, prostate *see* Destruction, Prostate 0V50
Third cranial nerve *use* Oculomotor Nerve
Third occipital nerve *use* Cervical Nerve
Third ventricle *use* Cerebral Ventricle
Thoracectomy *see* Excision, Anatomical Regions, General 0WB
Thoracentesis *see* Drainage, Anatomical Regions, General 0W9
Thoracic aortic plexus *use* Thoracic Sympathetic Nerve
Thoracic esophagus *use* Esophagus, Middle
Thoracic facet joint *use* Thoracic Vertebral Joint
Thoracic ganglion *use* Thoracic Sympathetic Nerve
Thoracoacromial artery
use Axillary Artery, Left
use Axillary Artery, Right
Thoracocentesis *see* Drainage, Anatomical Regions, General 0W9
Thoracolumbar facet joint *use* Thoracolumbar Vertebral Joint
Thoracoplasty
see Repair, Anatomical Regions, General 0WQ
see Supplement, Anatomical Regions, General 0WU
Thoracostomy, for lung collapse *see* Drainage, Respiratory System 0B9
Thoracostomy tube *use* Drainage Device
Thoracotomy *see* Drainage, Anatomical Regions, General 0W9
Thoratec IVAD (Implantable Ventricular Assist Device) *use* Implantable Heart Assist System in Heart and Great Vessels
Thoratec Paracorporeal Ventricular Assist Device *use* Short-term External Heart Assist System in Heart and Great Vessels
Thrombectomy *see* Extirpation

Thrombolysis, Ultrasound assisted *see* Fragmentation, Artery
Thymectomy
  see Excision, Lymphatic and Hemic Systems 07B
  see Resection, Lymphatic and Hemic Systems 07T
Thymopexy
  see Repair, Lymphatic and Hemic Systems 07Q
  see Reposition, Lymphatic and Hemic Systems 07S
Thymus gland *use* Thymus
Thyroarytenoid muscle
  use Neck Muscle, Left
  use Neck Muscle, Right
Thyrocervical trunk
  use Thyroid Artery, Left
  use Thyroid Artery, Right
Thyroid cartilage *use* Larynx
Thyroidectomy
  see Excision, Endocrine System 0GB
  see Resection, Endocrine System 0GT
Thyroidorrhaphy *see* Repair, Endocrine System 0GQ
Thyroidoscopy 0GJK4ZZ
Thyroidotomy *see* Drainage, Endocrine System 0G9
Tibial insert *use* Liner in Lower Joints
Tibialis anterior muscle
  use Lower Leg Muscle, Left
  use Lower Leg Muscle, Right
Tibialis posterior muscle
  use Lower Leg Muscle, Left
  use Lower Leg Muscle, Right
Tibiofemoral joint
  use Knee Joint, Left
  use Knee Joint, Right
  use Knee Joint, Tibial Surface, Left
  use Knee Joint, Tibial Surface, Right
Tibioperoneal trunk
  use Popliteal Artery, Left
  use Popliteal Artery, Right
Tisagenlecleucel *use* Engineered Autologous Chimeric Antigen Receptor T-cell Immunotherapy
Tissue bank graft *use* Nonautologous Tissue Substitute
Tissue expander (inflatable) (injectable)
  use Tissue Expander in Skin and Breast
  use Tissue Expander in Subcutaneous Tissue and Fascia
Tissue Expander
  Insertion of device in
    Breast
      Bilateral 0HHV
      Left 0HHU
      Right 0HHT
    Nipple
      Left 0HHX
      Right 0HHW
    Subcutaneous Tissue and Fascia
      Abdomen 0JH8
      Back 0JH7
      Buttock 0JH9
      Chest 0JH6
      Face 0JH1
      Foot
        Left 0JHR
        Right 0JHQ
      Hand
        Left 0JHK
        Right 0JHJ
      Lower Arm
        Left 0JHH
        Right 0JHG
      Lower Leg
        Left 0JHP
        Right 0JHN
      Neck
        Left 0JH5
        Right 0JH4
      Pelvic Region 0JHC
      Perineum 0JHB
      Scalp 0JH0
      Upper Arm
        Left 0JHF
        Right 0JHD
      Upper Leg
        Left 0JHM
        Right 0JHL
  Removal of device from
    Breast
      Left 0HPU
      Right 0HPT

Tissue Expander — *continued*
  Removal of device from — *continued*
    Subcutaneous Tissue and Fascia
      Head and Neck 0JPS
      Lower Extremity 0JPW
      Trunk 0JPT
      Upper Extremity 0JPV
  Revision of device in
    Breast
      Left 0HWU
      Right 0HWT
    Subcutaneous Tissue and Fascia
      Head and Neck 0JWS
      Lower Extremity 0JWW
      Trunk 0JWT
      Upper Extremity 0JWV
Tissue Plasminogen Activator (tPA) (r-tPA) *use* Other Thrombolytic
Titanium Sternal Fixation System (TSFS)
  use Internal Fixation Device, Rigid Plate in 0PS
  use Internal Fixation Device, Rigid Plate in 0PH
Tomographic (Tomo) Nuclear Medicine Imaging
  Abdomen CW20
  Abdomen and Chest CW24
  Abdomen and Pelvis CW21
  Anatomical Regions, Multiple CW2YYZZ
  Bladder, Kidneys and Ureters CT23
  Brain C020
  Breast CH2YYZZ
    Bilateral CH22
    Left CH21
    Right CH20
  Bronchi and Lungs CB22
  Central Nervous System C02YYZZ
  Cerebrospinal Fluid C025
  Chest CW23
  Chest and Abdomen CW24
  Chest and Neck CW26
  Digestive System CD2YYZZ
  Endocrine System CG2YYZZ
  Extremity
    Lower CW2D
      Bilateral CP2F
      Left CP2D
      Right CP2C
    Upper CW2M
      Bilateral CP2B
      Left CP29
      Right CP28
  Gallbladder CF24
  Gastrointestinal Tract CD27
  Gland, Parathyroid CG21
  Head and Neck CW2B
  Heart C22YYZZ
    Right and Left C226
  Hepatobiliary System and Pancreas CF2YYZZ
  Kidneys, Ureters and Bladder CT23
  Liver CF25
  Liver and Spleen CF26
  Lungs and Bronchi CB22
  Lymphatics and Hematologic System C72YYZZ
  Musculoskeletal System, Other CP2YYZZ
  Myocardium C22G
  Neck and Chest CW26
  Neck and Head CW2B
  Pancreas and Hepatobiliary System CF2YYZZ
  Pelvic Region CW2J
  Pelvis CP26
  Pelvis and Abdomen CW21
  Pelvis and Spine CP27
  Respiratory System CB2YYZZ
  Skin CH2YYZZ
  Skull CP21
  Skull and Cervical Spine CP23
  Spine
    Cervical CP22
    Cervical and Skull CP23
    Lumbar CP2H
    Thoracic CP2G
    Thoracolumbar CP2J
  Spine and Pelvis CP27
  Spleen C722
  Spleen and Liver CF26
  Subcutaneous Tissue CH2YYZZ
  Thorax CP24
  Ureters, Kidneys and Bladder CT23
  Urinary System CT2YYZZ
Tomography, computerized *see* Computerized Tomography (CT Scan)

Tongue, base of *use* Pharynx
Tonometry 4A07XBZ
Tonsillectomy
  see Excision, Mouth and Throat 0CB
  see Resection, Mouth and Throat 0CT
Tonsillotomy *see* Drainage, Mouth and Throat 0C9
Total Anomalous Pulmonary Venous Return (TAPVR) repair
  see Bypass, Atrium, Left 0217
  see Bypass, Vena Cava, Superior 021V
Total artificial (replacement) heart *use* Synthetic Substitute
Total parenteral nutrition (TPN) *see* Introduction of Nutritional Substance
Trachectomy
  see Excision, Trachea 0BB1
  see Resection, Trachea 0BT1
Trachelectomy
  see Excision, Cervix 0UBC
  see Resection, Cervix 0UTC
Trachelopexy
  see Repair, Cervix 0UQC
  see Reposition, Cervix 0USC
Tracheloplasty *see* Repair, Cervix 0UQC
Trachelorrhaphy *see* Repair, Cervix 0UQC
Trachelotomy *see* Drainage, Cervix 0U9C
Tracheobronchial lymph node *use* Lymphatic, Thorax
Tracheoesophageal fistulization 0B110D6
Tracheolysis *see* Release, Respiratory System 0BN
Tracheoplasty
  see Repair, Respiratory System 0BQ
  see Supplement, Respiratory System 0BU
Tracheorrhaphy *see* Repair, Respiratory System 0BQ
Tracheoscopy 0BJ18ZZ
Tracheostomy *see* Bypass, Respiratory System 0B1
Tracheostomy Device
  Bypass, Trachea 0B11
  Change device in, Trachea 0B21XFZ
  Removal of device from, Trachea 0BP1
  Revision of device in, Trachea 0BW1
Tracheostomy tube *use* Tracheostomy Device in Respiratory System
Tracheotomy *see* Drainage, Respiratory System 0B9
Traction
  Abdominal Wall 2W63X
  Arm
    Lower
      Left 2W6DX
      Right 2W6CX
    Upper
      Left 2W6BX
      Right 2W6AX
  Back 2W65X
  Chest Wall 2W64X
  Extremity
    Lower
      Left 2W6MX
      Right 2W6LX
    Upper
      Left 2W69X
      Right 2W68X
  Face 2W61X
  Finger
    Left 2W6KX
    Right 2W6JX
  Foot
    Left 2W6TX
    Right 2W6SX
  Hand
    Left 2W6FX
    Right 2W6EX
  Head 2W60X
  Inguinal Region
    Left 2W67X
    Right 2W66X
  Leg
    Lower
      Left 2W6RX
      Right 2W6QX
    Upper
      Left 2W6PX
      Right 2W6NX
  Neck 2W62X
  Thumb
    Left 2W6HX
    Right 2W6GX
  Toe
    Left 2W6VX

Traction — continued
   Toe — continued
      Right 2W6UX
Tractotomy see Division, Central Nervous System and Cranial Nerves 008
Tragus
   use External Ear, Bilateral
   use External Ear, Left
   use External Ear, Right
Training, caregiver see Caregiver Training
TRAM (transverse rectus abdominis myocutaneous) flap reconstruction
   Free see Replacement, Skin and Breast 0HR
   Pedicled see Transfer, Muscles 0KX
Transdermal Glomerular Filtration Rate (GFR) Measurement System XT25XE5
Transection see Division
Transfer
   Buccal Mucosa 0CX4
   Bursa and Ligament
     Abdomen
       Left 0MXJ
       Right 0MXH
     Ankle
       Left 0MXR
       Right 0MXQ
     Elbow
       Left 0MX4
       Right 0MX3
     Foot
       Left 0MXT
       Right 0MXS
     Hand
       Left 0MX8
       Right 0MX7
     Head and Neck 0MX0
     Hip
       Left 0MXM
       Right 0MXL
     Knee
       Left 0MXP
       Right 0MXN
     Lower Extremity
       Left 0MXW
       Right 0MXV
     Perineum 0MXK
     Rib(s) 0MXG
     Shoulder
       Left 0MX2
       Right 0MX1
     Spine
       Lower 0MXD
       Upper 0MXC
     Sternum 0MXF
     Upper Extremity
       Left 0MXB
       Right 0MX9
     Wrist
       Left 0MX6
       Right 0MX5
   Finger
     Left 0XXP0ZM
     Right 0XXN0ZL
   Gingiva
     Lower 0CX6
     Upper 0CX5
   Intestine
     Large 0DXE
     Small 0DX8
   Lip
     Lower 0CX1
     Upper 0CX0
   Muscle
     Abdomen
       Left 0KXL
       Right 0KXK
     Extraocular
       Left 08XM
       Right 08XL
     Facial 0KX1
     Foot
       Left 0KXW
       Right 0KXV
     Hand
       Left 0KXD
       Right 0KXC
     Head 0KX0

Transfer — continued
   Muscle — continued
     Hip
       Left 0KXP
       Right 0KXN
     Lower Arm and Wrist
       Left 0KXB
       Right 0KX9
     Lower Leg
       Left 0KXT
       Right 0KXS
     Neck
       Left 0KX3
       Right 0KX2
     Perineum 0KXM
     Shoulder
       Left 0KX6
       Right 0KX5
     Thorax
       Left 0KXJ
       Right 0KXH
     Tongue, Palate, Pharynx 0KX4
     Trunk
       Left 0KXG
       Right 0KXF
     Upper Arm
       Left 0KX8
       Right 0KX7
     Upper Leg
       Left 0KXR
       Right 0KXQ
   Nerve
     Abducens 00XL
     Accessory 00XR
     Acoustic 00XN
     Cervical 01X1
     Facial 00XM
     Femoral 01XD
     Glossopharyngeal 00XP
     Hypoglossal 00XS
     Lumbar 01XB
     Median 01X5
     Oculomotor 00XH
     Olfactory 00XF
     Optic 00XG
     Peroneal 01XH
     Phrenic 01X2
     Pudendal 01XC
     Radial 01X6
     Sciatic 01XF
     Thoracic 01X8
     Tibial 01XG
     Trigeminal 00XK
     Trochlear 00XJ
     Ulnar 01X4
     Vagus 00XQ
   Palate, Soft 0CX3
   Prepuce 0VXT
   Skin
     Abdomen 0HX7XZZ
     Back 0HX6XZZ
     Buttock 0HX8XZZ
     Chest 0HX5XZZ
     Ear
       Left 0HX3XZZ
       Right 0HX2XZZ
     Face 0HX1XZZ
     Foot
       Left 0HXNXZZ
       Right 0HXMXZZ
     Hand
       Left 0HXGXZZ
       Right 0HXFXZZ
     Inguinal 0HXAXZZ
     Lower Arm
       Left 0HXEXZZ
       Right 0HXDXZZ
     Lower Leg
       Left 0HXLXZZ
       Right 0HXKXZZ
     Neck 0HX4XZZ
     Perineum 0HX9XZZ
     Scalp 0HX0XZZ
     Upper Arm
       Left 0HXCXZZ
       Right 0HXBXZZ
     Upper Leg
       Left 0HXJXZZ
       Right 0HXHXZZ

Transfer — continued
   Stomach 0DX6
   Subcutaneous Tissue and Fascia
     Abdomen 0JX8
     Back 0JX7
     Buttock 0JX9
     Chest 0JX6
     Face 0JX1
     Foot
       Left 0JXR
       Right 0JXQ
     Hand
       Left 0JXK
       Right 0JXJ
     Lower Arm
       Left 0JXH
       Right 0JXG
     Lower Leg
       Left 0JXP
       Right 0JXN
     Neck
       Left 0JX5
       Right 0JX4
     Pelvic Region 0JXC
     Perineum 0JXB
     Scalp 0JX0
     Upper Arm
       Left 0JXF
       Right 0JXD
     Upper Leg
       Left 0JXM
       Right 0JXL
   Tendon
     Abdomen
       Left 0LXG
       Right 0LXF
     Ankle
       Left 0LXT
       Right 0LXS
     Foot
       Left 0LXW
       Right 0LXV
     Hand
       Left 0LX8
       Right 0LX7
     Head and Neck 0LX0
     Hip
       Left 0LXK
       Right 0LXJ
     Knee
       Left 0LXR
       Right 0LXQ
     Lower Arm and Wrist
       Left 0LX6
       Right 0LX5
     Lower Leg
       Left 0LXP
       Right 0LXN
     Perineum 0LXH
     Shoulder
       Left 0LX2
       Buttock 0LX1
     Thorax
       Left 0LXD
       Right 0LXC
     Trunk
       Left 0LXB
       Right 0LX9
     Upper Arm
       Left 0LX4
       Right 0LX3
     Upper Leg
       Left 0LXM
       Right 0LXL
   Tongue 0CX7
Transfusion
   Immunotherapy see New Technology, Anatomical Regions XW2
   Products of Conception
     Antihemophilic Factors 3027
     Blood
       Platelets 3027
       Red Cells 3027
         Frozen 3027
       White Cells 3027
       Whole 3027
     Factor IX 3027
     Fibrinogen 3027
     Globulin 3027

Transfusion — *continued*
  Products of Conception — *continued*
    Plasma
      Fresh 3027
      Frozen 3027
    Plasma Cryoprecipitate 3027
    Serum Albumin 3027
  Vein
    4-Factor Prothrombin Complex Concentrate 30280B1
    Central
      Antihemophilic Factors 3024
      Blood
        Platelets 3024
        Red Cells 3024
          Frozen 3024
        White Cells 3024
        Whole 3024
      Bone Marrow 3024
      Factor IX 3024
      Fibrinogen 3024
      Globulin 3024
      Hematopoietic Stem/Progenitor Cells (HSPC), Genetically Modified 3024
      Plasma
        Fresh 3024
        Frozen 3024
      Plasma Cryoprecipitate 3024
      Serum Albumin 3024
      Stem Cells
        Cord Blood 3024
        Embryonic 3024
        Hematopoietic 3024
        T-cell Depleted Hematopoietic 3024
    Peripheral
      Antihemophilic Factors 3023
      Blood
        Platelets 3023
        Red Cells 3023
          Frozen 3023
        White Cells 3023
        Whole 3023
      Bone Marrow 3023
      Factor IX 3023
      Fibrinogen 3023
      Globulin 3023
      Hematopoietic Stem/Progenitor Cells (HSPC), Genetically Modified 3023
      Plasma
        Fresh 3023
        Frozen 3023
      Plasma Cryoprecipitate 3023
      Serum Albumin 3023
      Stem Cells
        Cord Blood 3023
        Embryonic 3023
        Hematopoietic 3023
        T-cell Depleted Hematopoietic 3023
Transplant *see* Transplantation
Transplantation
  Bone marrow *see* Transfusion, Circulatory 302
  Esophagus 0DY50Z
  Face 0WY20Z
  Hand
    Left 0XYK0Z
    Right 0XYJ0Z
  Heart 02YA0Z
  Hematopoietic cell *see* Transfusion, Circulatory 302
  Intestine
    Large 0DYE0Z
    Small 0DY80Z
  Kidney
    Left 0TY10Z
    Right 0TY00Z
  Liver 0FY00Z
  Lung
    Bilateral 0BYM0Z
    Left 0BYL0Z
    Lower Lobe
      Left 0BYJ0Z
      Right 0BYF0Z
    Middle Lobe, Right 0BYD0Z
    Right 0BYK0Z

Transplantation — *continued*
  Lung — *continued*
    Upper Lobe
      Left 0BYG0Z
      Right 0BYC0Z
    Lung Lingula 0BYH0Z
  Ovary
    Left 0UY10Z
    Right 0UY00Z
  Pancreas 0FYG0Z
  Penis 0VYS0Z
  Products of Conception 10Y0
  Scrotum 0VY50Z
  Spleen 07YP0Z
  Stem cell *see* Transfusion, Circulatory 302
  Stomach 0DY60Z
  Thymus 07YM0Z
  Uterus 0UY90Z
Transposition
  see Bypass
  see Reposition
  see Transfer
Transversalis fascia *use* Subcutaneous Tissue and Fascia, Trunk
Transverse acetabular ligament
  use Hip Bursa and Ligament, Left
  use Hip Bursa and Ligament, Right
Transverse (cutaneous) cervical nerve *use* Cervical Plexus
Transverse facial artery
  use Temporal Artery, Left
  use Temporal Artery, Right
Transverse foramen *use* Cervical Vertebra
Transverse humeral ligament
  use Shoulder Bursa and Ligament, Left
  use Shoulder Bursa and Ligament, Right
Transverse ligament of atlas *use* Head and Neck Bursa and Ligament
Transverse process
  use Cervical Vertebra
  use Lumbar Vertebra
  use Thoracic Vertebra
Transverse Rectus Abdominis Myocutaneous Flap
  Replacement
    Bilateral 0HRV076
    Left 0HRU076
    Right 0HRT076
  Transfer
    Left 0KXL
    Right 0KXK
Transverse scapular ligament
  use Shoulder Bursa and Ligament, Left
  use Shoulder Bursa and Ligament, Right
Transverse thoracis muscle
  use Thorax Muscle, Left
  use Thorax Muscle, Right
Transversospinalis muscle
  use Trunk Muscle, Left
  use Trunk Muscle, Right
Transversus abdominis muscle
  use Abdomen Muscle, Left
  use Abdomen Muscle, Right
Trapezium bone
  use Carpal, Left
  use Carpal, Right
Trapezius muscle
  use Trunk Muscle, Left
  use Trunk Muscle, Right
Trapezoid bone
  use Carpal, Left
  use Carpal, Right
Triceps brachii muscle
  use Upper Arm Muscle, Left
  use Upper Arm Muscle, Right
Tricuspid annulus *use* Tricuspid Valve
Trifacial nerve *use* Trigeminal Nerve
Trifecta™ Valve (aortic) *use* Zooplastic Tissue in Heart and Great Vessels
Trigone of bladder *use* Bladder
TriGuard 3™ CEPD (cerebral embolic protection device) X2A6325
Trimming, excisional *see* Excision
Triquetral bone
  use Carpal, Left
  use Carpal, Right
Trochanteric bursa
  use Hip Bursa and Ligament, Left

Trochanteric bursa — *continued*
  use Hip Bursa and Ligament, Right
TUMT (transurethral microwave thermotherapy of prostate) 0V507ZZ
TUNA (transurethral needle ablation of prostate) 0V507ZZ
Tunneled central venous catheter *use* Vascular Access Device, Tunneled in Subcutaneous Tissue and Fascia
Tunneled spinal (intrathecal) catheter *use* Infusion Device
Turbinectomy
  see Excision, Ear, Nose, Sinus 09B
  see Resection, Ear, Nose, Sinus 09T
Turbinoplasty
  see Repair, Ear, Nose, Sinus 09Q
  see Replacement, Ear, Nose, Sinus 09R
  see Supplement, Ear, Nose, Sinus 09U
Turbinotomy
  see Division, Ear, Nose, Sinus 098
  see Drainage, Ear, Nose, Sinus 099
TURP (transurethral resection of prostate) 0VB07ZZ
  see Excision, Prostate 0VB0
  see Resection, Prostate 0VT0
Twelfth cranial nerve *use* Hypoglossal Nerve
Two lead pacemaker *use* Pacemaker, Dual Chamber in 0JH
Tympanic cavity
  use Middle Ear, Left
  use Middle Ear, Right
Tympanic nerve *use* Glossopharyngeal Nerve
Tympanic part of temporal bone
  use Temporal Bone, Left
  use Temporal Bone, Right
Tympanogram *see* Hearing Assessment, Diagnostic Audiology F13
Tympanoplasty
  see Repair, Ear, Nose, Sinus 09Q
  see Replacement, Ear, Nose, Sinus 09R
  see Supplement, Ear, Nose, Sinus 09U
Tympanosympathectomy *see* Excision, Nerve, Head and Neck Sympathetic 01BK
Tympanotomy *see* Drainage, Ear, Nose, Sinus 099
TYRX Antibacterial Envelope *use* Anti-Infective Envelope

U

Ulnar collateral carpal ligament
  use Wrist Bursa and Ligament, Left
  use Wrist Bursa and Ligament, Right
Ulnar collateral ligament
  use Elbow Bursa and Ligament, Left
  use Elbow Bursa and Ligament, Right
Ulnar notch
  use Radius, Left
  use Radius, Right
Ulnar vein
  use Brachial Vein, Left
  use Brachial Vein, Right
Ultrafiltration
  Hemodialysis *see* Performance, Urinary 5A1D
  Therapeutic plasmapheresis *see* Pheresis, Circulatory 6A55
Ultraflex™ Precision Colonic Stent System *use* Intraluminal Device
ULTRAPRO Hernia System (UHS) *use* Synthetic Substitute
ULTRAPRO Partially Absorbable Lightweight Mesh *use* Synthetic Substitute
ULTRAPRO Plug *use* Synthetic Substitute
Ultrasonic osteogenic stimulator
  use Bone Growth Stimulator in Head and Facial Bones
  use Bone Growth Stimulator in Lower Bones
  use Bone Growth Stimulator in Upper Bones
Ultrasonography
  Abdomen BW40ZZZ
  Abdomen and Pelvis BW41ZZZ
  Abdominal Wall BH49ZZZ
  Aorta
    Abdominal, Intravascular B440ZZ3
    Thoracic, Intravascular B340ZZ3
  Appendix BD48ZZZ

▽ **Subterms under main terms may continue to next column or page**

Ultrasonography — *continued*
  Artery
    Brachiocephalic-Subclavian, Right, Intravascular B341ZZ3
    Celiac and Mesenteric, Intravascular B44KZZ3
    Common Carotid
      Bilateral, Intravascular B345ZZ3
      Left, Intravascular B344ZZ3
      Right, Intravascular B343ZZ3
    Coronary
      Multiple B241YZZ
        Intravascular B241ZZ3
        Transesophageal B241ZZ4
      Single B240YZZ
        Intravascular B240ZZ3
        Transesophageal B240ZZ4
    Femoral, Intravascular B44LZZ3
    Inferior Mesenteric, Intravascular B445ZZ3
    Internal Carotid
      Bilateral, Intravascular B348ZZ3
      Left, Intravascular B347ZZ3
      Right, Intravascular B346ZZ3
    Intra-Abdominal, Other, Intravascular B44BZZ3
    Intracranial, Intravascular B34RZZ3
    Lower Extremity
      Bilateral, Intravascular B44HZZ3
      Left, Intravascular B44GZZ3
      Right, Intravascular B44FZZ3
    Mesenteric and Celiac, Intravascular B44KZZ3
    Ophthalmic, Intravascular B34VZZ3
    Penile, Intravascular B44NZZ3
    Pulmonary
      Left, Intravascular B34TZZ3
      Right, Intravascular B34SZZ3
    Renal
      Bilateral, Intravascular B448ZZ3
      Left, Intravascular B447ZZ3
      Right, Intravascular B446ZZ3
    Subclavian, Left, Intravascular B342ZZ3
    Superior Mesenteric, Intravascular B444ZZ3
    Upper Extremity
      Bilateral, Intravascular B34KZZ3
      Left, Intravascular B34JZZ3
      Right, Intravascular B34HZZ3
  Bile Duct BF40ZZZ
  Bile Duct and Gallbladder BF43ZZZ
  Bladder BT40ZZZ
    and Kidney BT4JZZZ
  Brain B040ZZZ
  Breast
    Bilateral BH42ZZZ
    Left BH41ZZZ
    Right BH40ZZZ
  Chest Wall BH4BZZZ
  Coccyx BR4FZZZ
  Connective Tissue
    Lower Extremity BL41ZZZ
    Upper Extremity BL40ZZZ
  Duodenum BD49ZZZ
  Elbow
    Left, Densitometry BP4HZZ1
    Right, Densitometry BP4GZZ1
  Esophagus BD41ZZZ
  Extremity
    Lower BH48ZZZ
    Upper BH47ZZZ
  Eye
    Bilateral B847ZZZ
    Left B846ZZZ
    Right B845ZZZ
  Fallopian Tube
    Bilateral BU42
    Left BU41
    Right BU40
  Fetal Umbilical Cord BY47ZZZ
  Fetus
    First Trimester, Multiple Gestation BY4BZZZ
    Second Trimester, Multiple Gestation BY4DZZZ
    Single
      First Trimester BY49ZZZ
      Second Trimester BY4CZZZ
      Third Trimester BY4FZZZ
    Third Trimester, Multiple Gestation BY4GZZZ
  Gallbladder BF42ZZZ
  Gallbladder and Bile Duct BF43ZZZ
  Gastrointestinal Tract BD47ZZZ

Ultrasonography — *continued*
  Gland
    Adrenal
      Bilateral BG42ZZZ
      Left BG41ZZZ
      Right BG40ZZZ
    Parathyroid BG43ZZZ
    Thyroid BG44ZZZ
  Hand
    Left, Densitometry BP4PZZ1
    Right, Densitometry BP4NZZ1
  Head and Neck BH4CZZZ
  Heart
    Left B245YZZ
      Intravascular B245ZZ3
      Transesophageal B245ZZ4
    Pediatric B24DYZZ
      Intravascular B24DZZ3
      Transesophageal B24DZZ4
    Right B244YZZ
      Intravascular B244ZZ3
      Transesophageal B244ZZ4
    Right and Left B246YZZ
      Intravascular B246ZZ3
      Transesophageal B246ZZ4
  Heart with Aorta B24BYZZ
    Intravascular B24BZZ3
    Transesophageal B24BZZ4
  Hepatobiliary System, All BF4CZZZ
  Hip
    Bilateral BQ42ZZZ
    Left BQ41ZZZ
    Right BQ40ZZZ
  Kidney
    and Bladder BT4JZZZ
    Bilateral BT43ZZZ
    Left BT42ZZZ
    Right BT41ZZZ
    Transplant BT49ZZZ
  Knee
    Bilateral BQ49ZZZ
    Left BQ48ZZZ
    Right BQ47ZZZ
  Liver BF45ZZZ
  Liver and Spleen BF46ZZZ
  Mediastinum BB4CZZZ
  Neck BW4FZZZ
  Ovary
    Bilateral BU45
    Left BU44
    Right BU43
  Ovary and Uterus BU4C
  Pancreas BF47ZZZ
  Pelvic Region BW4GZZZ
  Pelvis and Abdomen BW41ZZZ
  Penis BV4BZZZ
  Pericardium B24CYZZ
    Intravascular B24CZZ3
    Transesophageal B24CZZ4
  Placenta BY48ZZZ
  Pleura BB4BZZZ
  Prostate and Seminal Vesicle BV49ZZZ
  Rectum BD4CZZZ
  Sacrum BR4FZZZ
  Scrotum BV44ZZZ
  Seminal Vesicle and Prostate BV49ZZZ
  Shoulder
    Left, Densitometry BP49ZZ1
    Right, Densitometry BP48ZZ1
  Spinal Cord B04BZZZ
  Spine
    Cervical BR40ZZZ
    Lumbar BR49ZZZ
    Thoracic BR47ZZZ
  Spleen and Liver BF46ZZZ
  Stomach BD42ZZZ
  Tendon
    Lower Extremity BL43ZZZ
    Upper Extremity BL42ZZZ
  Ureter
    Bilateral BT48ZZZ
    Left BT47ZZZ
    Right BT46ZZZ
  Urethra BT45ZZZ
  Uterus BU46
  Uterus and Ovary BU4C
  Vein
    Jugular
      Left, Intravascular B544ZZ3

Ultrasonography — *continued*
  Vein — *continued*
    Jugular — *continued*
      Right, Intravascular B543ZZ3
    Lower Extremity
      Bilateral, Intravascular B54DZZ3
      Left, Intravascular B54CZZ3
      Right, Intravascular B54BZZ3
    Portal, Intravascular B54TZZ3
    Renal
      Bilateral, Intravascular B54LZZ3
      Left, Intravascular B54KZZ3
      Right, Intravascular B54JZZ3
    Spanchnic, Intravascular B54TZZ3
    Subclavian
      Left, Intravascular B547ZZ3
      Right, Intravascular B546ZZ3
    Upper Extremity
      Bilateral, Intravascular B54PZZ3
      Left, Intravascular B54NZZ3
      Right, Intravascular B54MZZ3
  Vena Cava
    Inferior, Intravascular B549ZZ3
    Superior, Intravascular B548ZZ3
  Wrist
    Left, Densitometry BP4MZZ1
    Right, Densitometry BP4LZZ1
Ultrasound bone healing system
  use Bone Growth Stimulator in Head and Facial Bones
  use Bone Growth Stimulator in Lower Bones
  use Bone Growth Stimulator in Upper Bones
Ultrasound Therapy
  Heart 6A75
  No Qualifier 6A75
  Vessels
    Head and Neck 6A75
    Other 6A75
    Peripheral 6A75
Ultraviolet Light Therapy, Skin 6A80
Umbilical artery
  use Internal Iliac Artery, Left
  use Internal Iliac Artery, Right
  use Lower Artery
Uniplanar external fixator
  use External Fixation Device, Monoplanar in 0PH
  use External Fixation Device, Monoplanar in 0PS
  use External Fixation Device, Monoplanar in 0QH
  use External Fixation Device, Monoplanar in 0QS
Upper GI series *see* Fluoroscopy, Gastrointestinal, Upper BD15
Ureteral orifice
  use Ureter
  use Ureter, Left
  use Ureter, Right
  use Ureters, Bilateral
Ureterectomy
  see Excision, Urinary System 0TB
  see Resection, Urinary System 0TT
Ureterocolostomy *see* Bypass, Urinary System 0T1
Ureterocystostomy *see* Bypass, Urinary System 0T1
Ureteroenterostomy *see* Bypass, Urinary System 0T1
Ureteroileostomy *see* Bypass, Urinary System 0T1
Ureterolithotomy *see* Extirpation, Urinary System 0TC
Ureterolysis *see* Release, Urinary System 0TN
Ureteroneocystostomy
  see Bypass, Urinary System 0T1
  see Reposition, Urinary System 0TS
Ureteropelvic junction (UPJ)
  use Kidney Pelvis, Left
  use Kidney Pelvis, Right
Ureteropexy
  see Repair, Urinary System 0TQ
  see Reposition, Urinary System 0TS
Ureteroplasty
  see Repair, Urinary System 0TQ
  see Replacement, Urinary System 0TR
  see Supplement, Urinary System 0TU
Ureteroplication *see* Restriction, Urinary System 0TV
Ureteropyelography *see* Fluoroscopy, Urinary System BT1
Ureterorrhaphy *see* Repair, Urinary System 0TQ
Ureteroscopy 0TJ98ZZ
Ureterostomy
  see Bypass, Urinary System 0T1
  see Drainage, Urinary System 0T9
Ureterotomy *see* Drainage, Urinary System 0T9

Ureteroureterostomy see Bypass, Urinary System ØT1
Ureterovesical orifice
   use Ureter
   use Ureter, Left
   use Ureter, Right
   use Ureters, Bilateral
Urethral catheterization, indwelling ØT9B7ØZ
Urethrectomy
   see Excision, Urethra ØTBD
   see Resection, Urethra ØTTD
Urethrolithotomy see Extirpation, Urethra ØTCD
Urethrolysis see Release, Urethra ØTND
Urethropexy
   see Repair, Urethra ØTQD
   see Reposition, Urethra ØTSD
Urethroplasty
   see Repair, Urethra ØTQD
   see Replacement, Urethra ØTRD
   see Supplement, Urethra ØTUD
Urethrorrhaphy see Repair, Urethra ØTQD
Urethroscopy ØTJD8ZZ
Urethrotomy see Drainage, Urethra ØT9D
Uridine Triacetate XWØDX82
Urinary incontinence stimulator lead use Stimulator
   Lead in Urinary System
Urography see Fluoroscopy, Urinary System BT1
Ustekinumab use Other New Technology Therapeutic
   Substance
Uterine Artery
   use Internal Iliac Artery, Left
   use Internal Iliac Artery, Right
Uterine artery embolization (UAE) see Occlusion,
   Lower Arteries Ø4L
Uterine cornu use Uterus
Uterine tube
   use Fallopian Tube, Left
   use Fallopian Tube, Right
Uterine vein
   use Hypogastric Vein, Left
   use Hypogastric Vein, Right
Uvulectomy
   see Excision, Uvula ØCBN
   see Resection, Uvula ØCTN
Uvulorrhaphy see Repair, Uvula ØCQN
Uvulotomy see Drainage, Uvula ØC9N

V

Vabomere™ use Meropenem-vaborbactam Anti-infective
Vaccination see Introduction of Serum, Toxoid, and
   Vaccine
Vacuum extraction, obstetric 1ØDØ7Z6
Vaginal artery
   use Internal Iliac Artery, Left
   use Internal Iliac Artery, Right
Vaginal pessary use Intraluminal Device, Pessary in
   Female Reproductive System
Vaginal vein
   use Hypogastric Vein, Left
   use Hypogastric Vein, Right
Vaginectomy
   see Excision, Vagina ØUBG
   see Resection, Vagina ØUTG
Vaginofixation
   see Repair, Vagina ØUQG
   see Reposition, Vagina ØUSG
Vaginoplasty
   see Repair, Vagina ØUQG
   see Supplement, Vagina ØUUG
Vaginorrhaphy see Repair, Vagina ØUQG
Vaginoscopy ØUJH8ZZ
Vaginotomy see Drainage, Female Reproductive System ØU9
Vagotomy see Division, Nerve, Vagus ØØ8Q
Valiant Thoracic Stent Graft use Intraluminal Device
Valvotomy, valvulotomy
   see Division, Heart and Great Vessels Ø28
   see Release, Heart and Great Vessels Ø2N
Valvuloplasty
   see Repair, Heart and Great Vessels Ø2Q
   see Replacement, Heart and Great Vessels Ø2R
   see Supplement, Heart and Great Vessels Ø2U
Valvuloplasty, Alfieri Stitch see Restriction, Valve,
   Mitral Ø2VG

Vascular Access Device
  Totally Implantable
    Insertion of device in
      Abdomen ØJH8
      Chest ØJH6
      Lower Arm
        Left ØJHH
        Right ØJHG
      Lower Leg
        Left ØJHP
        Right ØJHN
      Upper Arm
        Left ØJHF
        Right ØJHD
      Upper Leg
        Left ØJHM
        Right ØJHL
    Removal of device from
      Lower Extremity ØJPW
      Trunk ØJPT
      Upper Extremity ØJPV
    Revision of device in
      Lower Extremity ØJWW
      Trunk ØJWT
      Upper Extremity ØJWV
  Tunneled
    Insertion of device in
      Abdomen ØJH8
      Chest ØJH6
      Lower Arm
        Left ØJHH
        Right ØJHG
      Lower Leg
        Left ØJHP
        Right ØJHN
      Upper Arm
        Left ØJHF
        Right ØJHD
      Upper Leg
        Left ØJHM
        Right ØJHL
    Removal of device from
      Lower Extremity ØJPW
      Trunk ØJPT
      Upper Extremity ØJPV
    Revision of device in
      Lower Extremity ØJWW
      Trunk ØJWT
      Upper Extremity ØJWV
Vasectomy see Excision, Male Reproductive System ØVB
Vasography
   see Fluoroscopy, Male Reproductive System BV1
   see Plain Radiography, Male Reproductive System BVØ
Vasoligation see Occlusion, Male Reproductive System ØVL
Vasorrhaphy see Repair, Male Reproductive System ØVQ
Vasostomy see Bypass, Male Reproductive System ØV1
Vasotomy
   Drainage see Drainage, Male Reproductive System ØV9
   With ligation see Occlusion, Male Reproductive System ØVL
Vasovasostomy see Repair, Male Reproductive System ØVQ
Vastus intermedius muscle
   use Upper Leg Muscle, Left
   use Upper Leg Muscle, Right
Vastus lateralis muscle
   use Upper Leg Muscle, Left
   use Upper Leg Muscle, Right
Vastus medialis muscle
   use Upper Leg Muscle, Left
   use Upper Leg Muscle, Right
VCG (vectorcardiogram) see Measurement, Cardiac 4AØ2
Vectra® Vascular Access Graft use Vascular Access
   Device, Tunneled in Subcutaneous Tissue and
   Fascia
Venclexta® use Venetoclax Antineoplastic
Venectomy
   see Excision, Lower Veins Ø6B
   see Excision, Upper Veins Ø5B
Venetoclax Antineoplastic XWØDXR5
Venography
   see Fluoroscopy, Veins B51

Venography — continued
   see Plain Radiography, Veins B5Ø
Venorrhaphy
   see Repair, Lower Veins Ø6Q
   see Repair, Upper Veins Ø5Q
Venotripsy
   see Occlusion, Lower Veins Ø6L
   see Occlusion, Upper Veins Ø5L
Ventricular fold use Larynx
Ventriculoatriostomy see Bypass, Central Nervous
   System and Cranial Nerves ØØ1
Ventriculocisternostomy see Bypass, Central Nervous
   System and Cranial Nerves ØØ1
Ventriculogram, cardiac
   Combined left and right heart see Fluoroscopy,
     Heart, Right and Left B216
   Left ventricle see Fluoroscopy, Heart, Left B215
   Right ventricle see Fluoroscopy, Heart, Right B214
**Ventriculopuncture, through previously implanted
   catheter** 8CØ1X6J
Ventriculoscopy ØØJØ4ZZ
Ventriculostomy
   External drainage see Drainage, Cerebral Ventricle ØØ96
   Internal shunt see Bypass, Cerebral Ventricle ØØ16
Ventriculovenostomy see Bypass, Cerebral Ventricle ØØ16
Ventrio™ Hernia Patch use Synthetic Substitute
VEP (visual evoked potential) 4AØ7XØZ
Vermiform appendix use Appendix
Vermilion border
   use Lower Lip
   use Upper Lip
Versa use Pacemaker, Dual Chamber in ØJH
Version, obstetric
   External 1ØSØXZZ
   Internal 1ØSØ7ZZ
Vertebral arch
   use Cervical Vertebra
   use Lumbar Vertebra
   use Thoracic Vertebra
Vertebral body
   use Cervical Vertebra
   use Lumbar Vertebra
   use Thoracic Vertebra
Vertebral canal use Spinal Canal
Vertebral foramen
   use Cervical Vertebra
   use Lumbar Vertebra
   use Thoracic Vertebra
Vertebral lamina
   use Cervical Vertebra
   use Lumbar Vertebra
   use Thoracic Vertebra
Vertebral pedicle
   use Cervical Vertebra
   use Lumbar Vertebra
   use Thoracic Vertebra
Vesical vein
   use Hypogastric Vein, Left
   use Hypogastric Vein, Right
Vesicotomy see Drainage, Urinary System ØT9
Vesiculectomy
   see Excision, Male Reproductive System ØVB
   see Resection, Male Reproductive System ØVT
Vesiculogram, seminal see Plain Radiography, Male
   Reproductive System BVØ
Vesiculotomy see Drainage, Male Reproductive System ØV9
Vestibular Assessment F15Z
Vestibular (Scarpa's) ganglion use Acoustic Nerve
Vestibular nerve use Acoustic Nerve
Vestibular Treatment FØC
Vestibulocochlear nerve use Acoustic Nerve
**VH-IVUS (virtual histology intravascular ultra-
   sound)** see Ultrasonography, Heart B24
Virchow's (supraclavicular) lymph node
   use Lymphatic, Left Neck
   use Lymphatic, Right Neck
Virtuoso (II) (DR) (VR) use Defibrillator Generator in ØJH
Vistogard(R) use Uridine Triacetate
Vitrectomy
   see Excision, Eye Ø8B
   see Resection, Eye Ø8T

Vitreous body
  use Vitreous, Left
  use Vitreous, Right
Viva (XT) (S) *use* Cardiac Resynchronization Defibrillator
    Pulse Generator in ØJH
Vocal fold
  use Vocal Cord, Left
  use Vocal Cord, Right
Vocational
  Assessment *see* Activities of Daily Living Assess-
    ment, Rehabilitation FØ2
  Retraining *see* Activities of Daily Living Treatment,
    Rehabilitation FØ8
Volar (palmar) digital vein
  use Hand Vein, Left
  use Hand Vein, Right
Volar (palmar) metacarpal vein
  use Hand Vein, Left
  use Hand Vein, Right
Vomer bone *use* Nasal Septum
Vomer of nasal septum *use* Nasal Bone
Voraxaze *use* Glucarpidase
Vulvectomy
  see Excision, Female Reproductive System ØUB
  see Resection, Female Reproductive System ØUT
V-Wave Interatrial Shunt System *use* Synthetic
    Substitute
VYXEOS™ *use* Cytarabine and Daunorubicin Liposome
    Antineoplastic

W

WALLSTENT® Endoprosthesis *use* Intraluminal Device
Washing *see* Irrigation
WavelinQ EndoAVF system
  Radial Artery, Left Ø31C3ZF
  Radial Artery, Right Ø31B3ZF
  Ulnar Artery, Left Ø31A3ZF

WavelinQ EndoAVF system — *continued*
  Ulnar Artery, Right Ø3193ZF
Wedge resection, pulmonary *see* Excision, Respiratory
    System ØBB
Whole Blood Nucleic Acid-base Microbial Detection
    XXE5XM5
Window *see* Drainage
Wiring, dental 2W31X9Z

X

Xact Carotid Stent System *use* Intraluminal Device
XENLETA™ *use* Lefamulin Anti-infective
Xenograft *use* Zooplastic Tissue in Heart and Great
    Vessels
XIENCE Everolimus Eluting Coronary Stent System
  use Intraluminal Device, Drug-eluting in Heart
    and Great Vessels
Xiphoid process *use* Sternum
XLIF® System *use* Interbody Fusion Device in Lower
    Joints
XOSPATA® *use* Gilteritinib Antineoplastic
X-ray *see* Plain Radiography
X-STOP® Spacer
  use Spinal Stabilization Device, Interspinous Pro-
    cess in ØRH
  use Spinal Stabilization Device, Interspinous Pro-
    cess in ØSH

Y

Yoga Therapy 8EØZXY4

Z

Z-plasty, skin for scar contracture *see* Release, Skin
    and Breast ØHN

Zenith AAA Endovascular Graft *use* Intraluminal
    Device
Zenith® Fenestrated AAA Endovascular Graft
  use Intraluminal Device, Branched or Fenestrated,
    One or Two Arteries in Ø4V
  use Intraluminal Device, Branched or Fenestrated,
    Three or More Arteries in Ø4V
Zenith Flex® AAA Endovascular Graft *use* Intralumi-
    nal Device
Zenith® Renu™ AAA Ancillary Graft *use* Intraluminal
    Device
Zenith TX2® TAA Endovascular Graft *use* Intraluminal
    Device
ZERBAXA® *use* Ceftolozane/Tazobactam Anti-infective
**Zilver® PTX® (paclitaxel) Drug-Eluting Peripheral
    Stent**
  use Intraluminal Device, Drug-eluting in Lower
    Arteries
  use Intraluminal Device, Drug-eluting in Upper
    Arteries
Zimmer® NexGen® LPS Mobile Bearing Knee *use*
    Synthetic Substitute
Zimmer® NexGen® LPS-Flex Mobile Knee *use* Syn-
    thetic Substitute
ZINPLAVA™ use Bezlotoxumab Monoclonal Antibody
Zonule of Zinn
  use Lens, Left
  use Lens, Right
**Zooplastic Tissue, Rapid Deployment Technique,
    Replacement** X2RF
Zotarolimus-eluting Coronary Stent *use* Intraluminal
    Device, Drug-eluting in Heart and Great Vessels
ZULRESSO™ use Brexanolone
Zygomatic process of frontal bone *use* Frontal Bone
Zygomatic process of temporal bone
  use Temporal Bone, Left
  use Temporal Bone, Right
Zygomaticus muscle *use* Facial Muscle
Zyvox *use* Oxazolidinones

ICD-10-PCS Tables

Central Nervous System and Cranial Nerves 001–00X

Character Meanings

This Character Meaning table is provided as a guide to assist the user in the identification of character members that may be found in this section of code tables. It **SHOULD NOT** be used to build a PCS code.

Operation–Character 3	Body Part–Character 4	Approach–Character 5	Device–Character 6	Qualifier–Character 7
1 Bypass	0 Brain	0 Open	0 Drainage Device	0 Nasopharynx
2 Change	1 Cerebral Meninges	3 Percutaneous	1 Radioactive Element	1 Mastoid Sinus
5 Destruction	2 Dura Mater	4 Percutaneous Endoscopic	2 Monitoring Device	2 Atrium
7 Dilation	3 Epidural Space, Intracranial	X External	3 Infusion Device	3 Blood Vessel
8 Division	4 Subdural Space, Intracranial		4 Radioactive Element, Cesium-131 Collagen Implant	4 Pleural Cavity
9 Drainage	5 Subarachnoid Space, Intracranial		7 Autologous Tissue Substitute	5 Intestine
B Excision	6 Cerebral Ventricle		J Synthetic Substitute	6 Peritoneal Cavity
C Extirpation	7 Cerebral Hemisphere		K Nonautologous Tissue Substitute	7 Urinary Tract
D Extraction	8 Basal Ganglia		M Neurostimulator Lead	8 Bone Marrow
F Fragmentation	9 Thalamus		Y Other Device	9 Fallopian Tube
H Insertion	A Hypothalamus		Z No Device	A Subgaleal Space
J Inspection	B Pons			B Cerebral Cisterns
K Map	C Cerebellum			F Olfactory Nerve
N Release	D Medulla Oblongata			G Optic Nerve
P Removal	E Cranial Nerve			H Oculomotor Nerve
Q Repair	F Olfactory Nerve			J Trochlear Nerve
R Replacement	G Optic Nerve			K Trigeminal Nerve
S Reposition	H Oculomotor Nerve			L Abducens Nerve
T Resection	J Trochlear Nerve			M Facial Nerve
U Supplement	K Trigeminal Nerve			N Acoustic Nerve
W Revision	L Abducens Nerve			P Glossopharyngeal Nerve
X Transfer	M Facial Nerve			Q Vagus Nerve
	N Acoustic Nerve			R Accessory Nerve
	P Glossopharyngeal Nerve			S Hypoglossal Nerve
	Q Vagus Nerve			X Diagnostic
	R Accessory Nerve			Z No Qualifier
	S Hypoglossal Nerve			
	T Spinal Meninges			
	U Spinal Canal			
	V Spinal Cord			
	W Cervical Spinal Cord			
	X Thoracic Spinal Cord			
	Y Lumbar Spinal Cord			

AHA Coding Clinic for table 001

2019, 4Q, 21-22	Cerebral ventricle bypass Qualifier
2018, 4Q, 86	Placement of lumboatrial shunt
2017, 4Q, 39-41	Dilation and bypass of cerebral ventricle
2015, 2Q, 9	Revision of ventriculoperitoneal (VP) shunt
2013, 2Q, 36	Insertion of ventriculoperitoneal shunt with laparoscopic assistance

AHA Coding Clinic for table 007

2017, 4Q, 39-41	Dilation and bypass of cerebral ventricle

AHA Coding Clinic for table 009

2018, 4Q, 85	Externalization of lumboatrial shunt
2017, 1Q, 50	Failed lumbar puncture
2015, 3Q, 10	Open evacuation of subdural hematoma
2015, 3Q, 11	Percutaneous drainage of subdural hematoma
2015, 3Q, 12	Subdural evacuation portal system (SEPS) placement
2015, 3Q, 12	Placement of ventriculostomy catheter via burr hole
2015, 2Q, 30	Drainage of syrinx
2015, 1Q, 31	Intrathecal chemotherapy
2014, 1Q, 8	Diagnostic lumbar tap
2014, 1Q, 8	Lumbar drainage port aspiration

AHA Coding Clinic for table 00B

2017, 3Q, 17	Resection of schwannoma and placement of DuraGen and Lorenz cranial plating system
2016, 2Q, 12	Resection of malignant neoplasm of infratemporal fossa
2016, 2Q, 18	Amygdalohippocampectomy
2014, 4Q, 34	Resection of brain malignancy with implantation of chemotherapeutic wafer
2014, 3Q, 24	Repair of lipomyelomeningocele and tethered cord

AHA Coding Clinic for table 00C

2019, 3Q, 4	Evacuation of subdural hematoma and control of bleeding artery
2019, 2Q, 36	Evacuation of hematoma using NICO Brainpath® technology
2017, 4Q, 48	New and revised body part values - Extirpation spinal canal
2016, 2Q, 29	Decompressive craniectomy with cryopreservation and storage of bone flap
2015, 3Q, 10	Open evacuation of subdural hematoma
2015, 3Q, 11	Percutaneous drainage of subdural hematoma
2015, 3Q, 13	Evacuation of intracerebral hematoma

AHA Coding Clinic for table 00D

2015, 3Q, 13	Nonexcisional debridement of cranial wound with removal and replacement of hardware

AHA Coding Clinic for table 00H

2020, 2Q, 15	Ommaya Reservoir with Ventricular Catheter Placement
2020, 2Q, 16	Ommaya Reservoir Placement for Cerebrospinal Fluid Infusion Therapy
2017, 4Q, 30-31	Radiotherapeutic brain implant
2017, 3Q, 13	Implantation of bilateral neurostimulator electrodes
2014, 3Q, 19	End of life replacement of Baclofen pump

AHA Coding Clinic for table 00J

2019, 2Q, 36	Evacuation of hematoma using NICO Brainpath® technology
2017, 1Q, 50	Failed lumbar puncture

AHA Coding Clinic for table 00N

2019, 2Q, 19	Cervical spinal fusion, decompression and placement of interfacet stabilization device
2019, 1Q, 28	Decompressive laminectomy of both spinal cord and nerve roots
2018, 3Q, 30	Decompressive laminectomy (release of spinal cord versus release of spinal meninges)
2017, 3Q, 10	Repair of Chiari malformation
2017, 2Q, 23	Decompression of spinal cord and placement of instrumentation
2016, 2Q, 29	Decompressive craniectomy with cryopreservation and storage of bone flap
2015, 2Q, 20	Cervical laminoplasty
2015, 2Q, 21	Multiple decompressive cervical laminectomies
2015, 2Q, 34	Decompressive laminectomy
2014, 3Q, 24	Repair of lipomyelomeningocele and tethered cord

AHA Coding Clinic for table 00P

2014, 3Q, 19	End of life replacement of Baclofen pump

AHA Coding Clinic for table 00Q

2014, 3Q, 7	Hemi-cranioplasty for repair of cranial defect
2013, 3Q, 25	Fracture of frontal bone with repair and coagulation for hemostasis

AHA Coding Clinic for table 00S

2014, 4Q, 35	Reimplantation of buccal nerve

AHA Coding Clinic for table 00U

2018, 1Q, 9	Craniectomy with DuraGaurd placement
2017, 4Q, 62	Added and revised device values - Nerve substitutes
2017, 3Q, 10	Repair of Chiari malformation
2017, 3Q, 17	Resection of schwannoma and placement of DuraGen and Lorenz cranial plating system
2015, 4Q, 39	Dural patch graft
2014, 3Q, 24	Repair of lipomyelomeningocele and tethered cord

AHA Coding Clinic for table 00W

2018, 4Q, 86	Placement of lumboatrial shunt

Brain

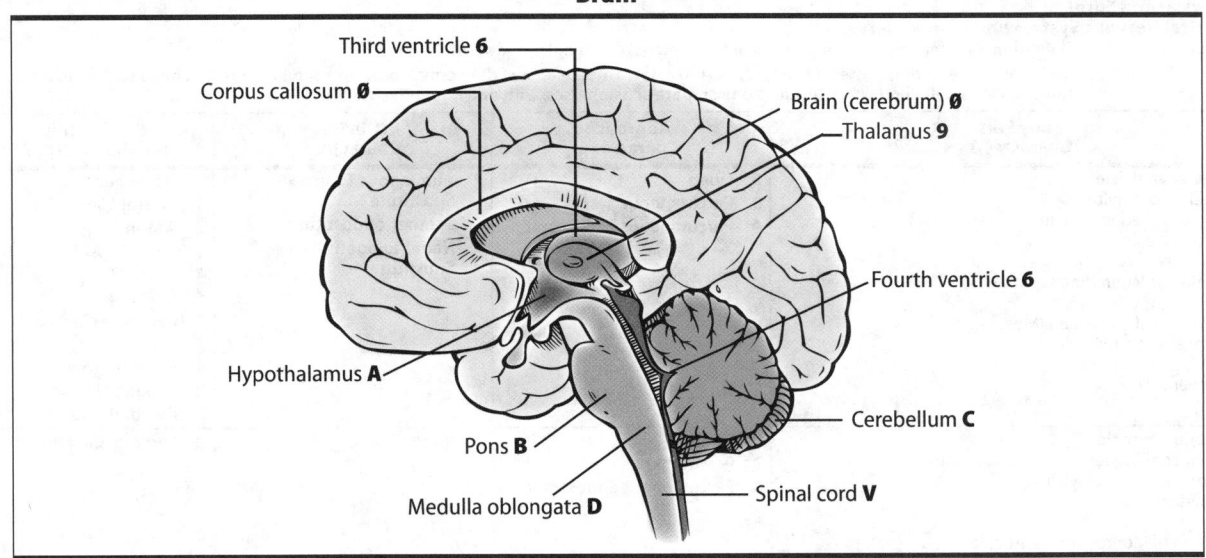

Third ventricle **6**

Corpus callosum **Ø**

Brain (cerebrum) **Ø**

Thalamus **9**

Fourth ventricle **6**

Hypothalamus **A**

Cerebellum **C**

Pons **B**

Spinal cord **V**

Medulla oblongata **D**

Cranial Nerves

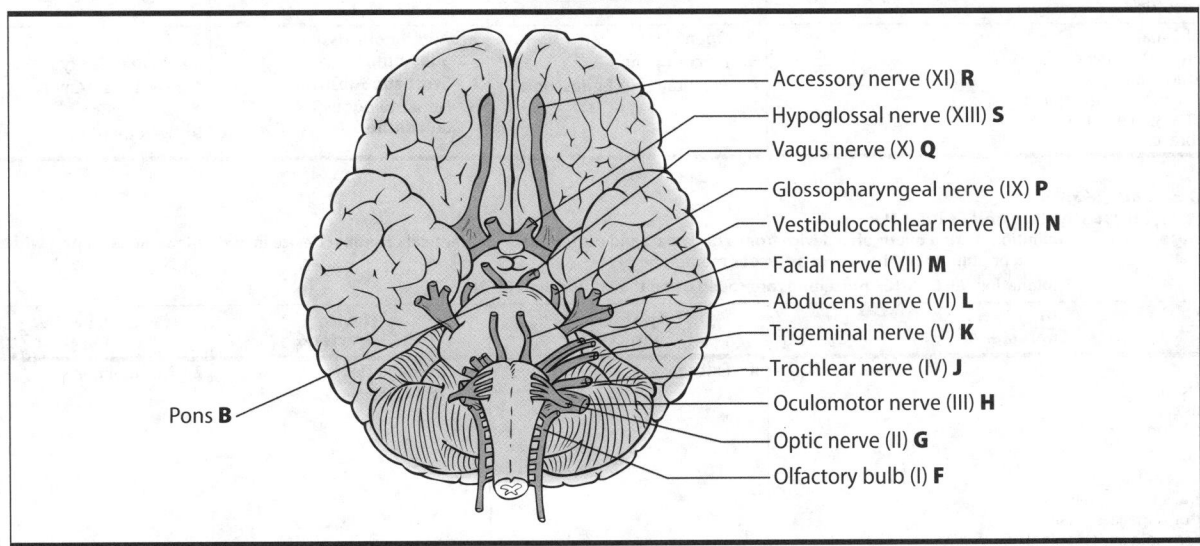

Accessory nerve (XI) **R**

Hypoglossal nerve (XIII) **S**

Vagus nerve (X) **Q**

Glossopharyngeal nerve (IX) **P**

Vestibulocochlear nerve (VIII) **N**

Facial nerve (VII) **M**

Abducens nerve (VI) **L**

Trigeminal nerve (V) **K**

Trochlear nerve (IV) **J**

Oculomotor nerve (III) **H**

Optic nerve (II) **G**

Olfactory bulb (I) **F**

Pons **B**

Ø   **Medical and Surgical**
Ø   **Central Nervous System and Cranial Nerves**
1   **Bypass**   Definition: Altering the route of passage of the contents of a tubular body part

            Explanation: Rerouting contents of a body part to a downstream area of the normal route, to a similar route and body part, or to an abnormal route and dissimilar body part. Includes one or more anastomoses, with or without the use of a device.

Body Part Character 4	Approach Character 5	Device Character 6	Qualifier Character 7

6 Cerebral Ventricle
Aqueduct of Sylvius
Cerebral aqueduct (Sylvius)
Choroid plexus
Ependyma
Foramen of Monro (intraventricular)
Fourth ventricle
Interventricular foramen (Monro)
Left lateral ventricle
Right lateral ventricle
Third ventricle
	Ø Open
	3 Percutaneous
	4 Percutaneous Endoscopic
		7 Autologous Tissue
		   Substitute
		J Synthetic Substitute
		K Nonautologous Tissue
		   Substitute
			Ø Nasopharynx
			1 Mastoid Sinus
			2 Atrium
			3 Blood Vessel
			4 Pleural Cavity
			5 Intestine
			6 Peritoneal Cavity
			7 Urinary Tract
			8 Bone Marrow
			A Subgaleal Space
			B Cerebral Cisterns

6 Cerebral Ventricle Aqueduct of Sylvius Cerebral aqueduct (Sylvius) Choroid plexus Ependyma Foramen of Monro (intraventricular) Fourth ventricle Interventricular foramen (Monro) Left lateral ventricle Right lateral ventricle Third ventricle	Ø Open 3 Percutaneous 4 Percutaneous Endoscopic	Z No Device	B Cerebral Cisterns

U Spinal Canal
Epidural space, spinal
Extradural space, spinal
Subarachnoid space, spinal
Subdural space, spinal
Vertebral canal
	Ø Open
	3 Percutaneous
	4 Percutaneous Endoscopic
		7 Autologous Tissue
		   Substitute
		J Synthetic Substitute
		K Nonautologous Tissue
		   Substitute
			2 Atrium
			4 Pleural Cavity
			6 Peritoneal Cavity
			7 Urinary Tract
			9 Fallopian Tube

Ø   **Medical and Surgical**
Ø   **Central Nervous System and Cranial Nerves**
2   **Change**   Definition: Taking out or off a device from a body part and putting back an identical or similar device in or on the same body part without cutting or puncturing the skin or a mucous membrane

            Explanation: All CHANGE procedures are coded using the approach EXTERNAL

Body Part Character 4	Approach Character 5	Device Character 6	Qualifier Character 7
Ø Brain Cerebrum Corpus callosum Encephalon **E Cranial Nerve** **U Spinal Canal** Epidural space, spinal Extradural space, spinal Subarachnoid space, spinal Subdural space, spinal Vertebral canal	X External	Ø Drainage Device Y Other Device	Z No Qualifier

Non-OR   All body part, approach, device, and qualifier values

Ø   Medical and Surgical
Ø   Central Nervous System and Cranial Nerves
5   Destruction   Definition: Physical eradication of all or a portion of a body part by the direct use of energy, force, or a destructive agent
                        Explanation: None of the body part is physically taken out

Body Part Character 4		Approach Character 5	Device Character 6	Qualifier Character 7

Ø Brain
Cerebrum
Corpus callosum
Encephalon
1 Cerebral Meninges
Arachnoid mater,
   intracranial
Leptomeninges,
   intracranial
Pia mater, intracranial
2 Dura Mater
Diaphragma sellae
Dura mater, intracranial
Falx cerebri
Tentorium cerebelli
6 Cerebral Ventricle
Aqueduct of Sylvius
Cerebral aqueduct (Sylvius)
Choroid plexus
Ependyma
Foramen of Monro
   (intraventricular)
Fourth ventricle
Interventricular foramen
   (Monro)
Left lateral ventricle
Right lateral ventricle
Third ventricle
7 Cerebral Hemisphere
Frontal lobe
Occipital lobe
Parietal lobe
Temporal lobe
8 Basal Ganglia
Basal nuclei
Claustrum
Corpus striatum
Globus pallidus
Substantia nigra
Subthalamic nucleus
9 Thalamus
Epithalamus
Geniculate nucleus
Metathalamus
Pulvinar
A Hypothalamus
Mammillary body
B Pons
Apneustic center
Basis pontis
Locus ceruleus
Pneumotaxic center
Pontine tegmentum
Superior olivary nucleus
C Cerebellum
Culmen
D Medulla Oblongata
Myelencephalon
F Olfactory Nerve
First cranial nerve
Olfactory bulb
G Optic Nerve
Optic chiasma
Second cranial nerve
	H Oculomotor Nerve
	Third cranial nerve
	J Trochlear Nerve
	Fourth cranial nerve
	K Trigeminal Nerve
	Fifth cranial nerve
	Gasserian ganglion
	Mandibular nerve
	Maxillary nerve
	Ophthalmic nerve
	Trifacial nerve
	L Abducens Nerve
	Sixth cranial nerve
	M Facial Nerve
	Chorda tympani
	Geniculate ganglion
	Greater superficial petrosal
	   nerve
	Nerve to the stapedius
	Parotid plexus
	Posterior auricular nerve
	Seventh cranial nerve
	Submandibular ganglion
	N Acoustic Nerve
	Cochlear nerve
	Eighth cranial nerve
	Scarpa's (vestibular)
	   ganglion
	Spiral ganglion
	Vestibular (Scarpa's)
	   ganglion
	Vestibular nerve
	Vestibulocochlear nerve
	P Glossopharyngeal Nerve
	Carotid sinus nerve
	Ninth cranial nerve
	Tympanic nerve
	Q Vagus Nerve
	Anterior vagal trunk
	Pharyngeal plexus
	Pneumogastric nerve
	Posterior vagal trunk
	Pulmonary plexus
	Recurrent laryngeal nerve
	Superior laryngeal nerve
	Tenth cranial nerve
	R Accessory Nerve
	Eleventh cranial nerve
	S Hypoglossal Nerve
	Twelfth cranial nerve
	T Spinal Meninges
	Arachnoid mater, spinal
	Denticulate (dentate)
	   ligament
	Dura mater, spinal
	Filum terminale
	Leptomeninges, spinal
	Pia mater, spinal
	W Cervical Spinal Cord
	X Thoracic Spinal Cord
	Y Lumbar Spinal Cord
	Cauda equina
	Conus medullaris
		Ø Open
		3 Percutaneous
		4 Percutaneous Endoscopic
			Z No Device	**Z No Qualifier**

Non-OR   ØØ5[F,G,H,J,K,L,M,N,P,Q,R,S][Ø,3,4]ZZ

LC Limited Coverage   NC Noncoverage   ⊞ Combination Member   HAC associated procedure   Combination Only   DRG Non-OR   Non-OR   New/Revised in GREEN

ICD-10-PCS 2021   135

Ø   **Medical and Surgical**
Ø   **Central Nervous System and Cranial Nerves**
7   **Dilation**   Definition: Expanding an orifice or the lumen of a tubular body part

Explanation: The orifice can be a natural orifice or an artificially created orifice. Accomplished by stretching a tubular body part using intraluminal pressure or by cutting part of the orifice or wall of the tubular body part.

Body Part Character 4	Approach Character 5	Device Character 6	Qualifier Character 7
6 **Cerebral Ventricle** Aqueduct of Sylvius Cerebral aqueduct (Sylvius) Choroid plexus Ependyma Foramen of Monro (intraventricular) Fourth ventricle Interventricular foramen (Monro) Left lateral ventricle Right lateral ventricle Third ventricle	**Ø** Open **3** Percutaneous **4** Percutaneous Endoscopic	**Z** No Device	**Z** No Qualifier

Ø   **Medical and Surgical**
Ø   **Central Nervous System and Cranial Nerves**
8   **Division**   Definition: Cutting into a body part, without draining fluids and/or gases from the body part, in order to separate or transect a body part

Explanation: All or a portion of the body part is separated into two or more portions

Body Part Character 4	Approach Character 5	Device Character 6	Qualifier Character 7
Ø **Brain** Cerebrum Corpus callosum Encephalon **7** **Cerebral Hemisphere** Frontal lobe Occipital lobe Parietal lobe Temporal lobe **8** **Basal Ganglia** Basal nuclei Claustrum Corpus striatum Globus pallidus Substantia nigra Subthalamic nucleus **F** **Olfactory Nerve** First cranial nerve Olfactory bulb **G** **Optic Nerve** Optic chiasma Second cranial nerve **H** **Oculomotor Nerve** Third cranial nerve **J** **Trochlear Nerve** Fourth cranial nerve **K** **Trigeminal Nerve** Fifth cranial nerve Gasserian ganglion Mandibular nerve Maxillary nerve Ophthalmic nerve Trifacial nerve **L** **Abducens Nerve** Sixth cranial nerve **M** **Facial Nerve** Chorda tympani Geniculate ganglion Greater superficial petrosal nerve Nerve to the stapedius Parotid plexus Posterior auricular nerve Seventh cranial nerve Submandibular ganglion **N** **Acoustic Nerve** Cochlear nerve Eighth cranial nerve Scarpa's (vestibular) ganglion Spiral ganglion Vestibular (Scarpa's) ganglion Vestibular nerve Vestibulocochlear nerve **P** **Glossopharyngeal Nerve** Carotid sinus nerve Ninth cranial nerve Tympanic nerve **Q** **Vagus Nerve** Anterior vagal trunk Pharyngeal plexus Pneumogastric nerve Posterior vagal trunk Pulmonary plexus Recurrent laryngeal nerve Superior laryngeal nerve Tenth cranial nerve **R** **Accessory Nerve** Eleventh cranial nerve **S** **Hypoglossal Nerve** Twelfth cranial nerve **W** **Cervical Spinal Cord** **X** **Thoracic Spinal Cord** **Y** **Lumbar Spinal Cord** Cauda equina Conus medullaris	**Ø** Open **3** Percutaneous **4** Percutaneous Endoscopic	**Z** No Device	**Z** No Qualifier

LC Limited Coverage   **NC** Noncovered   ⊞ Combination Member   HAC associated procedure   Combination Only   DRG Non-OR   Non-OR   New/Revised in **GREEN**

136   ICD-10-PCS 2021

Ø   **Medical and Surgical**
Ø   **Central Nervous System and Cranial Nerves**
9   **Drainage**   Definition: Taking or letting out fluids and/or gases from a body part
                  Explanation: The qualifier DIAGNOSTIC is used to identify drainage procedures that are biopsies

Body Part Character 4		Approach Character 5	Device Character 6	Qualifier Character 7

Ø Brain
Cerebrum
Corpus callosum
Encephalon
1 Cerebral Meninges
Arachnoid mater,
  intracranial
Leptomeninges,
  intracranial
Pia mater, intracranial
2 Dura Mater
Diaphragma sellae
Dura mater, intracranial
Falx cerebri
Tentorium cerebelli
3 Epidural Space,
  Intracranial
Extradural space,
  intracranial
4 Subdural Space,
  Intracranial
5 Subarachnoid Space,
  Intracranial
6 Cerebral Ventricle
Aqueduct of Sylvius
Cerebral aqueduct (Sylvius)
Choroid plexus
Ependyma
Foramen of Monro
  (intraventricular)
Fourth ventricle
Interventricular foramen
  (Monro)
Left lateral ventricle
Right lateral ventricle
Third ventricle
7 Cerebral Hemisphere
Frontal lobe
Occipital lobe
Parietal lobe
Temporal lobe
8 Basal Ganglia
Basal nuclei
Claustrum
Corpus striatum
Globus pallidus
Substantia nigra
Subthalamic nucleus
9 Thalamus
Epithalamus
Geniculate nucleus
Metathalamus
Pulvinar
A Hypothalamus
Mammillary body
B Pons
Apneustic center
Basis pontis
Locus ceruleus
Pneumotaxic center
Pontine tegmentum
Superior olivary nucleus
C Cerebellum
Culmen
D Medulla Oblongata
Myelencephalon
F Olfactory Nerve
First cranial nerve
Olfactory bulb
	G Optic Nerve
	Optic chiasma
	Second cranial nerve
	H Oculomotor Nerve
	Third cranial nerve
	J Trochlear Nerve
	Fourth cranial nerve
	K Trigeminal Nerve
	Fifth cranial nerve
	Gasserian ganglion
	Mandibular nerve
	Maxillary nerve
	Ophthalmic nerve
	Trifacial nerve
	L Abducens Nerve
	Sixth cranial nerve
	M Facial Nerve
	Chorda tympani
	Geniculate ganglion
	Greater superficial petrosal
	  nerve
	Nerve to the stapedius
	Parotid plexus
	Posterior auricular nerve
	Seventh cranial nerve
	Submandibular ganglion
	N Acoustic Nerve
	Cochlear nerve
	Eighth cranial nerve
	Scarpa's (vestibular) ganglion
	Spiral ganglion
	Vestibular (Scarpa's) ganglion
	Vestibular nerve
	Vestibulocochlear nerve
	P Glossopharyngeal Nerve
	Carotid sinus nerve
	Ninth cranial nerve
	Tympanic nerve
	Q Vagus Nerve
	Anterior vagal trunk
	Pharyngeal plexus
	Pneumogastric nerve
	Posterior vagal trunk
	Pulmonary plexus
	Recurrent laryngeal nerve
	Superior laryngeal nerve
	Tenth cranial nerve
	R Accessory Nerve
	Eleventh cranial nerve
	S Hypoglossal Nerve
	Twelfth cranial nerve
	T Spinal Meninges
	Arachnoid mater, spinal
	Denticulate (dentate)
	  ligament
	Dura mater, spinal
	Filum terminale
	Leptomeninges, spinal
	Pia mater, spinal
	U Spinal Canal
	Epidural space, spinal
	Extradural space, spinal
	Subarachnoid space, spinal
	Subdural space, spinal
	Vertebral canal
	W Cervical Spinal Cord
	X Thoracic Spinal Cord
	Y Lumbar Spinal Cord
	Cauda equina
	Conus medullaris
		Ø Open
		3 Percutaneous
		4 Percutaneous Endoscopic
			Ø Drainage Device	**Z No Qualifier**

Non-OR	009[T,W,X,Y]30Z
Non-OR	009U[3,4]0Z

009 Continued on next page

0 Medical and Surgical
0 Central Nervous System and Cranial Nerves
9 Drainage

009 Continued

Definition: Taking or letting out fluids and/or gases from a body part
Explanation: The qualifier DIAGNOSTIC is used to identify drainage procedures that are biopsies

Body Part Character 4		Approach Character 5	Device Character 6	Qualifier Character 7
0 Brain Cerebrum Corpus callosum Encephalon	**G Optic Nerve** Optic chiasma Second cranial nerve	**0 Open** **3 Percutaneous** **4 Percutaneous Endoscopic**	**Z No Device**	**X Diagnostic** **Z No Qualifier**
1 Cerebral Meninges Arachnoid mater, intracranial Leptomeninges, intracranial Pia mater, intracranial	**H Oculomotor Nerve** Third cranial nerve **J Trochlear Nerve** Fourth cranial nerve **K Trigeminal Nerve** Fifth cranial nerve Gasserian ganglion			
2 Dura Mater Diaphragma sellae Dura mater, intracranial Falx cerebri Tentorium cerebelli	Mandibular nerve Maxillary nerve Ophthalmic nerve Trifacial nerve			
3 Epidural Space, Intracranial Extradural space, intracranial	**L Abducens Nerve** Sixth cranial nerve **M Facial Nerve** Chorda tympani			
4 Subdural Space, Intracranial	Geniculate ganglion Greater superficial petrosal nerve			
5 Subarachnoid Space, Intracranial	Nerve to the stapedius Parotid plexus			
6 Cerebral Ventricle Aqueduct of Sylvius Cerebral aqueduct (Sylvius) Choroid plexus Ependyma Foramen of Monro (intraventricular) Fourth ventricle Interventricular foramen (Monro) Left lateral ventricle Right lateral ventricle Third ventricle	Posterior auricular nerve Seventh cranial nerve Submandibular ganglion **N Acoustic Nerve** Cochlear nerve Eighth cranial nerve Scarpa's (vestibular) ganglion Spiral ganglion Vestibular (Scarpa's) ganglion Vestibular nerve Vestibulocochlear nerve			
7 Cerebral Hemisphere Frontal lobe Occipital lobe Parietal lobe Temporal lobe	**P Glossopharyngeal Nerve** Carotid sinus nerve Ninth cranial nerve Tympanic nerve **Q Vagus Nerve** Anterior vagal trunk			
8 Basal Ganglia Basal nuclei Claustrum Corpus striatum Globus pallidus Substantia nigra Subthalamic nucleus	Pharyngeal plexus Pneumogastric nerve Posterior vagal trunk Pulmonary plexus Recurrent laryngeal nerve Superior laryngeal nerve Tenth cranial nerve			
9 Thalamus Epithalamus Geniculate nucleus Metathalamus Pulvinar	**R Accessory Nerve** Eleventh cranial nerve **S Hypoglossal Nerve** Twelfth cranial nerve **T Spinal Meninges**			
A Hypothalamus Mammillary body	Arachnoid mater, spinal Denticulate (dentate) ligament			
B Pons Apneustic center Basis pontis Locus ceruleus Pneumotaxic center Pontine tegmentum Superior olivary nucleus	Dura mater, spinal Filum terminale Leptomeninges, spinal Pia mater, spinal **U Spinal Canal** Epidural space, spinal			
C Cerebellum Culmen	Extradural space, spinal Subarachnoid space, spinal Subdural space, spinal			
D Medulla Oblongata Myelencephalon	Vertebral canal **W Cervical Spinal Cord**			
F Olfactory Nerve First cranial nerve Olfactory bulb	**X Thoracic Spinal Cord** **Y Lumbar Spinal Cord** Cauda equina Conus medullaris			

Non-OR   009[0,1,2,3,4,5,6,7,8,9,A,B,C,D,F,G,H,J,K,L,M,N,P,Q,R,S][3,4]ZX
Non-OR   009[T,W,X,Y]3Z[X,Z]
Non-OR   009U[3,4]Z[X,Z]

Ø   **Medical and Surgical**
Ø   **Central Nervous System and Cranial Nerves**
B   **Excision**   Definition: Cutting out or off, without replacement, a portion of a body part
                           Explanation: The qualifier DIAGNOSTIC is used to identify excision procedures that are biopsies

Body Part Character 4		Approach Character 5	Device Character 6	Qualifier Character 7

Ø **Brain**
Cerebrum
Corpus callosum
Encephalon
1 **Cerebral Meninges**
Arachnoid mater,
    intracranial
Leptomeninges,
    intracranial
Pia mater, intracranial
2 **Dura Mater**
Diaphragma sellae
Dura mater, intracranial
Falx cerebri
Tentorium cerebelli
6 **Cerebral Ventricle**
Aqueduct of Sylvius
Cerebral aqueduct (Sylvius)
Choroid plexus
Ependyma
Foramen of Monro
    (intraventricular)
Fourth ventricle
Interventricular foramen
    (Monro)
Left lateral ventricle
Right lateral ventricle
Third ventricle
7 **Cerebral Hemisphere**
Frontal lobe
Occipital lobe
Parietal lobe
Temporal lobe
8 **Basal Ganglia**
Basal nuclei
Claustrum
Corpus striatum
Globus pallidus
Substantia nigra
Subthalamic nucleus
9 **Thalamus**
Epithalamus
Geniculate nucleus
Metathalamus
Pulvinar
A **Hypothalamus**
Mammillary body
B **Pons**
Apneustic center
Basis pontis
Locus ceruleus
Pneumotaxic center
Pontine tegmentum
Superior olivary nucleus
C **Cerebellum**
Culmen
D **Medulla Oblongata**
Myelencephalon
F **Olfactory Nerve**
First cranial nerve
Olfactory bulb
G **Optic Nerve**
Optic chiasma
Second cranial nerve
	H **Oculomotor Nerve**
	Third cranial nerve
	J **Trochlear Nerve**
	Fourth cranial nerve
	K **Trigeminal Nerve**
	Fifth cranial nerve
	Gasserian ganglion
	Mandibular nerve
	Maxillary nerve
	Ophthalmic nerve
	Trifacial nerve
	L **Abducens Nerve**
	Sixth cranial nerve
	M **Facial Nerve**
	Chorda tympani
	Geniculate ganglion
	Greater superficial petrosal
	    nerve
	Nerve to the stapedius
	Parotid plexus
	Posterior auricular nerve
	Seventh cranial nerve
	Submandibular ganglion
	N **Acoustic Nerve**
	Cochlear nerve
	Eighth cranial nerve
	Scarpa's (vestibular)
	    ganglion
	Spiral ganglion
	Vestibular (Scarpa's)
	    ganglion
	Vestibular nerve
	Vestibulocochlear nerve
	P **Glossopharyngeal Nerve**
	Carotid sinus nerve
	Ninth cranial nerve
	Tympanic nerve
	Q **Vagus Nerve**
	Anterior vagal trunk
	Pharyngeal plexus
	Pneumogastric nerve
	Posterior vagal trunk
	Pulmonary plexus
	Recurrent laryngeal nerve
	Superior laryngeal nerve
	Tenth cranial nerve
	R **Accessory Nerve**
	Eleventh cranial nerve
	S **Hypoglossal Nerve**
	Twelfth cranial nerve
	T **Spinal Meninges**
	Arachnoid mater, spinal
	Denticulate (dentate)
	    ligament
	Dura mater, spinal
	Filum terminale
	Leptomeninges, spinal
	Pia mater, spinal
	W **Cervical Spinal Cord**
	X **Thoracic Spinal Cord**
	Y **Lumbar Spinal Cord**
	Cauda equina
	Conus medullaris
		Ø **Open**
		3 **Percutaneous**
		4 **Percutaneous Endoscopic**
			Z **No Device**	X **Diagnostic**
				Z **No Qualifier**

Non-OR   ØØB[F,G,H,J,K,L,M,N,P,Q,R,S][3,4]ZX

Central Nervous System and Cranial Nerves *(left margin)*

0 Medical and Surgical
0 Central Nervous System and Cranial Nerves
C Extirpation
Definition: Taking or cutting out solid matter from a body part
Explanation: The solid matter may be an abnormal byproduct of a biological function or a foreign body; it may be imbedded in a body part or in the lumen of a tubular body part. The solid matter may or may not have been previously broken into pieces.

Body Part Character 4		Approach Character 5	Device Character 6	Qualifier Character 7
0 Brain Cerebrum Corpus callosum Encephalon	**G** Optic Nerve Optic chiasma Second cranial nerve	**0** Open **3** Percutaneous **4** Percutaneous Endoscopic	**Z** No Device	**Z** No Qualifier
1 Cerebral Meninges Arachnoid mater, intracranial Leptomeninges, intracranial Pia mater, intracranial	**H** Oculomotor Nerve Third cranial nerve			
2 Dura Mater Diaphragma sellae Dura mater, intracranial Falx cerebri Tentorium cerebelli	**J** Trochlear Nerve Fourth cranial nerve			
3 Epidural Space, Intracranial Extradural space, intracranial	**K** Trigeminal Nerve Fifth cranial nerve Gasserian ganglion Mandibular nerve Maxillary nerve Ophthalmic nerve Trifacial nerve			
4 Subdural Space, Intracranial	**L** Abducens Nerve Sixth cranial nerve			
5 Subarachnoid Space, Intracranial	**M** Facial Nerve Chorda tympani Geniculate ganglion Greater superficial petrosal nerve Nerve to the stapedius Parotid plexus Posterior auricular nerve Seventh cranial nerve Submandibular ganglion			
6 Cerebral Ventricle Aqueduct of Sylvius Cerebral aqueduct (Sylvius) Choroid plexus Ependyma Foramen of Monro (intraventricular) Fourth ventricle Interventricular foramen (Monro) Left lateral ventricle Right lateral ventricle Third ventricle	**N** Acoustic Nerve Cochlear nerve Eighth cranial nerve Scarpa's (vestibular) ganglion Spiral ganglion Vestibular (Scarpa's) ganglion Vestibular nerve Vestibulocochlear nerve			
7 Cerebral Hemisphere Frontal lobe Occipital lobe Parietal lobe Temporal lobe	**P** Glossopharyngeal Nerve Carotid sinus nerve Ninth cranial nerve Tympanic nerve			
8 Basal Ganglia Basal nuclei Claustrum Corpus striatum Globus pallidus Substantia nigra Subthalamic nucleus	**Q** Vagus Nerve Anterior vagal trunk Pharyngeal plexus Pneumogastric nerve Posterior vagal trunk Pulmonary plexus Recurrent laryngeal nerve Superior laryngeal nerve Tenth cranial nerve			
9 Thalamus Epithalamus Geniculate nucleus Metathalamus Pulvinar	**R** Accessory Nerve Eleventh cranial nerve			
A Hypothalamus Mammillary body	**S** Hypoglossal Nerve Twelfth cranial nerve			
B Pons Apneustic center Basis pontis Locus ceruleus Pneumotaxic center Pontine tegmentum Superior olivary nucleus	**T** Spinal Meninges Arachnoid mater, spinal Denticulate (dentate) ligament Dura mater, spinal Filum terminale Leptomeninges, spinal Pia mater, spinal			
C Cerebellum Culmen	**U** Spinal Canal			
D Medulla Oblongata Myelencephalon	**W** Cervical Spinal Cord **X** Thoracic Spinal Cord **Y** Lumbar Spinal Cord Cauda equina Conus medullaris			
F Olfactory Nerve First cranial nerve Olfactory bulb				

Ø Medical and Surgical
Ø Central Nervous System and Cranial Nerves
D Extraction   Definition: Pulling or stripping out or off all or a portion of a body part by the use of force
        Explanation: The qualifier DIAGNOSTIC is used to identify extraction procedures that are biopsies

Body Part — Character 4	Approach — Character 5	Device — Character 6	Qualifier — Character 7
1 Cerebral Meninges Arachnoid mater, intracranial Leptomeninges, intracranial Pia mater, intracranial **2 Dura Mater** Diaphragma sellae Dura mater, intracranial Falx cerebri Tentorium cerebelli **F Olfactory Nerve** First cranial nerve Olfactory bulb **G Optic Nerve** Optic chiasma Second cranial nerve **H Oculomotor Nerve** Third cranial nerve **J Trochlear Nerve** Fourth cranial nerve **K Trigeminal Nerve** Fifth cranial nerve Gasserian ganglion Mandibular nerve Maxillary nerve Ophthalmic nerve Trifacial nerve **L Abducens Nerve** Sixth cranial nerve **M Facial Nerve** Chorda tympani Geniculate ganglion Greater superficial petrosal nerve Nerve to the stapedius Parotid plexus Posterior auricular nerve Seventh cranial nerve Submandibular ganglion **N Acoustic Nerve** Cochlear nerve Eighth cranial nerve Scarpa's (vestibular) ganglion Spiral ganglion Vestibular (Scarpa's) ganglion Vestibular nerve Vestibulocochlear nerve **P Glossopharyngeal Nerve** Carotid sinus nerve Ninth cranial nerve Tympanic nerve **Q Vagus Nerve** Anterior vagal trunk Pharyngeal plexus Pneumogastric nerve Posterior vagal trunk Pulmonary plexus Recurrent laryngeal nerve Superior laryngeal nerve Tenth cranial nerve **R Accessory Nerve** Eleventh cranial nerve **S Hypoglossal Nerve** Twelfth cranial nerve **T Spinal Meninges** Arachnoid mater, spinal Denticulate (dentate) ligament Dura mater, spinal Filum terminale Leptomeninges, spinal Pia mater, spinal	**Ø** Open **3** Percutaneous **4** Percutaneous Endoscopic	**Z** No Device	**Z** No Qualifier

Ø Medical and Surgical
Ø Central Nervous System and Cranial Nerves
F Fragmentation   Definition: Breaking solid matter in a body part into pieces
        Explanation: Physical force (e.g., manual, ultrasonic) applied directly or indirectly is used to break the solid matter into pieces. The solid matter may be an abnormal byproduct of a biological function or a foreign body. The pieces of solid matter are not taken out.

Body Part — Character 4	Approach — Character 5	Device — Character 6	Qualifier — Character 7
3 Epidural Space, Intracranial `NC` Extradural space, intracranial **4 Subdural Space, Intracranial** `NC` **5 Subarachnoid Space, Intracranial** `NC` **6 Cerebral Ventricle** `NC` Aqueduct of Sylvius Cerebral aqueduct (Sylvius) Choroid plexus Ependyma Foramen of Monro (intraventricular) Fourth ventricle Interventricular foramen (Monro) Left lateral ventricle Right lateral ventricle Third ventricle **U Spinal Canal** Epidural space, spinal Extradural space, spinal Subarachnoid space, spinal Subdural space, spinal Vertebral canal	**Ø** Open **3** Percutaneous **4** Percutaneous Endoscopic **X** External	**Z** No Device	**Z** No Qualifier

Non-OR ØØF[3,4,5,6]XZZ
`NC` ØØF[3,4,5,6]XZZ

`LC` Limited Coverage   `NC` Noncovered   ⊞ Combination Member   HAC associated procedure   Combination Only   DRG Non-OR   Non-OR   New/Revised in GREEN
ICD-10-PCS 2021   141

ØØD–ØØF

Ø   **Medical and Surgical**
Ø   **Central Nervous System and Cranial Nerves**
H   **Insertion**   Definition: Putting in a nonbiological appliance that monitors, assists, performs, or prevents a physiological function but does not physically take the place of a body part

                     Explanation: None

Body Part Character 4	Approach Character 5	Device Character 6	Qualifier Character 7
Ø **Brain** ⊞ Cerebrum Corpus callosum Encephalon	Ø Open	1 Radioactive Element 2 Monitoring Device 3 Infusion Device 4 Radioactive Element, Cesium-131 Collagen Implant M Neurostimulator Lead Y Other Device	Z No Qualifier
Ø **Brain** ⊞ Cerebrum Corpus callosum Encephalon	3 Percutaneous 4 Percutaneous Endoscopic	1 Radioactive Element 2 Monitoring Device 3 Infusion Device M Neurostimulator Lead Y Other Device	Z No Qualifier

6 **Cerebral Ventricle** ⊞
Aqueduct of Sylvius
Cerebral aqueduct (Sylvius)
Choroid plexus
Ependyma
Foramen of Monro (intraventricular)
Fourth ventricle Interventricular foramen (Monro)
Left lateral ventricle
Right lateral ventricle
Third ventricle
 	
E **Cranial Nerve** ⊞
U **Spinal Canal** ⊞
  Epidural space, spinal
  Extradural space, spinal
  Subarachnoid space, spinal
  Subdural space, spinal
  Vertebral canal
V **Spinal Cord** ⊞
	Ø Open
	3 Percutaneous
	4 Percutaneous Endoscopic
		1 Radioactive Element
		2 Monitoring Device
		3 Infusion Device
		M Neurostimulator Lead
		Y Other Device
			Z No Qualifier

DRG Non-OR	00H004Z	**See Appendix L for Procedure Combinations**
Non-OR	00H[E,U,V]32Z	⊞ 00H00MZ
Non-OR	00H[E,U][3,4]YZ	⊞ 00H0[3,4]MZ
Non-OR	00H[U,V][0,3,4]3Z	⊞ 00H[6,E,U,V][0,3,4]MZ

Ø   **Medical and Surgical**
Ø   **Central Nervous System and Cranial Nerves**
J   **Inspection**   Definition: Visually and/or manually exploring a body part

                     Explanation: Visual exploration may be performed with or without optical instrumentation. Manual exploration may be performed directly or through intervening body layers.

Body Part Character 4	Approach Character 5	Device Character 6	Qualifier Character 7

Ø **Brain**
Cerebrum
Corpus callosum
Encephalon
E **Cranial Nerve**
 	
U **Spinal Canal**
  Epidural space, spinal
  Extradural space, spinal
  Subarachnoid space, spinal
  Subdural space, spinal
  Vertebral canal
V **Spinal Cord**
	Ø Open
	3 Percutaneous
	4 Percutaneous Endoscopic
		Z No Device	Z No Qualifier

Non-OR	00J[0,E,U,V]3ZZ

Ø   **Medical and Surgical**
Ø   **Central Nervous System and Cranial Nerves**
K   **Map**   Definition: Locating the route of passage of electrical impulses and/or locating functional areas in a body part

                  Explanation: Applicable only to the cardiac conduction mechanism and the central nervous system

Body Part Character 4	Approach Character 5	Device Character 6	Qualifier Character 7
Ø **Brain** Cerebrum Corpus callosum Encephalon 7 **Cerebral Hemisphere** Frontal lobe Occipital lobe Parietal lobe Temporal lobe 8 **Basal Ganglia** Basal nuclei Claustrum Corpus striatum Globus pallidus Substantia nigra Subthalamic nucleus	9 **Thalamus** Epithalamus Geniculate nucleus Metathalamus Pulvinar A **Hypothalamus** Mammillary body B **Pons** Apneustic center Basis pontis Locus ceruleus Pneumotaxic center Pontine tegmentum Superior olivary nucleus C **Cerebellum** Culmen D **Medulla Oblongata** Myelencephalon	Ø Open 3 Percutaneous 4 Percutaneous Endoscopic	Z No Device	Z No Qualifier

LC Limited Coverage   NC Noncovered   ⊞ Combination Member   HAC associated procedure   Combination Only   DRG Non-OR   Non-OR   New/Revised in GREEN

142   ICD-10-PCS 2021

Ø   **Medical and Surgical**
Ø   **Central Nervous System and Cranial Nerves**
N   **Release**   Definition: Freeing a body part from an abnormal physical constraint by cutting or by the use of force
                          Explanation: Some of the restraining tissue may be taken out but none of the body part is taken out

Body Part Character 4		Approach Character 5	Device Character 6	Qualifier Character 7
Ø Brain Cerebrum Corpus callosum Encephalon **1 Cerebral Meninges** Arachnoid mater, intracranial Leptomeninges, intracranial Pia mater, intracranial **2 Dura Mater** Diaphragma sellae Dura mater, intracranial Falx cerebri Tentorium cerebelli **6 Cerebral Ventricle** Aqueduct of Sylvius Cerebral aqueduct (Sylvius) Choroid plexus Ependyma Foramen of Monro (intraventricular) Fourth ventricle Interventricular foramen (Monro) Left lateral ventricle Right lateral ventricle Third ventricle **7 Cerebral Hemisphere** Frontal lobe Occipital lobe Parietal lobe Temporal lobe **8 Basal Ganglia** Basal nuclei Claustrum Corpus striatum Globus pallidus Substantia nigra Subthalamic nucleus **9 Thalamus** Epithalamus Geniculate nucleus Metathalamus Pulvinar **A Hypothalamus** Mammillary body **B Pons** Apneustic center Basis pontis Locus ceruleus Pneumotaxic center Pontine tegmentum Superior olivary nucleus **C Cerebellum** Culmen **D Medulla Oblongata** Myelencephalon **F Olfactory Nerve** First cranial nerve Olfactory bulb **G Optic Nerve** Optic chiasma Second cranial nerve	**H Oculomotor Nerve** Third cranial nerve **J Trochlear Nerve** Fourth cranial nerve **K Trigeminal Nerve** Fifth cranial nerve Gasserian ganglion Mandibular nerve Maxillary nerve Ophthalmic nerve Trifacial nerve **L Abducens Nerve** Sixth cranial nerve **M Facial Nerve** Chorda tympani Geniculate ganglion Greater superficial petrosal nerve Nerve to the stapedius Parotid plexus Posterior auricular nerve Seventh cranial nerve Submandibular ganglion **N Acoustic Nerve** Cochlear nerve Eighth cranial nerve Scarpa's (vestibular) ganglion Spiral ganglion Vestibular (Scarpa's) ganglion Vestibular nerve Vestibulocochlear nerve **P Glossopharyngeal Nerve** Carotid sinus nerve Ninth cranial nerve Tympanic nerve **Q Vagus Nerve** Anterior vagal trunk Pharyngeal plexus Pneumogastric nerve Posterior vagal trunk Pulmonary plexus Recurrent laryngeal nerve Superior laryngeal nerve Tenth cranial nerve **R Accessory Nerve** Eleventh cranial nerve **S Hypoglossal Nerve** Twelfth cranial nerve **T Spinal Meninges** Arachnoid mater, spinal Denticulate (dentate) ligament Dura mater, spinal Filum terminale Leptomeninges, spinal Pia mater, spinal **W Cervical Spinal Cord** **X Thoracic Spinal Cord** **Y Lumbar Spinal Cord** Cauda equina Conus medullaris	**Ø Open** **3 Percutaneous** **4 Percutaneous Endoscopic**	**Z No Device**	**Z No Qualifier**

LC Limited Coverage   NC Noncovered   ⊞ Combination Member   HAC associated procedure   Combination Only   DRG Non-OR   Non-OR   New/Revised in GREEN

0   Medical and Surgical
0   Central Nervous System and Cranial Nerves
P   Removal   Definition: Taking out or off a device from a body part

Explanation: If a device is taken out and a similar device put in without cutting or puncturing the skin or mucous membrane, the procedure is coded to the root operation CHANGE. Otherwise, the procedure for taking out a device is coded to the root operation REMOVAL.

Body Part Character 4	Approach Character 5	Device Character 6	Qualifier Character 7
0 Brain Cerebrum Corpus callosum Encephalon **V Spinal Cord**	**0** Open **3** Percutaneous **4** Percutaneous Endoscopic	**0** Drainage Device **2** Monitoring Device **3** Infusion Device **7** Autologous Tissue Substitute **J** Synthetic Substitute **K** Nonautologous Tissue Substitute **M** Neurostimulator Lead **Y** Other Device	**Z** No Qualifier
0 Brain Cerebrum Corpus callosum Encephalon **V Spinal Cord**	**X** External	**0** Drainage Device **2** Monitoring Device **3** Infusion Device **M** Neurostimulator Lead	**Z** No Qualifier
6 Cerebral Ventricle Aqueduct of Sylvius Cerebral aqueduct (Sylvius) Choroid plexus Ependyma Foramen of Monro (intraventricular) Fourth ventricle Interventricular foramen (Monro) Left lateral ventricle Right lateral ventricle Third ventricle **U Spinal Canal** Epidural space, spinal Extradural space, spinal Subarachnoid space, spinal Subdural space, spinal Vertebral canal	**0** Open **3** Percutaneous **4** Percutaneous Endoscopic	**0** Drainage Device **2** Monitoring Device **3** Infusion Device **J** Synthetic Substitute **M** Neurostimulator Lead **Y** Other Device	**Z** No Qualifier
6 Cerebral Ventricle Aqueduct of Sylvius Cerebral aqueduct (Sylvius) Choroid plexus Ependyma Foramen of Monro (intraventricular) Fourth ventricle Interventricular foramen (Monro) Left lateral ventricle Right lateral ventricle Third ventricle **U Spinal Canal** Epidural space, spinal Extradural space, spinal Subarachnoid space, spinal Subdural space, spinal Vertebral canal	**X** External	**0** Drainage Device **2** Monitoring Device **3** Infusion Device **M** Neurostimulator Lead	**Z** No Qualifier
E Cranial Nerve	**0** Open **3** Percutaneous **4** Percutaneous Endoscopic	**0** Drainage Device **2** Monitoring Device **3** Infusion Device **7** Autologous Tissue Substitute **M** Neurostimulator Lead **Y** Other Device	**Z** No Qualifier
E Cranial Nerve	**X** External	**0** Drainage Device **2** Monitoring Device **3** Infusion Device **M** Neurostimulator Lead	**Z** No Qualifier

Non-OR	00P[0,V]3[0,2,3]Z
Non-OR	00P[0,V][3,4]YZ
Non-OR	00P[0,V]X[0,2,3,M]Z
Non-OR	00P[6,U]3[0,2,3]Z
Non-OR	00P[6,U][3,4]YZ
Non-OR	00P[6,U]X[0,2,3,M]Z
Non-OR	00PE3[0,2,3]Z
Non-OR	00PE[3,4]YZ
Non-OR	00PEX[0,2,3,M]Z

Ø   **Medical and Surgical**
Ø   **Central Nervous System and Cranial Nerves**
Q   **Repair**   Definition: Restoring, to the extent possible, a body part to its normal anatomic structure and function
                       Explanation: Used only when the method to accomplish the repair is not one of the other root operations

Body Part Character 4		Approach Character 5	Device Character 6	Qualifier Character 7

Ø Brain
  Cerebrum
  Corpus callosum
  Encephalon
1 Cerebral Meninges
  Arachnoid mater,
    intracranial
  Leptomeninges,
    intracranial
  Pia mater, intracranial
2 Dura Mater
  Diaphragma sellae
  Dura mater, intracranial
  Falx cerebri
  Tentorium cerebelli
6 Cerebral Ventricle
  Aqueduct of Sylvius
  Cerebral aqueduct (Sylvius)
  Choroid plexus
  Ependyma
  Foramen of Monro
    (intraventricular)
  Fourth ventricle
  Interventricular foramen
    (Monro)
  Left lateral ventricle
  Right lateral ventricle
  Third ventricle
7 Cerebral Hemisphere
  Frontal lobe
  Occipital lobe
  Parietal lobe
  Temporal lobe
8 Basal Ganglia
  Basal nuclei
  Claustrum
  Corpus striatum
  Globus pallidus
  Substantia nigra
  Subthalamic nucleus
9 Thalamus
  Epithalamus
  Geniculate nucleus
  Metathalamus
  Pulvinar
A Hypothalamus
  Mammillary body
B Pons
  Apneustic center
  Basis pontis
  Locus ceruleus
  Pneumotaxic center
  Pontine tegmentum
  Superior olivary nucleus
C Cerebellum
  Culmen
D Medulla Oblongata
  Myelencephalon
F Olfactory Nerve
  First cranial nerve
  Olfactory bulb
G Optic Nerve
  Optic chiasma
  Second cranial nerve
	H Oculomotor Nerve
	  Third cranial nerve
	J Trochlear Nerve
	  Fourth cranial nerve
	K Trigeminal Nerve
	  Fifth cranial nerve
	  Gasserian ganglion
	  Mandibular nerve
	  Maxillary nerve
	  Ophthalmic nerve
	  Trifacial nerve
	L Abducens Nerve
	  Sixth cranial nerve
	M Facial Nerve
	  Chorda tympani
	  Geniculate ganglion
	  Greater superficial petrosal
	    nerve
	  Nerve to the stapedius
	  Parotid plexus
	  Posterior auricular nerve
	  Seventh cranial nerve
	  Submandibular ganglion
	N Acoustic Nerve
	  Cochlear nerve
	  Eighth cranial nerve
	  Scarpa's (vestibular)
	    ganglion
	  Spiral ganglion
	  Vestibular (Scarpa's)
	    ganglion
	  Vestibular nerve
	  Vestibulocochlear nerve
	P Glossopharyngeal Nerve
	  Carotid sinus nerve
	  Ninth cranial nerve
	  Tympanic nerve
	Q Vagus Nerve
	  Anterior vagal trunk
	  Pharyngeal plexus
	  Pneumogastric nerve
	  Posterior vagal trunk
	  Pulmonary plexus
	  Recurrent laryngeal nerve
	  Superior laryngeal nerve
	  Tenth cranial nerve
	R Accessory Nerve
	  Eleventh cranial nerve
	S Hypoglossal Nerve
	  Twelfth cranial nerve
	T Spinal Meninges
	  Arachnoid mater, spinal
	  Denticulate (dentate)
	    ligament
	  Dura mater, spinal
	  Filum terminale
	  Leptomeninges, spinal
	  Pia mater, spinal
	W Cervical Spinal Cord
	X Thoracic Spinal Cord
	Y Lumbar Spinal Cord
	  Cauda equina
	  Conus medullaris
		Ø Open
		3 Percutaneous
		4 Percutaneous Endoscopic
			Z No Device	**Z No Qualifier**

Central Nervous System and Cranial Nerves *(side tab)*

Ø   **Medical and Surgical**
Ø   **Central Nervous System and Cranial Nerves**
R   **Replacement**   Definition: Putting in or on biological or synthetic material that physically takes the place and/or function of all or a portion of a body part

                                Explanation: The body part may have been taken out or replaced, or may be taken out, physically eradicated, or rendered nonfunctional during the REPLACEMENT procedure. A REMOVAL procedure is coded for taking out the device used in a previous replacement procedure.

Body Part Character 4		Approach Character 5	Device Character 6	Qualifier Character 7
1 Cerebral Meninges Arachnoid mater, intracranial Leptomeninges, intracranial Pia mater, intracranial **2 Dura Mater** Diaphragma sellae Dura mater, intracranial Falx cerebri Tentorium cerebelli **6 Cerebral Ventricle** Aqueduct of Sylvius Cerebral aqueduct (Sylvius) Choroid plexus Ependyma Foramen of Monro (intraventricular) Fourth ventricle Interventricular foramen (Monro) Left lateral ventricle Right lateral ventricle Third ventricle **F Olfactory Nerve** First cranial nerve Olfactory bulb **G Optic Nerve** Optic chiasma Second cranial nerve **H Oculomotor Nerve** Third cranial nerve **J Trochlear Nerve** Fourth cranial nerve **K Trigeminal Nerve** Fifth cranial nerve Gasserian ganglion Mandibular nerve Maxillary nerve Ophthalmic nerve Trifacial nerve **L Abducens Nerve** Sixth cranial nerve	**M Facial Nerve** Chorda tympani Geniculate ganglion Greater superficial petrosal nerve Nerve to the stapedius Parotid plexus Posterior auricular nerve Seventh cranial nerve Submandibular ganglion **N Acoustic Nerve** Cochlear nerve Eighth cranial nerve Scarpa's (vestibular) ganglion Spiral ganglion Vestibular (Scarpa's) ganglion Vestibular nerve Vestibulocochlear nerve **P Glossopharyngeal Nerve** Carotid sinus nerve Ninth cranial nerve Tympanic nerve **Q Vagus Nerve** Anterior vagal trunk Pharyngeal plexus Pneumogastric nerve Posterior vagal trunk Pulmonary plexus Recurrent laryngeal nerve Superior laryngeal nerve Tenth cranial nerve **R Accessory Nerve** Eleventh cranial nerve **S Hypoglossal Nerve** Twelfth cranial nerve **T Spinal Meninges** Arachnoid mater, spinal Denticulate (dentate) ligament Dura mater, spinal Filum terminale Leptomeninges, spinal Pia mater, spinal	**Ø Open** **4 Percutaneous Endoscopic**	**7 Autologous Tissue Substitute** **J Synthetic Substitute** **K Nonautologous Tissue Substitute**	**Z No Qualifier**

LC Limited Coverage NC Noncovered ⊞ Combination Member HAC associated procedure Combination Only DRG Non-OR Non-OR New/Revised in GREEN
146   ICD-10-PCS 2021

ØØR–ØØR *(side tab, bottom)*

Ø   **Medical and Surgical**
Ø   **Central Nervous System and Cranial Nerves**
S   **Reposition**   Definition: Moving to its normal location, or other suitable location, all or a portion of a body part

Explanation: The body part is moved to a new location from an abnormal location, or from a normal location where it is not functioning correctly. The body part may or may not be cut out or off to be moved to the new location.

Body Part Character 4		Approach Character 5	Device Character 6	Qualifier Character 7
F Olfactory Nerve First cranial nerve Olfactory bulb **G Optic Nerve** Optic chiasma Second cranial nerve **H Oculomotor Nerve** Third cranial nerve **J Trochlear Nerve** Fourth cranial nerve **K Trigeminal Nerve** Fifth cranial nerve Gasserian ganglion Mandibular nerve Maxillary nerve Ophthalmic nerve Trifacial nerve **L Abducens Nerve** Sixth cranial nerve **M Facial Nerve** Chorda tympani Geniculate ganglion Greater superficial petrosal nerve Nerve to the stapedius Parotid plexus Posterior auricular nerve Seventh cranial nerve Submandibular ganglion	**N Acoustic Nerve** Cochlear nerve Eighth cranial nerve Scarpa's (vestibular) ganglion Spiral ganglion Vestibular (Scarpa's) ganglion Vestibular nerve Vestibulocochlear nerve **P Glossopharyngeal Nerve** Carotid sinus nerve Ninth cranial nerve Tympanic nerve **Q Vagus Nerve** Anterior vagal trunk Pharyngeal plexus Pneumogastric nerve Posterior vagal trunk Pulmonary plexus Recurrent laryngeal nerve Superior laryngeal nerve Tenth cranial nerve **R Accessory Nerve** Eleventh cranial nerve **S Hypoglossal Nerve** Twelfth cranial nerve **W Cervical Spinal Cord** **X Thoracic Spinal Cord** **Y Lumbar Spinal Cord** Cauda equina Conus medullaris	Ø Open 3 Percutaneous 4 Percutaneous Endoscopic	Z No Device	Z No Qualifier

Ø   **Medical and Surgical**
Ø   **Central Nervous System and Cranial Nerves**
T   **Resection**   Definition: Cutting out or off, without replacement, all of a body part

Explanation: None

Body Part Character 4	Approach Character 5	Device Character 6	Qualifier Character 7
7 Cerebral Hemisphere Frontal lobe Occipital lobe Parietal lobe Temporal lobe	Ø Open 3 Percutaneous 4 Percutaneous Endoscopic	Z No Device	Z No Qualifier

LC Limited Coverage   NC Noncovered   ⊞ Combination Member   HAC associated procedure   Combination Only   DRG Non-OR   Non-OR   New/Revised in GREEN

ICD-10-PCS 2021   147

0   Medical and Surgical
0   Central Nervous System and Cranial Nerves
U   Supplement   Definition: Putting in or on biological or synthetic material that physically reinforces and/or augments the function of a portion of a body part
Explanation: The biological material is non-living, or is living and from the same individual. The body part may have been previously replaced, and the SUPPLEMENT procedure is performed to physically reinforce and/or augment the function of the replaced body part.

Body Part Character 4		Approach Character 5	Device Character 6	Qualifier Character 7

1 Cerebral Meninges
  Arachnoid mater,
    intracranial
  Leptomeninges,
    intracranial
  Pia mater, intracranial
2 Dura Mater
  Diaphragma sellae
  Dura mater, intracranial
  Falx cerebri
  Tentorium cerebelli
6 Cerebral Ventricle
  Aqueduct of Sylvius
  Cerebral aqueduct (Sylvius)
  Choroid plexus
  Ependyma
  Foramen of Monro
    (intraventricular)
  Fourth ventricle
  Interventricular foramen
    (Monro)
  Left lateral ventricle
  Right lateral ventricle
  Third ventricle
F Olfactory Nerve
  First cranial nerve
  Olfactory bulb
G Optic Nerve
  Optic chiasma
  Second cranial nerve
H Oculomotor Nerve
  Third cranial nerve
J Trochlear Nerve
  Fourth cranial nerve
K Trigeminal Nerve
  Fifth cranial nerve
  Gasserian ganglion
  Mandibular nerve
  Maxillary nerve
  Ophthalmic nerve
  Trifacial nerve
L Abducens Nerve
  Sixth cranial nerve
	M Facial Nerve
	  Chorda tympani
	  Geniculate ganglion
	  Greater superficial petrosal
	    nerve
	  Nerve to the stapedius
	  Parotid plexus
	  Posterior auricular nerve
	  Seventh cranial nerve
	  Submandibular ganglion
	N Acoustic Nerve
	  Cochlear nerve
	  Eighth cranial nerve
	  Scarpa's (vestibular)
	    ganglion
	  Spiral ganglion
	  Vestibular (Scarpa's)
	    ganglion
	  Vestibular nerve
	  Vestibulocochlear nerve
	P Glossopharyngeal Nerve
	  Carotid sinus nerve
	  Ninth cranial nerve
	  Tympanic nerve
	Q Vagus Nerve
	  Anterior vagal trunk
	  Pharyngeal plexus
	  Pneumogastric nerve
	  Posterior vagal trunk
	  Pulmonary plexus
	  Recurrent laryngeal nerve
	  Superior laryngeal nerve
	  Tenth cranial nerve
	R Accessory Nerve
	  Eleventh cranial nerve
	S Hypoglossal Nerve
	  Twelfth cranial nerve
	T Spinal Meninges
	  Arachnoid mater, spinal
	  Denticulate (dentate)
	    ligament
	  Dura mater, spinal
	  Filum terminale
	  Leptomeninges, spinal
	  Pia mater, spinal
		0 Open
		3 Percutaneous
		4 Percutaneous Endoscopic
			**7 Autologous Tissue
			    Substitute**
			J Synthetic Substitute
			**K Nonautologous Tissue
			    Substitute**
				Z No Qualifier

Ø **Medical and Surgical**
Ø **Central Nervous System and Cranial Nerves**
W **Revision** Definition: Correcting, to the extent possible, a portion of a malfunctioning device or the position of a displaced device
Explanation: Revision can include correcting a malfunctioning or displaced device by taking out or putting in components of the device such as a screw or pin

Body Part Character 4	Approach Character 5	Device Character 6	Qualifier Character 7
Ø Brain Cerebrum Corpus callosum Encephalon V Spinal Cord	Ø Open 3 Percutaneous 4 Percutaneous Endoscopic	Ø Drainage Device 2 Monitoring Device 3 Infusion Device 7 Autologous Tissue Substitute J Synthetic Substitute K Nonautologous Tissue Substitute M Neurostimulator Lead Y Other Device	Z No Qualifier
Ø Brain Cerebrum Corpus callosum Encephalon V Spinal Cord	X External	Ø Drainage Device 2 Monitoring Device 3 Infusion Device 7 Autologous Tissue Substitute J Synthetic Substitute K Nonautologous Tissue Substitute M Neurostimulator Lead	Z No Qualifier
6 Cerebral Ventricle Aqueduct of Sylvius Cerebral aqueduct (Sylvius) Choroid plexus Ependyma Foramen of Monro (intraventricular) Fourth ventricle Interventricular foramen (Monro) Left lateral ventricle Right lateral ventricle Third ventricle U Spinal Canal Epidural space, spinal Extradural space, spinal Subarachnoid space, spinal Subdural space, spinal Vertebral canal	Ø Open 3 Percutaneous 4 Percutaneous Endoscopic	Ø Drainage Device 2 Monitoring Device 3 Infusion Device J Synthetic Substitute M Neurostimulator Lead Y Other Device	Z No Qualifier
6 Cerebral Ventricle Aqueduct of Sylvius Cerebral aqueduct (Sylvius) Choroid plexus Ependyma Foramen of Monro (intraventricular) Fourth ventricle Interventricular foramen (Monro) Left lateral ventricle Right lateral ventricle Third ventricle U Spinal Canal Epidural space, spinal Extradural space, spinal Subarachnoid space, spinal Subdural space, spinal Vertebral canal	X External	Ø Drainage Device 2 Monitoring Device 3 Infusion Device J Synthetic Substitute M Neurostimulator Lead	Z No Qualifier
E Cranial Nerve	Ø Open 3 Percutaneous 4 Percutaneous Endoscopic	Ø Drainage Device 2 Monitoring Device 3 Infusion Device 7 Autologous Tissue Substitute M Neurostimulator Lead Y Other Device	Z No Qualifier
E Cranial Nerve	X External	Ø Drainage Device 2 Monitoring Device 3 Infusion Device 7 Autologous Tissue Substitute M Neurostimulator Lead	Z No Qualifier

Non-OR 00W[Ø,V][3,4]YZ
Non-OR 00W[Ø,V]X[Ø,2,3,7,J,K,M]Z
Non-OR 00W[6,U][3,4]YZ
Non-OR 00W[6,U]X[Ø,2,3,J,M]Z
Non-OR 00WE[3,4]YZ
Non-OR 00WEX[Ø,2,3,7,M]Z

LC Limited Coverage NC Noncovered ⊞ Combination Member HAC associated procedure Combination Only DRG Non-OR Non-OR New/Revised in GREEN

Ø   **Medical and Surgical**
Ø   **Central Nervous System and Cranial Nerves**
X   **Transfer**   Definition: Moving, without taking out, all or a portion of a body part to another location to take over the function of all or a portion of a body part
                    Explanation: The body part transferred remains connected to its vascular and nervous supply

Body Part Character 4	Approach Character 5	Device Character 6	Qualifier Character 7
F Olfactory Nerve First cranial nerve Olfactory bulb **G Optic Nerve** Optic chiasma Second cranial nerve **H Oculomotor Nerve** Third cranial nerve **J Trochlear Nerve** Fourth cranial nerve **K Trigeminal Nerve** Fifth cranial nerve Gasserian ganglion Mandibular nerve Maxillary nerve Ophthalmic nerve Trifacial nerve **L Abducens Nerve** Sixth cranial nerve **M Facial Nerve** Chorda tympani Geniculate ganglion Greater superficial petrosal nerve Nerve to the stapedius Parotid plexus Posterior auricular nerve Seventh cranial nerve Submandibular ganglion **N Acoustic Nerve** Cochlear nerve Eighth cranial nerve Scarpa's (vestibular) ganglion Spiral ganglion Vestibular (Scarpa's) ganglion Vestibular nerve Vestibulocochlear nerve **P Glossopharyngeal Nerve** Carotid sinus nerve Ninth cranial nerve Tympanic nerve **Q Vagus Nerve** Anterior vagal trunk Pharyngeal plexus Pneumogastric nerve Posterior vagal trunk Pulmonary plexus Recurrent laryngeal nerve Superior laryngeal nerve Tenth cranial nerve **R Accessory Nerve** Eleventh cranial nerve **S Hypoglossal Nerve** Twelfth cranial nerve	**Ø Open** **4 Percutaneous Endoscopic**	**Z No Device**	**F Olfactory Nerve** **G Optic Nerve** **H Oculomotor Nerve** **J Trochlear Nerve** **K Trigeminal Nerve** **L Abducens Nerve** **M Facial Nerve** **N Acoustic Nerve** **P Glossopharyngeal Nerve** **Q Vagus Nerve** **R Accessory Nerve** **S Hypoglossal Nerve**

LC Limited Coverage   NC Noncovered   ⊞ Combination Member   HAC associated procedure   Combination Only   DRG Non-OR   Non-OR   New/Revised in GREEN

150   ICD-10-PCS 2021

Peripheral Nervous System Ø12–Ø1X

Character Meanings

This Character Meaning table is provided as a guide to assist the user in the identification of character members that may be found in this section of code tables. It **SHOULD NOT** be used to build a PCS code.

Operation–Character 3	Body Part–Character 4	Approach–Character 5	Device–Character 6	Qualifier–Character 7
2 Change	Ø Cervical Plexus	Ø Open	Ø Drainage Device	1 Cervical Nerve
5 Destruction	1 Cervical Nerve	3 Percutaneous	1 Radioactive Element	2 Phrenic Nerve
8 Division	2 Phrenic Nerve	4 Percutaneous Endoscopic	2 Monitoring Device	4 Ulnar Nerve
9 Drainage	3 Brachial Plexus	X External	7 Autologous Tissue Substitute	5 Median Nerve
B Excision	4 Ulnar Nerve		M Neurostimulator Lead	6 Radial Nerve
C Extirpation	5 Median Nerve		Y Other Device	8 Thoracic Nerve
D Extraction	6 Radial Nerve		Z No Device	B Lumbar Nerve
H Insertion	8 Thoracic Nerve			C Perineal Nerve
J Inspection	9 Lumbar Plexus			D Femoral Nerve
N Release	A Lumbosacral Plexus			F Sciatic Nerve
P Removal	B Lumbar Nerve			G Tibial Nerve
Q Repair	C Pudendal Nerve			H Peroneal Nerve
R Replacement	D Femoral Nerve			X Diagnostic
S Reposition	F Sciatic Nerve			Z No Qualifier
U Supplement	G Tibial Nerve			
W Revision	H Peroneal Nerve			
X Transfer	K Head and Neck Sympathetic Nerve			
	L Thoracic Sympathetic Nerve			
	M Abdominal Sympathetic Nerve			
	N Lumbar Sympathetic Nerve			
	P Sacral Sympathetic Nerve			
	Q Sacral Plexus			
	R Sacral Nerve			
	Y Peripheral Nerve			

AHA Coding Clinic for table Ø1B
2018, 2Q, 22   Excision of synovial cyst
2017, 2Q, 19   Thoracic outlet decompression with sympathectomy

AHA Coding Clinic for table Ø1N
2019, 1Q, 28   Decompressive laminectomy of both spinal cord and nerve roots
2018, 2Q, 22   Excision of synovial cyst
2017, 2Q, 19   Thoracic outlet decompression with sympathectomy
2016, 2Q, 16   Decompressive laminectomy/foraminotomy and lumbar discectomy
2016, 2Q, 17   Removal of longitudinal ligament to decompress cervical nerve root
2016, 2Q, 23   Thoracic outlet syndrome and release of brachial plexus
2015, 2Q, 34   Decompressive laminectomy
2014, 3Q, 33   Radial fracture treatment with open reduction internal fixation, and release of carpal ligament

AHA Coding Clinic for table Ø1Q
2019, 3Q, 32   Breast reconstruction with neurotization

AHA Coding Clinic for table Ø1U
2019, 3Q, 32   Breast reconstruction with neurotization
2017, 4Q, 62   Added and revised device values - Nerve substitutes

Median and Ulnar Nerves

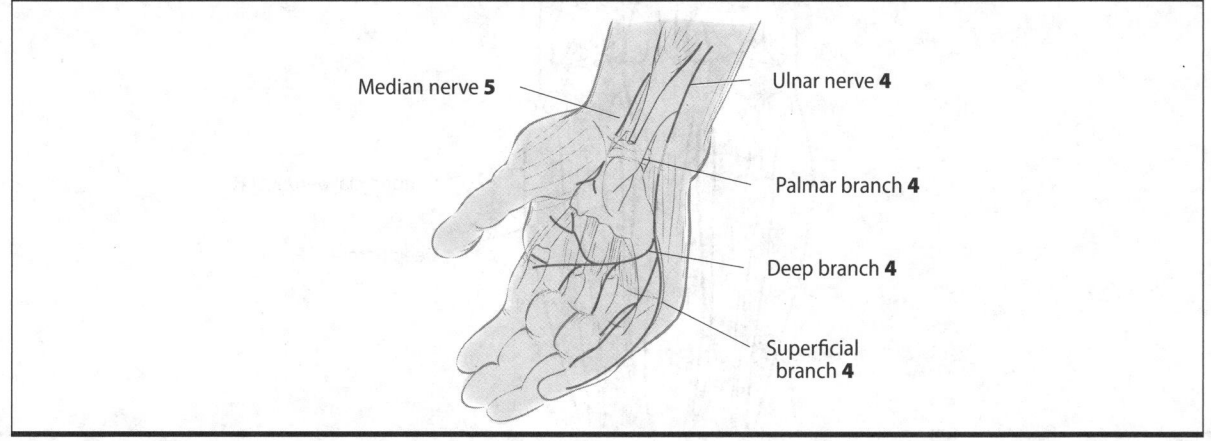

Median nerve **5**
Ulnar nerve **4**
Palmar branch **4**
Deep branch **4**
Superficial branch **4**

Peripheral Nervous System

- Great auricular — Cervical plexus **Ø**
- Lesser occiptial
- Greater occipital
- Suboccipital — Cervical nerve **1**
- 3rd occipital
- L. phrenic **2**
- Supraclavicular **Ø**
- Cervical plexus **Ø**
- Ansa cervicalis
- Transverse cervical
- Dorsal scapular
- First intercostal
- Subclavian
- Long thoracic — Brachial plexus **3**
- Axillary
- Musculocutaneous
- Median **5**
- Ulnar **4**
- Radial **6**
- Intercostal nerves **8**
- Thoracic splanchnic **L**
- Subcostal **8**
- Lumbar splanchnic **N**
- Genitofemoral
- Iliohypogastric
- Ilioinguinal
- Obturator — Lumbar plexus **9**
- Lateral femoral cutaneous
- Sacral **R**
- Accessory obturator
- Superior gluteal
- Inferior gluteal **Q**
- Sacral splanchnic **P**
- Pelvic splanchnic **P** — Sacral plexus and sacral sympathetic nerves
- Pudendal **Q**
- Posterior scrotal/labial **C**
- Posterior femoral cutaneous **Q**
- Femoral **D**
- Sciatic **F**
- Saphenous **D**
- Common peroneal **H**
- Tibial **G**
- Superficial peroneal **H**
- Deep peroneal **H**

Ø   Medical and Surgical
1   Peripheral Nervous System
2   Change
Definition: Taking out or off a device from a body part and putting back an identical or similar device in or on the same body part without cutting or puncturing the skin or a mucous membrane

Explanation: All CHANGE procedures are coded using the approach EXTERNAL

Body Part Character 4	Approach Character 5	Device Character 6	Qualifier Character 7
Y Peripheral Nerve	X External	Ø Drainage Device Y Other Device	Z No Qualifier

Non-OR   All body part, approach, device, and qualifier values

Ø   Medical and Surgical
1   Peripheral Nervous System
5   Destruction
Definition: Physical eradication of all or a portion of a body part by the direct use of energy, force, or a destructive agent

Explanation: None of the body part is physically taken out

Body Part Character 4		Approach Character 5	Device Character 6	Qualifier Character 7

Ø Cervical Plexus
   Ansa cervicalis
   Cutaneous (transverse) cervical nerve
   Great auricular nerve
   Lesser occipital nerve
   Supraclavicular nerve
   Transverse (cutaneous) cervical nerve
1 Cervical Nerve
   Greater occipital nerve
   Spinal nerve, cervical
   Suboccipital nerve
   Third occipital nerve
2 Phrenic Nerve
   Accessory phrenic nerve
3 Brachial Plexus
   Axillary nerve
   Dorsal scapular nerve
   First intercostal nerve
   Long thoracic nerve
   Musculocutaneous nerve
   Subclavius nerve
   Suprascapular nerve
4 Ulnar Nerve
   Cubital nerve
5 Median Nerve
   Anterior interosseous nerve
   Palmar cutaneous nerve
6 Radial Nerve
   Dorsal digital nerve
   Musculospiral nerve
   Palmar cutaneous nerve
   Posterior interosseous nerve
8 Thoracic Nerve
   Intercostal nerve
   Intercostobrachial nerve
   Spinal nerve, thoracic
   Subcostal nerve
9 Lumbar Plexus
   Accessory obturator nerve
   Genitofemoral nerve
   Iliohypogastric nerve
   Ilioinguinal nerve
   Lateral femoral cutaneous nerve
   Obturator nerve
   Superior gluteal nerve
A Lumbosacral Plexus
B Lumbar Nerve
   Lumbosacral trunk
   Spinal nerve, lumbar
   Superior clunic (cluneal) nerve
C Pudendal Nerve
   Posterior labial nerve
   Posterior scrotal nerve
D Femoral Nerve
   Anterior crural nerve
   Saphenous nerve
F Sciatic Nerve
   Ischiatic nerve
G Tibial Nerve
   Lateral plantar nerve
   Medial plantar nerve
   Medial popliteal nerve
   Medial sural cutaneous nerve
	H Peroneal Nerve
	   Common fibular nerve
	   Common peroneal nerve
	   External popliteal nerve
	   Lateral sural cutaneous nerve
	K Head and Neck Sympathetic Nerve
	   Cavernous plexus
	   Cervical ganglion
	   Ciliary ganglion
	   Internal carotid plexus
	   Otic ganglion
	   Pterygopalatine (sphenopalatine)
	      ganglion
	   Sphenopalatine (pterygopalatine)
	      ganglion
	   Stellate ganglion
	   Submandibular ganglion
	   Submaxillary ganglion
	L Thoracic Sympathetic Nerve
	   Cardiac plexus
	   Esophageal plexus
	   Greater splanchnic nerve
	   Inferior cardiac nerve
	   Least splanchnic nerve
	   Lesser splanchnic nerve
	   Middle cardiac nerve
	   Pulmonary plexus
	   Superior cardiac nerve
	   Thoracic aortic plexus
	   Thoracic ganglion
	M Abdominal Sympathetic Nerve
	   Abdominal aortic plexus
	   Auerbach's (myenteric) plexus
	   Celiac (solar) plexus
	   Celiac ganglion
	   Gastric plexus
	   Hepatic plexus
	   Inferior hypogastric plexus
	   Inferior mesenteric ganglion
	   Inferior mesenteric plexus
	   Meissner's (submucous) plexus
	   Myenteric (Auerbach's) plexus
	   Pancreatic plexus
	   Pelvic splanchnic nerve
	   Renal nerve
	   Renal plexus
	   Solar (celiac) plexus
	   Splenic plexus
	   Submucous (Meissner's) plexus
	   Superior hypogastric plexus
	   Superior mesenteric ganglion
	   Superior mesenteric plexus
	   Suprarenal plexus
	N Lumbar Sympathetic Nerve
	   Lumbar ganglion
	   Lumbar splanchnic nerve
	P Sacral Sympathetic Nerve
	   Ganglion impar (ganglion of
	      Walther)
	   Pelvic splanchnic nerve
	   Sacral ganglion
	   Sacral splanchnic nerve
	Q Sacral Plexus
	   Inferior gluteal nerve
	   Posterior femoral cutaneous nerve
	   Pudendal nerve
	R Sacral Nerve
	   Spinal nerve, sacral
		Ø Open
		3 Percutaneous
		4 Percutaneous
		       Endoscopic
			Z No Device	**Z** No Qualifier

Non-OR Ø15[Ø,2,3,4,5,6,9,A,C,D,F,G,H,Q][Ø,3,4]ZZ	**Non-OR** Ø15[1,8,B,R]3ZZ

LC Limited Coverage   NC Noncovered   ⊞ Combination Member   HAC associated procedure   Combination Only   DRG Non-OR   Non-OR   New/Revised in GREEN

ICD-10-PCS 2021   **153**

Peripheral Nervous System

Ø   **Medical and Surgical**
1   **Peripheral Nervous System**
8   **Division**   Definition: Cutting into a body part, without draining fluids and/or gases from the body part, in order to separate or transect a body part
Explanation: All or a portion of the body part is separated into two or more portions

Body Part Character 4		Approach Character 5	Device Character 6	Qualifier Character 7
Ø **Cervical Plexus** Ansa cervicalis Cutaneous (transverse) cervical nerve Great auricular nerve Lesser occipital nerve Supraclavicular nerve Transverse (cutaneous) cervical nerve 1 **Cervical Nerve** Greater occipital nerve Spinal nerve, cervical Suboccipital nerve Third occipital nerve 2 **Phrenic Nerve** Accessory phrenic nerve 3 **Brachial Plexus** Axillary nerve Dorsal scapular nerve First intercostal nerve Long thoracic nerve Musculocutaneous nerve Subclavius nerve Suprascapular nerve 4 **Ulnar Nerve** Cubital nerve 5 **Median Nerve** Anterior interosseous nerve Palmar cutaneous nerve 6 **Radial Nerve** Dorsal digital nerve Musculospiral nerve Palmar cutaneous nerve Posterior interosseous nerve 8 **Thoracic Nerve** Intercostal nerve Intercostobrachial nerve Spinal nerve, thoracic Subcostal nerve 9 **Lumbar Plexus** Accessory obturator nerve Genitofemoral nerve Iliohypogastric nerve Ilioinguinal nerve Lateral femoral cutaneous nerve Obturator nerve Superior gluteal nerve A **Lumbosacral Plexus** B **Lumbar Nerve** Lumbosacral trunk Spinal nerve, lumbar Superior clunic (cluneal) nerve C **Pudendal Nerve** Posterior labial nerve Posterior scrotal nerve D **Femoral Nerve** Anterior crural nerve Saphenous nerve F **Sciatic Nerve** Ischiatic nerve G **Tibial Nerve** Lateral plantar nerve Medial plantar nerve Medial popliteal nerve Medial sural cutaneous nerve	H **Peroneal Nerve** Common fibular nerve Common peroneal nerve External popliteal nerve Lateral sural cutaneous nerve K **Head and Neck Sympathetic Nerve** Cavernous plexus Cervical ganglion Ciliary ganglion Internal carotid plexus Otic ganglion Pterygopalatine (sphenopalatine) ganglion Sphenopalatine (pterygopalatine) ganglion Stellate ganglion Submandibular ganglion Submaxillary ganglion L **Thoracic Sympathetic Nerve** Cardiac plexus Esophageal plexus Greater splanchnic nerve Inferior cardiac nerve Least splanchnic nerve Lesser splanchnic nerve Middle cardiac nerve Pulmonary plexus Superior cardiac nerve Thoracic aortic plexus Thoracic ganglion M **Abdominal Sympathetic Nerve** Abdominal aortic plexus Auerbach's (myenteric) plexus Celiac (solar) plexus Celiac ganglion Gastric plexus Hepatic plexus Inferior hypogastric plexus Inferior mesenteric ganglion Inferior mesenteric plexus Meissner's (submucous) plexus Myenteric (Auerbach's) plexus Pancreatic plexus Pelvic splanchnic nerve Renal nerve Renal plexus Solar (celiac) plexus Splenic plexus Submucous (Meissner's) plexus Superior hypogastric plexus Superior mesenteric ganglion Superior mesenteric plexus Suprarenal plexus N **Lumbar Sympathetic Nerve** Lumbar ganglion Lumbar splanchnic nerve P **Sacral Sympathetic Nerve** Ganglion impar (ganglion of Walther) Pelvic splanchnic nerve Sacral ganglion Sacral splanchnic nerve Q **Sacral Plexus** Inferior gluteal nerve Posterior femoral cutaneous nerve Pudendal nerve R **Sacral Nerve** Spinal nerve, sacral	Ø Open 3 Percutaneous 4 Percutaneous Endoscopic	Z No Device	Z No Qualifier

Ø   Medical and Surgical
1   Peripheral Nervous System
9   Drainage   Definition: Taking or letting out fluids and/or gases from a body part

               Explanation: The qualifier DIAGNOSTIC is used to identify drainage procedures that are biopsies

Body Part Character 4		Approach Character 5	Device Character 6	Qualifier Character 7

Ø Cervical Plexus
Ansa cervicalis
Cutaneous (transverse) cervical
   nerve
Great auricular nerve
Lesser occipital nerve
Supraclavicular nerve
Transverse (cutaneous) cervical
   nerve
1 Cervical Nerve
Greater occipital nerve
Spinal nerve, cervical
Suboccipital nerve
Third occipital nerve
2 Phrenic Nerve
Accessory phrenic nerve
3 Brachial Plexus
Axillary nerve
Dorsal scapular nerve
First intercostal nerve
Long thoracic nerve
Musculocutaneous nerve
Subclavius nerve
Suprascapular nerve
4 Ulnar Nerve
Cubital nerve
5 Median Nerve
Anterior interosseous nerve
Palmar cutaneous nerve
6 Radial Nerve
Dorsal digital nerve
Musculospiral nerve
Palmar cutaneous nerve
Posterior interosseous nerve
8 Thoracic Nerve
Intercostal nerve
Intercostobrachial nerve
Spinal nerve, thoracic
Subcostal nerve
9 Lumbar Plexus
Accessory obturator nerve
Genitofemoral nerve
Iliohypogastric nerve
Ilioinguinal nerve
Lateral femoral cutaneous
   nerve
Obturator nerve
Superior gluteal nerve
A Lumbosacral Plexus
B Lumbar Nerve
Lumbosacral trunk
Spinal nerve, lumbar
Superior clunic (cluneal) nerve
C Pudendal Nerve
Posterior labial nerve
Posterior scrotal nerve
D Femoral Nerve
Anterior crural nerve
Saphenous nerve
F Sciatic Nerve
Ischiatic nerve
G Tibial Nerve
Lateral plantar nerve
Medial plantar nerve
Medial popliteal nerve
Medial sural cutaneous nerve
	H Peroneal Nerve
	Common fibular nerve
	Common peroneal nerve
	External popliteal nerve
	Lateral sural cutaneous nerve
	**K Head and Neck Sympathetic
	Nerve**
	Cavernous plexus
	Cervical ganglion
	Ciliary ganglion
	Internal carotid plexus
	Otic ganglion
	Pterygopalatine
	   (sphenopalatine) ganglion
	Sphenopalatine
	   (pterygopalatine) ganglion
	Stellate ganglion
	Submandibular ganglion
	Submaxillary ganglion
	L Thoracic Sympathetic Nerve
	Cardiac plexus
	Esophageal plexus
	Greater splanchnic nerve
	Inferior cardiac nerve
	Least splanchnic nerve
	Lesser splanchnic nerve
	Middle cardiac nerve
	Pulmonary plexus
	Superior cardiac nerve
	Thoracic aortic plexus
	Thoracic ganglion
	**M Abdominal Sympathetic
	Nerve**
	Abdominal aortic plexus
	Auerbach's (myenteric) plexus
	Celiac (solar) plexus
	Celiac ganglion
	Gastric plexus
	Hepatic plexus
	Inferior hypogastric plexus
	Inferior mesenteric ganglion
	Inferior mesenteric plexus
	Meissner's (submucous) plexus
	Myenteric (Auerbach's) plexus
	Pancreatic plexus
	Pelvic splanchnic nerve
	Renal nerve
	Renal plexus
	Solar (celiac) plexus
	Splenic plexus
	Submucous (Meissner's) plexus
	Superior hypogastric plexus
	Superior mesenteric ganglion
	Superior mesenteric plexus
	Suprarenal plexus
	N Lumbar Sympathetic Nerve
	Lumbar ganglion
	Lumbar splanchnic nerve
	P Sacral Sympathetic Nerve
	Ganglion impar (ganglion of
	   Walther)
	Pelvic splanchnic nerve
	Sacral ganglion
	Sacral splanchnic nerve
	Q Sacral Plexus
	Inferior gluteal nerve
	Posterior femoral cutaneous
	   nerve
	Pudendal nerve
	R Sacral Nerve
	Spinal nerve, sacral
		Ø Open
		3 Percutaneous
		4 Percutaneous Endoscopic
			Ø Drainage Device	**Z No Qualifier**

Non-OR   Ø19[Ø,1,2,3,4,5,6,8,9,A,B,C,D,F,G,H,K,L,M,N,P,Q,R]3ØZ

Ø19 Continued on next page

Peripheral Nervous System

Ø19–Ø19

Ø19 Continued

Ø Medical and Surgical
1 Peripheral Nervous System
9 Drainage   Definition: Taking or letting out fluids and/or gases from a body part

Explanation: The qualifier DIAGNOSTIC is used to identify drainage procedures that are biopsies

Body Part Character 4		Approach Character 5	Device Character 6	Qualifier Character 7

Ø Cervical Plexus
Ansa cervicalis
Cutaneous (transverse) cervical
  nerve
Great auricular nerve
Lesser occipital nerve
Supraclavicular nerve
Transverse (cutaneous) cervical
  nerve
1 Cervical Nerve
Greater occipital nerve
Spinal nerve, cervical
Suboccipital nerve
Third occipital nerve
2 Phrenic Nerve
Accessory phrenic nerve
3 Brachial Plexus
Axillary nerve
Dorsal scapular nerve
First intercostal nerve
Long thoracic nerve
Musculocutaneous nerve
Subclavius nerve
Suprascapular nerve
4 Ulnar Nerve
Cubital nerve
5 Median Nerve
Anterior interosseous nerve
Palmar cutaneous nerve
6 Radial Nerve
Dorsal digital nerve
Musculospiral nerve
Palmar cutaneous nerve
Posterior interosseous nerve
8 Thoracic Nerve
Intercostal nerve
Intercostobrachial nerve
Spinal nerve, thoracic
Subcostal nerve
9 Lumbar Plexus
Accessory obturator nerve
Genitofemoral nerve
Iliohypogastric nerve
Ilioinguinal nerve
Lateral femoral cutaneous
  nerve
Obturator nerve
Superior gluteal nerve
A Lumbosacral Plexus
B Lumbar Nerve
Lumbosacral trunk
Spinal nerve, lumbar
Superior clunic (cluneal) nerve
C Pudendal Nerve
Posterior labial nerve
Posterior scrotal nerve
D Femoral Nerve
Anterior crural nerve
Saphenous nerve
F Sciatic Nerve
Ischiatic nerve
G Tibial Nerve
Lateral plantar nerve
Medial plantar nerve
Medial popliteal nerve
Medial sural cutaneous nerve
	H Peroneal Nerve
	Common fibular nerve
	Common peroneal nerve
	External popliteal nerve
	Lateral sural cutaneous nerve
	K Head and Neck Sympathetic
	Nerve
	Cavernous plexus
	Cervical ganglion
	Ciliary ganglion
	Internal carotid plexus
	Otic ganglion
	Pterygopalatine
	  (sphenopalatine) ganglion
	Sphenopalatine
	  (pterygopalatine) ganglion
	Stellate ganglion
	Submandibular ganglion
	Submaxillary ganglion
	L Thoracic Sympathetic Nerve
	Cardiac plexus
	Esophageal plexus
	Greater splanchnic nerve
	Inferior cardiac nerve
	Least splanchnic nerve
	Lesser splanchnic nerve
	Middle cardiac nerve
	Pulmonary plexus
	Superior cardiac nerve
	Thoracic aortic plexus
	Thoracic ganglion
	M Abdominal Sympathetic
	Nerve
	Abdominal aortic plexus
	Auerbach's (myenteric) plexus
	Celiac (solar) plexus
	Celiac ganglion
	Gastric plexus
	Hepatic plexus
	Inferior hypogastric plexus
	Inferior mesenteric ganglion
	Inferior mesenteric plexus
	Meissner's (submucous) plexus
	Myenteric (Auerbach's) plexus
	Pancreatic plexus
	Pelvic splanchnic nerve
	Renal nerve
	Renal plexus
	Solar (celiac) plexus
	Splenic plexus
	Submucous (Meissner's) plexus
	Superior hypogastric plexus
	Superior mesenteric ganglion
	Superior mesenteric plexus
	Suprarenal plexus
	N Lumbar Sympathetic Nerve
	Lumbar ganglion
	Lumbar splanchnic nerve
	P Sacral Sympathetic Nerve
	Ganglion impar (ganglion of
	  Walther)
	Pelvic splanchnic nerve
	Sacral ganglion
	Sacral splanchnic nerve
	Q Sacral Plexus
	Inferior gluteal nerve
	Posterior femoral cutaneous
	  nerve
	Pudendal nerve
	R Sacral Nerve
	Spinal nerve, sacral
		Ø Open
		3 Percutaneous
		4 Percutaneous Endoscopic
			Z No Device	**X Diagnostic**
				Z No Qualifier

Non-OR	Ø19[Ø,1,2,3,4,5,6,8,9,A,B,C,D,F,G,H,Q,R][3,4]ZX
Non-OR	Ø19[Ø,1,2,3,4,5,6,8,9,A,B,C,D,F,G,H,K,L,M,N,P,Q,R]3ZZ

LC Limited Coverage   NC Noncovered   ⊞ Combination Member   HAC associated procedure   Combination Only   DRG Non-OR   Non-OR   New/Revised in GREEN

156   ICD-10-PCS 2021

Ø **Medical and Surgical**
1 **Peripheral Nervous System**
B **Excision**　　　　Definition: Cutting out or off, without replacement, a portion of a body part
　　　　　　　　　　　Explanation: The qualifier DIAGNOSTIC is used to identify excision procedures that are biopsies

Body Part Character 4		Approach Character 5	Device Character 6	Qualifier Character 7
Ø Cervical Plexus 　Ansa cervicalis 　Cutaneous (transverse) cervical 　　nerve 　Great auricular nerve 　Lesser occipital nerve 　Supraclavicular nerve 　Transverse (cutaneous) cervical 　　nerve **1** Cervical Nerve 　Greater occipital nerve 　Spinal nerve, cervical 　Suboccipital nerve 　Third occipital nerve **2** Phrenic Nerve 　Accessory phrenic nerve **3** Brachial Plexus 　Axillary nerve 　Dorsal scapular nerve 　First intercostal nerve 　Long thoracic nerve 　Musculocutaneous nerve 　Subclavius nerve 　Suprascapular nerve **4** Ulnar Nerve 　Cubital nerve **5** Median Nerve 　Anterior interosseous nerve 　Palmar cutaneous nerve **6** Radial Nerve 　Dorsal digital nerve 　Musculospiral nerve 　Palmar cutaneous nerve 　Posterior interosseous nerve **8** Thoracic Nerve 　Intercostal nerve 　Intercostobrachial nerve 　Spinal nerve, thoracic 　Subcostal nerve **9** Lumbar Plexus 　Accessory obturator nerve 　Genitofemoral nerve 　Iliohypogastric nerve 　Ilioinguinal nerve 　Lateral femoral cutaneous 　　nerve 　Obturator nerve 　Superior gluteal nerve **A** Lumbosacral Plexus **B** Lumbar Nerve 　Lumbosacral trunk 　Spinal nerve, lumbar 　Superior clunic (cluneal) nerve **C** Pudendal Nerve 　Posterior labial nerve 　Posterior scrotal nerve **D** Femoral Nerve 　Anterior crural nerve 　Saphenous nerve **F** Sciatic Nerve 　Ischiatic nerve **G** Tibial Nerve 　Lateral plantar nerve 　Medial plantar nerve 　Medial popliteal nerve 　Medial sural cutaneous nerve	**H** Peroneal Nerve 　Common fibular nerve 　Common peroneal nerve 　External popliteal nerve 　Lateral sural cutaneous nerve **K** Head and Neck Sympathetic 　Nerve 　Cavernous plexus 　Cervical ganglion 　Ciliary ganglion 　Internal carotid plexus 　Otic ganglion 　Pterygopalatine 　　(sphenopalatine) ganglion 　Sphenopalatine 　　(pterygopalatine) ganglion 　Stellate ganglion 　Submandibular ganglion 　Submaxillary ganglion **L** Thoracic Sympathetic 　Nerve 　Cardiac plexus 　Esophageal plexus 　Greater splanchnic nerve 　Inferior cardiac nerve 　Least splanchnic nerve 　Lesser splanchnic nerve 　Middle cardiac nerve 　Pulmonary plexus 　Superior cardiac nerve 　Thoracic aortic plexus 　Thoracic ganglion **M** Abdominal Sympathetic 　Nerve 　Abdominal aortic plexus 　Auerbach's (myenteric) plexus 　Celiac (solar) plexus 　Celiac ganglion 　Gastric plexus 　Hepatic plexus 　Inferior hypogastric plexus 　Inferior mesenteric ganglion 　Inferior mesenteric plexus 　Meissner's (submucous) plexus 　Myenteric (Auerbach's) plexus 　Pancreatic plexus 　Pelvic splanchnic nerve 　Renal nerve 　Renal plexus 　Solar (celiac) plexus 　Splenic plexus 　Submucous (Meissner's) plexus 　Superior hypogastric plexus 　Superior mesenteric ganglion 　Superior mesenteric plexus 　Suprarenal plexus **N** Lumbar Sympathetic Nerve 　Lumbar ganglion 　Lumbar splanchnic nerve **P** Sacral Sympathetic Nerve 　Ganglion impar (ganglion of 　　Walther) 　Pelvic splanchnic nerve 　Sacral ganglion 　Sacral splanchnic nerve **Q** Sacral Plexus 　Inferior gluteal nerve 　Posterior femoral cutaneous 　　nerve 　Pudendal nerve **R** Sacral Nerve 　Spinal nerve, sacral	**Ø** Open **3** Percutaneous **4** Percutaneous Endoscopic	**Z** No Device	**X** Diagnostic **Z** No Qualifier

Non-OR Ø1B[Ø,1,2,3,4,5,6,8,9,A,B,C,D,F,G,H,Q,R][3,4]ZX

LC Limited Coverage　**NC** Noncovered　⊞ Combination Member　HAC associated procedure　Combination Only　DRG Non-OR　Non-OR　New/Revised in **GREEN**

ICD-10-PCS 2021　　　　　　　　　　　　　　　　　　　　　　　　　　　　　　　　　　　　　　**157**

Peripheral Nervous System

0   **Medical and Surgical**
1   **Peripheral Nervous System**
C   **Extirpation**   Definition: Taking or cutting out solid matter from a body part

Explanation: The solid matter may be an abnormal byproduct of a biological function or a foreign body; it may be imbedded in a body part or in the lumen of a tubular body part. The solid matter may or may not have been previously broken into pieces.

Body Part Character 4		Approach Character 5	Device Character 6	Qualifier Character 7

0 Cervical Plexus
Ansa cervicalis
Cutaneous (transverse) cervical
  nerve
Great auricular nerve
Lesser occipital nerve
Supraclavicular nerve
Transverse (cutaneous) cervical
  nerve
1 Cervical Nerve
Greater occipital nerve
Spinal nerve, cervical
Suboccipital nerve
Third occipital nerve
2 Phrenic Nerve
Accessory phrenic nerve
3 Brachial Plexus
Axillary nerve
Dorsal scapular nerve
First intercostal nerve
Long thoracic nerve
Musculocutaneous nerve
Subclavius nerve
Suprascapular nerve
4 Ulnar Nerve
Cubital nerve
5 Median Nerve
Anterior interosseous nerve
Palmar cutaneous nerve
6 Radial Nerve
Dorsal digital nerve
Musculospiral nerve
Palmar cutaneous nerve
Posterior interosseous nerve
8 Thoracic Nerve
Intercostal nerve
Intercostobrachial nerve
Spinal nerve, thoracic
Subcostal nerve
9 Lumbar Plexus
Accessory obturator nerve
Genitofemoral nerve
Iliohypogastric nerve
Ilioinguinal nerve
Lateral femoral cutaneous
  nerve
Obturator nerve
Superior gluteal nerve
A Lumbosacral Plexus
B Lumbar Nerve
Lumbosacral trunk
Spinal nerve, lumbar
Superior clunic (cluneal) nerve
C Pudendal Nerve
Posterior labial nerve
Posterior scrotal nerve
D Femoral Nerve
Anterior crural nerve
Saphenous nerve
F Sciatic Nerve
Ischiatic nerve
G Tibial Nerve
Lateral plantar nerve
Medial plantar nerve
Medial popliteal nerve
Medial sural cutaneous nerve
	H Peroneal Nerve
	Common fibular nerve
	Common peroneal nerve
	External popliteal nerve
	Lateral sural cutaneous nerve
	K Head and Neck Sympathetic
	  Nerve
	Cavernous plexus
	Cervical ganglion
	Ciliary ganglion
	Internal carotid plexus
	Otic ganglion
	Pterygopalatine
	  (sphenopalatine) ganglion
	Sphenopalatine
	  (pterygopalatine) ganglion
	Stellate ganglion
	Submandibular ganglion
	Submaxillary ganglion
	L Thoracic Sympathetic Nerve
	Cardiac plexus
	Esophageal plexus
	Greater splanchnic nerve
	Inferior cardiac nerve
	Least splanchnic nerve
	Lesser splanchnic nerve
	Middle cardiac nerve
	Pulmonary plexus
	Superior cardiac nerve
	Thoracic aortic plexus
	Thoracic ganglion
	M Abdominal Sympathetic
	  Nerve
	Abdominal aortic plexus
	Auerbach's (myenteric) plexus
	Celiac (solar) plexus
	Celiac ganglion
	Gastric plexus
	Hepatic plexus
	Inferior hypogastric plexus
	Inferior mesenteric ganglion
	Inferior mesenteric plexus
	Meissner's (submucous) plexus
	Myenteric (Auerbach's) plexus
	Pancreatic plexus
	Pelvic splanchnic nerve
	Renal nerve
	Renal plexus
	Solar (celiac) plexus
	Splenic plexus
	Submucous (Meissner's) plexus
	Superior hypogastric plexus
	Superior mesenteric ganglion
	Superior mesenteric plexus
	Suprarenal plexus
	N Lumbar Sympathetic Nerve
	Lumbar ganglion
	Lumbar splanchnic nerve
	P Sacral Sympathetic Nerve
	Ganglion impar (ganglion of
	  Walther)
	Pelvic splanchnic nerve
	Sacral ganglion
	Sacral splanchnic nerve
	Q Sacral Plexus
	Inferior gluteal nerve
	Posterior femoral cutaneous
	  nerve
	Pudendal nerve
	R Sacral Nerve
	Spinal nerve, sacral
		0 Open
		3 Percutaneous
		4 Percutaneous Endoscopic
			Z No Device	**Z** No Qualifier

Ø   Medical and Surgical
1   Peripheral Nervous System
D   Extraction   Definition: Pulling or stripping out or off all or a portion of a body part by the use of force

                Explanation: The qualifier DIAGNOSTIC is used to identify extraction procedures that are biopsies

Body Part Character 4	Approach Character 5	Device Character 6	Qualifier Character 7
Ø Cervical Plexus Ansa cervicalis Cutaneous (transverse) cervical nerve Great auricular nerve Lesser occipital nerve Supraclavicular nerve Transverse (cutaneous) cervical nerve **1 Cervical Nerve** Greater occipital nerve Spinal nerve, cervical Suboccipital nerve Third occipital nerve **2 Phrenic Nerve** Accessory phrenic nerve **3 Brachial Plexus** Axillary nerve Dorsal scapular nerve First intercostal nerve Long thoracic nerve Musculocutaneous nerve Subclavius nerve Suprascapular nerve **4 Ulnar Nerve** Cubital nerve **5 Median Nerve** Anterior interosseous nerve Palmar cutaneous nerve **6 Radial Nerve** Dorsal digital nerve Musculospiral nerve Palmar cutaneous nerve Posterior interosseous nerve **8 Thoracic Nerve** Intercostal nerve Intercostobrachial nerve Spinal nerve, thoracic Subcostal nerve **9 Lumbar Plexus** Accessory obturator nerve Genitofemoral nerve Iliohypogastric nerve Ilioinguinal nerve Lateral femoral cutaneous nerve Obturator nerve Superior gluteal nerve **A Lumbosacral Plexus** **B Lumbar Nerve** Lumbosacral trunk Spinal nerve, lumbar Superior clunic (cluneal) nerve **C Pudendal Nerve]** Posterior labial nerve Posterior scrotal nerve **D Femoral Nerve** Anterior crural nerve Saphenous nerve **F Sciatic Nerve** Ischiatic nerve **G Tibial Nerve** Lateral plantar nerve Medial plantar nerve Medial popliteal nerve Medial sural cutaneous nerve	**Ø Open** **3 Percutaneous** **4 Percutaneous Endoscopic**	**Z No Device**	**Z No Qualifier**
H Peroneal Nerve Common fibular nerve Common peroneal nerve External popliteal nerve Lateral sural cutaneous nerve **K Head and Neck Sympathetic Nerve** Cavernous plexus Cervical ganglion Ciliary ganglion Internal carotid plexus Otic ganglion Pterygopalatine (sphenopalatine) ganglion Sphenopalatine (pterygopalatine) ganglion Stellate ganglion Submandibular ganglion Submaxillary ganglion **L Thoracic Sympathetic Nerve** Cardiac plexus Esophageal plexus Greater splanchnic nerve Inferior cardiac nerve Least splanchnic nerve Lesser splanchnic nerve Middle cardiac nerve Pulmonary plexus Superior cardiac nerve Thoracic aortic plexus Thoracic ganglion **M Abdominal Sympathetic Nerve** Abdominal aortic plexus Auerbach's (myenteric) plexus Celiac (solar) plexus Celiac ganglion Gastric plexus Hepatic plexus Inferior hypogastric plexus Inferior mesenteric ganglion Inferior mesenteric plexus Meissner's (submucous) plexus Myenteric (Auerbach's) plexus Pancreatic plexus Pelvic splanchnic nerve Renal nerve Renal plexus Solar (celiac) plexus Splenic plexus Submucous (Meissner's) plexus Superior hypogastric plexus Superior mesenteric ganglion Superior mesenteric plexus Suprarenal plexus **N Lumbar Sympathetic Nerve** Lumbar ganglion Lumbar splanchnic nerve **P Sacral Sympathetic Nerve** Ganglion impar (ganglion of Walther) Pelvic splanchnic nerve Sacral ganglion Sacral splanchnic nerve **Q Sacral Plexus** Inferior gluteal nerve Posterior femoral cutaneous nerve Pudendal nerve **R Sacral Nerve** Spinal nerve, sacral			

LC Limited Coverage   **NC** Noncovered   ⊞ Combination Member   HAC associated procedure   Combination Only   DRG Non-OR   Non-OR   New/Revised in **GREEN**

ICD-10-PCS 2021   159

Ø **Medical and Surgical**
1 **Peripheral Nervous System**
H **Insertion**   Definition: Putting in a nonbiological appliance that monitors, assists, performs, or prevents a physiological function but does not physically take the place of a body part

                 Explanation: None

Body Part Character 4	Approach Character 5	Device Character 6	Qualifier Character 7
Y Peripheral Nerve ⊞	Ø Open 3 Percutaneous 4 Percutaneous Endoscopic	1 Radioactive Element 2 Monitoring Device M Neurostimulator Lead Y Other Device	Z No Qualifier

Non-OR	Ø1HY[3,4]YZ		See Appendix L for Procedure Combinations ⊞ Ø1HY[Ø,3,4]MZ

Ø **Medical and Surgical**
1 **Peripheral Nervous System**
J **Inspection**   Definition: Visually and/or manually exploring a body part

                 Explanation: Visual exploration may be performed with or without optical instrumentation. Manual exploration may be performed directly or through intervening body layers.

Body Part Character 4	Approach Character 5	Device Character 6	Qualifier Character 7
Y Peripheral Nerve	Ø Open 3 Percutaneous 4 Percutaneous Endoscopic	Z No Device	Z No Qualifier

Non-OR	Ø1JY3ZZ

0   **Medical and Surgical**
1   **Peripheral Nervous System**
N   **Release**   Definition: Freeing a body part from an abnormal physical constraint by cutting or by the use of force
                        Explanation: Some of the restraining tissue may be taken out but none of the body part is taken out

Body Part Character 4		Approach Character 5	Device Character 6	Qualifier Character 7
0 **Cervical Plexus** Ansa cervicalis Cutaneous (transverse) cervical nerve Great auricular nerve Lesser occipital nerve Supraclavicular nerve Transverse (cutaneous) cervical nerve **1** **Cervical Nerve** Greater occipital nerve Spinal nerve, cervical Suboccipital nerve Third occipital nerve **2** **Phrenic Nerve** Accessory phrenic nerve **3** **Brachial Plexus** Axillary nerve Dorsal scapular nerve First intercostal nerve Long thoracic nerve Musculocutaneous nerve Subclavius nerve Suprascapular nerve **4** **Ulnar Nerve** Cubital nerve **5** **Median Nerve** Anterior interosseous nerve Palmar cutaneous nerve **6** **Radial Nerve** Dorsal digital nerve Musculospiral nerve Palmar cutaneous nerve Posterior interosseous nerve **8** **Thoracic Nerve** Intercostal nerve Intercostobrachial nerve Spinal nerve, thoracic Subcostal nerve **9** **Lumbar Plexus** Accessory obturator nerve Genitofemoral nerve Iliohypogastric nerve Ilioinguinal nerve Lateral femoral cutaneous nerve Obturator nerve Superior gluteal nerve **A** **Lumbosacral Plexus** **B** **Lumbar Nerve** Lumbosacral trunk Spinal nerve, lumbar Superior clunic (cluneal) nerve **C** **Pudendal Nerve** Posterior labial nerve Posterior scrotal nerve **D** **Femoral Nerve** Anterior crural nerve Saphenous nerve **F** **Sciatic Nerve** Ischiatic nerve **G** **Tibial Nerve** Lateral plantar nerve Medial plantar nerve Medial popliteal nerve Medial sural cutaneous nerve	**H** **Peroneal Nerve** Common fibular nerve Common peroneal nerve External popliteal nerve Lateral sural cutaneous nerve **K** **Head and Neck Sympathetic Nerve** Cavernous plexus Cervical ganglion Ciliary ganglion Internal carotid plexus Otic ganglion Pterygopalatine (sphenopalatine) ganglion Sphenopalatine (pterygopalatine) ganglion Stellate ganglion Submandibular ganglion Submaxillary ganglion **L** **Thoracic Sympathetic Nerve** Cardiac plexus Esophageal plexus Greater splanchnic nerve Inferior cardiac nerve Least splanchnic nerve Lesser splanchnic nerve Middle cardiac nerve Pulmonary plexus Superior cardiac nerve Thoracic aortic plexus Thoracic ganglion **M** **Abdominal Sympathetic Nerve** Abdominal aortic plexus Auerbach's (myenteric) plexus Celiac (solar) plexus Celiac ganglion Gastric plexus Hepatic plexus Inferior hypogastric plexus Inferior mesenteric ganglion Inferior mesenteric plexus Meissner's (submucous) plexus Myenteric (Auerbach's) plexus Pancreatic plexus Pelvic splanchnic nerve Renal nerve Renal plexus Solar (celiac) plexus Splenic plexus Submucous (Meissner's) plexus Superior hypogastric plexus Superior mesenteric ganglion Superior mesenteric plexus Suprarenal plexus **N** **Lumbar Sympathetic Nerve** Lumbar ganglion Lumbar splanchnic nerve **P** **Sacral Sympathetic Nerve** Ganglion impar (ganglion of Walther) Pelvic splanchnic nerve Sacral ganglion Sacral splanchnic nerve **Q** **Sacral Plexus** Inferior gluteal nerve Posterior femoral cutaneous nerve Pudendal nerve **R** **Sacral Nerve** Spinal nerve, sacral	**0** Open **3** Percutaneous **4** Percutaneous Endoscopic	**Z** No Device	**Z** No Qualifier

LC Limited Coverage   **NC** Noncovered   ⊞ Combination Member   HAC associated procedure   Combination Only   DRG Non-OR   Non-OR   New/Revised in GREEN

ICD-10-PCS 2021   161

Ø   Medical and Surgical
1   Peripheral Nervous System
P   Removal   Definition: Taking out or off a device from a body part

Explanation: If a device is taken out and a similar device put in without cutting or puncturing the skin or mucous membrane, the procedure is coded to the root operation CHANGE. Otherwise, the procedure for taking out a device is coded to the root operation REMOVAL.

Body Part Character 4	Approach Character 5	Device Character 6	Qualifier Character 7
Y Peripheral Nerve	**Ø** Open **3** Percutaneous **4** Percutaneous Endoscopic	**Ø** Drainage Device **2** Monitoring Device **7** Autologous Tissue Substitute **M** Neurostimulator Lead **Y** Other Device	**Z** No Qualifier
Y Peripheral Nerve	**X** External	**Ø** Drainage Device **2** Monitoring Device **M** Neurostimulator Lead	**Z** No Qualifier

Non-OR   Ø1PY3[Ø,2]Z
Non-OR   Ø1PY[3,4]YZ
Non-OR   Ø1PYX[Ø,2,M]Z

LC Limited Coverage   NC Noncovered   ⊞ Combination Member   HAC associated procedure   Combination Only   DRG Non-OR   Non-OR   New/Revised in GREEN

162   ICD-10-PCS 2021

Ø   Medical and Surgical
1   Peripheral Nervous System
Q   Repair   Definition: Restoring, to the extent possible, a body part to its normal anatomic structure and function
                           Explanation: Used only when the method to accomplish the repair is not one of the other root operations

Body Part Character 4		Approach Character 5	Device Character 6	Qualifier Character 7

Ø   Cervical Plexus
   Ansa cervicalis
   Cutaneous (transverse) cervical
     nerve
   Great auricular nerve
   Lesser occipital nerve
   Supraclavicular nerve
   Transverse (cutaneous) cervical
     nerve
1   Cervical Nerve
   Greater occipital nerve
   Spinal nerve, cervical
   Suboccipital nerve
   Third occipital nerve
2   Phrenic Nerve
   Accessory phrenic nerve
3   Brachial Plexus
   Axillary nerve
   Dorsal scapular nerve
   First intercostal nerve
   Long thoracic nerve
   Musculocutaneous nerve
   Subclavius nerve
   Suprascapular nerve
4   Ulnar Nerve
   Cubital nerve
5   Median Nerve
   Anterior interosseous nerve
   Palmar cutaneous nerve
6   Radial Nerve
   Dorsal digital nerve
   Musculospiral nerve
   Palmar cutaneous nerve
   Posterior interosseous nerve
8   Thoracic Nerve
   Intercostal nerve
   Intercostobrachial nerve
   Spinal nerve, thoracic
   Subcostal nerve
9   Lumbar Plexus
   Accessory obturator nerve
   Genitofemoral nerve
   Iliohypogastric nerve
   Ilioinguinal nerve
   Lateral femoral cutaneous
     nerve
   Obturator nerve
   Superior gluteal nerve
A   Lumbosacral Plexus
B   Lumbar Nerve
   Lumbosacral trunk
   Spinal nerve, lumbar
   Superior clunic (cluneal) nerve
C   Pudendal Nerve
   Posterior labial nerve
   Posterior scrotal nerve
D   Femoral Nerve
   Anterior crural nerve
   Saphenous nerve
F   Sciatic Nerve
   Ischiatic nerve
G   Tibial Nerve
   Lateral plantar nerve
   Medial plantar nerve
   Medial popliteal nerve
   Medial sural cutaneous nerve
	H Peroneal Nerve
	   Common fibular nerve
	   Common peroneal nerve
	   External popliteal nerve
	   Lateral sural cutaneous nerve
	K Head and Neck Sympathetic
	     Nerve
	   Cavernous plexus
	   Cervical ganglion
	   Ciliary ganglion
	   Internal carotid plexus
	   Otic ganglion
	   Pterygopalatine
	     (sphenopalatine) ganglion
	   Sphenopalatine
	     (pterygopalatine) ganglion
	   Stellate ganglion
	   Submandibular ganglion
	   Submaxillary ganglion
	L Thoracic Sympathetic Nerve
	   Cardiac plexus
	   Esophageal plexus
	   Greater splanchnic nerve
	   Inferior cardiac nerve
	   Least splanchnic nerve
	   Lesser splanchnic nerve
	   Middle cardiac nerve
	   Pulmonary plexus
	   Superior cardiac nerve
	   Thoracic aortic plexus
	   Thoracic ganglion
	M Abdominal Sympathetic
	     Nerve
	   Abdominal aortic plexus
	   Auerbach's (myenteric) plexus
	   Celiac (solar) plexus
	   Celiac ganglion
	   Gastric plexus
	   Hepatic plexus
	   Inferior hypogastric plexus
	   Inferior mesenteric ganglion
	   Inferior mesenteric plexus
	   Meissner's (submucous) plexus
	   Myenteric (Auerbach's) plexus
	   Pancreatic plexus
	   Pelvic splanchnic nerve
	   Renal nerve
	   Renal plexus
	   Solar (celiac) plexus
	   Splenic plexus
	   Submucous (Meissner's) plexus
	   Superior hypogastric plexus
	   Superior mesenteric ganglion
	   Superior mesenteric plexus
	   Suprarenal plexus
	N Lumbar Sympathetic Nerve
	   Lumbar ganglion
	   Lumbar splanchnic nerve
	P Sacral Sympathetic Nerve
	   Ganglion impar (ganglion of
	     Walther)
	   Pelvic splanchnic nerve
	   Sacral ganglion
	   Sacral splanchnic nerve
	Q Sacral Plexus
	   Inferior gluteal nerve
	   Posterior femoral cutaneous
	     nerve
	   Pudendal nerve
	R Sacral Nerve
	   Spinal nerve, sacral
		Ø Open
		3 Percutaneous
		4 Percutaneous Endoscopic
			Z No Device	**Z No Qualifier**

LC Limited Coverage   **NC** Noncovered   ⊞ Combination Member   HAC associated procedure   Combination Only   DRG Non-OR   Non-OR   New/Revised in GREEN

ICD-10-PCS 2021   163

Peripheral Nervous System

0   Medical and Surgical
1   Peripheral Nervous System
R   Replacement   Definition: Putting in or on biological or synthetic material that physically takes the place and/or function of all or a portion of a body part

Explanation: The body part may have been taken out or replaced, or may be taken out, physically eradicated, or rendered nonfunctional during the REPLACEMENT procedure. A REMOVAL procedure is coded for taking out the device used in a previous replacement procedure.

Body Part Character 4	Approach Character 5	Device Character 6	Qualifier Character 7
1 Cervical Nerve Greater occipital nerve Spinal nerve, cervical Suboccipital nerve Third occipital nerve **2 Phrenic Nerve** Accessory phrenic nerve **4 Ulnar Nerve** Cubital nerve **5 Median Nerve** Anterior interosseous nerve Palmar cutaneous nerve **6 Radial Nerve** Dorsal digital nerve Musculospiral nerve Palmar cutaneous nerve Posterior interosseous nerve **8 Thoracic Nerve** Intercostal nerve Intercostobrachial nerve Spinal nerve, thoracic Subcostal nerve **B Lumbar Nerve** Lumbosacral trunk Spinal nerve, lumbar Superior clunic (cluneal) nerve **C Pudendal Nerve** Posterior labial nerve Posterior scrotal nerve **D Femoral Nerve** Anterior crural nerve Saphenous nerve **F Sciatic Nerve** Ischiatic nerve **G Tibial Nerve** Lateral plantar nerve Medial plantar nerve Medial popliteal nerve Medial sural cutaneous nerve **H Peroneal Nerve** Common fibular nerve Common peroneal nerve External popliteal nerve Lateral sural cutaneous nerve **R Sacral Nerve** Spinal nerve, sacral	**0 Open** **4 Percutaneous Endoscopic**	**7 Autologous Tissue Substitute** **J Synthetic Substitute** **K Nonautologous Tissue Substitute**	**Z No Qualifier**

0   **Medical and Surgical**
1   **Peripheral Nervous System**
S   **Reposition**   Definition: Moving to its normal location, or other suitable location, all or a portion of a body part

Explanation: The body part is moved to a new location from an abnormal location, or from a normal location where it is not functioning correctly. The body part may or may not be cut out or off to be moved to the new location.

Body Part Character 4	Approach Character 5	Device Character 6	Qualifier Character 7
0 Cervical Plexus Ansa cervicalis Cutaneous (transverse) cervical nerve Great auricular nerve Lesser occipital nerve Supraclavicular nerve Transverse (cutaneous) cervical nerve **1 Cervical Nerve** Greater occipital nerve Spinal nerve, cervical Suboccipital nerve Third occipital nerve **2 Phrenic Nerve** Accessory phrenic nerve **3 Brachial Plexus** Axillary nerve Dorsal scapular nerve First intercostal nerve Long thoracic nerve Musculocutaneous nerve Subclavius nerve Suprascapular nerve **4 Ulnar Nerve** Cubital nerve **5 Median Nerve** Anterior interosseous nerve Palmar cutaneous nerve **6 Radial Nerve** Dorsal digital nerve Musculospiral nerve Palmar cutaneous nerve Posterior interosseous nerve **8 Thoracic Nerve** Intercostal nerve Intercostobrachial nerve Spinal nerve, thoracic Subcostal nerve **9 Lumbar Plexus** Accessory obturator nerve Genitofemoral nerve Iliohypogastric nerve Ilioinguinal nerve Lateral femoral cutaneous nerve Obturator nerve Superior gluteal nerve **A Lumbosacral Plexus** **B Lumbar Nerve** Lumbosacral trunk Spinal nerve, lumbar Superior clunic (cluneal) nerve **C Pudendal Nerve** Posterior labial nerve Posterior scrotal nerve **D Femoral Nerve** Anterior crural nerve Saphenous nerve **F Sciatic Nerve** Ischiatic nerve **G Tibial Nerve** Lateral plantar nerve Medial plantar nerve Medial popliteal nerve Medial sural cutaneous nerve **H Peroneal Nerve** Common fibular nerve Common peroneal nerve External popliteal nerve Lateral sural cutaneous nerve **Q Sacral Plexus** Inferior gluteal nerve Posterior femoral cutaneous nerve Pudendal nerve **R Sacral Nerve** Spinal nerve, sacral	**0 Open** **3 Percutaneous** **4 Percutaneous Endoscopic**	**Z No Device**	**Z No Qualifier**

LC Limited Coverage   **NC** Noncovered   ⊞ Combination Member   HAC associated procedure   Combination Only   DRG Non-OR   Non-OR   New/Revised in GREEN

ICD-10-PCS 2021   165

01S–01S

Peripheral Nervous System

Ø   Medical and Surgical
1   Peripheral Nervous System
U   Supplement   Definition: Putting in or on biological or synthetic material that physically reinforces and/or augments the function of a portion of a body part
                        Explanation: The biological material is non-living, or is living and from the same individual. The body part may have been previously replaced, and the SUPPLEMENT procedure is performed to physically reinforce and/or augment the function of the replaced body part.

Body Part Character 4	Approach Character 5	Device Character 6	Qualifier Character 7

1   Cervical Nerve
    Greater occipital nerve
    Spinal nerve, cervical
    Suboccipital nerve
    Third occipital nerve
2   Phrenic Nerve
    Accessory phrenic nerve
4   Ulnar Nerve
    Cubital nerve
5   Median Nerve
    Anterior interosseous nerve
    Palmar cutaneous nerve
6   Radial Nerve
    Dorsal digital nerve
    Musculospiral nerve
    Palmar cutaneous nerve
    Posterior interosseous nerve
8   Thoracic Nerve
    Intercostal nerve
    Intercostobrachial nerve
    Spinal nerve, thoracic
    Subcostal nerve
B   Lumbar Nerve
    Lumbosacral trunk
    Spinal nerve, lumbar
    Superior clunic (cluneal) nerve
C   Pudendal Nerve
    Posterior labial nerve
    Posterior scrotal nerve
D   Femoral Nerve
    Anterior crural nerve
    Saphenous nerve
F   Sciatic Nerve
    Ischiatic nerve
G   Tibial Nerve
    Lateral plantar nerve
    Medial plantar nerve
    Medial popliteal nerve
    Medial sural cutaneous nerve
H   Peroneal Nerve
    Common fibular nerve
    Common peroneal nerve
    External popliteal nerve
    Lateral sural cutaneous nerve
R   Sacral Nerve
    Spinal nerve, sacral
	Ø Open
	3 Percutaneous
	4 Percutaneous Endoscopic
		7 Autologous Tissue Substitute
		J Synthetic Substitute
		K Nonautologous Tissue Substitute
			Z No Qualifier

Ø   Medical and Surgical
1   Peripheral Nervous System
W   Revision   Definition: Correcting, to the extent possible, a portion of a malfunctioning device or the position of a displaced device
                      Explanation: Revision can include correcting a malfunctioning or displaced device by taking out or putting in components of the device such as a screw or pin

Body Part Character 4	Approach Character 5	Device Character 6	Qualifier Character 7
Y Peripheral Nerve	**Ø Open** **3 Percutaneous** **4 Percutaneous Endoscopic**	**Ø Drainage Device** **2 Monitoring Device** **7 Autologous Tissue Substitute** **M Neurostimulator Lead** **Y Other Device**	**Z No Qualifier**
Y Peripheral Nerve	**X External**	**Ø Drainage Device** **2 Monitoring Device** **7 Autologous Tissue Substitute** **M Neurostimulator Lead**	**Z No Qualifier**

Non-OR	Ø1WY[3,4]YZ
Non-OR	Ø1WYX[Ø,2,7,M]Z

0   **Medical and Surgical**
1   **Peripheral Nervous System**
X   **Transfer**   Definition: Moving, without taking out, all or a portion of a body part to another location to take over the function of all or a portion of a body part
                 Explanation: The body part transferred remains connected to its vascular and nervous supply

Body Part Character 4	Approach Character 5	Device Character 6	Qualifier Character 7

1 **Cervical Nerve**
   Greater occipital nerve
   Spinal nerve, cervical
   Suboccipital nerve
   Third occipital nerve
2 **Phrenic Nerve**
   Accessory phrenic nerve
	0 Open
	4 Percutaneous Endoscopic
		Z No Device	**1** Cervical Nerve
			2 Phrenic Nerve

4 **Ulnar Nerve**
   Cubital nerve
5 **Median Nerve**
   Anterior interosseous nerve
   Palmar cutaneous nerve
6 **Radial Nerve**
   Dorsal digital nerve
   Musculospiral nerve
   Palmar cutaneous nerve
   Posterior interosseous nerve
	0 Open
	4 Percutaneous Endoscopic
		Z No Device	**4** Ulnar Nerve
			5 Median Nerve
			6 Radial Nerve

8 **Thoracic Nerve**
   Intercostal nerve
   Intercostobrachial nerve
   Spinal nerve, thoracic
   Subcostal nerve
	0 Open
	4 Percutaneous Endoscopic
		Z No Device	**8** Thoracic Nerve

B **Lumbar Nerve**
   Lumbosacral trunk
   Spinal nerve, lumbar
   Superior clunic (cluneal) nerve
C **Pudendal Nerve**
   Posterior labial nerve
   Posterior scrotal nerve
	0 Open
	4 Percutaneous Endoscopic
		Z No Device	**B** Lumbar Nerve
			C Perineal Nerve

D **Femoral Nerve**
   Anterior crural nerve
   Saphenous nerve
F **Sciatic Nerve**
   Ischiatic nerve
G **Tibial Nerve**
   Lateral plantar nerve
   Medial plantar nerve
   Medial popliteal nerve
   Medial sural cutaneous nerve
H **Peroneal Nerve**
   Common fibular nerve
   Common peroneal nerve
   External popliteal nerve
   Lateral sural cutaneous nerve
	0 Open
	4 Percutaneous Endoscopic
		Z No Device	**D** Femoral Nerve
			F Sciatic Nerve
			G Tibial Nerve
			H Peroneal Nerve

Heart and Great Vessels Ø21–Ø2Y

Character Meanings

This Character Meaning table is provided as a guide to assist the user in the identification of character members that may be found in this section of code tables. It **SHOULD NOT** be used to build a PCS code.

Operation–Character 3	Body Part–Character 4	Approach–Character 5	Device–Character 6	Qualifier–Character 7
1 Bypass	Ø Coronary Artery, One Artery	Ø Open	Ø Monitoring Device, Pressure Sensor	Ø Allogeneic OR Ultrasonic
4 Creation	1 Coronary Artery, Two Arteries	3 Percutaneous	2 Monitoring Device	1 Syngeneic
5 Destruction	2 Coronary Artery, Three Arteries	4 Percutaneous Endoscopic	3 Infusion Device	2 Zooplastic OR Common Atrioventricular Valve
7 Dilation	3 Coronary Artery, Four or More Arteries	X External	4 Intraluminal Device, Drug-eluting	3 Coronary Artery
8 Division	4 Coronary Vein		5 Intraluminal Device, Drug-eluting, Two	4 Coronary Vein
B Excision	5 Atrial Septum		6 Intraluminal Device, Drug-eluting, Three	5 Coronary Circulation
C Extirpation	6 Atrium, Right		7 Intraluminal Device, Drug-eluting, Four or More OR Autologous Tissue Substitute	6 Bifurcation OR Atrium, Right
F Fragmentation	7 Atrium, Left		8 Zooplastic Tissue	7 Atrium, Left
H Insertion	8 Conduction Mechanism		9 Autologous Venous Tissue	8 Internal Mammary, Right
J Inspection	9 Chordae Tendineae		A Autologous Arterial Tissue	9 Internal Mammary, Left
K Map	A Heart		C Extraluminal Device	A Innominate Artery
L Occlusion	B Heart, Right		D Intraluminal Device	B Subclavian
N Release	C Heart, Left		E Intraluminal Device, Two OR Intraluminal Device, Branched or Fenestrated, One or Two Arteries	C Thoracic Artery
P Removal	D Papillary Muscle		F Intraluminal Device, Three OR Intraluminal Device, Branched or Fenestrated, Three or More Arteries	D Carotid
Q Repair	F Aortic Valve		G Intraluminal Device, Four or More	E Atrioventricular Valve, Left
R Replacement	G Mitral Valve		J Synthetic Substitute OR Cardiac Lead, Pacemaker	F Abdominal Artery
S Reposition	H Pulmonary Valve		K Nonautologous Tissue Substitute OR Cardiac Lead, Defibrillator	G Atrioventricular Valve, Right OR Axillary Artery
T Resection	J Tricuspid Valve		M Cardiac Lead	H Transapical OR Brachial Artery
U Supplement	K Ventricle, Right		N Intracardiac Pacemaker	J Truncal Valve OR Temporary OR Intraoperative
V Restriction	L Ventricle, Left		Q Implantable Heart Assist System	K Left Atrial Appendage
W Revision	M Ventricular Septum		R Short-term External Heart Assist System	P Pulmonary Trunk
Y Transplantation	N Pericardium		T Intraluminal Device, Radioactive	Q Pulmonary Artery, Right
	P Pulmonary Trunk		Y Other Device	R Pulmonary Artery, Left
	Q Pulmonary Artery, Right		Z No Device	S Pulmonary Vein, Right OR Biventricular
	R Pulmonary Artery, Left			T Pulmonary Vein, Left OR Ductus Arteriosus
	S Pulmonary Vein, Right			U Pulmonary Vein, Confluence
	T Pulmonary Vein, Left			V Lower Extremity Artery
	V Superior Vena Cava			W Aorta
	W Thoracic Aorta, Descending			X Diagnostic
	X Thoracic Aorta, Ascending/ Arch			Z No Qualifier
	Y Great Vessel			

Heart and Great Vessels

AHA Coding Clinic for table 021

2020, 1Q, 24	Pulmonary artery unifocalization
2020, 1Q, 37	Bypass of ascending aorta to brachiocephalic artery
2019, 4Q, 23	Bypass thoracic aorta to innominate artery
2019, 3Q, 30	Aortic aneurysm repair with debranching of common carotid and brachiocephalic arteries
2018, 4Q, 45-46	Descending thoracic aorta bypass
2018, 3Q, 8	Coronary artery bypass graft surgery (revision versus total redo)
2018, 3Q, 26	Coronary artery bypass graft surgery with endarterectomy
2017, 4Q, 56	Added approach values - Percutaneous heart valve procedures
2017, 1Q, 19	Norwood Sano procedure
2016, 4Q, 80-81	Thoracic aorta, ascending/arch and descending
2016, 4Q, 82-83	Coronary artery, number of arteries
2016, 4Q, 102-109	Correction of congenital heart defects
2016, 4Q, 144	Repair of atrial septal defect and anomalous pulmonary venous return
2016, 4Q, 145	Modified Warden procedure for repair of septal defect and right partial anomalous pulmonary venous return
2016, 1Q, 27	Aortocoronary bypass graft utilizing Y-graft
2015, 4Q, 22, 24	Congenital heart corrective procedures
2015, 3Q, 16	Revision of previous truncus arteriosus surgery with ventricle to pulmonary artery conduit
2014, 3Q, 3	Blalock-Taussig shunt procedure
2014, 3Q, 8	Coronary artery bypass graft utilizing internal mammary as pedicle graft
2014, 3Q, 20	MAZE procedure performed with coronary artery bypass graft
2014, 3Q, 29	Fontan completion procedure stage II
2014, 3Q, 30	Creation of conduit from right ventricle to pulmonary artery
2014, 1Q, 10	Repair of thoracic aortic aneurysm & coronary artery bypass graft
2013, 2Q, 37	Coronary artery release performed during coronary artery bypass graft

AHA Coding Clinic for table 024

2016, 4Q, 101	Root operation Creation
2016, 4Q, 102-109	Correction of congenital heart defects

AHA Coding Clinic for table 025

2020, 1Q, 32	Ablation convergent procedure (catheter-based and thoracoscopic ablations)
2018, 3Q, 27	Alcohol septal ablation
2016, 4Q, 80-81	Thoracic aorta, ascending/arch and descending
2016, 3Q, 43-44	Peri-pulmonary catheter ablation
2016, 3Q, 44-45	Maze procedure
2016, 2Q, 17	Photodynamic therapy for treatment of malignant mesothelioma
2014, 4Q, 47	Catheter ablation of peripulmonary veins
2014, 3Q, 19	Ablation of ventricular tachycardia with Impella® support
2014, 3Q, 20	MAZE procedure performed with coronary artery bypass graft
2013, 2Q, 38	Catheter ablation to treat atrial fibrillation

AHA Coding Clinic for table 027

2018, 3Q, 7	Coronary brachytherapy with angioplasty
2018, 3Q, 10	Disruption of perma-catheter fibrin sheath via angioplasty of superior vena cava
2018, 2Q, 24	Coronary artery bifurcation
2017, 4Q, 32-33	Corrective surgery of left ventricular outflow tract obstruction
2016, 4Q, 80-81	Thoracic aorta, ascending/arch and descending
2016, 4Q, 82-83	Coronary artery, number of arteries
2016, 4Q, 84-85	Coronary Artery, number of stents
2016, 4Q, 86-88	Coronary and peripheral artery bifurcation
2016, 1Q, 16	Pulmonary valvotomy and dilation of annulus
2015, 4Q, 13	New Section X codes—New Technology procedures
2015, 3Q, 9	Failed attempt to treat coronary artery occlusion
2015, 3Q, 10	Coronary angioplasty with unsuccessful stent insertion
2015, 3Q, 16	Revision of previous truncus arteriosus surgery with ventricle to pulmonary artery conduit
2015, 2Q, 3-5	Coronary artery intervention site
2014, 2Q, 4	Coronary angioplasty of bypassed vessel

AHA Coding Clinic for table 02B

2019, 3Q, 32	Endomyocardial biopsy and right heart catheterization
2019, 2Q, 20	Pericardiectomy for constrictive pericarditis
2017, 1Q, 38	Mitral valve repair and chordae tendineae transfer
2016, 4Q, 80-81	Thoracic aorta, ascending/arch and descending
2015, 2Q, 23	Annuloplasty ring

AHA Coding Clinic for table 02C

2019, 4Q, 25	Coronary artery to root operation Supplement
2018, 3Q, 26	Coronary artery bypass graft surgery with endarterectomy
2018, 2Q, 24	Coronary artery bifurcation
2017, 2Q, 23	Thrombectomy via Fogarty catheter
2016, 4Q, 80-81	Thoracic aorta, ascending/arch and descending
2016, 4Q, 82-83	Coronary artery, number of arteries
2016, 4Q, 86-87	Coronary and peripheral artery bifurcation
2016, 2Q, 24	Repair/decalcification of mitral valve
2016, 2Q, 25	Aortic valve surgery with excision of calcium deposits

AHA Coding Clinic for table 02H

2019, 4Q, 23-24	Coronary artery Body Part to root operation Insertion
2019, 3Q, 19	Insertion of left ventricular catheter
2019, 3Q, 23	Placement of pacemaker lead in Bundle of HIS
2019, 1Q, 24	Replacement of left ventricular assist device with retention of outflow graft
2018, 4Q, 94	Insertion and removal of failed Watchman™ device
2018, 2Q, 3-5	Intra-aortic balloon pump
2018, 2Q, 19	Pacing lead attached to automatic implantable cardioverter defibrillator
2017, 4Q, 42-45	Insertion of external heart assist devices
2017, 4Q, 63-64	Added and revised device values - Vascular access reservoir
2017, 4Q, 104	Placement of Watchman™ left atrial appendage device
2017, 3Q, 11	Placement of peripherally inserted central catheter using 3CG ECG technology
2017, 2Q, 24	Tunneled catheter versus totally implantable catheter
2017, 2Q, 26	Exchange of tunneled catheter
2017, 1Q, 10-11	External heart assist device
2016, 4Q, 80-81	Thoracic aorta, ascending/arch and descending
2016, 4Q, 95	Intracardiac pacemaker
2016, 4Q, 137-138	Heart assist device systems
2016, 2Q, 15	Removal and replacement of tunneled internal jugular catheter
2015, 4Q, 14	New Section X codes—New Technology procedures
2015, 4Q, 26-31	Vascular access devices
2015, 3Q, 35	Swan Ganz catheterization
2015, 2Q, 31	Leadless pacemaker insertion
2015, 2Q, 33	Totally implantable central venous access device (Port-a-Cath)
2013, 3Q, 18	Placement of peripherally inserted central catheter (PICC)

AHA Coding Clinic for table 02J

2015, 3Q, 9	Failed attempt to treat coronary artery occlusion

AHA Coding Clinic for table 02K

2020, 1Q, 32	Ablation convergent procedure (catheter-based and thoracoscopic ablations)

AHA Coding Clinic for table 02L

2018, 4Q, 94	Insertion and removal of failed Watchman™ device
2017, 4Q, 31	Resuscitative endovascular balloon occlusion of the aorta
2017, 4Q, 33-34	Occlusion/ligation of pulmonary trunk & right pulmonary artery
2016, 4Q, 102-109	Correction of congenital heart defects
2016, 2Q, 26	Embolization of pulmonary arteriovenous fistula
2015, 4Q, 23	Congenital heart corrective procedures
2014, 3Q, 20	MAZE procedure performed with coronary artery bypass graft

AHA Coding Clinic for table 02N

2019, 2Q, 13	Unroofing of anomalous coronary artery
2019, 2Q, 20	Pericardiectomy for constrictive pericarditis
2017, 4Q, 35	Release of myocardial bridge
2016, 4Q, 80-81	Thoracic aorta, ascending/arch and descending
2014, 3Q, 16	Repair of Tetralogy of Fallot

AHA Coding Clinic for table 02P

2019, 1Q, 24	Replacement of left ventricular assist device with retention of outflow graft
2018, 4Q, 52-54	Percutaneous extracorporeal membrane oxygenation
2018, 4Q, 85	Externalization of lumboatrial shunt
2018, 4Q, 94	Insertion and removal of failed Watchman™ device
2018, 2Q, 3-5	Intra-aortic balloon pump
2017, 4Q, 42-45	Insertion of external heart assist devices
2017, 4Q, 104	Placement of Watchman™ left atrial appendage device
2017, 3Q, 18	Intra-aortic balloon pump removal
2017, 2Q, 24	Tunneled catheter versus totally implantable catheter
2017, 2Q, 26	Exchange of tunneled catheter
2017, 1Q, 11	External heart assist device
2017, 1Q, 13	SynCardia total artificial heart
2016, 4Q, 95-96	Intracardiac pacemaker
2016, 4Q, 137-139	Heart assist device systems
2016, 3Q, 19	Nonoperative removal of peripherally inserted central catheter
2016, 2Q, 15	Removal and replacement of tunneled internal jugular catheter
2015, 4Q, 31	Vascular access devices
2015, 3Q, 33	Approach values for repositioning and removal of cardiac lead

AHA Coding Clinic for table 02Q

2018, 1Q, 12	Percutaneous balloon valvuloplasty & cardiac catheterization with ventriculogram
2017, 1Q, 18	Sutureless repair of pulmonary vein stenosis
2016, 4Q, 80-81	Thoracic aorta, ascending/arch and descending
2016, 4Q, 82-83	Coronary artery, number of arteries
2016, 4Q, 101	Root operation Creation
2016, 4Q, 102-109	Correction of congenital heart defects
2015, 4Q, 23	Congenital heart corrective procedures
2015, 3Q, 16	Vascular ring surgery and double aortic arch
2015, 2Q, 23	Annuloplasty ring
2013, 3Q, 26	Transcatheter replacement of heart valve (TAVR) with measurements

AHA Coding Clinic for table 02R

2020, 1Q, 25	Elephant trunk repair of aortic dissection
2019, 4Q, 24	Coronary artery Body Part to root operation Insertion
2019, 4Q, 46	Cerebral embolic filtration
2019, 3Q, 23	Replacement of atrioventricular valve
2019, 3Q, 24	Valve sparing aortic root replacement with modified Gleason Vascutek® graft to ascending aorta
2019, 1Q, 31	Transcatheter aortic valve in valve replacement
2018, 3Q, 11	Transcatheter aortic valve replacement via transaortic approach
2018, 1Q, 12	Percutaneous balloon valvuloplasty & cardiac catheterization with ventriculogram
2017, 4Q, 55-56	Added approach values - Percutaneous heart valve procedures
2017, 1Q, 13	SynCardia total artificial heart
2016, 4Q, 80-81	Thoracic aorta, ascending/arch and descending
2016, 3Q, 32	Transcatheter tricuspid valve replacement
2014, 1Q, 10	Repair of thoracic aortic aneurysm & coronary artery bypass graft

AHA Coding Clinic for table 02S

2016, 4Q, 80-81	Thoracic aorta, ascending/arch and descending
2016, 4Q, 82-83	Coronary artery, number of arteries
2016, 4Q, 102-109	Correction of congenital heart defects
2015, 4Q, 23	Congenital heart corrective procedures

AHA Coding Clinic for table 02U

2020, 1Q, 24	Pulmonary artery unifocalization
2019, 4Q, 25	Coronary artery to root operation Supplement
2018, 1Q, 12	Percutaneous balloon valvuloplasty & cardiac catheterization with ventriculogram
2017, 4Q, 36	Alfieri stitch procedure
2017, 3Q, 7	Senning procedure (arterial switch)
2017, 1Q, 19	Norwood Sano procedure
2016, 4Q, 80-81	Thoracic aorta, ascending/arch and descending
2016, 4Q, 101	Root operation Creation
2016, 4Q, 102-109	Correction of congenital heart defects
2016, 2Q, 23	Repair of tetralogy of Fallot with autologous pericardial patch graft
2016, 2Q, 26	Aortic valve replacement with aortic root enlargement
2015, 4Q, 22-24	Congenital heart corrective procedures
2015, 3Q, 16	Revision of previous truncus arteriosus surgery with ventricle to pulmonary artery conduit
2015, 2Q, 23	Annuloplasty ring
2014, 3Q, 16	Repair of Tetralogy of Fallot

AHA Coding Clinic for table 02V

2020, 1Q, 25	Elephant trunk repair of aortic dissection
2017, 4Q, 35-36	Alfieri stitch procedure
2016, 4Q, 80-81	Thoracic aorta, ascending/arch and descending
2016, 4Q, 89-92	Branched and fenestrated endograft repair of aneurysms

AHA Coding Clinic for table 02W

2019, 1Q, 24	Replacement of left ventricular assist device with retention of outflow graft
2018, 3Q, 8	Coronary artery bypass graft surgery (revision versus total redo)
2018, 3Q, 9	Fibrin sheath stripping of malfunctioning port-a-cath
2018, 1Q, 17	Repositioning of Impella short-term external heart assist device
2017, 4Q, 42-45	Insertion of external heart assist devices
2017, 4Q, 55-56	Added approach values - Percutaneous heart valve procedures
2016, 4Q, 85	Coronary Artery, number of stents
2016, 4Q, 95-96	Intracardiac pacemaker
2015, 3Q, 32	Approach values for repositioning and removal of cardiac lead
2014, 3Q, 31	Closure of paravalvular leak using Amplatzer® vascular plug

AHA Coding Clinic for table 02Y

2013, 3Q, 18	Heart transplant surgery

Coronary Arteries

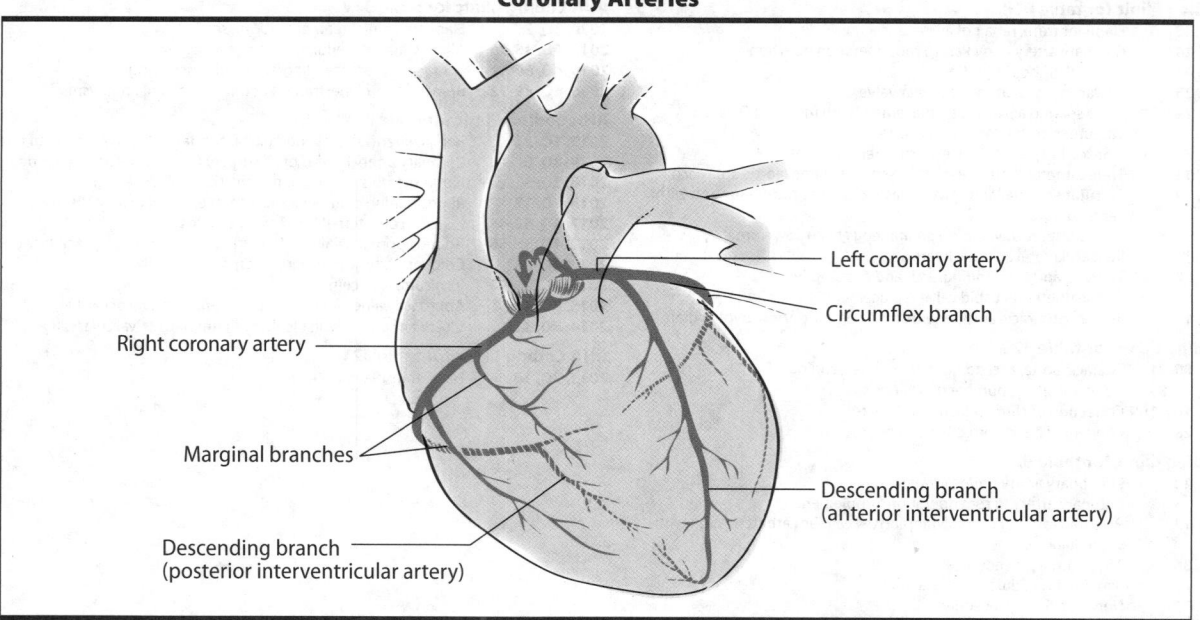

Left coronary artery

Circumflex branch

Right coronary artery

Marginal branches

Descending branch
(posterior interventricular artery)

Descending branch
(anterior interventricular artery)

Heart Anatomy

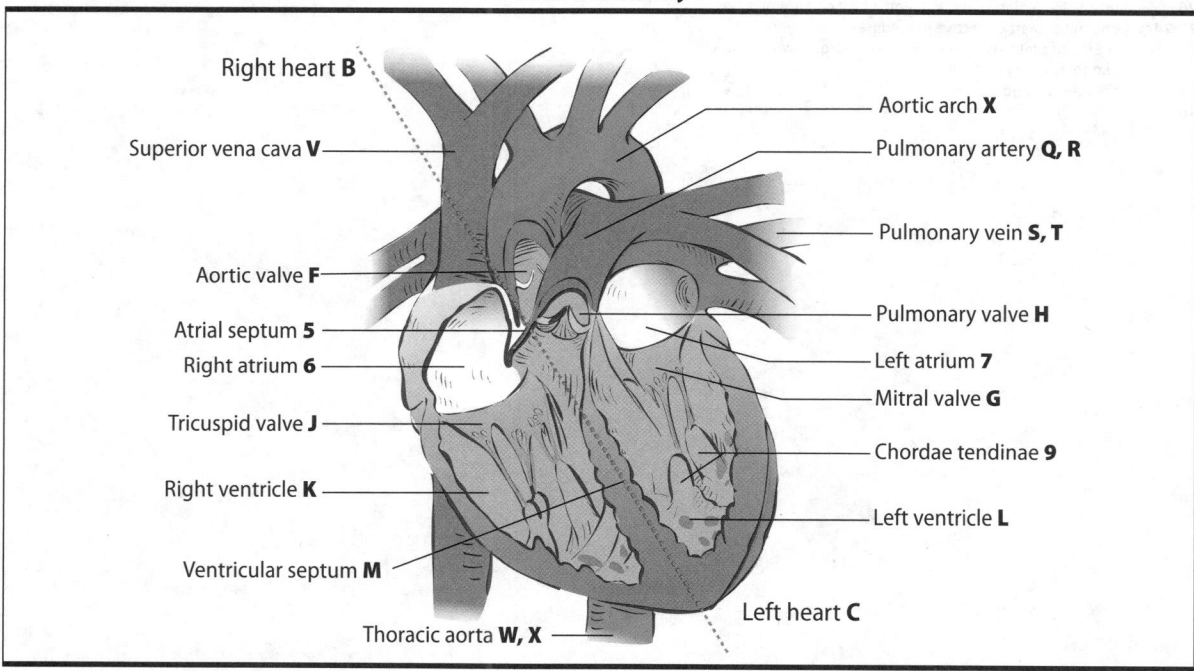

Right heart **B**

Superior vena cava **V**

Aortic valve **F**

Atrial septum **5**

Right atrium **6**

Tricuspid valve **J**

Right ventricle **K**

Ventricular septum **M**

Thoracic aorta **W, X**

Aortic arch **X**

Pulmonary artery **Q, R**

Pulmonary vein **S, T**

Pulmonary valve **H**

Left atrium **7**

Mitral valve **G**

Chordae tendinae **9**

Left ventricle **L**

Left heart **C**

Heart and Great Vessels

Ø   **Medical and Surgical**
2   **Heart and Great Vessels**
1   **Bypass**   Definition: Altering the route of passage of the contents of a tubular body part

                         Explanation: Rerouting contents of a body part to a downstream area of the normal route, to a similar route and body part, or to an abnormal route and dissimilar body part. Includes one or more anastomoses, with or without the use of a device.

Body Part Character 4	Approach Character 5	Device Character 6	Qualifier Character 7
Ø Coronary Artery, One Artery 1 Coronary Artery, Two Arteries 2 Coronary Artery, Three Arteries 3 Coronary Artery, Four or More Arteries	Ø Open	8 Zooplastic Tissue 9 Autologous Venous Tissue A Autologous Arterial Tissue J Synthetic Substitute K Nonautologous Tissue Substitute	3 Coronary Artery 8 Internal Mammary, Right 9 Internal Mammary, Left C Thoracic Artery F Abdominal Artery W Aorta
Ø Coronary Artery, One Artery 1 Coronary Artery, Two Arteries 2 Coronary Artery, Three Arteries 3 Coronary Artery, Four or More Arteries	Ø Open	Z No Device	3 Coronary Artery 8 Internal Mammary, Right 9 Internal Mammary, Left C Thoracic Artery F Abdominal Artery
Ø Coronary Artery, One Artery 1 Coronary Artery, Two Arteries 2 Coronary Artery, Three Arteries 3 Coronary Artery, Four or More Arteries	3 Percutaneous	4 Intraluminal Device, Drug-eluting D Intraluminal Device	4 Coronary Vein
Ø Coronary Artery, One Artery 1 Coronary Artery, Two Arteries 2 Coronary Artery, Three Arteries 3 Coronary Artery, Four or More Arteries	4 Percutaneous Endoscopic	4 Intraluminal Device, Drug-eluting D Intraluminal Device	4 Coronary Vein
Ø Coronary Artery, One Artery 1 Coronary Artery, Two Arteries 2 Coronary Artery, Three Arteries 3 Coronary Artery, Four or More Arteries	4 Percutaneous Endoscopic	8 Zooplastic Tissue 9 Autologous Venous Tissue A Autologous Arterial Tissue J Synthetic Substitute K Nonautologous Tissue Substitute	3 Coronary Artery 8 Internal Mammary, Right 9 Internal Mammary, Left C Thoracic Artery F Abdominal Artery W Aorta
Ø Coronary Artery, One Artery 1 Coronary Artery, Two Arteries 2 Coronary Artery, Three Arteries 3 Coronary Artery, Four or More Arteries	4 Percutaneous Endoscopic	Z No Device	3 Coronary Artery 8 Internal Mammary, Right 9 Internal Mammary, Left C Thoracic Artery F Abdominal Artery

6 Atrium, Right
   Atrium dextrum cordis
   Right auricular appendix
   Sinus venosus
	Ø Open
	4 Percutaneous Endoscopic
		8 Zooplastic Tissue
		9 Autologous Venous Tissue
		A Autologous Arterial Tissue
		J Synthetic Substitute
		K Nonautologous Tissue Substitute
			P Pulmonary Trunk
			Q Pulmonary Artery, Right
			R Pulmonary Artery, Left

6 Atrium, Right
   Atrium dextrum cordis
   Right auricular appendix
   Sinus venosus
	Ø Open
	4 Percutaneous Endoscopic
		Z No Device	7 Atrium, Left
			P Pulmonary Trunk
			Q Pulmonary Artery, Right
			R Pulmonary Artery, Left

6 Atrium, Right
   Atrium dextrum cordis
   Right auricular appendix
   Sinus venosus
	3 Percutaneous	Z No Device	7 Atrium, Left

7 Atrium, Left
   Atrium pulmonale
   Left auricular appendix
	Ø Open
	4 Percutaneous Endoscopic
		8 Zooplastic Tissue
		9 Autologous Venous Tissue
		A Autologous Arterial Tissue
		J Synthetic Substitute
		K Nonautologous Tissue Substitute
		Z No Device
			P Pulmonary Trunk
			Q Pulmonary Artery, Right
			R Pulmonary Artery, Left
			S Pulmonary Vein, Right
			T Pulmonary Vein, Left
			U Pulmonary Vein, Confluence

7 Atrium, Left
   Atrium pulmonale
   Left auricular appendix
	3 Percutaneous	J Synthetic Substitute	6 Atrium, Right

K Ventricle, Right Conus arteriosus L Ventricle, Left	Ø Open 4 Percutaneous Endoscopic	8 Zooplastic Tissue 9 Autologous Venous Tissue A Autologous Arterial Tissue J Synthetic Substitute K Nonautologous Tissue Substitute	P Pulmonary Trunk Q Pulmonary Artery, Right R Pulmonary Artery, Left

HAC   Ø21[Ø,1,2,3]Ø[8,9,A,J,K][3,8,9,C,F,W] when reported with SDx J98.51 or J98.59
HAC   Ø21[Ø,1,2,3]ØZ[3,8,9,C,F] when reported with SDx J98.51 or J98.59
HAC   Ø21[Ø,1,2,3]4[8,9,A,J,K][3,8,9,C,F,W] when reported with SDx J98.51 or J98.59
HAC   Ø21[Ø,1,2,3]4Z[3,8,9,C,F] when reported with SDx J98.51 or J98.59

Ø21 Continued on next page

LC Limited Coverage   NC Noncovered   ⊞ Combination Member   HAC associated procedure   Combination Only   DRG Non-OR   Non-OR   New/Revised in GREEN

Heart and Great Vessels

Ø   **Medical and Surgical**   *Ø21 Continued*
2   **Heart and Great Vessels**
1   **Bypass**   Definition: Altering the route of passage of the contents of a tubular body part

                 Explanation: Rerouting contents of a body part to a downstream area of the normal route, to a similar route and body part, or to an abnormal route and dissimilar body part. Includes one or more anastomoses, with or without the use of a device.

Body Part Character 4	Approach Character 5	Device Character 6	Qualifier Character 7
K Ventricle, Right Conus arteriosus **L** Ventricle, Left	**Ø** Open **4** Percutaneous Endoscopic	**Z** No Device	**5** Coronary Circulation **8** Internal Mammary, Right **9** Internal Mammary, Left **C** Thoracic Artery **F** Abdominal Artery **P** Pulmonary Trunk **Q** Pulmonary Artery, Right **R** Pulmonary Artery, Left **W** Aorta

P Pulmonary Trunk
Q Pulmonary Artery, Right
R Pulmonary Artery, Left
    Arterial canal (duct)
    Botallo's duct
    Pulmoaortic canal
	Ø Open
	4 Percutaneous Endoscopic
		8 Zooplastic Tissue
		9 Autologous Venous Tissue
		A Autologous Arterial Tissue
		J Synthetic Substitute
		K Nonautologous Tissue Substitute
		Z No Device
			A Innominate Artery
			B Subclavian
			D Carotid

V Superior Vena Cava Precava	**Ø** Open **4** Percutaneous Endoscopic	**8** Zooplastic Tissue **9** Autologous Venous Tissue **A** Autologous Arterial Tissue **J** Synthetic Substitute **K** Nonautologous Tissue Substitute **Z** No Device	**P** Pulmonary Trunk **Q** Pulmonary Artery, Right **R** Pulmonary Artery, Left **S** Pulmonary Vein, Right **T** Pulmonary Vein, Left **U** Pulmonary Vein, Confluence
W Thoracic Aorta, Descending	**Ø** Open	**8** Zooplastic Tissue **9** Autologous Venous Tissue **A** Autologous Arterial Tissue **J** Synthetic Substitute **K** Nonautologous Tissue Substitute	**A** Innominate Artery **B** Subclavian **D** Carotid **F** Abdominal Artery **G** Axillary Artery **H** Brachial Artery **P** Pulmonary Trunk **Q** Pulmonary Artery, Right **R** Pulmonary Artery, Left **V** Lower Extremity Artery
W Thoracic Aorta, Descending	**Ø** Open	**Z** No Device	**A** Innominate Artery **B** Subclavian **D** Carotid **P** Pulmonary Trunk **Q** Pulmonary Artery, Right **R** Pulmonary Artery, Left
W Thoracic Aorta, Descending	**4** Percutaneous Endoscopic	**8** Zooplastic Tissue **9** Autologous Venous Tissue **A** Autologous Arterial Tissue **J** Synthetic Substitute **K** Nonautologous Tissue Substitute **Z** No Device	**A** Innominate Artery **B** Subclavian **D** Carotid **P** Pulmonary Trunk **Q** Pulmonary Artery, Right **R** Pulmonary Artery, Left

X Thoracic Aorta, Ascending/Arch
    Aortic arch
    Ascending aorta
	Ø Open
	4 Percutaneous Endoscopic
		8 Zooplastic Tissue
		9 Autologous Venous Tissue
		A Autologous Arterial Tissue
		J Synthetic Substitute
		K Nonautologous Tissue Substitute
		Z No Device
			A Innominate Artery
			B Subclavian
			D Carotid
			P Pulmonary Trunk
			Q Pulmonary Artery, Right
			R Pulmonary Artery, Left

Ø   **Medical and Surgical**
2   **Heart and Great Vessels**
4   **Creation**   Definition: Putting in or on biological or synthetic material to form a new body part that to the extent possible replicates the anatomic structure or function of an absent body part

                 Explanation: Used for gender reassignment surgery and corrective procedures in individuals with congenital anomalies

Body Part Character 4	Approach Character 5	Device Character 6	Qualifier Character 7
F Aortic Valve Aortic annulus	**Ø** Open	**7** Autologous Tissue **8** Zooplastic Tissue **J** Synthetic Substitute **K** Nonautologous Tissue Substitute	**J** Truncal Valve

G Mitral Valve
    Bicuspid valve
    Left atrioventricular valve
    Mitral annulus
J Tricuspid Valve
    Right atrioventricular valve
    Tricuspid annulus
	Ø Open	**7** Autologous Tissue
		8 Zooplastic Tissue
		J Synthetic Substitute
		K Nonautologous Tissue Substitute
			2 Common Atrioventricular Valve

LC Limited Coverage   NC Noncovered   ⊞ Combination Member   HAC associated procedure   Combination Only   DRG Non-OR   Non-OR   New/Revised in GREEN

174   ICD-10-PCS 2021

Ø   Medical and Surgical
2   Heart and Great Vessels
5   Destruction   Definition: Physical eradication of all or a portion of a body part by the direct use of energy, force, or a destructive agent
                     Explanation: None of the body part is physically taken out

Body Part Character 4	Approach Character 5	Device Character 6	Qualifier Character 7

4 Coronary Vein
5 Atrial Septum
   Interatrial septum
6 Atrium, Right
   Atrium dextrum cordis
   Right auricular appendix
   Sinus venosus
8 Conduction Mechanism
   Atrioventricular node
   Bundle of His
   Bundle of Kent
   Sinoatrial node
9 Chordae Tendineae
D Papillary Muscle
F Aortic Valve
   Aortic annulus
G Mitral Valve
   Bicuspid valve
   Left atrioventricular valve
   Mitral annulus
H Pulmonary Valve
   Pulmonary annulus
   Pulmonic valve
J Tricuspid Valve
   Right atrioventricular valve
   Tricuspid annulus
K Ventricle, Right
   Conus arteriosus
L Ventricle, Left
M Ventricular Septum
   Interventricular septum
N Pericardium
P Pulmonary Trunk
Q Pulmonary Artery, Right
R Pulmonary Artery, Left
   Arterial canal (duct)
   Botallo's duct
   Pulmoaortic canal
S Pulmonary Vein, Right
   Right inferior pulmonary vein
   Right superior pulmonary vein
T Pulmonary Vein, Left
   Left inferior pulmonary vein
   Left superior pulmonary vein
V Superior Vena Cava
   Precava
W Thoracic Aorta, Descending
X Thoracic Aorta, Ascending/Arch
   Aortic arch
   Ascending aorta
	Ø Open
	3 Percutaneous
	4 Percutaneous Endoscopic
		Z No Device	**Z No Qualifier**

7 Atrium, Left
   Atrium pulmonale
   Left auricular appendix
	Ø Open
	3 Percutaneous
	4 Percutaneous Endoscopic
		Z No Device	**K Left Atrial Appendage**
			Z No Qualifier

DRG Non-OR   Ø257[Ø,3,4]ZK

Heart and Great Vessels

Ø   **Medical and Surgical**
2   **Heart and Great Vessels**
7   **Dilation**   Definition: Expanding an orifice or the lumen of a tubular body part

             Explanation: The orifice can be a natural orifice or an artificially created orifice. Accomplished by stretching a tubular body part using intraluminal pressure or by cutting part of the orifice or wall of the tubular body part.

Body Part Character 4	Approach Character 5	Device Character 6	Qualifier Character 7
Ø Coronary Artery, One Artery 1 Coronary Artery, Two Arteries 2 Coronary Artery, Three Arteries 3 Coronary Artery, Four or More Arteries	Ø Open 3 Percutaneous 4 Percutaneous Endoscopic	4 Intraluminal Device, Drug-eluting 5 Intraluminal Device, Drug-eluting, Two 6 Intraluminal Device, Drug-eluting, Three 7 Intraluminal Device, Drug-eluting, Four or More D Intraluminal Device E Intraluminal Device, Two F Intraluminal Device, Three G Intraluminal Device, Four or More T Intraluminal Device, Radioactive Z No Device	6 Bifurcation Z No Qualifier

F Aortic Valve
   Aortic annulus
G Mitral Valve
   Bicuspid valve
   Left atrioventricular valve
   Mitral annulus
H Pulmonary Valve
   Pulmonary annulus
   Pulmonic valve
J Tricuspid Valve
   Right atrioventricular valve
   Tricuspid annulus
K Ventricle, Right
   Conus arteriosus
L Ventricle, Left
P Pulmonary Trunk
Q Pulmonary Artery, Right
S Pulmonary Vein, Right
   Right inferior pulmonary vein
   Right superior pulmonary vein
T Pulmonary Vein, Left
   Left inferior pulmonary vein
   Left superior pulmonary vein
V Superior Vena Cava
   Precava
W Thoracic Aorta, Descending
X Thoracic Aorta, Ascending/Arch
   Aortic arch
   Ascending aorta
	Ø Open
	3 Percutaneous
	4 Percutaneous Endoscopic
		4 Intraluminal Device, Drug-eluting
		D Intraluminal Device
		Z No Device
			Z No Qualifier

R Pulmonary Artery, Left
   Arterial canal (duct)
   Botallo's duct
   Pulmoaortic canal
	Ø Open
	3 Percutaneous
	4 Percutaneous Endoscopic
		4 Intraluminal Device, Drug-eluting
		D Intraluminal Device
		Z No Device
			T Ductus Arteriosus
			Z No Qualifier

Ø   **Medical and Surgical**
2   **Heart and Great Vessels**
8   **Division**   Definition: Cutting into a body part, without draining fluids and/or gases from the body part, in order to separate or transect a body part

             Explanation: All or a portion of the body part is separated into two or more portions

Body Part Character 4	Approach Character 5	Device Character 6	Qualifier Character 7

8 Conduction Mechanism
   Atrioventricular node
   Bundle of His
   Bundle of Kent
   Sinoatrial node
9 Chordae Tendineae
D Papillary Muscle
	Ø Open
	3 Percutaneous
	4 Percutaneous Endoscopic
		Z No Device	Z No Qualifier

LC Limited Coverage   **NC** Noncovered   ⊞ Combination Member   HAC associated procedure   Combination Only   DRG Non-OR   Non-OR   New/Revised in GREEN

176   ICD-10-PCS 2021

Ø Medical and Surgical
2 Heart and Great Vessels
B Excision   Definition: Cutting out or off, without replacement, a portion of a body part
                      Explanation: The qualifier DIAGNOSTIC is used to identify excision procedures that are biopsies

Body Part Character 4	Approach Character 5	Device Character 6	Qualifier Character 7
4 Coronary Vein	**Ø Open**	**Z No Device**	**X Diagnostic**
5 Atrial Septum	**3 Percutaneous**		**Z No Qualifier**
Interatrial septum	**4 Percutaneous Endoscopic**		
6 Atrium, Right			
Atrium dextrum cordis			
Right auricular appendix			
Sinus venosus			
8 Conduction Mechanism			
Atrioventricular node			
Bundle of His			
Bundle of Kent			
Sinoatrial node			
9 Chordae Tendineae			
D Papillary Muscle			
F Aortic Valve			
Aortic annulus			
G Mitral Valve			
Bicuspid valve			
Left atrioventricular valve			
Mitral annulus			
H Pulmonary Valve			
Pulmonary annulus			
Pulmonic valve			
J Tricuspid Valve			
Right atrioventricular valve			
Tricuspid annulus			
K Ventricle, Right NC			
Conus arteriosus			
L Ventricle, Left NC			
M Ventricular Septum			
Interventricular septum			
N Pericardium			
P Pulmonary Trunk			
Q Pulmonary Artery, Right			
R Pulmonary Artery, Left			
Arterial canal (duct)			
Botallo's duct			
Pulmoaortic canal			
S Pulmonary Vein, Right			
Right inferior pulmonary vein			
Right superior pulmonary vein			
T Pulmonary Vein, Left			
Left inferior pulmonary vein			
Left superior pulmonary vein			
V Superior Vena Cava			
Precava			
W Thoracic Aorta, Descending			
X Thoracic Aorta, Ascending/Arch			
Aortic arch			
Ascending aorta			
7 Atrium, Left	**Ø Open**	**Z No Device**	**K Left Atrial Appendage**
Atrium pulmonale	**3 Percutaneous**		**X Diagnostic**
Left auricular appendix	**4 Percutaneous Endoscopic**		**Z No Qualifier**

DRG Non-OR	Ø2B7[Ø,3,4]ZK
Non-OR	Ø2B[4,5,6,8,9,D,F,G,H,J,K,L,M][Ø,3,4]ZX
NC	Ø2B[K,L][Ø,3,4]ZZ

LC Limited Coverage **NC** Noncovered ⊞ Combination Member HAC associated procedure Combination Only DRG Non-OR Non-OR New/Revised in GREEN

ICD-10-PCS 2021   **177**

Heart and Great Vessels *(left margin)*

Ø   Medical and Surgical
2   Heart and Great Vessels
C   Extirpation   Definition: Taking or cutting out solid matter from a body part

Explanation: The solid matter may be an abnormal byproduct of a biological function or a foreign body; it may be imbedded in a body part or in the lumen of a tubular body part. The solid matter may or may not have been previously broken into pieces.

Body Part Character 4	Approach Character 5	Device Character 6	Qualifier Character 7
Ø Coronary Artery, One Artery 1 Coronary Artery, Two Arteries 2 Coronary Artery, Three Arteries 3 Coronary Artery, Four or More Arteries	Ø Open 3 Percutaneous 4 Percutaneous Endoscopic	Z No Device	6 Bifurcation Z No Qualifier

4   Coronary Vein
5   Atrial Septum
     Interatrial septum
6   Atrium, Right
     Atrium dextrum cordis
     Right auricular appendix
     Sinus venosus
7   Atrium, Left
     Atrium pulmonale
     Left auricular appendix
8   Conduction Mechanism
     Atrioventricular node
     Bundle of His
     Bundle of Kent
     Sinoatrial node
9   Chordae Tendineae
D   Papillary Muscle
F   Aortic Valve
     Aortic annulus
G   Mitral Valve
     Bicuspid valve
     Left atrioventricular valve
     Mitral annulus
H   Pulmonary Valve
     Pulmonary annulus
     Pulmonic valve
J   Tricuspid Valve
     Right atrioventricular valve
     Tricuspid annulus
K   Ventricle, Right
     Conus arteriosus
L   Ventricle, Left
M   Ventricular Septum
     Interventricular septum
N   Pericardium
P   Pulmonary Trunk
Q   Pulmonary Artery, Right
R   Pulmonary Artery, Left
     Arterial canal (duct)
     Botallo's duct
     Pulmoaortic canal
S   Pulmonary Vein, Right
     Right inferior pulmonary vein
     Right superior pulmonary vein
T   Pulmonary Vein, Left
     Left inferior pulmonary vein
     Left superior pulmonary vein
V   Superior Vena Cava
     Precava
W   Thoracic Aorta, Descending
X   Thoracic Aorta, Ascending/Arch
     Aortic arch
     Ascending aorta
	Ø Open
	3 Percutaneous
	4 Percutaneous Endoscopic
		Z No Device	Z No Qualifier

LC Limited Coverage   NC Noncovered   ⊞ Combination Member   HAC associated procedure   Combination Only   DRG Non-OR   Non-OR   New/Revised in GREEN

178   ICD-10-PCS 2021

02C–02C *(left margin bottom)*

Ø   **Medical and Surgical**
2   **Heart and Great Vessels**
F   **Fragmentation**   Definition: Breaking solid matter in a body part into pieces

Explanation: Physical force (e.g., manual, ultrasonic) applied directly or indirectly is used to break the solid matter into pieces. The solid matter may be an abnormal byproduct of a biological function or a foreign body. The pieces of solid matter are not taken out.

Body Part Character 4	Approach Character 5	Device Character 6	Qualifier Character 7
N Pericardium NC	**Ø** Open **3** Percutaneous **4** Percutaneous Endoscopic **X** External	**Z** No Device	**Z** No Qualifier

P Pulmonary Trunk
Q Pulmonary Artery, Right
R Pulmonary Artery, Left
   Arterial canal (duct)
   Botallo's duct
   Pulmoaortic canal
S Pulmonary Vein, Right
   Right inferior pulmonary vein
   Right superior pulmonary vein
T Pulmonary Vein, Left
   Left inferior pulmonary vein
   Left superior pulmonary vein
	3 Percutaneous	**Z** No Device	**Ø** Ultrasonic
			Z No Qualifier

Non-OR   02FNXZZ
NC   02FNXZZ

Heart and Great Vessels

Ø   **Medical and Surgical**
2   **Heart and Great Vessels**
H   **Insertion**   Definition: Putting in a nonbiological appliance that monitors, assists, performs, or prevents a physiological function but does not physically take the place of a body part
                           Explanation: None

Body Part Character 4	Approach Character 5	Device Character 6	Qualifier Character 7
Ø Coronary Artery, One Artery 1 Coronary Artery, Two Arteries 2 Coronary Artery, Three Arteries 3 Coronary Artery, Four or More Arteries	Ø Open 3 Percutaneous 4 Percutaneous Endoscopic	D Intraluminal Device Y Other Device	Z No Qualifier

4 Coronary Vein ⊞
6 Atrium, Right ⊞
    Atrium dextrum cordis
    Right auricular appendix
    Sinus venosus
7 Atrium, Left ⊞
    Atrium pulmonale
    Left auricular appendix
K Ventricle, Right ⊞
    Conus arteriosus
L Ventricle, Left ⊞
	Ø Open
	3 Percutaneous
	4 Percutaneous Endoscopic
		Ø Monitoring Device, Pressure Sensor
		2 Monitoring Device
		3 Infusion Device
		D Intraluminal Device
		J Cardiac Lead, Pacemaker
		K Cardiac Lead, Defibrillator
		M Cardiac Lead
		N Intracardiac Pacemaker
		Y Other Device
			Z No Qualifier

A Heart LC NC	Ø Open 3 Percutaneous 4 Percutaneous Endoscopic	Q Implantable Heart Assist System Y Other Device	Z No Qualifier
A Heart ⊞	Ø Open 3 Percutaneous 4 Percutaneous Endoscopic	R Short-term External Heart Assist System	J Intraoperative S Biventricular Z No Qualifier
N Pericardium ⊞	Ø Open 3 Percutaneous 4 Percutaneous Endoscopic	Ø Monitoring Device, Pressure Sensor 2 Monitoring Device J Cardiac Lead, Pacemaker K Cardiac Lead, Defibrillator M Cardiac Lead Y Other Device	Z No Qualifier

P Pulmonary Trunk
Q Pulmonary Artery, Right
R Pulmonary Artery, Left
    Arterial canal (duct)
    Botallo's duct
    Pulmoaortic canal
S Pulmonary Vein, Right
    Right inferior pulmonary vein
    Right superior pulmonary vein
T Pulmonary Vein, Left
    Left inferior pulmonary vein
    Left superior pulmonary vein
V Superior Vena Cava
    Precava
W Thoracic Aorta, Descending
	Ø Open
	3 Percutaneous
	4 Percutaneous Endoscopic
		Ø Monitoring Device, Pressure Sensor
		2 Monitoring Device
		3 Infusion Device
		D Intraluminal Device
		Y Other Device
			Z No Qualifier

X Thoracic Aorta, Ascending/Arch
    Aortic arch
    Ascending aorta
	Ø Open
	3 Percutaneous
	4 Percutaneous Endoscopic
		Ø Monitoring Device, Pressure Sensor
		2 Monitoring Device
		3 Infusion Device
		D Intraluminal Device
			Z No Qualifier

DRG Non-OR Ø2H[4,6,7,K,L][Ø,3,4][J,M]Z	**HAC** Ø2H43[J,K,M]Z when reported with SDx K68.11 or T81.4Ø-T81.49, T82.6-T82.7 with 7th character A
DRG Non-OR Ø2HK32Z	**HAC** Ø2H[6,K]33Z when reported with SDx J95.811
DRG Non-OR Ø2HN[Ø,3,4][J,M]Z	**HAC** Ø2H[6,7]3[J,M]Z when reported with SDx K68.11 or T81.4Ø-T81.49, T82.6-T82.7 with 7th character A
Non-OR Ø2H[4,6,7,L]3[2,3]Z	
Non-OR Ø2H[6,7]3MZ	**HAC** Ø2H[K,L]3JZ when reported with SDx K68.11 or T81.4Ø-T81.49, T82.6-T82.7 with 7th character A
Non-OR Ø2HK3[Ø,3]Z	
Non-OR Ø2HN32Z	**HAC** Ø2HN[Ø,3,4][J,M]Z when reported with SDx K68.11 or T81.4Ø-T81.49, T82.6-T82.7 with 7th character A
Non-OR Ø2HP[Ø,3,4][Ø,2,3]Z	
Non-OR Ø2H[Q,R][Ø,3,4][2,3]Z	**HAC** Ø2H[S,T,V][3,4]3Z when reported with SDx J95.811
Non-OR Ø2H[S,T,V,W][Ø,3,4]3Z	LC Ø2HAØQZ
Non-OR Ø2H[S,T,V,W]32Z	NC Ø2HA[3,4]QZ
Non-OR Ø2HW[Ø,3]ØZ	**See Appendix L for Procedure Combinations**
Non-OR Ø2HX[Ø,3,4][Ø,3]Z	⊞ Ø2H[4,6,7,K,L][Ø,3,4][J,K,M]Z
	⊞ Ø2HA[Ø,4]R[S,Z]
	⊞ Ø2HA3RS
	⊞ Ø2HN[Ø,3,4][J,K,M]Z

LC Limited Coverage   NC Noncovered   ⊞ Combination Member   HAC associated procedure   Combination Only   DRG Non-OR   Non-OR   New/Revised in GREEN

Ø   Medical and Surgical
2   Heart and Great Vessels
J   Inspection   Definition: Visually and/or manually exploring a body part

Explanation: Visual exploration may be performed with or without optical instrumentation. Manual exploration may be performed directly or through intervening body layers.

Body Part Character 4	Approach Character 5	Device Character 6	Qualifier Character 7
A Heart **Y** Great Vessel	**Ø** Open **3** Percutaneous **4** Percutaneous Endoscopic	**Z** No Device	**Z** No Qualifier

Non-OR   Ø2J[A,Y]3ZZ

Ø   Medical and Surgical
2   Heart and Great Vessels
K   Map   Definition: Locating the route of passage of electrical impulses and/or locating functional areas in a body part

Explanation: Applicable only to the cardiac conduction mechanism and the central nervous system

Body Part Character 4	Approach Character 5	Device Character 6	Qualifier Character 7
8 Conduction Mechanism Atrioventricular node Bundle of His Bundle of Kent Sinoatrial node	**Ø** Open **3** Percutaneous **4** Percutaneous Endoscopic	**Z** No Device	**Z** No Qualifier

DRG Non-OR   Ø2K8[Ø,3,4]ZZ

Ø   Medical and Surgical
2   Heart and Great Vessels
L   Occlusion   Definition: Completely closing an orifice or the lumen of a tubular body part

Explanation: The orifice can be a natural orifice or an artificially created orifice

Body Part Character 4	Approach Character 5	Device Character 6	Qualifier Character 7
7 Atrium, Left Atrium pulmonale Left auricular appendix	**Ø** Open **3** Percutaneous **4** Percutaneous Endoscopic	**C** Extraluminal Device **D** Intraluminal Device **Z** No Device	**K** Left Atrial Appendage
H Pulmonary Valve Pulmonary annulus Pulmonic valve **P** Pulmonary Trunk **Q** Pulmonary Artery, Right **S** Pulmonary Vein, Right Right inferior pulmonary vein Right superior pulmonary vein **T** Pulmonary Vein, Left Left inferior pulmonary vein Left superior pulmonary vein **V** Superior Vena Cava Precava	**Ø** Open **3** Percutaneous **4** Percutaneous Endoscopic	**C** Extraluminal Device **D** Intraluminal Device **Z** No Device	**Z** No Qualifier
R Pulmonary Artery, Left Arterial canal (duct) Botallo's duct Pulmoaortic canal	**Ø** Open **3** Percutaneous **4** Percutaneous Endoscopic	**C** Extraluminal Device **D** Intraluminal Device **Z** No Device	**T** Ductus Arteriosus **Z** No Qualifier
W Thoracic Aorta, Descending	**3** Percutaneous	**D** Intraluminal Device	**J** Temporary

DRG Non-OR   Ø2L7[Ø,3,4][C,D,Z]K

LC Limited Coverage   **NC** Noncovered   ⊞ Combination Member   HAC associated procedure   Combination Only   DRG Non-OR   Non-OR   New/Revised in GREEN

ICD-10-PCS 2021   181

Heart and Great Vessels

Ø   Medical and Surgical
2   Heart and Great Vessels
N   Release   Definition: Freeing a body part from an abnormal physical constraint by cutting or by the use of force

                         Explanation: Some of the restraining tissue may be taken out but none of the body part is taken out

Body Part Character 4	Approach Character 5	Device Character 6	Qualifier Character 7

Ø   **Coronary Artery, One Artery**
1   **Coronary Artery, Two Arteries**
2   **Coronary Artery, Three Arteries**
3   **Coronary Artery, Four or More Arteries**
4   **Coronary Vein**
5   **Atrial Septum**
     Interatrial septum
6   **Atrium, Right**
     Atrium dextrum cordis
     Right auricular appendix
     Sinus venosus
7   **Atrium, Left**
     Atrium pulmonale
     Left auricular appendix
8   **Conduction Mechanism**
     Atrioventricular node
     Bundle of His
     Bundle of Kent
     Sinoatrial node
9   **Chordae Tendineae**
D   **Papillary Muscle**
F   **Aortic Valve**
     Aortic annulus
G   **Mitral Valve**
     Bicuspid valve
     Left atrioventricular valve
     Mitral annulus
H   **Pulmonary Valve**
     Pulmonary annulus
     Pulmonic valve
J   **Tricuspid Valve**
     Right atrioventricular valve
     Tricuspid annulus
K   **Ventricle, Right**
     Conus arteriosus
L   **Ventricle, Left**
M   **Ventricular Septum**
     Interventricular septum
N   **Pericardium**
P   **Pulmonary Trunk**
Q   **Pulmonary Artery, Right**
R   **Pulmonary Artery, Left**
     Arterial canal (duct)
     Botallo's duct
     Pulmoaortic canal
S   **Pulmonary Vein, Right**
     Right inferior pulmonary vein
     Right superior pulmonary vein
T   **Pulmonary Vein, Left**
     Left inferior pulmonary vein
     Left superior pulmonary vein
V   **Superior Vena Cava**
     Precava
W   **Thoracic Aorta, Descending**
X   **Thoracic Aorta, Ascending/Arch**
     Aortic arch
     Ascending aorta
	Ø **Open**
	3 **Percutaneous**
	4 **Percutaneous Endoscopic**
		Z **No Device**	Z **No Qualifier**

LC Limited Coverage   NC Noncovered   ⊞ Combination Member   HAC associated procedure   Combination Only   DRG Non-OR   Non-OR   New/Revised in GREEN

182   ICD-10-PCS 2021

Ø Medical and Surgical
2 Heart and Great Vessels
P Removal   Definition: Taking out or off a device from a body part

Explanation: If a device is taken out and a similar device put in without cutting or puncturing the skin or mucous membrane, the procedure is coded to the root operation CHANGE. Otherwise, the procedure for taking out a device is coded to the root operation REMOVAL.

Body Part Character 4	Approach Character 5	Device Character 6	Qualifier Character 7
A Heart	Ø Open 3 Percutaneous 4 Percutaneous Endoscopic	2 Monitoring Device 3 Infusion Device 7 Autologous Tissue Substitute 8 Zooplastic Tissue C Extraluminal Device D Intraluminal Device J Synthetic Substitute K Nonautologous Tissue Substitute M Cardiac Lead N Intracardiac Pacemaker Q Implantable Heart Assist System Y Other Device	Z No Qualifier
A Heart ⊞	Ø Open 3 Percutaneous 4 Percutaneous Endoscopic	R Short-term External Heart Assist System	S Biventricular Z No Qualifier
A Heart	X External	2 Monitoring Device 3 Infusion Device D Intraluminal Device M Cardiac Lead	Z No Qualifier
Y Great Vessel	Ø Open 3 Percutaneous 4 Percutaneous Endoscopic	2 Monitoring Device 3 Infusion Device 7 Autologous Tissue Substitute 8 Zooplastic Tissue C Extraluminal Device D Intraluminal Device J Synthetic Substitute K Nonautologous Tissue Substitute Y Other Device	Z No Qualifier
Y Great Vessel	X External	2 Monitoring Device 3 Infusion Device D Intraluminal Device	Z No Qualifier

Non-OR	Ø2PA3[2,3,D]Z	
Non-OR	Ø2PA[3,4]YZ	
Non-OR	Ø2PAX[2,3,D,M]Z	
Non-OR	Ø2PY3[2,3,D]Z	
Non-OR	Ø2PY[3,4]YZ	
Non-OR	Ø2PYX[2,3,D]Z	
HAC	Ø2PA[Ø,3,4]MZ when reported with SDx K68.11 or T81.4Ø-T81.49, T82.6- T82.7 with 7th character A	
HAC	Ø2PAXMZ when reported with SDx K68.11 or T81.4Ø-T81.49, T82.6-T82.7 with 7th character A	

See Appendix L for Procedure Combinations
⊞   Ø2PA[Ø,3,4]RZ

LC Limited Coverage   NC Noncovered   ⊞ Combination Member   HAC associated procedure   Combination Only   DRG Non-OR   Non-OR   New/Revised in GREEN

ICD-10-PCS 2021   183

Heart and Great Vessels *(left margin)*

0 Medical and Surgical
2 Heart and Great Vessels
Q Repair   Definition: Restoring, to the extent possible, a body part to its normal anatomic structure and function
                     Explanation: Used only when the method to accomplish the repair is not one of the other root operations

Body Part Character 4	Approach Character 5	Device Character 6	Qualifier Character 7

0 Coronary Artery, One Artery
1 Coronary Artery, Two Arteries
2 Coronary Artery, Three Arteries
3 Coronary Artery, Four or More
   Arteries
4 Coronary Vein
5 Atrial Septum
   Interatrial septum
6 Atrium, Right
   Atrium dextrum cordis
   Right auricular appendix
   Sinus venosus
7 Atrium, Left
   Atrium pulmonale
   Left auricular appendix
8 Conduction Mechanism
   Atrioventricular node
   Bundle of His
   Bundle of Kent
   Sinoatrial node
9 Chordae Tendineae
A Heart
B Heart, Right
   Right coronary sulcus
C Heart, Left
   Left coronary sulcus
   Obtuse margin
D Papillary Muscle
H Pulmonary Valve
   Pulmonary annulus
   Pulmonic valve
K Ventricle, Right
   Conus arteriosus
L Ventricle, Left
M Ventricular Septum
   Interventricular septum
N Pericardium
P Pulmonary Trunk
Q Pulmonary Artery, Right
R Pulmonary Artery, Left
   Arterial canal (duct)
   Botallo's duct
   Pulmoaortic canal
S Pulmonary Vein, Right
   Right inferior pulmonary vein
   Right superior pulmonary vein
T Pulmonary Vein, Left
   Left inferior pulmonary vein
   Left superior pulmonary vein
V Superior Vena Cava
   Precava
W Thoracic Aorta, Descending
X Thoracic Aorta, Ascending/Arch
   Aortic arch
   Ascending aorta
	0 Open
	3 Percutaneous
	4 Percutaneous Endoscopic
		Z No Device	Z No Qualifier

F Aortic Valve Aortic annulus	0 Open 3 Percutaneous 4 Percutaneous Endoscopic	Z No Device	J Truncal Valve Z No Qualifier

G Mitral Valve
   Bicuspid valve
   Left atrioventricular valve
   Mitral annulus
	0 Open
	3 Percutaneous
	4 Percutaneous Endoscopic
		Z No Device	E Atrioventricular Valve, Left
			Z No Qualifier

J Tricuspid Valve
   Right atrioventricular valve
   Tricuspid annulus
	0 Open
	3 Percutaneous
	4 Percutaneous Endoscopic
		Z No Device	G Atrioventricular Valve, Right
			Z No Qualifier

Ø   Medical and Surgical
2   Heart and Great Vessels
R   Replacement   Definition: Putting in or on biological or synthetic material that physically takes the place and/or function of all or a portion of a body part

Explanation: The body part may have been taken out or replaced, or may be taken out, physically eradicated, or rendered nonfunctional during the REPLACEMENT procedure. A REMOVAL procedure is coded for taking out the device used in a previous replacement procedure.

Body Part Character 4	Approach Character 5	Device Character 6	Qualifier Character 7
5 Atrial Septum Interatrial septum **6 Atrium, Right** Atrium dextrum cordis Right auricular appendix Sinus venosus **7 Atrium, Left** Atrium pulmonale Left auricular appendix **9 Chordae Tendineae** **D Papillary Muscle** **K Ventricle, Right** LC NC ⊞ Conus arteriosus **L Ventricle, Left** LC NC ⊞ **M Ventricular Septum** Interventricular septum **N Pericardium** **P Pulmonary Trunk** **Q Pulmonary Artery, Right** **R Pulmonary Artery, Left** Arterial canal (duct) Botallo's duct Pulmoaortic canal **S Pulmonary Vein, Right** Right inferior pulmonary vein Right superior pulmonary vein **T Pulmonary Vein, Left** Left inferior pulmonary vein Left superior pulmonary vein **V Superior Vena Cava** Precava **W Thoracic Aorta, Descending** **X Thoracic Aorta, Ascending/Arch** Aortic arch Ascending aorta	**Ø Open** **4 Percutaneous Endoscopic**	**7 Autologous Tissue Substitute** **8 Zooplastic Tissue** **J Synthetic Substitute** **K Nonautologous Tissue Substitute**	**Z No Qualifier**
F Aortic Valve Aortic annulus **G Mitral Valve** Bicuspid valve Left atrioventricular valve Mitral annulus **H Pulmonary Valve** Pulmonary annulus Pulmonic valve **J Tricuspid Valve** Right atrioventricular valve Tricuspid annulus	**Ø Open** **4 Percutaneous Endoscopic**	**7 Autologous Tissue Substitute** **8 Zooplastic Tissue** **J Synthetic Substitute** **K Nonautologous Tissue Substitute**	**Z No Qualifier**
F Aortic Valve Aortic annulus **G Mitral Valve** Bicuspid valve Left atrioventricular valve Mitral annulus **H Pulmonary Valve** Pulmonary annulus Pulmonic valve **J Tricuspid Valve** Right atrioventricular valve Tricuspid annulus	**3 Percutaneous**	**7 Autologous Tissue Substitute** **8 Zooplastic Tissue** **J Synthetic Substitute** **K Nonautologous Tissue Substitute**	**H Transapical** **Z No Qualifier**

LC Ø2RKØJZ with Ø2RLØJZ with diagnosis code ZØØ.6	**See Appendix L for Procedure Combinations**	
NC Ø2RKØJZ with Ø2RLØJZ without diagnosis code ZØØ.6	⊞ Ø2R[K,L]ØJZ	

LC Limited Coverage   NC Noncovered   ⊞ Combination Member   HAC associated procedure   Combination Only   DRG Non-OR   Non-OR   New/Revised in GREEN

ICD-10-PCS 2021   185

Heart and Great Vessels

Ø2R–Ø2R

Ø   **Medical and Surgical**
2   **Heart and Great Vessels**
S   **Reposition**   Definition: Moving to its normal location, or other suitable location, all or a portion of a body part

                       Explanation: The body part is moved to a new location from an abnormal location, or from a normal location where it is not functioning correctly. The body part may or may not be cut out or off to be moved to the new location.

Body Part Character 4	Approach Character 5	Device Character 6	Qualifier Character 7
Ø **Coronary Artery, One Artery**	**Ø** Open	**Z** No Device	**Z** No Qualifier
1 **Coronary Artery, Two Arteries**			
P **Pulmonary Trunk**			
Q **Pulmonary Artery, Right**			
R **Pulmonary Artery, Left**			
Arterial canal (duct)			
Botallo's duct			
Pulmoaortic canal			
S **Pulmonary Vein, Right**			
Right inferior pulmonary vein			
Right superior pulmonary vein			
T **Pulmonary Vein, Left**			
Left inferior pulmonary vein			
Left superior pulmonary vein			
V **Superior Vena Cava**			
Precava			
W **Thoracic Aorta, Descending**			
X **Thoracic Aorta, Ascending/Arch**			
Aortic arch			
Ascending aorta			

Ø   **Medical and Surgical**
2   **Heart and Great Vessels**
T   **Resection**   Definition: Cutting out or off, without replacement, all of a body part

                       Explanation: None

Body Part Character 4	Approach Character 5	Device Character 6	Qualifier Character 7
5 **Atrial Septum**	**Ø** Open	**Z** No Device	**Z** No Qualifier
Interatrial septum	**3** Percutaneous		
8 **Conduction Mechanism**	**4** Percutaneous Endoscopic		
Atrioventricular node			
Bundle of His			
Bundle of Kent			
Sinoatrial node			
9 **Chordae Tendineae**			
D **Papillary Muscle**			
H **Pulmonary Valve**			
Pulmonary annulus			
Pulmonic valve			
M **Ventricular Septum**			
Interventricular septum			
N **Pericardium**			

Heart and Great Vessels

Ø   **Medical and Surgical**
2   **Heart and Great Vessels**
U   **Supplement**   Definition: Putting in or on biological or synthetic material that physically reinforces and/or augments the function of a portion of a body part
                          Explanation: The biological material is non-living, or is living and from the same individual. The body part may have been previously replaced, and the SUPPLEMENT procedure is performed to physically reinforce and/or augment the function of the replaced body part.

Body Part Character 4	Approach Character 5	Device Character 6	Qualifier Character 7

Ø   **Coronary Artery, One Artery**
 1   **Coronary Artery, Two Arteries**
 2   **Coronary Artery, Three Arteries**
 3   **Coronary Artery, Four or More Arteries**
 5   **Atrial Septum**
      Interatrial septum
 6   **Atrium, Right**
      Atrium dextrum cordis
      Right auricular appendix
      Sinus venosus
 7   **Atrium, Left**
      Atrium pulmonale
      Left auricular appendix
 9   **Chordae Tendineae**
 A   **Heart**
 D   **Papillary Muscle**
 H   **Pulmonary Valve**
      Pulmonary annulus
      Pulmonic valve
 K   **Ventricle, Right**
      Conus arteriosus
 L   **Ventricle, Left**
 M   **Ventricular Septum**
      Interventricular septum
 N   **Pericardium**
 P   **Pulmonary Trunk**
 Q   **Pulmonary Artery, Right**
 R   **Pulmonary Artery, Left**
      Arterial canal (duct)
      Botallo's duct
      Pulmoaortic canal
 S   **Pulmonary Vein, Right**
      Right inferior pulmonary vein
      Right superior pulmonary vein
 T   **Pulmonary Vein, Left**
      Left inferior pulmonary vein
      Left superior pulmonary vein
 V   **Superior Vena Cava**
      Precava
 W   **Thoracic Aorta, Descending**
 X   **Thoracic Aorta, Ascending/Arch**
      Aortic arch
      Ascending aorta
	Ø **Open**
	 3 **Percutaneous**
	 4 **Percutaneous Endoscopic**
		7 **Autologous Tissue Substitute**
		 8 **Zooplastic Tissue**
		 J **Synthetic Substitute**
		 K **Nonautologous Tissue Substitute**
			Z **No Qualifier**

F **Aortic Valve** Aortic annulus	Ø **Open** 3 **Percutaneous** 4 **Percutaneous Endoscopic**	7 **Autologous Tissue Substitute** 8 **Zooplastic Tissue** J **Synthetic Substitute** K **Nonautologous Tissue Substitute**	J **Truncal Valve** Z **No Qualifier**

G   **Mitral Valve**
      Bicuspid valve
      Left atrioventricular valve
      Mitral annulus
	Ø **Open**
	 4 **Percutaneous Endoscopic**
		7 **Autologous Tissue Substitute**
		 8 **Zooplastic Tissue**
		 J **Synthetic Substitute**
		 K **Nonautologous Tissue Substitute**
			E **Atrioventricular Valve, Left**
			 Z **No Qualifier**

G   Mitral Valve
      Bicuspid valve
      Left atrioventricular valve
      Mitral annulus
	3 Percutaneous	7 Autologous Tissue Substitute
		 8 Zooplastic Tissue
		 K Nonautologous Tissue Substitute
			E Atrioventricular Valve, Left
			 Z No Qualifier

G   Mitral Valve
      Bicuspid valve
      Left atrioventricular valve
      Mitral annulus
	3 Percutaneous	J Synthetic Substitute	E Atrioventricular Valve, Left
			 H Transapical
			 Z No Qualifier

J   **Tricuspid Valve**
      Right atrioventricular valve
      Tricuspid annulus
	Ø **Open**
	 3 **Percutaneous**
	 4 **Percutaneous Endoscopic**
		7 **Autologous Tissue Substitute**
		 8 **Zooplastic Tissue**
		 J **Synthetic Substitute**
		 K **Nonautologous Tissue Substitute**
			G **Atrioventricular Valve, Right**
			 Z **No Qualifier**

DRG Non-OR   Ø2U7[3,4]JZ

Heart and Great Vessels

Ø   **Medical and Surgical**
2   **Heart and Great Vessels**
V   **Restriction**   Definition: Partially closing an orifice or the lumen of a tubular body part
                       Explanation: The orifice can be a natural orifice or an artificially created orifice

Body Part Character 4	Approach Character 5	Device Character 6	Qualifier Character 7
A Heart	**Ø** Open **3** Percutaneous **4** Percutaneous Endoscopic	**C** Extraluminal Device **Z** No Device	**Z** No Qualifier

G Mitral Valve
    Bicuspid valve
    Left atrioventricular valve
    Mitral annulus
	Ø Open
	3 Percutaneous
	4 Percutaneous Endoscopic
		Z No Device	**Z** No Qualifier

P Pulmonary Trunk
Q Pulmonary Artery, Right
S Pulmonary Vein, Right
    Right inferior pulmonary vein
    Right superior pulmonary vein
T Pulmonary Vein, Left
    Left inferior pulmonary vein
    Left superior pulmonary vein
V Superior Vena Cava
    Precava
	Ø Open
	3 Percutaneous
	4 Percutaneous Endoscopic
		C Extraluminal Device
		D Intraluminal Device
		Z No Device
			Z No Qualifier

R Pulmonary Artery, Left
    Arterial canal (duct)
    Botallo's duct
    Pulmoaortic canal
	Ø Open
	3 Percutaneous
	4 Percutaneous Endoscopic
		C Extraluminal Device
		D Intraluminal Device
		Z No Device
			T Ductus Arteriosus
			Z No Qualifier

W Thoracic Aorta, Descending
X Thoracic Aorta, Ascending/Arch
    Aortic arch
    Ascending aorta
	Ø Open
	3 Percutaneous
	4 Percutaneous Endoscopic
		C Extraluminal Device
		D Intraluminal Device
		E Intraluminal Device, Branched or
		    Fenestrated, One or Two Arteries
		F Intraluminal Device, Branched or
		    Fenestrated, Three or More Arteries
		Z No Device
			Z No Qualifier

0 Medical and Surgical
2 Heart and Great Vessels
W Revision   Definition: Correcting, to the extent possible, a portion of a malfunctioning device or the position of a displaced device
                     Explanation: Revision can include correcting a malfunctioning or displaced device by taking out or putting in components of the device such as a screw or pin

Body Part Character 4	Approach Character 5	Device Character 6	Qualifier Character 7

5 Atrial Septum
  Interatrial septum
M Ventricular Septum
  Interventricular septum
	0 Open
	4 Percutaneous Endoscopic
		J Synthetic Substitute	Z No Qualifier

A Heart LC NC ⊞	0 Open 3 Percutaneous 4 Percutaneous Endoscopic	2 Monitoring Device 3 Infusion Device 7 Autologous Tissue Substitute 8 Zooplastic Tissue C Extraluminal Device D Intraluminal Device J Synthetic Substitute K Nonautologous Tissue Substitute M Cardiac Lead N Intracardiac Pacemaker Q Implantable Heart Assist System Y Other Device	Z No Qualifier
A Heart ⊞	0 Open 3 Percutaneous 4 Percutaneous Endoscopic	R Short-term External Heart Assist System	S Biventricular Z No Qualifier
A Heart	X External	2 Monitoring Device 3 Infusion Device 7 Autologous Tissue Substitute 8 Zooplastic Tissue C Extraluminal Device D Intraluminal Device J Synthetic Substitute K Nonautologous Tissue Substitute M Cardiac Lead N Intracardiac Pacemaker Q Implantable Heart Assist System	Z No Qualifier
A Heart	X External	R Short-term External Heart Assist System	S Biventricular Z No Qualifier

F Aortic Valve
  Aortic annulus
G Mitral Valve
  Bicuspid valve
  Left atrioventricular valve
  Mitral annulus
H Pulmonary Valve
  Pulmonary annulus
  Pulmonic valve
J Tricuspid Valve
  Right atrioventricular valve
  Tricuspid annulus
	0 Open
	3 Percutaneous
	4 Percutaneous Endoscopic
		7 Autologous Tissue Substitute
		8 Zooplastic Tissue
		J Synthetic Substitute
		K Nonautologous Tissue Substitute
			Z No Qualifier

Y Great Vessel	0 Open 3 Percutaneous 4 Percutaneous Endoscopic	2 Monitoring Device 3 Infusion Device 7 Autologous Tissue Substitute 8 Zooplastic Tissue C Extraluminal Device D Intraluminal Device J Synthetic Substitute K Nonautologous Tissue Substitute Y Other Device	Z No Qualifier
Y Great Vessel	X External	2 Monitoring Device 3 Infusion Device 7 Autologous Tissue Substitute 8 Zooplastic Tissue C Extraluminal Device D Intraluminal Device J Synthetic Substitute K Nonautologous Tissue Substitute	Z No Qualifier

Non-OR   02WA3[2,3,D]Z
Non-OR   02WA[3,4]YZ
Non-OR   02WAX[2,3,7,8,C,D,J,K,M,N,Q]Z
Non-OR   02WAXRZ
Non-OR   02WY3[2,3,D]Z
Non-OR   02WY[3,4]YZ
Non-OR   02WYX[2,3,7,8,C,D,J,K]Z

HAC   02WA[0,3,4]MZ when reported with T81.40–T81.49, T82.6–T82.7 with 7th character A
LC   02WA0[J,Q]Z
NC   02WA[3,4]QZ

See Appendix L for Procedure Combinations
⊞   02WA[0,3,4]QZ
⊞   02WA[0,3,4]RZ

LC Limited Coverage   NC Noncovered   ⊞ Combination Member   HAC HAC associated procedure   Combination Only   DRG Non-OR   Non-OR   New/Revised in GREEN
ICD-10-PCS 2021   189

02W–02W

Ø   Medical and Surgical
2   Heart and Great Vessels
Y   Transplantation   Definition: Putting in or on all or a portion of a living body part taken from another individual or animal to physically take the place and/or function of all or a portion of a similar body part

Explanation: The native body part may or may not be taken out, and the transplanted body part may take over all or a portion of its function

Body Part Character 4	Approach Character 5	Device Character 6	Qualifier Character 7
A Heart LC	Ø Open	Z No Device	Ø Allogeneic 1 Syngeneic 2 Zooplastic

     LC   Ø2YAØZ[Ø,1,2]

LC Limited Coverage   NC Noncovered   ⊞ Combination Member   HAC associated procedure   Combination Only   DRG Non-OR   Non-OR   New/Revised in GREEN

190   ICD-10-PCS 2021

Upper Arteries Ø31–Ø3W

Character Meanings

This Character Meaning table is provided as a guide to assist the user in the identification of character members that may be found in this section of code tables. It **SHOULD NOT** be used to build a PCS code.

Operation–Character 3	Body Part–Character 4	Approach–Character 5	Device–Character 6	Qualifier–Character 7
1 Bypass	Ø Internal Mammary Artery, Right	Ø Open	Ø Drainage Device	Ø Upper Arm Artery, Right OR Ultrasonic
5 Destruction	1 Internal Mammary Artery, Left	3 Percutaneous	2 Monitoring Device	1 Upper Arm Artery, Left OR Drug-Coated Balloon
7 Dilation	2 Innominate Artery	4 Percutaneous Endoscopic	3 Infusion Device	2 Upper Arm Artery, Bilateral
9 Drainage	3 Subclavian Artery, Right	X External	4 Intraluminal Device, Drug-eluting	3 Lower Arm Artery, Right
B Excision	4 Subclavian Artery, Left		5 Intraluminal Device, Drug-eluting, Two	4 Lower Arm Artery, Left
C Extirpation	5 Axillary Artery, Right		6 Intraluminal Device, Drug-eluting, Three	5 Lower Arm Artery, Bilateral
F Fragmentation	6 Axillary Artery, Left		7 Intraluminal Device, Drug-eluting, Four or More OR Autologous Tissue Substitute	6 Upper Leg Artery, Right
H Insertion	7 Brachial Artery, Right		9 Autologous Venous Tissue	7 Upper Leg Artery, Left OR Stent Retriever
J Inspection	8 Brachial Artery, Left		A Autologous Arterial Tissue	8 Upper Leg Artery, Bilateral
L Occlusion	9 Ulnar Artery, Right		B Intraluminal Device, Bioactive	9 Lower Leg Artery, Right
N Release	A Ulnar Artery, Left		C Extraluminal Device	B Lower Leg Artery, Left
P Removal	B Radial Artery, Right		D Intraluminal Device	C Lower Leg Artery, Bilateral
Q Repair	C Radial Artery, Left		E Intraluminal Device, Two	D Upper Arm Vein
R Replacement	D Hand Artery, Right		F Intraluminal Device, Three	F Lower Arm Vein
S Reposition	F Hand Artery, Left		G Intraluminal Device, Four or More	G Intracranial Artery
U Supplement	G Intracranial Artery		H Intraluminal Device, Flow Diverter	J Extracranial Artery, Right
V Restriction	H Common Carotid Artery, Right		J Synthetic Substitute	K Extracranial Artery, Left
W Revision	J Common Carotid Artery, Left		K Nonautologous Tissue Substitute	M Pulmonary Artery, Right
	K Internal Carotid Artery, Right		M Stimulator Lead	N Pulmonary Artery, Left
	L Internal Carotid Artery, Left		Y Other Device	T Abdominal Artery
	M External Carotid Artery, Right		Z No Device	V Superior Vena Cava
	N External Carotid Artery, Left			W Lower Extremity Vein
	P Vertebral Artery, Right			X Diagnostic
	Q Vertebral Artery, Left			Y Upper Artery
	R Face Artery			Z No Qualifier
	S Temporal Artery, Right			
	T Temporal Artery, Left			
	U Thyroid Artery, Right			
	V Thyroid Artery, Left			
	Y Upper Artery			

AHA Coding Clinic for table Ø31

2019, 4Q, 26	Upper artery bypass Qualifier
2019, 4Q, 26	Percutaneous approach upper artery bypass
2017, 4Q, 64-65	New qualifier values - Left to right carotid bypass
2017, 2Q, 22	Carotid artery to subclavian artery transposition
2017, 1Q, 31	Left to right common carotid artery bypass
2016, 3Q, 37	Insertion of arteriovenous graft using HeRO device
2016, 3Q, 39	Revision of arteriovenous graft
2013, 4Q, 125	Stage II cephalic vein transposition (superficialization) of arteriovenous fistula
2013, 1Q, 27	Creation of radial artery fistula

AHA Coding Clinic for table Ø37

2019, 4Q, 27	Bifurcation Qualifier
2019, 3Q, 29	Transcarotid arterial catheterization
2018, 2Q, 24	Coronary artery bifurcation
2016, 4Q, 86	Peripheral artery, number of stents
2016, 4Q, 86-87	Coronary and peripheral artery bifurcation
2015, 1Q, 32	Deployment of stent for herniated/migrated coil in basilar artery

AHA Coding Clinic for table Ø3B

2016, 2Q, 12	Resection of malignant neoplasm of infratemporal fossa

AHA Coding Clinic for table Ø3C

2019, 4Q, 27	Bifurcation Qualifier
2018, 4Q, 47-48	Endovascular thrombectomy with stent retriever
2018, 2Q, 24	Coronary artery bifurcation
2017, 4Q, 64-65	New qualifier values - Left to right carotid bypass
2017, 2Q, 23	Thrombectomy via Fogarty catheter
2016, 4Q, 86-87	Coronary and peripheral artery bifurcation
2016, 2Q, 11	Carotid endarterectomy with patch angioplasty
2015, 1Q, 29	Discontinued carotid endarterectomy

AHA Coding Clinic for table Ø3H

2020, 1Q, 25	Elephant trunk repair of aortic dissection
2016, 2Q, 32	Arterial catheter placement

AHA Coding Clinic for table Ø3J

2015, 1Q, 29	Discontinued carotid endarterectomy

AHA Coding Clinic for table Ø3L

2016, 2Q, 30	Clipping (occlusion) of cerebral artery, decompressive craniectomy and storage of bone flap in abdominal wall
2014, 4Q, 20	Control of epistaxis
2014, 4Q, 37	Endovascular embolization of arteriovenous malformation using Onyx-18 liquid

AHA Coding Clinic for table Ø3Q

2017, 1Q, 31	Left to right common carotid artery bypass

AHA Coding Clinic for table Ø3S

2017, 2Q, 22	Carotid artery to subclavian artery transposition
2015, 3Q, 27	Moyamoya disease and hemispheric pial synagiosis with craniotomy

AHA Coding Clinic for table Ø3U

2019, 1Q, 22	Cerebral artery fusiform aneurysm repair via wrapping
2016, 2Q, 11	Carotid endarterectomy with patch angioplasty

AHA Coding Clinic for table Ø3V

2019, 4Q, 27-28	Aneurysm treatment using flow diverter stent
2019, 1Q, 22	Cerebral artery fusiform aneurysm repair via wrapping
2016, 1Q, 19	Embolization of superior hypophyseal aneurysm using stent-assisted coil

AHA Coding Clinic for table Ø3W

2016, 3Q, 39	Revision of arteriovenous graft
2015, 1Q, 32	Deployment of stent for herniated/migrated coil in basilar artery

Upper Arteries

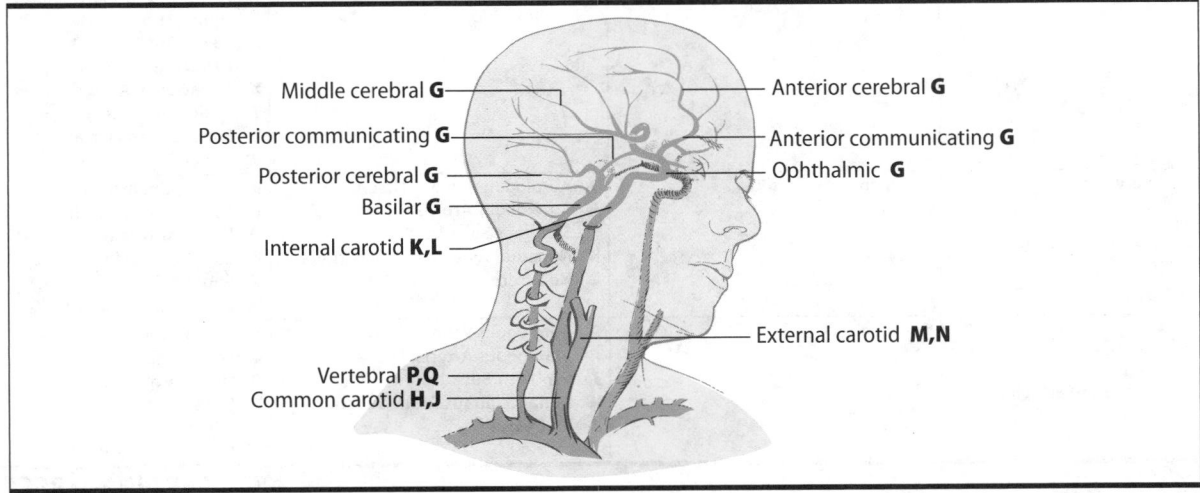

Middle temporal **S, T**
Transverse facial **S, T**
Superficial temporal **S, T**
Face **R**
External carotid **M, N**
Internal carotid **K, L**
Common carotid **H, J**
Superior thyroid **U, V**
Vertebral **P, Q**
Inferior thyroid **U, V**
Subclavian **3, 4**
Innominate **2**
Axillary **5, 6**
Internal thoracic (mammary) **Ø, 1**
Brachial **7, 8**
Radial **B, C**
Ulnar **9, A**
Deep palmar arch **D, F**
Superficial palmar arch **D, F**

Head and Neck Arteries

Middle cerebral **G**
Anterior cerebral **G**
Posterior communicating **G**
Anterior communicating **G**
Posterior cerebral **G**
Ophthalmic **G**
Basilar **G**
Internal carotid **K,L**
External carotid **M,N**
Vertebral **P,Q**
Common carotid **H,J**

Ø   **Medical and Surgical**
3   **Upper Arteries**
1   **Bypass**   Definition: Altering the route of passage of the contents of a tubular body part

Explanation: Rerouting contents of a body part to a downstream area of the normal route, to a similar route and body part, or to an abnormal route and dissimilar body part. Includes one or more anastomoses, with or without the use of a device.

Body Part Character 4	Approach Character 5	Device Character 6	Qualifier Character 7
2 **Innominate Artery** Brachiocephalic artery Brachiocephalic trunk	Ø Open	9 Autologous Venous Tissue A Autologous Arterial Tissue J Synthetic Substitute K Nonautologous Tissue Substitute Z No Device	Ø Upper Arm Artery, Right 1 Upper Arm Artery, Left 2 Upper Arm Artery, Bilateral 3 Lower Arm Artery, Right 4 Lower Arm Artery, Left 5 Lower Arm Artery, Bilateral 6 Upper Leg Artery, Right 7 Upper Leg Artery, Left 8 Upper Leg Artery, Bilateral 9 Lower Leg Artery, Right B Lower Leg Artery, Left C Lower Leg Artery, Bilateral D Upper Arm Vein F Lower Arm Vein J Extracranial Artery, Right K Extracranial Artery, Left W Lower Extremity Vein
3 **Subclavian Artery, Right** Costocervical trunk Dorsal scapular artery Internal thoracic artery **4** **Subclavian Artery, Left** *See 3 Subclavian Artery, Right*	Ø Open	9 Autologous Venous Tissue A Autologous Arterial Tissue J Synthetic Substitute K Nonautologous Tissue Substitute Z No Device	Ø Upper Arm Artery, Right 1 Upper Arm Artery, Left 2 Upper Arm Artery, Bilateral 3 Lower Arm Artery, Right 4 Lower Arm Artery, Left 5 Lower Arm Artery, Bilateral 6 Upper Leg Artery, Right 7 Upper Leg Artery, Left 8 Upper Leg Artery, Bilateral 9 Lower Leg Artery, Right B Lower Leg Artery, Left C Lower Leg Artery, Bilateral D Upper Arm Vein F Lower Arm Vein J Extracranial Artery, Right K Extracranial Artery, Left M Pulmonary Artery, Right N Pulmonary Artery, Left W Lower Extremity Vein
5 **Axillary Artery, Right** Anterior circumflex humeral artery Lateral thoracic artery Posterior circumflex humeral artery Subscapular artery Superior thoracic artery Thoracoacromial artery **6** **Axillary Artery, Left** *See 5 Axillary Artery, Right*	Ø Open	9 Autologous Venous Tissue A Autologous Arterial Tissue J Synthetic Substitute K Nonautologous Tissue Substitute Z No Device	Ø Upper Arm Artery, Right 1 Upper Arm Artery, Left 2 Upper Arm Artery, Bilateral 3 Lower Arm Artery, Right 4 Lower Arm Artery, Left 5 Lower Arm Artery, Bilateral 6 Upper Leg Artery, Right 7 Upper Leg Artery, Left 8 Upper Leg Artery, Bilateral 9 Lower Leg Artery, Right B Lower Leg Artery, Left C Lower Leg Artery, Bilateral D Upper Arm Vein F Lower Arm Vein J Extracranial Artery, Right K Extracranial Artery, Left T Abdominal Artery V Superior Vena Cava W Lower Extremity Vein
7 **Brachial Artery, Right** Inferior ulnar collateral artery Profunda brachii Superior ulnar collateral artery	Ø Open	9 Autologous Venous Tissue A Autologous Arterial Tissue J Synthetic Substitute K Nonautologous Tissue Substitute Z No Device	Ø Upper Arm Artery, Right 3 Lower Arm Artery, Right D Upper Arm Vein F Lower Arm Vein V Superior Vena Cava W Lower Extremity Vein
8 **Brachial Artery, Left** Inferior ulnar collateral artery Profunda brachii Superior ulnar collateral artery	Ø Open	9 Autologous Venous Tissue A Autologous Arterial Tissue J Synthetic Substitute K Nonautologous Tissue Substitute Z No Device	1 Upper Arm Artery, Left 4 Lower Arm Artery, Left D Upper Arm Vein F Lower Arm Vein V Superior Vena Cava W Lower Extremity Vein

Ø31 Continued on next page

LC Limited Coverage **NC** Noncovered ⊞ Combination Member HAC associated procedure Combination Only DRG Non-OR Non-OR New/Revised in **GREEN**
194   ICD-10-PCS 2021

Ø31–Ø31

Ø   **Medical and Surgical**   *031 Continued*
3   **Upper Arteries**
1   **Bypass**   Definition: Altering the route of passage of the contents of a tubular body part

                     Explanation: Rerouting contents of a body part to a downstream area of the normal route, to a similar route and body part, or to an abnormal route and dissimilar body part. Includes one or more anastomoses, with or without the use of a device.

Body Part Character 4	Approach Character 5	Device Character 6	Qualifier Character 7

9 **Ulnar Artery, Right**
   Anterior ulnar recurrent artery
   Common interosseous artery
   Posterior ulnar recurrent artery
B **Radial Artery, Right**
   Radial recurrent artery
	Ø Open	**9** Autologous Venous Tissue
		A Autologous Arterial Tissue
		J Synthetic Substitute
		K Nonautologous Tissue Substitute
		Z No Device
			3 Lower Arm Artery, Right
			F Lower Arm Vein

9 **Ulnar Artery, Right**
   Anterior ulnar recurrent artery
   Common interosseous artery
   Posterior ulnar recurrent artery
B **Radial Artery, Right**
   Radial recurrent artery
	3 Percutaneous	**Z** No Device	**F** Lower Arm Vein

A **Ulnar Artery, Left**
   Anterior ulnar recurrent artery
   Common interosseous artery
   Posterior ulnar recurrent artery
C **Radial Artery, Left**
   Radial recurrent artery
	Ø Open	**9** Autologous Venous Tissue
		A Autologous Arterial Tissue
		J Synthetic Substitute
		K Nonautologous Tissue Substitute
		Z No Device
			4 Lower Arm Artery, Left
			F Lower Arm Vein

A **Ulnar Artery, Left**
   Anterior ulnar recurrent artery
   Common interosseous artery
   Posterior ulnar recurrent artery
C **Radial Artery, Left**
   Radial recurrent artery
	3 Percutaneous	**Z** No Device	**F** Lower Arm Vein

G **Intracranial Artery**
   Anterior cerebral artery
   Anterior choroidal artery
   Anterior communicating artery
   Basilar artery
   Circle of Willis
   Internal carotid artery, intracranial
     portion
   Middle cerebral artery
   Ophthalmic artery
   Posterior cerebral artery
   Posterior communicating artery
   Posterior inferior cerebellar artery
     (PICA)
S **Temporal Artery, Right**
   Middle temporal artery
   Superficial temporal artery
   Transverse facial artery
T **Temporal Artery, Left**
   See S Temporal Artery, Right
	Ø Open	**9** Autologous Venous Tissue
		A Autologous Arterial Tissue
		J Synthetic Substitute
		K Nonautologous Tissue Substitute
		Z No Device
			G Intracranial Artery

H **Common Carotid Artery, Right** **J** **Common Carotid Artery, Left**	**Ø** Open	**9** Autologous Venous Tissue **A** Autologous Arterial Tissue **J** Synthetic Substitute **K** Nonautologous Tissue Substitute **Z** No Device	**G** Intracranial Artery **J** Extracranial Artery, Right **K** Extracranial Artery, Left **Y** Upper Artery

K **Internal Carotid Artery, Right**
   Caroticotympanic artery
   Carotid sinus
L **Internal Carotid Artery, Left**
   Caroticotympanic artery
   Carotid sinus
M **External Carotid Artery, Right**
   Ascending pharyngeal artery
   Internal maxillary artery
   Lingual artery
   Maxillary artery
   Occipital artery
   Posterior auricular artery
   Superior thyroid artery
N **External Carotid Artery, Left**
   Ascending pharyngeal artery
   Internal maxillary artery
   Lingual artery
   Maxillary artery
   Occipital artery
   Posterior auricular artery
   Superior thyroid artery
	Ø Open	**9** Autologous Venous Tissue
		A Autologous Arterial Tissue
		J Synthetic Substitute
		K Nonautologous Tissue Substitute
		Z No Device
			J Extracranial Artery, Right
			K Extracranial Artery, Left

LC Limited Coverage   **NC** Noncovered   ⊞ Combination Member   HAC associated procedure   Combination Only   DRG Non-OR   Non-OR   New/Revised in GREEN

ICD-10-PCS 2021   195

031–031

Upper Arteries

Ø   Medical and Surgical
3   Upper Arteries
5   Destruction   Definition: Physical eradication of all or a portion of a body part by the direct use of energy, force, or a destructive agent

Explanation: None of the body part is physically taken out

Body Part Character 4	Approach Character 5	Device Character 6	Qualifier Character 7
Ø Internal Mammary Artery, Right Anterior intercostal artery Internal thoracic artery Musculophrenic artery Pericardiophrenic artery Superior epigastric artery **1 Internal Mammary Artery, Left** *See Ø Internal Mammary Artery, Right* **2 Innominate Artery** Brachiocephalic artery Brachiocephalic trunk **3 Subclavian Artery, Right** Costocervical trunk Dorsal scapular artery Internal thoracic artery **4 Subclavian Artery, Left** *See 3 Subclavian Artery, Right* **5 Axillary Artery, Right** Anterior circumflex humeral artery Lateral thoracic artery Posterior circumflex humeral artery Subscapular artery Superior thoracic artery Thoracoacromial artery **6 Axillary Artery, Left** *See 5 Axillary Artery, Right* **7 Brachial Artery, Right** Inferior ulnar collateral artery Profunda brachii Superior ulnar collateral artery **8 Brachial Artery, Left** *See 7 Brachial Artery, Right* **9 Ulnar Artery, Right** Anterior ulnar recurrent artery Common interosseous artery Posterior ulnar recurrent artery **A Ulnar Artery, Left** *See 9 Ulnar Artery, Right* **B Radial Artery, Right** Radial recurrent artery **C Radial Artery, Left** *See B Radial Artery, Right* **D Hand Artery, Right** Deep palmar arch Princeps pollicis artery Radialis indicis Superficial palmar arch **F Hand Artery, Left** *See D Hand Artery, Right* **G Intracranial Artery** Anterior cerebral artery Anterior choroidal artery Anterior communicating artery Basilar artery Circle of Willis Internal carotid artery, intracranial portion Middle cerebral artery Ophthalmic artery Posterior cerebral artery Posterior communicating artery Posterior inferior cerebellar artery (PICA) **H Common Carotid Artery, Right** **J Common Carotid Artery, Left** **K Internal Carotid Artery, Right** Caroticotympanic artery Carotid sinus **L Internal Carotid Artery, Left** *See K Internal Carotid Artery, Right* **M External Carotid Artery, Right** Ascending pharyngeal artery Internal maxillary artery Lingual artery Maxillary artery Occipital artery Posterior auricular artery Superior thyroid artery **N External Carotid Artery, Left** *See M External Carotid Artery, Right* **P Vertebral Artery, Right** Anterior spinal artery Posterior spinal artery **Q Vertebral Artery, Left** *See P Vertebral Artery, Right* **R Face Artery** Angular artery Ascending palatine artery External maxillary artery Facial artery Inferior labial artery Submental artery Superior labial artery **S Temporal Artery, Right** Middle temporal artery Superficial temporal artery Transverse facial artery **T Temporal Artery, Left** *See S Temporal Artery, Right* **U Thyroid Artery, Right** Cricothyroid artery Hyoid artery Sternocleidomastoid artery Superior laryngeal artery Superior thyroid artery Thyrocervical trunk **V Thyroid Artery, Left** *See U Thyroid Artery, Right* **Y Upper Artery** Aortic intercostal artery Bronchial artery Esophageal artery Subcostal artery	**Ø Open** **3 Percutaneous** **4 Percutaneous Endoscopic**	**Z No Device**	**Z No Qualifier**

LC Limited Coverage   **NC** Noncovered   ⊞ Combination Member   HAC associated procedure   Combination Only   DRG Non-OR   Non-OR   New/Revised in **GREEN**

196   ICD-10-PCS 2021

Ø   **Medical and Surgical**
3   **Upper Arteries**
7   **Dilation**   Definition: Expanding an orifice or the lumen of a tubular body part

Explanation: The orifice can be a natural orifice or an artificially created orifice. Accomplished by stretching a tubular body part using intraluminal pressure or by cutting part of the orifice or wall of the tubular body part.

Body Part Character 4		Approach Character 5	Device Character 6	Qualifier Character 7

Ø Internal Mammary Artery, Right
  Anterior intercostal artery
  Internal thoracic artery
  Musculophrenic artery
  Pericardiophrenic artery
  Superior epigastric artery
1 Internal Mammary Artery, Left
  See Ø Internal Mammary Artery, Right
2 Innominate Artery
  Brachiocephalic artery
  Brachiocephalic trunk
3 Subclavian Artery, Right
  Costocervical trunk
  Dorsal scapular artery
  Internal thoracic artery
4 Subclavian Artery, Left
  See 3 Subclavian Artery, Right
5 Axillary Artery, Right
  Anterior circumflex humeral artery
  Lateral thoracic artery
  Posterior circumflex humeral artery
  Subscapular artery
  Superior thoracic artery
  Thoracoacromial artery
	6 Axillary Artery, Left
	  See 5 Axillary Artery, Right
	7 Brachial Artery, Right
	  Inferior ulnar collateral artery
	  Profunda brachii
	  Superior ulnar collateral artery
	8 Brachial Artery, Left
	  See 7 Brachial Artery, Right
	9 Ulnar Artery, Right
	  Anterior ulnar recurrent artery
	  Common interosseous artery
	  Posterior ulnar recurrent artery
	A Ulnar Artery, Left
	  See 9 Ulnar Artery, Right
	B Radial Artery, Right
	  Radial recurrent artery
	C Radial Artery, Left
	  See B Radial Artery, Right
		Ø Open
		3 Percutaneous
		4 Percutaneous Endoscopic
			4 Intraluminal Device, Drug-eluting
			5 Intraluminal Device, Drug-eluting, Two
			6 Intraluminal Device, Drug-eluting, Three
			7 Intraluminal Device, Drug-eluting, Four or More
			E Intraluminal Device, Two
			F Intraluminal Device, Three
			G Intraluminal Device, Four or More
				Z No Qualifier

Ø Internal Mammary Artery, Right
  Anterior intercostal artery
  Internal thoracic artery
  Musculophrenic artery
  Pericardiophrenic artery
  Superior epigastric artery
1 Internal Mammary Artery, Left
  See Ø Internal Mammary Artery, Right
2 Innominate Artery
  Brachiocephalic artery
  Brachiocephalic trunk
3 Subclavian Artery, Right
  Costocervical trunk
  Dorsal scapular artery
  Internal thoracic artery
4 Subclavian Artery, Left
  See 3 Subclavian Artery, Right
5 Axillary Artery, Right
  Anterior circumflex humeral artery
  Lateral thoracic artery
  Posterior circumflex humeral artery
  Subscapular artery
  Superior thoracic artery
  Thoracoacromial artery
	6 Axillary Artery, Left
	  See 5 Axillary Artery, Right
	7 Brachial Artery, Right
	  Inferior ulnar collateral artery
	  Profunda brachii
	  Superior ulnar collateral artery
	8 Brachial Artery, Left
	  See 7 Brachial Artery, Right
	9 Ulnar Artery, Right
	  Anterior ulnar recurrent artery
	  Common interosseous artery
	  Posterior ulnar recurrent artery
	A Ulnar Artery, Left
	  See 9 Ulnar Artery, Right
	B Radial Artery, Right
	  Radial recurrent artery
	C Radial Artery, Left
	  See B Radial Artery, Right
		Ø Open
		3 Percutaneous
		4 Percutaneous Endoscopic
			D Intraluminal Device
			Z No Device
				1 Drug-Coated Balloon
				Z No Qualifier

Ø37 Continued on next page

LC Limited Coverage   NC Noncovered   ⊞ Combination Member   HAC associated procedure   Combination Only   DRG Non-OR   Non-OR   New/Revised in GREEN

Ø　Medical and Surgical
3　Upper Arteries
7　Dilation

Definition: Expanding an orifice or the lumen of a tubular body part

Explanation: The orifice can be a natural orifice or an artificially created orifice. Accomplished by stretching a tubular body part using intraluminal pressure or by cutting part of the orifice or wall of the tubular body part.

Body Part Character 4		Approach Character 5	Device Character 6	Qualifier Character 7
D Hand Artery, Right Deep palmar arch Princeps pollicis artery Radialis indicis Superficial palmar arch **F Hand Artery, Left** *See D Hand Artery, Right* **G Intracranial Artery** NC Anterior cerebral artery Anterior choroidal artery Anterior communicating artery Basilar artery Circle of Willis Internal carotid artery, intracranial portion Middle cerebral artery Ophthalmic artery Posterior cerebral artery Posterior communicating artery Posterior inferior cerebellar artery (PICA) **H Common Carotid Artery, Right** **J Common Carotid Artery, Left** **K Internal Carotid Artery, Right** Caroticotympanic artery Carotid sinus **L Internal Carotid Artery, Left** *See K Internal Carotid Artery, Right* **M External Carotid Artery, Right** Ascending pharyngeal artery Internal maxillary artery Lingual artery Maxillary artery Occipital artery Posterior auricular artery Superior thyroid artery	**N External Carotid Artery, Left** *See M External Carotid Artery, Right* **P Vertebral Artery, Right** Anterior spinal artery Posterior spinal artery **Q Vertebral Artery, Left** *See P Vertebral Artery, Right* **R Face Artery** Angular artery Ascending palatine artery External maxillary artery Facial artery Inferior labial artery Submental artery Superior labial artery **S Temporal Artery, Right** Middle temporal artery Superficial temporal artery Transverse facial artery **T Temporal Artery, Left** *See S Temporal Artery, Right* **U Thyroid Artery, Right** Cricothyroid artery Hyoid artery Sternocleidomastoid artery Superior laryngeal artery Superior thyroid artery Thyrocervical trunk **V Thyroid Artery, Left** *See U Thyroid Artery, Right* **Y Upper Artery** Aortic intercostal artery Bronchial artery Esophageal artery Subcostal artery	**Ø Open** **3 Percutaneous** **4 Percutaneous Endoscopic**	**4 Intraluminal Device, Drug-eluting** **5 Intraluminal Device, Drug-eluting, Two** **6 Intraluminal Device, Drug-eluting, Three** **7 Intraluminal Device, Drug-eluting, Four or More** **D Intraluminal Device** **E Intraluminal Device, Two** **F Intraluminal Device, Three** **G Intraluminal Device, Four or More** **Z No Device**	**Z No Qualifier**

NC　　Ø37G[3,4]ZZ

LC Limited Coverage　NC Noncovered　⊞ Combination Member　HAC associated procedure　Combination Only　DRG Non-OR　Non-OR　New/Revised in GREEN

198　　　　　　　　　　　　　　　　　　　　　　　　　　　　　　　ICD-10-PCS 2021

037–037

Ø   Medical and Surgical
3   Upper Arteries
9   Drainage   Definition: Taking or letting out fluids and/or gases from a body part

Explanation: The qualifier DIAGNOSTIC is used to identify drainage procedures that are biopsies

Body Part Character 4		Approach Character 5	Device Character 6	Qualifier Character 7
Ø Internal Mammary Artery, Right Anterior intercostal artery Internal thoracic artery Musculophrenic artery Pericardiophrenic artery Superior epigastric artery **1 Internal Mammary Artery, Left** *See Ø Internal Mammary Artery, Right above* **2 Innominate Artery** Brachiocephalic artery Brachiocephalic trunk **3 Subclavian Artery, Right** Costocervical trunk Dorsal scapular artery Internal thoracic artery **4 Subclavian Artery, Left** *See 3 Subclavian Artery, Right* **5 Axillary Artery, Right** Anterior circumflex humeral artery Lateral thoracic artery Posterior circumflex humeral artery Subscapular artery Superior thoracic artery Thoracoacromial artery **6 Axillary Artery, Left** *See 5 Axillary Artery, Right* **7 Brachial Artery, Right** Inferior ulnar collateral artery Profunda brachii Superior ulnar collateral artery **8 Brachial Artery, Left** *See 7 Brachial Artery, Right* **9 Ulnar Artery, Right** Anterior ulnar recurrent artery Common interosseous artery Posterior ulnar recurrent artery **A Ulnar Artery, Left** *See 9 Ulnar Artery, Right* **B Radial Artery, Right** Radial recurrent artery **C Radial Artery, Left** *See B Radial Artery, Right* **D Hand Artery, Right** Deep palmar arch Princeps pollicis artery Radialis indicis Superficial palmar arch **F Hand Artery, Left** *See D Hand Artery, Right* **G Intracranial Artery** Anterior cerebral artery Anterior choroidal artery Anterior communicating artery Basilar artery Circle of Willis Internal carotid artery, intracranial portion Middle cerebral artery Ophthalmic artery Posterior cerebral artery Posterior communicating artery Posterior inferior cerebellar artery (PICA)	**H Common Carotid Artery, Right** **J Common Carotid Artery, Left** **K Internal Carotid Artery, Right** Caroticotympanic artery Carotid sinus **L Internal Carotid Artery, Left** *See K Internal Carotid Artery, Right* **M External Carotid Artery, Right** Ascending pharyngeal artery Internal maxillary artery Lingual artery Maxillary artery Occipital artery Posterior auricular artery Superior thyroid artery **N External Carotid Artery, Left** *See M External Carotid Artery, Right* **P Vertebral Artery, Right** Anterior spinal artery Posterior spinal artery **Q Vertebral Artery, Left** *See P Vertebral Artery, Right* **R Face Artery** Angular artery Ascending palatine artery External maxillary artery Facial artery Inferior labial artery Submental artery Superior labial artery **S Temporal Artery, Right** Middle temporal artery Superficial temporal artery Transverse facial artery **T Temporal Artery, Left** *See S Temporal Artery, Right* **U Thyroid Artery, Right** Cricothyroid artery Hyoid artery Sternocleidomastoid artery Superior laryngeal artery Superior thyroid artery Thyrocervical trunk **V Thyroid Artery, Left** *See U Thyroid Artery, Right* **Y Upper Artery** Aortic intercostal artery Bronchial artery Esophageal artery Subcostal artery	**Ø Open** **3 Percutaneous** **4 Percutaneous Endoscopic**	**Ø Drainage Device**	**Z No Qualifier**

Non-OR   Ø39[Ø,1,2,3,4,5,6,7,8,9,A,B,C,D,F,G,H,J,K,L,M,N,P,Q,R,S,T,U,V,Y][Ø,3,4]ØZ

Ø39 Continued on next page

LC Limited Coverage   NC Noncovered   ⊞ Combination Member   HAC associated procedure   Combination Only   DRG Non-OR   Non-OR   New/Revised in GREEN

Upper Arteries *(side tab)*

Ø	**Medical and Surgical**
3	**Upper Arteries**
9	**Drainage**

Ø39 Continued

Definition: Taking or letting out fluids and/or gases from a body part

Explanation: The qualifier DIAGNOSTIC is used to identify drainage procedures that are biopsies

Body Part Character 4		Approach Character 5	Device Character 6	Qualifier Character 7
Ø Internal Mammary Artery, Right 　Anterior intercostal artery 　Internal thoracic artery 　Musculophrenic artery 　Pericardiophrenic artery 　Superior epigastric artery **1 Internal Mammary Artery, Left** 　*See Ø Internal Mammary Artery, Right* **2 Innominate Artery** 　Brachiocephalic artery 　Brachiocephalic trunk **3 Subclavian Artery, Right** 　Costocervical trunk 　Dorsal scapular artery 　Internal thoracic artery **4 Subclavian Artery, Left** 　*See 3 Subclavian Artery, Right* **5 Axillary Artery, Right** 　Anterior circumflex humeral 　　artery 　Lateral thoracic artery 　Posterior circumflex humeral 　　artery 　Subscapular artery 　Superior thoracic artery 　Thoracoacromial artery **6 Axillary Artery, Left** 　*See 5 Axillary Artery, Right* **7 Brachial Artery, Right** 　Inferior ulnar collateral artery 　Profunda brachii 　Superior ulnar collateral artery **8 Brachial Artery, Left** 　*See 7 Brachial Artery, Right* **9 Ulnar Artery, Right** 　Anterior ulnar recurrent artery 　Common interosseous artery 　Posterior ulnar recurrent artery **A Ulnar Artery, Left** 　*See 9 Ulnar Artery, Right* **B Radial Artery, Right** 　Radial recurrent artery **C Radial Artery, Left** 　*See B Radial Artery, Right* **D Hand Artery, Right** 　Deep palmar arch 　Princeps pollicis artery 　Radialis indicis 　Superficial palmar arch **F Hand Artery, Left** 　*See D Hand Artery, Right* **G Intracranial Artery** 　Anterior cerebral artery 　Anterior choroidal artery 　Anterior communicating artery 　Basilar artery 　Circle of Willis 　Internal carotid artery, 　　intracranial portion 　Middle cerebral artery 　Ophthalmic artery 　Posterior cerebral artery 　Posterior communicating artery 　Posterior inferior cerebellar 　　artery (PICA)	**H Common Carotid Artery, Right** **J Common Carotid Artery, Left** **K Internal Carotid Artery, Right** 　Caroticotympanic artery 　Carotid sinus **L Internal Carotid Artery, Left** 　*See K Internal Carotid Artery, Right* **M External Carotid Artery, Right** 　Ascending pharyngeal artery 　Internal maxillary artery 　Lingual artery 　Maxillary artery 　Occipital artery 　Posterior auricular artery 　Superior thyroid artery **N External Carotid Artery, Left** 　*See M External Carotid Artery, Right* **P Vertebral Artery, Right** 　Anterior spinal artery 　Posterior spinal artery **Q Vertebral Artery, Left** 　*See P Vertebral Artery, Right* **R Face Artery** 　Angular artery 　Ascending palatine artery 　External maxillary artery 　Facial artery 　Inferior labial artery 　Submental artery 　Superior labial artery **S Temporal Artery, Right** 　Middle temporal artery 　Superficial temporal artery 　Transverse facial artery **T Temporal Artery, Left** 　*See S Temporal Artery, Right* **U Thyroid Artery, Right** 　Cricothyroid artery 　Hyoid artery 　Sternocleidomastoid artery 　Superior laryngeal artery 　Superior thyroid artery 　Thyrocervical trunk **V Thyroid Artery, Left** 　*See U Thyroid Artery, Right* **Y Upper Artery** 　Aortic intercostal artery 　Bronchial artery 　Esophageal artery 　Subcostal artery	**Ø Open** **3 Percutaneous** **4 Percutaneous Endoscopic**	**Z No Device**	**X Diagnostic** **Z No Qualifier**

Non-OR　Ø39[Ø,1,2,3,4,5,6,7,8,9,A,B,C,D,F,G,H,J,K,L,M,N,P,Q,R,S,T,U,V,Y]3ZX
Non-OR　Ø39[Ø,1,2,3,4,5,6,7,8,9,A,B,C,D,F,G,H,J,K,L,M,N,P,Q,R,S,T,U,V,Y][Ø,3,4]ZZ

0   Medical and Surgical
3   Upper Arteries
B   Excision   Definition: Cutting out or off, without replacement, a portion of a body part
                  Explanation: The qualifier DIAGNOSTIC is used to identify excision procedures that are biopsies

Body Part Character 4	Approach Character 5	Device Character 6	Qualifier Character 7

0 Internal Mammary Artery, Right
  Anterior intercostal artery
  Internal thoracic artery
  Musculophrenic artery
  Pericardiophrenic artery
  Superior epigastric artery
1 Internal Mammary Artery, Left
  See 0 Internal Mammary Artery, Right
2 Innominate Artery
  Brachiocephalic artery
  Brachiocephalic trunk
3 Subclavian Artery, Right
  Costocervical trunk
  Dorsal scapular artery
  Internal thoracic artery
4 Subclavian Artery, Left
  See 3 Subclavian Artery, Right
5 Axillary Artery, Right
  Anterior circumflex humeral artery
  Lateral thoracic artery
  Posterior circumflex humeral artery
  Subscapular artery
  Superior thoracic artery
  Thoracoacromial artery
6 Axillary Artery, Left
  See 5 Axillary Artery, Right
7 Brachial Artery, Right
  Inferior ulnar collateral artery
  Profunda brachii
  Superior ulnar collateral artery
8 Brachial Artery, Left
  See 7 Brachial Artery, Right
9 Ulnar Artery, Right
  Anterior ulnar recurrent artery
  Common interosseous artery
  Posterior ulnar recurrent artery
A Ulnar Artery, Left
  See 9 Ulnar Artery, Right
B Radial Artery, Right
  Radial recurrent artery
C Radial Artery, Left
  See B Radial Artery, Right
D Hand Artery, Right
  Deep palmar arch
  Princeps pollicis artery
  Radialis indicis
  Superficial palmar arch
F Hand Artery, Left
  See D Hand Artery, Right
G Intracranial Artery
  Anterior cerebral artery
  Anterior choroidal artery
  Anterior communicating artery
  Basilar artery
  Circle of Willis
  Internal carotid artery, intracranial portion
  Middle cerebral artery
  Ophthalmic artery
  Posterior cerebral artery
  Posterior communicating artery
  Posterior inferior cerebellar artery (PICA)
 	
H Common Carotid Artery, Right
J Common Carotid Artery, Left
K Internal Carotid Artery, Right
  Caroticotympanic artery
  Carotid sinus
L Internal Carotid Artery, Left
  See K Internal Carotid Artery, Right
M External Carotid Artery, Right
  Ascending pharyngeal artery
  Internal maxillary artery
  Lingual artery
  Maxillary artery
  Occipital artery
  Posterior auricular artery
  Superior thyroid artery
N External Carotid Artery, Left
  See M External Carotid Artery, Right
P Vertebral Artery, Right
  Anterior spinal artery
  Posterior spinal artery
Q Vertebral Artery, Left
  See P Vertebral Artery, Right
R Face Artery
  Angular artery
  Ascending palatine artery
  External maxillary artery
  Facial artery
  Inferior labial artery
  Submental artery
  Superior labial artery
S Temporal Artery, Right
  Middle temporal artery
  Superficial temporal artery
  Transverse facial artery
T Temporal Artery, Left
  See S Temporal Artery, Right
U Thyroid Artery, Right
  Cricothyroid artery
  Hyoid artery
  Sternocleidomastoid artery
  Superior laryngeal artery
  Superior thyroid artery
  Thyrocervical trunk
V Thyroid Artery, Left
  See U Thyroid Artery, Right
Y Upper Artery
  Aortic intercostal artery
  Bronchial artery
  Esophageal artery
  Subcostal artery
	0 Open
	3 Percutaneous
	4 Percutaneous Endoscopic
		Z No Device	**X Diagnostic**
			Z No Qualifier

LC Limited Coverage   NC Noncovered   ⊞ Combination Member   HAC associated procedure   Combination Only   DRG Non-OR   Non-OR   New/Revised in GREEN

ICD-10-PCS 2021   201

03B–03B

Upper Arteries

Ø   **Medical and Surgical**
3   **Upper Arteries**
C   **Extirpation**   Definition: Taking or cutting out solid matter from a body part

Explanation: The solid matter may be an abnormal byproduct of a biological function or a foreign body; it may be imbedded in a body part or in the lumen of a tubular body part. The solid matter may or may not have been previously broken into pieces.

Body Part Character 4		Approach Character 5	Device Character 6	Qualifier Character 7
Ø Internal Mammary Artery, Right Anterior intercostal artery Internal thoracic artery Musculophrenic artery Pericardiophrenic artery Superior epigastric artery **1 Internal Mammary Artery, Left** *See Ø Internal Mammary Artery, Right* **2 Innominate Artery** Brachiocephalic artery Brachiocephalic trunk **3 Subclavian Artery, Right** Costocervical trunk Dorsal scapular artery Internal thoracic artery **4 Subclavian Artery, Left** *See 3 Subclavian Artery, Right* **5 Axillary Artery, Right** Anterior circumflex humeral artery Lateral thoracic artery Posterior circumflex humeral artery Subscapular artery Superior thoracic artery Thoracoacromial artery **6 Axillary Artery, Left** *See 5 Axillary Artery, Right* **7 Brachial Artery, Right** Inferior ulnar collateral artery Profunda brachii Superior ulnar collateral artery **8 Brachial Artery, Left** *See 7 Brachial Artery, Right* **9 Ulnar Artery, Right** Anterior ulnar recurrent artery Common interosseous artery Posterior ulnar recurrent artery	**A Ulnar Artery, Left** *See 9 Ulnar Artery, Right* **B Radial Artery, Right** Radial recurrent artery **C Radial Artery, Left** *See B Radial Artery, Right* **D Hand Artery, Right** Deep palmar arch Princeps pollicis artery Radialis indicis Superficial palmar arch **F Hand Artery, Left** *See D Hand Artery, Right* **R Face Artery** Angular artery Ascending palatine artery External maxillary artery Facial artery Inferior labial artery Submental artery Superior labial artery **S Temporal Artery, Right** Middle temporal artery Superficial temporal artery Transverse facial artery **T Temporal Artery, Left** *See S Temporal Artery, Right* **U Thyroid Artery, Right** Cricothyroid artery Hyoid artery Sternocleidomastoid artery Superior laryngeal artery Superior thyroid artery Thyrocervical trunk **V Thyroid Artery, Left** *See U Thyroid Artery, Right* **Y Upper Artery** Aortic intercostal artery Bronchial artery Esophageal artery Subcostal artery	**Ø Open** **3 Percutaneous** **4 Percutaneous Endoscopic**	**Z No Device**	**Z No Qualifier**
G Intracranial Artery Anterior cerebral artery Anterior choroidal artery Anterior communicating artery Basilar artery Circle of Willis Internal carotid artery, intracranial portion Middle cerebral artery Ophthalmic artery Posterior cerebral artery Posterior communicating artery Posterior inferior cerebellar artery (PICA) **H Common Carotid Artery, Right** **J Common Carotid Artery, Left** **K Internal Carotid Artery, Right** Caroticotympanic artery Carotid sinus	**L Internal Carotid Artery, Left** *See K Internal Carotid Artery, Right* **M External Carotid Artery, Right** Ascending pharyngeal artery Internal maxillary artery Lingual artery Maxillary artery Occipital artery Posterior auricular artery Superior thyroid artery **N External Carotid Artery, Left** *See M External Carotid Artery, Right* **P Vertebral Artery, Right** Anterior spinal artery Posterior spinal artery **Q Vertebral Artery, Left** *See P Vertebral Artery, Right*	**Ø Open** **4 Percutaneous Endoscopic**	**Z No Device**	**Z No Qualifier**

Ø3C Continued on next page

LC Limited Coverage   **NC** Noncovered   ⊞ Combination Member   HAC associated procedure   Combination Only   DRG Non-OR   Non-OR   New/Revised in GREEN

202   ICD-10-PCS 2021

Ø   **Medical and Surgical**   *Ø3C Continued*
3   **Upper Arteries**
C   **Extirpation**   Definition: Taking or cutting out solid matter from a body part

                         Explanation: The solid matter may be an abnormal byproduct of a biological function or a foreign body; it may be imbedded in a body part or in the lumen of a tubular body part. The solid matter may or may not have been previously broken into pieces.

Body Part Character 4		Approach Character 5	Device Character 6	Qualifier Character 7

G Intracranial Artery
Anterior cerebral artery
Anterior choroidal artery
Anterior communicating
   artery
Basilar artery
Circle of Willis
Internal carotid artery,
   intracranial portion
Middle cerebral artery
Ophthalmic artery
Posterior cerebral artery
Posterior communicating
   artery
Posterior inferior cerebellar
   artery (PICA)
**H Common Carotid Artery,
   Right**
J Common Carotid Artery, Left
K Internal Carotid Artery, Right
Caroticotympanic artery
Carotid sinus
	L Internal Carotid Artery, Left
	*See K Internal Carotid Artery,
	   Right*
	M External Carotid Artery, Right
	Ascending pharyngeal artery
	Internal maxillary artery
	Lingual artery
	Maxillary artery
	Occipital artery
	Posterior auricular artery
	Superior thyroid artery
	N External Carotid Artery, Left
	*See M External Carotid Artery,
	   Right*
	P Vertebral Artery, Right
	Anterior spinal artery
	Posterior spinal artery
	Q Vertebral Artery, Left
	See P Vertebral Artery, Right
		3 Percutaneous	**Z** No Device	**7** Stent Retriever
				Z No Qualifier

Ø   **Medical and Surgical**
3   **Upper Arteries**
F   **Fragmentation**   Definition: Breaking solid matter in a body part into pieces

                       Explanation: Physical force (e.g., manual, ultrasonic) applied directly or indirectly is used to break the solid matter into pieces. The solid matter may be an abnormal byproduct of a biological function or a foreign body. The pieces of solid matter are not taken out.

Body Part Character 4		Approach Character 5	Device Character 6	Qualifier Character 7

2 Innominate Artery
Brachiocephalic artery
Brachiocephalic trunk
3 Subclavian Artery, Right
Costocervical trunk
Dorsal scapular artery
Internal thoracic artery
4 Subclavian Artery, Left
See 3 Subclavian Artery, Right
5 Axillary Artery, Right
Anterior circumflex humeral
   artery
Lateral thoracic artery
Posterior circumflex humeral
   artery
Subscapular artery
Superior thoracic artery
Thoracoacromial artery
6 Axillary Artery, Left
See 5 Axillary Artery, Right
7 Brachial Artery, Right
Inferior ulnar collateral artery
Profunda brachii
Superior ulnar collateral artery
8 Brachial Artery, Left
See 7 Brachial Artery, Right
	9 Ulnar Artery, Right
	Anterior ulnar recurrent artery
	Common interosseous artery
	Posterior ulnar recurrent artery
	A Ulnar Artery, Left
	See 9 Ulnar Artery, Right
	B Radial Artery, Right
	Radial recurrent artery
	C Radial Artery, Left
	See B Radial Artery, Right
	Y Upper Artery
	Aortic intercostal artery
	Bronchial artery
	Esophageal artery
	Subcostal artery
		3 Percutaneous	**Z** No Device	**Ø** Ultrasonic
				Z No Qualifier

Ø   **Medical and Surgical**
3   **Upper Arteries**
H   **Insertion**   Definition: Putting in a nonbiological appliance that monitors, assists, performs, or prevents a physiological function but does not physically take the place of a body part
              Explanation: None

Body Part Character 4		Approach Character 5	Device Character 6	Qualifier Character 7
Ø Internal Mammary Artery, Right Anterior intercostal artery Internal thoracic artery Musculophrenic artery Pericardiophrenic artery Superior epigastric artery **1 Internal Mammary Artery, Left** *See Ø Internal Mammary Artery, Right* **2 Innominate Artery** Brachiocephalic artery Brachiocephalic trunk **3 Subclavian Artery, Right** Costocervical trunk Dorsal scapular artery Internal thoracic artery **4 Subclavian Artery, Left** *See 3 Subclavian Artery, Right* **5 Axillary Artery, Right** Anterior circumflex humeral artery Lateral thoracic artery Posterior circumflex humeral artery Subscapular artery Superior thoracic artery Thoracoacromial artery **6 Axillary Artery, Left** *See 5 Axillary Artery, Right* **7 Brachial Artery, Right** Inferior ulnar collateral artery Profunda brachii Superior ulnar collateral artery **8 Brachial Artery, Left** *See 7 Brachial Artery, Right* **9 Ulnar Artery, Right** Anterior ulnar recurrent artery Common interosseous artery Posterior ulnar recurrent artery **A Ulnar Artery, Left** *See 9 Ulnar Artery, Right* **B Radial Artery, Right** Radial recurrent artery **C Radial Artery, Left** *See B Radial Artery, Right* **D Hand Artery, Right** Deep palmar arch Princeps pollicis artery Radialis indicis Superficial palmar arch **F Hand Artery, Left** *See D Hand Artery, Right*	**G Intracranial Artery** Anterior cerebral artery Anterior choroidal artery Anterior communicating artery Basilar artery Circle of Willis Internal carotid artery, intracranial portion Middle cerebral artery Ophthalmic artery Posterior cerebral artery Posterior communicating artery Posterior inferior cerebellar artery (PICA) **H Common Carotid Artery, Right** **J Common Carotid Artery, Left** **M External Carotid Artery, Right** Ascending pharyngeal artery Internal maxillary artery Lingual artery Maxillary artery Occipital artery Posterior auricular artery Superior thyroid artery **N External Carotid Artery, Left** *See M External Carotid Artery, Right* **P Vertebral Artery, Right** Anterior spinal artery Posterior spinal artery **Q Vertebral Artery, Left** *See P Vertebral Artery, Right* **R Face Artery** Angular artery Ascending palatine artery External maxillary artery Facial artery Inferior labial artery Submental artery Superior labial artery **S Temporal Artery, Right** Middle temporal artery Superficial temporal artery Transverse facial artery **T Temporal Artery, Left** *See S Temporal Artery, Right* **U Thyroid Artery, Right** Cricothyroid artery Hyoid artery Sternocleidomastoid artery Superior laryngeal artery Superior thyroid artery Thyrocervical trunk **V Thyroid Artery, Left** *See U Thyroid Artery, Right*	**Ø Open** **3 Percutaneous** **4 Percutaneous Endoscopic**	**3 Infusion Device** **D Intraluminal Device**	**Z No Qualifier**
K Internal Carotid Artery, Right Caroticotympanic artery Carotid sinus **L Internal Carotid Artery, Left** *See K Internal Carotid Artery, Right*		**Ø Open** **3 Percutaneous** **4 Percutaneous Endoscope**	**3 Infusion Device** **D Intraluminal Device** **M Stimulator Lead**	**Z No Qualifier**
Y Upper Artery Aortic intercostal artery Bronchial artery Esophageal artery Subcostal artery		**Ø Open** **3 Percutaneous** **4 Percutaneous Endoscopic**	**2 Monitoring Device** **3 Infusion Device** **D Intraluminal Device** **Y Other Device**	**Z No Qualifier**

Non-OR	Ø3H[Ø,1,2,3,4,5,6,7,8,9,A,B,C,D,F,G,H,J,M,N,P,Q,R,S,T,U,V][Ø,3,4]3Z
Non-OR	Ø3H[K,L][Ø,3,4]3Z
Non-OR	Ø3HY[Ø,3,4]3Z
Non-OR	Ø3HY32Z
Non-OR	Ø3HY[3,4]YZ

LC Limited Coverage   **NC** Noncovered   ⊞ Combination Member   HAC associated procedure   Combination Only   DRG Non-OR   Non-OR   New/Revised in GREEN

204   ICD-10-PCS 2021

0   Medical and Surgical
3   Upper Arteries
J   Inspection   Definition: Visually and/or manually exploring a body part

Explanation: Visual exploration may be performed with or without optical instrumentation. Manual exploration may be performed directly or through intervening body layers.

Body Part Character 4	Approach Character 5	Device Character 6	Qualifier Character 7
Y Upper Artery Aortic intercostal artery Bronchial artery Esophageal artery Subcostal artery	**0** Open **3** Percutaneous **4** Percutaneous Endoscopic **X** External	**Z** No Device	**Z** No Qualifier

Non-OR   03JY[3,4,X]ZZ

Upper Arteries

Ø   Medical and Surgical
3   Upper Arteries
L   Occlusion   Definition: Completely closing an orifice or the lumen of a tubular body part
Explanation: The orifice can be a natural orifice or an artificially created orifice

Body Part Character 4		Approach Character 5	Device Character 6	Qualifier Character 7
Ø Internal Mammary Artery, Right Anterior intercostal artery Internal thoracic artery Musculophrenic artery Pericardiophrenic artery Superior epigastric artery **1** Internal Mammary Artery, Left *See Ø Internal Mammary Artery, Left* **2** Innominate Artery Brachiocephalic artery Brachiocephalic trunk **3** Subclavian Artery, Right Costocervical trunk Dorsal scapular artery Internal thoracic artery **4** Subclavian Artery, Left *See 3 Subclavian Artery, Right* **5** Axillary Artery, Right Anterior circumflex humeral artery Lateral thoracic artery Posterior circumflex humeral artery Subscapular artery Superior thoracic artery Thoracoacromial artery **6** Axillary Artery, Left *See 5 Axillary Artery, Right* **7** Brachial Artery, Right Inferior ulnar collateral artery Profunda brachii Superior ulnar collateral artery **8** Brachial Artery, Left *See 7 Brachial Artery, Right* **9** Ulnar Artery, Right Anterior ulnar recurrent artery Common interosseous artery Posterior ulnar recurrent artery	**A** Ulnar Artery, Left *See 9 Ulnar Artery, Right* **B** Radial Artery, Right Radial recurrent artery **C** Radial Artery, Left *See B Radial Artery, Right* **D** Hand Artery, Right Deep palmar arch Princeps pollicis artery Radialis indicis Superficial palmar arch **F** Hand Artery, Left *See D Hand Artery, Right* **R** Face Artery Angular artery Ascending palatine artery External maxillary artery Facial artery Inferior labial artery Submental artery Superior labial artery **S** Temporal Artery, Right Middle temporal artery Superficial temporal artery Transverse facial artery **T** Temporal Artery, Left *See S Temporal Artery, Right* **U** Thyroid Artery, Right Cricothyroid artery Hyoid artery Sternocleidomastoid artery Superior laryngeal artery Superior thyroid artery Thyrocervical trunk **V** Thyroid Artery, Left *See U Thyroid Artery, Right* **Y** Upper Artery Aortic intercostal artery Bronchial artery Esophageal artery Subcostal artery	**Ø** Open **3** Percutaneous **4** Percutaneous Endoscopic	**C** Extraluminal Device **D** Intraluminal Device **Z** No Device	**Z** No Qualifier
G Intracranial Artery Anterior cerebral artery Anterior choroidal artery Anterior communicating artery Basilar artery Circle of Willis Internal carotid artery, intracranial portion Middle cerebral artery Ophthalmic artery Posterior cerebral artery Posterior communicating artery Posterior inferior cerebellar artery (PICA) **H** Common Carotid Artery, Right **J** Common Carotid Artery, Left **K** Internal Carotid Artery, Right Caroticotympanic artery Carotid sinus	**L** Internal Carotid Artery, Left *See K Internal Carotid Artery, Right* **M** External Carotid Artery, Right Ascending pharyngeal artery Internal maxillary artery Lingual artery Maxillary artery Occipital artery Posterior auricular artery Superior thyroid artery **N** External Carotid Artery, Left *See M External Carotid Artery, Right* **P** Vertebral Artery, Right Anterior spinal artery Posterior spinal artery **Q** Vertebral Artery, Left *See P Vertebral Artery, Right*	**Ø** Open **3** Percutaneous **4** Percutaneous Endoscopic	**B** Intraluminal Device, Bioactive **C** Extraluminal Device **D** Intraluminal Device **Z** No Device	**Z** No Qualifier

Ø   **Medical and Surgical**
3   **Upper Arteries**
N   **Release**   Definition: Freeing a body part from an abnormal physical constraint by cutting or by the use of force

Explanation: Some of the restraining tissue may be taken out but none of the body part is taken out

Body Part Character 4		Approach Character 5	Device Character 6	Qualifier Character 7
Ø **Internal Mammary Artery, Right** Anterior intercostal artery Internal thoracic artery Musculophrenic artery Pericardiophrenic artery Superior epigastric artery **1** **Internal Mammary Artery, Left** *See Ø Internal Mammary Artery, Right* **2** **Innominate Artery** Brachiocephalic artery Brachiocephalic trunk **3** **Subclavian Artery, Right** Costocervical trunk Dorsal scapular artery Internal thoracic artery **4** **Subclavian Artery, Left** *See 3 Subclavian Artery, Right* **5** **Axillary Artery, Right** Anterior circumflex humeral artery Lateral thoracic artery Posterior circumflex humeral artery Subscapular artery Superior thoracic artery Thoracoacromial artery **6** **Axillary Artery, Left** *See 5 Axillary Artery, Right* **7** **Brachial Artery, Right** Inferior ulnar collateral artery Profunda brachii Superior ulnar collateral artery **8** **Brachial Artery, Left** *See 7 Brachial Artery, Right* **9** **Ulnar Artery, Right** Anterior ulnar recurrent artery Common interosseous artery Posterior ulnar recurrent artery **A** **Ulnar Artery, Left** *See 9 Ulnar Artery, Right* **B** **Radial Artery, Right** Radial recurrent artery **C** **Radial Artery, Left** *See B Radial Artery, Right* **D** **Hand Artery, Right** Deep palmar arch Princeps pollicis artery Radialis indicis Superficial palmar arch **F** **Hand Artery, Left** *See D Hand Artery, Right* **G** **Intracranial Artery** Anterior cerebral artery Anterior choroidal artery Anterior communicating artery Basilar artery Circle of Willis Internal carotid artery, intracranial portion Middle cerebral artery Ophthalmic artery Posterior cerebral artery Posterior communicating artery Posterior inferior cerebellar artery (PICA)	**H** **Common Carotid Artery, Right** **J** **Common Carotid Artery, Left** **K** **Internal Carotid Artery, Right** Caroticotympanic artery Carotid sinus **L** **Internal Carotid Artery, Left** *See K Internal Carotid Artery, Right* **M** **External Carotid Artery, Right** Ascending pharyngeal artery Internal maxillary artery Lingual artery Maxillary artery Occipital artery Posterior auricular artery Superior thyroid artery **N** **External Carotid Artery, Left** *See M External Carotid Artery, Right* **P** **Vertebral Artery, Right** Anterior spinal artery Posterior spinal artery **Q** **Vertebral Artery, Left** *See P Vertebral Artery, Right* **R** **Face Artery** Angular artery Ascending palatine artery External maxillary artery Facial artery Inferior labial artery Submental artery Superior labial artery **S** **Temporal Artery, Right** Middle temporal artery Superficial temporal artery Transverse facial artery **T** **Temporal Artery, Left** *See S Temporal Artery, Right* **U** **Thyroid Artery, Right** Cricothyroid artery Hyoid artery Sternocleidomastoid artery Superior laryngeal artery Superior thyroid artery Thyrocervical trunk **V** **Thyroid Artery, Left** *See U Thyroid Artery, Right* **Y** **Upper Artery** Aortic intercostal artery Bronchial artery Esophageal artery Subcostal artery	**Ø** Open **3** Percutaneous **4** Percutaneous Endoscopic	**Z** No Device	**Z** No Qualifier

LC Limited Coverage   **NC** Noncovered   ⊞ Combination Member   HAC associated procedure   Combination Only   DRG Non-OR   Non-OR   New/Revised in GREEN

ICD-10-PCS 2021   **207**

Upper Arteries (side tab)

Ø   Medical and Surgical
3   Upper Arteries
P   Removal

Definition: Taking out or off a device from a body part

Explanation: If a device is taken out and a similar device put in without cutting or puncturing the skin or mucous membrane, the procedure is coded to the root operation CHANGE. Otherwise, the procedure for taking out a device is coded to the root operation REMOVAL.

Body Part Character 4	Approach Character 5	Device Character 6	Qualifier Character 7
Y Upper Artery Aortic intercostal artery Bronchial artery Esophageal artery Subcostal artery	**Ø** Open **3** Percutaneous **4** Percutaneous Endoscopic	**Ø** Drainage Device **2** Monitoring Device **3** Infusion Device **7** Autologous Tissue Substitute **C** Extraluminal Device **D** Intraluminal Device **J** Synthetic Substitute **K** Nonautologous Tissue Substitute **M** Stimulator Lead **Y** Other Device	**Z** No Qualifier
Y Upper Artery Aortic intercostal artery Bronchial artery Esophageal artery Subcostal artery	**X** External	**Ø** Drainage Device **2** Monitoring Device **3** Infusion Device **D** Intraluminal Device **M** Stimulator Lead	**Z** No Qualifier

Non-OR   Ø3PY3[Ø,2,3,D]Z
Non-OR   Ø3PY[3,4]YZ
Non-OR   Ø3PYX[Ø,2,3,D,M]Z

0   Medical and Surgical
3   Upper Arteries
Q   Repair   Definition: Restoring, to the extent possible, a body part to its normal anatomic structure and function

                       Explanation: Used only when the method to accomplish the repair is not one of the other root operations

Body Part Character 4	Approach Character 5	Device Character 6	Qualifier Character 7
0 Internal Mammary Artery, Right Anterior intercostal artery Internal thoracic artery Musculophrenic artery Pericardiophrenic artery Superior epigastric artery **1 Internal Mammary Artery, Left** *See 0 Internal Mammary Artery, Right* **2 Innominate Artery** Brachiocephalic artery Brachiocephalic trunk **3 Subclavian Artery, Right** Costocervical trunk Dorsal scapular artery Internal thoracic artery **4 Subclavian Artery, Left** *See 3 Subclavian Artery, Right* **5 Axillary Artery, Right** Anterior circumflex humeral artery Lateral thoracic artery Posterior circumflex humeral artery Subscapular artery Superior thoracic artery Thoracoacromial artery **6 Axillary Artery, Left** *See 5 Axillary Artery, Right* **7 Brachial Artery, Right** Inferior ulnar collateral artery Profunda brachii Superior ulnar collateral artery **8 Brachial Artery, Left** *See 7 Brachial Artery, Right* **9 Ulnar Artery, Right** Anterior ulnar recurrent artery Common interosseous artery Posterior ulnar recurrent artery **A Ulnar Artery, Left** *See 9 Ulnar Artery, Right* **B Radial Artery, Right** Radial recurrent artery **C Radial Artery, Left** *See B Radial Artery, Right* **D Hand Artery, Right** Deep palmar arch Princeps pollicis artery Radialis indicis Superficial palmar arch **F Hand Artery, Left** *See D Hand Artery, Right* **G Intracranial Artery** Anterior cerebral artery Anterior choroidal artery Anterior communicating artery Basilar artery Circle of Willis Internal carotid artery, intracranial portion Middle cerebral artery Ophthalmic artery Posterior cerebral artery Posterior communicating artery Posterior inferior cerebellar artery (PICA)	**H Common Carotid Artery, Right** **J Common Carotid Artery, Left** **K Internal Carotid Artery, Right** Caroticotympanic artery Carotid sinus **L Internal Carotid Artery, Left** *See K Internal Carotid Artery, Right* **M External Carotid Artery, Right** Ascending pharyngeal artery Internal maxillary artery Lingual artery Maxillary artery Occipital artery Posterior auricular artery Superior thyroid artery **N External Carotid Artery, Left** *See M External Carotid Artery, Right* **P Vertebral Artery, Right** Anterior spinal artery Posterior spinal artery **Q Vertebral Artery, Left** *See P Vertebral Artery, Right* **R Face Artery** Angular artery Ascending palatine artery External maxillary artery Facial artery Inferior labial artery Submental artery Superior labial artery **S Temporal Artery, Right** Middle temporal artery Superficial temporal artery Transverse facial artery **T Temporal Artery, Left** *See S Temporal Artery, Right* **U Thyroid Artery, Right** Cricothyroid artery Hyoid artery Sternocleidomastoid artery Superior laryngeal artery Superior thyroid artery Thyrocervical trunk **V Thyroid Artery, Left** *See U Thyroid Artery, Right* **Y Upper Artery** Aortic intercostal artery Bronchial artery Esophageal artery Subcostal artery	**0 Open** **3 Percutaneous** **4 Percutaneous Endoscopic**	**Z No Device**	**Z No Qualifier**

LC Limited Coverage   **NC** Noncovered   ⊞ Combination Member   HAC associated procedure   Combination Only   DRG Non-OR   Non-OR   New/Revised in GREEN

ICD-10-PCS 2021   209

03Q–03Q

Ø   **Medical and Surgical**
3   **Upper Arteries**
R   **Replacement**   Definition: Putting in or on biological or synthetic material that physically takes the place and/or function of all or a portion of a body part
                 Explanation: The body part may have been taken out or replaced, or may be taken out, physically eradicated, or rendered nonfunctional during the REPLACEMENT procedure. A REMOVAL procedure is coded for taking out the device used in a previous replacement procedure.

Body Part Character 4		Approach Character 5	Device Character 6	Qualifier Character 7
Ø Internal Mammary Artery, Right Anterior intercostal artery Internal thoracic artery Musculophrenic artery Pericardiophrenic artery Superior epigastric artery **1 Internal Mammary Artery, Left** *See Ø Internal Mammary Artery, Right* **2 Innominate Artery** Brachiocephalic artery Brachiocephalic trunk **3 Subclavian Artery, Right** Costocervical trunk Dorsal scapular artery Internal thoracic artery **4 Subclavian Artery, Left** *See 3 Subclavian Artery, Right* **5 Axillary Artery, Right** Anterior circumflex humeral artery Lateral thoracic artery Posterior circumflex humeral artery Subscapular artery Superior thoracic artery Thoracoacromial artery **6 Axillary Artery, Left** *See 5 Axillary Artery, Right* **7 Brachial Artery, Right** Inferior ulnar collateral artery Profunda brachii Superior ulnar collateral artery **8 Brachial Artery, Left** *See 7 Brachial Artery, Right* **9 Ulnar Artery, Right** Anterior ulnar recurrent artery Common interosseous artery Posterior ulnar recurrent artery **A Ulnar Artery, Left** *See 9 Ulnar Artery, Right* **B Radial Artery, Right** Radial recurrent artery **C Radial Artery, Left** *See B Radial Artery, Right* **D Hand Artery, Right** Deep palmar arch Princeps pollicis artery Radialis indicis Superficial palmar arch **F Hand Artery, Left** *See D Hand Artery, Right* **G Intracranial Artery** Anterior cerebral artery Anterior choroidal artery Anterior communicating artery Basilar artery Circle of Willis Internal carotid artery, intracranial portion Middle cerebral artery Ophthalmic artery Posterior cerebral artery Posterior communicating artery Posterior inferior cerebellar artery (PICA)	**H Common Carotid Artery, Right** **J Common Carotid Artery, Left** **K Internal Carotid Artery, Right** Caroticotympanic artery Carotid sinus **L Internal Carotid Artery, Left** *See K Internal Carotid Artery, Right* **M External Carotid Artery, Right** Ascending pharyngeal artery Internal maxillary artery Lingual artery Maxillary artery Occipital artery Posterior auricular artery Superior thyroid artery **N External Carotid Artery, Left** *See M External Carotid Artery, Right* **P Vertebral Artery, Right** Anterior spinal artery Posterior spinal artery **Q Vertebral Artery, Left** *See P Vertebral Artery, Right* **R Face Artery** Angular artery Ascending palatine artery External maxillary artery Facial artery Inferior labial artery Submental artery Superior labial artery **S Temporal Artery, Right** Middle temporal artery Superficial temporal artery Transverse facial artery **T Temporal Artery, Left** *See S Temporal Artery, Right* **U Thyroid Artery, Right** Cricothyroid artery Hyoid artery Sternocleidomastoid artery Superior laryngeal artery Superior thyroid artery Thyrocervical trunk **V Thyroid Artery, Left** *See U Thyroid Artery, Right* **Y Upper Artery** Aortic intercostal artery Bronchial artery Esophageal artery Subcostal artery	**Ø Open** **4 Percutaneous Endoscopic**	**7 Autologous Tissue Substitute** **J Synthetic Substitute** **K Nonautologous Tissue Substitute**	**Z No Qualifier**

0   **Medical and Surgical**
3   **Upper Arteries**
S   **Reposition**   Definition: Moving to its normal location, or other suitable location, all or a portion of a body part

                       Explanation: The body part is moved to a new location from an abnormal location, or from a normal location where it is not functioning correctly. The body part may or may not be cut out or off to be moved to the new location.

Body Part Character 4		Approach Character 5	Device Character 6	Qualifier Character 7
0 Internal Mammary Artery, Right Anterior intercostal artery Internal thoracic artery Musculophrenic artery Pericardiophrenic artery Superior epigastric artery **1 Internal Mammary Artery, Left** *See 0 Internal Mammary Artery, Right* **2 Innominate Artery** Brachiocephalic artery Brachiocephalic trunk **3 Subclavian Artery, Right** Costocervical trunk Dorsal scapular artery Internal thoracic artery **4 Subclavian Artery, Left** *See 3 Subclavian Artery, Right* **5 Axillary Artery, Right** Anterior circumflex humeral artery Lateral thoracic artery Posterior circumflex humeral artery Subscapular artery Superior thoracic artery Thoracoacromial artery **6 Axillary Artery, Left** *See 5 Axillary Artery, Right* **7 Brachial Artery, Right** Inferior ulnar collateral artery Profunda brachii Superior ulnar collateral artery **8 Brachial Artery, Left** *See 7 Brachial Artery, Right* **9 Ulnar Artery, Right** Anterior ulnar recurrent artery Common interosseous artery Posterior ulnar recurrent artery **A Ulnar Artery, Left** *See 9 Ulnar Artery, Right* **B Radial Artery, Right** Radial recurrent artery **C Radial Artery, Left** *See B Radial Artery, Right* **D Hand Artery, Right** Deep palmar arch Princeps pollicis artery Radialis indicis Superficial palmar arch **F Hand Artery, Left** *See D Hand Artery, Right* **G Intracranial Artery** Anterior cerebral artery Anterior choroidal artery Anterior communicating artery Basilar artery Circle of Willis Internal carotid artery, intracranial portion Middle cerebral artery Ophthalmic artery Posterior cerebral artery Posterior communicating artery Posterior inferior cerebellar artery (PICA)	**H Common Carotid Artery, Right** **J Common Carotid Artery, Left** **K Internal Carotid Artery, Right** Caroticotympanic artery Carotid sinus **L Internal Carotid Artery, Left** *See K Internal Carotid Artery, Right* **M External Carotid Artery, Right** Ascending pharyngeal artery Internal maxillary artery Lingual artery Maxillary artery Occipital artery Posterior auricular artery Superior thyroid artery **N External Carotid Artery, Left** *See M External Carotid Artery, Right* **P Vertebral Artery, Right** Anterior spinal artery Posterior spinal artery **Q Vertebral Artery, Left** *See P Vertebral Artery, Right* **R Face Artery** Angular artery Ascending palatine artery External maxillary artery Facial artery Inferior labial artery Submental artery Superior labial artery **S Temporal Artery, Right** Middle temporal artery Superficial temporal artery Transverse facial artery **T Temporal Artery, Left** *See S Temporal Artery, Right* **U Thyroid Artery, Right** Cricothyroid artery Hyoid artery Sternocleidomastoid artery Superior laryngeal artery Superior thyroid artery Thyrocervical trunk **V Thyroid Artery, Left** *See U Thyroid Artery, Right* **Y Upper Artery** Aortic intercostal artery Bronchial artery Esophageal artery Subcostal artery	**0 Open** **3 Percutaneous** **4 Percutaneous Endoscopic**	**Z No Device**	**Z No Qualifier**

LC Limited Coverage   NC Noncovered   ⊞ Combination Member   HAC associated procedure   Combination Only   DRG Non-OR   Non-OR   New/Revised in GREEN

ICD-10-PCS 2021   211

03S–03S

Ø Medical and Surgical
3 Upper Arteries
U Supplement

Definition: Putting in or on biological or synthetic material that physically reinforces and/or augments the function of a portion of a body part

Explanation: The biological material is non-living, or is living and from the same individual. The body part may have been previously replaced, and the SUPPLEMENT procedure is performed to physically reinforce and/or augment the function of the replaced body part.

Body Part Character 4	Approach Character 5	Device Character 6	Qualifier Character 7
Ø Internal Mammary Artery, Right Anterior intercostal artery; Internal thoracic artery; Musculophrenic artery; Pericardiophrenic artery; Superior epigastric artery	**Ø Open** **3 Percutaneous** **4 Percutaneous Endoscopic**	**7 Autologous Tissue Substitute** **J Synthetic Substitute** **K Nonautologous Tissue Substitute**	**Z No Qualifier**
1 Internal Mammary Artery, Left See Ø Internal Mammary Artery, Right			
2 Innominate Artery Brachiocephalic artery; Brachiocephalic trunk			
3 Subclavian Artery, Right Costocervical trunk; Dorsal scapular artery; Internal thoracic artery			
4 Subclavian Artery, Left See 3 Subclavian Artery, Right			
5 Axillary Artery, Right Anterior circumflex humeral artery; Lateral thoracic artery; Posterior circumflex humeral artery; Subscapular artery; Superior thoracic artery; Thoracoacromial artery			
6 Axillary Artery, Left See 5 Axillary Artery, Right			
7 Brachial Artery, Right Inferior ulnar collateral artery; Profunda brachii; Superior ulnar collateral artery			
8 Brachial Artery, Left See 7 Brachial Artery, Right			
9 Ulnar Artery, Right Anterior ulnar recurrent artery; Common interosseous artery; Posterior ulnar recurrent artery			
A Ulnar Artery, Left See 9 Ulnar Artery, Right			
B Radial Artery, Right Radial recurrent artery			
C Radial Artery, Left See B Radial Artery, Right			
D Hand Artery, Right Deep palmar arch; Princeps pollicis artery; Radialis indicis; Superficial palmar arch			
F Hand Artery, Left See D Hand Artery, Right			
G Intracranial Artery Anterior cerebral artery; Anterior choroidal artery; Anterior communicating artery; Basilar artery; Circle of Willis; Internal carotid artery, intracranial portion; Middle cerebral artery; Ophthalmic artery; Posterior cerebral artery; Posterior communicating artery; Posterior inferior cerebellar artery (PICA)			
H Common Carotid Artery, Right			
J Common Carotid Artery, Left			
K Internal Carotid Artery, Right Caroticotympanic artery; Carotid sinus			
L Internal Carotid Artery, Left See K Internal Carotid Artery, Right			
M External Carotid Artery, Right Ascending pharyngeal artery; Internal maxillary artery; Lingual artery; Maxillary artery; Occipital artery; Posterior auricular artery; Superior thyroid artery			
N External Carotid Artery, Left See M External Carotid Artery, Right			
P Vertebral Artery, Right Anterior spinal artery; Posterior spinal artery			
Q Vertebral Artery, Left See P Vertebral Artery, Right			
R Face Artery Angular artery; Ascending palatine artery; External maxillary artery; Facial artery; Inferior labial artery; Submental artery; Superior labial artery			
S Temporal Artery, Right Middle temporal artery; Superficial temporal artery; Transverse facial artery			
T Temporal Artery, Left See S Temporal Artery, Right			
U Thyroid Artery, Right Cricothyroid artery; Hyoid artery; Sternocleidomastoid artery; Superior laryngeal artery; Superior thyroid artery; Thyrocervical trunk			
V Thyroid Artery, Left See U Thyroid Artery, Right			
Y Upper Artery Aortic intercostal artery; Bronchial artery; Esophageal artery; Subcostal artery			

LC Limited Coverage   NC Noncovered   ⊞ Combination Member   HAC associated procedure   Combination Only   DRG Non-OR   Non-OR   New/Revised in GREEN

212   ICD-10-PCS 2021

Ø   **Medical and Surgical**
3   **Upper Arteries**
V   **Restriction**   Definition: Partially closing an orifice or the lumen of a tubular body part
                     Explanation: The orifice can be a natural orifice or an artificially created orifice

Body Part Character 4		Approach Character 5	Device Character 6	Qualifier Character 7

Ø **Internal Mammary Artery, Right**
   Anterior intercostal artery
   Internal thoracic artery
   Musculophrenic artery
   Pericardiophrenic artery
   Superior epigastric artery
1 **Internal Mammary Artery, Left**
   See Ø Internal Mammary Artery,
   Right
2 **Innominate Artery**
   Brachiocephalic artery
   Brachiocephalic trunk
3 **Subclavian Artery, Right**
   Costocervical trunk
   Dorsal scapular artery
   Internal thoracic artery
4 **Subclavian Artery, Left**
   See 3 Subclavian Artery, Right
5 **Axillary Artery, Right**
   Anterior circumflex humeral artery
   Lateral thoracic artery
   Posterior circumflex humeral artery
   Subscapular artery
   Superior thoracic artery
   Thoracoacromial artery
6 **Axillary Artery, Left**
   See 5 Axillary Artery, Right
7 **Brachial Artery, Right**
   Inferior ulnar collateral artery
   Profunda brachii
   Superior ulnar collateral artery
8 **Brachial Artery, Left**
   See 7 Brachial Artery, Right
9 **Ulnar Artery, Right**
   Anterior ulnar recurrent artery
   Common interosseous artery
   Posterior ulnar recurrent artery
A **Ulnar Artery, Left**
   See 9 Ulnar Artery, Right
	B **Radial Artery, Right**
	   Radial recurrent artery
	C **Radial Artery, Left**
	   See B Radial Artery, Right
	D **Hand Artery, Right**
	   Deep palmar arch
	   Princeps pollicis artery
	   Radialis indicis
	   Superficial palmar arch
	F **Hand Artery, Left**
	   See D Hand Artery, Right
	R **Face Artery**
	   Angular artery
	   Ascending palatine artery
	   External maxillary artery
	   Facial artery
	   Inferior labial artery
	   Submental artery
	   Superior labial artery
	S **Temporal Artery, Right**
	   Middle temporal artery
	   Superficial temporal artery
	   Transverse facial artery
	T **Temporal Artery, Left**
	   See S Temporal Artery, Right
	U **Thyroid Artery, Right**
	   Cricothyroid artery
	   Hyoid artery
	   Sternocleidomastoid artery
	   Superior laryngeal artery
	   Superior thyroid artery
	   Thyrocervical trunk
	V **Thyroid Artery, Left**
	   See U Thyroid Artery, Right
	Y **Upper Artery**
	   Aortic intercostal artery
	   Bronchial artery
	   Esophageal artery
	   Subcostal artery
		Ø Open
		3 Percutaneous
		4 Percutaneous
		   Endoscopic
			C Extraluminal Device
			D Intraluminal Device
			Z No Device
				Z No Qualifier

G **Intracranial Artery**
   Anterior cerebral artery
   Anterior choroidal artery
   Anterior communicating artery
   Basilar artery
   Circle of Willis
   Internal carotid artery,
     intracranial portion
   Middle cerebral artery
   Ophthalmic artery
   Posterior cerebral artery
   Posterior communicating artery
   Posterior inferior cerebellar artery
     (PICA)
H **Common Carotid Artery, Right**
J **Common Carotid Artery, Left**
K **Internal Carotid Artery, Right**
   Caroticotympanic artery
   Carotid sinus
	L **Internal Carotid Artery, Left**
	   See K Internal Carotid Artery, Right
	M **External Carotid Artery, Right**
	   Ascending pharyngeal artery
	   Internal maxillary artery
	   Lingual artery
	   Maxillary artery
	   Occipital artery
	   Posterior auricular artery
	   Superior thyroid artery
	N **External Carotid Artery, Left**
	   See M External Carotid Artery, Right
	P **Vertebral Artery, Right**
	   Anterior spinal artery
	   Posterior spinal artery
	Q **Vertebral Artery, Left**
	   See P Vertebral Artery, Right
		Ø Open
		3 Percutaneous
		4 Percutaneous
		   Endoscopic
			B Intraluminal Device,
			   Bioactive
			C Extraluminal Device
			D Intraluminal Device
			H Intraluminal Device,
			   Flow Diverter
			Z No Device
				Z No Qualifier

LC Limited Coverage   NC Noncovered   ⊞ Combination Member   HAC associated procedure   Combination Only   DRG Non-OR   Non-OR   New/Revised in GREEN

ICD-10-PCS 2021   213

03V–03V

Ø   Medical and Surgical
3   Upper Arteries
W   Revision   Definition: Correcting, to the extent possible, a portion of a malfunctioning device or the position of a displaced device

Explanation: Revision can include correcting a malfunctioning or displaced device by taking out or putting in components of the device such as a screw or pin

Body Part Character 4	Approach Character 5	Device Character 6	Qualifier Character 7

Y   Upper Artery
    Aortic intercostal artery
    Bronchial artery
    Esophageal artery
    Subcostal artery
	Ø Open
	3 Percutaneous
	4 Percutaneous Endoscopic
		Ø Drainage Device
		2 Monitoring Device
		3 Infusion Device
		7 Autologous Tissue Substitute
		C Extraluminal Device
		D Intraluminal Device
		J Synthetic Substitute
		K Nonautologous Tissue Substitute
		M Stimulator Lead
		Y Other Device
			Z No Qualifier

Y   Upper Artery
    Aortic intercostal artery
    Bronchial artery
    Esophageal artery
    Subcostal artery
	X External	**Ø** Drainage Device
		2 Monitoring Device
		3 Infusion Device
		7 Autologous Tissue Substitute
		C Extraluminal Device
		D Intraluminal Device
		J Synthetic Substitute
		K Nonautologous Tissue Substitute
		M Stimulator Lead
			Z No Qualifier

Non-OR   Ø3WY3[Ø,2,3,D]Z
Non-OR   Ø3WY[3,4]YZ
Non-OR   Ø3WYX[Ø,2,3,7,C,D,J,K,M]Z

LC Limited Coverage   NC Noncovered   ⊞ Combination Member   HAC associated procedure   Combination Only   DRG Non-OR   Non-OR   New/Revised in GREEN

214   ICD-10-PCS 2021

Lower Arteries Ø41–Ø4W

Character Meanings

This Character Meaning table is provided as a guide to assist the user in the identification of character members that may be found in this section of code tables. It **SHOULD NOT** be used to build a PCS code.

Operation–Character 3	Body Part–Character 4	Approach–Character 5	Device–Character 6	Qualifier–Character 7
1 Bypass	Ø Abdominal Aorta	Ø Open	Ø Drainage Device	Ø Abdominal Aorta OR Ultrasonic
5 Destruction	1 Celiac Artery	3 Percutaneous	1 Radioactive Element	1 Celiac Artery OR Drug-Coated Balloon
7 Dilation	2 Gastric Artery	4 Percutaneous Endoscopic	2 Monitoring Device	2 Mesenteric Artery
9 Drainage	3 Hepatic Artery	X External	3 Infusion Device	3 Renal Artery, Right
B Excision	4 Splenic Artery		4 Intraluminal Device, Drug-eluting	4 Renal Artery, Left
C Extirpation	5 Superior Mesenteric Artery		5 Intraluminal Device, Drug-eluting, Two	5 Renal Artery, Bilateral
F Fragmentation	6 Colic Artery, Right		6 Intraluminal Device, Drug-eluting, Three	6 Common Iliac Artery, Right
H Insertion	7 Colic Artery, Left		7 Intraluminal Device, Drug-eluting, Four or More OR Autologous Tissue Substitute	7 Common Iliac Artery, Left
J Inspection	8 Colic Artery, Middle		9 Autologous Venous Tissue	8 Common Iliac Arteries, Bilateral
L Occlusion	9 Renal Artery, Right		A Autologous Arterial Tissue	9 Internal Iliac Artery, Right
N Release	A Renal Artery, Left		C Extraluminal Device	B Internal Iliac Artery, Left
P Removal	B Inferior Mesenteric Artery		D Intraluminal Device	C Internal Iliac Arteries, Bilateral
Q Repair	C Common Iliac Artery, Right		E Intraluminal Device, Two OR Intraluminal Device, Branched or Fenestrated, One or Two Arteries	D External Iliac Artery, Right
R Replacement	D Common Iliac Artery, Left		F Intraluminal Device, Three OR Intraluminal Device, Branched or Fenestrated, Three or More Arteries	F External Iliac Artery, Left
S Reposition	E Internal Iliac Artery, Right		G Intraluminal Device, Four or More	G External Iliac Arteries, Bilateral
U Supplement	F Internal Iliac Artery, Left		J Synthetic Substitute	H Femoral Artery, Right
V Restriction	H External Iliac Artery, Right		K Nonautologous Tissue Substitute	J Femoral Artery, Left OR Temporary
W Revision	J External Iliac Artery, Left		Y Other Device	K Femoral Arteries, Bilateral
	K Femoral Artery, Right		Z No Device	L Popliteal Artery
	L Femoral Artery, Left			M Peroneal Artery
	M Popliteal Artery, Right			N Posterior Tibial Artery
	N Popliteal Artery, Left			P Foot Artery
	P Anterior Tibial Artery, Right			Q Lower Extremity Artery
	Q Anterior Tibial Artery, Left			R Lower Artery
	R Posterior Tibial Artery, Right			S Lower Extremity Vein
	S Posterior Tibial Artery, Left			T Uterine Artery, Right
	T Peroneal Artery, Right			U Uterine Artery, Left
	U Peroneal Artery, Left			X Diagnostic
	V Foot Artery, Right			Z No Qualifier
	W Foot Artery, Left			
	Y Lower Artery			

AHA Coding Clinic for table Ø41

2019, 1Q, 23	Endovascular repair of shaggy aorta and deployment of chimney stent grafts
2018, 3Q, 25	Femoral artery to tibioperoneal trunk bypass
2017, 4Q, 46-47	New and revised body part values - Bypass hepatic artery to renal artery
2017, 3Q, 5	Femoral artery to posterior tibial artery bypass using autologous and synthetic grafts
2017, 3Q, 16	Abdominal aortic debranching with bypass of external iliac artery to bilateral renal arteries and superior mesenteric artery
2017, 1Q, 32	Peroneal artery to dorsalis pedis artery bypass using saphenous vein graft
2016, 2Q, 18	Femoral-tibial artery bypass and saphenous vein graft
2015, 3Q, 28	Bilateral renal artery bypass

AHA Coding Clinic for table Ø47

2019, 4Q, 27	Bifurcation Qualifier
2019, 2Q, 14	Revision of occluded femoral-popliteal bypass graft
2018, 2Q, 24	Coronary artery bifurcation
2016, 4Q, 86	Peripheral artery, number of stents
2016, 4Q, 86-88	Coronary and peripheral artery bifurcation
2016, 3Q, 39	Infrarenal abdominal aortic aneurysm repair with iliac graft extension
2015, 4Q, 4-7, 15	Drug-coated balloon angioplasty in peripheral vessels
2015, 3Q, 9	Aborted endovascular stenting of superficial femoral artery

AHA Coding Clinic for table Ø4C

2019, 4Q, 27	Bifurcation Qualifier
2019, 1Q, 23	Endovascular repair of shaggy aorta and deployment of chimney stent grafts
2018, 2Q, 24	Coronary artery bifurcation
2017, 2Q, 23	Thrombectomy via Fogarty catheter
2016, 4Q, 86-88	Coronary and peripheral artery bifurcation
2016, 1Q, 31	Iliofemoral endarterectomy with patch repair
2015, 1Q, 29	Discontinued carotid endarterectomy
2015, 1Q, 36	Percutaneous mechanical thrombectomy of femoropopliteal bypass graft

AHA Coding Clinic for table Ø4H

2019, 3Q, 20	Removal and revision of ECMO component
2019, 1Q, 23	Endovascular repair of shaggy aorta and deployment of chimney stent grafts
2017, 1Q, 30	Insertion of umbilical artery catheter

AHA Coding Clinic for table Ø4L

2018, 2Q, 18	Transverse rectus abdominis myocutaneous (TRAM) delay
2017, 4Q, 31	Resuscitative endovascular balloon occlusion of the aorta
2015, 2Q, 27	Uterine artery embolization using Gelfoam
2014, 3Q, 26	Coil embolization of gastroduodenal artery with chemoembolization of hepatic artery
2014, 1Q, 24	Endovascular embolization for gastrointestinal bleeding

AHA Coding Clinic for table Ø4N

2015, 2Q, 28	Release and replacement of celiac artery

AHA Coding Clinic for table Ø4P

2019, 3Q, 20	Removal and revision of ECMO component

AHA Coding Clinic for table Ø4Q

2014, 1Q, 21	Repair of femoral artery pseudoaneurysm

AHA Coding Clinic for table Ø4R

2019, 1Q, 22	Abdominal aortic aneurysm repair using tube graft
2015, 2Q, 28	Release and replacement of celiac artery

AHA Coding Clinic for table Ø4U

2019, 1Q, 22	Abdominal aortic aneurysm repair using tube graft
2016, 2Q, 18	Femoral-tibial artery bypass and saphenous vein graft
2016, 1Q, 31	Iliofemoral endarterectomy with patch repair
2014, 4Q, 37	Bovine patch arterioplasty
2014, 1Q, 22	Repair of pseudoaneurysm of femoral-popliteal bypass graft

AHA Coding Clinic for table Ø4V

2019, 4Q, 27	Bifurcation Qualifier
2019, 1Q, 22	Abdominal aortic aneurysm repair using tube graft
2018, 2Q, 24	Coronary artery bifurcation
2016, 4Q, 86-87	Coronary and peripheral artery bifurcation
2016, 4Q, 89-93	Branched and fenestrated endograft repair of aneurysms
2016, 3Q, 39	Infrarenal abdominal aortic aneurysm repair with iliac graft extension
2014, 1Q, 9	Endovascular repair of abdominal aortic aneurysm

AHA Coding Clinic for table Ø4W

2019, 2Q, 14	Revision of occluded femoral-popliteal bypass graft
2015, 1Q, 36	Revision of femoropopliteal bypass graft
2014, 1Q, 9	Endovascular repair of endoleak
2014, 1Q, 22	Repair of pseudoaneurysm of femoral-popliteal bypass graft

Lower Arteries

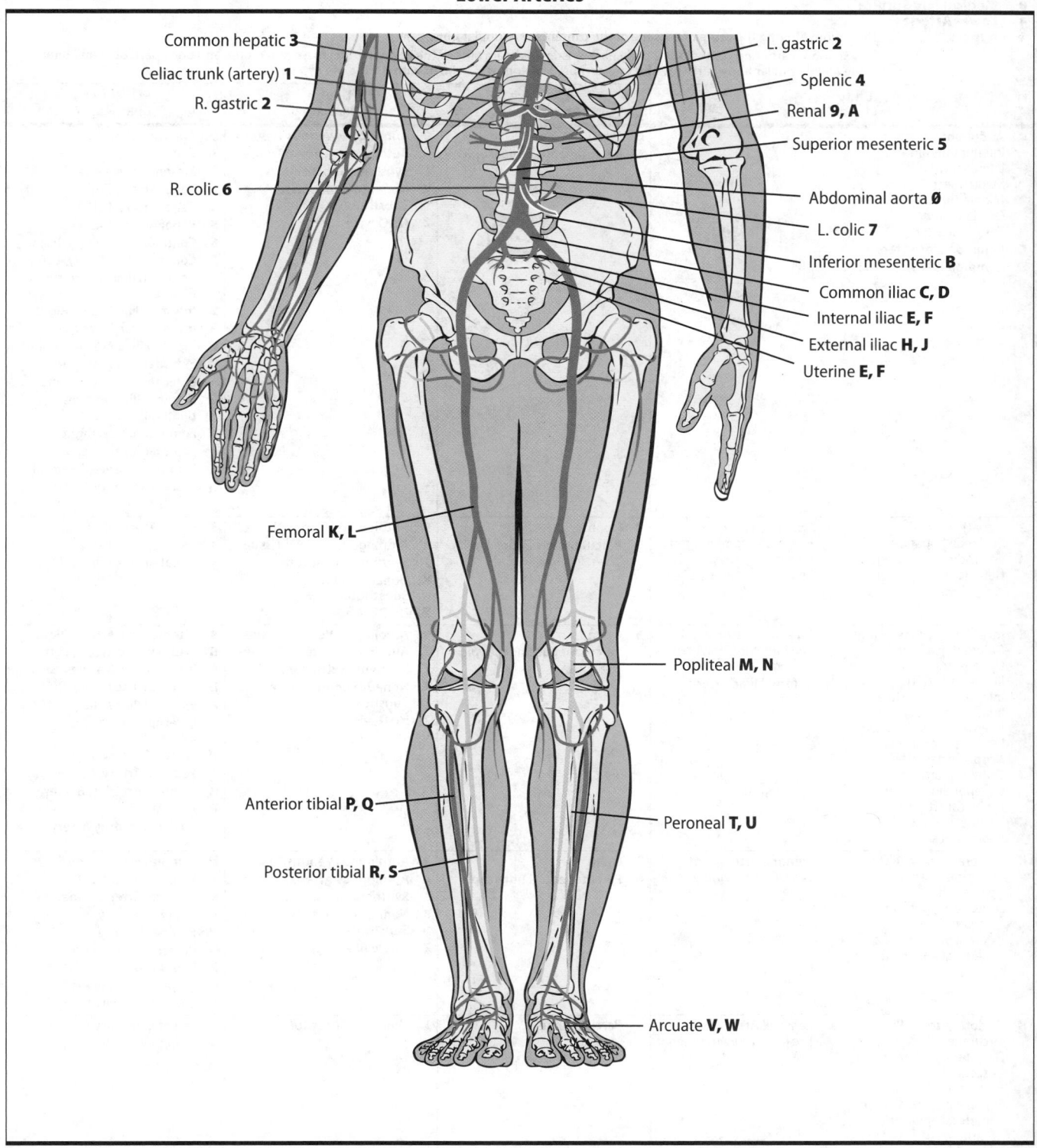

Common hepatic **3**
Celiac trunk (artery) **1**
R. gastric **2**

R. colic **6**

L. gastric **2**
Splenic **4**
Renal **9, A**
Superior mesenteric **5**

Abdominal aorta **Ø**
L. colic **7**
Inferior mesenteric **B**
Common iliac **C, D**
Internal iliac **E, F**
External iliac **H, J**
Uterine **E, F**

Femoral **K, L**

Popliteal **M, N**

Anterior tibial **P, Q**

Peroneal **T, U**

Posterior tibial **R, S**

Arcuate **V, W**

Lower Arteries

Ø   **Medical and Surgical**
4   **Lower Arteries**
1   **Bypass**   Definition: Altering the route of passage of the contents of a tubular body part

                 Explanation: Rerouting contents of a body part to a downstream area of the normal route, to a similar route and body part, or to an abnormal route and dissimilar body part. Includes one or more anastomoses, with or without the use of a device.

Body Part Character 4		Approach Character 5	Device Character 6	Qualifier Character 7

Ø **Abdominal Aorta**
  Inferior phrenic artery
  Lumbar artery
  Median sacral artery
  Middle suprarenal artery
  Ovarian artery
  Testicular artery
C **Common Iliac Artery, Right**
D **Common Iliac Artery, Left**
		Ø Open
		4 Percutaneous Endoscopic
			9 Autologous Venous Tissue
			A Autologous Arterial Tissue
			J Synthetic Substitute
			K Nonautologous Tissue
			   Substitute
			Z No Device
				Ø Abdominal Aorta
				1 Celiac Artery
				2 Mesenteric Artery
				3 Renal Artery, Right
				4 Renal Artery, Left
				5 Renal Artery, Bilateral
				6 Common Iliac Artery, Right
				7 Common Iliac Artery, Left
				8 Common Iliac Arteries,
				   Bilateral
				9 Internal Iliac Artery, Right
				B Internal Iliac Artery, Left
				C Internal Iliac Arteries, Bilateral
				D External Iliac Artery, Right
				F External Iliac Artery, Left
				G External Iliac Arteries,
				   Bilateral
				H Femoral Artery, Right
				J Femoral Artery, Left
				K Femoral Arteries, Bilateral
				Q Lower Extremity Artery
				R Lower Artery

3 **Hepatic Artery**
  Common hepatic artery
  Gastroduodenal artery
  Hepatic artery proper
	4 **Splenic Artery**
	  Left gastroepiploic artery
	  Pancreatic artery
	  Short gastric artery
		Ø Open
		4 Percutaneous Endoscopic
			9 Autologous Venous Tissue
			A Autologous Arterial Tissue
			J Synthetic Substitute
			K Nonautologous Tissue
			   Substitute
			Z No Device
				3 Renal Artery, Right
				4 Renal Artery, Left
				5 Renal Artery, Bilateral

E **Internal Iliac Artery, Right**
  Deferential artery
  Hypogastric artery
  Iliolumbar artery
  Inferior gluteal artery
  Inferior vesical artery
  Internal pudendal artery
  Lateral sacral artery
  Middle rectal artery
  Obturator artery
  Superior gluteal artery
  Umbilical artery
  Uterine artery
  Vaginal artery
	F **Internal Iliac Artery, Left**
	  See E Internal Iliac Artery,
	  Right
	H **External Iliac Artery,**
	  Right
	  Deep circumflex iliac
	    artery
	  Inferior epigastric artery
	J **External Iliac Artery, Left**
	  See H External Iliac Artery,
	  Right
		Ø Open
		4 Percutaneous Endoscopic
			9 Autologous Venous Tissue
			A Autologous Arterial Tissue
			J Synthetic Substitute
			K Nonautologous Tissue
			   Substitute
			Z No Device
				9 Internal Iliac Artery, Right
				B Internal Iliac Artery, Left
				C Internal Iliac Arteries, Bilateral
				D External Iliac Artery, Right
				F External Iliac Artery, Left
				G External Iliac Arteries,
				   Bilateral
				H Femoral Artery, Right
				J Femoral Artery, Left
				K Femoral Arteries, Bilateral
				P Foot Artery
				Q Lower Extremity Artery

K **Femoral Artery, Right**
  Circumflex iliac artery
  Deep femoral artery
  Descending genicular
    artery
  External pudendal artery
  Superficial epigastric
    artery
	L **Femoral Artery, Left**
	  See K Femoral Artery, Right
		Ø Open
		4 Percutaneous Endoscopic
			9 Autologous Venous Tissue
			A Autologous Arterial Tissue
			J Synthetic Substitute
			K Nonautologous Tissue
			   Substitute
			Z No Device
				H Femoral Artery, Right
				J Femoral Artery, Left
				K Femoral Arteries, Bilateral
				L Popliteal Artery
				M Peroneal Artery
				N Posterior Tibial Artery
				P Foot Artery
				Q Lower Extremity Artery
				S Lower Extremity Vein

K **Femoral Artery, Right**
  Circumflex iliac artery
  Deep femoral artery
  Descending genicular
    artery
  External pudendal artery
  Superficial epigastric
    artery
	L **Femoral Artery, Left**
	  See K Femoral Artery, Right
		3 Percutaneous	J Synthetic Substitute	Q Lower Extremity Artery
				S Lower Extremity Vein

M **Popliteal Artery, Right**
  Inferior genicular artery
  Middle genicular artery
  Superior genicular artery
  Sural artery
  Tibioperoneal trunk
	N **Popliteal Artery, Left**
	  See M Popliteal Artery,
	  Right
		Ø Open
		4 Percutaneous Endoscopic
			9 Autologous Venous Tissue
			A Autologous Arterial Tissue
			J Synthetic Substitute
			K Nonautologous Tissue
			   Substitute
			Z No Device
				L Popliteal Artery
				M Peroneal Artery
				P Foot Artery
				Q Lower Extremity Artery
				S Lower Extremity Vein

Ø41 Continued on next page

LC Limited Coverage   NC Noncovered   ⊞ Combination Member   HAC associated procedure   Combination Only   DRG Non-OR   Non-OR   New/Revised in GREEN

218   ICD-10-PCS 2021

Ø Medical and Surgical
4 Lower Arteries
1 Bypass

041 Continued

Definition: Altering the route of passage of the contents of a tubular body part

Explanation: Rerouting contents of a body part to a downstream area of the normal route, to a similar route and body part, or to an abnormal route and dissimilar body part. Includes one or more anastomoses, with or without the use of a device.

Body Part Character 4		Approach Character 5	Device Character 6	Qualifier Character 7
M Popliteal Artery, Right Inferior genicular artery Middle genicular artery Superior genicular artery Sural artery Tibioperoneal trunk	**N Popliteal Artery, Left** *See M Popliteal Artery, Right*	**3** Percutaneous	**J** Synthetic Substitute	**Q** Lower Extremity Artery **S** Lower Extremity Vein
P Anterior Tibial Artery, Right Anterior lateral malleolar artery Anterior medial malleolar artery Anterior tibial recurrent artery Dorsalis pedis artery Posterior tibial recurrent artery	**Q Anterior Tibial Artery, Left** *See P Anterior Tibial Artery, Right* **R Posterior Tibial Artery, Right** **S Posterior Tibial Artery, Left**	**Ø** Open **3** Percutaneous **4** Percutaneous Endoscopic	**J** Synthetic Substitute	**Q** Lower Extremity Artery **S** Lower Extremity Vein
T Peroneal Artery, Right Fibular artery **U Peroneal Artery, Left** *See T Peroneal Artery, Right*	**V Foot Artery, Right** Arcuate artery Dorsal metatarsal artery Lateral plantar artery Lateral tarsal artery Medial plantar artery **W Foot Artery, Left** *See V Foot Artery, Right*	**Ø** Open **4** Percutaneous Endoscopic	**9** Autologous Venous Tissue **A** Autologous Arterial Tissue **J** Synthetic Substitute **K** Nonautologous Tissue Substitute **Z** No Device	**P** Foot Artery **Q** Lower Extremity Artery **S** Lower Extremity Vein
T Peroneal Artery, Right Fibular artery **U Peroneal Artery, Left** *See T Peroneal Artery, Right*	**V Foot Artery, Right** Arcuate artery Dorsal metatarsal artery Lateral plantar artery Lateral tarsal artery Medial plantar artery **W Foot Artery, Left** *See V Foot Artery, Right*	**3** Percutaneous	**J** Synthetic Substitute	**Q** Lower Extremity Artery **S** Lower Extremity Vein

LC Limited Coverage   NC Noncovered   ⊞ Combination Member   HAC associated procedure   Combination Only   DRG Non-OR   Non-OR   New/Revised in GREEN

ICD-10-PCS 2021   219

041–041

Lower Arteries

Ø   **Medical and Surgical**
4   **Lower Arteries**
5   **Destruction**   Definition: Physical eradication of all or a portion of a body part by the direct use of energy, force, or a destructive agent
                 Explanation: None of the body part is physically taken out

Body Part Character 4		Approach Character 5	Device Character 6	Qualifier Character 7

Ø Abdominal Aorta
  Inferior phrenic artery
  Lumbar artery
  Median sacral artery
  Middle suprarenal artery
  Ovarian artery
  Testicular artery
1 Celiac Artery
  Celiac trunk
2 Gastric Artery
  Left gastric artery
  Right gastric artery
3 Hepatic Artery
  Common hepatic artery
  Gastroduodenal artery
  Hepatic artery proper
4 Splenic Artery
  Left gastroepiploic artery
  Pancreatic artery
  Short gastric artery
5 Superior Mesenteric Artery
  Ileal artery
  Ileocolic artery
  Inferior pancreaticoduodenal
    artery
  Jejunal artery
6 Colic Artery, Right
7 Colic Artery, Left
8 Colic Artery, Middle
9 Renal Artery, Right
  Inferior suprarenal artery
  Renal segmental artery
A Renal Artery, Left
  See 9 Renal Artery, Right
B Inferior Mesenteric Artery
  Sigmoid artery
  Superior rectal artery
C Common Iliac Artery, Right
D Common Iliac Artery, Left
E Internal Iliac Artery, Right
  Deferential artery
  Hypogastric artery
  Iliolumbar artery
  Inferior gluteal artery
  Inferior vesical artery
  Internal pudendal artery
  Lateral sacral artery
  Middle rectal artery
  Obturator artery
  Superior gluteal artery
  Umbilical artery
  Uterine artery
  Vaginal artery
	F Internal Iliac Artery, Left
	  See E Internal Iliac Artery, Right
	H External Iliac Artery, Right
	  Deep circumflex iliac artery
	  Inferior epigastric artery
	J External Iliac Artery, Left
	  See H External Iliac Artery, Right
	K Femoral Artery, Right
	  Circumflex iliac artery
	  Deep femoral artery
	  Descending genicular artery
	  External pudendal artery
	  Superficial epigastric artery
	L Femoral Artery, Left
	  See K Femoral Artery, Right
	M Popliteal Artery, Right
	  Inferior genicular artery
	  Middle genicular artery
	  Superior genicular artery
	  Sural artery
	  Tibioperoneal trunk
	N Popliteal Artery, Left
	  See M Popliteal Artery, Right
	P Anterior Tibial Artery, Right
	  Anterior lateral malleolar
	    artery
	  Anterior medial malleolar
	    artery
	  Anterior tibial recurrent artery
	  Dorsalis pedis artery
	  Posterior tibial recurrent artery
	Q Anterior Tibial Artery, Left
	  See P Anterior Tibial Artery,
	    Right
	R Posterior Tibial Artery, Right
	S Posterior Tibial Artery, Left
	T Peroneal Artery, Right
	  Fibular artery
	U Peroneal Artery, Left
	  See T Peroneal Artery, Right
	V Foot Artery, Right
	  Arcuate artery
	  Dorsal metatarsal artery
	  Lateral plantar artery
	  Lateral tarsal artery
	  Medial plantar artery
	W Foot Artery, Left
	  See V Foot Artery, Right
	Y Lower Artery
	  Umbilical artery
		Ø Open
		3 Percutaneous
		4 Percutaneous Endoscopic
			Z No Device	**Z No Qualifier**

Ø Medical and Surgical
4 Lower Arteries
7 Dilation   Definition: Expanding an orifice or the lumen of a tubular body part

Explanation: The orifice can be a natural orifice or an artificially created orifice. Accomplished by stretching a tubular body part using intraluminal pressure or by cutting part of the orifice or wall of the tubular body part.

Body Part Character 4		Approach Character 5	Device Character 6	Qualifier Character 7

Ø Abdominal Aorta
Inferior phrenic artery
Lumbar artery
Median sacral artery
Middle suprarenal artery
Ovarian artery
Testicular artery
1 Celiac Artery
Celiac trunk
2 Gastric Artery
Left gastric artery
Right gastric artery
3 Hepatic Artery
Common hepatic artery
Gastroduodenal artery
Hepatic artery proper
4 Splenic Artery
Left gastroepiploic artery
Pancreatic artery
Short gastric artery
5 Superior Mesenteric Artery
Ileal artery
Ileocolic artery
Inferior pancreaticoduodenal
   artery
Jejunal artery
6 Colic Artery, Right
7 Colic Artery, Left
8 Colic Artery, Middle
9 Renal Artery, Right
Inferior suprarenal artery
Renal segmental artery
A Renal Artery, Left
See 9 Renal Artery, Right
B Inferior Mesenteric Artery
Sigmoid artery
Superior rectal artery
C Common Iliac Artery, Right
D Common Iliac Artery, Left
E Internal Iliac Artery, Right
Deferential artery
Hypogastric artery
Iliolumbar artery
Inferior gluteal artery
Inferior vesical artery
Internal pudendal artery
Lateral sacral artery
Middle rectal artery
Obturator artery
Superior gluteal artery
Umbilical artery
Uterine artery
Vaginal artery
	F Internal Iliac Artery, Left
	See E Internal Iliac Artery, Right
	H External Iliac Artery, Right
	Deep circumflex iliac artery
	Inferior epigastric artery
	J External Iliac Artery, Left
	See H External Iliac Artery, Right
	K Femoral Artery, Right
	Circumflex iliac artery
	Deep femoral artery
	Descending genicular artery
	External pudendal artery
	Superficial epigastric artery
	L Femoral Artery, Left
	See K Femoral Artery, Right
	M Popliteal Artery, Right
	Inferior genicular artery
	Middle genicular artery
	Superior genicular artery
	Sural artery
	Tibioperoneal trunk
	N Popliteal Artery, Left
	See M Popliteal Artery, Right
	P Anterior Tibial Artery, Right
	Anterior lateral malleolar
	   artery
	Anterior medial malleolar
	   artery
	Anterior tibial recurrent artery
	Dorsalis pedis artery
	Posterior tibial recurrent artery
	Q Anterior Tibial Artery, Left
	See P Anterior Tibial Artery,
	   Right
	R Posterior Tibial Artery, Right
	S Posterior Tibial Artery, Left
	T Peroneal Artery, Right
	Fibular artery
	U Peroneal Artery, Left
	See T Peroneal Artery, Right
	V Foot Artery, Right
	Arcuate artery
	Dorsal metatarsal artery
	Lateral plantar artery
	Lateral tarsal artery
	Medial plantar artery
	W Foot Artery, Left
	See V Foot Artery, Right
	Y Lower Artery
	Umbilical artery
		Ø Open
		3 Percutaneous
		4 Percutaneous Endoscopic
			4 Intraluminal Device, Drug-eluting
			D Intraluminal Device
			Z No Device
				1 Drug-Coated Balloon
				Z No Qualifier

Ø47 Continued on next page

LC Limited Coverage   NC Noncovered   ⊞ Combination Member   HAC associated procedure   Combination Only   DRG Non-OR   Non-OR   New/Revised in GREEN

ICD-10-PCS 2021   221

Ø47–Ø47

Ø　**Medical and Surgical**　　　　　　　　　　　　　　　　　　　　　　　　*047 Continued*
4　**Lower Arteries**
7　**Dilation**　　Definition: Expanding an orifice or the lumen of a tubular body part

Explanation: The orifice can be a natural orifice or an artificially created orifice. Accomplished by stretching a tubular body part using intraluminal pressure or by cutting part of the orifice or wall of the tubular body part.

Body Part Character 4		Approach Character 5	Device Character 6	Qualifier Character 7
Ø **Abdominal Aorta** 　Inferior phrenic artery 　Lumbar artery 　Median sacral artery 　Middle suprarenal artery 　Ovarian artery 　Testicular artery 1 **Celiac Artery** 　Celiac trunk 2 **Gastric Artery** 　Left gastric artery 　Right gastric artery 3 **Hepatic Artery** 　Common hepatic artery 　Gastroduodenal artery 　Hepatic artery proper 4 **Splenic Artery** 　Left gastroepiploic artery 　Pancreatic artery 　Short gastric artery 5 **Superior Mesenteric Artery** 　Ileal artery 　Ileocolic artery 　Inferior pancreaticoduodenal 　　artery 　Jejunal artery 6 **Colic Artery, Right** 7 **Colic Artery, Left** 8 **Colic Artery, Middle** 9 **Renal Artery, Right** 　Inferior suprarenal artery 　Renal segmental artery A **Renal Artery, Left** 　*See 9 Renal Artery, Right* B **Inferior Mesenteric Artery** 　Sigmoid artery 　Superior rectal artery C **Common Iliac Artery, Right** D **Common Iliac Artery, Left** E **Internal Iliac Artery, Right** 　Deferential artery 　Hypogastric artery 　Iliolumbar artery 　Inferior gluteal artery 　Inferior vesical artery 　Internal pudendal artery 　Lateral sacral artery 　Middle rectal artery 　Obturator artery 　Superior gluteal artery 　Umbilical artery 　Uterine artery 　Vaginal artery	F **Internal Iliac Artery, Left** 　*See E Internal Iliac Artery, Right* H **External Iliac Artery, Right** 　Deep circumflex iliac artery 　Inferior epigastric artery J **External Iliac Artery, Left** 　*See H External Iliac Artery, Right* K **Femoral Artery, Right** 　Circumflex iliac artery 　Deep femoral artery 　Descending genicular artery 　External pudendal artery 　Superficial epigastric artery L **Femoral Artery, Left** 　*See K Femoral Artery, Right* M **Popliteal Artery, Right** 　Inferior genicular artery 　Middle genicular artery 　Superior genicular artery 　Sural artery 　Tibioperoneal trunk N **Popliteal Artery, Left** 　*See M Popliteal Artery, Right* P **Anterior Tibial Artery, Right** 　Anterior lateral malleolar 　　artery 　Anterior medial malleolar 　　artery 　Anterior tibial recurrent artery 　Dorsalis pedis artery 　Posterior tibial recurrent artery Q **Anterior Tibial Artery, Left** 　*See P Anterior Tibial Artery, 　Right* R **Posterior Tibial Artery, Right** S **Posterior Tibial Artery, Left** T **Peroneal Artery, Right** 　Fibular artery U **Peroneal Artery, Left** 　*See T Peroneal Artery, Right* V **Foot Artery, Right** 　Arcuate artery 　Dorsal metatarsal artery 　Lateral plantar artery 　Lateral tarsal artery 　Medial plantar artery W **Foot Artery, Left** 　*See V Foot Artery, Right* Y **Lower Artery** 　Umbilical artery	Ø **Open** 3 **Percutaneous** 4 **Percutaneous Endoscopic**	5 **Intraluminal Device, Drug- 　eluting, Two** 6 **Intraluminal Device, Drug- 　eluting, Three** 7 **Intraluminal Device, Drug- 　eluting, Four or More** E **Intraluminal Device, Two** F **Intraluminal Device, Three** G **Intraluminal Device, Four 　or More**	Z **No Qualifier**

LC Limited Coverage　　NC Noncovered　　⊞ Combination Member　　HAC associated procedure　　Combination Only　　DRG Non-OR　　Non-OR　　New/Revised in GREEN

222　　ICD-10-PCS 2021

Ø   Medical and Surgical
4   Lower Arteries
9   Drainage   Definition: Taking or letting out fluids and/or gases from a body part

Explanation: The qualifier DIAGNOSTIC is used to identify drainage procedures that are biopsies

Body Part Character 4		Approach Character 5	Device Character 6	Qualifier Character 7

Ø Abdominal Aorta
Inferior phrenic artery
Lumbar artery
Median sacral artery
Middle suprarenal artery
Ovarian artery
Testicular artery
1 Celiac Artery
Celiac trunk
2 Gastric Artery
Left gastric artery
Right gastric artery
3 Hepatic Artery
Common hepatic artery
Gastroduodenal artery
Hepatic artery proper
4 Splenic Artery
Left gastroepiploic artery
Pancreatic artery
Short gastric artery
5 Superior Mesenteric Artery
Ileal artery
Ileocolic artery
Inferior pancreaticoduodenal
   artery
Jejunal artery
6 Colic Artery, Right
7 Colic Artery, Left
8 Colic Artery, Middle
9 Renal Artery, Right
Inferior suprarenal artery
Renal segmental artery
A Renal Artery, Left
See 9 Renal Artery, Right
B Inferior Mesenteric Artery
Sigmoid artery
Superior rectal artery
C Common Iliac Artery, Right
D Common Iliac Artery, Left
E Internal Iliac Artery, Right
Deferential artery
Hypogastric artery
Iliolumbar artery
Inferior gluteal artery
Inferior vesical artery
Internal pudendal artery
Lateral sacral artery
Middle rectal artery
Obturator artery
Superior gluteal artery
Umbilical artery
Uterine artery
Vaginal artery
	F Internal Iliac Artery, Left
	See E Internal Iliac Artery, Right
	H External Iliac Artery, Right
	Deep circumflex iliac artery
	Inferior epigastric artery
	J External Iliac Artery, Left
	See H External Iliac Artery, Right
	K Femoral Artery, Right
	Circumflex iliac artery
	Deep femoral artery
	Descending genicular artery
	External pudendal artery
	Superficial epigastric artery
	L Femoral Artery, Left
	See K Femoral Artery, Right
	M Popliteal Artery, Right
	Inferior genicular artery
	Middle genicular artery
	Superior genicular artery
	Sural artery
	Tibioperoneal trunk
	N Popliteal Artery, Left
	See M Popliteal Artery, Right
	P Anterior Tibial Artery, Right
	Anterior lateral malleolar
	   artery
	Anterior medial malleolar
	   artery
	Anterior tibial recurrent artery
	Dorsalis pedis artery
	Posterior tibial recurrent artery
	Q Anterior Tibial Artery, Left
	See P Anterior Tibial Artery,
	Right
	R Posterior Tibial Artery, Right
	S Posterior Tibial Artery, Left
	T Peroneal Artery, Right
	Fibular artery
	U Peroneal Artery, Left
	See T Peroneal Artery, Right
	V Foot Artery, Right
	Arcuate artery
	Dorsal metatarsal artery
	Lateral plantar artery
	Lateral tarsal artery
	Medial plantar artery
	W Foot Artery, Left
	See V Foot Artery, Right
	Y Lower Artery
	Umbilical artery
		Ø Open
		3 Percutaneous
		4 Percutaneous Endoscopic
			Ø Drainage Device	**Z No Qualifier**

Non-OR   Ø49[Ø,1,2,3,4,5,6,7,8,9,A,B,C,D,E,F,H,J,K,L,M,N,P,Q,R,S,T,U,V,W,Y][Ø,3,4]ØZ

Ø49 Continued on next page

LC Limited Coverage   **NC** Noncovered   ⊞ Combination Member   HAC associated procedure   Combination Only   DRG Non-OR   Non-OR   New/Revised in GREEN

ICD-10-PCS 2021   223

Lower Arteries

Ø   **Medical and Surgical**
4   **Lower Arteries**
9   **Drainage**

Ø49 Continued

Definition: Taking or letting out fluids and/or gases from a body part

Explanation: The qualifier DIAGNOSTIC is used to identify drainage procedures that are biopsies

Body Part Character 4		Approach Character 5	Device Character 6	Qualifier Character 7
Ø Abdominal Aorta Inferior phrenic artery Lumbar artery Median sacral artery Middle suprarenal artery Ovarian artery Testicular artery **1 Celiac Artery** Celiac trunk **2 Gastric Artery** Left gastric artery Right gastric artery **3 Hepatic Artery** Common hepatic artery Gastroduodenal artery Hepatic artery proper **4 Splenic Artery** Left gastroepiploic artery Pancreatic artery Short gastric artery **5 Superior Mesenteric Artery** Ileal artery Ileocolic artery Inferior pancreaticoduodenal artery Jejunal artery **6 Colic Artery, Right** **7 Colic Artery, Left** **8 Colic Artery, Middle** **9 Renal Artery, Right** Inferior suprarenal artery Renal segmental artery **A Renal Artery, Left** *See 9 Renal Artery, Right* **B Inferior Mesenteric Artery** Sigmoid artery Superior rectal artery **C Common Iliac Artery, Right** **D Common Iliac Artery, Left** **E Internal Iliac Artery, Right** Deferential artery Hypogastric artery Iliolumbar artery Inferior gluteal artery Inferior vesical artery Internal pudendal artery Lateral sacral artery Middle rectal artery Obturator artery Superior gluteal artery Umbilical artery Uterine artery Vaginal artery	**F Internal Iliac Artery, Left** *See E Internal Iliac Artery, Right* **H External Iliac Artery, Right** Deep circumflex iliac artery Inferior epigastric artery **J External Iliac Artery, Left** *See H External Iliac Artery, Right* **K Femoral Artery, Right** Circumflex iliac artery Deep femoral artery Descending genicular artery External pudendal artery Superficial epigastric artery **L Femoral Artery, Left** *See K Femoral Artery, Right* **M Popliteal Artery, Right** Inferior genicular artery Middle genicular artery Superior genicular artery Sural artery Tibioperoneal trunk **N Popliteal Artery, Left** *See M Popliteal Artery, Right* **P Anterior Tibial Artery, Right** Anterior lateral malleolar artery Anterior medial malleolar artery Anterior tibial recurrent artery Dorsalis pedis artery Posterior tibial recurrent artery **Q Anterior Tibial Artery, Left** *See P Anterior Tibial Artery, Right* **R Posterior Tibial Artery, Right** **S Posterior Tibial Artery, Left** **T Peroneal Artery, Right** Fibular artery **U Peroneal Artery, Left** *See T Peroneal Artery, Right* **V Foot Artery, Right** Arcuate artery Dorsal metatarsal artery Lateral plantar artery Lateral tarsal artery Medial plantar artery **W Foot Artery, Left** *See V Foot Artery, Right* **Y Lower Artery** Umbilical artery	**Ø Open** **3 Percutaneous** **4 Percutaneous Endoscopic**	**Z No Device**	**X Diagnostic** **Z No Qualifier**

Non-OR   Ø49[Ø,1,2,3,4,5,6,7,8,9,A,B,C,D,E,F,H,J,K,L,M,N,P,Q,R,S,T,U,V,W,Y]3ZX
Non-OR   Ø49[Ø,1,2,3,4,5,6,7,8,9,A,B,C,D,E,F,H,J,K,L,M,N,P,Q,R,S,T,U,V,W,Y][Ø,3,4]ZZ

LC Limited Coverage   NC Noncovered   ⊞ Combination Member   HAC associated procedure   Combination Only   DRG Non-OR   Non-OR   New/Revised in GREEN

224   ICD-10-PCS 2021

0   **Medical and Surgical**
4   **Lower Arteries**
B   **Excision**   Definition: Cutting out or off, without replacement, a portion of a body part
                       Explanation: The qualifier DIAGNOSTIC is used to identify excision procedures that are biopsies

Body Part Character 4		Approach Character 5	Device Character 6	Qualifier Character 7
0 **Abdominal Aorta** Inferior phrenic artery Lumbar artery Median sacral artery Middle suprarenal artery Ovarian artery Testicular artery **1** **Celiac Artery** Celiac trunk **2** **Gastric Artery** Left gastric artery Right gastric artery **3** **Hepatic Artery** Common hepatic artery Gastroduodenal artery Hepatic artery proper **4** **Splenic Artery** Left gastroepiploic artery Pancreatic artery Short gastric artery **5** **Superior Mesenteric Artery** Ileal artery Ileocolic artery Inferior pancreaticoduodenal artery Jejunal artery **6** **Colic Artery, Right** **7** **Colic Artery, Left** **8** **Colic Artery, Middle** **9** **Renal Artery, Right** Inferior suprarenal artery Renal segmental artery **A** **Renal Artery, Left** *See 9 Renal Artery, Right* **B** **Inferior Mesenteric Artery** Sigmoid artery Superior rectal artery **C** **Common Iliac Artery, Right** **D** **Common Iliac Artery, Left** **E** **Internal Iliac Artery, Right** Deferential artery Hypogastric artery Iliolumbar artery Inferior gluteal artery Inferior vesical artery Internal pudendal artery Lateral sacral artery Middle rectal artery Obturator artery Superior gluteal artery Umbilical artery Uterine artery Vaginal artery	**F** **Internal Iliac Artery, Left** *See E Internal Iliac Artery, Right* **H** **External Iliac Artery, Right** Deep circumflex iliac artery Inferior epigastric artery **J** **External Iliac Artery, Left** *See H External Iliac Artery, Right* **K** **Femoral Artery, Right** Circumflex iliac artery Deep femoral artery Descending genicular artery External pudendal artery Superficial epigastric artery **L** **Femoral Artery, Left** *See K Femoral Artery, Right* **M** **Popliteal Artery, Right** Inferior genicular artery Middle genicular artery Superior genicular artery Sural artery Tibioperoneal trunk **N** **Popliteal Artery, Left** *See M Popliteal Artery, Right* **P** **Anterior Tibial Artery, Right** Anterior lateral malleolar artery Anterior medial malleolar artery Anterior tibial recurrent artery Dorsalis pedis artery Posterior tibial recurrent artery **Q** **Anterior Tibial Artery, Left** *See P Anterior Tibial Artery, Right* **R** **Posterior Tibial Artery, Right** **S** **Posterior Tibial Artery, Left** **T** **Peroneal Artery, Right** Fibular artery **U** **Peroneal Artery, Left** *See T Peroneal Artery, Right* **V** **Foot Artery, Right** Arcuate artery Dorsal metatarsal artery Lateral plantar artery Lateral tarsal artery Medial plantar artery **W** **Foot Artery, Left** *See V Foot Artery, Right* **Y** **Lower Artery** Umbilical artery	**0** Open **3** Percutaneous **4** Percutaneous Endoscopic	**Z** No Device	**X** Diagnostic **Z** No Qualifier

Ø Medical and Surgical
4 Lower Arteries
C Extirpation   Definition: Taking or cutting out solid matter from a body part

Explanation: The solid matter may be an abnormal byproduct of a biological function or a foreign body; it may be imbedded in a body part or in the lumen of a tubular body part. The solid matter may or may not have been previously broken into pieces.

Body Part Character 4		Approach Character 5	Device Character 6	Qualifier Character 7
Ø Abdominal Aorta Inferior phrenic artery Lumbar artery Median sacral artery Middle suprarenal artery Ovarian artery Testicular artery **1 Celiac Artery** Celiac trunk **2 Gastric Artery** Left gastric artery Right gastric artery **3 Hepatic Artery** Common hepatic artery Gastroduodenal artery Hepatic artery proper **4 Splenic Artery** Left gastroepiploic artery Pancreatic artery Short gastric artery **5 Superior Mesenteric Artery** Ileal artery Ileocolic artery Inferior pancreaticoduodenal artery Jejunal artery **6 Colic Artery, Right** **7 Colic Artery, Left** **8 Colic Artery, Middle** **9 Renal Artery, Right** Inferior suprarenal artery Renal segmental artery **A Renal Artery, Left** *See 9 Renal Artery, Right* **B Inferior Mesenteric Artery** Sigmoid artery Superior rectal artery **C Common Iliac Artery, Right** **D Common Iliac Artery, Left** **E Internal Iliac Artery, Right** Deferential artery Hypogastric artery Iliolumbar artery Inferior gluteal artery Inferior vesical artery Internal pudendal artery Lateral sacral artery Middle rectal artery Obturator artery Superior gluteal artery Umbilical artery Uterine artery Vaginal artery	**F Internal Iliac Artery, Left** *See E Internal Iliac Artery, Right* **H External Iliac Artery, Right** Deep circumflex iliac artery Inferior epigastric artery **J External Iliac Artery, Left** *See H External Iliac Artery, Right* **K Femoral Artery, Right** Circumflex iliac artery Deep femoral artery Descending genicular artery External pudendal artery Superficial epigastric artery **L Femoral Artery, Left** *See K Femoral Artery, Right* **M Popliteal Artery, Right** Inferior genicular artery Middle genicular artery Superior genicular artery Sural artery Tibioperoneal trunk **N Popliteal Artery, Left** *See M Popliteal Artery, Right* **P Anterior Tibial Artery, Right** Anterior lateral malleolar artery Anterior medial malleolar artery Anterior tibial recurrent artery Dorsalis pedis artery Posterior tibial recurrent artery **Q Anterior Tibial Artery, Left** *See P Anterior Tibial Artery,* *Right* **R Posterior Tibial Artery, Right** **S Posterior Tibial Artery, Left** **T Peroneal Artery, Right** Fibular artery **U Peroneal Artery, Left** *See T Peroneal Artery, Right* **V Foot Artery, Right** Arcuate artery Dorsal metatarsal artery Lateral plantar artery Lateral tarsal artery Medial plantar artery **W Foot Artery, Left** *See V Foot Artery, Right* **Y Lower Artery** Umbilical artery	**Ø Open** **3 Percutaneous** **4 Percutaneous Endoscopic**	**Z No Device**	**Z No Qualifier**

LC Limited Coverage   NC Noncovered   ⊞ Combination Member   HAC associated procedure   Combination Only   DRG Non-OR   Non-OR   New/Revised in GREEN

226   ICD-10-PCS 2021

Ø   **Medical and Surgical**
4   **Lower Arteries**
F   **Fragmentation**   Definition: Breaking solid matter in a body part into pieces
                     Explanation: Physical force (e.g., manual, ultrasonic) applied directly or indirectly is used to break the solid matter into pieces. The solid matter may be an abnormal byproduct of a biological function or a foreign body. The pieces of solid matter are not taken out.

Body Part Character 4	Approach Character 5	Device Character 6	Qualifier Character 7

C Common Iliac Artery, Right
D Common Iliac Artery, Left
E Internal Iliac Artery, Right
    Deferential artery
    Hypogastric artery
    Iliolumbar artery
    Inferior gluteal artery
    Inferior vesical artery
    Internal pudendal artery
    Lateral sacral artery
    Middle rectal artery
    Obturator artery
    Superior gluteal artery
    Umbilical artery
    Uterine artery
    Vaginal artery
F Internal Iliac Artery, Left
    See E Internal Iliac Artery, Right
H External Iliac Artery, Right
    Deep circumflex iliac artery
    Inferior epigastric artery
J External Iliac Artery, Left
    See H External Iliac Artery, Right
K Femoral Artery, Right
    Circumflex iliac artery
    Deep femoral artery
    Descending genicular artery
    External pudendal artery
    Superficial epigastric artery
 	
L Femoral Artery, Left
    See K Femoral Artery, Right
M Popliteal Artery, Right
    Inferior genicular artery
    Middle genicular artery
    Superior genicular artery
    Sural artery
    Tibioperoneal trunk
N Popliteal Artery, Left
    See M Popliteal Artery, Right
P Anterior Tibial Artery, Right
    Anterior lateral malleolar artery
    Anterior medial malleolar artery
    Anterior tibial recurrent artery
    Dorsalis pedis artery
    Posterior tibial recurrent artery
Q Anterior Tibial Artery, Left
    See P Anterior Tibial Artery, Right
R Posterior Tibial Artery, Right
S Posterior Tibial Artery, Left
T Peroneal Artery, Right
    Fibular artery
U Peroneal Artery, Left
    See T Peroneal Artery, Right
Y Lower Artery
    Umbilical artery
	3 Percutaneous	**Z** No Device	**Ø** Ultrasonic
			Z No Qualifier

LC Limited Coverage   NC Noncovered   ⊞ Combination Member   HAC associated procedure   Combination Only   DRG Non-OR   Non-OR   New/Revised in GREEN

ICD-10-PCS 2021   227

04F–04F

Ø   Medical and Surgical
4   Lower Arteries
H   Insertion   Definition: Putting in a nonbiological appliance that monitors, assists, performs, or prevents a physiological function but does not physically take the place of a body part
Explanation: None

Body Part Character 4		Approach Character 5	Device Character 6	Qualifier Character 7
Ø Abdominal Aorta Inferior phrenic artery Lumbar artery Median sacral artery Middle suprarenal artery Ovarian artery Testicular artery		**Ø Open** **3 Percutaneous** **4 Percutaneous Endoscopic**	**2 Monitoring Device** **3 Infusion Device** **D Intraluminal Device**	**Z No Qualifier**
1 Celiac Artery Celiac trunk	**F Internal Iliac Artery, Left** *See E Internal Iliac Artery, Right*	**Ø Open** **3 Percutaneous** **4 Percutaneous Endoscopic**	**3 Infusion Device** **D Intraluminal Device**	**Z No Qualifier**
2 Gastric Artery Left gastric artery Right gastric artery	**H External Iliac Artery, Right** Deep circumflex iliac artery Inferior epigastric artery			
3 Hepatic Artery Common hepatic artery Gastroduodenal artery Hepatic artery proper	**J External Iliac Artery, Left** *See H External Iliac Artery, Right*			
4 Splenic Artery Left gastroepiploic artery Pancreatic artery Short gastric artery	**K Femoral Artery, Right** Circumflex iliac artery Deep femoral artery Descending genicular artery External pudendal artery Superficial epigastric artery			
5 Superior Mesenteric Artery Ileal artery Ileocolic artery Inferior pancreaticoduodenal artery Jejunal artery	**L Femoral Artery, Left** *See K Femoral Artery, Right* **M Popliteal Artery, Right** Inferior genicular artery Middle genicular artery Superior genicular artery Sural artery Tibioperoneal trunk			
6 Colic Artery, Right **7 Colic Artery, Left** **8 Colic Artery, Middle** **9 Renal Artery, Right** Inferior suprarenal artery Renal segmental artery	**N Popliteal Artery, Left** *See M Popliteal Artery, Right* **P Anterior Tibial Artery, Right** Anterior lateral malleolar artery Anterior medial malleolar artery Anterior tibial recurrent artery Dorsalis pedis artery Posterior tibial recurrent artery			
A Renal Artery, Left *See 9 Renal Artery, Right* **B Inferior Mesenteric Artery** Sigmoid artery Superior rectal artery	**Q Anterior Tibial Artery, Left** *See P Anterior Tibial Artery, Right*			
C Common Iliac Artery, Right **D Common Iliac Artery, Left** **E Internal Iliac Artery, Right** Deferential artery Hypogastric artery Iliolumbar artery Inferior gluteal artery Inferior vesical artery Internal pudendal artery Lateral sacral artery Middle rectal artery Obturator artery Superior gluteal artery Umbilical artery Uterine artery Vaginal artery	**R Posterior Tibial Artery, Right** **S Posterior Tibial Artery, Left** **T Peroneal Artery, Right** Fibular artery **U Peroneal Artery, Left** *See T Peroneal Artery, Right* **V Foot Artery, Right** Arcuate artery Dorsal metatarsal artery Lateral plantar artery Lateral tarsal artery Medial plantar artery **W Foot Artery, Left** *See V Foot Artery, Right*			
Y Lower Artery Umbilical artery		**Ø Open** **3 Percutaneous** **4 Percutaneous Endoscopic**	**2 Monitoring Device** **3 Infusion Device** **D Intraluminal Device** **Y Other Device**	**Z No Qualifier**

Non-OR   04HØ[Ø,3,4][2,3]Z
Non-OR   04H[1,2,3,4,5,6,7,8,9,A,B,C,D,E,F,H,J,K,L,M,N,P,Q,R,S,T,U,V,W][Ø,3,4]3Z
Non-OR   04HY32Z
Non-OR   04HY[Ø,3,4]3Z
Non-OR   04HY[3,4]YZ

Ø   Medical and Surgical
4   Lower Arteries
J   Inspection   Definition: Visually and/or manually exploring a body part

Explanation: Visual exploration may be performed with or without optical instrumentation. Manual exploration may be performed directly or through intervening body layers.

Body Part Character 4	Approach Character 5	Device Character 6	Qualifier Character 7
Y Lower Artery Umbilical artery	**Ø** Open **3** Percutaneous **4** Percutaneous Endoscopic **X** External	**Z** No Device	**Z** No Qualifier

Non-OR   Ø4JY[3,4,X]ZZ

Ø   Medical and Surgical
4   Lower Arteries
L   Occlusion   Definition: Completely closing an orifice or the lumen of a tubular body part

Explanation: The orifice can be a natural orifice or an artificially created orifice

Body Part Character 4	Approach Character 5	Device Character 6	Qualifier Character 7

Ø   Abdominal Aorta
     Inferior phrenic artery
     Lumbar artery
     Median sacral artery
     Middle suprarenal artery
     Ovarian artery
     Testicular artery
	Ø Open
	4 Percutaneous Endoscopic
		C Extraluminal Device
		D Intraluminal Device
		Z No Device
			Z No Qualifier

Ø   Abdominal Aorta
     Inferior phrenic artery
     Lumbar artery
     Median sacral artery
     Middle suprarenal artery
     Ovarian artery
     Testicular artery
	3 Percutaneous	**C** Extraluminal Device
		Z No Device
			Z No Qualifier

Ø   Abdominal Aorta
     Inferior phrenic artery
     Lumbar artery
     Median sacral artery
     Middle suprarenal artery
     Ovarian artery
     Testicular artery
	3 Percutaneous	**D** Intraluminal Device	**J** Temporary
			Z No Qualifier

Ø4L Continued on next page

LC Limited Coverage   NC Noncovered   ⊞ Combination Member   HAC associated procedure   Combination Only   DRG Non-OR   Non-OR   New/Revised in GREEN

ICD-10-PCS 2021   229

Ø4J–Ø4L

0 Medical and Surgical
4 Lower Arteries
L Occlusion   Definition: Completely closing an orifice or the lumen of a tubular body part
                  Explanation: The orifice can be a natural orifice or an artificially created orifice

Body Part Character 4	Approach Character 5	Device Character 6	Qualifier Character 7
1 Celiac Artery Celiac trunk	**0 Open**	**C Extraluminal Device**	**Z No Qualifier**
2 Gastric Artery Left gastric artery Right gastric artery	**3 Percutaneous**	**D Intraluminal Device**	
3 Hepatic Artery Common hepatic artery Gastroduodenal artery Hepatic artery proper	**4 Percutaneous Endoscopic**	**Z No Device**	

K Femoral Artery, Right
    Circumflex iliac artery
    Deep femoral artery
    Descending genicular artery
    External pudendal artery
    Superficial epigastric artery
L Femoral Artery, Left
    See K Femoral Artery, Right
M Popliteal Artery, Right
    Inferior genicular artery
    Middle genicular artery
    Superior genicular artery
    Sural artery
    Tibioperoneal trunk
N Popliteal Artery, Left
    See M Popliteal Artery, Right
P Anterior Tibial Artery, Right
    Anterior lateral malleolar artery
    Anterior medial malleolar artery
    Anterior tibial recurrent artery
    Dorsalis pedis artery
    Posterior tibial recurrent artery
Q Anterior Tibial Artery, Left
    See P Anterior Tibial Artery, Right
R Posterior Tibial Artery, Right
S Posterior Tibial Artery, Left
T Peroneal Artery, Right
    Fibular artery
U Peroneal Artery, Left
    See T Peroneal Artery, Right
V Foot Artery, Right
    Arcuate artery
    Dorsal metatarsal artery
    Lateral plantar artery
    Lateral tarsal artery
    Medial plantar artery
W Foot Artery, Left
    See V Foot Artery, Right
Y Lower Artery
    Umbilical artery

4 Splenic Artery
    Left gastroepiploic artery
    Pancreatic artery
    Short gastric artery
5 Superior Mesenteric Artery
    Ileal artery
    Ileocolic artery
    Inferior pancreaticoduodenal artery
    Jejunal artery
6 Colic Artery, Right
7 Colic Artery, Left
8 Colic Artery, Middle
9 Renal Artery, Right
    Inferior suprarenal artery
    Renal segmental artery
A Renal Artery, Left
    See 9 Renal Artery, Right
B Inferior Mesenteric Artery
    Sigmoid artery
    Superior rectal artery
C Common Iliac Artery, Right
D Common Iliac Artery, Left
H External Iliac Artery, Right
    Deep circumflex iliac artery
    Inferior epigastric artery
J External Iliac Artery, Left
    See H External Iliac Artery, Right

Body Part Character 4	Approach Character 5	Device Character 6	Qualifier Character 7
E Internal Iliac Artery, Right Deferential artery Hypogastric artery Iliolumbar artery Inferior gluteal artery Inferior vesical artery Internal pudendal artery Lateral sacral artery Middle rectal artery Obturator artery Superior gluteal artery Umbilical artery Uterine artery Vaginal artery	**0 Open** **3 Percutaneous** **4 Percutaneous Endoscopic**	**C Extraluminal Device** **D Intraluminal Device** **Z No Device**	**T Uterine Artery, Right** ♀ **Z No Qualifier**
F Internal Iliac Artery, Left Deferential artery Hypogastric artery Iliolumbar artery Inferior gluteal artery Inferior vesical artery Internal pudendal artery Lateral sacral artery Middle rectal artery Obturator artery Superior gluteal artery Umbilical artery Uterine Artery Vaginal artery	**0 Open** **3 Percutaneous** **4 Percutaneous Endoscopic**	**C Extraluminal Device** **D Intraluminal Device** **Z No Device**	**U Uterine Artery, Left** ♀ **Z No Qualifier**

♀   04LE[0,3,4][C,D,Z]T
♀   04LF[0,3,4][C,D,Z]U

LC Limited Coverage   NC Noncovered   ⊞ Combination Member   HAC associated procedure   Combination Only   DRG Non-OR   Non-OR   New/Revised in GREEN

230

04L–04L

ICD-10-PCS 2021

Ø   Medical and Surgical
4   Lower Arteries
N   Release   Definition: Freeing a body part from an abnormal physical constraint by cutting or by the use of force
                    Explanation: Some of the restraining tissue may be taken out but none of the body part is taken out

Body Part Character 4		Approach Character 5	Device Character 6	Qualifier Character 7

Ø Abdominal Aorta
Inferior phrenic artery
Lumbar artery
Median sacral artery
Middle suprarenal artery
Ovarian artery
Testicular artery
1 Celiac Artery
Celiac trunk
2 Gastric Artery
Left gastric artery
Right gastric artery
3 Hepatic Artery
Common hepatic artery
Gastroduodenal artery
Hepatic artery proper
4 Splenic Artery
Left gastroepiploic artery
Pancreatic artery
Short gastric artery
5 Superior Mesenteric Artery
Ileal artery
Ileocolic artery
Inferior pancreaticoduodenal artery
Jejunal artery
6 Colic Artery, Right
7 Colic Artery, Left
8 Colic Artery, Middle
9 Renal Artery, Right
Inferior suprarenal artery
Renal segmental artery
A Renal Artery, Left
See 9 Renal Artery, Right
B Inferior Mesenteric Artery
Sigmoid artery
Superior rectal artery
C Common Iliac Artery, Right
D Common Iliac Artery, Left
E Internal Iliac Artery, Right
Deferential artery
Hypogastric artery
Iliolumbar artery
Inferior gluteal artery
Inferior vesical artery
Internal pudendal artery
Lateral sacral artery
Middle rectal artery
Obturator artery
Superior gluteal artery
Umbilical artery
Uterine artery
Vaginal artery
	F Internal Iliac Artery, Left
	See E Internal Iliac Artery, Right
	H External Iliac Artery, Right
	Deep circumflex iliac artery
	Inferior epigastric artery
	J External Iliac Artery, Left
	See H External Iliac Artery, Right
	K Femoral Artery, Right
	Circumflex iliac artery
	Deep femoral artery
	Descending genicular artery
	External pudendal artery
	Superficial epigastric artery
	L Femoral Artery, Left
	See K Femoral Artery, Right
	M Popliteal Artery, Right
	Inferior genicular artery
	Middle genicular artery
	Superior genicular artery
	Sural artery
	Tibioperoneal trunk
	N Popliteal Artery, Left
	See M Popliteal Artery, Right
	P Anterior Tibial Artery, Right
	Anterior lateral malleolar
	  artery
	Anterior medial malleolar
	  artery
	Anterior tibial recurrent
	  artery
	Dorsalis pedis artery
	Posterior tibial recurrent
	  artery
	Q Anterior Tibial Artery, Left
	See P Anterior Tibial Artery, Right
	R Posterior Tibial Artery, Right
	S Posterior Tibial Artery, Left
	T Peroneal Artery, Right
	Fibular artery
	U Peroneal Artery, Left
	See T Peroneal Artery, Right
	V Foot Artery, Right
	Arcuate artery
	Dorsal metatarsal artery
	Lateral plantar artery
	Lateral tarsal artery
	Medial plantar artery
	W Foot Artery, Left
	See V Foot Artery, Right
	Y Lower Artery
	Umbilical artery
		Ø Open
		3 Percutaneous
		4 Percutaneous Endoscopic
			Z No Device	**Z No Qualifier**

LC Limited Coverage   **NC** Noncovered   ⊞ Combination Member   HAC associated procedure   Combination Only   DRG Non-OR   Non-OR   New/Revised in GREEN

ICD-10-PCS 2021   231

Ø Medical and Surgical
4 Lower Arteries
P Removal

Definition: Taking out or off a device from a body part

Explanation: If a device is taken out and a similar device put in without cutting or puncturing the skin or mucous membrane, the procedure is coded to the root operation CHANGE. Otherwise, the procedure for taking out a device is coded to the root operation REMOVAL.

Body Part Character 4	Approach Character 5	Device Character 6	Qualifier Character 7
Y Lower Artery Umbilical artery	Ø Open 3 Percutaneous 4 Percutaneous Endoscopic	Ø Drainage Device 2 Monitoring Device 3 Infusion Device 7 Autologous Tissue Substitute C Extraluminal Device D Intraluminal Device J Synthetic Substitute K Nonautologous Tissue Substitute Y Other Device	Z No Qualifier
Y Lower Artery Umbilical artery	X External	Ø Drainage Device 1 Radioactive Element 2 Monitoring Device 3 Infusion Device D Intraluminal Device	Z No Qualifier

Non-OR   04PY3[Ø,2,3,D]Z
Non-OR   04PY[3,4]YZ
Non-OR   04PYX[Ø,1,2,3,D]Z

Ø   **Medical and Surgical**
4   **Lower Arteries**
Q   **Repair**   Definition: Restoring, to the extent possible, a body part to its normal anatomic structure and function

                 Explanation: Used only when the method to accomplish the repair is not one of the other root operations

Body Part Character 4		Approach Character 5	Device Character 6	Qualifier Character 7

Ø Abdominal Aorta
Inferior phrenic artery
Lumbar artery
Median sacral artery
Middle suprarenal artery
Ovarian artery
Testicular artery
1 Celiac Artery
Celiac trunk
2 Gastric Artery
Left gastric artery
Right gastric artery
3 Hepatic Artery
Common hepatic artery
Gastroduodenal artery
Hepatic artery proper
4 Splenic Artery
Left gastroepiploic artery
Pancreatic artery
Short gastric artery
5 Superior Mesenteric Artery
Ileal artery
Ileocolic artery
Inferior pancreaticoduodenal
  artery
Jejunal artery
6 Colic Artery, Right
7 Colic Artery, Left
8 Colic Artery, Middle
9 Renal Artery, Right
Inferior suprarenal artery
Renal segmental artery
A Renal Artery, Left
See 9 Renal Artery, Right
B Inferior Mesenteric Artery
Sigmoid artery
Superior rectal artery
C Common Iliac Artery, Right
D Common Iliac Artery, Left
E Internal Iliac Artery, Right
Deferential artery
Hypogastric artery
Iliolumbar artery
Inferior gluteal artery
Inferior vesical artery
Internal pudendal artery
Lateral sacral artery
Middle rectal artery
Obturator artery
Superior gluteal artery
Umbilical artery
Uterine artery
Vaginal artery
	F Internal Iliac Artery, Left
	*See E Internal Iliac Artery,
	Right*
	H External Iliac Artery, Right
	Deep circumflex iliac artery
	Inferior epigastric artery
	J External Iliac Artery, Left
	*See H External Iliac Artery,
	Right*
	K Femoral Artery, Right
	Circumflex iliac artery
	Deep femoral artery
	Descending genicular artery
	External pudendal artery
	Superficial epigastric artery
	L Femoral Artery, Left
	See K Femoral Artery, Right
	M Popliteal Artery, Right
	Inferior genicular artery
	Middle genicular artery
	Superior genicular artery
	Sural artery
	Tibioperoneal trunk
	N Popliteal Artery, Left
	See M Popliteal Artery, Right
	P Anterior Tibial Artery, Right
	Anterior lateral malleolar
	  artery
	Anterior medial malleolar
	  artery
	Anterior tibial recurrent
	  artery
	Dorsalis pedis artery
	Posterior tibial recurrent
	  artery
	Q Anterior Tibial Artery, Left
	*See P Anterior Tibial Artery,
	Right*
	**R Posterior Tibial Artery,
	Right**
	S Posterior Tibial Artery, Left
	T Peroneal Artery, Right
	Fibular artery
	U Peroneal Artery, Left
	See T Peroneal Artery, Right
	V Foot Artery, Right
	Arcuate artery
	Dorsal metatarsal artery
	Lateral plantar artery
	Lateral tarsal artery
	Medial plantar artery
	W Foot Artery, Left
	See V Foot Artery, Right
	Y Lower Artery
	Umbilical artery
		Ø Open
		3 Percutaneous
		4 Percutaneous Endoscopic
			Z No Device	**Z No Qualifier**

[LC] Limited Coverage   [NC] Noncovered   ⊞ Combination Member   HAC associated procedure   Combination Only   DRG Non-OR   Non-OR   New/Revised in GREEN

ICD-10-PCS 2021   233

04Q–04Q

0 Medical and Surgical
4 Lower Arteries
R Replacement Definition: Putting in or on biological or synthetic material that physically takes the place and/or function of all or a portion of a body part

Explanation: The body part may have been taken out or replaced, or may be taken out, physically eradicated, or rendered nonfunctional during the REPLACEMENT procedure. A REMOVAL procedure is coded for taking out the device used in a previous replacement procedure.

Body Part Character 4		Approach Character 5	Device Character 6	Qualifier Character 7
0 Abdominal Aorta Inferior phrenic artery Lumbar artery Median sacral artery Middle suprarenal artery Ovarian artery Testicular artery **1 Celiac Artery** Celiac trunk **2 Gastric Artery** Left gastric artery Right gastric artery **3 Hepatic Artery** Common hepatic artery Gastroduodenal artery Hepatic artery proper **4 Splenic Artery** Left gastroepiploic artery Pancreatic artery Short gastric artery **5 Superior Mesenteric Artery** Ileal artery Ileocolic artery Inferior pancreaticoduodenal artery Jejunal artery **6 Colic Artery, Right** **7 Colic Artery, Left** **8 Colic Artery, Middle** **9 Renal Artery, Right** Inferior suprarenal artery Renal segmental artery **A Renal Artery, Left** *See 9 Renal Artery, Right* **B Inferior Mesenteric Artery** Sigmoid artery Superior rectal artery **C Common Iliac Artery, Right** **D Common Iliac Artery, Left** **E Internal Iliac Artery, Right** Deferential artery Hypogastric artery Iliolumbar artery Inferior gluteal artery Inferior vesical artery Internal pudendal artery Lateral sacral artery Middle rectal artery Obturator artery Superior gluteal artery Umbilical artery Uterine artery Vaginal artery	**F Internal Iliac Artery, Left** *See E Internal Iliac Artery, Right* **H External Iliac Artery, Right** Deep circumflex iliac artery Inferior epigastric artery **J External Iliac Artery, Left** *See H External Iliac Artery, Right* **K Femoral Artery, Right** Circumflex iliac artery Deep femoral artery Descending genicular artery External pudendal artery Superficial epigastric artery **L Femoral Artery, Left** *See K Femoral Artery, Right* **M Popliteal Artery, Right** Inferior genicular artery Middle genicular artery Superior genicular artery Sural artery Tibioperoneal trunk **N Popliteal Artery, Left** *See M Popliteal Artery, Right* **P Anterior Tibial Artery, Right** Anterior lateral malleolar artery Anterior medial malleolar artery Anterior tibial recurrent artery Dorsalis pedis artery Posterior tibial recurrent artery **Q Anterior Tibial Artery, Left** *See P Anterior Tibial Artery, Right* **R Posterior Tibial Artery, Right** **S Posterior Tibial Artery, Left** **T Peroneal Artery, Right** Fibular artery **U Peroneal Artery, Left** *See T Peroneal Artery, Right* **V Foot Artery, Right** Arcuate artery Dorsal metatarsal artery Lateral plantar artery Lateral tarsal artery Medial plantar artery **W Foot Artery, Left** *See V Foot Artery, Right* **Y Lower Artery** Umbilical artery	**0 Open** **4 Percutaneous Endoscopic**	**7 Autologous Tissue Substitute** **J Synthetic Substitute** **K Nonautologous Tissue Substitute**	**Z No Qualifier**

Lower Arteries *(side tab)*

Ø Medical and Surgical
4 Lower Arteries
S Reposition

Definition: Moving to its normal location, or other suitable location, all or a portion of a body part

Explanation: The body part is moved to a new location from an abnormal location, or from a normal location where it is not functioning correctly. The body part may or may not be cut out or off to be moved to the new location.

Body Part Character 4		Approach Character 5	Device Character 6	Qualifier Character 7
Ø Abdominal Aorta Inferior phrenic artery Lumbar artery Median sacral artery Middle suprarenal artery Ovarian artery Testicular artery **1 Celiac Artery** Celiac trunk **2 Gastric Artery** Left gastric artery Right gastric artery **3 Hepatic Artery** Common hepatic artery Gastroduodenal artery Hepatic artery proper **4 Splenic Artery** Left gastroepiploic artery Pancreatic artery Short gastric artery **5 Superior Mesenteric Artery** Ileal artery Ileocolic artery Inferior pancreaticoduodenal artery Jejunal artery **6 Colic Artery, Right** **7 Colic Artery, Left** **8 Colic Artery, Middle** **9 Renal Artery, Right** Inferior suprarenal artery Renal segmental artery **A Renal Artery, Left** *See 9 Renal Artery, Right* **B Inferior Mesenteric Artery** Sigmoid artery Superior rectal artery **C Common Iliac Artery, Right** **D Common Iliac Artery, Left** **E Internal Iliac Artery, Right** Deferential artery Hypogastric artery Iliolumbar artery Inferior gluteal artery Inferior vesical artery Internal pudendal artery Lateral sacral artery Middle rectal artery Obturator artery Superior gluteal artery Umbilical artery Uterine artery Vaginal artery	**F Internal Iliac Artery, Left** *See E Internal Iliac Artery, Right* **H External Iliac Artery, Right** Deep circumflex iliac artery Inferior epigastric artery **J External Iliac Artery, Left** *See H External Iliac Artery, Right* **K Femoral Artery, Right** Circumflex iliac artery Deep femoral artery Descending genicular artery External pudendal artery Superficial epigastric artery **L Femoral Artery, Left** *See K Femoral Artery, Right* **M Popliteal Artery, Right** Inferior genicular artery Middle genicular artery Superior genicular artery Sural artery Tibioperoneal trunk **N Popliteal Artery, Left** *See M Popliteal Artery, Right* **P Anterior Tibial Artery, Right** Anterior lateral malleolar artery Anterior medial malleolar artery Anterior tibial recurrent artery Dorsalis pedis artery Posterior tibial recurrent artery **Q Anterior Tibial Artery, Left** *See P Anterior Tibial Artery, Right* **R Posterior Tibial Artery, Right** **S Posterior Tibial Artery, Left** **T Peroneal Artery, Right** Fibular artery **U Peroneal Artery, Left** *See T Peroneal Artery, Right* **V Foot Artery, Right** Arcuate artery Dorsal metatarsal artery Lateral plantar artery Lateral tarsal artery Medial plantar artery **W Foot Artery, Left** *See V Foot Artery, Right* **Y Lower Artery** Umbilical artery	**Ø Open** **3 Percutaneous** **4 Percutaneous Endoscopic**	**Z No Device**	**Z No Qualifier**

Ø   **Medical and Surgical**
4   **Lower Arteries**
U   **Supplement**   Definition: Putting in or on biological or synthetic material that physically reinforces and/or augments the function of a portion of a body part

Explanation: The biological material is non-living, or is living and from the same individual. The body part may have been previously replaced, and the SUPPLEMENT procedure is performed to physically reinforce and/or augment the function of the replaced body part.

Body Part Character 4		Approach Character 5	Device Character 6	Qualifier Character 7
Ø **Abdominal Aorta** Inferior phrenic artery Lumbar artery Median sacral artery Middle suprarenal artery Ovarian artery Testicular artery **1** **Celiac Artery** Celiac trunk **2** **Gastric Artery** Left gastric artery Right gastric artery **3** **Hepatic Artery** Common hepatic artery Gastroduodenal artery Hepatic artery proper **4** **Splenic Artery** Left gastroepiploic artery Pancreatic artery Short gastric artery **5** **Superior Mesenteric Artery** Ileal artery Ileocolic artery Inferior pancreaticoduodenal artery Jejunal artery **6** **Colic Artery, Right** **7** **Colic Artery, Left** **8** **Colic Artery, Middle** **9** **Renal Artery, Right** Inferior suprarenal artery Renal segmental artery **A** **Renal Artery, Left** *See 9 Renal Artery, Right* **B** **Inferior Mesenteric Artery** Sigmoid artery Superior rectal artery **C** **Common Iliac Artery, Right** **D** **Common Iliac Artery, Left** **E** **Internal Iliac Artery, Right** Deferential artery Hypogastric artery Iliolumbar artery Inferior gluteal artery Inferior vesical artery Internal pudendal artery Lateral sacral artery Middle rectal artery Obturator artery Superior gluteal artery Umbilical artery Uterine artery Vaginal artery	**F** **Internal Iliac Artery, Left** *See E Internal Iliac Artery, Right* **H** **External Iliac Artery, Right** Deep circumflex iliac artery Inferior epigastric artery **J** **External Iliac Artery, Left** *See H External Iliac Artery, Right* **K** **Femoral Artery, Right** Circumflex iliac artery Deep femoral artery Descending genicular artery External pudendal artery Superficial epigastric artery **L** **Femoral Artery, Left** *See K Femoral Artery, Right* **M** **Popliteal Artery, Right** Inferior genicular artery Middle genicular artery Superior genicular artery Sural artery Tibioperoneal trunk **N** **Popliteal Artery, Left** *See M Popliteal Artery, Right* **P** **Anterior Tibial Artery, Right** Anterior lateral malleolar artery Anterior medial malleolar artery Anterior tibial recurrent artery Dorsalis pedis artery Posterior tibial recurrent artery **Q** **Anterior Tibial Artery, Left** *See P Anterior Tibial Artery, Right* **R** **Posterior Tibial Artery, Right** **S** **Posterior Tibial Artery, Left** **T** **Peroneal Artery, Right** Fibular artery **U** **Peroneal Artery, Left** *See T Peroneal Artery, Right* **V** **Foot Artery, Right** Arcuate artery Dorsal metatarsal artery Lateral plantar artery Lateral tarsal artery Medial plantar artery **W** **Foot Artery, Left** *See V Foot Artery, Right* **Y** **Lower Artery** Umbilical artery	**Ø** Open **3** Percutaneous **4** Percutaneous Endoscopic	**7** Autologous Tissue Substitute **J** Synthetic Substitute **K** Nonautologous Tissue Substitute	**Z** No Qualifier

LC Limited Coverage   NC Noncovered   ⊞ Combination Member   HAC associated procedure   Combination Only   DRG Non-OR   Non-OR   New/Revised in GREEN

236   ICD-10-PCS 2021

04U–04U

Ø   **Medical and Surgical**
4   **Lower Arteries**
V   **Restriction**   Definition: Partially closing an orifice or the lumen of a tubular body part
                             Explanation: The orifice can be a natural orifice or an artificially created orifice

Body Part Character 4		Approach Character 5	Device Character 6	Qualifier Character 7
Ø Abdominal Aorta Inferior phrenic artery Lumbar artery Median sacral artery Middle suprarenal artery Ovarian artery Testicular artery		**Ø** Open **3** Percutaneous **4** Percutaneous Endoscopic	**C** Extraluminal Device **E** Intraluminal Device, Branched or Fenestrated, One or Two Arteries **F** Intraluminal Device, Branched or Fenestrated, Three or More Arteries **Z** No Device	**Z** No Qualifier
Ø Abdominal Aorta Inferior phrenic artery Lumbar artery Median sacral artery Middle suprarenal artery Ovarian artery Testicular artery		**Ø** Open **3** Percutaneous **4** Percutaneous Endoscopic	**D** Intraluminal Device	**J** Temporary **Z** No Qualifier
1 Celiac Artery Celiac trunk **2 Gastric Artery** Left gastric artery Right gastric artery **3 Hepatic Artery** Common hepatic artery Gastroduodenal artery Hepatic artery proper **4 Splenic Artery** Left gastroepiploic artery Pancreatic artery Short gastric artery **5 Superior Mesenteric Artery** Ileal artery Ileocolic artery Inferior pancreaticoduodenal artery Jejunal artery **6 Colic Artery, Right** **7 Colic Artery, Left** **8 Colic Artery, Middle** **9 Renal Artery, Right** Inferior suprarenal artery Renal segmental artery **A Renal Artery, Left** *See 9 Renal Artery, Right* **B Inferior Mesenteric Artery** Sigmoid artery Superior rectal artery **E Internal Iliac Artery, Right** Deferential artery Hypogastric artery Iliolumbar artery Inferior gluteal artery Inferior vesical artery Internal pudendal artery Lateral sacral artery Middle rectal artery Obturator artery Superior gluteal artery Umbilical artery Uterine artery Vaginal artery **F Internal Iliac Artery, Left** *See E Internal Iliac Artery, Right*	**H External Iliac Artery, Right** Deep circumflex iliac artery Inferior epigastric artery **J External Iliac Artery, Left** *See H External Iliac Artery, Right* **K Femoral Artery, Right** Circumflex iliac artery Deep femoral artery Descending genicular artery External pudendal artery Superficial epigastric artery **L Femoral Artery, Left** *See K Femoral Artery, Right* **M Popliteal Artery, Right** Inferior genicular artery Middle genicular artery Superior genicular artery Sural artery Tibioperoneal trunk **N Popliteal Artery, Left** *See M Popliteal Artery, Right* **P Anterior Tibial Artery, Right** Anterior lateral malleolar artery Anterior medial malleolar artery Anterior tibial recurrent artery Dorsalis pedis artery Posterior tibial recurrent artery **Q Anterior Tibial Artery, Left** *See P Anterior Tibial Artery, Right* **R Posterior Tibial Artery, Right** **S Posterior Tibial Artery, Left** **T Peroneal Artery, Right** Fibular artery **U Peroneal Artery, Left** *See T Peroneal Artery, Right* **V Foot Artery, Right** Arcuate artery Dorsal metatarsal artery Lateral plantar artery Lateral tarsal artery Medial plantar artery **W Foot Artery, Left** *See V Foot Artery, Right* **Y Lower Artery** Umbilical artery	**Ø** Open **3** Percutaneous **4** Percutaneous Endoscopic	**C** Extraluminal Device **D** Intraluminal Device **Z** No Device	**Z** No Qualifier
C Common Iliac Artery, Right **D Common Iliac Artery, Left**		**Ø** Open **3** Percutaneous **4** Percutaneous Endoscopic	**C** Extraluminal Device **D** Intraluminal Device **E** Intraluminal Device, Branched or Fenestrated, One or Two Arteries **Z** No Device	**Z** No Qualifier

LC Limited Coverage **NC** Noncovered ⊞ Combination Member HAC associated procedure Combination Only DRG Non-OR Non-OR New/Revised in GREEN

ICD-10-PCS 2021   237

04V–04V

Ø   Medical and Surgical
4   Lower Arteries
W   Revision

Definition: Correcting, to the extent possible, a portion of a malfunctioning device or the position of a displaced device

Explanation: Revision can include correcting a malfunctioning or displaced device by taking out or putting in components of the device such as a screw or pin

Body Part Character 4	Approach Character 5	Device Character 6	Qualifier Character 7
Y Lower Artery Umbilical artery	**Ø** Open **3** Percutaneous **4** Percutaneous Endoscopic	**Ø** Drainage Device **2** Monitoring Device **3** Infusion Device **7** Autologous Tissue Substitute **C** Extraluminal Device **D** Intraluminal Device **J** Synthetic Substitute **K** Nonautologous Tissue Substitute **Y** Other Device	**Z** No Qualifier
Y Lower Artery Umbilical artery	**X** External	**Ø** Drainage Device **2** Monitoring Device **3** Infusion Device **7** Autologous Tissue Substitute **C** Extraluminal Device **D** Intraluminal Device **J** Synthetic Substitute **K** Nonautologous Tissue Substitute	**Z** No Qualifier

Non-OR 04WY3[Ø,2,3,D]Z
Non-OR 04WY[3,4]YZ
Non-OR 04WYX[Ø,2,3,7,C,D,J,K]Z

Upper Veins Ø51–Ø5W

Character Meanings

This Character Meaning table is provided as a guide to assist the user in the identification of character members that may be found in this section of code tables. It **SHOULD NOT** be used to build a PCS code.

Operation–Character 3		Body Part–Character 4		Approach–Character 5		Device–Character 6		Qualifier–Character 7	
1	Bypass	Ø	Azygos Vein	Ø	Open	Ø	Drainage Device	Ø	Ultrasonic
5	Destruction	1	Hemiazygos Vein	3	Percutaneous	2	Monitoring Device	1	Drug-Coated Balloon
7	Dilation	3	Innominate Vein, Right	4	Percutaneous Endoscopic	3	Infusion Device	X	Diagnostic
9	Drainage	4	Innominate Vein, Left	X	External	7	Autologous Tissue Substitute	Y	Upper Vein
B	Excision	5	Subclavian Vein, Right			9	Autologous Venous Tissue	Z	No Qualifier
C	Extirpation	6	Subclavian Vein, Left			A	Autologous Arterial Tissue		
D	Extraction	7	Axillary Vein, Right			C	Extraluminal Device		
F	Fragmentation	8	Axillary Vein, Left			D	Intraluminal Device		
H	Insertion	9	Brachial Vein, Right			J	Synthetic Substitute		
J	Inspection	A	Brachial Vein, Left			K	Nonautologous Tissue Substitute		
L	Occlusion	B	Basilic Vein, Right			M	Neurostimulator Lead		
N	Release	C	Basilic Vein, Left			Y	Other Device		
P	Removal	D	Cephalic Vein, Right			Z	No Device		
Q	Repair	F	Cephalic Vein, Left						
R	Replacement	G	Hand Vein, Right						
S	Reposition	H	Hand Vein, Left						
U	Supplement	L	Intracranial Vein						
V	Restriction	M	Internal Jugular Vein, Right						
W	Revision	N	Internal Jugular Vein, Left						
		P	External Jugular Vein, Right						
		Q	External Jugular Vein, Left						
		R	Vertebral Vein, Right						
		S	Vertebral Vein, Left						
		T	Face Vein, Right						
		V	Face Vein, Left						
		Y	Upper Vein						

AHA Coding Clinic for table Ø51
2020, 1Q, 28   Free flap microvascular breast reconstruction
2017, 3Q, 15   Bypass of innominate vein to atrial appendage

AHA Coding Clinic for table Ø59
2018, 3Q, 7   Catheter placement for treatment of congestive heart failure

AHA Coding Clinic for table Ø5B
2020, 1Q, 24   Resection of vascular malformation, likely cavernoma
2016, 2Q, 12   Resection of malignant neoplasm of infratemporal fossa

AHA Coding Clinic for table Ø5H
2016, 4Q, 97-98   Phrenic neurostimulator

AHA Coding Clinic for table Ø5P
2016, 4Q, 97-98   Phrenic neurostimulator

AHA Coding Clinic for table Ø5Q
2017, 3Q, 15   Bypass of innominate vein to atrial appendage

AHA Coding Clinic for table Ø5S
2013, 4Q, 125   Stage II cephalic vein transposition (superficialization) of arteriovenous fistula

AHA Coding Clinic for table Ø5W
2016, 4Q, 97-98   Phrenic neurostimulator

Head and Neck Veins

Superficial temporal **L**

Superior ophthalmic **L**

Retromandibular **T, V**

Facial **T, V**

Lingual **T, V**

Thyroid **P, Q**

Anterior jugular **P, Q**

External jugular **P, Q**

Bracheocephalic **3, 4**

Superior sagittal sinus **L**

Inferior sagittal sinus **L**

Straight sinus **L**

Transverse sinus **L**

Occipital sinus **L**

Posterior auricular **P, Q**

Deep cervical **R, S**

External jugular **P, Q**

Vertebral **R, S**

Subclavian **5, 6**

Upper Veins

Superficial temporal **L**

Vertebral **R, S**

Internal jugular **M, N**

External jugular **P, Q**

Subclavian **5, 6**

Innominate **3, 4**

Azygos **Ø**

Axillary **7, 8**

Hemiazygos **1**

Brachial **9, A**

Cephalic **D, F**

Basilic **B, C**

Radial **9, A**

Ulnar **9, A**

Digital **G, H**

Ø   **Medical and Surgical**
5   **Upper Veins**
1   **Bypass**   Definition: Altering the route of passage of the contents of a tubular body part

                 Explanation: Rerouting contents of a body part to a downstream area of the normal route, to a similar route and body part, or to an abnormal route and dissimilar body part. Includes one or more anastomoses, with or without the use of a device.

Body Part Character 4	Approach Character 5	Device Character 6	Qualifier Character 7

Ø **Azygos Vein**
    Right ascending lumbar vein
    Right subcostal vein
1 **Hemiazygos Vein**
    Left ascending lumbar vein
    Left subcostal vein
3 **Innominate Vein, Right**
    Brachiocephalic vein
    Inferior thyroid vein
4 **Innominate Vein, Left**
    See 3 Innominate Vein, Right
5 **Subclavian Vein, Right**
6 **Subclavian Vein, Left**
7 **Axillary Vein, Right**
8 **Axillary Vein, Left**
9 **Brachial Vein, Right**
    Radial vein
    Ulnar vein
A **Brachial Vein, Left**
    See 9 Brachial Vein, Right
B **Basilic Vein, Right**
    Median antebrachial vein
    Median cubital vein
C **Basilic Vein, Left**
    See B Basilic Vein, Right
D **Cephalic Vein, Right**
    Accessory cephalic vein
F **Cephalic Vein, Left**
    See D Cephalic Vein, Right
G **Hand Vein, Right**
    Dorsal metacarpal vein
    Palmar (volar) digital vein
    Palmar (volar) metacarpal vein
    Superficial palmar venous arch
    Volar (palmar) digital vein
    Volar (palmar) metacarpal vein
	Ø **Open**
	4 **Percutaneous Endoscopic**
		7 **Autologous Tissue Substitute**
		9 **Autologous Venous Tissue**
		A **Autologous Arterial Tissue**
		J **Synthetic Substitute**
		K **Nonautologous Tissue Substitute**
		Z **No Device**
			Y **Upper Vein**

H **Hand Vein, Left**
    See G Hand Vein, Right
L **Intracranial Vein**
    Anterior cerebral vein
    Basal (internal) cerebral vein
    Dural venous sinus
    Great cerebral vein
    Inferior cerebellar vein
    Inferior cerebral vein
    Internal (basal) cerebral vein
    Middle cerebral vein
    Ophthalmic vein
    Superior cerebellar vein
    Superior cerebral vein
M **Internal Jugular Vein, Right**
N **Internal Jugular Vein, Left**
P **External Jugular Vein, Right**
    Posterior auricular vein
Q **External Jugular Vein, Left**
    See P External Jugular Vein,
       Right
R **Vertebral Vein, Right**
    Deep cervical vein
    Suboccipital venous plexus
S **Vertebral Vein, Left**
    See R Vertebral Vein, Right
T **Face Vein, Right**
    Angular vein
    Anterior facial vein
    Common facial vein
    Deep facial vein
    Frontal vein
    Posterior facial
       (retromandibular) vein
    Supraorbital vein
V **Face Vein, Left**
    See T Face Vein, Right			

LC Limited Coverage   NC Noncovered   ⊞ Combination Member   HAC associated procedure   Combination Only   DRG Non-OR   Non-OR   New/Revised in GREEN

Ø   **Medical and Surgical**
5   **Upper Veins**
5   **Destruction**   Definition: Physical eradication of all or a portion of a body part by the direct use of energy, force, or a destructive agent
                          Explanation: None of the body part is physically taken out

Body Part Character 4		Approach Character 5	Device Character 6	Qualifier Character 7
Ø Azygos Vein Right ascending lumbar vein Right subcostal vein **1 Hemiazygos Vein** Left ascending lumbar vein Left subcostal vein **3 Innominate Vein, Right** Brachiocephalic vein Inferior thyroid vein **4 Innominate Vein, Left** *See 3 Innominate Vein, Right* **5 Subclavian Vein, Right** **6 Subclavian Vein, Left** **7 Axillary Vein, Right** **8 Axillary Vein, Left** **9 Brachial Vein, Right** Radial vein Ulnar vein **A Brachial Vein, Left** *See 9 Brachial Vein, Right* **B Basilic Vein, Right** Median antebrachial vein Median cubital vein **C Basilic Vein, Left** *See B Basilic Vein, Right* **D Cephalic Vein, Right** Accessory cephalic vein **F Cephalic Vein, Left** *See D Cephalic Vein, Right* **G Hand Vein, Right** Dorsal metacarpal vein Palmar (volar) digital vein Palmar (volar) metacarpal vein Superficial palmar venous arch Volar (palmar) digital vein Volar (palmar) metacarpal vein	**H Hand Vein, Left** *See G Hand Vein, Right* **L Intracranial Vein** Anterior cerebral vein Basal (internal) cerebral vein Dural venous sinus Great cerebral vein Inferior cerebellar vein Inferior cerebral vein Internal (basal) cerebral vein Middle cerebral vein Ophthalmic vein Superior cerebellar vein Superior cerebral vein **M Internal Jugular Vein, Right** **N Internal Jugular Vein, Left** **P External Jugular Vein, Right** Posterior auricular vein **Q External Jugular Vein, Left** *See P External Jugular Vein, Right* **R Vertebral Vein, Right** Deep cervical vein Suboccipital venous plexus **S Vertebral Vein, Left** *See R Vertebral Vein, Right* **T Face Vein, Right** Angular vein Anterior facial vein Common facial vein Deep facial vein Frontal vein Posterior facial (retromandibular) vein Supraorbital vein **V Face Vein, Left** *See T Face Vein, Right* **Y Upper Vein**	**Ø Open** **3 Percutaneous** **4 Percutaneous Endoscopic**	**Z No Device**	**Z No Qualifier**

LC Limited Coverage   NC Noncovered   ⊞ Combination Member   HAC associated procedure   Combination Only   DRG Non-OR   Non-OR   New/Revised in GREEN
242   ICD-10-PCS 2021

Ø55–Ø55

Ø   **Medical and Surgical**
5   **Upper Veins**
7   **Dilation**   Definition: Expanding an orifice or the lumen of a tubular body part

Explanation: The orifice can be a natural orifice or an artificially created orifice. Accomplished by stretching a tubular body part using intraluminal pressure or by cutting part of the orifice or wall of the tubular body part.

Body Part Character 4		Approach Character 5	Device Character 6	Qualifier Character 7

Ø **Azygos Vein**
  Right ascending lumbar vein
  Right subcostal vein
1 **Hemiazygos Vein**
  Left ascending lumbar vein
  Left subcostal vein
G **Hand Vein, Right**
  Dorsal metacarpal vein
  Palmar (volar) digital vein
  Palmar (volar) metacarpal vein
  Superficial palmar venous arch
  Volar (palmar) digital vein
  Volar (palmar) metacarpal vein
H **Hand Vein, Left**
  See G Hand Vein, Right
L **Intracranial Vein** [NC]
  Anterior cerebral vein
  Basal (internal) cerebral vein
  Dural venous sinus
  Great cerebral vein
  Inferior cerebellar vein
  Inferior cerebral vein
  Internal (basal) cerebral vein
  Middle cerebral vein
  Ophthalmic vein
  Superior cerebellar vein
  Superior cerebral vein
	M **Internal Jugular Vein, Right**
	N **Internal Jugular Vein, Left**
	P **External Jugular Vein, Right**
	  Posterior auricular vein
	Q **External Jugular Vein, Left**
	  See P External Jugular Vein,
	    Right
	R **Vertebral Vein, Right**
	  Deep cervical vein
	  Suboccipital venous plexus
	S **Vertebral Vein, Left**
	  See R Vertebral Vein, Right
	T **Face Vein, Right**
	  Angular vein
	  Anterior facial vein
	  Common facial vein
	  Deep facial vein
	  Frontal vein
	  Posterior facial
	    (retromandibular) vein
	  Supraorbital vein
	V **Face Vein, Left**
	  See T Face Vein, Right
	Y **Upper Vein**
		Ø Open
		3 Percutaneous
		4 Percutaneous Endoscopic
			D Intraluminal Device
			Z No Device
				Z No Qualifier

3 **Innominate Vein, Right**
  Brachiocephalic vein
  Inferior thyroid vein
4 **Innominate Vein, Left**
  See 3 Innominate Vein, Right
5 **Subclavian Vein, Right**
6 **Subclavian Vein, Left**
7 **Axillary Vein, Right**
8 **Axillary Vein, Left**
9 **Brachial Vein, Right**
  Radial vein
  Ulnar vein
	A **Brachial Vein, Left**
	  See 9 Brachial Vein, Right
	B **Basilic Vein, Right**
	  Median antebrachial vein
	  Median cubital vein
	C **Basilic Vein, Left**
	  See B Basilic Vein, Right
	D **Cephalic Vein, Right**
	  Accessory cephalic vein
	F **Cephalic Vein, Left**
	  See D Cephalic Vein, Right
		Ø Open
		3 Percutaneous
		4 Percutaneous Endoscopic
			D Intraluminal Device
			Z No Device
				1 Drug-Coated Balloon
				Z No Qualifier

[NC]   Ø57L[3,4]ZZ

[LC] Limited Coverage   [NC] Noncovered   ⊞ Combination Member   HAC associated procedure   Combination Only   DRG Non-OR   Non-OR   New/Revised in GREEN

ICD-10-PCS 2021   **243**

Ø57–Ø57

Ø   **Medical and Surgical**
5   **Upper Veins**
9   **Drainage**   Definition: Taking or letting out fluids and/or gases from a body part

Explanation: The qualifier DIAGNOSTIC is used to identify drainage procedures that are biopsies

Body Part Character 4		Approach Character 5	Device Character 6	Qualifier Character 7
Ø Azygos Vein Right ascending lumbar vein Right subcostal vein **1 Hemiazygos Vein** Left ascending lumbar vein Left subcostal vein **3 Innominate Vein, Right** Brachiocephalic vein Inferior thyroid vein **4 Innominate Vein, Left** *See 3 Innominate Vein, Right* **5 Subclavian Vein, Right** **6 Subclavian Vein, Left** **7 Axillary Vein, Right** **8 Axillary Vein, Left** **9 Brachial Vein, Right** Radial vein Ulnar vein **A Brachial Vein, Left** *See 9 Brachial Vein, Right* **B Basilic Vein, Right** Median antebrachial vein Median cubital vein **C Basilic Vein, Left** *See B Basilic Vein, Right* **D Cephalic Vein, Right** Accessory cephalic vein **F Cephalic Vein, Left** *See D Cephalic Vein, Right* **G Hand Vein, Right** Dorsal metacarpal vein Palmar (volar) digital vein Palmar (volar) metacarpal vein Superficial palmar venous arch Volar (palmar) digital vein Volar (palmar) metacarpal vein	**H Hand Vein, Left** *See G Hand Vein, Right* **L Intracranial Vein** Anterior cerebral vein Basal (internal) cerebral vein Dural venous sinus Great cerebral vein Inferior cerebellar vein Inferior cerebral vein Internal (basal) cerebral vein Middle cerebral vein Ophthalmic vein Superior cerebellar vein Superior cerebral vein **M Internal Jugular Vein, Right** **N Internal Jugular Vein, Left** **P External Jugular Vein, Right** Posterior auricular vein **Q External Jugular Vein, Left** *See P External Jugular Vein, Right* **R Vertebral Vein, Right** Deep cervical vein Suboccipital venous plexus **S Vertebral Vein, Left** *See R Vertebral Vein, Right* **T Face Vein, Right** Angular vein Anterior facial vein Common facial vein Deep facial vein Frontal vein Posterior facial (retromandibular) vein Supraorbital vein **V Face Vein, Left** *See T Face Vein, Right* **Y Upper Vein**	**Ø Open** **3 Percutaneous** **4 Percutaneous Endoscopic**	**Ø Drainage Device**	**Z No Qualifier**
Ø Azygos Vein Right ascending lumbar vein Right subcostal vein **1 Hemiazygos Vein** Left ascending lumbar vein Left subcostal vein **3 Innominate Vein, Right** Brachiocephalic vein Inferior thyroid vein **4 Innominate Vein, Left** *See 3 Innominate Vein, Right* **5 Subclavian Vein, Right** **6 Subclavian Vein, Left** **7 Axillary Vein, Right** **8 Axillary Vein, Left** **9 Brachial Vein, Right** Radial vein Ulnar vein **A Brachial Vein, Left** *See 9 Brachial Vein, Right* **B Basilic Vein, Right** Median antebrachial vein Median cubital vein **C Basilic Vein, Left** *See B Basilic Vein, Right* **D Cephalic Vein, Right** Accessory cephalic vein **F Cephalic Vein, Left** *See D Cephalic Vein, Right* **G Hand Vein, Right** Dorsal metacarpal vein Palmar (volar) digital vein Palmar (volar) metacarpal vein Superficial palmar venous arch Volar (palmar) digital vein Volar (palmar) metacarpal vein	**H Hand Vein, Left** *See G Hand Vein, Right* **L Intracranial Vein** Anterior cerebral vein Basal (internal) cerebral vein Dural venous sinus Great cerebral vein Inferior cerebellar vein Inferior cerebral vein Internal (basal) cerebral vein Middle cerebral vein Ophthalmic vein Superior cerebellar vein Superior cerebral vein **M Internal Jugular Vein, Right** **N Internal Jugular Vein, Left** **P External Jugular Vein, Right** Posterior auricular vein **Q External Jugular Vein, Left** *See P External Jugular Vein, Right* **R Vertebral Vein, Right** Deep cervical vein Suboccipital venous plexus **S Vertebral Vein, Left** *See R Vertebral Vein, Right* **T Face Vein, Right** Angular vein Anterior facial vein Common facial vein Deep facial vein Frontal vein Posterior facial (retromandibular) vein Supraorbital vein **V Face Vein, Left** *See T Face Vein, Right* **Y Upper Vein**	**Ø Open** **3 Percutaneous** **4 Percutaneous Endoscopic**	**Z No Device**	**X Diagnostic** **Z No Qualifier**

Non-OR   059[Ø,1,3,4,5,6,7,8,9,A,B,C,D,F,G,H,L,M,N,P,Q,R,S,T,V,Y][Ø,3,4]ØZ
Non-OR   059[Ø,1,3,4,5,6,7,8,9,A,B,C,D,F,G,H,L,M,N,P,Q,R,S,T,V,Y]3ZX
Non-OR   059[Ø,1,3,4,5,6,7,8,9,A,B,C,D,F,G,H,L,M,N,P,Q,R,S,T,V,Y][Ø,3,4]ZZ

LC Limited Coverage   NC Noncovered   ⊞ Combination Member   HAC associated procedure   Combination Only   DRG Non-OR   Non-OR   New/Revised in GREEN

244   ICD-10-PCS 2021

Ø　**Medical and Surgical**
5　**Upper Veins**
B　**Excision**　　　　　Definition: Cutting out or off, without replacement, a portion of a body part
　　　　　　　　　　　　　Explanation: The qualifier DIAGNOSTIC is used to identify excision procedures that are biopsies

Body Part Character 4		Approach Character 5	Device Character 6	Qualifier Character 7
Ø **Azygos Vein** 　Right ascending lumbar vein 　Right subcostal vein 1 **Hemiazygos Vein** 　Left ascending lumbar vein 　Left subcostal vein 3 **Innominate Vein, Right** 　Brachiocephalic vein 　Inferior thyroid vein 4 **Innominate Vein, Left** 　*See 3 Innominate Vein, Right* 5 **Subclavian Vein, Right** 6 **Subclavian Vein, Left** 7 **Axillary Vein, Right** 8 **Axillary Vein, Left** 9 **Brachial Vein, Right** 　Radial vein 　Ulnar vein A **Brachial Vein, Left** 　*See 9 Brachial Vein, Right* B **Basilic Vein, Right** 　Median antebrachial vein 　Median cubital vein C **Basilic Vein, Left** 　*See B Basilic Vein, Right* D **Cephalic Vein, Right** 　Accessory cephalic vein F **Cephalic Vein, Left** 　*See D Cephalic Vein, Right* G **Hand Vein, Right** 　Dorsal metacarpal vein 　Palmar (volar) digital vein 　Palmar (volar) metacarpal vein 　Superficial palmar venous arch 　Volar (palmar) digital vein 　Volar (palmar) metacarpal vein	H **Hand Vein, Left** 　*See G Hand Vein, Right* L **Intracranial Vein** 　Anterior cerebral vein 　Basal (internal) cerebral vein 　Dural venous sinus 　Great cerebral vein 　Inferior cerebellar vein 　Inferior cerebral vein 　Internal (basal) cerebral vein 　Middle cerebral vein 　Ophthalmic vein 　Superior cerebellar vein 　Superior cerebral vein M **Internal Jugular Vein, Right** N **Internal Jugular Vein, Left** P **External Jugular Vein, Right** 　Posterior auricular vein Q **External Jugular Vein, Left** 　*See P External Jugular Vein, 　　Right* R **Vertebral Vein, Right** 　Deep cervical vein 　Suboccipital venous plexus S **Vertebral Vein, Left** 　*See R Vertebral Vein, Right* T **Face Vein, Right** 　Angular vein 　Anterior facial vein 　Common facial vein 　Deep facial vein 　Frontal vein 　Posterior facial 　　(retromandibular) vein 　Supraorbital vein V **Face Vein, Left** 　*See T Face Vein, Right* Y **Upper Vein**	Ø **Open** 3 **Percutaneous** 4 **Percutaneous Endoscopic**	Z **No Device**	X **Diagnostic** Z **No Qualifier**

LC Limited Coverage　**NC** Noncovered　⊞ Combination Member　HAC associated procedure　Combination Only　DRG Non-OR　Non-OR　New/Revised in GREEN

ICD-10-PCS 2021　　　　　　　　　　　　　　　　　　　　　　　　　　　　　　　　　　　　　　　**245**

Ø5B–Ø5B

Ø   **Medical and Surgical**
5   **Upper Veins**
C   **Extirpation**   Definition: Taking or cutting out solid matter from a body part

Explanation: The solid matter may be an abnormal byproduct of a biological function or a foreign body; it may be imbedded in a body part or in the lumen of a tubular body part. The solid matter may or may not have been previously broken into pieces.

Body Part Character 4		Approach Character 5	Device Character 6	Qualifier Character 7
Ø Azygos Vein Right ascending lumbar vein Right subcostal vein **1 Hemiazygos Vein** Left ascending lumbar vein Left subcostal vein **3 Innominate Vein, Right** Brachiocephalic vein Inferior thyroid vein **4 Innominate Vein, Left** *See 3 Innominate Vein, Right* **5 Subclavian Vein, Right** **6 Subclavian Vein, Left** **7 Axillary Vein, Right** **8 Axillary Vein, Left** **9 Brachial Vein, Right** Radial vein Ulnar vein **A Brachial Vein, Left** *See 9 Brachial Vein, Right* **B Basilic Vein, Right** Median antebrachial vein Median cubital vein **C Basilic Vein, Left** *See B Basilic Vein, Right* **D Cephalic Vein, Right** Accessory cephalic vein **F Cephalic Vein, Left** *See D Cephalic Vein, Right* **G Hand Vein, Right** Dorsal metacarpal vein Palmar (volar) digital vein Palmar (volar) metacarpal vein Superficial palmar venous arch Volar (palmar) digital vein Volar (palmar) metacarpal vein	**H Hand Vein, Left** *See G Hand Vein, Right* **L Intracranial Vein** Anterior cerebral vein Basal (internal) cerebral vein Dural venous sinus Great cerebral vein Inferior cerebellar vein Inferior cerebral vein Internal (basal) cerebral vein Middle cerebral vein Ophthalmic vein Superior cerebellar vein Superior cerebral vein **M Internal Jugular Vein, Right** **N Internal Jugular Vein, Left** **P External Jugular Vein, Right** Posterior auricular vein **Q External Jugular Vein, Left** *See P External Jugular Vein, Right* **R Vertebral Vein, Right** Deep cervical vein Suboccipital venous plexus **S Vertebral Vein, Left** *See R Vertebral Vein, Right* **T Face Vein, Right** Angular vein Anterior facial vein Common facial vein Deep facial vein Frontal vein Posterior facial (retromandibular) vein Supraorbital vein **V Face Vein, Left** *See T Face Vein, Right* **Y Upper Vein**	**Ø Open** **3 Percutaneous** **4 Percutaneous Endoscopic**	**Z No Device**	**Z No Qualifier**

Ø   **Medical and Surgical**
5   **Upper Veins**
D   **Extraction**   Definition: Pulling or stripping out or off all or a portion of a body part by the use of force

Explanation: The qualifier DIAGNOSTIC is used to identify extraction procedures that are biopsies

Body Part Character 4		Approach Character 5	Device Character 6	Qualifier Character 7
9 Brachial Vein, Right Radial vein Ulnar vein **A Brachial Vein, Left** *See 9 Brachial Vein, Right* **B Basilic Vein, Right** Median antebrachial vein Median cubital vein **C Basilic Vein, Left** *See B Basilic Vein, Right* **D Cephalic Vein, Right** Accessory cephalic vein	**F Cephalic Vein, Left** *See D Cephalic Vein, Right* **G Hand Vein, Right** Dorsal metacarpal vein Palmar (volar) digital vein Palmar (volar) metacarpal vein Superficial palmar venous arch Volar (palmar) digital vein Volar (palmar) metacarpal vein **H Hand Vein, Left** *See G Hand Vein, Right* **Y Upper Vein**	**Ø Open** **3 Percutaneous**	**Z No Device**	**Z No Qualifier**

LC Limited Coverage   NC Noncovered   ⊞ Combination Member   HAC associated procedure   Combination Only   DRG Non-OR   Non-OR   New/Revised in GREEN

246   ICD-10-PCS 2021

Upper Veins

Ø   **Medical and Surgical**
5   **Upper Veins**
F   **Fragmentation**   Definition: Breaking solid matter in a body part into pieces

Explanation: Physical force (e.g., manual, ultrasonic) applied directly or indirectly is used to break the solid matter into pieces. The solid matter may be an abnormal byproduct of a biological function or a foreign body. The pieces of solid matter are not taken out.

Body Part Character 4		Approach Character 5	Device Character 6	Qualifier Character 7

3   Innominate Vein, Right
     Brachiocephalic vein
     Inferior thyroid vein
4   Innominate Vein, Left
     See 3 Innominate Vein, Right
5   Subclavian Vein, Right
6   Subclavian Vein, Left
7   Axillary Vein, Right
8   Axillary Vein, Left
9   Brachial Vein, Right
     Radial vein
     Ulnar vein
	A Brachial Vein, Left
	     See 9 Brachial Vein, Right
	B Basilic Vein, Right
	     Median antebrachial vein
	     Median cubital vein
	C Basilic Vein, Left
	     See B Basilic Vein, Right
	D Cephalic Vein, Right
	     Accessory cephalic vein
	F Cephalic Vein, Left
	     See D Cephalic Vein, Right
	Y Upper Vein
		3 Percutaneous	Z No Device	Ø Ultrasonic
				Z No Qualifier

LC Limited Coverage   **NC** Noncovered   ⊞ Combination Member   HAC associated procedure   Combination Only   DRG Non-OR   Non-OR   New/Revised in GREEN

ICD-10-PCS 2021   **247**

Ø   **Medical and Surgical**
5   **Upper Veins**
H   **Insertion**   Definition: Putting in a nonbiological appliance that monitors, assists, performs, or prevents a physiological function but does not physically take the place of a body part
                        Explanation: None

Body Part Character 4		Approach Character 5	Device Character 6	Qualifier Character 7
Ø Azygos Vein ⊞ Right ascending lumbar vein Right subcostal vein		**Ø** Open **3** Percutaneous **4** Percutaneous Endoscopic	**2** Monitoring Device **3** Infusion Device **D** Intraluminal Device **M** Neurostimulator Lead	**Z** No Qualifier
1 Hemiazygos Vein Left ascending lumbar vein Left subcostal vein **5 Subclavian Vein, Right** **6 Subclavian Vein, Left** **7 Axillary Vein, Right** **8 Axillary Vein, Left** **9 Brachial Vein, Right** Radial vein Ulnar vein **A Brachial Vein, Left** *See 9 Brachial Vein, Right* **B Basilic Vein, Right** Median antebrachial vein Median cubital vein **C Basilic Vein, Left** *See B Basilic Vein, Right* **D Cephalic Vein, Right** Accessory cephalic vein **F Cephalic Vein, Left** *See D Cephalic Vein, Right* **G Hand Vein, Right** Dorsal metacarpal vein Palmar (volar) digital vein Palmar (volar) metacarpal vein Superficial palmar venous arch Volar (palmar) digital vein Volar (palmar) metacarpal vein **H Hand Vein, Left** *See G Hand Vein, Right*	**L Intracranial Vein** Anterior cerebral vein Basal (internal) cerebral vein Dural venous sinus Great cerebral vein Inferior cerebellar vein Inferior cerebral vein Internal (basal) cerebral vein Middle cerebral vein Ophthalmic vein Superior cerebellar vein Superior cerebral vein **M Internal Jugular Vein, Right** **N Internal Jugular Vein, Left** **P External Jugular Vein, Right** Posterior auricular vein **Q External Jugular Vein, Left** *See P External Jugular Vein, Right* **R Vertebral Vein, Right** Deep cervical vein Suboccipital venous plexus **S Vertebral Vein, Left** *See R Vertebral Vein, Right* **T Face Vein, Right** Angular vein Anterior facial vein Common facial vein Deep facial vein Frontal vein Posterior facial (retromandibular) vein Supraorbital vein **V Face Vein, Left** *See T Face Vein, Right*	**Ø** Open **3** Percutaneous **4** Percutaneous Endoscopic	**3** Infusion Device **D** Intraluminal Device	**Z** No Qualifier
3 Innominate Vein, Right ⊞ Brachiocephalic vein Inferior thyroid vein **4 Innominate Vein, Left** ⊞ *See 3 Innominate Vein, Right*		**Ø** Open **3** Percutaneous **4** Percutaneous Endoscopic	**3** Infusion Device **D** Intraluminal Device **M** Neurostimulator Lead	**Z** No Qualifier
Y Upper Vein		**Ø** Open **3** Percutaneous **4** Percutaneous Endoscopic	**2** Monitoring Device **3** Infusion Device **D** Intraluminal Device **Y** Other Device	**Z** No Qualifier

Non-OR	Ø5HØ[Ø,3,4]3Z	
Non-OR	Ø5H[1,5,6,7,8,9,A,B,C,D,F,G,H,L,M,N,P,Q,R,S,T,V][Ø,3,4]3Z	
Non-OR	Ø5H[3,4][Ø,3,4]3Z	
Non-OR	Ø5HY[Ø,3,4]3Z	
Non-OR	Ø5HY32Z	
Non-OR	Ø5HY[3,4]YZ	
HAC	Ø5HØ[3,4]3Z when reported with SDx J95.811	
HAC	Ø5H[1,5,6][3,4]3Z when reported with SDx J95.811	
HAC	Ø5H[M,N,P,Q]33Z when reported with SDx J95.811	
HAC	Ø5H[3,4][3,4]3Z when reported with SDx J95.811	

See Appendix L for Procedure Combinations
⊞   Ø5HØ[Ø,3,4]MZ
⊞   Ø5H[3,4][Ø,3,4]MZ

LC Limited Coverage   **NC** Noncovered   ⊞ Combination Member   HAC associated procedure   Combination Only   DRG Non-OR   Non-OR   New/Revised in **GREEN**

248

ICD-10-PCS 2021

Ø   Medical and Surgical
5   Upper Veins
J   Inspection   Definition: Visually and/or manually exploring a body part

Explanation: Visual exploration may be performed with or without optical instrumentation. Manual exploration may be performed directly or through intervening body layers.

Body Part Character 4	Approach Character 5	Device Character 6	Qualifier Character 7
Y Upper Vein	Ø Open 3 Percutaneous 4 Percutaneous Endoscopic X External	Z No Device	Z No Qualifier

Non-OR   Ø5JY[3,X]ZZ

Ø   Medical and Surgical
5   Upper Veins
L   Occlusion   Definition: Completely closing an orifice or the lumen of a tubular body part

Explanation: The orifice can be a natural orifice or an artificially created orifice

Body Part Character 4	Approach Character 5	Device Character 6	Qualifier Character 7

Ø   **Azygos Vein**
     Right ascending lumbar vein
     Right subcostal vein
1   **Hemiazygos Vein**
     Left ascending lumbar vein
     Left subcostal vein
3   **Innominate Vein, Right**
     Brachiocephalic vein
     Inferior thyroid vein
4   **Innominate Vein, Left**
     See 3 Innominate Vein, Right
5   **Subclavian Vein, Right**
6   **Subclavian Vein, Left**
7   **Axillary Vein, Right**
8   **Axillary Vein, Left**
9   **Brachial Vein, Right**
     Radial vein
     Ulnar vein
A   **Brachial Vein, Left**
     See 9 Brachial Vein, Right
B   **Basilic Vein, Right**
     Median antebrachial vein
     Median cubital vein
C   **Basilic Vein, Left**
     See B Basilic Vein, Right
D   **Cephalic Vein, Right**
     Accessory cephalic vein
F   **Cephalic Vein, Left**
     See D Cephalic Vein, Right
G   **Hand Vein, Right**
     Dorsal metacarpal vein
     Palmar (volar) digital vein
     Palmar (volar) metacarpal vein
     Superficial palmar venous arch
     Volar (palmar) digital vein
     Volar (palmar) metacarpal vein
	H **Hand Vein, Left**
	     See G Hand Vein, Right
	L **Intracranial Vein**
	     Anterior cerebral vein
	     Basal (internal) cerebral vein
	     Dural venous sinus
	     Great cerebral vein
	     Inferior cerebellar vein
	     Inferior cerebral vein
	     Internal (basal) cerebral vein
	     Middle cerebral vein
	     Ophthalmic vein
	     Superior cerebellar vein
	     Superior cerebral vein
	M **Internal Jugular Vein, Right**
	N **Internal Jugular Vein, Left**
	P **External Jugular Vein, Right**
	     Posterior auricular vein
	Q **External Jugular Vein, Left**
	     See P External Jugular Vein,
	     Right
	R **Vertebral Vein, Right**
	     Deep cervical vein
	     Suboccipital venous plexus
	S **Vertebral Vein, Left**
	     See R Vertebral Vein, Right
	T **Face Vein, Right**
	     Angular vein
	     Anterior facial vein
	     Common facial vein
	     Deep facial vein
	     Frontal vein
	     Posterior facial
	        (retromandibular) vein
	     Supraorbital vein
	V **Face Vein, Left**
	     See T Face Vein, Right
	Y **Upper Vein**
		Ø Open
		3 Percutaneous
		4 Percutaneous Endoscopic
			C Extraluminal Device
			D Intraluminal Device
			Z No Device
				Z No Qualifier

LC Limited Coverage   **NC** Noncovered   ⊞ Combination Member   HAC associated procedure   Combination Only   DRG Non-OR   Non-OR   New/Revised in GREEN

ICD-10-PCS 2021   **249**

Ø   **Medical and Surgical**
5   **Upper Veins**
N   **Release**   Definition: Freeing a body part from an abnormal physical constraint by cutting or by the use of force
               Explanation: Some of the restraining tissue may be taken out but none of the body part is taken out

Body Part Character 4		Approach Character 5	Device Character 6	Qualifier Character 7
Ø Azygos Vein Right ascending lumbar vein Right subcostal vein **1 Hemiazygos Vein** Left ascending lumbar vein Left subcostal vein **3 Innominate Vein, Right** Brachiocephalic vein Inferior thyroid vein **4 Innominate Vein, Left** *See 3 Innominate Vein, Right* **5 Subclavian Vein, Right** **6 Subclavian Vein, Left** **7 Axillary Vein, Right** **8 Axillary Vein, Left** **9 Brachial Vein, Right** Radial vein Ulnar vein **A Brachial Vein, Left** *See 9 Brachial Vein, Right* **B Basilic Vein, Right** Median antebrachial vein Median cubital vein **C Basilic Vein, Left** *See B Basilic Vein, Right* **D Cephalic Vein, Right** Accessory cephalic vein **F Cephalic Vein, Left** *See D Cephalic Vein, Right* **G Hand Vein, Right** Dorsal metacarpal vein Palmar (volar) digital vein Palmar (volar) metacarpal vein Superficial palmar venous arch Volar (palmar) digital vein Volar (palmar) metacarpal vein	**H Hand Vein, Left** *See G Hand Vein, Right* **L Intracranial Vein** Anterior cerebral vein Basal (internal) cerebral vein Dural venous sinus Great cerebral vein Inferior cerebellar vein Inferior cerebral vein Internal (basal) cerebral vein Middle cerebral vein Ophthalmic vein Superior cerebellar vein Superior cerebral vein **M Internal Jugular Vein, Right** **N Internal Jugular Vein, Left** **P External Jugular Vein, Right** Posterior auricular vein **Q External Jugular Vein, Left** *See P External Jugular Vein, Right* **R Vertebral Vein, Right** Deep cervical vein Suboccipital venous plexus **S Vertebral Vein, Left** *See R Vertebral Vein, Right* **T Face Vein, Right** Angular vein Anterior facial vein Common facial vein Deep facial vein Frontal vein Posterior facial (retromandibular) vein Supraorbital vein **V Face Vein, Left** *See T Face Vein, Right* **Y Upper Vein**	**Ø Open** **3 Percutaneous** **4 Percutaneous Endoscopic**	**Z No Device**	**Z No Qualifier**

LC Limited Coverage   NC Noncovered   ⊞ Combination Member   HAC associated procedure   Combination Only   DRG Non-OR   Non-OR   New/Revised in GREEN

250   ICD-10-PCS 2021

Ø5N–Ø5N

Ø Medical and Surgical
5 Upper Veins
P Removal   Definition: Taking out or off a device from a body part

                Explanation: If a device is taken out and a similar device put in without cutting or puncturing the skin or mucous membrane, the procedure is coded to the root operation CHANGE. Otherwise, the procedure for taking out a device is coded to the root operation REMOVAL.

Body Part Character 4	Approach Character 5	Device Character 6	Qualifier Character 7
Ø Azygos Vein Right ascending lumbar vein Right subcostal vein	**Ø** Open **3** Percutaneous **4** Percutaneous Endoscopic **X** External	**2** Monitoring Device **M** Neurostimulator Lead	**Z** No Qualifier
3 Innominate Vein, Right Brachiocephalic vein Inferior thyroid vein **4 Innominate Vein, Left** *See 3 Innominate Vein, Right*	**Ø** Open **3** Percutaneous **4** Percutaneous Endoscopic **X** External	**M** Neurostimulator Lead	**Z** No Qualifier
Y Upper Vein	**Ø** Open **3** Percutaneous **4** Percutaneous Endoscopic	**Ø** Drainage Device **2** Monitoring Device **3** Infusion Device **7** Autologous Tissue Substitute **C** Extraluminal Device **D** Intraluminal Device **J** Synthetic Substitute **K** Nonautologous Tissue Substitute **Y** Other Device	**Z** No Qualifier
Y Upper Vein	**X** External	**Ø** Drainage Device **2** Monitoring Device **3** Infusion Device **D** Intraluminal Device	**Z** No Qualifier

Non-OR Ø5PØ[Ø,3,4,X]2Z
Non-OR Ø5PY3[Ø,2,3]Z
Non-OR Ø5PY[3,4]YZ
Non-OR Ø5PYX[Ø,2,3,D]Z

LC Limited Coverage   NC Noncovered   ⊞ Combination Member   HAC associated procedure   Combination Only   DRG Non-OR   Non-OR   New/Revised in GREEN

Ø Medical and Surgical
5 Upper Veins
Q Repair   Definition: Restoring, to the extent possible, a body part to its normal anatomic structure and function

Explanation: Used only when the method to accomplish the repair is not one of the other root operations

Body Part Character 4		Approach Character 5	Device Character 6	Qualifier Character 7
Ø Azygos Vein Right ascending lumbar vein Right subcostal vein **1 Hemiazygos Vein** Left ascending lumbar vein Left subcostal vein **3 Innominate Vein, Right** Brachiocephalic vein Inferior thyroid vein **4 Innominate Vein, Left** *See 3 Innominate Vein, Right* **5 Subclavian Vein, Right** **6 Subclavian Vein, Left** **7 Axillary Vein, Right** **8 Axillary Vein, Left** **9 Brachial Vein, Right** Radial vein Ulnar vein **A Brachial Vein, Left** *See 9 Brachial Vein, Right* **B Basilic Vein, Right** Median antebrachial vein Median cubital vein **C Basilic Vein, Left** *See B Basilic Vein, Right* **D Cephalic Vein, Right** Accessory cephalic vein **F Cephalic Vein, Left** *See D Cephalic Vein, Right* **G Hand Vein, Right** Dorsal metacarpal vein Palmar (volar) digital vein Palmar (volar) metacarpal vein Superficial palmar venous arch Volar (palmar) digital vein Volar (palmar) metacarpal vein	**H Hand Vein, Left** *See G Hand Vein, Right* **L Intracranial Vein** Anterior cerebral vein Basal (internal) cerebral vein Dural venous sinus Great cerebral vein Inferior cerebellar vein Inferior cerebral vein Internal (basal) cerebral vein Middle cerebral vein Ophthalmic vein Superior cerebellar vein Superior cerebral vein **M Internal Jugular Vein, Right** **N Internal Jugular Vein, Left** **P External Jugular Vein, Right** Posterior auricular vein **Q External Jugular Vein, Left** *See P External Jugular Vein,* *Right* **R Vertebral Vein, Right** Deep cervical vein Suboccipital venous plexus **S Vertebral Vein, Left** *See R Vertebral Vein, Right* **T Face Vein, Right** Angular vein Anterior facial vein Common facial vein Deep facial vein Frontal vein Posterior facial (retromandibular) vein Supraorbital vein **V Face Vein, Left** *See T Face Vein, Right* **Y Upper Vein**	**Ø Open** **3 Percutaneous** **4 Percutaneous Endoscopic**	**Z No Device**	**Z No Qualifier**

LC Limited Coverage **NC** Noncovered ⊞ Combination Member HAC associated procedure Combination Only DRG Non-OR Non-OR New/Revised in GREEN

252   ICD-10-PCS 2021

Ø　**Medical and Surgical**
5　**Upper Veins**
R　**Replacement**　　Definition: Putting in or on biological or synthetic material that physically takes the place and/or function of all or a portion of a body part

Explanation: The body part may have been taken out or replaced, or may be taken out, physically eradicated, or rendered nonfunctional during the REPLACEMENT procedure. A REMOVAL procedure is coded for taking out the device used in a previous replacement procedure.

Body Part Character 4		Approach Character 5	Device Character 6	Qualifier Character 7
Ø **Azygos Vein** Right ascending lumbar vein Right subcostal vein **1** **Hemiazygos Vein** Left ascending lumbar vein Left subcostal vein **3** **Innominate Vein, Right** Brachiocephalic vein Inferior thyroid vein **4** **Innominate Vein, Left** *See 3 Innominate Vein, Right* **5** **Subclavian Vein, Right** **6** **Subclavian Vein, Left** **7** **Axillary Vein, Right** **8** **Axillary Vein, Left** **9** **Brachial Vein, Right** Radial vein Ulnar vein **A** **Brachial Vein, Left** *See 9 Brachial Vein, Right* **B** **Basilic Vein, Right** Median antebrachial vein Median cubital vein **C** **Basilic Vein, Left** *See B Basilic Vein, Right* **D** **Cephalic Vein, Right** Accessory cephalic vein **F** **Cephalic Vein, Left** *See D Cephalic Vein, Right* **G** **Hand Vein, Right** Dorsal metacarpal vein Palmar (volar) digital vein Palmar (volar) metacarpal vein Superficial palmar venous arch Volar (palmar) digital vein Volar (palmar) metacarpal vein	**H** **Hand Vein, Left** *See G Hand Vein, Right* **L** **Intracranial Vein** Anterior cerebral vein Basal (internal) cerebral vein Dural venous sinus Great cerebral vein Inferior cerebellar vein Inferior cerebral vein Internal (basal) cerebral vein Middle cerebral vein Ophthalmic vein Superior cerebellar vein Superior cerebral vein **M** **Internal Jugular Vein, Right** **N** **Internal Jugular Vein, Left** **P** **External Jugular Vein, Right** Posterior auricular vein **Q** **External Jugular Vein, Left** *See P External Jugular Vein, Right* **R** **Vertebral Vein, Right** Deep cervical vein Suboccipital venous plexus **S** **Vertebral Vein, Left** *See R Vertebral Vein, Right* **T** **Face Vein, Right** Angular vein Anterior facial vein Common facial vein Deep facial vein Frontal vein Posterior facial (retromandibular) vein Supraorbital vein **V** **Face Vein, Left** *See T Face Vein, Right* **Y** **Upper Vein**	**Ø** Open **4** Percutaneous Endoscopic	**7** Autologous Tissue Substitute **J** Synthetic Substitute **K** Nonautologous Tissue Substitute	**Z** No Qualifier

LC Limited Coverage　**NC** Noncovered　⊞ Combination Member　HAC associated procedure　Combination Only　DRG Non-OR　Non-OR　New/Revised in GREEN

ICD-10-PCS 2021　　　　　　　　　　　　　　　　　　　　　　　　　　　　　　　　　253

Ø5R–Ø5R

Upper Veins

Ø **Medical and Surgical**
5 **Upper Veins**
S **Reposition**   Definition: Moving to its normal location, or other suitable location, all or a portion of a body part

Explanation: The body part is moved to a new location from an abnormal location, or from a normal location where it is not functioning correctly. The body part may or may not be cut out or off to be moved to the new location.

Body Part Character 4		Approach Character 5	Device Character 6	Qualifier Character 7

Ø **Azygos Vein**
   Right ascending lumbar vein
   Right subcostal vein
1 **Hemiazygos Vein**
   Left ascending lumbar vein
   Left subcostal vein
3 **Innominate Vein, Right**
   Brachiocephalic vein
   Inferior thyroid vein
4 **Innominate Vein, Left**
   See 3 Innominate Vein, Right
5 **Subclavian Vein, Right**
6 **Subclavian Vein, Left**
7 **Axillary Vein, Right**
8 **Axillary Vein, Left**
9 **Brachial Vein, Right**
   Radial vein
   Ulnar vein
A **Brachial Vein, Left**
   See 9 Brachial Vein, Right
B **Basilic Vein, Right**
   Median antebrachial vein
   Median cubital vein
C **Basilic Vein, Left**
   See B Basilic Vein, Right
D **Cephalic Vein, Right**
   Accessory cephalic vein
F **Cephalic Vein, Left**
   See D Cephalic Vein, Right
G **Hand Vein, Right**
   Dorsal metacarpal vein
   Palmar (volar) digital vein
   Palmar (volar) metacarpal vein
   Superficial palmar venous arch
   Volar (palmar) digital vein
   Volar (palmar) metacarpal vein
	H **Hand Vein, Left**
	   See G Hand Vein, Right
	L **Intracranial Vein**
	   Anterior cerebral vein
	   Basal (internal) cerebral vein
	   Dural venous sinus
	   Great cerebral vein
	   Inferior cerebellar vein
	   Inferior cerebral vein
	   Internal (basal) cerebral vein
	   Middle cerebral vein
	   Ophthalmic vein
	   Superior cerebellar vein
	   Superior cerebral vein
	M **Internal Jugular Vein, Right**
	N **Internal Jugular Vein, Left**
	P **External Jugular Vein, Right**
	   Posterior auricular vein
	Q **External Jugular Vein, Left**
	   See P External Jugular Vein,
	   Right
	R **Vertebral Vein, Right**
	   Deep cervical vein
	   Suboccipital venous plexus
	S **Vertebral Vein, Left**
	   See R Vertebral Vein, Right
	T **Face Vein, Right**
	   Angular vein
	   Anterior facial vein
	   Common facial vein
	   Deep facial vein
	   Frontal vein
	   Posterior facial
	      (retromandibular) vein
	   Supraorbital vein
	V **Face Vein, Left**
	   See T Face Vein, Right
	Y **Upper Vein**
		Ø Open
		3 Percutaneous
		4 Percutaneous Endoscopic
			Z No Device	**Z** No Qualifier

LC Limited Coverage   **NC** Noncovered   ⊞ Combination Member   HAC associated procedure   Combination Only   DRG Non-OR   Non-OR   New/Revised in GREEN

254   ICD-10-PCS 2021

Ø   Medical and Surgical
5   Upper Veins
U   Supplement   Definition: Putting in or on biological or synthetic material that physically reinforces and/or augments the function of a portion of a body part

Explanation: The biological material is non-living, or is living and from the same individual. The body part may have been previously replaced, and the SUPPLEMENT procedure is performed to physically reinforce and/or augment the function of the replaced body part.

Body Part Character 4		Approach Character 5	Device Character 6	Qualifier Character 7
Ø Azygos Vein Right ascending lumbar vein Right subcostal vein **1 Hemiazygos Vein** Left ascending lumbar vein Left subcostal vein **3 Innominate Vein, Right** Brachiocephalic vein Inferior thyroid vein **4 Innominate Vein, Left** *See 3 Innominate Vein, Right* **5 Subclavian Vein, Right** **6 Subclavian Vein, Left** **7 Axillary Vein, Right** **8 Axillary Vein, Left** **9 Brachial Vein, Right** Radial vein Ulnar vein **A Brachial Vein, Left** *See 9 Brachial Vein, Right* **B Basilic Vein, Right** Median antebrachial vein Median cubital vein **C Basilic Vein, Left** *See B Basilic Vein, Right* **D Cephalic Vein, Right** Accessory cephalic vein **F Cephalic Vein, Left** *See D Cephalic Vein, Right* **G Hand Vein, Right** Dorsal metacarpal vein Palmar (volar) digital vein Palmar (volar) metacarpal vein Superficial palmar venous arch Volar (palmar) digital vein Volar (palmar) metacarpal vein	**H Hand Vein, Left** *See G Hand Vein, Right* **L Intracranial Vein** Anterior cerebral vein Basal (internal) cerebral vein Dural venous sinus Great cerebral vein Inferior cerebellar vein Inferior cerebral vein Internal (basal) cerebral vein Middle cerebral vein Ophthalmic vein Superior cerebellar vein Superior cerebral vein **M Internal Jugular Vein, Right** **N Internal Jugular Vein, Left** **P External Jugular Vein, Right** Posterior auricular vein **Q External Jugular Vein, Left** *See P External Jugular Vein,* *Right* **R Vertebral Vein, Right** Deep cervical vein Suboccipital venous plexus **S Vertebral Vein, Left** *See R Vertebral Vein, Right* **T Face Vein, Right** Angular vein Anterior facial vein Common facial vein Deep facial vein Frontal vein Posterior facial (retromandibular) vein Supraorbital vein **V Face Vein, Left** *See T Face Vein, Right* **Y Upper Vein**	**Ø Open** **3 Percutaneous** **4 Percutaneous Endoscopic**	**7 Autologous Tissue** **Substitute** **J Synthetic Substitute** **K Nonautologous Tissue** **Substitute**	**Z No Qualifier**

Ø   **Medical and Surgical**
5   **Upper Veins**
V   **Restriction**   Definition: Partially closing an orifice or the lumen of a tubular body part
                        Explanation: The orifice can be a natural orifice or an artificially created orifice

Body Part Character 4		Approach Character 5	Device Character 6	Qualifier Character 7

Ø   **Azygos Vein**
    Right ascending lumbar vein
    Right subcostal vein
1   **Hemiazygos Vein**
    Left ascending lumbar vein
    Left subcostal vein
3   **Innominate Vein, Right**
    Brachiocephalic vein
    Inferior thyroid vein
4   **Innominate Vein, Left**
    See 3 Innominate Vein, Right
5   **Subclavian Vein, Right**
6   **Subclavian Vein, Left**
7   **Axillary Vein, Right**
8   **Axillary Vein, Left**
9   **Brachial Vein, Right**
    Radial vein
    Ulnar vein
A   **Brachial Vein, Left**
    See 9 Brachial Vein, Right
B   **Basilic Vein, Right**
    Median antebrachial vein
    Median cubital vein
C   **Basilic Vein, Left**
    See B Basilic Vein, Right
D   **Cephalic Vein, Right**
    Accessory cephalic vein
F   **Cephalic Vein, Left**
    See D Cephalic Vein, Right
G   **Hand Vein, Right**
    Dorsal metacarpal vein
    Palmar (volar) digital vein
    Palmar (volar) metacarpal vein
    Superficial palmar venous arch
    Volar (palmar) digital vein
    Volar (palmar) metacarpal vein
	H **Hand Vein, Left**
	    See G Hand Vein, Right
	L **Intracranial Vein**
	    Anterior cerebral vein
	    Basal (internal) cerebral vein
	    Dural venous sinus
	    Great cerebral vein
	    Inferior cerebellar vein
	    Inferior cerebral vein
	    Internal (basal) cerebral vein
	    Middle cerebral vein
	    Ophthalmic vein
	    Superior cerebellar vein
	    Superior cerebral vein
	M **Internal Jugular Vein, Right**
	N **Internal Jugular Vein, Left**
	P **External Jugular Vein, Right**
	    Posterior auricular vein
	Q **External Jugular Vein, Left**
	    See P External Jugular Vein,
	      Right
	R **Vertebral Vein, Right**
	    Deep cervical vein
	    Suboccipital venous plexus
	S **Vertebral Vein, Left**
	    See R Vertebral Vein, Right
	T **Face Vein, Right**
	    Angular vein
	    Anterior facial vein
	    Common facial vein
	    Deep facial vein
	    Frontal vein
	    Posterior facial
	      (retromandibular) vein
	    Supraorbital vein
	V **Face Vein, Left**
	    See T Face Vein, Right
	Y **Upper Vein**
		Ø Open
		3 Percutaneous
		4 Percutaneous Endoscopic
			C Extraluminal Device
			D Intraluminal Device
			Z No Device
				Z No Qualifier

LC Limited Coverage   NC Noncovered   ⊞ Combination Member   HAC associated procedure   Combination Only   DRG Non-OR   Non-OR   New/Revised in GREEN
256   ICD-10-PCS 2021

Ø5V–Ø5V

Ø   Medical and Surgical
5   Upper Veins
W   Revision   Definition: Correcting, to the extent possible, a portion of a malfunctioning device or the position of a displaced device

                        Explanation: Revision can include correcting a malfunctioning or displaced device by taking out or putting in components of the device such as a screw or pin

Body Part Character 4	Approach Character 5	Device Character 6	Qualifier Character 7

Ø   Azygos Vein
    Right ascending lumbar vein
    Right subcostal vein
	Ø Open
	3 Percutaneous
	4 Percutaneous Endoscopic
	X External
		2 Monitoring Device
		M Neurostimulator Lead
			Z No Qualifier

3   Innominate Vein, Right
    Brachiocephalic vein
    Inferior thyroid vein
4   Innominate Vein, Left
    See 3 Innominate Vein, Right
	Ø Open
	3 Percutaneous
	4 Percutaneous Endoscopic
	X External
		M Neurostimulator Lead	**Z No Qualifier**

Y Upper Vein	**Ø Open** **3 Percutaneous** **4 Percutaneous Endoscopic**	**Ø Drainage Device** **2 Monitoring Device** **3 Infusion Device** **7 Autologous Tissue Substitute** **C Extraluminal Device** **D Intraluminal Device** **J Synthetic Substitute** **K Nonautologous Tissue Substitute** **Y Other Device**	**Z No Qualifier**
Y Upper Vein	**X External**	**Ø Drainage Device** **2 Monitoring Device** **3 Infusion Device** **7 Autologous Tissue Substitute** **C Extraluminal Device** **D Intraluminal Device** **J Synthetic Substitute** **K Nonautologous Tissue Substitute**	**Z No Qualifier**

Non-OR   Ø5WØXMZ
Non-OR   Ø5W[3,4]XMZ
Non-OR   Ø5WY3[Ø,2,3,D]Z
Non-OR   Ø5WY[3,4]YZ
Non-OR   Ø5WYX[Ø,2,3,7,C,D,J,K]Z

LC Limited Coverage   NC Noncovered   ⊞ Combination Member   HAC associated procedure   Combination Only   DRG Non-OR   Non-OR   New/Revised in GREEN

ICD-10-PCS 2021   257

Lower Veins Ø61–Ø6W

Character Meanings

This Character Meaning table is provided as a guide to assist the user in the identification of character members that may be found in this section of code tables. It **SHOULD NOT** be used to build a PCS code.

Operation–Character 3	Body Part–Character 4	Approach–Character 5	Device–Character 6	Qualifier–Character 7
1 Bypass	Ø Inferior Vena Cava	Ø Open	Ø Drainage Device	Ø Ultrasonic
5 Destruction	1 Splenic Vein	3 Percutaneous	2 Monitoring Device	4 Hepatic Vein
7 Dilation	2 Gastric Vein	4 Percutaneous Endoscopic	3 Infusion Device	5 Superior Mesenteric Vein
9 Drainage	3 Esophageal Vein	7 Via Natural or Artificial Opening	7 Autologous Tissue Substitute	6 Inferior Mesenteric Vein
B Excision	4 Hepatic Vein	8 Via Natural or Artificial Opening Endoscopic	9 Autologous Venous Tissue	9 Renal Vein, Right
C Extirpation	5 Superior Mesenteric Vein	X External	A Autologous Arterial Tissue	B Renal Vein, Left
D Extraction	6 Inferior Mesenteric Vein		C Extraluminal Device	C Hemorrhoidal Plexus
F Fragmentation	7 Colic Vein		D Intraluminal Device	P Pulmonary Trunk
H Insertion	8 Portal Vein		J Synthetic Substitute	Q Pulmonary Artery, Right
J Inspection	9 Renal Vein, Right		K Nonautologous Tissue Substitute	R Pulmonary Artery, Left
L Occlusion	B Renal Vein, Left		Y Other Device	T Via Umbilical Vein
N Release	C Common Iliac Vein, Right		Z No Device	X Diagnostic
P Removal	D Common Iliac Vein, Left			Y Lower Vein
Q Repair	F External Iliac Vein, Right			Z No Qualifier
R Replacement	G External Iliac Vein, Left			
S Reposition	H Hypogastric Vein, Right			
U Supplement	J Hypogastric Vein, Left			
V Restriction	M Femoral Vein, Right			
W Revision	N Femoral Vein, Left			
	P Saphenous Vein, Right			
	Q Saphenous Vein, Left			
	T Foot Vein, Right			
	V Foot Vein, Left			
	Y Lower Vein			

AHA Coding Clinic for table Ø61
2017, 4Q, 36-38   Fontan completion procedure
2017, 4Q, 66-67   New qualifier values - Portal to hepatic shunt

AHA Coding Clinic for table Ø6B
2020, 1Q, 28   Free flap microvascular breast reconstruction
2017, 3Q, 5   Femoral artery to posterior tibial artery bypass using autologous and synthetic grafts
2017, 1Q, 31   Left to right common carotid artery bypass
2017, 1Q, 32   Peroneal artery to dorsalis pedis artery bypass using saphenous vein graft
2016, 3Q, 31   Femoral to peroneal artery bypass with in-situ saphenous vein graft and lysis of valves
2016, 2Q, 18   Femoral-tibial artery bypass and saphenous vein graft
2016, 1Q, 27   Aortocoronary bypass graft utilizing Y-graft
2014, 3Q, 8   Excision of saphenous vein for coronary artery bypass graft
2014, 3Q, 20   MAZE procedure performed with coronary artery bypass graft
2014, 1Q, 10   Repair of thoracic aortic aneurysm & coronary artery bypass graft

AHA Coding Clinic for table Ø6H
2017, 3Q, 11   Placement of peripherally inserted central catheter using 3CG ECG technology
2017, 1Q, 31   Umbilical vein catheterization
2017, 1Q, 31   Central catheter placement in femoral vein
2013, 3Q, 18   Heart transplant surgery

AHA Coding Clinic for table Ø6L
2019, 4Q, 28   Transorifice occlusion of gastric varices
2018, 2Q, 18   Transverse rectus abdominis myocutaneous (TRAM) delay
2017, 4Q, 57-58   Added approach values - Transorifice esophageal vein banding
2013, 4Q, 112   Endoscopic banding of esophageal varices

AHA Coding Clinic for table Ø6V
2018, 3Q, 11   Transvenous transcatheter placement of valve in inferior vena cava
2018, 1Q, 10   Revision of transjugular intrahepatic portosystemic shunt

AHA Coding Clinic for table Ø6W
2019, 2Q, 39   Transjugular intrahepatic portosystemic shunt revision
2018, 1Q, 10   Revision of transjugular intrahepatic portosystemic shunt
2014, 3Q, 25   Revision of transjugular intrahepatic portosystemic shunt (TIPS)

Lower Veins

Inferior vena cava **Ø**
Common hepatic **4**
Portal **B**
Colic **7**
Internal pudendal **H, J**
Femoral **M, N**
Greater saphenous **P, Q**
Lesser saphenous **P, Q**
Anterior tibial **M, N**
Posterior tibial **M, N**
Digital **T, V**

Esophageal **3**
Gastric **2**
Splenic **1**
Renal **9, B**
Inferior mesenteric **6**
Superior mesenteric **5**
Common iliac **C, D**
Internal iliac (Hypogastric) **H, J**
External iliac **F, G**
Rectal venous plexus **H, J**
Popliteal **M, N**
Lesser saphenous **P, Q**
Greater saphenous **P, Q**
Dorsal venous arch **T, V**

Portal Venous Circulation

Inferior vena cava **Ø**
Portal **8**
Superior mesenteric **5**
Right colic **7**
Ileocolic **7**
Inferior mesenteric **6**
Gastric **2**
Splenic **1**
Left colic **7**

Ø Medical and Surgical
6 Lower Veins
1 Bypass   Definition: Altering the route of passage of the contents of a tubular body part

Explanation: Rerouting contents of a body part to a downstream area of the normal route, to a similar route and body part, or to an abnormal route and dissimilar body part. Includes one or more anastomoses, with or without the use of a device.

Body Part Character 4		Approach Character 5	Device Character 6	Qualifier Character 7
Ø Inferior Vena Cava Postcava Right inferior phrenic vein Right ovarian vein Right second lumbar vein Right suprarenal vein Right testicular vein		**Ø** Open **4** Percutaneous Endoscopic	**7** Autologous Tissue Substitute **9** Autologous Venous Tissue **A** Autologous Arterial Tissue **J** Synthetic Substitute **K** Nonautologous Tissue Substitute **Z** No Device	**5** Superior Mesenteric Vein **6** Inferior Mesenteric Vein **P** Pulmonary Trunk **Q** Pulmonary Artery, Right **R** Pulmonary Artery, Left **Y** Lower Vein
1 Splenic Vein Left gastroepiploic vein Pancreatic vein		**Ø** Open **4** Percutaneous Endoscopic	**7** Autologous Tissue Substitute **9** Autologous Venous Tissue **A** Autologous Arterial Tissue **J** Synthetic Substitute **K** Nonautologous Tissue Substitute **Z** No Device	**9** Renal Vein, Right **B** Renal Vein, Left **Y** Lower Vein
2 Gastric Vein **3 Esophageal Vein** **4 Hepatic Vein** **5 Superior Mesenteric Vein** Right gastroepiploic vein **6 Inferior Mesenteric Vein** Sigmoid vein Superior rectal vein **7 Colic Vein** Ileocolic vein Left colic vein Middle colic vein Right colic vein **9 Renal Vein, Right** **B Renal Vein, Left** Left inferior phrenic vein Left ovarian vein Left second lumbar vein Left suprarenal vein Left testicular vein **C Common Iliac Vein, Right** **D Common Iliac Vein, Left** **F External Iliac Vein, Right** **G External Iliac Vein, Left** **H Hypogastric Vein, Right** Gluteal vein Internal iliac vein Internal pudendal vein Lateral sacral vein Middle hemorrhoidal vein Obturator vein Uterine vein Vaginal vein Vesical vein	**J Hypogastric Vein, Left** *See H Hypogastric Vein, Right* **M Femoral Vein, Right** Deep femoral (profunda femoris) vein Popliteal vein Profunda femoris (deep femoral) vein **N Femoral Vein, Left** *See M Femoral Vein, Right* **P Saphenous Vein, Right** External pudendal vein Great(er) saphenous vein Lesser saphenous vein Small saphenous vein Superficial circumflex iliac vein Superficial epigastric vein **Q Saphenous Vein, Left** *See P Saphenous Vein, Right* **T Foot Vein, Right** Common digital vein Dorsal metatarsal vein Dorsal venous arch Plantar digital vein Plantar metatarsal vein Plantar venous arch **V Foot Vein, Left** *See T Foot Vein, Right*	**Ø** Open **4** Percutaneous Endoscopic	**7** Autologous Tissue Substitute **9** Autologous Venous Tissue **A** Autologous Arterial Tissue **J** Synthetic Substitute **K** Nonautologous Tissue Substitute **Z** No Device	**Y** Lower Vein
8 Portal Vein Hepatic portal vein		**Ø** Open	**7** Autologous Tissue Substitute **9** Autologous Venous Tissue **A** Autologous Arterial Tissue **J** Synthetic Substitute **K** Nonautologous Tissue Substitute **Z** No Device	**9** Renal Vein, Right **B** Renal Vein, Left **Y** Lower Vein
8 Portal Vein Hepatic portal vein		**3** Percutaneous	**J** Synthetic Substitute	**4** Hepatic Vein **Y** Lower Vein
8 Portal Vein Hepatic portal vein		**4** Percutaneous Endoscopic	**7** Autologous Tissue Substitute **9** Autologous Venous Tissue **A** Autologous Arterial Tissue **K** Nonautologous Tissue Substitute **Z** No Device	**9** Renal Vein, Right **B** Renal Vein, Left **Y** Lower Vein
8 Portal Vein Hepatic portal vein		**4** Percutaneous Endoscopic	**J** Synthetic Substitute	**4** Hepatic Vein **9** Renal Vein, Right **B** Renal Vein, Left **Y** Lower Vein

LC Limited Coverage   NC Noncovered   ⊞ Combination Member   HAC associated procedure   Combination Only   DRG Non-OR   Non-OR   New/Revised in GREEN

ICD-10-PCS 2021   261

Ø61–Ø61

Ø   Medical and Surgical
6   Lower Veins
5   Destruction   Definition: Physical eradication of all or a portion of a body part by the direct use of energy, force, or a destructive agent
                          Explanation: None of the body part is physically taken out

Body Part Character 4	Approach Character 5	Device Character 6	Qualifier Character 7
Ø Inferior Vena Cava Postcava Right inferior phrenic vein Right ovarian vein Right second lumbar vein Right suprarenal vein Right testicular vein **1 Splenic Vein** Left gastroepiploic vein Pancreatic vein **2 Gastric Vein** **3 Esophageal Vein** **4 Hepatic Vein** **5 Superior Mesenteric Vein** Right gastroepiploic vein **6 Inferior Mesenteric Vein** Sigmoid vein Superior rectal vein **7 Colic Vein** Ileocolic vein Left colic vein Middle colic vein Right colic vein **8 Portal Vein** Hepatic portal vein **9 Renal Vein, Right** **B Renal Vein, Left** Left inferior phrenic vein Left ovarian vein Left second lumbar vein Left suprarenal vein Left testicular vein **C Common Iliac Vein, Right** **D Common Iliac Vein, Left** **F External Iliac Vein, Right** **G External Iliac Vein, Left** **H Hypogastric Vein, Right** Gluteal vein Internal iliac vein Internal pudendal vein Lateral sacral vein Middle hemorrhoidal vein Obturator vein Uterine vein Vaginal vein Vesical vein **J Hypogastric Vein, Left** *See H Hypogastric Vein, Right* **M Femoral Vein, Right** Deep femoral (profunda femoris) vein Popliteal vein Profunda femoris (deep femoral) vein **N Femoral Vein, Left** *See M Femoral Vein, Right* **P Saphenous Vein, Right** External pudendal vein Great(er) saphenous vein Lesser saphenous vein Small saphenous vein Superficial circumflex iliac vein Superficial epigastric vein **Q Saphenous Vein, Left** *See P Saphenous Vein, Right* **T Foot Vein, Right** Common digital vein Dorsal metatarsal vein Dorsal venous arch Plantar digital vein Plantar metatarsal vein Plantar venous arch **V Foot Vein, Left** *See T Foot Vein, Right*	**Ø** Open **3** Percutaneous **4** Percutaneous Endoscopic	**Z** No Device	**Z** No Qualifier
Y Lower Vein	**Ø** Open **3** Percutaneous **4** Percutaneous Endoscopic	**Z** No Device	**C** Hemorrhoidal Plexus **Z** No Qualifier

LC Limited Coverage   NC Noncovered   ⊞ Combination Member   HAC associated procedure   Combination Only   DRG Non-OR   Non-OR   New/Revised in GREEN

0　Medical and Surgical
6　Lower Veins
7　Dilation　　Definition: Expanding an orifice or the lumen of a tubular body part

Explanation: The orifice can be a natural orifice or an artificially created orifice. Accomplished by stretching a tubular body part using intraluminal pressure or by cutting part of the orifice or wall of the tubular body part.

Body Part Character 4	Approach Character 5	Device Character 6	Qualifier Character 7
0　Inferior Vena Cava 　　Postcava 　　Right inferior phrenic vein 　　Right ovarian vein 　　Right second lumbar vein 　　Right suprarenal vein 　　Right testicular vein **1　Splenic Vein** 　　Left gastroepiploic vein 　　Pancreatic vein **2　Gastric Vein** **3　Esophageal Vein** **4　Hepatic Vein** **5　Superior Mesenteric Vein** 　　Right gastroepiploic vein **6　Inferior Mesenteric Vein** 　　Sigmoid vein 　　Superior rectal vein **7　Colic Vein** 　　Ileocolic vein 　　Left colic vein 　　Middle colic vein 　　Right colic vein **8　Portal Vein** 　　Hepatic portal vein **9　Renal Vein, Right** **B　Renal Vein, Left** 　　Left inferior phrenic vein 　　Left ovarian vein 　　Left second lumbar vein 　　Left suprarenal vein 　　Left testicular vein **C　Common Iliac Vein, Right** **D　Common Iliac Vein, Left** **F　External Iliac Vein, Right** **G　External Iliac Vein, Left** **H　Hypogastric Vein, Right** 　　Gluteal vein 　　Internal iliac vein 　　Internal pudendal vein 　　Lateral sacral vein 　　Middle hemorrhoidal vein 　　Obturator vein 　　Uterine vein 　　Vaginal vein 　　Vesical vein **J　Hypogastric Vein, Left** 　　*See H Hypogastric Vein, Right* **M　Femoral Vein, Right** 　　Deep femoral (profunda femoris) vein 　　Popliteal vein 　　Profunda femoris (deep femoral) vein **N　Femoral Vein, Left** 　　*See M Femoral Vein, Right* **P　Saphenous Vein, Right** 　　External pudendal vein 　　Great(er) saphenous vein 　　Lesser saphenous vein 　　Small saphenous vein 　　Superficial circumflex iliac vein 　　Superficial epigastric vein **Q　Saphenous Vein, Left** 　　*See P Saphenous Vein, Right* **T　Foot Vein, Right** 　　Common digital vein 　　Dorsal metatarsal vein 　　Dorsal venous arch 　　Plantar digital vein 　　Plantar metatarsal vein 　　Plantar venous arch **V　Foot Vein, Left** 　　*See T Foot Vein, Right* **Y　Lower Vein**	**0　Open** **3　Percutaneous** **4　Percutaneous Endoscopic**	**D　Intraluminal Device** **Z　No Device**	**Z　No Qualifier**

Lower Veins

0   **Medical and Surgical**
6   **Lower Veins**
9   **Drainage**   Definition: Taking or letting out fluids and/or gases from a body part

Explanation: The qualifier DIAGNOSTIC is used to identify drainage procedures that are biopsies

Body Part Character 4		Approach Character 5	Device Character 6	Qualifier Character 7

0 **Inferior Vena Cava**
   Postcava
   Right inferior phrenic vein
   Right ovarian vein
   Right second lumbar vein
   Right suprarenal vein
   Right testicular vein
1 **Splenic Vein**
   Left gastroepiploic vein
   Pancreatic vein
2 **Gastric Vein**
3 **Esophageal Vein**
4 **Hepatic Vein**
5 **Superior Mesenteric Vein**
   Right gastroepiploic vein
6 **Inferior Mesenteric Vein**
   Sigmoid vein
   Superior rectal vein
7 **Colic Vein**
   Ileocolic vein
   Left colic vein
   Middle colic vein
   Right colic vein
8 **Portal Vein**
   Hepatic portal vein
9 **Renal Vein, Right**
B **Renal Vein, Left**
   Left inferior phrenic vein
   Left ovarian vein
   Left second lumbar vein
   Left suprarenal vein
   Left testicular vein
C **Common Iliac Vein, Right**
D **Common Iliac Vein, Left**
F **External Iliac Vein, Right**
G **External Iliac Vein, Left**
	H **Hypogastric Vein, Right**
	   Gluteal vein
	   Internal iliac vein
	   Internal pudendal vein
	   Lateral sacral vein
	   Middle hemorrhoidal vein
	   Obturator vein
	   Uterine vein
	   Vaginal vein
	   Vesical vein
	J **Hypogastric Vein, Left**
	   See H Hypogastric Vein, Right
	M **Femoral Vein, Right**
	   Deep femoral (profunda
	     femoris) vein
	   Popliteal vein
	   Profunda femoris (deep
	     femoral) vein
	N **Femoral Vein, Left**
	   See M Femoral Vein, Right
	P **Saphenous Vein, Right**
	   External pudendal vein
	   Great(er) saphenous vein
	   Lesser saphenous vein
	   Small saphenous vein
	   Superficial circumflex iliac vein
	   Superficial epigastric vein
	Q **Saphenous Vein, Left**
	   See P Saphenous Vein, Right
	T **Foot Vein, Right**
	   Common digital vein
	   Dorsal metatarsal vein
	   Dorsal venous arch
	   Plantar digital vein
	   Plantar metatarsal vein
	   Plantar venous arch
	V **Foot Vein, Left**
	   See T Foot Vein, Right
	Y **Lower Vein**
		0 Open
		3 Percutaneous
		4 Percutaneous Endoscopic
			0 Drainage Device	**Z** No Qualifier

Non-OR   069[0,1,2,4,5,6,7,8,9,B,C,D,F,G,H,J,M,N,P,Q,T,V,Y][0,3,4]0Z
Non-OR   069330Z

069 Continued on next page

Ø   Medical and Surgical
6   Lower Veins
9   Drainage

Ø69 Continued

Definition: Taking or letting out fluids and/or gases from a body part
Explanation: The qualifier DIAGNOSTIC is used to identify drainage procedures that are biopsies

Body Part Character 4		Approach Character 5	Device Character 6	Qualifier Character 7
Ø Inferior Vena Cava Postcava Right inferior phrenic vein Right ovarian vein Right second lumbar vein Right suprarenal vein Right testicular vein **1 Splenic Vein** Left gastroepiploic vein Pancreatic vein **2 Gastric Vein** **3 Esophageal Vein** **4 Hepatic Vein** **5 Superior Mesenteric Vein** Right gastroepiploic vein **6 Inferior Mesenteric Vein** Sigmoid vein Superior rectal vein **7 Colic Vein** Ileocolic vein Left colic vein Middle colic vein Right colic vein **8 Portal Vein** Hepatic portal vein **9 Renal Vein, Right** **B Renal Vein, Left** Left inferior phrenic vein Left ovarian vein Left second lumbar vein Left suprarenal vein Left testicular vein **C Common Iliac Vein, Right** **D Common Iliac Vein, Left** **F External Iliac Vein, Right** **G External Iliac Vein, Left**	**H Hypogastric Vein, Right** Gluteal vein Internal iliac vein Internal pudendal vein Lateral sacral vein Middle hemorrhoidal vein Obturator vein Uterine vein Vaginal vein Vesical vein **J Hypogastric Vein, Left** *See H Hypogastric Vein, Right* **M Femoral Vein, Right** Deep femoral (profunda femoris) vein Popliteal vein Profunda femoris (deep femoral) vein **N Femoral Vein, Left** *See M Femoral Vein, Right* **P Saphenous Vein, Right** External pudendal vein Great(er) saphenous vein Lesser saphenous vein Small saphenous vein Superficial circumflex iliac vein Superficial epigastric vein **Q Saphenous Vein, Left** *See P Saphenous Vein, Right* **T Foot Vein, Right** Common digital vein Dorsal metatarsal vein Dorsal venous arch Plantar digital vein Plantar metatarsal vein Plantar venous arch **V Foot Vein, Left** *See T Foot Vein, Right* **Y Lower Vein**	**Ø Open** **3 Percutaneous** **4 Percutaneous Endoscopic**	**Z No Device**	**X Diagnostic** **Z No Qualifier**

Non-OR	Ø69[Ø,1,2,3,4,5,6,7,8,9,B,C,D,F,G,H,J,M,N,P,Q,T,V,Y]3ZX
Non-OR	Ø69[Ø,1,2,4,5,6,7,8,9,B,C,D,F,G,H,J,M,N,P,Q,T,V,Y][Ø,3,4]ZZ
Non-OR	Ø6933ZZ

LC Limited Coverage   NC Noncovered   ⊞ Combination Member   HAC associated procedure   Combination Only   DRG Non-OR   Non-OR   New/Revised in GREEN

ICD-10-PCS 2021   265

Ø69–Ø69

0 Medical and Surgical
6 Lower Veins
B Excision

Definition: Cutting out or off, without replacement, a portion of a body part

Explanation: The qualifier DIAGNOSTIC is used to identify excision procedures that are biopsies

Body Part Character 4		Approach Character 5	Device Character 6	Qualifier Character 7
0 Inferior Vena Cava Postcava Right inferior phrenic vein Right ovarian vein Right second lumbar vein Right suprarenal vein Right testicular vein **1 Splenic Vein** Left gastroepiploic vein Pancreatic vein **2 Gastric Vein** **3 Esophageal Vein** **4 Hepatic Vein** **5 Superior Mesenteric Vein** Right gastroepiploic vein **6 Inferior Mesenteric Vein** Sigmoid vein Superior rectal vein **7 Colic Vein** Ileocolic vein Left colic vein Middle colic vein Right colic vein **8 Portal Vein** Hepatic portal vein **9 Renal Vein, Right** **B Renal Vein, Left** Left inferior phrenic vein Left ovarian vein Left second lumbar vein Left suprarenal vein Left testicular vein **C Common Iliac Vein, Right** **D Common Iliac Vein, Left** **F External Iliac Vein, Right** **G External Iliac Vein, Left**	**H Hypogastric Vein, Right** Gluteal vein Internal iliac vein Internal pudendal vein Lateral sacral vein Middle hemorrhoidal vein Obturator vein Uterine vein Vaginal vein Vesical vein **J Hypogastric Vein, Left** *See H Hypogastric Vein, Right* **M Femoral Vein, Right** Deep femoral (profunda femoris) vein Popliteal vein Profunda femoris (deep femoral) vein **N Femoral Vein, Left** *See M Femoral Vein, Right* **P Saphenous Vein, Right** External pudendal vein Great(er) saphenous vein Lesser saphenous vein Small saphenous vein Superficial circumflex iliac vein Superficial epigastric vein **Q Saphenous Vein, Left** *See P Saphenous Vein, Right* **T Foot Vein, Right** Common digital vein Dorsal metatarsal vein Dorsal venous arch Plantar digital vein Plantar metatarsal vein Plantar venous arch **V Foot Vein, Left** *See T Foot Vein, Right*	**0 Open** **3 Percutaneous** **4 Percutaneous Endoscopic**	**Z No Device**	**X Diagnostic** **Z No Qualifier**
Y Lower Vein		**0 Open** **3 Percutaneous** **4 Percutaneous Endoscopic**	**Z No Device**	**C Hemorrhoidal Plexus** **X Diagnostic** **Z No Qualifier**

LC Limited Coverage   NC Noncovered   ⊞ Combination Member   HAC associated procedure   Combination Only   DRG Non-OR   Non-OR   New/Revised in GREEN

266   ICD-10-PCS 2021

06B–06B

Ø   **Medical and Surgical**
6   **Lower Veins**
C   **Extirpation**   Definition: Taking or cutting out solid matter from a body part

Explanation: The solid matter may be an abnormal byproduct of a biological function or a foreign body; it may be imbedded in a body part or in the lumen of a tubular body part. The solid matter may or may not have been previously broken into pieces.

Body Part Character 4		Approach Character 5	Device Character 6	Qualifier Character 7

Ø Inferior Vena Cava
Postcava
Right inferior phrenic vein
Right ovarian vein
Right second lumbar vein
Right suprarenal vein
Right testicular vein
1 Splenic Vein
Left gastroepiploic vein
Pancreatic vein
2 Gastric Vein
3 Esophageal Vein
4 Hepatic Vein
5 Superior Mesenteric Vein
Right gastroepiploic vein
6 Inferior Mesenteric Vein
Sigmoid vein
Superior rectal vein
7 Colic Vein
Ileocolic vein
Left colic vein
Middle colic vein
Right colic vein
8 Portal Vein
Hepatic portal vein
9 Renal Vein, Right
B Renal Vein, Left
Left inferior phrenic vein
Left ovarian vein
Left second lumbar vein
Left suprarenal vein
Left testicular vein
C Common Iliac Vein, Right
D Common Iliac Vein, Left
F External Iliac Vein, Right
G External Iliac Vein, Left
	H Hypogastric Vein, Right
	Gluteal vein
	Internal iliac vein
	Internal pudendal vein
	Lateral sacral vein
	Middle hemorrhoidal vein
	Obturator vein
	Uterine vein
	Vaginal vein
	Vesical vein
	J Hypogastric Vein, Left
	See H Hypogastric Vein, Right
	M Femoral Vein, Right
	Deep femoral (profunda
	   femoris) vein
	Popliteal vein
	Profunda femoris (deep
	   femoral) vein
	N Femoral Vein, Left
	See M Femoral Vein, Right
	P Saphenous Vein, Right
	External pudendal vein
	Great(er) saphenous vein
	Lesser saphenous vein
	Small saphenous vein
	Superficial circumflex iliac vein
	Superficial epigastric vein
	Q Saphenous Vein, Left
	See P Saphenous Vein, Right
	T Foot Vein, Right
	Common digital vein
	Dorsal metatarsal vein
	Dorsal venous arch
	Plantar digital vein
	Plantar metatarsal vein
	Plantar venous arch
	V Foot Vein, Left
	See T Foot Vein, Right
	Y Lower Vein
		Ø Open
		3 Percutaneous
		4 Percutaneous Endoscopic
			Z No Device	**Z No Qualifier**

Ø   **Medical and Surgical**
6   **Lower Veins**
D   **Extraction**   Definition: Pulling or stripping out or off all or a portion of a body part by the use of force

Explanation: The qualifier DIAGNOSTIC is used to identify extraction procedures that are biopsies

Body Part Character 4		Approach Character 5	Device Character 6	Qualifier Character 7

M Femoral Vein, Right
Deep femoral (profunda
   femoris) vein
Popliteal vein
Profunda femoris (deep
   femoral) vein
N Femoral Vein, Left
See M Femoral Vein, Right
P Saphenous Vein, Right
External pudendal vein
Great(er) saphenous vein
Lesser saphenous vein
Small saphenous vein
Superficial circumflex iliac vein
Superficial epigastric vein
Q Saphenous Vein, Left
See P Saphenous Vein, Right
	T Foot Vein, Right
	Common digital vein
	Dorsal metatarsal vein
	Dorsal venous arch
	Plantar digital vein
	Plantar metatarsal vein
	Plantar venous arch
	V Foot Vein, Left
	See T Foot Vein, Right
	Y Lower Vein
		Ø Open
		3 Percutaneous
		4 Percutaneous Endoscopic
			Z No Device	**Z No Qualifier**

LC Limited Coverage   **NC** Noncovered   ⊞ Combination Member   HAC associated procedure   Combination Only   DRG Non-OR   Non-OR   New/Revised in GREEN

ICD-10-PCS 2021   267

06C–06D

Ø   **Medical and Surgical**
6   **Lower Veins**
F   **Fragmentation**   Definition: Breaking solid matter in a body part into pieces

Explanation: Physical force (e.g., manual, ultrasonic) applied directly or indirectly is used to break the solid matter into pieces. The solid matter may be an abnormal byproduct of a biological function or a foreign body. The pieces of solid matter are not taken out.

Body Part Character 4		Approach Character 5	Device Character 6	Qualifier Character 7

C Common Iliac Vein, Right
D Common Iliac Vein, Left
F External Iliac Vein, Right
G External Iliac Vein, Left
H Hypogastric Vein, Right
   Gluteal vein
   Internal iliac vein
   Internal pudendal vein
   Lateral sacral vein
   Middle hemorrhoidal vein
   Obturator vein
   Uterine vein
   Vaginal vein
   Vesical vein
J Hypogastric Vein, Left
   See H Hypogastric Vein, Right
	M Femoral Vein, Right
	   Deep femoral (profunda
	     femoris) vein
	   Popliteal vein
	   Profunda femoris (deep
	     femoral) vein
	N Femoral Vein, Left
	   See M Femoral Vein, Right
	P Saphenous Vein, Right
	   External pudendal vein
	   Great(er) saphenous vein
	   Lesser saphenous vein
	   Small saphenous vein
	   Superficial circumflex iliac vein
	   Superficial epigastric vein
	Q Saphenous Vein, Left
	   See P Saphenous Vein, Right
	Y Lower Vein
		3 Percutaneous	**Z** No Device	**Ø** Ultrasonic
				Z No Qualifier

LC Limited Coverage   **NC** Noncovered   ⊞ Combination Member   HAC associated procedure   Combination Only   DRG Non-OR   Non-OR   New/Revised in **GREEN**

268

ICD-10-PCS 2021

Ø6F–Ø6F

Ø   Medical and Surgical
6   Lower Veins
H   Insertion   Definition: Putting in a nonbiological appliance that monitors, assists, performs, or prevents a physiological function but does not physically take the place of a body part
                 Explanation: None

Body Part Character 4		Approach Character 5	Device Character 6	Qualifier Character 7
Ø Inferior Vena Cava Postcava Right inferior phrenic vein Right ovarian vein Right second lumbar vein Right suprarenal vein Right testicular vein		**Ø** Open **3** Percutaneous	**3** Infusion Device	**T** Via Umbilical Vein **Z** No Qualifier
Ø Inferior Vena Cava Postcava Right inferior phrenic vein Right ovarian vein Right second lumbar vein Right suprarenal vein Right testicular vein		**Ø** Open **3** Percutaneous	**D** Intraluminal Device	**Z** No Qualifier
Ø Inferior Vena Cava Postcava Right inferior phrenic vein Right ovarian vein Right second lumbar vein Right suprarenal vein Right testicular vein		**4** Percutaneous Endoscopic	**3** Infusion Device **D** Intraluminal Device	**Z** No Qualifier
1 Splenic Vein Left gastroepiploic vein Pancreatic vein **2 Gastric Vein** **3 Esophageal Vein** **4 Hepatic Vein** **5 Superior Mesenteric Vein** Right gastroepiploic vein **6 Inferior Mesenteric Vein** Sigmoid vein Superior rectal vein **7 Colic Vein** Ileocolic vein Left colic vein Middle colic vein Right colic vein **8 Portal Vein** Hepatic portal vein **9 Renal Vein, Right** **B Renal Vein, Left** Left inferior phrenic vein Left ovarian vein Left second lumbar vein Left suprarenal vein Left testicular vein **C Common Iliac Vein, Right** **D Common Iliac Vein, Left** **F External Iliac Vein, Right** **G External Iliac Vein, Left**	**H Hypogastric Vein, Right** Gluteal vein Internal iliac vein Internal pudendal vein Lateral sacral vein Middle hemorrhoidal vein Obturator vein Uterine vein Vaginal vein Vesical vein **J Hypogastric Vein, Left** *See H Hypogastric Vein, Right* **M Femoral Vein, Right** Deep femoral (profunda femoris) vein Popliteal vein Profunda femoris (deep femoral) vein **N Femoral Vein, Left** *See M Femoral Vein, Right* **P Saphenous Vein, Right** External pudendal vein Great(er) saphenous vein Lesser saphenous vein Small saphenous vein Superficial circumflex iliac vein Superficial epigastric vein **Q Saphenous Vein, Left** *See P Saphenous Vein, Right* **T Foot Vein, Right** Common digital vein Dorsal metatarsal vein Dorsal venous arch Plantar digital vein Plantar metatarsal vein Plantar venous arch **V Foot Vein, Left** *See T Foot Vein, Right*	**Ø** Open **3** Percutaneous **4** Percutaneous Endoscopic	**3** Infusion Device **D** Intraluminal Device	**Z** No Qualifier
Y Lower Vein		**Ø** Open **3** Percutaneous **4** Percutaneous Endoscopic	**2** Monitoring Device **3** Infusion Device **D** Intraluminal Device **Y** Other Device	**Z** No Qualifier

Non-OR	06HØ[Ø,3]3[T,Z]
Non-OR	06HØ[Ø,3]DZ
Non-OR	06HØ4[3,D]Z
Non-OR	06H[1,2,3,4,5,6,7,8,9,B,C,D,F,G,H,J,M,N,P,Q,T,V][Ø,3,4]3Z
Non-OR	06HY[Ø,3,4]3Z
Non-OR	06HY32Z
Non-OR	06HY[3,4]YZ

LC Limited Coverage   **NC** Noncovered   ⊞ Combination Member   HAC associated procedure   Combination Only   DRG Non-OR   Non-OR   New/Revised in GREEN

ICD-10-PCS 2021   269

06H–06H

Ø   Medical and Surgical
6   Lower Veins
J   Inspection   Definition: Visually and/or manually exploring a body part

Explanation: Visual exploration may be performed with or without optical instrumentation. Manual exploration may be performed directly or through intervening body layers.

Body Part Character 4	Approach Character 5	Device Character 6	Qualifier Character 7
Y Lower Vein	Ø Open 3 Percutaneous 4 Percutaneous Endoscopic X External	Z No Device	Z No Qualifier

Non-OR   Ø6JY[3,X]ZZ

Ø   Medical and Surgical
6   Lower Veins
L   Occlusion   Definition: Completely closing an orifice or the lumen of a tubular body part

Explanation: The orifice can be a natural orifice or an artificially created orifice

Body Part Character 4	Approach Character 5	Device Character 6	Qualifier Character 7

Ø **Inferior Vena Cava**
   Postcava
   Right inferior phrenic vein
   Right ovarian vein
   Right second lumbar vein
   Right suprarenal vein
   Right testicular vein
1 **Splenic Vein**
   Left gastroepiploic vein
   Pancreatic vein
4 **Hepatic Vein**
5 **Superior Mesenteric Vein**
   Right gastroepiploic vein
6 **Inferior Mesenteric Vein**
   Sigmoid vein
   Superior rectal vein
7 **Colic Vein**
   Ileocolic vein
   Left colic vein
   Middle colic vein
   Right colic vein
8 **Portal Vein**
   Hepatic portal vein
9 **Renal Vein, Right**
B **Renal Vein, Left**
   Left inferior phrenic vein
   Left ovarian vein
   Left second lumbar vein
   Left suprarenal vein
   Left testicular vein
C **Common Iliac Vein, Right**
D **Common Iliac Vein, Left**
F **External Iliac Vein, Right**
G **External Iliac Vein, Left**
	H **Hypogastric Vein, Right**
	   Gluteal vein
	   Internal iliac vein
	   Internal pudendal vein
	   Lateral sacral vein
	   Middle hemorrhoidal vein
	   Obturator vein
	   Uterine vein
	   Vaginal vein
	   Vesical vein
	J **Hypogastric Vein, Left**
	   See H Hypogastric Vein, Right
	M **Femoral Vein, Right**
	   Deep femoral (profunda
	     femoris) vein
	   Popliteal vein
	   Profunda femoris (deep
	     femoral) vein
	N **Femoral Vein, Left**
	   See M Femoral Vein, Right
	P **Saphenous Vein, Right**
	   External pudendal vein
	   Great(er) saphenous vein
	   Lesser saphenous vein
	   Small saphenous vein
	   Superficial circumflex iliac vein
	   Superficial epigastric vein
	Q **Saphenous Vein, Left**
	   See P Saphenous Vein, Right
	T **Foot Vein, Right**
	   Common digital vein
	   Dorsal metatarsal vein
	   Dorsal venous arch
	   Plantar digital vein
	   Plantar metatarsal vein
	   Plantar venous arch
	V **Foot Vein, Left**
	   See T Foot Vein, Right
		Ø Open
		3 Percutaneous
		4 Percutaneous Endoscopic
			C Extraluminal Device
			D Intraluminal Device
			Z No Device
				Z No Qualifier

2 **Gastric Vein**
3 **Esophageal Vein**
		Ø Open
		3 Percutaneous
		4 Percutaneous Endoscopic
		7 Via Natural or Artificial
		   Opening
		8 Via Natural or Artificial
		   Opening Endoscopic
			C Extraluminal Device
			D Intraluminal Device
			Z No Device
				Z No Qualifier

Y Lower Vein		Ø Open 3 Percutaneous 4 Percutaneous Endoscopic	C Extraluminal Device D Intraluminal Device Z No Device	C Hemorrhoidal Plexus Z No Qualifier

Non-OR   Ø6L2[7,8][C,D,Z]Z
Non-OR   Ø6L3[3,4,7,8][C,D,Z]Z

LC Limited Coverage   NC Noncovered   ⊞ Combination Member   HAC associated procedure   Combination Only   DRG Non-OR   Non-OR   New/Revised in GREEN

270   ICD-10-PCS 2021

0   **Medical and Surgical**
6   **Lower Veins**
N   **Release**   Definition: Freeing a body part from an abnormal physical constraint by cutting or by the use of force

                            Explanation: Some of the restraining tissue may be taken out but none of the body part is taken out

Body Part Character 4		Approach Character 5	Device Character 6	Qualifier Character 7

0 **Inferior Vena Cava**
  Postcava
  Right inferior phrenic vein
  Right ovarian vein
  Right second lumbar vein
  Right suprarenal vein
  Right testicular vein
1 **Splenic Vein**
  Left gastroepiploic vein
  Pancreatic vein
2 **Gastric Vein**
3 **Esophageal Vein**
4 **Hepatic Vein**
5 **Superior Mesenteric Vein**
  Right gastroepiploic vein
6 **Inferior Mesenteric Vein**
  Sigmoid vein
  Superior rectal vein
7 **Colic Vein**
  Ileocolic vein
  Left colic vein
  Middle colic vein
  Right colic vein
8 **Portal Vein**
  Hepatic portal vein
9 **Renal Vein, Right**
B **Renal Vein, Left**
  Left inferior phrenic vein
  Left ovarian vein
  Left second lumbar vein
  Left suprarenal vein
  Left testicular vein
C **Common Iliac Vein, Right**
D **Common Iliac Vein, Left**
F **External Iliac Vein, Right**
G **External Iliac Vein, Left**
	H **Hypogastric Vein, Right**
	  Gluteal vein
	  Internal iliac vein
	  Internal pudendal vein
	  Lateral sacral vein
	  Middle hemorrhoidal vein
	  Obturator vein
	  Uterine vein
	  Vaginal vein
	  Vesical vein
	J **Hypogastric Vein, Left**
	  See H Hypogastric Vein, Right
	M **Femoral Vein, Right**
	  Deep femoral (profunda
	    femoris) vein
	  Popliteal vein
	  Profunda femoris (deep
	    femoral) vein
	N **Femoral Vein, Left**
	  See M Femoral Vein, Right
	P **Saphenous Vein, Right**
	  External pudendal vein
	  Great(er) saphenous vein
	  Lesser saphenous vein
	  Small saphenous vein
	  Superficial circumflex iliac vein
	  Superficial epigastric vein
	Q **Saphenous Vein, Left**
	  See P Saphenous Vein, Right
	T **Foot Vein, Right**
	  Common digital vein
	  Dorsal metatarsal vein
	  Dorsal venous arch
	  Plantar digital vein
	  Plantar metatarsal vein
	  Plantar venous arch
	V **Foot Vein, Left**
	  See T Foot Vein, Right
	Y **Lower Vein**
		0 Open
		3 Percutaneous
		4 Percutaneous Endoscopic
			Z No Device	**Z** No Qualifier

0   **Medical and Surgical**
6   **Lower Veins**
P   **Removal**   Definition: Taking out or off a device from a body part

                           Explanation: If a device is taken out and a similar device put in without cutting or puncturing the skin or mucous membrane, the procedure is coded to the root operation CHANGE. Otherwise, the procedure for taking out a device is coded to the root operation REMOVAL.

Body Part Character 4	Approach Character 5	Device Character 6	Qualifier Character 7

Y Lower Vein	**0** Open
	3 Percutaneous
	4 Percutaneous Endoscopic
		0 Drainage Device
		2 Monitoring Device
		3 Infusion Device
		7 Autologous Tissue
		    Substitute
		C Extraluminal Device
		D Intraluminal Device
		J Synthetic Substitute
		K Nonautologous Tissue
		    Substitute
		Y Other Device
			Z No Qualifier

Y Lower Vein	**X** External	**0** Drainage Device **2** Monitoring Device **3** Infusion Device **D** Intraluminal Device	**Z** No Qualifier

Non-OR   06PY3[0,2,3]Z
Non-OR   06PY[3,4]YZ
Non-OR   06PYX[0,2,3,D]Z

LC Limited Coverage   **NC** Noncovered   ⊞ Combination Member   HAC associated procedure   Combination Only   DRG Non-OR   Non-OR   New/Revised in GREEN

ICD-10-PCS 2021   **271**

06N–06P

0   **Medical and Surgical**
6   **Lower Veins**
Q   **Repair**   Definition: Restoring, to the extent possible, a body part to its normal anatomic structure and function
                     Explanation: Used only when the method to accomplish the repair is not one of the other root operations

Body Part Character 4	Approach Character 5	Device Character 6	Qualifier Character 7

0   **Inferior Vena Cava**
    Postcava
    Right inferior phrenic vein
    Right ovarian vein
    Right second lumbar vein
    Right suprarenal vein
    Right testicular vein
1   **Splenic Vein**
    Left gastroepiploic vein
    Pancreatic vein
2   **Gastric Vein**
3   **Esophageal Vein**
4   **Hepatic Vein**
5   **Superior Mesenteric Vein**
    Right gastroepiploic vein
6   **Inferior Mesenteric Vein**
    Sigmoid vein
    Superior rectal vein
7   **Colic Vein**
    Ileocolic vein
    Left colic vein
    Middle colic vein
    Right colic vein
8   **Portal Vein**
    Hepatic portal vein
9   **Renal Vein, Right**
B   **Renal Vein, Left**
    Left inferior phrenic vein
    Left ovarian vein
    Left second lumbar vein
    Left suprarenal vein
    Left testicular vein
C   **Common Iliac Vein, Right**
D   **Common Iliac Vein, Left**
F   **External Iliac Vein, Right**
G   **External Iliac Vein, Left**
H   **Hypogastric Vein, Right**
    Gluteal vein
    Internal iliac vein
    Internal pudendal vein
    Lateral sacral vein
    Middle hemorrhoidal vein
    Obturator vein
    Uterine vein
    Vaginal vein
    Vesical vein
J   **Hypogastric Vein, Left**
    See H Hypogastric Vein, Right
M   **Femoral Vein, Right**
    Deep femoral (profunda femoris) vein
    Popliteal vein
    Profunda femoris (deep femoral) vein
N   **Femoral Vein, Left**
    See M Femoral Vein, Right
P   **Saphenous Vein, Right**
    External pudendal vein
    Great(er) saphenous vein
    Lesser saphenous vein
    Small saphenous vein
    Superficial circumflex iliac vein
    Superficial epigastric vein
Q   **Saphenous Vein, Left**
    See P Saphenous Vein, Right
T   **Foot Vein, Right**
    Common digital vein
    Dorsal metatarsal vein
    Dorsal venous arch
    Plantar digital vein
    Plantar metatarsal vein
    Plantar venous arch
V   **Foot Vein, Left**
    See T Foot Vein, Right
Y   **Lower Vein**
	0 Open
	3 Percutaneous
	4 Percutaneous Endoscopic
		Z No Device	**Z** No Qualifier

LC Limited Coverage   **NC** Noncovered   ⊞ Combination Member   HAC associated procedure   Combination Only   DRG Non-OR   Non-OR   New/Revised in GREEN

272   ICD-10-PCS 2021

06Q–06Q

0   **Medical and Surgical**
6   **Lower Veins**
R   **Replacement**   Definition: Putting in or on biological or synthetic material that physically takes the place and/or function of all or a portion of a body part

                                Explanation: The body part may have been taken out or replaced, or may be taken out, physically eradicated, or rendered nonfunctional during the REPLACEMENT procedure. A REMOVAL procedure is coded for taking out the device used in a previous replacement procedure.

Body Part Character 4	Approach Character 5	Device Character 6	Qualifier Character 7

0   **Inferior Vena Cava**
     Postcava
     Right inferior phrenic vein
     Right ovarian vein
     Right second lumbar vein
     Right suprarenal vein
     Right testicular vein
1   **Splenic Vein**
     Left gastroepiploic vein
     Pancreatic vein
2   **Gastric Vein**
3   **Esophageal Vein**
4   **Hepatic Vein**
5   **Superior Mesenteric Vein**
     Right gastroepiploic vein
6   **Inferior Mesenteric Vein**
     Sigmoid vein
     Superior rectal vein
7   **Colic Vein**
     Ileocolic vein
     Left colic vein
     Middle colic vein
     Right colic vein
8   **Portal Vein**
     Hepatic portal vein
9   **Renal Vein, Right**
B   **Renal Vein, Left**
     Left inferior phrenic vein
     Left ovarian vein
     Left second lumbar vein
     Left suprarenal vein
     Left testicular vein
C   **Common Iliac Vein, Right**
D   **Common Iliac Vein, Left**
F   **External Iliac Vein, Right**
G   **External Iliac Vein, Left**
H   **Hypogastric Vein, Right**
     Gluteal vein
     Internal iliac vein
     Internal pudendal vein
     Lateral sacral vein
     Middle hemorrhoidal vein
     Obturator vein
     Uterine vein
     Vaginal vein
     Vesical vein
J   **Hypogastric Vein, Left**
     See H Hypogastric Vein, Right
M   **Femoral Vein, Right**
     Deep femoral (profunda femoris) vein
     Popliteal vein
     Profunda femoris (deep femoral) vein
N   **Femoral Vein, Left**
     See M Femoral Vein, Right
P   **Saphenous Vein, Right**
     External pudendal vein
     Great(er) saphenous vein
     Lesser saphenous vein
     Small saphenous vein
     Superficial circumflex iliac vein
     Superficial epigastric vein
Q   **Saphenous Vein, Left**
     See P Saphenous Vein, Right
T   **Foot Vein, Right**
     Common digital vein
     Dorsal metatarsal vein
     Dorsal venous arch
     Plantar digital vein
     Plantar metatarsal vein
     Plantar venous arch
V   **Foot Vein, Left**
     See T Foot Vein, Right
Y   **Lower Vein**
	0 Open
	4 Percutaneous Endoscopic
		7 Autologous Tissue Substitute
		J Synthetic Substitute
		K Nonautologous Tissue Substitute
			Z No Qualifier

LC Limited Coverage   NC Noncovered   ⊞ Combination Member   HAC associated procedure   Combination Only   DRG Non-OR   Non-OR   New/Revised in GREEN

ICD-10-PCS 2021   273

0   **Medical and Surgical**
6   **Lower Veins**
S   **Reposition**   Definition: Moving to its normal location, or other suitable location, all or a portion of a body part

                     Explanation: The body part is moved to a new location from an abnormal location, or from a normal location where it is not functioning correctly. The body part may or may not be cut out or off to be moved to the new location.

Body Part Character 4	Approach Character 5	Device Character 6	Qualifier Character 7

0 Inferior Vena Cava
   Postcava
   Right inferior phrenic vein
   Right ovarian vein
   Right second lumbar vein
   Right suprarenal vein
   Right testicular vein
1 Splenic Vein
   Left gastroepiploic vein
   Pancreatic vein
2 Gastric Vein
3 Esophageal Vein
4 Hepatic Vein
5 Superior Mesenteric Vein
   Right gastroepiploic vein
6 Inferior Mesenteric Vein
   Sigmoid vein
   Superior rectal vein
7 Colic Vein
   Ileocolic vein
   Left colic vein
   Middle colic vein
   Right colic vein
8 Portal Vein
   Hepatic portal vein
9 Renal Vein, Right
B Renal Vein, Left
   Left inferior phrenic vein
   Left ovarian vein
   Left second lumbar vein
   Left suprarenal vein
   Left testicular vein
C Common Iliac Vein, Right
D Common Iliac Vein, Left
F External Iliac Vein, Right
G External Iliac Vein, Left
H Hypogastric Vein, Right
   Gluteal vein
   Internal iliac vein
   Internal pudendal vein
   Lateral sacral vein
   Middle hemorrhoidal vein
   Obturator vein
   Uterine vein
   Vaginal vein
   Vesical vein
J Hypogastric Vein, Left
   See H Hypogastric Vein, Right
M Femoral Vein, Right
   Deep femoral (profunda femoris) vein
   Popliteal vein
   Profunda femoris (deep femoral) vein
N Femoral Vein, Left
   See M Femoral Vein, Right
P Saphenous Vein, Right
   External pudendal vein
   Great(er) saphenous vein
   Lesser saphenous vein
   Small saphenous vein
   Superficial circumflex iliac vein
   Superficial epigastric vein
Q Saphenous Vein, Left
   See P Saphenous Vein, Right
T Foot Vein, Right
   Common digital vein
   Dorsal metatarsal vein
   Dorsal venous arch
   Plantar digital vein
   Plantar metatarsal vein
   Plantar venous arch
V Foot Vein, Left
   See T Foot Vein, Right
Y Lower Vein
	0 Open
	3 Percutaneous
	4 Percutaneous Endoscopic
		Z No Device	**Z** No Qualifier

LC Limited Coverage   **NC** Noncovered   ⊞ Combination Member   HAC associated procedure   Combination Only   DRG Non-OR   Non-OR   New/Revised in GREEN

274   ICD-10-PCS 2021

0   **Medical and Surgical**
6   **Lower Veins**
U   **Supplement**   Definition: Putting in or on biological or synthetic material that physically reinforces and/or augments the function of a portion of a body part

Explanation: The biological material is non-living, or is living and from the same individual. The body part may have been previously replaced, and the SUPPLEMENT procedure is performed to physically reinforce and/or augment the function of the replaced body part.

Body Part Character 4	Approach Character 5	Device Character 6	Qualifier Character 7

0   **Inferior Vena Cava**
    Postcava
    Right inferior phrenic vein
    Right ovarian vein
    Right second lumbar vein
    Right suprarenal vein
    Right testicular vein
1   **Splenic Vein**
    Left gastroepiploic vein
    Pancreatic vein
2   **Gastric Vein**
3   **Esophageal Vein**
4   **Hepatic Vein**
5   **Superior Mesenteric Vein**
    Right gastroepiploic vein
6   **Inferior Mesenteric Vein**
    Sigmoid vein
    Superior rectal vein
7   **Colic Vein**
    Ileocolic vein
    Left colic vein
    Middle colic vein
    Right colic vein
8   **Portal Vein**
    Hepatic portal vein
9   **Renal Vein, Right**
B   **Renal Vein, Left**
    Left inferior phrenic vein
    Left ovarian vein
    Left second lumbar vein
    Left suprarenal vein
    Left testicular vein
C   **Common Iliac Vein, Right**
D   **Common Iliac Vein, Left**
F   **External Iliac Vein, Right**
G   **External Iliac Vein, Left**
H   **Hypogastric Vein, Right**
    Gluteal vein
    Internal iliac vein
    Internal pudendal vein
    Lateral sacral vein
    Middle hemorrhoidal vein
    Obturator vein
    Uterine vein
    Vaginal vein
    Vesical vein
J   **Hypogastric Vein, Left**
    See H Hypogastric Vein, Right
M   **Femoral Vein, Right**
    Deep femoral (profunda femoris) vein
    Popliteal vein
    Profunda femoris (deep femoral) vein
N   **Femoral Vein, Left**
    See M Femoral Vein, Right
P   **Saphenous Vein, Right**
    External pudendal vein
    Great(er) saphenous vein
    Lesser saphenous vein
    Small saphenous vein
    Superficial circumflex iliac vein
    Superficial epigastric vein
Q   **Saphenous Vein, Left**
    See P Saphenous Vein, Right
T   **Foot Vein, Right**
    Common digital vein
    Dorsal metatarsal vein
    Dorsal venous arch
    Plantar digital vein
    Plantar metatarsal vein
    Plantar venous arch
V   **Foot Vein, Left**
    See T Foot Vein, Right
Y   **Lower Vein**
	0 Open
	3 Percutaneous
	4 Percutaneous Endoscopic
		7 Autologous Tissue Substitute
		J Synthetic Substitute
		K Nonautologous Tissue Substitute
			Z No Qualifier

LC Limited Coverage   **NC** Noncovered   ⊞ Combination Member   HAC associated procedure   Combination Only   DRG Non-OR   Non-OR   New/Revised in GREEN

ICD-10-PCS 2021   275

06U–06U

Ø   **Medical and Surgical**
6   **Lower Veins**
V   **Restriction**   Definition: Partially closing an orifice or the lumen of a tubular body part
                          Explanation: The orifice can be a natural orifice or an artificially created orifice

Body Part Character 4	Approach Character 5	Device Character 6	Qualifier Character 7

Ø **Inferior Vena Cava**
    Postcava
    Right inferior phrenic vein
    Right ovarian vein
    Right second lumbar vein
    Right suprarenal vein
    Right testicular vein
1 **Splenic Vein**
    Left gastroepiploic vein
    Pancreatic vein
2 **Gastric Vein**
3 **Esophageal Vein**
4 **Hepatic Vein**
5 **Superior Mesenteric Vein**
    Right gastroepiploic vein
6 **Inferior Mesenteric Vein**
    Sigmoid vein
    Superior rectal vein
7 **Colic Vein**
    Ileocolic vein
    Left colic vein
    Middle colic vein
    Right colic vein
8 **Portal Vein**
    Hepatic portal vein
9 **Renal Vein, Right**
B **Renal Vein, Left**
    Left inferior phrenic vein
    Left ovarian vein
    Left second lumbar vein
    Left suprarenal vein
    Left testicular vein
C **Common Iliac Vein, Right**
D **Common Iliac Vein, Left**
F **External Iliac Vein, Right**
G **External Iliac Vein, Left**
H **Hypogastric Vein, Right**
    Gluteal vein
    Internal iliac vein
    Internal pudendal vein
    Lateral sacral vein
    Middle hemorrhoidal vein
    Obturator vein
    Uterine vein
    Vaginal vein
    Vesical vein
J **Hypogastric Vein, Left**
    See H Hypogastric Vein, Right
M **Femoral Vein, Right**
    Deep femoral (profunda femoris) vein
    Popliteal vein
    Profunda femoris (deep femoral) vein
N **Femoral Vein, Left**
    See M Femoral Vein, Right
P **Saphenous Vein, Right**
    External pudendal vein
    Great(er) saphenous vein
    Lesser saphenous vein
    Small saphenous vein
    Superficial circumflex iliac vein
    Superficial epigastric vein
Q **Saphenous Vein, Left**
    See P Saphenous Vein, Right
T **Foot Vein, Right**
    Common digital vein
    Dorsal metatarsal vein
    Dorsal venous arch
    Plantar digital vein
    Plantar metatarsal vein
    Plantar venous arch
V **Foot Vein, Left**
    See T Foot Vein, Right
Y **Lower Vein**
	Ø Open
	3 Percutaneous
	4 Percutaneous Endoscopic
		C Extraluminal Device
		D Intraluminal Device
		Z No Device
			Z No Qualifier

LC Limited Coverage   NC Noncovered   ⊞ Combination Member   HAC associated procedure   Combination Only   DRG Non-OR   Non-OR   New/Revised in GREEN

276   ICD-10-PCS 2021

Ø   Medical and Surgical
6   Lower Veins
W   Revision

Definition: Correcting, to the extent possible, a portion of a malfunctioning device or the position of a displaced device

Explanation: Revision can include correcting a malfunctioning or displaced device by taking out or putting in components of the device such as a screw or pin

Body Part Character 4	Approach Character 5	Device Character 6	Qualifier Character 7
Y Lower Vein	Ø Open 3 Percutaneous 4 Percutaneous Endoscopic	Ø Drainage Device 2 Monitoring Device 3 Infusion Device 7 Autologous Tissue Substitute C Extraluminal Device D Intraluminal Device J Synthetic Substitute K Nonautologous Tissue Substitute Y Other Device	Z No Qualifier
Y Lower Vein	X External	Ø Drainage Device 2 Monitoring Device 3 Infusion Device 7 Autologous Tissue Substitute C Extraluminal Device D Intraluminal Device J Synthetic Substitute K Nonautologous Tissue Substitute	Z No Qualifier

Non-OR   06WY3[Ø,2,3,D]Z
Non-OR   06WY[3,4]YZ
Non-OR   06WYX[Ø,2,3,7,C,D,J,K]Z

LC Limited Coverage   NC Noncovered   ⊞ Combination Member   HAC associated procedure   Combination Only   DRG Non-OR   Non-OR   New/Revised in GREEN

ICD-10-PCS 2021   277

Lymphatic and Hemic Systems Ø72–Ø7Y

Character Meanings*

This Character Meaning table is provided as a guide to assist the user in the identification of character members that may be found in this section of code tables. It **SHOULD NOT** be used to build a PCS code.

Operation–Character 3	Body Part–Character 4	Approach–Character 5	Device–Character 6	Qualifier–Character 7
2　Change	Ø　Lymphatic, Head	Ø　Open	Ø　Drainage Device	Ø　Allogeneic
5　Destruction	1　Lymphatic, Right Neck	3　Percutaneous	1　Radioactive Element	1　Syngeneic
9　Drainage	2　Lymphatic, Left Neck	4　Percutaneous Endoscopic	3　Infusion Device	2　Zooplastic
B　Excision	3　Lymphatic, Right Upper Extremity	8　Via Natural or Artificial Opening Endoscopic	7　Autologous Tissue Substitute	X　Diagnostic
C　Extirpation	4　Lymphatic, Left Upper Extremity	X　External	C　Extraluminal Device	Z　No Qualifier
D　Extraction	5　Lymphatic, Right Axillary		D　Intraluminal Device	
H　Insertion	6　Lymphatic, Left Axillary		J　Synthetic Substitute	
J　Inspection	7　Lymphatic, Thorax		K　Nonautologous Tissue Substitute	
L　Occlusion	8　Lymphatic, Internal Mammary, Right		Y　Other Device	
N　Release	9　Lymphatic, Internal Mammary, Left		Z　No Device	
P　Removal	B　Lymphatic, Mesenteric			
Q　Repair	C　Lymphatic, Pelvis			
S　Reposition	D　Lymphatic, Aortic			
T　Resection	F　Lymphatic, Right Lower Extremity			
U　Supplement	G　Lymphatic, Left Lower Extremity			
V　Restriction	H　Lymphatic, Right Inguinal			
W　Revision	J　Lymphatic, Left Inguinal			
Y　Transplantation	K　Thoracic Duct			
	L　Cisterna Chyli			
	M　Thymus			
	N　Lymphatic			
	P　Spleen			
	Q　Bone Marrow, Sternum			
	R　Bone Marrow, Iliac			
	S　Bone Marrow, Vertebral			
	T　Bone Marrow			

* Includes lymph vessels and lymph nodes.

AHA Coding Clinic for table Ø79
2018, 4Q, 84	Fine needle aspiration biopsy of lymphatic tissue
2017, 1Q, 34	Lymphovenous bypass following mastectomy
2014, 1Q, 26	Transbronchial needle aspiration lymph node biopsy
2013, 4Q, 111	Transbronchial needle aspiration lymph node biopsy

AHA Coding Clinic for table Ø7B
2019, 1Q, 3-8	Whipple procedure
2018, 4Q, 84	Fine needle aspiration biopsy of lymphatic tissue
2018, 1Q, 22	Resection of lymph node chains
2016, 1Q, 30	Axillary lymph node resection with modified radical mastectomy
2014, 3Q, 10	Selective excision of paratracheal lymph nodes
2014, 1Q, 20	Fiducial marker placement
2014, 1Q, 26	Transbronchial endoscopic lymph node aspiration biopsy

AHA Coding Clinic for table Ø7D
2018, 4Q, 84	Fine needle aspiration biopsy of lymphatic tissue
2013, 4Q, 111	Root operation for bone marrow biopsy

AHA Coding Clinic for table Ø7Q
2017, 1Q, 34	Lymphovenous bypass following mastectomy

AHA Coding Clinic for table Ø7S
2019, 3Q, 29	Thymus transplant for T-Cell production

AHA Coding Clinic for table Ø7T
2018, 1Q, 22	Resection of lymph node chains
2016, 2Q, 12	Resection of malignant neoplasm of infratemporal fossa
2016, 1Q, 30	Axillary lymph node resection with modified radical mastectomy
2015, 4Q, 13	New Section X codes—New Technology procedures
2014, 3Q, 9	Radical resection of level I lymph nodes
2014, 3Q, 16	Repair of Tetralogy of Fallot

AHA Coding Clinic for table Ø7Y
2019, 3Q, 29	Thymus transplant for T-Cell production

Lymphatic System

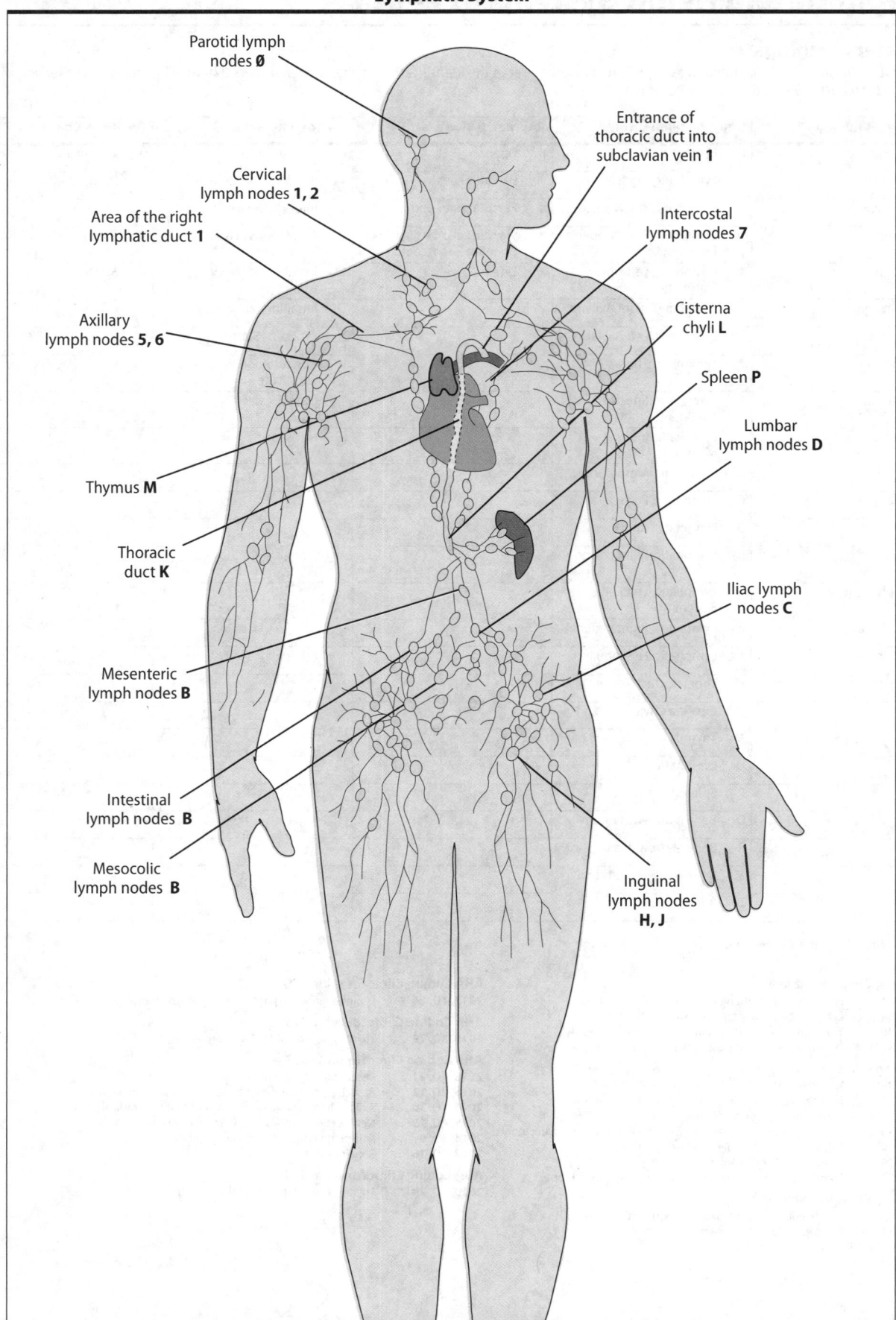

Parotid lymph nodes **Ø**

Entrance of thoracic duct into subclavian vein **1**

Cervical lymph nodes **1, 2**

Intercostal lymph nodes **7**

Area of the right lymphatic duct **1**

Cisterna chyli **L**

Axillary lymph nodes **5, 6**

Spleen **P**

Lumbar lymph nodes **D**

Thymus **M**

Thoracic duct **K**

Iliac lymph nodes **C**

Mesenteric lymph nodes **B**

Intestinal lymph nodes **B**

Inguinal lymph nodes **H, J**

Mesocolic lymph nodes **B**

Ø   Medical and Surgical
7   Lymphatic and Hemic Systems
2   Change   Definition: Taking out or off a device from a body part and putting back an identical or similar device in or on the same body part without cutting or puncturing the skin or a mucous membrane

                               Explanation: All CHANGE procedures are coded using the approach EXTERNAL

Body Part Character 4		Approach Character 5	Device Character 6	Qualifier Character 7

K   Thoracic Duct
     Left jugular trunk
     Left subclavian trunk
L   Cisterna Chyli
     Intestinal lymphatic trunk
     Lumbar lymphatic trunk
	M Thymus
	     Thymus gland
	N Lymphatic
	P Spleen
	     Accessory spleen
	T Bone Marrow
		X External	**Ø** Drainage Device
			Y Other Device
				Z No Qualifier

Non-OR   All body part, approach, device, and qualifier values

Ø   Medical and Surgical
7   Lymphatic and Hemic Systems
5   Destruction   Definition: Physical eradication of all or a portion of a body part by the direct use of energy, force, or a destructive agent

                               Explanation: None of the body part is physically taken out

Body Part Character 4		Approach Character 5	Device Character 6	Qualifier Character 7

Ø   Lymphatic, Head
     Buccinator lymph node
     Infraauricular lymph node
     Infraparotid lymph node
     Parotid lymph node
     Preauricular lymph node
     Submandibular lymph node
     Submaxillary lymph node
     Submental lymph node
     Subparotid lymph node
     Suprahyoid lymph node
1   Lymphatic, Right Neck
     Cervical lymph node
     Jugular lymph node
     Mastoid (postauricular) lymph node
     Occipital lymph node
     Postauricular (mastoid) lymph node
     Retropharyngeal lymph node
     Right jugular trunk
     Right lymphatic duct
     Right subclavian trunk
     Supraclavicular (Virchow's) lymph node
     Virchow's (supraclavicular) lymph node
2   Lymphatic, Left Neck
     Cervical lymph node
     Jugular lymph node
     Mastoid (postauricular) lymph node
     Occipital lymph node
     Postauricular (mastoid) lymph node
     Retropharyngeal lymph node
     Supraclavicular (Virchow's) lymph node
     Virchow's (supraclavicular) lymph node
3   Lymphatic, Right Upper Extremity
     Cubital lymph node
     Deltopectoral (infraclavicular) lymph
        node
     Epitrochlear lymph node
     Infraclavicular (deltopectoral) lymph
        node
     Supratrochlear lymph node
4   Lymphatic, Left Upper Extremity
     See 3 Lymphatic, Right Upper Extremity
5   Lymphatic, Right Axillary
     Anterior (pectoral) lymph node
     Apical (subclavicular) lymph node
     Brachial (lateral) lymph node
     Central axillary lymph node
     Lateral (brachial) lymph node
     Pectoral (anterior) lymph node
     Posterior (subscapular) lymph node
     Subclavicular (apical) lymph node
     Subscapular (posterior) lymph node
	6 Lymphatic, Left Axillary
	     See 5 Lymphatic, Right Axillary
	7 Lymphatic, Thorax
	     Intercostal lymph node
	     Mediastinal lymph node
	     Parasternal lymph node
	     Paratracheal lymph node
	     Tracheobronchial lymph node
	8 Lymphatic, Internal Mammary, Right
	9 Lymphatic, Internal Mammary, Left
	B Lymphatic, Mesenteric
	     Inferior mesenteric lymph node
	     Pararectal lymph node
	     Superior mesenteric lymph node
	C Lymphatic, Pelvis
	     Common iliac (subaortic) lymph node
	     Gluteal lymph node
	     Iliac lymph node
	     Inferior epigastric lymph node
	     Obturator lymph node
	     Sacral lymph node
	     Subaortic (common iliac) lymph node
	     Suprainguinal lymph node
	D Lymphatic, Aortic
	     Celiac lymph node
	     Gastric lymph node
	     Hepatic lymph node
	     Lumbar lymph node
	     Pancreaticosplenic lymph node
	     Paraaortic lymph node
	     Retroperitoneal lymph node
	F Lymphatic, Right Lower Extremity
	     Femoral lymph node
	     Popliteal lymph node
	G Lymphatic, Left Lower Extremity
	     See F Lymphatic, Right Lower Extremity
	H Lymphatic, Right Inguinal
	J Lymphatic, Left Inguinal
	K Thoracic Duct
	     Left jugular trunk
	     Left subclavian trunk
	L Cisterna Chyli
	     Intestinal lymphatic trunk
	     Lumbar lymphatic trunk
	M Thymus
	     Thymus gland
	P Spleen
	     Accessory spleen
		Ø Open
		3 Percutaneous
		4 Percutaneous Endoscopic
			Z No Device	**Z** No Qualifier

Ø   Medical and Surgical
7   Lymphatic and Hemic Systems
9   Drainage   Definition: Taking or letting out fluids and/or gases from a body part
                   Explanation: The qualifier DIAGNOSTIC is used to identify drainage procedures that are biopsies

Body Part Character 4		Approach Character 5	Device Character 6	Qualifier Character 7

Ø Lymphatic, Head
 Buccinator lymph node
 Infraauricular lymph node
 Infraparotid lymph node
 Parotid lymph node
 Preauricular lymph node
 Submandibular lymph node
 Submaxillary lymph node
 Submental lymph node
 Subparotid lymph node
 Suprahyoid lymph node
 1 Lymphatic, Right Neck
 Cervical lymph node
 Jugular lymph node
 Mastoid (postauricular) lymph node
 Occipital lymph node
 Postauricular (mastoid) lymph node
 Retropharyngeal lymph node
 Right jugular trunk
 Right lymphatic duct
 Right subclavian trunk
 Supraclavicular (Virchow's) lymph
     node
 Virchow's (supraclavicular) lymph
     node
 2 Lymphatic, Left Neck
 Cervical lymph node
 Jugular lymph node
 Mastoid (postauricular) lymph node
 Occipital lymph node
 Postauricular (mastoid) lymph node
 Retropharyngeal lymph node
 Supraclavicular (Virchow's) lymph
     node
 Virchow's (supraclavicular) lymph
     node
 3 Lymphatic, Right Upper Extremity
 Cubital lymph node
 Deltopectoral (infraclavicular) lymph
     node
 Epitrochlear lymph node
 Infraclavicular (deltopectoral) lymph
     node
 Supratrochlear lymph node
 4 Lymphatic, Left Upper Extremity
 See 3 Lymphatic, Right Upper Extremity
 5 Lymphatic, Right Axillary
 Anterior (pectoral) lymph node
 Apical (subclavicular) lymph node
 Brachial (lateral) lymph node
 Central axillary lymph node
 Lateral (brachial) lymph node
 Pectoral (anterior) lymph node
 Posterior (subscapular) lymph node
 Subclavicular (apical) lymph node
 Subscapular (posterior) lymph node
	6 Lymphatic, Left Axillary
	 See 5 Lymphatic, Right Axillary
	 7 Lymphatic, Thorax
	 Intercostal lymph node
	 Mediastinal lymph node
	 Parasternal lymph node
	 Paratracheal lymph node
	 Tracheobronchial lymph node
	 8 Lymphatic, Internal Mammary, Right
	 9 Lymphatic, Internal Mammary, Left
	 B Lymphatic, Mesenteric
	 Inferior mesenteric lymph node
	 Pararectal lymph node
	 Superior mesenteric lymph node
	 C Lymphatic, Pelvis
	 Common iliac (subaortic) lymph node
	 Gluteal lymph node
	 Iliac lymph node
	 Inferior epigastric lymph node
	 Obturator lymph node
	 Sacral lymph node
	 Subaortic (common iliac) lymph node
	 Suprainguinal lymph node
	 D Lymphatic, Aortic
	 Celiac lymph node
	 Gastric lymph node
	 Hepatic lymph node
	 Lumbar lymph node
	 Pancreaticosplenic lymph node
	 Paraaortic lymph node
	 Retroperitoneal lymph node
	 F Lymphatic, Right Lower Extremity
	 Femoral lymph node
	 Popliteal lymph node
	 G Lymphatic, Left Lower Extremity
	 See F Lymphatic, Right Lower Extremity
	 H Lymphatic, Right Inguinal
	 J Lymphatic, Left Inguinal
	 K Thoracic Duct
	 Left jugular trunk
	 Left subclavian trunk
	 L Cisterna Chyli
	 Intestinal lymphatic trunk
	 Lumbar lymphatic trunk
		Ø Open
		 3 Percutaneous
		 4 Percutaneous Endoscopic
		 8 Via Natural or Artificial Opening Endoscopic
			Ø Drainage Device	**Z No Qualifier**

Non-OR	Ø79[Ø,1,2,3,4,5,6,7,8,9,B,C,D,F,G,H,J,K,L][3,8]ØZ

Ø79 Continued on next page

Ø79 Continued

Ø   Medical and Surgical
7   Lymphatic and Hemic Systems
9   Drainage   Definition: Taking or letting out fluids and/or gases from a body part
                            Explanation: The qualifier DIAGNOSTIC is used to identify drainage procedures that are biopsies

Body Part Character 4		Approach Character 5	Device Character 6	Qualifier Character 7

Ø Lymphatic, Head
 Buccinator lymph node
 Infraauricular lymph node
 Infraparotid lymph node
 Parotid lymph node
 Preauricular lymph node
 Submandibular lymph node
 Submaxillary lymph node
 Submental lymph node
 Subparotid lymph node
 Suprahyoid lymph node
 1 Lymphatic, Right Neck
 Cervical lymph node
 Jugular lymph node
 Mastoid (postauricular) lymph node
 Occipital lymph node
 Postauricular (mastoid) lymph node
 Retropharyngeal lymph node
 Right jugular trunk
 Right lymphatic duct
 Right subclavian trunk
 Supraclavicular (Virchow's) lymph
       node
 Virchow's (supraclavicular) lymph
       node
 2 Lymphatic, Left Neck
 Cervical lymph node
 Jugular lymph node
 Mastoid (postauricular) lymph node
 Occipital lymph node
 Postauricular (mastoid) lymph node
 Retropharyngeal lymph node
 Supraclavicular (Virchow's) lymph
       node
 Virchow's (supraclavicular) lymph
       node
 3 Lymphatic, Right Upper Extremity
 Cubital lymph node
 Deltopectoral (infraclavicular) lymph
       node
 Epitrochlear lymph node
 Infraclavicular (deltopectoral) lymph
       node
 Supratrochlear lymph node
 4 Lymphatic, Left Upper Extremity
 See 3 Lymphatic, Right Upper Extremity
 5 Lymphatic, Right Axillary
 Anterior (pectoral) lymph node
 Apical (subclavicular) lymph node
 Brachial (lateral) lymph node
 Central axillary lymph node
 Lateral (brachial) lymph node
 Pectoral (anterior) lymph node
 Posterior (subscapular) lymph node
 Subclavicular (apical) lymph node
 Subscapular (posterior) lymph node
	6 Lymphatic, Left Axillary
	 See 5 Lymphatic, Right Axillary
	 7 Lymphatic, Thorax
	 Intercostal lymph node
	 Mediastinal lymph node
	 Parasternal lymph node
	 Paratracheal lymph node
	 Tracheobronchial lymph node
	 8 Lymphatic, Internal Mammary, Right
	 9 Lymphatic, Internal Mammary, Left
	 B Lymphatic, Mesenteric
	 Inferior mesenteric lymph node
	 Pararectal lymph node
	 Superior mesenteric lymph node
	 C Lymphatic, Pelvis
	 Common iliac (subaortic) lymph node
	 Gluteal lymph node
	 Iliac lymph node
	 Inferior epigastric lymph node
	 Obturator lymph node
	 Sacral lymph node
	 Subaortic (common iliac) lymph node
	 Suprainguinal lymph node
	 D Lymphatic, Aortic
	 Celiac lymph node
	 Gastric lymph node
	 Hepatic lymph node
	 Lumbar lymph node
	 Pancreaticosplenic lymph node
	 Paraaortic lymph node
	 Retroperitoneal lymph node
	 F Lymphatic, Right Lower Extremity
	 Femoral lymph node
	 Popliteal lymph node
	 G Lymphatic, Left Lower Extremity
	 See F Lymphatic, Right Lower Extremity
	 H Lymphatic, Right Inguinal
	 J Lymphatic, Left Inguinal
	 K Thoracic Duct
	 Left jugular trunk
	 Left subclavian trunk
	 L Cisterna Chyli
	 Intestinal lymphatic trunk
	 Lumbar lymphatic trunk
		Ø Open
		 3 Percutaneous
		 4 Percutaneous
		      Endoscopic
		 8 Via Natural or
		      Artificial Opening
		      Endoscopic
			Z No Device	**X** Diagnostic
				 Z No Qualifier

M Thymus Thymus gland **P Spleen** Accessory spleen **T Bone Marrow**		**Ø** Open **3** Percutaneous **4** Percutaneous Endoscopic	**Ø** Drainage Device	**Z** No Qualifier
M Thymus Thymus gland **P Spleen** Accessory spleen **T Bone Marrow**		**Ø** Open **3** Percutaneous **4** Percutaneous Endoscopic	**Z** No Device	**X** Diagnostic **Z** No Qualifier

Non-OR	Ø79[Ø,1,2,3,4,5,6,7,8,9,B,C,D,F,G,H,J,K,L]8ZX
Non-OR	Ø79[Ø,1,2,3,4,5,6,7,8,9,B,C,D,F,G,H,J,K,L][3,8]ZZ
Non-OR	Ø79M3ØZ
Non-OR	Ø79P[3,4]ØZ
Non-OR	Ø79T[Ø,3,4]ØZ
Non-OR	Ø79M3ZZ
Non-OR	Ø79P[3,4]Z[X,Z]
Non-OR	Ø79T[Ø,3,4]Z[X,Z]

Ø   Medical and Surgical
7   Lymphatic and Hemic Systems
B   Excision   Definition: Cutting out or off, without replacement, a portion of a body part
                     Explanation: The qualifier DIAGNOSTIC is used to identify excision procedures that are biopsies

Body Part Character 4		Approach Character 5	Device Character 6	Qualifier Character 7

Ø Lymphatic, Head
Buccinator lymph node
Infraauricular lymph node
Infraparotid lymph node
Parotid lymph node
Preauricular lymph node
Submandibular lymph node
Submaxillary lymph node
Submental lymph node
Subparotid lymph node
Suprahyoid lymph node
1 Lymphatic, Right Neck
Cervical lymph node
Jugular lymph node
Mastoid (postauricular) lymph node
Occipital lymph node
Postauricular (mastoid) lymph node
Retropharyngeal lymph node
Right jugular trunk
Right lymphatic duct
Right subclavian trunk
Supraclavicular (Virchow's) lymph
    node
Virchow's (supraclavicular) lymph
    node
2 Lymphatic, Left Neck
Cervical lymph node
Jugular lymph node
Mastoid (postauricular) lymph node
Occipital lymph node
Postauricular (mastoid) lymph node
Retropharyngeal lymph node
Supraclavicular (Virchow's) lymph
    node
Virchow's (supraclavicular) lymph
    node
3 Lymphatic, Right Upper Extremity
Cubital lymph node
Deltopectoral (infraclavicular) lymph
    node
Epitrochlear lymph node
Infraclavicular (deltopectoral) lymph
    node
Supratrochlear lymph node
4 Lymphatic, Left Upper Extremity
See 3 Lymphatic, Right Upper Extremity
5 Lymphatic, Right Axillary
Anterior (pectoral) lymph node
Apical (subclavicular) lymph node
Brachial (lateral) lymph node
Central axillary lymph node
Lateral (brachial) lymph node
Pectoral (anterior) lymph node
Posterior (subscapular) lymph node
Subclavicular (apical) lymph node
Subscapular (posterior) lymph node
	6 Lymphatic, Left Axillary
	See 5 Lymphatic, Right Axillary
	7 Lymphatic, Thorax
	Intercostal lymph node
	Mediastinal lymph node
	Parasternal lymph node
	Paratracheal lymph node
	Tracheobronchial lymph node
	8 Lymphatic, Internal Mammary, Right
	9 Lymphatic, Internal Mammary, Left
	B Lymphatic, Mesenteric
	Inferior mesenteric lymph node
	Pararectal lymph node
	Superior mesenteric lymph node
	C Lymphatic, Pelvis
	Common iliac (subaortic) lymph node
	Gluteal lymph node
	Iliac lymph node
	Inferior epigastric lymph node
	Obturator lymph node
	Sacral lymph node
	Subaortic (common iliac) lymph node
	Suprainguinal lymph node
	D Lymphatic, Aortic
	Celiac lymph node
	Gastric lymph node
	Hepatic lymph node
	Lumbar lymph node
	Pancreaticosplenic lymph node
	Paraaortic lymph node
	Retroperitoneal lymph node
	F Lymphatic, Right Lower Extremity
	Femoral lymph node
	Popliteal lymph node
	G Lymphatic, Left Lower Extremity
	See F Lymphatic, Right Lower Extremity
	H Lymphatic, Right Inguinal ⊞
	J Lymphatic, Left Inguinal ⊞
	K Thoracic Duct
	Left jugular trunk
	Left subclavian trunk
	L Cisterna Chyli
	Intestinal lymphatic trunk
	Lumbar lymphatic trunk
	M Thymus
	Thymus gland
	P Spleen
	Accessory spleen
		Ø Open
		3 Percutaneous
		**4 Percutaneous
		    Endoscopic**
			Z No Device	**X Diagnostic**
				Z No Qualifier

Non-OR   Ø7BP[3,4]ZX

See Appendix L for Procedure Combinations
    ⊞   Ø7B[H,J][Ø,4]ZZ

Ø   **Medical and Surgical**
7   **Lymphatic and Hemic Systems**
C   **Extirpation**   Definition: Taking or cutting out solid matter from a body part

                        Explanation: The solid matter may be an abnormal byproduct of a biological function or a foreign body; it may be imbedded in a body part or in the lumen of a tubular body part. The solid matter may or may not have been previously broken into pieces.

Body Part Character 4		Approach Character 5	Device Character 6	Qualifier Character 7

Ø **Lymphatic, Head**
   Buccinator lymph node
   Infraauricular lymph node
   Infraparotid lymph node
   Parotid lymph node
   Preauricular lymph node
   Submandibular lymph node
   Submaxillary lymph node
   Submental lymph node
   Subparotid lymph node
   Suprahyoid lymph node
1 **Lymphatic, Right Neck**
   Cervical lymph node
   Jugular lymph node
   Mastoid (postauricular) lymph node
   Occipital lymph node
   Postauricular (mastoid) lymph node
   Retropharyngeal lymph node
   Right jugular trunk
   Right lymphatic duct
   Right subclavian trunk
   Supraclavicular (Virchow's) lymph node
   Virchow's (supraclavicular) lymph node
2 **Lymphatic, Left Neck**
   Cervical lymph node
   Jugular lymph node
   Mastoid (postauricular) lymph node
   Occipital lymph node
   Postauricular (mastoid) lymph node
   Retropharyngeal lymph node
   Supraclavicular (Virchow's) lymph node
   Virchow's (supraclavicular) lymph node
3 **Lymphatic, Right Upper Extremity**
   Cubital lymph node
   Deltopectoral (infraclavicular) lymph node
   Epitrochlear lymph node
   Infraclavicular (deltopectoral) lymph node
   Supratrochlear lymph node
4 **Lymphatic, Left Upper Extremity**
   See 3 Lymphatic, Right Upper Extremity
5 **Lymphatic, Right Axillary**
   Anterior (pectoral) lymph node
   Apical (subclavicular) lymph node
   Brachial (lateral) lymph node
   Central axillary lymph node
   Lateral (brachial) lymph node
   Pectoral (anterior) lymph node
   Posterior (subscapular) lymph node
   Subclavicular (apical) lymph node
   Subscapular (posterior) lymph node
	6 **Lymphatic, Left Axillary**
	   See 5 Lymphatic, Right Axillary
	7 **Lymphatic, Thorax**
	   Intercostal lymph node
	   Mediastinal lymph node
	   Parasternal lymph node
	   Paratracheal lymph node
	   Tracheobronchial lymph node
	8 **Lymphatic, Internal Mammary, Right**
	9 **Lymphatic, Internal Mammary, Left**
	B **Lymphatic, Mesenteric**
	   Inferior mesenteric lymph node
	   Pararectal lymph node
	   Superior mesenteric lymph node
	C **Lymphatic, Pelvis**
	   Common iliac (subaortic) lymph node
	   Gluteal lymph node
	   Iliac lymph node
	   Inferior epigastric lymph node
	   Obturator lymph node
	   Sacral lymph node
	   Subaortic (common iliac) lymph node
	   Suprainguinal lymph node
	D **Lymphatic, Aortic**
	   Celiac lymph node
	   Gastric lymph node
	   Hepatic lymph node
	   Lumbar lymph node
	   Pancreaticosplenic lymph node
	   Paraaortic lymph node
	   Retroperitoneal lymph node
	F **Lymphatic, Right Lower Extremity**
	   Femoral lymph node
	   Popliteal lymph node
	G **Lymphatic, Left Lower Extremity**
	   See F Lymphatic, Right Lower Extremity
	H **Lymphatic, Right Inguinal**
	J **Lymphatic, Left Inguinal**
	K **Thoracic Duct**
	   Left jugular trunk
	   Left subclavian trunk
	L **Cisterna Chyli**
	   Intestinal lymphatic trunk
	   Lumbar lymphatic trunk
	M **Thymus**
	   Thymus gland
	P **Spleen**
	   Accessory spleen
		Ø Open
		3 Percutaneous
		4 Percutaneous Endoscopic
			Z No Device	**Z** No Qualifier

Non-OR   Ø7CP[3,4]ZZ

Lymphatic and Hemic Systems *(side tab)*

Ø   **Medical and Surgical**
7   **Lymphatic and Hemic Systems**
D   **Extraction**   Definition: Pulling or stripping out or off all or a portion of a body part by the use of force
                             Explanation: The qualifier DIAGNOSTIC is used to identify extraction procedures that are biopsies

Body Part Character 4		Approach Character 5	Device Character 6	Qualifier Character 7

Ø **Lymphatic, Head**
   Buccinator lymph node
   Infraauricular lymph node
   Infraparotid lymph node
   Parotid lymph node
   Preauricular lymph node
   Submandibular lymph node
   Submaxillary lymph node
   Submental lymph node
   Subparotid lymph node
   Suprahyoid lymph node
1 **Lymphatic, Right Neck**
   Cervical lymph node
   Jugular lymph node
   Mastoid (postauricular) lymph
     node
   Occipital lymph node
   Postauricular (mastoid) lymph
     node
   Retropharyngeal lymph node
   Right jugular trunk
   Right lymphatic duct
   Right subclavian trunk
   Supraclavicular (Virchow's)
     lymph node
   Virchow's (supraclavicular)
     lymph node
2 **Lymphatic, Left Neck**
   Cervical lymph node
   Jugular lymph node
   Mastoid (postauricular) lymph
     node
   Occipital lymph node
   Postauricular (mastoid) lymph
     node
   Retropharyngeal lymph node
   Supraclavicular (Virchow's)
     lymph node
   Virchow's (supraclavicular)
     lymph node
3 **Lymphatic, Right Upper**
   Extremity
   Cubital lymph node
   Deltopectoral (infraclavicular)
     lymph node
   Epitrochlear lymph node
   Infraclavicular (deltopectoral)
     lymph node
   Supratrochlear lymph node
4 **Lymphatic, Left Upper**
   Extremity
   See 3 Lymphatic, Right Upper
     Extremity
5 **Lymphatic, Right Axillary**
   Anterior (pectoral) lymph node
   Apical (subclavicular) lymph
     node
   Brachial (lateral) lymph node
   Central axillary lymph node
   Lateral (brachial) lymph node
   Pectoral (anterior) lymph node
   Posterior (subscapular) lymph
     node
   Subclavicular (apical) lymph
     node
   Subscapular (posterior) lymph
     node
	6 **Lymphatic, Left Axillary**
	   See 5 Lymphatic, Right Axillary
	7 **Lymphatic, Thorax**
	   Intercostal lymph node
	   Mediastinal lymph node
	   Parasternal lymph node
	   Paratracheal lymph node
	   Tracheobronchial lymph node
	8 **Lymphatic, Internal**
	   Mammary, Right
	9 **Lymphatic, Internal**
	   Mammary, Left
	B **Lymphatic, Mesenteric**
	   Inferior mesenteric lymph
	     node
	   Pararectal lymph node
	   Superior mesenteric lymph
	     node
	C **Lymphatic, Pelvis**
	   Common iliac (subaortic)
	     lymph node
	   Gluteal lymph node
	   Iliac lymph node
	   Inferior epigastric lymph node
	   Obturator lymph node
	   Sacral lymph node
	   Subaortic (common iliac)
	     lymph node
	   Suprainguinal lymph node
	D **Lymphatic, Aortic**
	   Celiac lymph node
	   Gastric lymph node
	   Hepatic lymph node
	   Lumbar lymph node
	   Pancreaticosplenic lymph
	     node
	   Paraaortic lymph node
	   Retroperitoneal lymph node
	F **Lymphatic, Right Lower**
	   Extremity
	   Femoral lymph node
	   Popliteal lymph node
	G **Lymphatic, Left Lower**
	   Extremity
	   See F Lymphatic, Right Lower
	     Extremity
	H **Lymphatic, Right Inguinal**
	J **Lymphatic, Left Inguinal**
	K **Thoracic Duct**
	   Left jugular trunk
	   Left subclavian trunk
	L **Cisterna Chyli**
	   Intestinal lymphatic trunk
	   Lumbar lymphatic trunk
		3 Percutaneous
		4 Percutaneous Endoscopic
		8 Via Natural or Artificial
		   Opening Endoscopic
			Z No Device	**X** Diagnostic

M **Thymus**
   Thymus gland
P **Spleen**
   Accessory spleen
		3 Percutaneous
		4 Percutaneous Endoscopic
			Z No Device	**X** Diagnostic

Q **Bone Marrow, Sternum** **R** **Bone Marrow, Iliac** **S** **Bone Marrow, Vertebral**		**Ø** Open **3** Percutaneous	**Z** No Device	**X** Diagnostic **Z** No Qualifier

Non-OR   All body part, approach, device, and qualifier values

---

0 **Medical and Surgical**
7 **Lymphatic and Hemic Systems**
H **Insertion**   Definition: Putting in a nonbiological appliance that monitors, assists, performs, or prevents a physiological function but does not physically take the place of a body part
   Explanation: None

Body Part Character 4	Approach Character 5	Device Character 6	Qualifier Character 7

K Thoracic Duct
  Left jugular trunk
  Left subclavian trunk
L Cisterna Chyli
  Intestinal lymphatic trunk
  Lumbar lymphatic trunk
M Thymus
  Thymus gland
N Lymphatic
P Spleen
  Accessory spleen
T Bone Marrow
	0 Open
	3 Percutaneous
	4 Percutaneous Endoscopic
		1 Radioactive Element
		3 Infusion Device
		Y Other Device
			Z No Qualifier

Non-OR	07H[K,L,M,N,P][0,3,4]3Z
Non-OR	07H[K,L,M]3YZ
Non-OR	07H[N,P][3,4]YZ

0 **Medical and Surgical**
7 **Lymphatic and Hemic Systems**
J **Inspection**   Definition: Visually and/or manually exploring a body part
   Explanation: Visual exploration may be performed with or without optical instrumentation. Manual exploration may be performed directly or through intervening body layers.

Body Part Character 4	Approach Character 5	Device Character 6	Qualifier Character 7

K Thoracic Duct
  Left jugular trunk
  Left subclavian trunk
L Cisterna Chyli
  Intestinal lymphatic trunk
  Lumbar lymphatic trunk
M Thymus
  Thymus gland
T Bone Marrow
	0 Open
	3 Percutaneous
	4 Percutaneous Endoscopic
		Z No Device	**Z** No Qualifier

N Lymphatic	**0** Open **3** Percutaneous **4** Percutaneous Endoscopic **8** Via Natural or Artificial Opening Endoscopic **X** External	**Z** No Device	**Z** No Qualifier
P Spleen Accessory spleen	**0** Open **3** Percutaneous **4** Percutaneous Endoscopic **X** External	**Z** No Device	**Z** No Qualifier

Non-OR	07J[K,L,M]3ZZ
Non-OR	07JT[0,3,4]ZZ
Non-OR	07JN[3,8,X]ZZ
Non-OR	07JP[3,4,X]ZZ

Ø   Medical and Surgical
7   Lymphatic and Hemic Systems
L   Occlusion   Definition: Completely closing an orifice or the lumen of a tubular body part

Explanation: The orifice can be a natural orifice or an artificially created orifice

Body Part Character 4		Approach Character 5	Device Character 6	Qualifier Character 7

Ø Lymphatic, Head
Buccinator lymph node
Infraauricular lymph node
Infraparotid lymph node
Parotid lymph node
Preauricular lymph node
Submandibular lymph node
Submaxillary lymph node
Submental lymph node
Subparotid lymph node
Suprahyoid lymph node
1 Lymphatic, Right Neck
Cervical lymph node
Jugular lymph node
Mastoid (postauricular) lymph node
Occipital lymph node
Postauricular (mastoid) lymph node
Retropharyngeal lymph node
Right jugular trunk
Right lymphatic duct
Right subclavian trunk
Supraclavicular (Virchow's) lymph
   node
Virchow's (supraclavicular) lymph
   node
2 Lymphatic, Left Neck
Cervical lymph node
Jugular lymph node
Mastoid (postauricular) lymph node
Occipital lymph node
Postauricular (mastoid) lymph node
Retropharyngeal lymph node
Supraclavicular (Virchow's) lymph
   node
Virchow's (supraclavicular) lymph
   node
3 Lymphatic, Right Upper Extremity
Cubital lymph node
Deltopectoral (infraclavicular) lymph
   node
Epitrochlear lymph node
Infraclavicular (deltopectoral) lymph
   node
Supratrochlear lymph node
4 Lymphatic, Left Upper Extremity
See 3 Lymphatic, Right Upper Extremity
5 Lymphatic, Right Axillary
Anterior (pectoral) lymph node
Apical (subclavicular) lymph node
Brachial (lateral) lymph node
Central axillary lymph node
Lateral (brachial) lymph node
Pectoral (anterior) lymph node
Posterior (subscapular) lymph node
Subclavicular (apical) lymph node
Subscapular (posterior) lymph node
	6 Lymphatic, Left Axillary
	See 5 Lymphatic, Right Axillary
	7 Lymphatic, Thorax
	Intercostal lymph node
	Mediastinal lymph node
	Parasternal lymph node
	Paratracheal lymph node
	Tracheobronchial lymph node
	8 Lymphatic, Internal Mammary, Right
	9 Lymphatic, Internal Mammary, Left
	B Lymphatic, Mesenteric
	Inferior mesenteric lymph node
	Pararectal lymph node
	Superior mesenteric lymph node
	C Lymphatic, Pelvis
	Common iliac (subaortic) lymph node
	Gluteal lymph node
	Iliac lymph node
	Inferior epigastric lymph node
	Obturator lymph node
	Sacral lymph node
	Subaortic (common iliac) lymph node
	Suprainguinal lymph node
	D Lymphatic, Aortic
	Celiac lymph node
	Gastric lymph node
	Hepatic lymph node
	Lumbar lymph node
	Pancreaticosplenic lymph node
	Paraaortic lymph node
	Retroperitoneal lymph node
	F Lymphatic, Right Lower Extremity
	Femoral lymph node
	Popliteal lymph node
	G Lymphatic, Left Lower Extremity
	See F Lymphatic, Right Lower Extremity
	H Lymphatic, Right Inguinal
	J Lymphatic, Left Inguinal
	K Thoracic Duct
	Left jugular trunk
	Left subclavian trunk
	L Cisterna Chyli
	Intestinal lymphatic trunk
	Lumbar lymphatic trunk
		Ø Open
		3 Percutaneous
		**4 Percutaneous
		   Endoscopic**
			C Extraluminal Device
			D Intraluminal Device
			Z No Device
				Z No Qualifier

Ø   **Medical and Surgical**
7   **Lymphatic and Hemic Systems**
N   **Release**   Definition: Freeing a body part from an abnormal physical constraint by cutting or by the use of force
                         Explanation: Some of the restraining tissue may be taken out but none of the body part is taken out

Body Part Character 4		Approach Character 5	Device Character 6	Qualifier Character 7
Ø **Lymphatic, Head** Buccinator lymph node Infraauricular lymph node Infraparotid lymph node Parotid lymph node Preauricular lymph node Submandibular lymph node Submaxillary lymph node Submental lymph node Subparotid lymph node Suprahyoid lymph node 1 **Lymphatic, Right Neck** Cervical lymph node Jugular lymph node Mastoid (postauricular) lymph node Occipital lymph node Postauricular (mastoid) lymph node Retropharyngeal lymph node Right jugular trunk Right lymphatic duct Right subclavian trunk Supraclavicular (Virchow's) lymph node Virchow's (supraclavicular) lymph node 2 **Lymphatic, Left Neck** Cervical lymph node Jugular lymph node Mastoid (postauricular) lymph node Occipital lymph node Postauricular (mastoid) lymph node Retropharyngeal lymph node Supraclavicular (Virchow's) lymph node Virchow's (supraclavicular) lymph node 3 **Lymphatic, Right Upper Extremity** Cubital lymph node Deltopectoral (infraclavicular) lymph node Epitrochlear lymph node Infraclavicular (deltopectoral) lymph node Supratrochlear lymph node 4 **Lymphatic, Left Upper Extremity** *See 3 Lymphatic, Right Upper Extremity* 5 **Lymphatic, Right Axillary** Anterior (pectoral) lymph node Apical (subclavicular) lymph node Brachial (lateral) lymph node Central axillary lymph node Lateral (brachial) lymph node Pectoral (anterior) lymph node Posterior (subscapular) lymph node Subclavicular (apical) lymph node Subscapular (posterior) lymph node	6 **Lymphatic, Left Axillary** *See 5 Lymphatic, Right Axillary* 7 **Lymphatic, Thorax** Intercostal lymph node Mediastinal lymph node Parasternal lymph node Paratracheal lymph node Tracheobronchial lymph node 8 **Lymphatic, Internal Mammary, Right** 9 **Lymphatic, Internal Mammary, Left** B **Lymphatic, Mesenteric** Inferior mesenteric lymph node Pararectal lymph node Superior mesenteric lymph node C **Lymphatic, Pelvis** Common iliac (subaortic) lymph node Gluteal lymph node Iliac lymph node Inferior epigastric lymph node Obturator lymph node Sacral lymph node Subaortic (common iliac) lymph node Suprainguinal lymph node D **Lymphatic, Aortic** Celiac lymph node Gastric lymph node Hepatic lymph node Lumbar lymph node Pancreaticosplenic lymph node Paraaortic lymph node Retroperitoneal lymph node F **Lymphatic, Right Lower Extremity** Femoral lymph node Popliteal lymph node G **Lymphatic, Left Lower Extremity** *See F Lymphatic, Right Lower Extremity* H **Lymphatic, Right Inguinal** J **Lymphatic, Left Inguinal** K **Thoracic Duct** Left jugular trunk Left subclavian trunk L **Cisterna Chyli** Intestinal lymphatic trunk Lumbar lymphatic trunk M **Thymus** Thymus gland P **Spleen** Accessory spleen	Ø Open 3 Percutaneous 4 Percutaneous Endoscopic	Z No Device	Z No Qualifier

Ø   Medical and Surgical
7   Lymphatic and Hemic Systems
P   Removal   Definition: Taking out or off a device from a body part

Explanation: If a device is taken out and a similar device put in without cutting or puncturing the skin or mucous membrane, the procedure is coded to the root operation CHANGE. Otherwise, the procedure for taking out a device is coded to the root operation REMOVAL.

Body Part Character 4	Approach Character 5	Device Character 6	Qualifier Character 7
K Thoracic Duct Left jugular trunk Left subclavian trunk **L Cisterna Chyli** Intestinal lymphatic trunk Lumbar lymphatic trunk **N Lymphatic**	**Ø** Open **3** Percutaneous **4** Percutaneous Endoscopic	**Ø** Drainage Device **3** Infusion Device **7** Autologous Tissue Substitute **C** Extraluminal Device **D** Intraluminal Device **J** Synthetic Substitute **K** Nonautologous Tissue Substitute **Y** Other Device	**Z** No Qualifier
K Thoracic Duct Left jugular trunk Left subclavian trunk **L Cisterna Chyli** Intestinal lymphatic trunk Lumbar lymphatic trunk **N Lymphatic**	**X** External	**Ø** Drainage Device **3** Infusion Device **D** Intraluminal Device	**Z** No Qualifier
M Thymus Thymus gland **P Spleen** Accessory spleen	**Ø** Open **3** Percutaneous **4** Percutaneous Endoscopic	**Ø** Drainage Device **3** Infusion Device **Y** Other Device	**Z** No Qualifier
M Thymus Thymus gland **P Spleen** Accessory spleen	**X** External	**Ø** Drainage Device **3** Infusion Device	**Z** No Qualifier
T Bone Marrow	**Ø** Open **3** Percutaneous **4** Percutaneous Endoscopic **X** External	**Ø** Drainage Device	**Z** No Qualifier

Non-OR	Ø7P[K,L,N][3,4]YZ
Non-OR	Ø7P[K,L,N]X[Ø,3,D]Z
Non-OR	Ø7P[M,P][3,4]YZ
Non-OR	Ø7P[M,P]X[Ø,3]Z
Non-OR	Ø7PT[Ø,3,4,X]ØZ

Ø   Medical and Surgical
7   Lymphatic and Hemic Systems
Q   Repair   Definition: Restoring, to the extent possible, a body part to its normal anatomic structure and function
              Explanation: Used only when the method to accomplish the repair is not one of the other root operations

Body Part Character 4		Approach Character 5	Device Character 6	Qualifier Character 7
Ø Lymphatic, Head Buccinator lymph node Infraauricular lymph node Infraparotid lymph node Parotid lymph node Preauricular lymph node Submandibular lymph node Submaxillary lymph node Submental lymph node Subparotid lymph node Suprahyoid lymph node **1 Lymphatic, Right Neck** Cervical lymph node Jugular lymph node Mastoid (postauricular) lymph node Occipital lymph node Postauricular (mastoid) lymph node Retropharyngeal lymph node Right jugular trunk Right lymphatic duct Right subclavian trunk Supraclavicular (Virchow's) lymph node Virchow's (supraclavicular) lymph node **2 Lymphatic, Left Neck** Cervical lymph node Jugular lymph node Mastoid (postauricular) lymph node Occipital lymph node Postauricular (mastoid) lymph node Retropharyngeal lymph node Supraclavicular (Virchow's) lymph node Virchow's (supraclavicular) lymph node **3 Lymphatic, Right Upper Extremity** Cubital lymph node Deltopectoral (infraclavicular) lymph node Epitrochlear lymph node Infraclavicular (deltopectoral) lymph node Supratrochlear lymph node **4 Lymphatic, Left Upper Extremity** *See 3 Lymphatic, Right Upper Extremity* **5 Lymphatic, Right Axillary** Anterior (pectoral) lymph node Apical (subclavicular) lymph node Brachial (lateral) lymph node Central axillary lymph node Lateral (brachial) lymph node Pectoral (anterior) lymph node Posterior (subscapular) lymph node Subclavicular (apical) lymph node Subscapular (posterior) lymph node	**6 Lymphatic, Left Axillary** *See 5 Lymphatic, Right Axillary* **7 Lymphatic, Thorax** Intercostal lymph node Mediastinal lymph node Parasternal lymph node Paratracheal lymph node Tracheobronchial lymph node **8 Lymphatic, Internal Mammary, Right** **9 Lymphatic, Internal Mammary, Left** **B Lymphatic, Mesenteric** Inferior mesenteric lymph node Pararectal lymph node Superior mesenteric lymph node **C Lymphatic, Pelvis** Common iliac (subaortic) lymph node Gluteal lymph node Iliac lymph node Inferior epigastric lymph node Obturator lymph node Sacral lymph node Subaortic (common iliac) lymph node Suprainguinal lymph node **D Lymphatic, Aortic** Celiac lymph node Gastric lymph node Hepatic lymph node Lumbar lymph node Pancreaticosplenic lymph node Paraaortic lymph node Retroperitoneal lymph node **F Lymphatic, Right Lower Extremity** Femoral lymph node Popliteal lymph node **G Lymphatic, Left Lower Extremity** *See F Lymphatic, Right Lower Extremity* **H Lymphatic, Right Inguinal** **J Lymphatic, Left Inguinal** **K Thoracic Duct** Left jugular trunk Left subclavian trunk **L Cisterna Chyli** Intestinal lymphatic trunk Lumbar lymphatic trunk	**Ø Open** **3 Percutaneous** **4 Percutaneous Endoscopic** **8 Via Natural or Artificial Opening Endoscopic**	**Z No Device**	**Z No Qualifier**
M Thymus Thymus gland **P Spleen** Accessory spleen		**Ø Open** **3 Percutaneous** **4 Percutaneous Endoscopic**	**Z No Device**	**Z No Qualifier**

Lymphatic and Hemic Systems

Ø **Medical and Surgical**
7 **Lymphatic and Hemic Systems**
S **Reposition**   Definition: Moving to its normal location, or other suitable location, all or a portion of a body part

Explanation: The body part is moved to a new location from an abnormal location, or from a normal location where it is not functioning correctly. The body part may or may not be cut out or off to be moved to the new location.

Body Part Character 4	Approach Character 5	Device Character 6	Qualifier Character 7

M Thymus
  Thymus gland
P Spleen
  Accessory spleen
	Ø Open	**Z** No Device	**Z** No Qualifier

Ø **Medical and Surgical**
7 **Lymphatic and Hemic Systems**
T **Resection**   Definition: Cutting out or off, without replacement, all of a body part

Explanation: None

Body Part Character 4		Approach Character 5	Device Character 6	Qualifier Character 7

Ø Lymphatic, Head
  Buccinator lymph node
  Infraauricular lymph node
  Infraparotid lymph node
  Parotid lymph node
  Preauricular lymph node
  Submandibular lymph node
  Submaxillary lymph node
  Submental lymph node
  Subparotid lymph node
  Suprahyoid lymph node
1 Lymphatic, Right Neck
  Cervical lymph node
  Jugular lymph node
  Mastoid (postauricular) lymph node
  Occipital lymph node
  Postauricular (mastoid) lymph node
  Retropharyngeal lymph node
  Right jugular trunk
  Right lymphatic duct
  Right subclavian trunk
  Supraclavicular (Virchow's) lymph
    node
  Virchow's (supraclavicular) lymph
    node
2 Lymphatic, Left Neck
  Cervical lymph node
  Jugular lymph node
  Mastoid (postauricular) lymph node
  Occipital lymph node
  Postauricular (mastoid) lymph node
  Retropharyngeal lymph node
  Supraclavicular (Virchow's) lymph
    node
  Virchow's (supraclavicular) lymph
    node
3 Lymphatic, Right Upper Extremity
  Cubital lymph node
  Deltopectoral (infraclavicular) lymph
    node
  Epitrochlear lymph node
  Infraclavicular (deltopectoral) lymph
    node
  Supratrochlear lymph node
4 Lymphatic, Left Upper Extremity
  See 3 Lymphatic, Right Upper Extremity
5 Lymphatic, Right Axillary ⊞
  Anterior (pectoral) lymph node
  Apical (subclavicular) lymph node
  Brachial (lateral) lymph node
  Central axillary lymph node
  Lateral (brachial) lymph node
  Pectoral (anterior) lymph node
  Posterior (subscapular) lymph node
  Subclavicular (apical) lymph node
  Subscapular (posterior) lymph node
	6 Lymphatic, Left Axillary ⊞
	  See 5 Lymphatic, Right Axillary
	7 Lymphatic, Thorax ⊞
	  Intercostal lymph node
	  Mediastinal lymph node
	  Parasternal lymph node
	  Paratracheal lymph node
	  Tracheobronchial lymph node
	8 Lymphatic, Internal ⊞
	  Mammary, Right
	9 Lymphatic, Internal ⊞
	  Mammary, Left
	B Lymphatic, Mesenteric
	  Inferior mesenteric lymph node
	  Pararectal lymph node
	  Superior mesenteric lymph node
	C Lymphatic, Pelvis
	  Common iliac (subaortic) lymph node
	  Gluteal lymph node
	  Iliac lymph node
	  Inferior epigastric lymph node
	  Obturator lymph node
	  Sacral lymph node
	  Subaortic (common iliac) lymph node
	  Suprainguinal lymph node
	D Lymphatic, Aortic
	  Celiac lymph node
	  Gastric lymph node
	  Hepatic lymph node
	  Lumbar lymph node
	  Pancreaticosplenic lymph node
	  Paraaortic lymph node
	  Retroperitoneal lymph node
	F Lymphatic, Right Lower Extremity
	  Femoral lymph node
	  Popliteal lymph node
	G Lymphatic, Left Lower Extremity
	  See F Lymphatic, Right Lower Extremity
	H Lymphatic, Right Inguinal
	J Lymphatic, Left Inguinal
	K Thoracic Duct
	  Left jugular trunk
	  Left subclavian trunk
	L Cisterna Chyli
	  Intestinal lymphatic trunk
	  Lumbar lymphatic trunk
	M Thymus
	  Thymus gland
	P Spleen
	  Accessory spleen
		Ø Open
		4 Percutaneous
		  Endoscopic
			Z No Device	**Z** No Qualifier

See Appendix L for Procedure Combinations
  ⊞   07T[5,6,7,8,9]ØZZ

LC Limited Coverage   **NC** Noncovered   ⊞ Combination Member   HAC associated procedure   Combination Only   DRG Non-OR   Non-OR   New/Revised in GREEN

292   ICD-10-PCS 2021

Ø   **Medical and Surgical**
7   **Lymphatic and Hemic Systems**
U   **Supplement**   Definition: Putting in or on biological or synthetic material that physically reinforces and/or augments the function of a portion of a body part
                   Explanation: The biological material is non-living, or is living and from the same individual. The body part may have been previously replaced, and the SUPPLEMENT procedure is performed to physically reinforce and/or augment the function of the replaced body part.

Body Part Character 4		Approach Character 5	Device Character 6	Qualifier Character 7

Ø Lymphatic, Head
Buccinator lymph node
Infraauricular lymph node
Infraparotid lymph node
Parotid lymph node
Preauricular lymph node
Submandibular lymph node
Submaxillary lymph node
Submental lymph node
Subparotid lymph node
Suprahyoid lymph node
1 Lymphatic, Right Neck
Cervical lymph node
Jugular lymph node
Mastoid (postauricular) lymph node
Occipital lymph node
Postauricular (mastoid) lymph node
Retropharyngeal lymph node
Right jugular trunk
Right lymphatic duct
Right subclavian trunk
Supraclavicular (Virchow's) lymph
    node
Virchow's (supraclavicular) lymph
    node
2 Lymphatic, Left Neck
Cervical lymph node
Jugular lymph node
Mastoid (postauricular) lymph node
Occipital lymph node
Postauricular (mastoid) lymph node
Retropharyngeal lymph node
Supraclavicular (Virchow's) lymph
    node
Virchow's (supraclavicular) lymph
    node
3 Lymphatic, Right Upper Extremity
Cubital lymph node
Deltopectoral (infraclavicular) lymph
    node
Epitrochlear lymph node
Infraclavicular (deltopectoral) lymph
    node
Supratrochlear lymph node
4 Lymphatic, Left Upper Extremity
See 3 Lymphatic, Right Upper Extremity
5 Lymphatic, Right Axillary
Anterior (pectoral) lymph node
Apical (subclavicular) lymph node
Brachial (lateral) lymph node
Central axillary lymph node
Lateral (brachial) lymph node
Pectoral (anterior) lymph node
Posterior (subscapular) lymph node
Subclavicular (apical) lymph node
Subscapular (posterior) lymph node
	6 Lymphatic, Left Axillary
	See 5 Lymphatic, Right Axillary
	7 Lymphatic, Thorax
	Intercostal lymph node
	Mediastinal lymph node
	Parasternal lymph node
	Paratracheal lymph node
	Tracheobronchial lymph node
	8 Lymphatic, Internal Mammary, Right
	9 Lymphatic, Internal Mammary, Left
	B Lymphatic, Mesenteric
	Inferior mesenteric lymph node
	Pararectal lymph node
	Superior mesenteric lymph node
	C Lymphatic, Pelvis
	Common iliac (subaortic) lymph node
	Gluteal lymph node
	Iliac lymph node
	Inferior epigastric lymph node
	Obturator lymph node
	Sacral lymph node
	Subaortic (common iliac) lymph node
	Suprainguinal lymph node
	D Lymphatic, Aortic
	Celiac lymph node
	Gastric lymph node
	Hepatic lymph node
	Lumbar lymph node
	Pancreaticosplenic lymph node
	Paraaortic lymph node
	Retroperitoneal lymph node
	F Lymphatic, Right Lower Extremity
	Femoral lymph node
	Popliteal lymph node
	G Lymphatic, Left Lower Extremity
	See F Lymphatic, Right Lower Extremity
	H Lymphatic, Right Inguinal
	J Lymphatic, Left Inguinal
	K Thoracic Duct
	Left jugular trunk
	Left subclavian trunk
	L Cisterna Chyli
	Intestinal lymphatic trunk
	Lumbar lymphatic trunk
		Ø Open
		4 Percutaneous Endoscopic
			7 Autologous Tissue Substitute
			J Synthetic Substitute
			K Nonautologous Tissue Substitute
				Z No Qualifier

Ø Medical and Surgical
7 Lymphatic and Hemic Systems
V Restriction Definition: Partially closing an orifice or the lumen of a tubular body part
Explanation: The orifice can be a natural orifice or an artificially created orifice

Body Part Character 4		Approach Character 5	Device Character 6	Qualifier Character 7
Ø Lymphatic, Head Buccinator lymph node Infraauricular lymph node Infraparotid lymph node Parotid lymph node Preauricular lymph node Submandibular lymph node Submaxillary lymph node Submental lymph node Subparotid lymph node Suprahyoid lymph node **1 Lymphatic, Right Neck** Cervical lymph node Jugular lymph node Mastoid (postauricular) lymph node Occipital lymph node Postauricular (mastoid) lymph node Retropharyngeal lymph node Right jugular trunk Right lymphatic duct Right subclavian trunk Supraclavicular (Virchow's) lymph node Virchow's (supraclavicular) lymph node **2 Lymphatic, Left Neck** Cervical lymph node Jugular lymph node Mastoid (postauricular) lymph node Occipital lymph node Postauricular (mastoid) lymph node Retropharyngeal lymph node Supraclavicular (Virchow's) lymph node Virchow's (supraclavicular) lymph node **3 Lymphatic, Right Upper Extremity** Cubital lymph node Deltopectoral (infraclavicular) lymph node Epitrochlear lymph node Infraclavicular (deltopectoral) lymph node Supratrochlear lymph node **4 Lymphatic, Left Upper Extremity** *See 3 Lymphatic, Right Upper Extremity* **5 Lymphatic, Right Axillary** Anterior (pectoral) lymph node Apical (subclavicular) lymph node Brachial (lateral) lymph node Central axillary lymph node Lateral (brachial) lymph node Pectoral (anterior) lymph node Posterior (subscapular) lymph node Subclavicular (apical) lymph node Subscapular (posterior) lymph node	**6 Lymphatic, Left Axillary** *See 5 Lymphatic, Right Axillary* **7 Lymphatic, Thorax** Intercostal lymph node Mediastinal lymph node Parasternal lymph node Paratracheal lymph node Tracheobronchial lymph node **8 Lymphatic, Internal Mammary, Right** **9 Lymphatic, Internal Mammary, Left** **B Lymphatic, Mesenteric** Inferior mesenteric lymph node Pararectal lymph node Superior mesenteric lymph node **C Lymphatic, Pelvis** Common iliac (subaortic) lymph node Gluteal lymph node Iliac lymph node Inferior epigastric lymph node Obturator lymph node Sacral lymph node Subaortic (common iliac) lymph node Suprainguinal lymph node **D Lymphatic, Aortic** Celiac lymph node Gastric lymph node Hepatic lymph node Lumbar lymph node Pancreaticosplenic lymph node Paraaortic lymph node Retroperitoneal lymph node **F Lymphatic, Right Lower Extremity** Femoral lymph node Popliteal lymph node **G Lymphatic, Left Lower Extremity** *See F Lymphatic, Right Lower Extremity* **H Lymphatic, Right Inguinal** **J Lymphatic, Left Inguinal** **K Thoracic Duct** Left jugular trunk Left subclavian trunk **L Cisterna Chyli** Intestinal lymphatic trunk Lumbar lymphatic trunk	**Ø Open** **3 Percutaneous** **4 Percutaneous Endoscopic**	**C Extraluminal Device** **D Intraluminal Device** **Z No Device**	**Z No Qualifier**

Ø   **Medical and Surgical**
7   **Lymphatic and Hemic Systems**
W   **Revision**   Definition: Correcting, to the extent possible, a portion of a malfunctioning device or the position of a displaced device

Explanation: Revision can include correcting a malfunctioning or displaced device by taking out or putting in components of the device such as a screw or pin

Body Part Character 4	Approach Character 5	Device Character 6	Qualifier Character 7

K Thoracic Duct
   Left jugular trunk
   Left subclavian trunk
L Cisterna Chyli
   Intestinal lymphatic trunk
   Lumbar lymphatic trunk
N Lymphatic
	Ø Open
	3 Percutaneous
	4 Percutaneous Endoscopic
		Ø Drainage Device
		3 Infusion Device
		7 Autologous Tissue Substitute
		C Extraluminal Device
		D Intraluminal Device
		J Synthetic Substitute
		K Nonautologous Tissue Substitute
		Y Other Device
			Z No Qualifier

K Thoracic Duct
   Left jugular trunk
   Left subclavian trunk
L Cisterna Chyli
   Intestinal lymphatic trunk
   Lumbar lymphatic trunk
N Lymphatic
	X External	**Ø** Drainage Device
		3 Infusion Device
		7 Autologous Tissue Substitute
		C Extraluminal Device
		D Intraluminal Device
		J Synthetic Substitute
		K Nonautologous Tissue Substitute
			Z No Qualifier

M Thymus
   Thymus gland
P Spleen
   Accessory spleen
	Ø Open
	3 Percutaneous
	4 Percutaneous Endoscopic
		Ø Drainage Device
		3 Infusion Device
		Y Other Device
			Z No Qualifier

M Thymus
   Thymus gland
P Spleen
   Accessory spleen
	X External	**Ø** Drainage Device
		3 Infusion Device
			Z No Qualifier

T Bone Marrow	**Ø** Open **3** Percutaneous **4** Percutaneous Endoscopic **X** External	**Ø** Drainage Device	**Z** No Qualifier

Non-OR	07W[K,L,N][3,4]YZ
Non-OR	07W[K,L,N]X[Ø,3,7,C,D,J,K]Z
Non-OR	07W[M,P][3,4]YZ
Non-OR	07W[M,P]X[Ø,3]Z
Non-OR	07WT[Ø,3,4,X]ØZ

Ø   **Medical and Surgical**
7   **Lymphatic and Hemic Systems**
Y   **Transplantation**   Definition: Putting in or on all or a portion of a living body part taken from another individual or animal to physically take the place and/or function of all or a portion of a similar body part

Explanation: The native body part may or may not be taken out, and the transplanted body part may take over all or a portion of its function

Body Part Character 4	Approach Character 5	Device Character 6	Qualifier Character 7

M Thymus
   Thymus gland
P Spleen
   Accessory spleen
	Ø Open	**Z** No Device	**Ø** Allogeneic
			1 Syngeneic
			2 Zooplastic

LC Limited Coverage   **NC** Noncovered   ⊞ Combination Member   HAC associated procedure   Combination Only   DRG Non-OR   Non-OR   New/Revised in GREEN

ICD-10-PCS 2021   295

07W–07Y

Eye Ø8Ø–Ø8X

Character Meanings

This Character Meaning table is provided as a guide to assist the user in the identification of character members that may be found in this section of code tables. It **SHOULD NOT** be used to build a PCS code.

Operation–Character 3	Body Part–Character 4	Approach–Character 5	Device–Character 6	Qualifier–Character 7
Ø Alteration	Ø Eye, Right	Ø Open	Ø Drainage Device OR Synthetic Substitute, Intraocular Telescope	3 Nasal Cavity
1 Bypass	1 Eye, Left	3 Percutaneous	1 Radioactive Element	4 Sclera
2 Change	2 Anterior Chamber, Right	7 Via Natural or Artificial Opening	3 Infusion Device	X Diagnostic
5 Destruction	3 Anterior Chamber, Left	8 Via Natural or Artificial Opening Endoscopic	5 Epiretinal Visual Prosthesis	Z No Qualifier
7 Dilation	4 Vitreous, Right	X External	7 Autologous Tissue Substitute	
9 Drainage	5 Vitreous, Left		C Extraluminal Device	
B Excision	6 Sclera, Right		D Intraluminal Device	
C Extirpation	7 Sclera, Left		J Synthetic Substitute	
D Extraction	8 Cornea, Right		K Nonautologous Tissue Substitute	
F Fragmentation	9 Cornea, Left		Y Other Device	
H Insertion	A Choroid, Right		Z No Device	
J Inspection	B Choroid, Left			
L Occlusion	C Iris, Right			
M Reattachment	D Iris, Left			
N Release	E Retina, Right			
P Removal	F Retina, Left			
Q Repair	G Retinal Vessel, Right			
R Replacement	H Retinal Vessel, Left			
S Reposition	J Lens, Right			
T Resection	K Lens, Left			
U Supplement	L Extraocular Muscle, Right			
V Restriction	M Extraocular Muscle, Left			
W Revision	N Upper Eyelid, Right			
X Transfer	P Upper Eyelid, Left			
	Q Lower Eyelid, Right			
	R Lower Eyelid, Left			
	S Conjunctiva, Right			
	T Conjunctiva, Left			
	V Lacrimal Gland, Right			
	W Lacrimal Gland, Left			
	X Lacrimal Duct, Right			
	Y Lacrimal Duct, Left			

AHA Coding Clinic for table Ø81
2019, 1Q, 27   Glaucoma tube shunt

AHA Coding Clinic for table Ø89
2016, 2Q, 21   Laser trabeculoplasty

AHA Coding Clinic for table Ø8B
2014, 4Q, 35   Vitrectomy with air/fluid exchange
2014, 4Q, 36   Pars plans vitrectomy without mention of instillation of oil, air or fluid

AHA Coding Clinic for table Ø8J
2015, 1Q, 35   Attempted removal of foreign body from cornea

AHA Coding Clinic for table Ø8N
2015, 2Q, 24   Penetrating keratoplasty and anterior segment reconstruction

AHA Coding Clinic for table Ø8Q
2018, 3Q, 13   Repair of ruptured globe

AHA Coding Clinic for table Ø8R
2015, 2Q, 24   Penetrating keratoplasty and anterior segment reconstruction
2015, 2Q, 25   Penetrating keratoplasty and placement of viscoelastic eye with paracentesis

AHA Coding Clinic for table Ø8T
2015, 2Q, 12   Orbital exenteration

AHA Coding Clinic for table Ø8U
2014, 3Q, 31   Corneal amniotic membrane transplantation

Eye

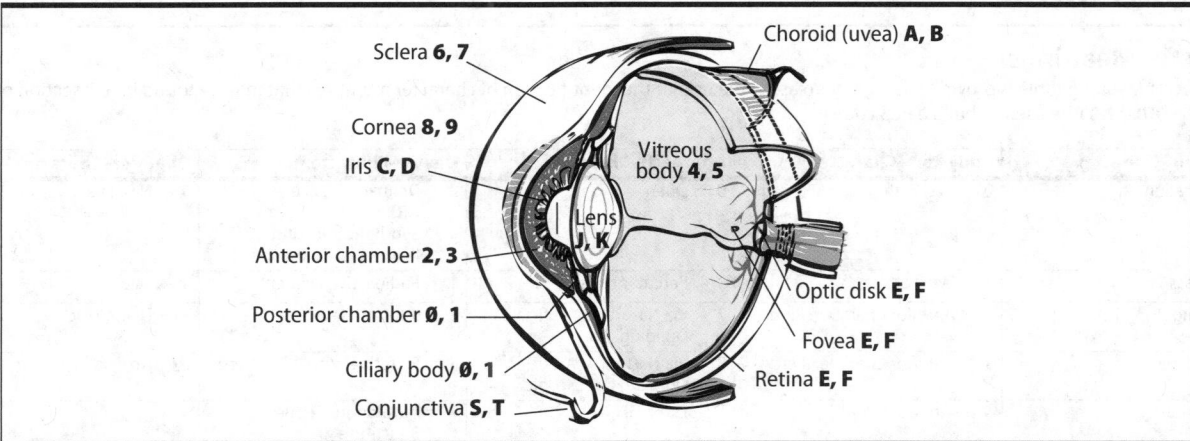

Sclera **6, 7**
Cornea **8, 9**
Iris **C, D**
Anterior chamber **2, 3**
Posterior chamber **Ø, 1**
Ciliary body **Ø, 1**
Conjunctiva **S, T**
Choroid (uvea) **A, B**
Vitreous body **4, 5**
Lens **J, K**
Optic disk **E, F**
Fovea **E, F**
Retina **E, F**

Eye Musculature

Superior rectus
Superior oblique
Lateral rectus
Medial rectus
Inferior oblique
Inferior rectus
Muscles and actions (right eye) **L, M**

Lacrimal System

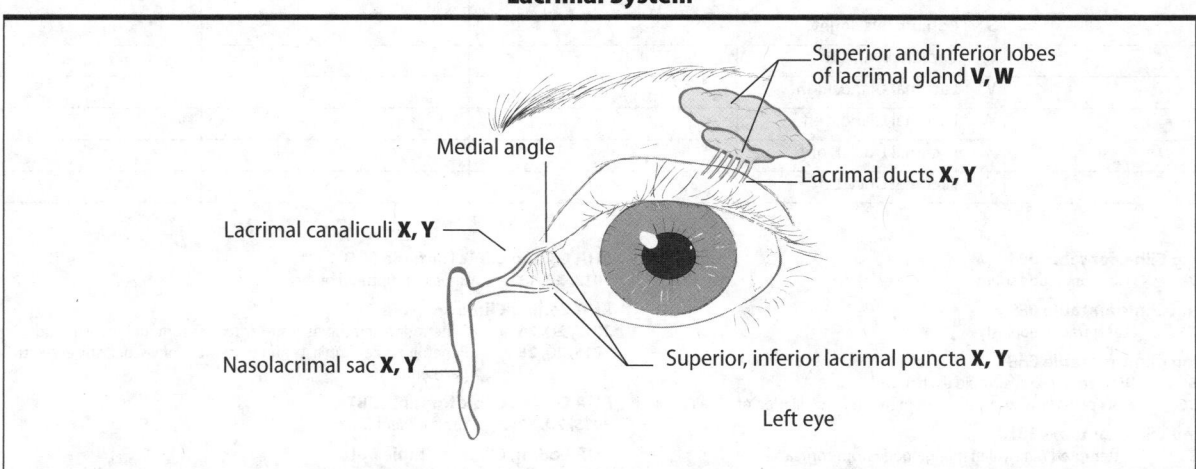

Superior and inferior lobes of lacrimal gland **V, W**
Medial angle
Lacrimal ducts **X, Y**
Lacrimal canaliculi **X, Y**
Nasolacrimal sac **X, Y**
Superior, inferior lacrimal puncta **X, Y**
Left eye

Ø Medical and Surgical
8 Eye
Ø Alteration   Definition: Modifying the anatomic structure of a body part without affecting the function of the body part

Explanation: Principal purpose is to improve appearance

Body Part Character 4	Approach Character 5	Device Character 6	Qualifier Character 7
N Upper Eyelid, Right Lateral canthus Levator palpebrae superioris muscle Orbicularis oculi muscle Superior tarsal plate **P** Upper Eyelid, Left *See N Upper Eyelid, Right* **Q** Lower Eyelid, Right Inferior tarsal plate Medial canthus **R** Lower Eyelid, Left *See Q Lower Eyelid, Right*	**Ø** Open **3** Percutaneous **X** External	**7** Autologous Tissue Substitute **J** Synthetic Substitute **K** Nonautologous Tissue Substitute **Z** No Device	**Z** No Qualifier

Non-OR   All body part, approach, device, and qualifier values

Ø Medical and Surgical
8 Eye
1 Bypass   Definition: Altering the route of passage of the contents of a tubular body part

Explanation: Rerouting contents of a body part to a downstream area of the normal route, to a similar route and body part, or to an abnormal route and dissimilar body part. Includes one or more anastomoses, with or without the use of a device.

Body Part Character 4	Approach Character 5	Device Character 6	Qualifier Character 7
2 Anterior Chamber, Right Aqueous humour **3** Anterior Chamber, Left *See 2 Anterior Chamber, Right*	**3** Percutaneous	**J** Synthetic Substitute **K** Nonautologous Tissue Substitute **Z** No Device	**4** Sclera
X Lacrimal Duct, Right Lacrimal canaliculus Lacrimal punctum Lacrimal sac Nasolacrimal duct **Y** Lacrimal Duct, Left *See X Lacrimal Duct, Right*	**Ø** Open **3** Percutaneous	**J** Synthetic Substitute **K** Nonautologous Tissue Substitute **Z** No Device	**3** Nasal Cavity

Ø Medical and Surgical
8 Eye
2 Change   Definition: Taking out or off a device from a body part and putting back an identical or similar device in or on the same body part without cutting or puncturing the skin or a mucous membrane

Explanation: All CHANGE procedures are coded using the approach EXTERNAL

Body Part Character 4	Approach Character 5	Device Character 6	Qualifier Character 7
Ø Eye, Right Ciliary body Posterior chamber **1** Eye, Left *See Ø Eye, Right*	**X** External	**Ø** Drainage Device **Y** Other Device	**Z** No Qualifier

Non-OR   All body part, approach, device, and qualifier values

LC Limited Coverage   NC Noncovered   ⊞ Combination Member   HAC associated procedure   Combination Only   DRG Non-OR   Non-OR   New/Revised in GREEN

ICD-10-PCS 2021   299   080–082

Ø   **Medical and Surgical**
8   **Eye**
5   **Destruction**   Definition: Physical eradication of all or a portion of a body part by the direct use of energy, force, or a destructive agent

Explanation: None of the body part is physically taken out

Body Part Character 4		Approach Character 5	Device Character 6	Qualifier Character 7
Ø **Eye, Right** Ciliary body Posterior chamber **1** **Eye, Left** *See Ø Eye, Right* **6** **Sclera, Right** **7** **Sclera, Left**	**8** **Cornea, Right** **9** **Cornea, Left** **S** **Conjunctiva, Right** Plica semilunaris **T** **Conjunctiva, Left** *See S Conjunctiva, Right*	**X** External	**Z** No Device	**Z** No Qualifier
2 **Anterior Chamber, Right** Aqueous humour **3** **Anterior Chamber, Left** *See 2 Anterior Chamber, Right* **4** **Vitreous, Right** Vitreous body **5** **Vitreous, Left** *See 4 Vitreous, Right* **C** **Iris, Right** **D** **Iris, Left**	**E** **Retina, Right** Fovea Macula Optic disc **F** **Retina, Left** *See E Retina, Right* **G** **Retinal Vessel, Right** **H** **Retinal Vessel, Left** **J** **Lens, Right** Zonule of Zinn **K** **Lens, Left** *See J Lens, Right*	**3** Percutaneous	**Z** No Device	**Z** No Qualifier
A **Choroid, Right** **B** **Choroid, Left** **L** **Extraocular Muscle, Right** Inferior oblique muscle Inferior rectus muscle Lateral rectus muscle Medial rectus muscle Superior oblique muscle Superior rectus muscle	**M** **Extraocular Muscle, Left** *See L Extraocular Muscle, Right* **V** **Lacrimal Gland, Right** **W** **Lacrimal Gland, Left**	**Ø** Open **3** Percutaneous	**Z** No Device	**Z** No Qualifier
N **Upper Eyelid, Right** Lateral canthus Levator palpebrae superioris muscle Orbicularis oculi muscle Superior tarsal plate **P** **Upper Eyelid, Left** *See N Upper Eyelid, Right*	**Q** **Lower Eyelid, Right** Inferior tarsal plate Medial canthus **R** **Lower Eyelid, Left** *See Q Lower Eyelid, Right*	**Ø** Open **3** Percutaneous **X** External	**Z** No Device	**Z** No Qualifier

X **Lacrimal Duct, Right**
Lacrimal canaliculus
Lacrimal punctum
Lacrimal sac
Nasolacrimal duct
	Y **Lacrimal Duct, Left**
	See X Lacrimal Duct, Right
		Ø Open
		3 Percutaneous
		7 Via Natural or Artificial
		  Opening
		8 Via Natural or Artificial
		  Opening Endoscopic
			Z No Device	**Z** No Qualifier

Non-OR   Ø85[E,F]3ZZ

Ø   **Medical and Surgical**
8   **Eye**
7   **Dilation**   Definition: Expanding an orifice or the lumen of a tubular body part

Explanation: The orifice can be a natural orifice or an artificially created orifice. Accomplished by stretching a tubular body part using intraluminal pressure or by cutting part of the orifice or wall of the tubular body part.

Body Part Character 4	Approach Character 5	Device Character 6	Qualifier Character 7

X **Lacrimal Duct, Right**
Lacrimal canaliculus
Lacrimal punctum
Lacrimal sac
Nasolacrimal duct
Y **Lacrimal Duct, Left**
See X Lacrimal Duct, Right
	Ø Open
	3 Percutaneous
	7 Via Natural or Artificial
	  Opening
	8 Via Natural or Artificial
	  Opening Endoscopic
		D Intraluminal Device
		Z No Device
			Z No Qualifier

LC Limited Coverage   **NC** Noncovered   ⊞ Combination Member   HAC associated procedure   Combination Only   DRG Non-OR   Non-OR   New/Revised in GREEN

300

Ø85–Ø87

ICD-10-PCS 2021

Ø   **Medical and Surgical**
8   **Eye**
9   **Drainage**   Definition: Taking or letting out fluids and/or gases from a body part

                       Explanation: The qualifier DIAGNOSTIC is used to identify drainage procedures that are biopsies

Body Part Character 4		Approach Character 5	Device Character 6	Qualifier Character 7
Ø Eye, Right Ciliary body Posterior chamber **1 Eye, Left** *See Ø Eye, Right* **6 Sclera, Right** **7 Sclera, Left**	**8 Cornea, Right** **9 Cornea, Left** **S Conjunctiva, Right** Plica semilunaris **T Conjunctiva, Left** *See S Conjunctiva, Right*	**X External**	**Ø Drainage Device**	**Z No Qualifier**
Ø Eye, Right Ciliary body Posterior chamber **1 Eye, Left** *See Ø Eye, Right* **6 Sclera, Right** **7 Sclera, Left**	**8 Cornea, Right** **9 Cornea, Left** **S Conjunctiva, Right** Plica semilunaris **T Conjunctiva, Left** *See S Conjunctiva, Right*	**X External**	**Z No Device**	**X Diagnostic** **Z No Qualifier**
2 Anterior Chamber, Right Aqueous humour **3 Anterior Chamber, Left** *See 2 Anterior Chamber, Right* **4 Vitreous, Right** Vitreous body **5 Vitreous, Left** *See 4 Vitreous, Right* **C Iris, Right** **D Iris, Left**	**E Retina, Right** Fovea Macula Optic disc **F Retina, Left** *See E Retina, Right* **G Retinal Vessel, Right** **H Retinal Vessel, Left** **J Lens, Right** Zonule of Zinn **K Lens, Left** *See J Lens, Right*	**3 Percutaneous**	**Ø Drainage Device**	**Z No Qualifier**
2 Anterior Chamber, Right Aqueous humour **3 Anterior Chamber, Left** *See 2 Anterior Chamber, Right* **4 Vitreous, Right** Vitreous body **5 Vitreous, Left** *See 4 Vitreous, Right* **C Iris, Right** **D Iris, Left**	**E Retina, Right** Fovea Macula Optic disc **F Retina, Left** *See E Retina, Right* **G Retinal Vessel, Right** **H Retinal Vessel, Left** **J Lens, Right** Zonule of Zinn **K Lens, Left** *See J Lens, Right*	**3 Percutaneous**	**Z No Device**	**X Diagnostic** **Z No Qualifier**
A Choroid, Right **B Choroid, Left** **L Extraocular Muscle, Right** Inferior oblique muscle Inferior rectus muscle Lateral rectus muscle Medial rectus muscle Superior oblique muscle Superior rectus muscle	**M Extraocular Muscle, Left** *See L Extraocular Muscle, Right* **V Lacrimal Gland, Right** **W Lacrimal Gland, Left**	**Ø Open** **3 Percutaneous**	**Ø Drainage Device**	**Z No Qualifier**
A Choroid, Right **B Choroid, Left** **L Extraocular Muscle, Right** Inferior oblique muscle Inferior rectus muscle Lateral rectus muscle Medial rectus muscle Superior oblique muscle Superior rectus muscle	**M Extraocular Muscle, Left** *See L Extraocular Muscle, Right* **V Lacrimal Gland, Right** **W Lacrimal Gland, Left**	**Ø Open** **3 Percutaneous**	**Z No Device**	**X Diagnostic** **Z No Qualifier**
N Upper Eyelid, Right Lateral canthus Levator palpebrae superioris muscle Orbicularis oculi muscle Superior tarsal plate **P Upper Eyelid, Left** *See N Upper Eyelid, Right*	**Q Lower Eyelid, Right** Inferior tarsal plate Medial canthus **R Lower Eyelid, Left** *See Q Lower Eyelid, Right*	**Ø Open** **3 Percutaneous** **X External**	**Ø Drainage Device**	**Z No Qualifier**

Non-OR	Ø89[Ø,1,6,7,8,9,S,T]XZ[X,Z]
Non-OR	Ø89[N,P,Q,R][Ø,3,X]ØZ

Ø89 Continued on next page

LC Limited Coverage   NC Noncovered   ⊞ Combination Member   HAC associated procedure   Combination Only   DRG Non-OR   Non-OR   New/Revised in GREEN

ICD-10-PCS 2021   301   Ø89–Ø89

Ø89 Continued

Ø   **Medical and Surgical**
8   **Eye**
9   **Drainage**   Definition: Taking or letting out fluids and/or gases from a body part

                      Explanation: The qualifier DIAGNOSTIC is used to identify drainage procedures that are biopsies

Body Part Character 4		Approach Character 5	Device Character 6	Qualifier Character 7

N **Upper Eyelid, Right**
   Lateral canthus
   Levator palpebrae superioris
     muscle
   Orbicularis oculi muscle
   Superior tarsal plate
P **Upper Eyelid, Left**
   See N Upper Eyelid, Right
	Q **Lower Eyelid, Right**
	   Inferior tarsal plate
	   Medial canthus
	R **Lower Eyelid, Left**
	   See Q Lower Eyelid, Right
		Ø Open
		3 Percutaneous
		X External
			Z No Device	**X** Diagnostic
				Z No Qualifier

X **Lacrimal Duct, Right**
   Lacrimal canaliculus
   Lacrimal punctum
   Lacrimal sac
   Nasolacrimal duct
	Y **Lacrimal Duct, Left**
	   See X Lacrimal Duct, Right
		Ø Open
		3 Percutaneous
		7 Via Natural or Artificial
		   Opening
		8 Via Natural or Artificial
		   Opening Endoscopic
			Ø Drainage Device	**Z** No Qualifier

X **Lacrimal Duct, Right**
   Lacrimal canaliculus
   Lacrimal punctum
   Lacrimal sac
   Nasolacrimal duct
	Y **Lacrimal Duct, Left**
	   See X Lacrimal Duct, Right
		Ø Open
		3 Percutaneous
		7 Via Natural or Artificial
		   Opening
		8 Via Natural or Artificial
		   Opening Endoscopic
			Z No Device	**X** Diagnostic
				Z No Qualifier

Non-OR	Ø89[N,P,Q,R]ØZZ
Non-OR	Ø89[N,P,Q,R][3,X]Z[X,Z]

Ø   **Medical and Surgical**
8   **Eye**
B   **Excision**   Definition: Cutting out or off, without replacement, a portion of a body part

                      Explanation: The qualifier DIAGNOSTIC is used to identify excision procedures that are biopsies

Body Part Character 4		Approach Character 5	Device Character 6	Qualifier Character 7

Ø **Eye, Right**
   Ciliary body
   Posterior chamber
1 **Eye, Left**
   See Ø Eye, Right
N **Upper Eyelid, Right**
   Lateral canthus
   Levator palpebrae superioris
     muscle
   Orbicularis oculi muscle
   Superior tarsal plate
	P **Upper Eyelid, Left**
	   See N Upper Eyelid, Right
	Q **Lower Eyelid, Right**
	   Inferior tarsal plate
	   Medial canthus
	R **Lower Eyelid, Left**
	   See Q Lower Eyelid, Right
		Ø Open
		3 Percutaneous
		X External
			Z No Device	**X** Diagnostic
				Z No Qualifier

4 **Vitreous, Right**
   Vitreous body
5 **Vitreous, Left**
   See 4 Vitreous, Right
C **Iris, Right**
D **Iris, Left**
E **Retina, Right**
   Fovea
   Macula
   Optic disc
	F **Retina, Left**
	   See E Retina, Right
	J **Lens, Right**
	   Zonule of Zinn
	K **Lens, Left**
	   See J Lens, Right
		3 Percutaneous	**Z** No Device	**X** Diagnostic
				Z No Qualifier

6 **Sclera, Right**
7 **Sclera, Left**
8 **Cornea, Right**
9 **Cornea, Left**
	S **Conjunctiva, Right**
	   Plica semilunaris
	T **Conjunctiva, Left**
	   See S Conjunctiva, Right
		X External	**Z** No Device	**X** Diagnostic
				Z No Qualifier

A **Choroid, Right**
B **Choroid, Left**
L **Extraocular Muscle, Right**
   Inferior oblique muscle
   Inferior rectus muscle
   Lateral rectus muscle
   Medial rectus muscle
   Superior oblique muscle
   Superior rectus muscle
	M **Extraocular Muscle, Left**
	   See L Extraocular Muscle, Right
	V **Lacrimal Gland, Right**
	W **Lacrimal Gland, Left**
		Ø Open
		3 Percutaneous
			Z No Device	**X** Diagnostic
				Z No Qualifier

X **Lacrimal Duct, Right**
   Lacrimal canaliculus
   Lacrimal punctum
   Lacrimal sac
   Nasolacrimal duct
	Y **Lacrimal Duct, Left**
	   See X Lacrimal Duct, Right
		Ø Open
		3 Percutaneous
		7 Via Natural or Artificial
		   Opening
		8 Via Natural or Artificial
		   Opening Endoscopic
			Z No Device	**X** Diagnostic
				Z No Qualifier

LC Limited Coverage   **NC** Noncovered   ⊞ Combination Member   HAC associated procedure   Combination Only   DRG Non-OR   Non-OR   New/Revised in **GREEN**

302   ICD-10-PCS 2021

Eye   Ø89–Ø8B

Ø　Medical and Surgical
8　Eye
C　Extirpation　　Definition: Taking or cutting out solid matter from a body part

Explanation: The solid matter may be an abnormal byproduct of a biological function or a foreign body; it may be imbedded in a body part or in the lumen of a tubular body part. The solid matter may or may not have been previously broken into pieces.

Body Part Character 4	Approach Character 5	Device Character 6	Qualifier Character 7
Ø　Eye, Right 　　Ciliary body 　　Posterior chamber 1　Eye, Left 　　*See* Ø Eye, Right 6　Sclera, Right 7　Sclera, Left 8　Cornea, Right 9　Cornea, Left S　Conjunctiva, Right 　　Plica semilunaris T　Conjunctiva, Left 　　*See* S Conjunctiva, Right	X　External	Z　No Device	Z　No Qualifier
2　Anterior Chamber, Right 　　Aqueous humour 3　Anterior Chamber, Left 　　*See* 2 Anterior Chamber, Right 4　Vitreous, Right 　　Vitreous body 5　Vitreous, Left 　　*See* 4 Vitreous, Right C　Iris, Right D　Iris, Left E　Retina, Right 　　Fovea 　　Macula 　　Optic disc F　Retina, Left 　　*See* E Retina, Right G　Retinal Vessel, Right H　Retinal Vessel, Left J　Lens, Right 　　Zonule of Zinn K　Lens, Left 　　*See* J Lens, Right	3　Percutaneous X　External	Z　No Device	Z　No Qualifier
A　Choroid, Right B　Choroid, Left L　Extraocular Muscle, Right 　　Inferior oblique muscle 　　Inferior rectus muscle 　　Lateral rectus muscle 　　Medial rectus muscle 　　Superior oblique muscle 　　Superior rectus muscle M　Extraocular Muscle, Left 　　*See* L Extraocular Muscle, Right N　Upper Eyelid, Right 　　Lateral canthus 　　Levator palpebrae superioris muscle 　　Orbicularis oculi muscle 　　Superior tarsal plate P　Upper Eyelid, Left 　　*See* N Upper Eyelid, Right Q　Lower Eyelid, Right 　　Inferior tarsal plate 　　Medial canthus R　Lower Eyelid, Left 　　*See* Q Lower Eyelid, Right V　Lacrimal Gland, Right W　Lacrimal Gland, Left	Ø　Open 3　Percutaneous X　External	Z　No Device	Z　No Qualifier
X　Lacrimal Duct, Right 　　Lacrimal canaliculus 　　Lacrimal punctum 　　Lacrimal sac 　　Nasolacrimal duct Y　Lacrimal Duct, Left 　　*See* X Lacrimal Duct, Right	Ø　Open 3　Percutaneous 7　Via Natural or Artificial Opening 8　Via Natural or Artificial Opening 　　Endoscopic	Z　No Device	Z　No Qualifier

Non-OR　Ø8C[Ø,1,6,7,S,T]XZZ
Non-OR　Ø8C[2,3]XZZ
Non-OR　Ø8C[N,P,Q,R][Ø,3,X]ZZ

LC Limited Coverage　**NC** Noncovered　⊞ Combination Member　HAC associated procedure　Combination Only　DRG Non-OR　Non-OR　New/Revised in GREEN
ICD-10-PCS 2021　　　　　　　　　　　　　　　　　　　　　　　　　　　　　　　　　　　　303

Ø8C–Ø8C

Ø   **Medical and Surgical**
8   **Eye**
D   **Extraction**   Definition: Pulling or stripping out or off all or a portion of a body part by the use of force
                              Explanation: The qualifier DIAGNOSTIC is used to identify extraction procedures that are biopsies

Body Part Character 4	Approach Character 5	Device Character 6	Qualifier Character 7
8 Cornea, Right **9** Cornea, Left	**X** External	**Z** No Device	**X** Diagnostic **Z** No Qualifier
J Lens, Right Zonule of Zinn **K** Lens, Left *See J Lens, Right*	**3** Percutaneous	**Z** No Device	**Z** No Qualifier

Ø   **Medical and Surgical**
8   **Eye**
F   **Fragmentation**   Definition: Breaking solid matter in a body part into pieces
                              Explanation: Physical force (e.g., manual, ultrasonic) applied directly or indirectly is used to break the solid matter into pieces. The solid matter may be an abnormal byproduct of a biological function or a foreign body. The pieces of solid matter are not taken out.

Body Part Character 4	Approach Character 5	Device Character 6	Qualifier Character 7
4 Vitreous, Right NC Vitreous body **5** Vitreous, Left NC *See 4 Vitreous, Right*	**3** Percutaneous **X** External	**Z** No Device	**Z** No Qualifier

Non-OR   Ø8F[4,5]XZZ
NC   Ø8F[4,5]XZZ

Ø   **Medical and Surgical**
8   **Eye**
H   **Insertion**   Definition: Putting in a nonbiological appliance that monitors, assists, performs, or prevents a physiological function but does not physically take the place of a body part
                            Explanation: None

Body Part Character 4	Approach Character 5	Device Character 6	Qualifier Character 7
Ø Eye, Right Ciliary body Posterior chamber **1** Eye, Left *See Ø Eye, Right*	**Ø** Open	**5** Epiretinal Visual Prosthesis **Y** Other Device	**Z** No Qualifier
Ø Eye, Right Ciliary body Posterior chamber **1** Eye, Left *See Ø Eye, Right*	**3** Percutaneous	**1** Radioactive Element **3** Infusion Device **Y** Other Device	**Z** No Qualifier
Ø Eye, Right Ciliary body Posterior chamber **1** Eye, Left *See Ø Eye, Right*	**7** Via Natural or Artificial Opening **8** Via Natural or Artificial Opening Endoscopic	**Y** Other Device	**Z** No Qualifier
Ø Eye, Right Ciliary body Posterior chamber **1** Eye, Left *See Ø Eye, Right*	**X** External	**1** Radioactive Element **3** Infusion Device	**Z** No Qualifier

Non-OR   Ø8H[Ø,1]3YZ
Non-OR   Ø8H[Ø,1][7,8]YZ

LC Limited Coverage   NC Noncovered   ⊞ Combination Member   HAC associated procedure   Combination Only   DRG Non-OR   Non-OR   New/Revised in GREEN

304   ICD-10-PCS 2021

Ø Medical and Surgical
8 Eye
J Inspection   Definition: Visually and/or manually exploring a body part

Explanation: Visual exploration may be performed with or without optical instrumentation. Manual exploration may be performed directly or through intervening body layers.

Body Part Character 4	Approach Character 5	Device Character 6	Qualifier Character 7
Ø Eye, Right Ciliary body Posterior chamber **1 Eye, Left** *See Ø Eye, Right* **J Lens, Right** Zonule of Zinn **K Lens, Left** *See J Lens, Right*	**X** External	**Z** No Device	**Z** No Qualifier
L Extraocular Muscle, Right Inferior oblique muscle Inferior rectus muscle Lateral rectus muscle Medial rectus muscle Superior oblique muscle Superior rectus muscle **M Extraocular Muscle, Left** *See L Extraocular Muscle, Right*	**Ø** Open **X** External	**Z** No Device	**Z** No Qualifier

Non-OR Ø8J[Ø,1,J,K]XZZ
Non-OR Ø8J[L,M]XZZ

Ø Medical and Surgical
8 Eye
L Occlusion   Definition: Completely closing an orifice or the lumen of a tubular body part

Explanation: The orifice can be a natural orifice or an artificially created orifice

Body Part Character 4	Approach Character 5	Device Character 6	Qualifier Character 7
X Lacrimal Duct, Right Lacrimal canaliculus Lacrimal punctum Lacrimal sac Nasolacrimal duct **Y Lacrimal Duct, Left** *See X Lacrimal Duct, Right*	**Ø** Open **3** Percutaneous	**C** Extraluminal Device **D** Intraluminal Device **Z** No Device	**Z** No Qualifier
X Lacrimal Duct, Right Lacrimal canaliculus Lacrimal punctum Lacrimal sac Nasolacrimal duct **Y Lacrimal Duct, Left** *See X Lacrimal Duct, Right*	**7** Via Natural or Artificial Opening **8** Via Natural or Artificial Opening Endoscopic	**D** Intraluminal Device **Z** No Device	**Z** No Qualifier

Ø Medical and Surgical
8 Eye
M Reattachment   Definition: Putting back in or on all or a portion of a separated body part to its normal location or other suitable location

Explanation: Vascular circulation and nervous pathways may or may not be reestablished

Body Part Character 4	Approach Character 5	Device Character 6	Qualifier Character 7
N Upper Eyelid, Right Lateral canthus Levator palpebrae superioris muscle Orbicularis oculi muscle Superior tarsal plate **P Upper Eyelid, Left** *See N Upper Eyelid, Right* **Q Lower Eyelid, Right** Inferior tarsal plate Medial canthus **R Lower Eyelid, Left** *See Q Lower Eyelid, Right*	**X** External	**Z** No Device	**Z** No Qualifier

Ø   Medical and Surgical
8   Eye
N   Release   Definition: Freeing a body part from an abnormal physical constraint by cutting or by the use of force
                  Explanation: Some of the restraining tissue may be taken out but none of the body part is taken out

Body Part Character 4	Approach Character 5	Device Character 6	Qualifier Character 7

Ø   Eye, Right
      Ciliary body
      Posterior chamber
1   Eye, Left
      See Ø Eye, Right
6   Sclera, Right
7   Sclera, Left
8   Cornea, Right
9   Cornea, Left
S   Conjunctiva, Right
      Plica semilunaris
T   Conjunctiva, Left
      See S Conjunctiva, Right
	X External	**Z No Device**	**Z No Qualifier**

2   Anterior Chamber, Right
      Aqueous humour
3   Anterior Chamber, Left
      See 2 Anterior Chamber, Right
4   Vitreous, Right
      Vitreous body
5   Vitreous, Left
      See 4 Vitreous, Right
C   Iris, Right
D   Iris, Left
E   Retina, Right
      Fovea
      Macula
      Optic disc
F   Retina, Left
      See E Retina, Right
G   Retinal Vessel, Right
H   Retinal Vessel, Left
J   Lens, Right
      Zonule of Zinn
K   Lens, Left
      See J Lens, Right
	3 Percutaneous	**Z No Device**	**Z No Qualifier**

A   Choroid, Right
B   Choroid, Left
L   Extraocular Muscle, Right
      Inferior oblique muscle
      Inferior rectus muscle
      Lateral rectus muscle
      Medial rectus muscle
      Superior oblique muscle
      Superior rectus muscle
M   Extraocular Muscle, Left
      See L Extraocular Muscle, Right
V   Lacrimal Gland, Right
W   Lacrimal Gland, Left
	Ø Open
	3 Percutaneous
		Z No Device	**Z No Qualifier**

N   Upper Eyelid, Right
      Lateral canthus
      Levator palpebrae superioris muscle
      Orbicularis oculi muscle
      Superior tarsal plate
P   Upper Eyelid, Left
      See N Upper Eyelid, Right
Q   Lower Eyelid, Right
      Inferior tarsal plate
      Medial canthus
R   Lower Eyelid, Left
      See Q Lower Eyelid, Right
	Ø Open
	3 Percutaneous
	X External
		Z No Device	**Z No Qualifier**

X   Lacrimal Duct, Right
      Lacrimal canaliculus
      Lacrimal punctum
      Lacrimal sac
      Nasolacrimal duct
Y   Lacrimal Duct, Left
      See X Lacrimal Duct, Right
	Ø Open
	3 Percutaneous
	7 Via Natural or Artificial Opening
	**8 Via Natural or Artificial Opening
	      Endoscopic**
		Z No Device	**Z No Qualifier**

LC Limited Coverage   NC Noncovered   ⊞ Combination Member   HAC associated procedure   Combination Only   DRG Non-OR   Non-OR   New/Revised in GREEN
306   ICD-10-PCS 2021

Ø8N–Ø8N

Ø   Medical and Surgical
8   Eye
P   Removal   Definition: Taking out or off a device from a body part

Explanation: If a device is taken out and a similar device put in without cutting or puncturing the skin or mucous membrane, the procedure is coded to the root operation CHANGE. Otherwise, the procedure for taking out a device is coded to the root operation REMOVAL.

Body Part Character 4	Approach Character 5	Device Character 6	Qualifier Character 7

Ø   **Eye, Right**
    Ciliary body
    Posterior chamber
1   **Eye, Left**
    See Ø Eye, Right
	Ø Open
	3 Percutaneous
	7 Via Natural or Artificial Opening
	8 Via Natural or Artificial Opening
	    Endoscopic
		Ø Drainage Device
		1 Radioactive Element
		3 Infusion Device
		7 Autologous Tissue Substitute
		C Extraluminal Device
		D Intraluminal Device
		J Synthetic Substitute
		K Nonautologous Tissue Substitute
		Y Other Device
			Z No Qualifier

Ø   **Eye, Right**
    Ciliary body
    Posterior chamber
1   **Eye, Left**
    See Ø Eye, Right
	X External	**Ø** Drainage Device
		1 Radioactive Element
		3 Infusion Device
		7 Autologous Tissue Substitute
		C Extraluminal Device
		D Intraluminal Device
		J Synthetic Substitute
		K Nonautologous Tissue Substitute
			Z No Qualifier

J   **Lens, Right**
    Zonule of Zinn
K   **Lens, Left**
    See J Lens, Right
	3 Percutaneous	**J** Synthetic Substitute
		Y Other Device
			Z No Qualifier

L   **Extraocular Muscle, Right**
    Inferior oblique muscle
    Inferior rectus muscle
    Lateral rectus muscle
    Medial rectus muscle
    Superior oblique muscle
    Superior rectus muscle
M   **Extraocular Muscle, Left**
    See L Extraocular Muscle, Right
	Ø Open
	3 Percutaneous
		Ø Drainage Device
		7 Autologous Tissue Substitute
		J Synthetic Substitute
		K Nonautologous Tissue Substitute
		Y Other Device
			Z No Qualifier

Non-OR	08P[Ø,1]3YZ
Non-OR	08P[Ø,1][7,8][Ø,3,D,Y]Z
Non-OR	08P[Ø,1]X[Ø,1,3,C,D,J]Z
Non-OR	08P[J,K]3YZ
Non-OR	08P[L,M]3YZ

LC Limited Coverage   NC Noncovered   ⊞ Combination Member   HAC associated procedure   Combination Only   DRG Non-OR   Non-OR   New/Revised in GREEN

ICD-10-PCS 2021   307

Ø   Medical and Surgical
8   Eye
Q   Repair   Definition: Restoring, to the extent possible, a body part to its normal anatomic structure and function
                       Explanation: Used only when the method to accomplish the repair is not one of the other root operations

Body Part Character 4	Approach Character 5	Device Character 6	Qualifier Character 7

Ø Eye, Right
   Ciliary body
   Posterior chamber
1 Eye, Left
   See Ø Eye, Right
6 Sclera, Right
7 Sclera, Left
8 Cornea, Right NC
9 Cornea, Left NC
S Conjunctiva, Right
   Plica semilunaris
T Conjunctiva, Left
   See S Conjunctiva, Right
	X External	**Z No Device**	**Z No Qualifier**

2 Anterior Chamber, Right
   Aqueous humour
3 Anterior Chamber, Left
   See 2 Anterior Chamber, Right
4 Vitreous, Right
   Vitreous body
5 Vitreous, Left
   See 4 Vitreous, Right
C Iris, Right
D Iris, Left
E Retina, Right
   Fovea
   Macula
   Optic disc
F Retina, Left
   See E Retina, Right
G Retinal Vessel, Right
H Retinal Vessel, Left
J Lens, Right
   Zonule of Zinn
K Lens, Left
   See J Lens, Right
	3 Percutaneous	**Z No Device**	**Z No Qualifier**

A Choroid, Right
B Choroid, Left
L Extraocular Muscle, Right
   Inferior oblique muscle
   Inferior rectus muscle
   Lateral rectus muscle
   Medial rectus muscle
   Superior oblique muscle
   Superior rectus muscle
M Extraocular Muscle, Left
   See L Extraocular Muscle, Right
V Lacrimal Gland, Right
W Lacrimal Gland, Left
	Ø Open
	3 Percutaneous
		Z No Device	**Z No Qualifier**

N Upper Eyelid, Right
   Lateral canthus
   Levator palpebrae superioris muscle
   Orbicularis oculi muscle
   Superior tarsal plate
P Upper Eyelid, Left
   See N Upper Eyelid, Right
Q Lower Eyelid, Right
   Inferior tarsal plate
   Medial canthus
R Lower Eyelid, Left
   See Q Lower Eyelid, Right
	Ø Open
	3 Percutaneous
	X External
		Z No Device	**Z No Qualifier**

X Lacrimal Duct, Right
   Lacrimal canaliculus
   Lacrimal punctum
   Lacrimal sac
   Nasolacrimal duct
Y Lacrimal Duct, Left
   See X Lacrimal Duct, Right
	Ø Open
	3 Percutaneous
	7 Via Natural or Artificial Opening
	**8 Via Natural or Artificial Opening
	   Endoscopic**
		Z No Device	**Z No Qualifier**

Non-OR   Ø8Q[N,P,Q,R][Ø,3,X]ZZ
NC   Ø8Q[8,9]XZZ

LC Limited Coverage NC Noncovered ⊞ Combination Member HAC associated procedure Combination Only DRG Non-OR Non-OR New/Revised in GREEN
308   ICD-10-PCS 2021

Ø8Q–Ø8Q

Ø   **Medical and Surgical**
8   **Eye**
R   **Replacement**   Definition: Putting in or on biological or synthetic material that physically takes the place and/or function of all or a portion of a body part
                                Explanation: The body part may have been taken out or replaced, or may be taken out, physically eradicated, or rendered nonfunctional during the REPLACEMENT procedure. A REMOVAL procedure is coded for taking out the device used in a previous replacement procedure.

Body Part Character 4	Approach Character 5	Device Character 6	Qualifier Character 7

Ø   **Eye, Right**
     Ciliary body
     Posterior chamber
1   **Eye, Left**
     See Ø Eye, Right
A   **Choroid, Right**
B   **Choroid, Left**
	Ø Open
	3 Percutaneous
		7 Autologous Tissue Substitute
		J Synthetic Substitute
		K Nonautologous Tissue Substitute
			Z No Qualifier

4   **Vitreous, Right**
     Vitreous body
5   **Vitreous, Left**
     See 4 Vitreous, Right
C   **Iris, Right**
D   **Iris, Left**
G   **Retinal Vessel, Right**
H   **Retinal Vessel, Left**
	3 Percutaneous	**7** Autologous Tissue Substitute
		J Synthetic Substitute
		K Nonautologous Tissue Substitute
			Z No Qualifier

6   **Sclera, Right**
7   **Sclera, Left**
S   **Conjunctiva, Right**
     Plica semilunaris
T   **Conjunctiva, Left**
     See S Conjunctiva, Right
	X External	**7** Autologous Tissue Substitute
		J Synthetic Substitute
		K Nonautologous Tissue Substitute
			Z No Qualifier

8 **Cornea, Right** **9** **Cornea, Left**	**3** Percutaneous **X** External	**7** Autologous Tissue Substitute **J** Synthetic Substitute **K** Nonautologous Tissue Substitute	**Z** No Qualifier

J   **Lens, Right**
     Zonule of Zinn
K   **Lens, Left**
     See J Lens, Right
	3 Percutaneous	**Ø** Synthetic Substitute, Intraocular Telescope
		7 Autologous Tissue Substitute
		J Synthetic Substitute
		K Nonautologous Tissue Substitute
			Z No Qualifier

N   **Upper Eyelid, Right**
     Lateral canthus
     Levator palpebrae superioris muscle
     Orbicularis oculi muscle
     Superior tarsal plate
P   **Upper Eyelid, Left**
     See N Upper Eyelid, Right
Q   **Lower Eyelid, Right**
     Inferior tarsal plate
     Medial canthus
R   **Lower Eyelid, Left**
     See Q Lower Eyelid, Right
	Ø Open
	3 Percutaneous
	X External
		7 Autologous Tissue Substitute
		J Synthetic Substitute
		K Nonautologous Tissue Substitute
			Z No Qualifier

X   **Lacrimal Duct, Right**
     Lacrimal canaliculus
     Lacrimal punctum
     Lacrimal sac
     Nasolacrimal duct
Y   **Lacrimal Duct, Left**
     See X Lacrimal Duct, Right
	Ø Open
	3 Percutaneous
	7 Via Natural or Artificial Opening
	8 Via Natural or Artificial Opening Endoscopic
		7 Autologous Tissue Substitute
		J Synthetic Substitute
		K Nonautologous Tissue Substitute
			Z No Qualifier

LC Limited Coverage   NC Noncovered   ⊞ Combination Member   HAC associated procedure   Combination Only   DRG Non-OR   Non-OR   New/Revised in GREEN

ICD-10-PCS 2021   309

Ø8R–Ø8R

Ø   **Medical and Surgical**
8   **Eye**
S   **Reposition**   Definition: Moving to its normal location, or other suitable location, all or a portion of a body part

Explanation: The body part is moved to a new location from an abnormal location, or from a normal location where it is not functioning correctly. The body part may or may not be cut out or off to be moved to the new location.

Body Part Character 4	Approach Character 5	Device Character 6	Qualifier Character 7

C **Iris, Right**
D **Iris, Left**
G **Retinal Vessel, Right**
H **Retinal Vessel, Left**
J **Lens, Right**
    Zonule of Zinn
K **Lens, Left**
    See J Lens, Right
	3 Percutaneous	**Z** No Device	**Z** No Qualifier

L **Extraocular Muscle, Right**
    Inferior oblique muscle
    Inferior rectus muscle
    Lateral rectus muscle
    Medial rectus muscle
    Superior oblique muscle
    Superior rectus muscle
M **Extraocular Muscle, Left**
    See L Extraocular Muscle, Right
V **Lacrimal Gland, Right**
W **Lacrimal Gland, Left**
	Ø Open
	3 Percutaneous
		Z No Device	**Z** No Qualifier

N **Upper Eyelid, Right**
    Lateral canthus
    Levator palpebrae superioris muscle
    Orbicularis oculi muscle
    Superior tarsal plate
P **Upper Eyelid, Left**
    See N Upper Eyelid, Right
Q **Lower Eyelid, Right**
    Inferior tarsal plate
    Medial canthus
R **Lower Eyelid, Left**
    See Q Lower Eyelid, Right
	Ø Open
	3 Percutaneous
	X External
		Z No Device	**Z** No Qualifier

X **Lacrimal Duct, Right**
    Lacrimal canaliculus
    Lacrimal punctum
    Lacrimal sac
    Nasolacrimal duct
Y **Lacrimal Duct, Left**
    See X Lacrimal Duct, Right
	Ø Open
	3 Percutaneous
	7 Via Natural or Artificial Opening
	8 Via Natural or Artificial Opening Endoscopic
		Z No Device	**Z** No Qualifier

LC Limited Coverage   NC Noncovered   ⊞ Combination Member   HAC associated procedure   Combination Only   DRG Non-OR   Non-OR   New/Revised in GREEN

310   ICD-10-PCS 2021

Ø **Medical and Surgical**
8 **Eye**
T **Resection**   Definition: Cutting out or off, without replacement, all of a body part
                        Explanation: None

Body Part Character 4	Approach Character 5	Device Character 6	Qualifier Character 7
Ø **Eye, Right** Ciliary body Posterior chamber **1** **Eye, Left** *See Ø Eye, Right* **8** **Cornea, Right** **9** **Cornea, Left**	**X** **External**	**Z** **No Device**	**Z** **No Qualifier**
4 **Vitreous, Right** Vitreous body **5** **Vitreous, Left** *See 4 Vitreous, Right* **C** **Iris, Right** **D** **Iris, Left** **J** **Lens, Right** Zonule of Zinn **K** **Lens, Left** *See J Lens, Right*	**3** **Percutaneous**	**Z** **No Device**	**Z** **No Qualifier**
L **Extraocular Muscle, Right** Inferior oblique muscle Inferior rectus muscle Lateral rectus muscle Medial rectus muscle Superior oblique muscle Superior rectus muscle **M** **Extraocular Muscle, Left** *See L Extraocular Muscle, Right* **V** **Lacrimal Gland, Right** **W** **Lacrimal Gland, Left**	**Ø** **Open** **3** **Percutaneous**	**Z** **No Device**	**Z** **No Qualifier**
N **Upper Eyelid, Right** Lateral canthus Levator palpebrae superioris muscle Orbicularis oculi muscle Superior tarsal plate **P** **Upper Eyelid, Left** *See N Upper Eyelid, Right* **Q** **Lower Eyelid, Right** Inferior tarsal plate Medial canthus **R** **Lower Eyelid, Left** *See Q Lower Eyelid, Right*	**Ø** **Open** **X** **External**	**Z** **No Device**	**Z** **No Qualifier**
X **Lacrimal Duct, Right** Lacrimal canaliculus Lacrimal punctum Lacrimal sac Nasolacrimal duct **Y** **Lacrimal Duct, Left** *See X Lacrimal Duct, Right*	**Ø** **Open** **3** **Percutaneous** **7** **Via Natural or Artificial Opening** **8** **Via Natural or Artificial Opening** **Endoscopic**	**Z** **No Device**	**Z** **No Qualifier**

LC Limited Coverage   NC Noncovered   ⊞ Combination Member   HAC associated procedure   Combination Only   DRG Non-OR   Non-OR   New/Revised in GREEN
ICD-10-PCS 2021   311

08T–08T

Ø Medical and Surgical
8 Eye
U Supplement

Definition: Putting in or on biological or synthetic material that physically reinforces and/or augments the function of a portion of a body part

Explanation: The biological material is non-living, or is living and from the same individual. The body part may have been previously replaced, and the SUPPLEMENT procedure is performed to physically reinforce and/or augment the function of the replaced body part.

Body Part Character 4	Approach Character 5	Device Character 6	Qualifier Character 7

Ø Eye, Right
  Ciliary body
  Posterior chamber
1 Eye, Left
  See Ø Eye, Right
C Iris, Right
D Iris, Left
E Retina, Right
  Fovea
  Macula
  Optic disc
F Retina, Left
  See E Retina, Right
G Retinal Vessel, Right
H Retinal Vessel, Left
L Extraocular Muscle, Right
  Inferior oblique muscle
  Inferior rectus muscle
  Lateral rectus muscle
  Medial rectus muscle
  Superior oblique muscle
  Superior rectus muscle
M Extraocular Muscle, Left
  See L Extraocular Muscle, Right
	Ø Open
	3 Percutaneous
		7 Autologous Tissue Substitute
		J Synthetic Substitute
		K Nonautologous Tissue Substitute
			Z No Qualifier

8 Cornea, Right NC
9 Cornea, Left NC
N Upper Eyelid, Right
  Lateral canthus
  Levator palpebrae superioris muscle
  Orbicularis oculi muscle
  Superior tarsal plate
P Upper Eyelid, Left
  See N Upper Eyelid, Right
Q Lower Eyelid, Right
  Inferior tarsal plate
  Medial canthus
R Lower Eyelid, Left
  See Q Lower Eyelid, Right
	Ø Open
	3 Percutaneous
	X External
		7 Autologous Tissue Substitute
		J Synthetic Substitute
		K Nonautologous Tissue Substitute
			Z No Qualifier

X Lacrimal Duct, Right
  Lacrimal canaliculus
  Lacrimal punctum
  Lacrimal sac
  Nasolacrimal duct
Y Lacrimal Duct, Left
  See X Lacrimal Duct, Right
	Ø Open
	3 Percutaneous
	7 Via Natural or Artificial Opening
	8 Via Natural or Artificial Opening Endoscopic
		7 Autologous Tissue Substitute
		J Synthetic Substitute
		K Nonautologous Tissue Substitute
			Z No Qualifier

NC Ø8U[8,9][Ø,3,X]KZ

Ø Medical and Surgical
8 Eye
V Restriction

Definition: Partially closing an orifice or the lumen of a tubular body part

Explanation: The orifice can be a natural orifice or an artificially created orifice

Body Part Character 4	Approach Character 5	Device Character 6	Qualifier Character 7

X Lacrimal Duct, Right
  Lacrimal canaliculus
  Lacrimal punctum
  Lacrimal sac
  Nasolacrimal duct
Y Lacrimal Duct, Left
  See X Lacrimal Duct, Right
	Ø Open
	3 Percutaneous
		C Extraluminal Device
		D Intraluminal Device
		Z No Device
			Z No Qualifier

X Lacrimal Duct, Right
  Lacrimal canaliculus
  Lacrimal punctum
  Lacrimal sac
  Nasolacrimal duct
Y Lacrimal Duct, Left
  See X Lacrimal Duct, Right
	7 Via Natural or Artificial Opening
	8 Via Natural or Artificial Opening Endoscopic
		D Intraluminal Device
		Z No Device
			Z No Qualifier

Ø Medical and Surgical
8 Eye
W Revision   Definition: Correcting, to the extent possible, a portion of a malfunctioning device or the position of a displaced device

Explanation: Revision can include correcting a malfunctioning or displaced device by taking out or putting in components of the device such as a screw or pin

Body Part Character 4	Approach Character 5	Device Character 6	Qualifier Character 7

Ø Eye, Right
  Ciliary body
  Posterior chamber
1 Eye, Left
  See Ø Eye, Right
	Ø Open
	3 Percutaneous
	7 Via Natural or Artificial Opening
	8 Via Natural or Artificial Opening Endoscopic
		Ø Drainage Device
		3 Infusion Device
		7 Autologous Tissue Substitute
		C Extraluminal Device
		D Intraluminal Device
		J Synthetic Substitute
		K Nonautologous Tissue Substitute
		Y Other Device
			Z No Qualifier

Ø Eye, Right
  Ciliary body
  Posterior chamber
1 Eye, Left
  See Ø Eye, Right
	X External	Ø Drainage Device
		3 Infusion Device
		7 Autologous Tissue Substitute
		C Extraluminal Device
		D Intraluminal Device
		J Synthetic Substitute
		K Nonautologous Tissue Substitute
			Z No Qualifier

J Lens, Right
  Zonule of Zinn
K Lens, Left
  See J Lens, Right
	3 Percutaneous	J Synthetic Substitute
		Y Other Device
			Z No Qualifier

J Lens, Right
  Zonule of Zinn
K Lens, Left
  See J Lens, Right
	X External	J Synthetic Substitute	Z No Qualifier

L Extraocular Muscle, Right
  Inferior oblique muscle
  Inferior rectus muscle
  Lateral rectus muscle
  Medial rectus muscle
  Superior oblique muscle
  Superior rectus muscle
M Extraocular Muscle, Left
  See L Extraocular Muscle, Right
	Ø Open
	3 Percutaneous
		Ø Drainage Device
		7 Autologous Tissue Substitute
		J Synthetic Substitute
		K Nonautologous Tissue Substitute
		Y Other Device
			Z No Qualifier

Non-OR	Ø8W[Ø,1][3,7,8]YZ
Non-OR	Ø8W[Ø,1]X[Ø,3,7,C,D,J,K]Z
Non-OR	Ø8W[J,K]3YZ
Non-OR	Ø8W[J,K]XJZ
Non-OR	Ø8W[L,M]3YZ

Ø Medical and Surgical
8 Eye
X Transfer   Definition: Moving, without taking out, all or a portion of a body part to another location to take over the function of all or a portion of a body part

Explanation: The body part transferred remains connected to its vascular and nervous supply

Body Part Character 4	Approach Character 5	Device Character 6	Qualifier Character 7

L Extraocular Muscle, Right
  Inferior oblique muscle
  Inferior rectus muscle
  Lateral rectus muscle
  Medial rectus muscle
  Superior oblique muscle
  Superior rectus muscle
M Extraocular Muscle, Left
  See L Extraocular Muscle, Right
	Ø Open
	3 Percutaneous
		Z No Device	Z No Qualifier

LC Limited Coverage   NC Noncovered   ⊞ Combination Member   HAC associated procedure   Combination Only   DRG Non-OR   Non-OR   New/Revised in GREEN

ICD-10-PCS 2021   313

Ø8W–Ø8X

Ear, Nose, Sinus Ø9Ø–Ø9W

Character Meanings*

This Character Meaning table is provided as a guide to assist the user in the identification of character members that may be found in this section of code tables. It **SHOULD NOT** be used to build a PCS code.

Operation–Character 3		Body Part–Character 4		Approach–Character 5		Device–Character 6		Qualifier–Character 7	
Ø	Alteration	Ø	External Ear, Right	Ø	Open	Ø	Drainage Device	Ø	Endolymphatic
1	Bypass	1	External Ear, Left	3	Percutaneous	1	Radioactive Element	X	Diagnostic
2	Change	2	External Ear, Bilateral	4	Percutaneous Endoscopic	4	Hearing Device, Bone Conduction	Z	No Qualifier
3	Control	3	External Auditory Canal, Right	7	Via Natural or Artificial Opening	5	Hearing Device, Single Channel Cochlear Prosthesis		
5	Destruction	4	External Auditory Canal, Left	8	Via Natural or Artificial Opening Endoscopic	6	Hearing Device, Multiple Channel Cochlear Prosthesis		
7	Dilation	5	Middle Ear, Right	X	External	7	Autologous Tissue Substitute		
8	Division	6	Middle Ear, Left			B	Intraluminal Device, Airway		
9	Drainage	7	Tympanic Membrane, Right			D	Intraluminal Device		
B	Excision	8	Tympanic Membrane, Left			J	Synthetic Substitute		
C	Extirpation	9	Auditory Ossicle, Right			K	Nonautologous Tissue Substitute		
D	Extraction	A	Auditory Ossicle, Left			S	Hearing Device		
H	Insertion	B	Mastoid Sinus, Right			Y	Other Device		
J	Inspection	C	Mastoid Sinus, Left			Z	No Device		
M	Reattachment	D	Inner Ear, Right						
N	Release	E	Inner Ear, Left						
P	Removal	F	Eustachian Tube, Right						
Q	Repair	G	Eustachian Tube, Left						
R	Replacement	H	Ear, Right						
S	Reposition	J	Ear, Left						
T	Resection	K	Nasal Mucosa and Soft Tissue						
U	Supplement	L	Nasal Turbinate						
W	Revision	M	Nasal Septum						
		N	Nasopharynx						
		P	Accessory Sinus						
		Q	Maxillary Sinus, Right						
		R	Maxillary Sinus, Left						
		S	Frontal Sinus, Right						
		T	Frontal Sinus, Left						
		U	Ethmoid Sinus, Right						
		V	Ethmoid Sinus, Left						
		W	Sphenoid Sinus, Right						
		X	Sphenoid Sinus, Left						
		Y	Sinus						

* Includes sinus ducts.

AHA Coding Clinic for table Ø93
2018, 4Q, 38   Control of epistaxis

AHA Coding Clinic for table Ø95
2018, 1Q, 19   Control of epistaxis via silver nitrate cauterization

AHA Coding Clinic for table Ø9Q
2018, 1Q, 19   Control of epistaxis via silver nitrate cauterization
2017, 4Q, 106   Control of bleeding of external naris using suture
2014, 4Q, 20   Control of epistaxis
2014, 3Q, 22   Transsphenoidal removal of pituitary tumor and fat graft placement
2013, 4Q, 114   Balloon sinuplasty

AHA Coding Clinic for table Ø9U
2019, 4Q, 28-29   Sinus supplement

Ear Anatomy

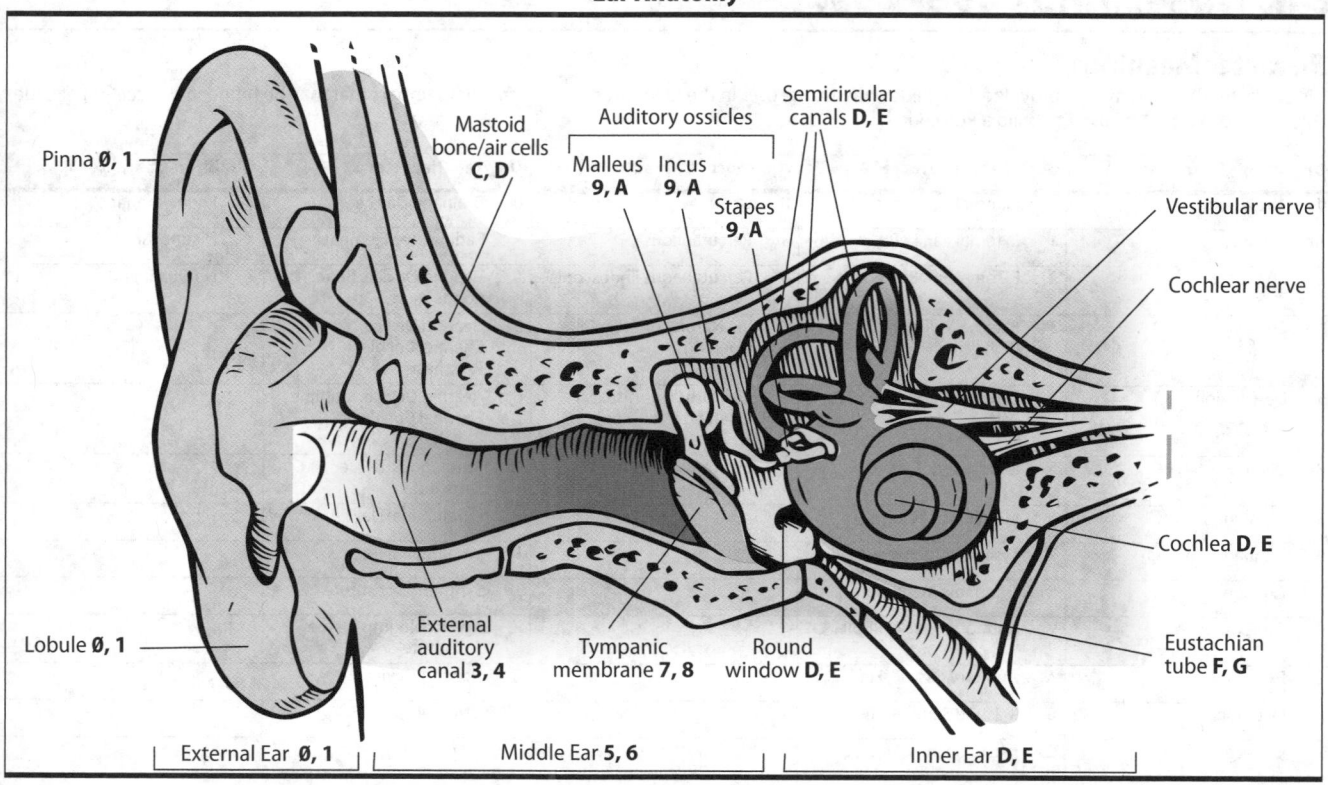

Pinna Ø, 1

Mastoid bone/air cells C, D

Auditory ossicles
Malleus 9, A   Incus 9, A

Stapes 9, A

Semicircular canals D, E

Vestibular nerve

Cochlear nerve

Cochlea D, E

Eustachian tube F, G

Round window D, E

Tympanic membrane 7, 8

External auditory canal 3, 4

Lobule Ø, 1

External Ear Ø, 1   Middle Ear 5, 6   Inner Ear D, E

Nasal Turbinates

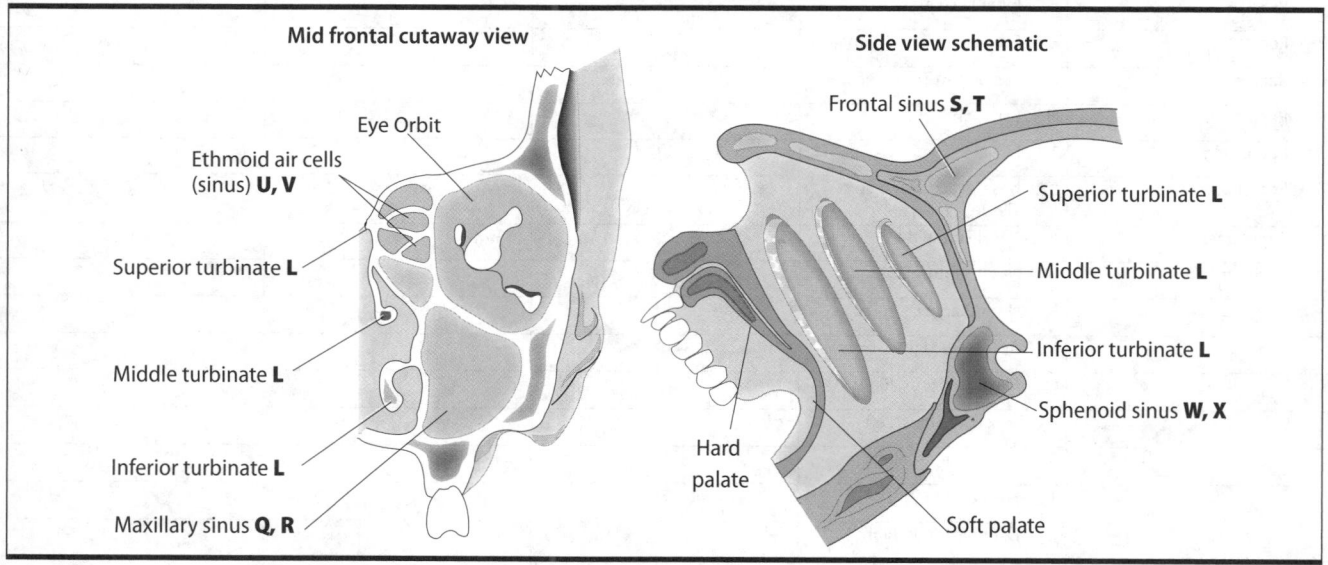

Mid frontal cutaway view

Eye Orbit

Ethmoid air cells (sinus) U, V

Superior turbinate L

Middle turbinate L

Inferior turbinate L

Maxillary sinus Q, R

Side view schematic

Frontal sinus S, T

Superior turbinate L

Middle turbinate L

Inferior turbinate L

Sphenoid sinus W, X

Hard palate

Soft palate

Paranasal Sinuses

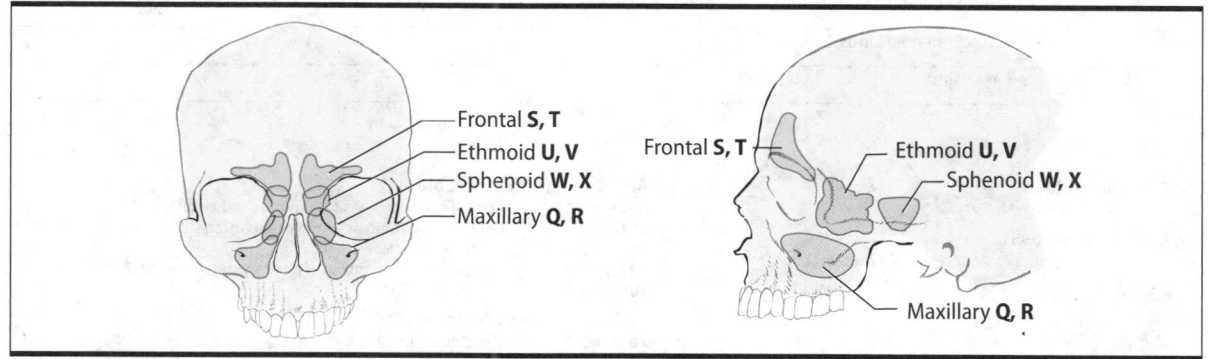

Frontal S, T
Ethmoid U, V
Sphenoid W, X
Maxillary Q, R

Frontal S, T

Ethmoid U, V
Sphenoid W, X

Maxillary Q, R

Ø   **Medical and Surgical**
9   **Ear, Nose, Sinus**
Ø   **Alteration**   Definition: Modifying the anatomic structure of a body part without affecting the function of the body part
                     Explanation: Principal purpose is to improve appearance

Body Part Character 4		Approach Character 5	Device Character 6	Qualifier Character 7

Ø **External Ear, Right**
  Antihelix
  Antitragus
  Auricle
  Earlobe
  Helix
  Pinna
  Tragus
1 **External Ear, Left**
  See Ø External Ear, Right
	2 **External Ear, Bilateral**
	  See Ø External Ear, Right
	K **Nasal Mucosa and Soft Tissue**
	  Columella
	  External naris
	  Greater alar cartilage
	  Internal naris
	  Lateral nasal cartilage
	  Lesser alar cartilage
	  Nasal cavity
	  Nostril
		Ø **Open**
		3 **Percutaneous**
		4 **Percutaneous Endoscopic**
		X **External**
			7 **Autologous Tissue Substitute**
			J **Synthetic Substitute**
			K **Nonautologous Tissue Substitute**
			Z **No Device**
				Z **No Qualifier**

Ø   **Medical and Surgical**
9   **Ear, Nose, Sinus**
1   **Bypass**   Definition: Altering the route of passage of the contents of a tubular body part
                Explanation: Rerouting contents of a body part to a downstream area of the normal route, to a similar route and body part, or to an abnormal route and dissimilar body part. Includes one or more anastomoses, with or without the use of a device.

Body Part Character 4	Approach Character 5	Device Character 6	Qualifier Character 7

D **Inner Ear, Right**
  Bony labyrinth
  Bony vestibule
  Cochlea
  Round window
  Semicircular canal
E **Inner Ear, Left**
  See D Inner Ear, Right
	Ø **Open**	7 **Autologous Tissue Substitute**
		J **Synthetic Substitute**
		K **Nonautologous Tissue Substitute**
		Z **No Device**
			Ø **Endolymphatic**

Ø   **Medical and Surgical**
9   **Ear, Nose, Sinus**
2   **Change**   Definition: Taking out or off a device from a body part and putting back an identical or similar device in or on the same body part without cutting or puncturing the skin or a mucous membrane
               Explanation: All CHANGE procedures are coded using the approach EXTERNAL

Body Part Character 4	Approach Character 5	Device Character 6	Qualifier Character 7

H **Ear, Right**
J **Ear, Left**
K **Nasal Mucosa and Soft Tissue**
  Columella
  External naris
  Greater alar cartilage
  Internal naris
  Lateral nasal cartilage
  Lesser alar cartilage
  Nasal cavity
  Nostril
Y **Sinus**
	X **External**	Ø **Drainage Device**
		Y **Other Device**
			Z **No Qualifier**

Non-OR   All body part, approach, device, and qualifier values

Ø   **Medical and Surgical**
9   **Ear, Nose, Sinus**
3   **Control**   Definition: Stopping, or attempting to stop, postprocedural or other acute bleeding
              Explanation: None

Body Part Character 4	Approach Character 5	Device Character 6	Qualifier Character 7

K **Nasal Mucosa and Soft Tissue**
  Columella
  External naris
  Greater alar cartilage
  Internal naris
  Lateral nasal cartilage
  Lesser alar cartilage
  Nasal cavity
  Nostril
	7 **Via Natural or Artificial Opening**
	8 **Via Natural or Artificial Opening Endoscopic**
		Z **No Device**	Z **No Qualifier**

Non-OR   Ø93K[7,8]ZZ

LC Limited Coverage   NC Noncovered   ⊞ Combination Member   HAC associated procedure   Combination Only   DRG Non-OR   Non-OR   New/Revised in GREEN

ICD-10-PCS 2021   317

Ø9Ø–Ø93

Ear, Nose, Sinus

Ø **Medical and Surgical**
9 **Ear, Nose, Sinus**
5 **Destruction**   Definition: Physical eradication of all or a portion of a body part by the direct use of energy, force, or a destructive agent
     Explanation: None of the body part is physically taken out

Body Part Character 4		Approach Character 5	Device Character 6	Qualifier Character 7
Ø **External Ear, Right** Antihelix Antitragus Auricle Earlobe Helix Pinna Tragus	**1** **External Ear, Left** *See Ø External Ear, Right*	**Ø** Open **3** Percutaneous **4** Percutaneous Endoscopic **X** External	**Z** No Device	**Z** No Qualifier
3 **External Auditory Canal, Right** External auditory meatus	**4** **External Auditory Canal, Left** *See 3 External Auditory Canal, Right*	**Ø** Open **3** Percutaneous **4** Percutaneous Endoscopic **7** Via Natural or Artificial Opening **8** Via Natural or Artificial Opening Endoscopic **X** External	**Z** No Device	**Z** No Qualifier
5 **Middle Ear, Right** Oval window Tympanic cavity **6** **Middle Ear, Left** *See 5 Middle Ear, Right* **9** **Auditory Ossicle, Right** Incus Malleus Stapes **A** **Auditory Ossicle, Left** *See 9 Auditory Ossicle, Right*	**D** **Inner Ear, Right** Bony labyrinth Bony vestibule Cochlea Round window Semicircular canal **E** **Inner Ear, Left** *See D Inner Ear, Right*	**Ø** Open **8** Via Natural or Artificial Opening Endoscopic	**Z** No Device	**Z** No Qualifier
7 **Tympanic Membrane, Right** Pars flaccida **8** **Tympanic Membrane, Left** *See 7 Tympanic Membrane, Right* **F** **Eustachian Tube, Right** Auditory tube Pharyngotympanic tube **G** **Eustachian Tube, Left** *See F Eustachian Tube, Right*	**L** **Nasal Turbinate** Inferior turbinate Middle turbinate Nasal concha Superior turbinate **N** **Nasopharynx** Choana Fossa of Rosenmuller Pharyngeal recess Rhinopharynx	**Ø** Open **3** Percutaneous **4** Percutaneous Endoscopic **7** Via Natural or Artificial Opening **8** Via Natural or Artificial Opening Endoscopic	**Z** No Device	**Z** No Qualifier
B **Mastoid Sinus, Right** Mastoid air cells **C** **Mastoid Sinus, Left** *See B Mastoid Sinus, Right* **M** **Nasal Septum** Quadrangular cartilage Septal cartilage Vomer bone **P** **Accessory Sinus** **Q** **Maxillary Sinus, Right** Antrum of Highmore	**R** **Maxillary Sinus, Left** *See Q Maxillary Sinus, Right* **S** **Frontal Sinus, Right** **T** **Frontal Sinus, Left** **U** **Ethmoid Sinus, Right** Ethmoidal air cell **V** **Ethmoid Sinus, Left** *See U Ethmoid Sinus, Right* **W** **Sphenoid Sinus, Right** **X** **Sphenoid Sinus, Left**	**Ø** Open **3** Percutaneous **4** Percutaneous Endoscopic **8** Via Natural or Artificial Opening Endoscopic	**Z** No Device	**Z** No Qualifier
K **Nasal Mucosa and Soft Tissue** Columella External naris Greater alar cartilage Internal naris Lateral nasal cartilage Lesser alar cartilage Nasal cavity Nostril		**Ø** Open **3** Percutaneous **4** Percutaneous Endoscopic **8** Via Natural or Artificial Opening Endoscopic **X** External	**Z** No Device	**Z** No Qualifier

Non-OR	Ø95[Ø,1][Ø,3,4,X]ZZ
Non-OR	Ø95[3,4][Ø,3,4,7,8,X]ZZ
Non-OR	Ø95[F,G][Ø,3,4,7,8]ZZ
Non-OR	Ø95M[Ø,3,4,8]ZZ
Non-OR	Ø95K[Ø,3,4,8,X]ZZ

Ø   **Medical and Surgical**
9   **Ear, Nose, Sinus**
7   **Dilation**   Definition: Expanding an orifice or the lumen of a tubular body part

Explanation: The orifice can be a natural orifice or an artificially created orifice. Accomplished by stretching a tubular body part using intraluminal pressure or by cutting part of the orifice or wall of the tubular body part.

Body Part Character 4	Approach Character 5	Device Character 6	Qualifier Character 7

F   Eustachian Tube, Right
    Auditory tube
    Pharyngotympanic tube
G   Eustachian Tube, Left
    See F Eustachian Tube, Right
	Ø Open
	7 Via Natural or Artificial Opening
	8 Via Natural or Artificial Opening
	    Endoscopic
		D Intraluminal Device
		Z No Device
			Z No Qualifier

F   Eustachian Tube, Right
    Auditory tube
    Pharyngotympanic tube
G   Eustachian Tube, Left
    See F Eustachian Tube, Right
	3 Percutaneous
	4 Percutaneous Endoscopic
		Z No Device	**Z** No Qualifier

Non-OR   All body part, approach, device, and qualifier values

Ø   **Medical and Surgical**
9   **Ear, Nose, Sinus**
8   **Division**   Definition: Cutting into a body part, without draining fluids and/or gases from the body part, in order to separate or transect a body part

Explanation: All or a portion of the body part is separated into two or more portions

Body Part Character 4	Approach Character 5	Device Character 6	Qualifier Character 7

L   Nasal Turbinate
    Inferior turbinate
    Middle turbinate
    Nasal concha
    Superior turbinate
	Ø Open
	3 Percutaneous
	4 Percutaneous Endoscopic
	7 Via Natural or Artificial Opening
	8 Via Natural or Artificial Opening
	    Endoscopic
		Z No Device	**Z** No Qualifier

Ø **Medical and Surgical**
9 **Ear, Nose, Sinus**
9 **Drainage**　　Definition: Taking or letting out fluids and/or gases from a body part
　　　　Explanation: The qualifier DIAGNOSTIC is used to identify drainage procedures that are biopsies

Body Part Character 4		Approach Character 5	Device Character 6	Qualifier Character 7
Ø External Ear, Right Antihelix Antitragus Auricle Earlobe Helix Pinna Tragus	1 External Ear, Left *See Ø External Ear, Right*	Ø Open 3 Percutaneous 4 Percutaneous Endoscopic X External	Ø Drainage Device	Z No Qualifier
Ø External Ear, Right Antihelix Antitragus Auricle Earlobe Helix Pinna Tragus	1 External Ear, Left *See Ø External Ear, Right*	Ø Open 3 Percutaneous 4 Percutaneous Endoscopic X External	Z No Device	X Diagnostic Z No Qualifier
3 External Auditory Canal, Right External auditory meatus 4 External Auditory Canal, Left *See 3 External Auditory Canal, Right*	K Nasal Mucosa and Soft Tissue Columella External naris Greater alar cartilage Internal naris Lateral nasal cartilage Lesser alar cartilage Nasal cavity Nostril	Ø Open 3 Percutaneous 4 Percutaneous Endoscopic 7 Via Natural or Artificial Opening 8 Via Natural or Artificial Opening Endoscopic X External	Ø Drainage Device	Z No Qualifier
3 External Auditory Canal, Right External auditory meatus 4 External Auditory Canal, Left *See 3 External Auditory Canal, Right*	K Nasal Mucosa and Soft Tissue Columella External naris Greater alar cartilage Internal naris Lateral nasal cartilage Lesser alar cartilage Nasal cavity Nostril	Ø Open 3 Percutaneous 4 Percutaneous Endoscopic 7 Via Natural or Artificial Opening 8 Via Natural or Artificial Opening Endoscopic X External	Z No Device	X Diagnostic Z No Qualifier
5 Middle Ear, Right Oval window Tympanic cavity 6 Middle Ear, Left *See 5 Middle Ear, Right* 9 Auditory Ossicle, Right Incus Malleus Stapes	A Auditory Ossicle, Left *See 9 Auditory Ossicle, Right* D Inner Ear, Right Bony labyrinth Bony vestibule Cochlea Round window Semicircular canal E Inner Ear, Left *See D Inner Ear, Right*	Ø Open 7 Via Natural or Artificial Opening 8 Via Natural or Artificial Opening Endoscopic	Ø Drainage Device	Z No Qualifier
5 Middle Ear, Right Oval window Tympanic cavity 6 Middle Ear, Left *See 5 Middle Ear, Right* 9 Auditory Ossicle, Right Incus Malleus Stapes	A Auditory Ossicle, Left *See 9 Auditory Ossicle, Right* D Inner Ear, Right Bony labyrinth Bony vestibule Cochlea Round window Semicircular canal E Inner Ear, Left *See D Inner Ear, Right*	Ø Open 7 Via Natural or Artificial Opening 8 Via Natural or Artificial Opening Endoscopic	Z No Device	X Diagnostic Z No Qualifier

Non-OR　Ø99[Ø,1][Ø,3,4,X]ØZ
Non-OR　Ø99[Ø,1][Ø,3,4,X]Z[X,Z]
Non-OR　Ø99[3,4,K][Ø,3,4,7,8,X]ØZ
Non-OR　Ø99[3,4,K][Ø,3,4,7,8,X]Z[X,Z]
Non-OR　Ø99[5,6]8ØZ
Non-OR　Ø99[9,A,D,E][7,8]ØZ
Non-OR　Ø99[5,6]ØZZ
Non-OR　Ø99[5,6,9,A,D,E][7,8]Z[X,Z]

Ø99 Continued on next page

Ø   **Medical and Surgical**   *Ø99 Continued*
9   **Ear, Nose, Sinus**
9   **Drainage**   Definition: Taking or letting out fluids and/or gases from a body part
                           Explanation: The qualifier DIAGNOSTIC is used to identify drainage procedures that are biopsies

Body Part Character 4		Approach Character 5	Device Character 6	Qualifier Character 7
7 Tympanic Membrane, Right Pars flaccida **8 Tympanic Membrane, Left** *See 7 Tympanic Membrane, Right* **B Mastoid Sinus, Right** Mastoid air cells **C Mastoid Sinus, Left** *See B Mastoid Sinus, Right* **F Eustachian Tube, Right** Auditory tube Pharyngotympanic tube **G Eustachian Tube, Left** *See F Eustachian Tube, Right* **L Nasal Turbinate** Inferior turbinate Middle turbinate Nasal concha Superior turbinate **M Nasal Septum** Quadrangular cartilage Septal cartilage Vomer bone	**N Nasopharynx** Choana Fossa of Rosenmuller Pharyngeal recess Rhinopharynx **P Accessory Sinus** **Q Maxillary Sinus, Right** Antrum of Highmore **R Maxillary Sinus, Left** *See Q Maxillary Sinus, Right* **S Frontal Sinus, Right** **T Frontal Sinus, Left** **U Ethmoid Sinus, Right** Ethmoidal air cell **V Ethmoid Sinus, Left** *See U Ethmoid Sinus, Right* **W Sphenoid Sinus, Right** **X Sphenoid Sinus, Left**	**Ø Open** **3 Percutaneous** **4 Percutaneous Endoscopic** **7 Via Natural or Artificial Opening** **8 Via Natural or Artificial Opening Endoscopic**	**Ø Drainage Device**	**Z No Qualifier**
7 Tympanic Membrane, Right Pars flaccida **8 Tympanic Membrane, Left** *See 7 Tympanic Membrane, Right* **B Mastoid Sinus, Right** Mastoid air cells **C Mastoid Sinus, Left** *See B Mastoid Sinus, Right* **F Eustachian Tube, Right** Auditory tube Pharyngotympanic tube **G Eustachian Tube, Left** *See F Eustachian Tube, Right* **L Nasal Turbinate** Inferior turbinate Middle turbinate Nasal concha Superior turbinate **M Nasal Septum** Quadrangular cartilage Septal cartilage Vomer bone	**N Nasopharynx** Choana Fossa of Rosenmuller Pharyngeal recess Rhinopharynx **P Accessory Sinus** **Q Maxillary Sinus, Right** Antrum of Highmore **R Maxillary Sinus, Left** *See Q Maxillary Sinus, Right* **S Frontal Sinus, Right** **T Frontal Sinus, Left** **U Ethmoid Sinus, Right** Ethmoidal air cell **V Ethmoid Sinus, Left** *See U Ethmoid Sinus, Right* **W Sphenoid Sinus, Right** **X Sphenoid Sinus, Left**	**Ø Open** **3 Percutaneous** **4 Percutaneous Endoscopic** **7 Via Natural or Artificial Opening** **8 Via Natural or Artificial Opening Endoscopic**	**Z No Device**	**X Diagnostic** **Z No Qualifier**

Non-OR	Ø99[B,C][3,7,8]ØZ
Non-OR	Ø99[F,G,L,M][Ø,3,4,7,8]ØZ
Non-OR	Ø99N3ØZ
Non-OR	Ø99[P,Q,R,S,T,U,V,W,X][3,4,7,8]ØZ
Non-OR	Ø99[7,8][Ø,3,4,7,8]ZZ
Non-OR	Ø99[7,8][7,8]ZX
Non-OR	Ø99[B,C]3ZZ
Non-OR	Ø99[B,C][7,8]Z[X,Z]
Non-OR	Ø99[F,G][Ø,3,4,7,8]ZZ
Non-OR	Ø99[F,G][7,8]ZX
Non-OR	Ø99[L,M][Ø,3,4,7,8]Z[X,Z]
Non-OR	Ø99N[Ø,3,4,7,8]ZX
Non-OR	Ø99N3ZZ
Non-OR	Ø99[P,Q,R,S,T,U,V,W,X][3,4,7,8]Z[X,Z]

LC Limited Coverage   NC Noncovered   ⊞ Combination Member   HAC associated procedure   Combination Only   DRG Non-OR   Non-OR   New/Revised in GREEN

ICD-10-PCS 2021   321

Ø99–Ø99

Ear, Nose, Sinus

- Ø   **Medical and Surgical**
- 9   **Ear, Nose, Sinus**
- B   **Excision**   Definition: Cutting out or off, without replacement, a portion of a body part

Explanation: The qualifier DIAGNOSTIC is used to identify excision procedures that are biopsies

Body Part Character 4		Approach Character 5	Device Character 6	Qualifier Character 7
Ø **External Ear, Right** Antihelix Antitragus Auricle Earlobe Helix Pinna Tragus	1 **External Ear, Left** *See Ø External Ear, Right*	Ø Open 3 Percutaneous 4 Percutaneous Endoscopic X External	Z No Device	X Diagnostic Z No Qualifier
3 **External Auditory Canal, Right** External auditory meatus	4 **External Auditory Canal, Left** *See 3 External Auditory Canal, Right*	Ø Open 3 Percutaneous 4 Percutaneous Endoscopic 7 Via Natural or Artificial Opening 8 Via Natural or Artificial Opening Endoscopic X External	Z No Device	X Diagnostic Z No Qualifier
5 **Middle Ear, Right** Oval window Tympanic cavity 6 **Middle Ear, Left** *See 5 Middle Ear, Right* 9 **Auditory Ossicle, Right** Incus Malleus Stapes	A **Auditory Ossicle, Left** *See 9 Auditory Ossicle, Right* D **Inner Ear, Right** Bony labyrinth Bony vestibule Cochlea Round window Semicircular canal E **Inner Ear, Left** *See D Inner Ear, Right*	Ø Open 8 Via Natural or Artificial Opening Endoscopic	Z No Device	X Diagnostic Z No Qualifier
7 **Tympanic Membrane, Right** Pars flaccida 8 **Tympanic Membrane, Left** *See 7 Tympanic Membrane, Right* F **Eustachian Tube, Right** Auditory tube Pharyngotympanic tube G **Eustachian Tube, Left** *See F Eustachian Tube, Right*	L **Nasal Turbinate** Inferior turbinate Middle turbinate Nasal concha Superior turbinate N **Nasopharynx** Choana Fossa of Rosenmuller Pharyngeal recess Rhinopharynx	Ø Open 3 Percutaneous 4 Percutaneous Endoscopic 7 Via Natural or Artificial Opening 8 Via Natural or Artificial Opening Endoscopic	Z No Device	X Diagnostic Z No Qualifier
B **Mastoid Sinus, Right** Mastoid air cells C **Mastoid Sinus, Left** *See B Mastoid Sinus, Right* M **Nasal Septum** Quadrangular cartilage Septal cartilage Vomer bone P **Accessory Sinus** Q **Maxillary Sinus, Right** Antrum of Highmore	R **Maxillary Sinus, Left** *See Q Maxillary Sinus, Right* S **Frontal Sinus, Right** T **Frontal Sinus, Left** U **Ethmoid Sinus, Right** Ethmoidal air cell V **Ethmoid Sinus, Left** *See U Ethmoid Sinus, Right* W **Sphenoid Sinus, Right** X **Sphenoid Sinus, Left**	Ø Open 3 Percutaneous 4 Percutaneous Endoscopic 8 Via Natural or Artificial Opening Endoscopic	Z No Device	X Diagnostic Z No Qualifier
K **Nasal Mucosa and Soft Tissue** Columella External naris Greater alar cartilage Internal naris Lateral nasal cartilage Lesser alar cartilage Nasal cavity Nostril		Ø Open 3 Percutaneous 4 Percutaneous Endoscopic 8 Via Natural or Artificial Opening Endoscopic X External	Z No Device	X Diagnostic Z No Qualifier

Non-OR   Ø9B[Ø,1][Ø,3,4,X]Z[X,Z]
Non-OR   Ø9B[3,4][Ø,3,4,7,8,X]Z[X,Z]
Non-OR   Ø9B[F,G,L,N][Ø,3,4,7,8]Z[X,Z]
Non-OR   Ø9BM[Ø,3,4,8]ZX
Non-OR   Ø9B[P,Q,R,S,T,U,V,W,X][3,4,8]ZX
Non-OR   Ø9BK8Z[X,Z]

LC Limited Coverage   **NC** Noncovered   ⊞ Combination Member   HAC associated procedure   Combination Only   DRG Non-OR   Non-OR   New/Revised in GREEN

322   ICD-10-PCS 2021

Ø   **Medical and Surgical**
9   **Ear, Nose, Sinus**
C   **Extirpation**   Definition: Taking or cutting out solid matter from a body part

Explanation: The solid matter may be an abnormal byproduct of a biological function or a foreign body; it may be imbedded in a body part or in the lumen of a tubular body part. The solid matter may or may not have been previously broken into pieces.

Body Part Character 4		Approach Character 5	Device Character 6	Qualifier Character 7
Ø External Ear, Right Antihelix Antitragus Auricle Earlobe Helix Pinna Tragus	**1 External Ear, Left** *See Ø External Ear, Right*	**Ø** Open **3** Percutaneous **4** Percutaneous Endoscopic **X** External	**Z** No Device	**Z** No Qualifier
3 External Auditory Canal, Right External auditory meatus	**4 External Auditory Canal, Left** *See 3 External Auditory Canal, Right*	**Ø** Open **3** Percutaneous **4** Percutaneous Endoscopic **7** Via Natural or Artificial Opening **8** Via Natural or Artificial Opening Endoscopic **X** External	**Z** No Device	**Z** No Qualifier
5 Middle Ear, Right Oval window Tympanic cavity **6 Middle Ear, Left** *See 5 Middle Ear, Right* **9 Auditory Ossicle, Right** Incus Malleus Stapes	**A Auditory Ossicle, Left** *See 9 Auditory Ossicle, Right* **D Inner Ear, Right** Bony labyrinth Bony vestibule Cochlea Round window Semicircular canal **E Inner Ear, Left** *See D Inner Ear, Right*	**Ø** Open **8** Via Natural or Artificial Opening Endoscopic	**Z** No Device	**Z** No Qualifier
7 Tympanic Membrane, Right Pars flaccida **8 Tympanic Membrane, Left** *See 7 Tympanic Membrane, Right* **F Eustachian Tube, Right** Auditory tube Pharyngotympanic tube **G Eustachian Tube, Left** *See F Eustachian Tube, Right*	**L Nasal Turbinate** Inferior turbinate Middle turbinate Nasal concha Superior turbinate **N Nasopharynx** Choana Fossa of Rosenmuller Pharyngeal recess Rhinopharynx	**Ø** Open **3** Percutaneous **4** Percutaneous Endoscopic **7** Via Natural or Artificial Opening **8** Via Natural or Artificial Opening Endoscopic	**Z** No Device	**Z** No Qualifier
B Mastoid Sinus, Right Mastoid air cells **C Mastoid Sinus, Left** *See B Mastoid Sinus, Right* **M Nasal Septum** Quadrangular cartilage Septal cartilage Vomer bone **P Accessory Sinus** **Q Maxillary Sinus, Right** Antrum of Highmore	**R Maxillary Sinus, Left** *See Q Maxillary Sinus, Right* **S Frontal Sinus, Right** **T Frontal Sinus, Left** **U Ethmoid Sinus, Right** Ethmoidal air cell **V Ethmoid Sinus, Left** *See U Ethmoid Sinus, Right* **W Sphenoid Sinus, Right** **X Sphenoid Sinus, Left**	**Ø** Open **3** Percutaneous **4** Percutaneous Endoscopic **8** Via Natural or Artificial Opening Endoscopic	**Z** No Device	**Z** No Qualifier
K Nasal Mucosa and Soft Tissue Columella External naris Greater alar cartilage Internal naris Lateral nasal cartilage Lesser alar cartilage Nasal cavity Nostril		**Ø** Open **3** Percutaneous **4** Percutaneous Endoscopic **8** Via Natural or Artificial Opening Endoscopic **X** External	**Z** No Device	**Z** No Qualifier

Non-OR   09C[Ø,1][Ø,3,4,X]ZZ
Non-OR   09C[3,4][Ø,3,4,7,8,X]ZZ
Non-OR   09C[7,8,F,G,L][Ø,3,4,7,8]ZZ
Non-OR   09CM[Ø,3,4,8]ZZ
Non-OR   09CK8ZZ

LC Limited Coverage   **NC** Noncovered   ⊞ Combination Member   HAC associated procedure   Combination Only   DRG Non-OR   Non-OR   New/Revised in GREEN

ICD-10-PCS 2021   323

09C–09C

Ø   **Medical and Surgical**
9   **Ear, Nose, Sinus**
D   **Extraction**   Definition: Pulling or stripping out or off all or a portion of a body part by the use of force

                              Explanation: The qualifier DIAGNOSTIC is used to identify extraction procedures that are biopsies

Body Part Character 4	Approach Character 5	Device Character 6	Qualifier Character 7
7 Tympanic Membrane, Right Pars flaccida **8 Tympanic Membrane, Left** *See 7 Tympanic Membrane, Right* **L Nasal Turbinate** Inferior turbinate Middle turbinate Nasal concha Superior turbinate	**Ø Open** **3 Percutaneous** **4 Percutaneous Endoscopic** **7 Via Natural or Artificial Opening** **8 Via Natural or Artificial Opening Endoscopic**	**Z No Device**	**Z No Qualifier**
9 Auditory Ossicle, Right Incus Malleus Stapes **A Auditory Ossicle, Left** *See 9 Auditory Ossicle, Right*	**Ø Open**	**Z No Device**	**Z No Qualifier**
B Mastoid Sinus, Right Mastoid air cells **C Mastoid Sinus, Left** *See B Mastoid Sinus, Right* **M Nasal Septum** Quadrangular cartilage Septal cartilage Vomer bone **P Accessory Sinus** **Q Maxillary Sinus, Right** Antrum of Highmore **R Maxillary Sinus, Left** *See Q Maxillary Sinus, Right* **S Frontal Sinus, Right** **T Frontal Sinus, Left** **U Ethmoid Sinus, Right** Ethmoidal air cell **V Ethmoid Sinus, Left** *See U Ethmoid Sinus, Right* **W Sphenoid Sinus, Right** **X Sphenoid Sinus, Left**	**Ø Open** **3 Percutaneous** **4 Percutaneous Endoscopic**	**Z No Device**	**Z No Qualifier**

Ø   **Medical and Surgical**
9   **Ear, Nose, Sinus**
H   **Insertion**   Definition: Putting in a nonbiological appliance that monitors, assists, performs, or prevents a physiological function but does not physically take the place of a body part

                              Explanation: None

Body Part Character 4	Approach Character 5	Device Character 6	Qualifier Character 7
D Inner Ear, Right Bony labyrinth Bony vestibule Cochlea Round window Semicircular canal **E Inner Ear, Left** *See D Inner Ear, Right*	**Ø Open** **3 Percutaneous** **4 Percutaneous Endoscopic**	**1 Radioactive Element** **4 Hearing Device, Bone Conduction** **5 Hearing Device, Single Channel Cochlear Prosthesis** **6 Hearing Device, Multiple Channel Cochlear Prosthesis** **S Hearing Device**	**Z No Qualifier**
H Ear, Right **J Ear, Left** **K Nasal Mucosa and Soft Tissue** Columella External naris Greater alar cartilage Internal naris Lateral nasal cartilage Lesser alar cartilage Nasal cavity Nostril **Y Sinus**	**Ø Open** **3 Percutaneous** **4 Percutaneous Endoscopic** **7 Via Natural or Artificial Opening** **8 Via Natural or Artificial Opening Endoscopic**	**1 Radioactive Element** **Y Other Device**	**Z No Qualifier**
N Nasopharynx Choana Fossa of Rosenmuller Pharyngeal recess Rhinopharynx	**7 Via Natural or Artificial Opening** **8 Via Natural or Artificial Opening Endoscopic**	**1 Radioactive Element** **B Intraluminal Device, Airway**	**Z No Qualifier**

Non-OR   Ø9H[H,J][3,4,7,8]YZ
Non-OR   Ø9H[K,Y][Ø,3,4,7,8]YZ
Non-OR   Ø9HN[7,8]BZ

LC Limited Coverage   **NC** Noncovered   ⊞ Combination Member   HAC associated procedure   Combination Only   DRG Non-OR   Non-OR   New/Revised in GREEN

324   ICD-10-PCS 2021

Ø Medical and Surgical
9 Ear, Nose, Sinus
J Inspection Definition: Visually and/or manually exploring a body part

Explanation: Visual exploration may be performed with or without optical instrumentation. Manual exploration may be performed directly or through intervening body layers.

Body Part Character 4	Approach Character 5	Device Character 6	Qualifier Character 7

7 Tympanic Membrane, Right
  Pars flaccida
8 Tympanic Membrane, Left
  See 7 Tympanic Membrane, Right
H Ear, Right
J Ear, Left
	Ø Open
	3 Percutaneous
	4 Percutaneous Endoscopic
	7 Via Natural or Artificial Opening
	8 Via Natural or Artificial Opening
	  Endoscopic
	X External
		Z No Device	Z No Qualifier

D Inner Ear, Right
  Bony labyrinth
  Bony vestibule
  Cochlea
  Round window
  Semicircular canal
E Inner Ear, Left
  See D Inner Ear, Right
K Nasal Mucosa and Soft Tissue
  Columella
  External naris
  Greater alar cartilage
  Internal naris
  Lateral nasal cartilage
  Lesser alar cartilage
  Nasal cavity
  Nostril
Y Sinus
	Ø Open
	3 Percutaneous
	4 Percutaneous Endoscopic
	8 Via Natural or Artificial Opening
	  Endoscopic
	X External
		Z No Device	Z No Qualifier

Non-OR   Ø9J[7,8][3,7,8,X]ZZ
Non-OR   Ø9J[H,J][Ø,3,4,7,8,X]ZZ
Non-OR   Ø9J[D,E][3,8,X]ZZ
Non-OR   Ø9J[K,Y][Ø,3,4,8,X]ZZ

Ø Medical and Surgical
9 Ear, Nose, Sinus
M Reattachment Definition: Putting back in or on all or a portion of a separated body part to its normal location or other suitable location

Explanation: Vascular circulation and nervous pathways may or may not be reestablished

Body Part Character 4	Approach Character 5	Device Character 6	Qualifier Character 7

Ø External Ear, Right
  Antihelix
  Antitragus
  Auricle
  Earlobe
  Helix
  Pinna
  Tragus
1 External Ear, Left
  See Ø External Ear, Right
K Nasal Mucosa and Soft Tissue
  Columella
  External naris
  Greater alar cartilage
  Internal naris
  Lateral nasal cartilage
  Lesser alar cartilage
  Nasal cavity
  Nostril
	X External	Z No Device	Z No Qualifier

LC Limited Coverage   NC Noncovered   ⊞ Combination Member   HAC associated procedure   Combination Only   DRG Non-OR   Non-OR   New/Revised in GREEN

ICD-10-PCS 2021   325

Ø9J–Ø9M

Ear, Nose, Sinus

Ø Medical and Surgical
9 Ear, Nose, Sinus
N Release

Definition: Freeing a body part from an abnormal physical constraint by cutting or by the use of force

Explanation: Some of the restraining tissue may be taken out but none of the body part is taken out

Body Part Character 4		Approach Character 5	Device Character 6	Qualifier Character 7
Ø External Ear, Right Antihelix Antitragus Auricle Earlobe Helix Pinna Tragus	**1 External Ear, Left** *See Ø External Ear, Right*	**Ø** Open **3** Percutaneous **4** Percutaneous Endoscopic **X** External	**Z** No Device	**Z** No Qualifier
3 External Auditory Canal, Right External auditory meatus	**4 External Auditory Canal, Left** *See 3 External Auditory Canal, Right*	**Ø** Open **3** Percutaneous **4** Percutaneous Endoscopic **7** Via Natural or Artificial Opening **8** Via Natural or Artificial Opening Endoscopic **X** External	**Z** No Device	**Z** No Qualifier
5 Middle Ear, Right Oval window Tympanic cavity **6 Middle Ear, Left** *See 5 Middle Ear, Right* **9 Auditory Ossicle, Right** Incus Malleus Stapes	**A Auditory Ossicle, Left** *See 9 Auditory Ossicle, Right* **D Inner Ear, Right** Bony labyrinth Bony vestibule Cochlea Round window Semicircular canal **E Inner Ear, Left** *See D Inner Ear, Right*	**Ø** Open **8** Via Natural or Artificial Opening Endoscopic	**Z** No Device	**Z** No Qualifier
7 Tympanic Membrane, Right Pars flaccida **8 Tympanic Membrane, Left** *See 7 Tympanic Membrane, Right* **F Eustachian Tube, Right** Auditory tube Pharyngotympanic tube **G Eustachian Tube, Left** *See F Eustachian Tube, Right*	**L Nasal Turbinate** Inferior turbinate Middle turbinate Nasal concha Superior turbinate **N Nasopharynx** Choana Fossa of Rosenmuller Pharyngeal recess Rhinopharynx	**Ø** Open **3** Percutaneous **4** Percutaneous Endoscopic **7** Via Natural or Artificial Opening **8** Via Natural or Artificial Opening Endoscopic	**Z** No Device	**Z** No Qualifier
B Mastoid Sinus, Right Mastoid air cells **C Mastoid Sinus, Left** *See B Mastoid Sinus, Right* **M Nasal Septum** Quadrangular cartilage Septal cartilage Vomer bone **P Accessory Sinus** **Q Maxillary Sinus, Right** Antrum of Highmore	**R Maxillary Sinus, Left** *See Q Maxillary Sinus, Right* **S Frontal Sinus, Right** **T Frontal Sinus, Left** **U Ethmoid Sinus, Right** Ethmoidal air cell **V Ethmoid Sinus, Left** *See U Ethmoid Sinus, Right* **W Sphenoid Sinus, Right** **X Sphenoid Sinus, Left**	**Ø** Open **3** Percutaneous **4** Percutaneous Endoscopic **8** Via Natural or Artificial Opening Endoscopic	**Z** No Device	**Z** No Qualifier
K Nasal Mucosa and Soft Tissue Columella External naris Greater alar cartilage Internal naris Lateral nasal cartilage Lesser alar cartilage Nasal cavity Nostril		**Ø** Open **3** Percutaneous **4** Percutaneous Endoscopic **8** Via Natural or Artificial Opening Endoscopic **X** External	**Z** No Device	**Z** No Qualifier

Non-OR	Ø9N[Ø,1]XZZ
Non-OR	Ø9N[3,4]XZZ
Non-OR	Ø9N[F,G,L][Ø,3,4,7,8]ZZ
Non-OR	Ø9NM[Ø,3,4,8]ZZ
Non-OR	Ø9NK[Ø,3,4,8,X]ZZ

LC Limited Coverage   **NC** Noncovered   ⊞ Combination Member   HAC associated procedure   Combination Only   DRG Non-OR   Non-OR   New/Revised in **GREEN**

326   ICD-10-PCS 2021

Ø **Medical and Surgical**
9 **Ear, Nose, Sinus**
P **Removal**   Definition: Taking out or off a device from a body part

Explanation: If a device is taken out and a similar device put in without cutting or puncturing the skin or mucous membrane, the procedure is coded to the root operation CHANGE. Otherwise, the procedure for taking out a device is coded to the root operation REMOVAL.

Body Part Character 4	Approach Character 5	Device Character 6	Qualifier Character 7
7 Tympanic Membrane, Right Pars flaccida **8 Tympanic Membrane, Left** *See 7 Tympanic Membrane, Right*	**Ø** Open **7** Via Natural or Artificial Opening **8** Via Natural or Artificial Opening Endoscopic **X** External	**Ø** Drainage Device	**Z** No Qualifier
D Inner Ear, Right Bony labyrinth Bony vestibule Cochlea Round window Semicircular canal **E Inner Ear, Left** *See D Inner Ear, Right*	**Ø** Open **7** Via Natural or Artificial Opening **8** Via Natural or Artificial Opening Endoscopic	**S** Hearing Device	**Z** No Qualifier
H Ear, Right **J Ear, Left** **K Nasal Mucosa and Soft Tissue** Columella External naris Greater alar cartilage Internal naris Lateral nasal cartilage Lesser alar cartilage Nasal cavity Nostril	**Ø** Open **3** Percutaneous **4** Percutaneous Endoscopic **7** Via Natural or Artificial Opening **8** Via Natural or Artificial Opening Endoscopic	**Ø** Drainage Device **7** Autologous Tissue Substitute **D** Intraluminal Device **J** Synthetic Substitute **K** Nonautologous Tissue Substitute **Y** Other Device	**Z** No Qualifier
H Ear, Right **J Ear, Left** **K Nasal Mucosa and Soft Tissue** Columella External naris Greater alar cartilage Internal naris Lateral nasal cartilage Lesser alar cartilage Nasal cavity Nostril	**X** External	**Ø** Drainage Device **7** Autologous Tissue Substitute **D** Intraluminal Device **J** Synthetic Substitute **K** Nonautologous Tissue Substitute	**Z** No Qualifier
Y Sinus	**Ø** Open **3** Percutaneous **4** Percutaneous Endoscopic	**Ø** Drainage Device **Y** Other Device	**Z** No Qualifier
Y Sinus	**7** Via Natural or Artificial Opening **8** Via Natural or Artificial Opening Endoscopic	**Y** Other Device	**Z** No Qualifier
Y Sinus	**X** External	**Ø** Drainage Device	**Z** No Qualifier

Non-OR   Ø9P[7,8][Ø,7,8,X]ØZ
Non-OR   Ø9P[H,J][3,4][Ø,J,K,Y]Z
Non-OR   Ø9P[H,J][7,8][Ø,D,Y]Z
Non-OR   Ø9PK[Ø,3,4,7,8][Ø,7,D,J,K,Y]Z
Non-OR   Ø9P[H,J]X[Ø,7,D,J,K]Z
Non-OR   Ø9PKX[Ø,7,D,J,K]Z
Non-OR   Ø9PY[3,4]YZ
Non-OR   Ø9PY[7,8]YZ
Non-OR   Ø9PYXØZ

LC Limited Coverage   NC Noncovered   ⊞ Combination Member   HAC associated procedure   Combination Only   DRG Non-OR   Non-OR   New/Revised in GREEN

Ear, Nose, Sinus

Ø   **Medical and Surgical**
9   **Ear, Nose, Sinus**
Q   **Repair**   Definition: Restoring, to the extent possible, a body part to its normal anatomic structure and function
                 Explanation: Used only when the method to accomplish the repair is not one of the other root operations

Body Part Character 4		Approach Character 5	Device Character 6	Qualifier Character 7

Ø **External Ear, Right**
  Antihelix
  Antitragus
  Auricle
  Earlobe
  Helix
  Pinna
  Tragus
	1 **External Ear, Left**
	  See Ø External Ear, Right
	2 **External Ear, Bilateral**
	  See Ø External Ear, Right
		Ø Open
		3 Percutaneous
		4 Percutaneous Endoscopic
		X External
			Z No Device	Z No Qualifier

3 **External Auditory Canal,
Right**
  External auditory meatus
4 **External Auditory Canal, Left**
  *See 3 External Auditory Canal,
  Right*
	F **Eustachian Tube, Right**
	  Auditory tube
	  Pharyngotympanic tube
	G **Eustachian Tube, Left**
	  See F Eustachian Tube, Right
		Ø Open
		3 Percutaneous
		4 Percutaneous Endoscopic
		7 Via Natural or Artificial
		   Opening
		8 Via Natural or Artificial
		   Opening Endoscopic
		X External
			Z No Device	Z No Qualifier

5 **Middle Ear, Right**
  Oval window
  Tympanic cavity
6 **Middle Ear, Left**
  See 5 Middle Ear, Right
9 **Auditory Ossicle, Right**
  Incus
  Malleus
  Stapes
	A **Auditory Ossicle, Left**
	  See 9 Auditory Ossicle, Right
	D **Inner Ear, Right**
	  Bony labyrinth
	  Bony vestibule
	  Cochlea
	  Round window
	  Semicircular canal
	E **Inner Ear, Left**
	  See D Inner Ear, Right
		Ø Open
		8 Via Natural or Artificial
		   Opening Endoscopic
			Z No Device	Z No Qualifier

7 **Tympanic Membrane, Right**
  Pars flaccida
8 **Tympanic Membrane, Left**
  *See 7 Tympanic Membrane,
  Right*
L **Nasal Turbinate**
  Inferior turbinate
  Middle turbinate
  Nasal concha
  Superior turbinate
	N **Nasopharynx**
	  Choana
	  Fossa of Rosenmuller
	  Pharyngeal recess
	  Rhinopharynx
		Ø Open
		3 Percutaneous
		4 Percutaneous Endoscopic
		7 Via Natural or Artificial
		   Opening
		8 Via Natural or Artificial
		   Opening Endoscopic
			Z No Device	Z No Qualifier

B **Mastoid Sinus, Right**
  Mastoid air cells
C **Mastoid Sinus, Left**
  See B Mastoid Sinus, Right
M **Nasal Septum**
  Quadrangular cartilage
  Septal cartilage
  Vomer bone
P **Accessory Sinus**
Q **Maxillary Sinus, Right**
  Antrum of Highmore
	R **Maxillary Sinus, Left**
	  See Q Maxillary Sinus, Right
	S **Frontal Sinus, Right**
	T **Frontal Sinus, Left**
	U **Ethmoid Sinus, Right**
	  Ethmoidal air cell
	V **Ethmoid Sinus, Left**
	  See U Ethmoid Sinus, Right
	W **Sphenoid Sinus, Right**
	X **Sphenoid Sinus, Left**
		Ø Open
		3 Percutaneous
		4 Percutaneous Endoscopic
		8 Via Natural or Artificial
		   Opening Endoscopic
			Z No Device	Z No Qualifier

K **Nasal Mucosa and Soft Tissue**
  Columella
  External naris
  Greater alar cartilage
  Internal naris
  Lateral nasal cartilage
  Lesser alar cartilage
  Nasal cavity
  Nostril
		Ø Open
		3 Percutaneous
		4 Percutaneous Endoscopic
		8 Via Natural or Artificial
		   Opening Endoscopic
		X External
			Z No Device	Z No Qualifier

Non-OR   Ø9Q[Ø,1,2]XZZ
Non-OR   Ø9Q[3,4]XZZ
Non-OR   Ø9Q[F,G][Ø,3,4,7,8,X]ZZ
Non-OR   Ø9QKXZZ

Ø   **Medical and Surgical**
9   **Ear, Nose, Sinus**
R   **Replacement**   Definition: Putting in or on biological or synthetic material that physically takes the place and/or function of all or a portion of a body part
                                Explanation: The body part may have been taken out or replaced, or may be taken out, physically eradicated, or rendered nonfunctional during
                                the REPLACEMENT procedure. A REMOVAL procedure is coded for taking out the device used in a previous replacement procedure.

Body Part Character 4	Approach Character 5	Device Character 6	Qualifier Character 7
Ø **External Ear, Right** Antihelix Antitragus Auricle Earlobe Helix Pinna Tragus **1** **External Ear, Left** *See Ø External Ear, Right* **2** **External Ear, Bilateral** *See Ø External Ear, Right* **K** **Nasal Mucosa and Soft Tissue** Columella External naris Greater alar cartilage Internal naris Lateral nasal cartilage Lesser alar cartilage Nasal cavity Nostril	**Ø** Open **X** External	**7** Autologous Tissue Substitute **J** Synthetic Substitute **K** Nonautologous Tissue Substitute	**Z** No Qualifier
5 **Middle Ear, Right** Oval window Tympanic cavity **6** **Middle Ear, Left** *See 5 Middle Ear, Right* **9** **Auditory Ossicle, Right** Incus Malleus Stapes **A** **Auditory Ossicle, Left** *See 9 Auditory Ossicle, Right* **D** **Inner Ear, Right** Bony labyrinth Bony vestibule Cochlea Round window Semicircular canal **E** **Inner Ear, Left** *See D Inner Ear, Right*	**Ø** Open	**7** Autologous Tissue Substitute **J** Synthetic Substitute **K** Nonautologous Tissue Substitute	**Z** No Qualifier
7 **Tympanic Membrane, Right** Pars flaccida **8** **Tympanic Membrane, Left** *See 7 Tympanic Membrane, Right* **N** **Nasopharynx** Choana Fossa of Rosenmuller Pharyngeal recess Rhinopharynx	**Ø** Open **7** Via Natural or Artificial Opening **8** Via Natural or Artificial Opening Endoscopic	**7** Autologous Tissue Substitute **J** Synthetic Substitute **K** Nonautologous Tissue Substitute	**Z** No Qualifier
L **Nasal Turbinate** Inferior turbinate Middle turbinate Nasal concha Superior turbinate	**Ø** Open **3** Percutaneous **4** Percutaneous Endoscopic **7** Via Natural or Artificial Opening **8** Via Natural or Artificial Opening Endoscopic	**7** Autologous Tissue Substitute **J** Synthetic Substitute **K** Nonautologous Tissue Substitute	**Z** No Qualifier
M **Nasal Septum** Quadrangular cartilage Septal cartilage Vomer bone	**Ø** Open **3** Percutaneous **4** Percutaneous Endoscopic	**7** Autologous Tissue Substitute **J** Synthetic Substitute **K** Nonautologous Tissue Substitute	**Z** No Qualifier

LC Limited Coverage   NC Noncovered   ⊞ Combination Member   HAC associated procedure   Combination Only   DRG Non-OR   Non-OR   New/Revised in GREEN
ICD-10-PCS 2021   329

Ø9R–Ø9R

Ear, Nose, Sinus

0 Medical and Surgical
9 Ear, Nose, Sinus
S Reposition   Definition: Moving to its normal location, or other suitable location, all or a portion of a body part

Explanation: The body part is moved to a new location from an abnormal location, or from a normal location where it is not functioning correctly. The body part may or may not be cut out or off to be moved to the new location.

Body Part Character 4	Approach Character 5	Device Character 6	Qualifier Character 7
0 External Ear, Right Antihelix Antitragus Auricle Earlobe Helix Pinna Tragus **1 External Ear, Left** *See 0 External Ear, Right* **2 External Ear, Bilateral** *See 0 External Ear, Right* **K Nasal Mucosa and Soft Tissue** Columella External naris Greater alar cartilage Internal naris Lateral nasal cartilage Lesser alar cartilage Nasal cavity Nostril	**0 Open** **4 Percutaneous Endoscopic** **X External**	**Z No Device**	**Z No Qualifier**
7 Tympanic Membrane, Right Pars flaccida **8 Tympanic Membrane, Left** *See 7 Tympanic Membrane, Right* **F Eustachian Tube, Right** Auditory tube Pharyngotympanic tube **G Eustachian Tube, Left** *See F Eustachian Tube, Right* **L Nasal Turbinate** Inferior turbinate Middle turbinate Nasal concha Superior turbinate	**0 Open** **4 Percutaneous Endoscopic** **7 Via Natural or Artificial Opening** **8 Via Natural or Artificial Opening Endoscopic**	**Z No Device**	**Z No Qualifier**
9 Auditory Ossicle, Right Incus Malleus Stapes **A Auditory Ossicle, Left** *See 9 Auditory Ossicle, Right* **M Nasal Septum** Quadrangular cartilage Septal cartilage Vomer bone	**0 Open** **4 Percutaneous Endoscopic**	**Z No Device**	**Z No Qualifier**

Non-OR   09S[F,G][0,4,7,8]ZZ

0   **Medical and Surgical**
9   **Ear, Nose, Sinus**
T   **Resection**   Definition: Cutting out or off, without replacement, all of a body part
           Explanation: None

Body Part Character 4		Approach Character 5	Device Character 6	Qualifier Character 7
0 External Ear, Right Antihelix Antitragus Auricle Earlobe Helix Pinna Tragus	**1 External Ear, Left** *See 0 External Ear, Right*	**0** Open **4** Percutaneous Endoscopic **X** External	**Z** No Device	**Z** No Qualifier
5 Middle Ear, Right Oval window Tympanic cavity **6 Middle Ear, Left** *See 5 Middle Ear, Right* **9 Auditory Ossicle, Right** Incus Malleus Stapes	**A Auditory Ossicle, Left** *See 9 Auditory Ossicle, Right* **D Inner Ear, Right** Bony labyrinth Bony vestibule Cochlea Round window Semicircular canal **E Inner Ear, Left** *See D Inner Ear, Right*	**0** Open **8** Via Natural or Artificial Opening Endoscopic	**Z** No Device	**Z** No Qualifier
7 Tympanic Membrane, Right Pars flaccida **8 Tympanic Membrane, Left** *See 7 Tympanic Membrane, Right* **F Eustachian Tube, Right** Auditory tube Pharyngotympanic tube **G Eustachian Tube, Left** *See F Eustachian Tube, Right*	**L Nasal Turbinate** Inferior turbinate Middle turbinate Nasal concha Superior turbinate **N Nasopharynx** Choana Fossa of Rosenmuller Pharyngeal recess Rhinopharynx	**0** Open **4** Percutaneous Endoscopic **7** Via Natural or Artificial Opening **8** Via Natural or Artificial Opening Endoscopic	**Z** No Device	**Z** No Qualifier
B Mastoid Sinus, Right Mastoid air cells **C Mastoid Sinus, Left** *See B Mastoid Sinus, Right* **M Nasal Septum** Quadrangular cartilage Septal cartilage Vomer bone **P Accessory Sinus** **Q Maxillary Sinus, Right** Antrum of Highmore	**R Maxillary Sinus, Left** *See Q Maxillary Sinus, Right* **S Frontal Sinus, Right** **T Frontal Sinus, Left** **U Ethmoid Sinus, Right** Ethmoidal air cell **V Ethmoid Sinus, Left** *See U Ethmoid Sinus, Right* **W Sphenoid Sinus, Right** **X Sphenoid Sinus, Left**	**0** Open **4** Percutaneous Endoscopic **8** Via Natural or Artificial Opening Endoscopic	**Z** No Device	**Z** No Qualifier
K Nasal Mucosa and Soft Tissue Columella External naris Greater alar cartilage Internal naris Lateral nasal cartilage Lesser alar cartilage Nasal cavity Nostril		**0** Open **4** Percutaneous Endoscopic **8** Via Natural or Artificial Opening Endoscopic **X** External	**Z** No Device	**Z** No Qualifier

Non-OR   09T[F,G][0,4,7,8]ZZ

LC Limited Coverage   NC Noncovered   ⊞ Combination Member   HAC associated procedure   Combination Only   DRG Non-OR   Non-OR   New/Revised in GREEN

ICD-10-PCS 2021   331

09T–09T

Ø   Medical and Surgical
9   Ear, Nose, Sinus
U   Supplement

Definition: Putting in or on biological or synthetic material that physically reinforces and/or augments the function of a portion of a body part

Explanation: The biological material is non-living, or is living and from the same individual. The body part may have been previously replaced, and the SUPPLEMENT procedure is performed to physically reinforce and/or augment the function of the replaced body part.

Body Part Character 4		Approach Character 5	Device Character 6	Qualifier Character 7
Ø External Ear, Right Antihelix Antitragus Auricle Earlobe Helix Pinna Tragus	**1 External Ear, Left** *See Ø External Ear, Right* **2 External Ear, Bilateral** *See Ø External Ear, Right*	**Ø Open** **X External**	**7 Autologous Tissue Substitute** **J Synthetic Substitute** **K Nonautologous Tissue Substitute**	**Z No Qualifier**
5 Middle Ear, Right Oval window Tympanic cavity **6 Middle Ear, Left** *See 5 Middle Ear, Right* **9 Auditory Ossicle, Right** Incus Malleus Stapes **A Auditory Ossicle, Left** *See 9 Auditory Ossicle, Right*	**D Inner Ear, Right** Bony labyrinth Bony vestibule Cochlea Round window Semicircular canal **E Inner Ear, Left** *See D Inner Ear, Right*	**Ø Open** **8 Via Natural or Artificial Opening Endoscopic**	**7 Autologous Tissue Substitute** **J Synthetic Substitute** **K Nonautologous Tissue Substitute**	**Z No Qualifier**
7 Tympanic Membrane, Right Pars flaccida **8 Tympanic Membrane, Left** *See 7 Tympanic Membrane, Right*	**N Nasopharynx** Choana Fossa of Rosenmuller Pharyngeal recess Rhinopharynx	**Ø Open** **7 Via Natural or Artificial Opening** **8 Via Natural or Artificial Opening Endoscopic**	**7 Autologous Tissue Substitute** **J Synthetic Substitute** **K Nonautologous Tissue Substitute**	**Z No Qualifier**
B Mastoid Sinus, Right Mastoid air cells **C Mastoid Sinus, Left** *See B Mastoid Sinus, Right* **L Nasal Turbinate** Inferior turbinate Middle turbinate Nasal concha Superior turbinate **P Accessory Sinus** **Q Maxillary Sinus, Right** Antrum of Highmore	**R Maxillary Sinus, Left** *See Q Maxillary Sinus, Right* **S Frontal Sinus, Right** **T Frontal Sinus, Left** **U Ethmoid Sinus, Right** Ethmoidal air cell **V Ethmoid Sinus, Left** *See U Ethmoid Sinus, Right* **W Sphenoid Sinus, Right** **X Sphenoid Sinus, Left**	**Ø Open** **3 Percutaneous** **4 Percutaneous Endoscopic** **7 Via Natural or Artificial Opening** **8 Via Natural or Artificial Opening Endoscopic**	**7 Autologous Tissue Substitute** **J Synthetic Substitute** **K Nonautologous Tissue Substitute**	**Z No Qualifier**
K Nasal Mucosa and Soft Tissue Columella External naris Greater alar cartilage Internal naris Lateral nasal cartilage Lesser alar cartilage Nasal cavity Nostril		**Ø Open** **8 Via Natural or Artificial Opening Endoscopic** **X External**	**7 Autologous Tissue Substitute** **J Synthetic Substitute** **K Nonautologous Tissue Substitute**	**Z No Qualifier**
M Nasal Septum Quadrangular cartilage Septal cartilage Vomer bone		**Ø Open** **3 Percutaneous** **4 Percutaneous Endoscopic** **8 Via Natural or Artificial Opening Endoscopic**	**7 Autologous Tissue Substitute** **J Synthetic Substitute** **K Nonautologous Tissue Substitute**	**Z No Qualifier**

LC Limited Coverage   NC Noncovered   ⊞ Combination Member   HAC associated procedure   Combination Only   DRG Non-OR   Non-OR   New/Revised in GREEN

332   ICD-10-PCS 2021

Ø9U–Ø9U

Ø Medical and Surgical
9 Ear, Nose, Sinus
W Revision

Definition: Correcting, to the extent possible, a portion of a malfunctioning device or the position of a displaced device

Explanation: Revision can include correcting a malfunctioning or displaced device by taking out or putting in components of the device such as a screw or pin

Body Part Character 4	Approach Character 5	Device Character 6	Qualifier Character 7
7 Tympanic Membrane, Right Pars flaccida **8 Tympanic Membrane, Left** *See 7 Tympanic Membrane, Right* **9 Auditory Ossicle, Right** Incus Malleus Stapes **A Auditory Ossicle, Left** *See 9 Auditory Ossicle, Right*	**Ø Open** **7 Via Natural or Artificial Opening** **8 Via Natural or Artificial Opening Endoscopic**	**7 Autologous Tissue Substitute** **J Synthetic Substitute** **K Nonautologous Tissue Substitute**	**Z No Qualifier**
D Inner Ear, Right Bony labyrinth Bony vestibule Cochlea Round window Semicircular canal **E Inner Ear, Left** *See D Inner Ear, Right*	**Ø Open** **7 Via Natural or Artificial Opening** **8 Via Natural or Artificial Opening Endoscopic**	**S Hearing Device**	**Z No Qualifier**
H Ear, Right **J Ear, Left** **K Nasal Mucosa and Soft Tissue** Columella External naris Greater alar cartilage Internal naris Lateral nasal cartilage Lesser alar cartilage Nasal cavity Nostril	**Ø Open** **3 Percutaneous** **4 Percutaneous Endoscopic** **7 Via Natural or Artificial Opening** **8 Via Natural or Artificial Opening Endoscopic**	**Ø Drainage Device** **7 Autologous Tissue Substitute** **D Intraluminal Device** **J Synthetic Substitute** **K Nonautologous Tissue Substitute** **Y Other Device**	**Z No Qualifier**
H Ear, Right **J Ear, Left** **K Nasal Mucosa and Soft Tissue** Columella External naris Greater alar cartilage Internal naris Lateral nasal cartilage Lesser alar cartilage Nasal cavity Nostril	**X External**	**Ø Drainage Device** **7 Autologous Tissue Substitute** **D Intraluminal Device** **J Synthetic Substitute** **K Nonautologous Tissue Substitute**	**Z No Qualifier**
Y Sinus	**Ø Open** **3 Percutaneous** **4 Percutaneous Endoscopic**	**Ø Drainage Device** **Y Other Device**	**Z No Qualifier**
Y Sinus	**7 Via Natural or Artificial Opening** **8 Via Natural or Artificial Opening Endoscopic**	**Y Other Device**	**Z No Qualifier**
Y Sinus	**X External**	**Ø Drainage Device**	**Z No Qualifier**

Non-OR	Ø9W[H,J][3,4][J,K,Y]Z
Non-OR	Ø9W[H,J][7,8][D,Y]Z
Non-OR	Ø9WK[Ø,3,4,7,8][Ø,7,D,J,K,Y]Z
Non-OR	Ø9W[H,J,K]X[Ø,7,D,J,K]Z
Non-OR	Ø9WY[3,4]YZ
Non-OR	Ø9WY[7,8]YZ
Non-OR	Ø9WYXØZ

Respiratory System ØB1–ØBY

Character Meanings

This Character Meaning table is provided as a guide to assist the user in the identification of character members that may be found in this section of code tables. It **SHOULD NOT** be used to build a PCS code.

Operation–Character 3	Body Part–Character 4	Approach–Character 5	Device–Character 6	Qualifier–Character 7
1 Bypass	Ø Tracheobronchial Tree	Ø Open	Ø Drainage Device	Ø Allogeneic
2 Change	1 Trachea	3 Percutaneous	1 Radioactive Element	1 Syngeneic
5 Destruction	2 Carina	4 Percutaneous Endoscopic	2 Monitoring Device	2 Zooplastic
7 Dilation	3 Main Bronchus, Right	7 Via Natural or Artificial Opening	3 Infusion Device	4 Cutaneous
9 Drainage	4 Upper Lobe Bronchus, Right	8 Via Natural or Artificial Opening Endoscopic	7 Autologous Tissue Substitute	6 Esophagus
B Excision	5 Middle Lobe Bronchus, Right	X External	C Extraluminal Device	X Diagnostic
C Extirpation	6 Lower Lobe Bronchus, Right		D Intraluminal Device	Z No Qualifier
D Extraction	7 Main Bronchus, Left		E Intraluminal Device, Endotracheal Airway	
F Fragmentation	8 Upper Lobe Bronchus, Left		F Tracheostomy Device	
H Insertion	9 Lingula Bronchus		G Intraluminal Device, Endobronchial Valve	
J Inspection	B Lower Lobe Bronchus, Left		J Synthetic Substitute	
L Occlusion	C Upper Lung Lobe, Right		K Nonautologous Tissue Substitute	
M Reattachment	D Middle Lung Lobe, Right		M Diaphragmatic Pacemaker Lead	
N Release	F Lower Lung Lobe, Right		Y Other Device	
P Removal	G Upper Lung Lobe, Left		Z No Device	
Q Repair	H Lung Lingula			
R Replacement	J Lower Lung Lobe, Left			
S Reposition	K Lung, Right			
T Resection	L Lung, Left			
U Supplement	M Lungs, Bilateral			
V Restriction	N Pleura, Right			
W Revision	P Pleura, Left			
Y Transplantation	Q Pleura			
	T Diaphragm			

AHA Coding Clinic for table ØB5
2016, 2Q, 17   Photodynamic therapy for treatment of malignant mesothelioma
2015, 2Q, 31   Thoracoscopic talc pleurodesis

AHA Coding Clinic for table ØB9
2017, 3Q, 15   Bronchoscopy with suctioning for removal of retained secretions
2017, 1Q, 51   Bronchoalveolar lavage
2016, 1Q, 26   Bronchoalveolar lavage, endobronchial biopsy and transbronchial biopsy
2016, 1Q, 27   Fiberoptic bronchoscopy with brushings and bronchoalveolar lavage

AHA Coding Clinic for table ØBB
2016, 1Q, 26   Bronchoalveolar lavage, endobronchial biopsy and transbronchial biopsy
2016, 1Q, 27   Fiberoptic bronchoscopy with brushings and bronchoalveolar lavage
2014, 1Q, 20   Fiducial marker placement

AHA Coding Clinic for table ØBC
2017, 3Q, 14   Bronchoscopy with suctioning and washings for removal of mucus plug

AHA Coding Clinic for table ØBD
2018, 3Q, 28   Lung decortication for empyema

AHA Coding Clinic for table ØBH
2019, 3Q, 33   Insertion of endobronchial valve
2014, 4Q, 3-10   Mechanical ventilation

AHA Coding Clinic for table ØBJ
2015, 2Q, 31   Thoracoscopic talc pleurodesis
2014, 1Q, 20   Fiducial marker placement

AHA Coding Clinic for table ØBL
2019, 3Q, 33   Insertion of endobronchial valve

AHA Coding Clinic for table ØBN
2019, 2Q, 20   Pericardiectomy for constrictive pericarditis
2018, 3Q, 28   Lung decortication
2018, 3Q, 28   Lung decortication for empyema
2015, 3Q, 15   Vascular ring surgery with release of esophagus and trachea

AHA Coding Clinic for table ØBQ
2016, 2Q, 22   Esophageal lengthening Collis gastroplasty with Nissen fundoplication and hiatal hernia
2014, 3Q, 28   Laparoscopic Nissen fundoplication and diaphragmatic hernia repair

AHA Coding Clinic for table ØBU
2015, 1Q, 28   Repair of bronchopleural fistula using omental pedicle graft

Respiratory System

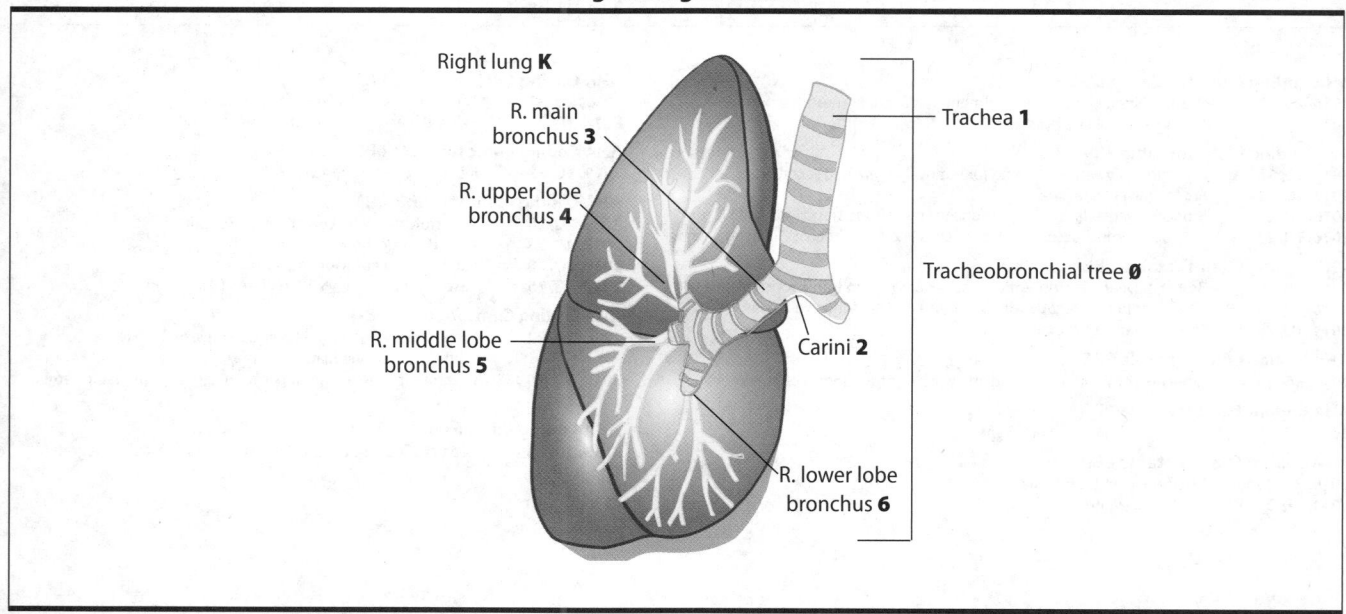

Trachea **1**

Right lung **K**

Right main/
primary
bronchus **3**

Diaphragm **T**

Pleura **N, P, Q**

Left lung **L**

Carina of trachea **2**

Left main/
primary
bronchus **7**

Right Lung Bronchi

Right lung **K**

R. main
bronchus **3**

R. upper lobe
bronchus **4**

R. middle lobe
bronchus **5**

R. lower lobe
bronchus **6**

Trachea **1**

Tracheobronchial tree **Ø**

Carini **2**

Ø   Medical and Surgical
B   Respiratory System
1   Bypass   Definition: Altering the route of passage of the contents of a tubular body part

Explanation: Rerouting contents of a body part to a downstream area of the normal route, to a similar route and body part, or to an abnormal route and dissimilar body part. Includes one or more anastomoses, with or without the use of a device.

Body Part Character 4	Approach Character 5	Device Character 6	Qualifier Character 7
1 Trachea Cricoid cartilage	**Ø** Open	**D** Intraluminal Device	**6** Esophagus
1 Trachea Cricoid cartilage	**Ø** Open	**F** Tracheostomy Device **Z** No Device	**4** Cutaneous
1 Trachea Cricoid cartilage	**3** Percutaneous **4** Percutaneous Endoscopic	**F** Tracheostomy Device **Z** No Device	**4** Cutaneous

DRG Non-OR   ØB113[F,Z]4
Non-OR   ØB11ØD6

Ø   Medical and Surgical
B   Respiratory System
2   Change   Definition: Taking out or off a device from a body part and putting back an identical or similar device in or on the same body part without cutting or puncturing the skin or a mucous membrane

Explanation: All CHANGE procedures are coded using the approach EXTERNAL

Body Part Character 4	Approach Character 5	Device Character 6	Qualifier Character 7
Ø Tracheobronchial Tree **K** Lung, Right **L** Lung, Left **Q** Pleura **T** Diaphragm	**X** External	**Ø** Drainage Device **Y** Other Device	**Z** No Qualifier
1 Trachea Cricoid cartilage	**X** External	**Ø** Drainage Device **E** Intraluminal Device, Endotracheal Airway **F** Tracheostomy Device **Y** Other Device	**Z** No Qualifier

Non-OR   All body part, approach, device, and qualifier values

Ø   Medical and Surgical
B   Respiratory System
5   Destruction   Definition: Physical eradication of all or a portion of a body part by the direct use of energy, force, or a destructive agent

Explanation: None of the body part is physically taken out

Body Part Character 4	Approach Character 5	Device Character 6	Qualifier Character 7

1 Trachea
    Cricoid cartilage
2 Carina
3 Main Bronchus, Right
    Bronchus intermedius
    Intermediate bronchus
4 Upper Lobe Bronchus, Right
5 Middle Lobe Bronchus, Right
6 Lower Lobe Bronchus, Right
7 Main Bronchus, Left
8 Upper Lobe Bronchus, Left
9 Lingula Bronchus
B Lower Lobe Bronchus, Left
C Upper Lung Lobe, Right
D Middle Lung Lobe, Right
F Lower Lung Lobe, Right
G Upper Lung Lobe, Left
H Lung Lingula
J Lower Lung Lobe, Left
K Lung, Right
L Lung, Left
M Lungs, Bilateral
	Ø Open
	3 Percutaneous
	4 Percutaneous Endoscopic
	7 Via Natural or Artificial Opening
	8 Via Natural or Artificial Opening Endoscopic
		Z No Device	**Z** No Qualifier

N Pleura, Right **P** Pleura, Left **T** Diaphragm	**Ø** Open **3** Percutaneous **4** Percutaneous Endoscopic	**Z** No Device	**Z** No Qualifier

Non-OR   ØB5[3,4,5,6,7,8,9,B][4,8]ZZ
Non-OR   ØB5[C,D,F,G,H,J,K,L,M]8ZZ

LC Limited Coverage   NC Noncovered   ⊞ Combination Member   HAC associated procedure   Combination Only   DRG Non-OR   Non-OR   New/Revised in GREEN

Respiratory System

Ø   **Medical and Surgical**
B   **Respiratory System**
7   **Dilation**   Definition: Expanding an orifice or the lumen of a tubular body part

Explanation: The orifice can be a natural orifice or an artificially created orifice. Accomplished by stretching a tubular body part using intraluminal pressure or by cutting part of the orifice or wall of the tubular body part.

Body Part Character 4	Approach Character 5	Device Character 6	Qualifier Character 7
1 Trachea Cricoid cartilage 2 Carina 3 Main Bronchus, Right Bronchus intermedius Intermediate bronchus 4 Upper Lobe Bronchus, Right 5 Middle Lobe Bronchus, Right 6 Lower Lobe Bronchus, Right 7 Main Bronchus, Left 8 Upper Lobe Bronchus, Left 9 Lingula Bronchus B Lower Lobe Bronchus, Left	Ø Open 3 Percutaneous 4 Percutaneous Endoscopic 7 Via Natural or Artificial Opening 8 Via Natural or Artificial Opening Endoscopic	D Intraluminal Device Z No Device	Z No Qualifier

Non-OR   ØB7[3,4,5,6,7,8,9,B][Ø,3,4,7,8][D,Z]Z

Ø   **Medical and Surgical**
B   **Respiratory System**
9   **Drainage**   Definition: Taking or letting out fluids and/or gases from a body part

Explanation: The qualifier DIAGNOSTIC is used to identify drainage procedures that are biopsies

Body Part Character 4		Approach Character 5	Device Character 6	Qualifier Character 7
1 Trachea Cricoid cartilage 2 Carina 3 Main Bronchus, Right Bronchus intermedius Intermediate bronchus 4 Upper Lobe Bronchus, Right 5 Middle Lobe Bronchus, Right 6 Lower Lobe Bronchus, Right 7 Main Bronchus, Left	8 Upper Lobe Bronchus, Left 9 Lingula Bronchus B Lower Lobe Bronchus, Left C Upper Lung Lobe, Right D Middle Lung Lobe, Right F Lower Lung Lobe, Right G Upper Lung Lobe, Left H Lung Lingula J Lower Lung Lobe, Left K Lung, Right L Lung, Left M Lungs, Bilateral	Ø Open 3 Percutaneous 4 Percutaneous Endoscopic 7 Via Natural or Artificial Opening 8 Via Natural or Artificial Opening Endoscopic	Ø Drainage Device	Z No Qualifier
1 Trachea Cricoid cartilage 2 Carina 3 Main Bronchus, Right Bronchus intermedius Intermediate bronchus 4 Upper Lobe Bronchus, Right 5 Middle Lobe Bronchus, Right 6 Lower Lobe Bronchus, Right 7 Main Bronchus, Left	8 Upper Lobe Bronchus, Left 9 Lingula Bronchus B Lower Lobe Bronchus, Left C Upper Lung Lobe, Right D Middle Lung Lobe, Right F Lower Lung Lobe, Right G Upper Lung Lobe, Left H Lung Lingula J Lower Lung Lobe, Left K Lung, Right L Lung, Left M Lungs, Bilateral	Ø Open 3 Percutaneous 4 Percutaneous Endoscopic 7 Via Natural or Artificial Opening 8 Via Natural or Artificial Opening Endoscopic	Z No Device	X Diagnostic Z No Qualifier
N Pleura, Right P Pleura, Left		Ø Open 3 Percutaneous 4 Percutaneous Endoscopic 8 Via Natural or Artificial Opening Endoscopic	Ø Drainage Device	Z No Qualifier
N Pleura, Right P Pleura, Left		Ø Open 3 Percutaneous 4 Percutaneous Endoscopic 8 Via Natural or Artificial Opening Endoscopic	Z No Device	X Diagnostic Z No Qualifier
T Diaphragm		Ø Open 3 Percutaneous 4 Percutaneous Endoscopic	Ø Drainage Device	Z No Qualifier
T Diaphragm		Ø Open 3 Percutaneous 4 Percutaneous Endoscopic	Z No Device	X Diagnostic Z No Qualifier

Non-OR   ØB9[1,2,3,4,5,6,7,8,9,B][7,8]ØZ
Non-OR   ØB9[1,2,3,4,5,6,7,8,9,B][3,4]ZX
Non-OR   ØB9[1,2,3,4,5,6,7,8,9,B][7,8]Z[X,Z]
Non-OR   ØB9[C,D,F,G,H,J,K,L,M][3,4,7]ZX
Non-OR   ØB9[C,D,F,G,H,J,K,L,M]8Z[X,Z]

Non-OR   ØB9[N,P][Ø,3,8]ØZ
Non-OR   ØB9[N,P][Ø,3,8]Z[X,Z]
Non-OR   ØB9[N,P]4ZX
Non-OR   ØB9T[3,4]ØZ
Non-OR   ØB9T[3,4]Z[X,Z]

LC Limited Coverage   NC Noncovered   ⊞ Combination Member   HAC associated procedure   Combination Only   DRG Non-OR   Non-OR   New/Revised in GREEN
338   ICD-10-PCS 2021

ØB7–ØB9

Respiratory System

Ø   **Medical and Surgical**
B   **Respiratory System**
B   **Excision**   Definition: Cutting out or off, without replacement, a portion of a body part

            Explanation: The qualifier DIAGNOSTIC is used to identify excision procedures that are biopsies

Body Part Character 4	Approach Character 5	Device Character 6	Qualifier Character 7

1 Trachea
   Cricoid cartilage
2 Carina
3 Main Bronchus, Right
   Bronchus intermedius
   Intermediate bronchus
4 Upper Lobe Bronchus, Right
5 Middle Lobe Bronchus, Right
6 Lower Lobe Bronchus, Right
7 Main Bronchus, Left
8 Upper Lobe Bronchus, Left
9 Lingula Bronchus
B Lower Lobe Bronchus, Left
C Upper Lung Lobe, Right
D Middle Lung Lobe, Right
F Lower Lung Lobe, Right
G Upper Lung Lobe, Left
H Lung Lingula
J Lower Lung Lobe, Left
K Lung, Right
L Lung, Left
M Lungs, Bilateral
	Ø Open
	3 Percutaneous
	4 Percutaneous Endoscopic
	7 Via Natural or Artificial Opening
	8 Via Natural or Artificial Opening Endoscopic
		Z No Device	X Diagnostic
			Z No Qualifier

N Pleura, Right P Pleura, Left	Ø Open 3 Percutaneous 4 Percutaneous Endoscopic 8 Via Natural or Artificial Opening Endoscopic	Z No Device	X Diagnostic Z No Qualifier
T Diaphragm	Ø Open 3 Percutaneous 4 Percutaneous Endoscopic	Z No Device	X Diagnostic Z No Qualifier

Non-OR   ØBB[1,2,3,4,5,6,7,8,9,B][3,4,7,8]ZX
Non-OR   ØBB[3,4,5,6,7,8,9,B,M][4,8]ZZ
Non-OR   ØBB[C,D,F,G,H,J,K,L,M]3ZX

Non-OR   ØBB[C,D,F,G,H,J,K,L]8ZZ
Non-OR   ØBB[N,P][Ø,3]ZX

Ø   **Medical and Surgical**
B   **Respiratory System**
C   **Extirpation**   Definition: Taking or cutting out solid matter from a body part

            Explanation: The solid matter may be an abnormal byproduct of a biological function or a foreign body; it may be imbedded in a body part or in the lumen of a tubular body part. The solid matter may or may not have been previously broken into pieces.

Body Part Character 4	Approach Character 5	Device Character 6	Qualifier Character 7

1 Trachea
   Cricoid cartilage
2 Carina
3 Main Bronchus, Right
   Bronchus intermedius
   Intermediate bronchus
4 Upper Lobe Bronchus, Right
5 Middle Lobe Bronchus, Right
6 Lower Lobe Bronchus, Right
7 Main Bronchus, Left
8 Upper Lobe Bronchus, Left
9 Lingula Bronchus
B Lower Lobe Bronchus, Left
C Upper Lung Lobe, Right
D Middle Lung Lobe, Right
F Lower Lung Lobe, Right
G Upper Lung Lobe, Left
H Lung Lingula
J Lower Lung Lobe, Left
K Lung, Right
L Lung, Left
M Lungs, Bilateral
	Ø Open
	3 Percutaneous
	4 Percutaneous Endoscopic
	7 Via Natural or Artificial Opening
	8 Via Natural or Artificial Opening Endoscopic
		Z No Device	Z No Qualifier

N Pleura, Right P Pleura, Left T Diaphragm	Ø Open 3 Percutaneous 4 Percutaneous Endoscopic	Z No Device	Z No Qualifier

Non-OR   ØBC[1,2,3,4,5,6,7,8,9,B][7,8]ZZ
Non-OR   ØBC[N,P]3ZZ

LC Limited Coverage   **NC** Noncovered   ⊞ Combination Member   HAC associated procedure   Combination Only   DRG Non-OR   Non-OR   New/Revised in GREEN

Respiratory System

Ø   **Medical and Surgical**
B   **Respiratory System**
D   **Extraction**   Definition: Pulling or stripping out or off all or a portion of a body part by the use of force

Explanation: The qualifier DIAGNOSTIC is used to identify extraction procedures that are biopsies

Body Part Character 4	Approach Character 5	Device Character 6	Qualifier Character 7

1 Trachea
   Cricoid cartilage
2 Carina
3 Main Bronchus, Right
   Bronchus intermedius
   Intermediate bronchus
4 Upper Lobe Bronchus, Right
5 Middle Lobe Bronchus, Right
6 Lower Lobe Bronchus, Right
7 Main Bronchus, Left
8 Upper Lobe Bronchus, Left
9 Lingula Bronchus
B Lower Lobe Bronchus, Left
C Upper Lung Lobe, Right
D Middle Lung Lobe, Right
F Lower Lung Lobe, Right
G Upper Lung Lobe, Left
H Lung Lingula
J Lower Lung Lobe, Left
K Lung, Right
L Lung, Left
M Lungs, Bilateral
	4 Percutaneous Endoscopic
	8 Via Natural or Artificial Opening
	   Endoscopic
		Z No Device	X Diagnostic

N Pleura, Right P Pleura, Left	Ø Open 3 Percutaneous 4 Percutaneous Endoscopic	Z No Device	X Diagnostic Z No Qualifier

Non-OR   ØBD[1,2,3,4,5,6,7,8,9,B,C,D,F,G,H,J,K,L,M][4,8]ZX

Ø   **Medical and Surgical**
B   **Respiratory System**
F   **Fragmentation**   Definition: Breaking solid matter in a body part into pieces

Explanation: Physical force (e.g., manual, ultrasonic) applied directly or indirectly is used to break the solid matter into pieces. The solid matter may be an abnormal byproduct of a biological function or a foreign body. The pieces of solid matter are not taken out.

Body Part Character 4	Approach Character 5	Device Character 6	Qualifier Character 7

1 Trachea NC
   Cricoid cartilage
2 Carina NC
3 Main Bronchus, Right NC
   Bronchus intermedius
   Intermediate bronchus
4 Upper Lobe Bronchus, Right NC
5 Middle Lobe Bronchus, Right NC
6 Lower Lobe Bronchus, Right NC
7 Main Bronchus, Left NC
8 Upper Lobe Bronchus, Left NC
9 Lingula Bronchus NC
B Lower Lobe Bronchus, Left NC
	Ø Open
	3 Percutaneous
	4 Percutaneous Endoscopic
	7 Via Natural or Artificial Opening
	8 Via Natural or Artificial Opening
	   Endoscopic
	X External
		Z No Device	Z No Qualifier

Non-OR   ØBF[1,2,3,4,5,6,7,8,9,B]XZZ
Non-OR   ØBF[3,4,5,6,7,8,9,B][7,8]ZZ
NC   ØBF[1,2,3,4,5,6,7,8,9,B]XZZ

Ø   **Medical and Surgical**
B   **Respiratory System**
H   **Insertion**   Definition: Putting in a nonbiological appliance that monitors, assists, performs, or prevents a physiological function but does not physically take the place of a body part
                   Explanation: None

Body Part Character 4	Approach Character 5	Device Character 6	Qualifier Character 7
Ø Tracheobronchial Tree	**Ø** Open **3** Percutaneous **4** Percutaneous Endoscopic **7** Via Natural or Artificial Opening **8** Via Natural or Artificial Opening Endoscopic	**1** Radioactive Element **2** Monitoring Device **3** Infusion Device **D** Intraluminal Device **Y** Other Device	**Z** No Qualifier
1 Trachea Cricoid cartilage	**Ø** Open	**2** Monitoring Device **D** Intraluminal Device **Y** Other Device	**Z** No Qualifier
1 Trachea Cricoid cartilage	**3** Percutaneous	**D** Intraluminal Device **E** Intraluminal Device, Endotracheal Airway **Y** Other Device	**Z** No Qualifier
1 Trachea Cricoid cartilage	**4** Percutaneous Endoscopic	**D** Intraluminal Device **Y** Other Device	**Z** No Qualifier
1 Trachea Cricoid cartilage	**7** Via Natural or Artificial Opening **8** Via Natural or Artificial Opening Endoscopic	**2** Monitoring Device **D** Intraluminal Device **E** Intraluminal Device, Endotracheal Airway **Y** Other Device	**Z** No Qualifier
3 Main Bronchus, Right Bronchus intermedius Intermediate bronchus **4** Upper Lobe Bronchus, Right **5** Middle Lobe Bronchus, Right **6** Lower Lobe Bronchus, Right **7** Main Bronchus, Left **8** Upper Lobe Bronchus, Left **9** Lingula Bronchus **B** Lower Lobe Bronchus, Left	**Ø** Open **3** Percutaneous **4** Percutaneous Endoscopic **7** Via Natural or Artificial Opening **8** Via Natural or Artificial Opening Endoscopic	**G** Intraluminal Device, Endobronchial Valve	**Z** No Qualifier
K Lung, Right **L** Lung, Left	**Ø** Open **3** Percutaneous **4** Percutaneous Endoscopic **7** Via Natural or Artificial Opening **8** Via Natural or Artificial Opening Endoscopic	**1** Radioactive Element **2** Monitoring Device **3** Infusion Device **Y** Other Device	**Z** No Qualifier
Q Pleura	**Ø** Open **3** Percutaneous **4** Percutaneous Endoscopic **7** Via Natural or Artificial Opening **8** Via Natural or Artificial Opening Endoscopic	**Y** Other Device	**Z** No Qualifier
T Diaphragm	**Ø** Open **3** Percutaneous **4** Percutaneous Endoscopic	**2** Monitoring Device **M** Diaphragmatic Pacemaker Lead **Y** Other Device	**Z** No Qualifier
T Diaphragm	**7** Via Natural or Artificial Opening **8** Via Natural or Artificial Opening Endoscopic	**Y** Other Device	**Z** No Qualifier

DRG Non-OR	ØBH[3,4,5,6,7,8,9,B]8GZ
Non-OR	ØBHØ3YZ
Non-OR	ØBHØ[7,8][2,3,D,Y]Z
Non-OR	ØBH13[E,Y]Z
Non-OR	ØBH1[7,8][2,D,E,Y]Z
Non-OR	ØBH[K,L]3YZ
Non-OR	ØBH[K,L]7[2,3,Y]Z
Non-OR	ØBH[K,L]8[2,3]Z
Non-OR	ØBHQ[3,7]YZ
Non-OR	ØBHT3YZ
Non-OR	ØBHT[7,8]YZ

LC Limited Coverage   NC Noncovered   ⊞ Combination Member   HAC associated procedure   Combination Only   DRG Non-OR   Non-OR   New/Revised in GREEN

ICD-10-PCS 2021   **341**

ØBH–ØBH

Respiratory System

Ø **Medical and Surgical**
B **Respiratory System**
J **Inspection**   Definition: Visually and/or manually exploring a body part

         Explanation: Visual exploration may be performed with or without optical instrumentation. Manual exploration may be performed directly or through intervening body layers.

Body Part Character 4	Approach Character 5	Device Character 6	Qualifier Character 7

Ø   Tracheobronchial Tree
1   Trachea
     Cricoid cartilage
K   Lung, Right
L   Lung, Left
Q   Pleura
T   Diaphragm
	Ø Open
	3 Percutaneous
	4 Percutaneous Endoscopic
	7 Via Natural or Artificial Opening
	8 Via Natural or Artificial Opening
	     Endoscopic
	X External
		Z No Device	Z No Qualifier

Non-OR   ØBJ[Ø,K,L,Q,T][3,7,8,X]ZZ
Non-OR   ØBJ1[3,4,7,8,X]ZZ

Ø **Medical and Surgical**
B **Respiratory System**
L **Occlusion**   Definition: Completely closing an orifice or the lumen of a tubular body part

         Explanation: The orifice can be a natural orifice or an artificially created orifice

Body Part Character 4	Approach Character 5	Device Character 6	Qualifier Character 7

1   Trachea
     Cricoid cartilage
2   Carina
3   Main Bronchus, Right
     Bronchus intermedius
     Intermediate bronchus
4   Upper Lobe Bronchus, Right
5   Middle Lobe Bronchus, Right
6   Lower Lobe Bronchus, Right
7   Main Bronchus, Left
8   Upper Lobe Bronchus, Left
9   Lingula Bronchus
B   Lower Lobe Bronchus, Left
	Ø Open
	3 Percutaneous
	4 Percutaneous Endoscopic
		C Extraluminal Device
		D Intraluminal Device
		Z No Device
			Z No Qualifier

1   Trachea
     Cricoid cartilage
2   Carina
3   Main Bronchus, Right
     Bronchus intermedius
     Intermediate bronchus
4   Upper Lobe Bronchus, Right
5   Middle Lobe Bronchus, Right
6   Lower Lobe Bronchus, Right
7   Main Bronchus, Left
8   Upper Lobe Bronchus, Left
9   Lingula Bronchus
B   Lower Lobe Bronchus, Left
	7 Via Natural or Artificial Opening
	8 Via Natural or Artificial Opening
	     Endoscopic
		D Intraluminal Device
		Z No Device
			Z No Qualifier

LC Limited Coverage   NC Noncovered   ⊞ Combination Member   HAC associated procedure   Combination Only   DRG Non-OR   Non-OR   New/Revised in GREEN

342   ICD-10-PCS 2021

Ø   Medical and Surgical
B   Respiratory System
M   Reattachment   Definition: Putting back in or on all or a portion of a separated body part to its normal location or other suitable location
                 Explanation: Vascular circulation and nervous pathways may or may not be reestablished

Body Part Character 4	Approach Character 5	Device Character 6	Qualifier Character 7

1   Trachea
    Cricoid cartilage
2   Carina
3   Main Bronchus, Right
    Bronchus intermedius
    Intermediate bronchus
4   Upper Lobe Bronchus, Right
5   Middle Lobe Bronchus, Right
6   Lower Lobe Bronchus, Right
7   Main Bronchus, Left
8   Upper Lobe Bronchus, Left
9   Lingula Bronchus
B   Lower Lobe Bronchus, Left
C   Upper Lung Lobe, Right
D   Middle Lung Lobe, Right
F   Lower Lung Lobe, Right
G   Upper Lung Lobe, Left
H   Lung Lingula
J   Lower Lung Lobe, Left
K   Lung, Right
L   Lung, Left
T   Diaphragm
	Ø Open	Z No Device	Z No Qualifier

Ø   Medical and Surgical
B   Respiratory System
N   Release   Definition: Freeing a body part from an abnormal physical constraint by cutting or by the use of force
                 Explanation: Some of the restraining tissue may be taken out but none of the body part is taken out

Body Part Character 4	Approach Character 5	Device Character 6	Qualifier Character 7

1   Trachea
    Cricoid cartilage
2   Carina
3   Main Bronchus, Right
    Bronchus intermedius
    Intermediate bronchus
4   Upper Lobe Bronchus, Right
5   Middle Lobe Bronchus, Right
6   Lower Lobe Bronchus, Right
7   Main Bronchus, Left
8   Upper Lobe Bronchus, Left
9   Lingula Bronchus
B   Lower Lobe Bronchus, Left
C   Upper Lung Lobe, Right
D   Middle Lung Lobe, Right
F   Lower Lung Lobe, Right
G   Upper Lung Lobe, Left
H   Lung Lingula
J   Lower Lung Lobe, Left
K   Lung, Right
L   Lung, Left
M   Lungs, Bilateral
	Ø Open
	3 Percutaneous
	4 Percutaneous Endoscopic
	7 Via Natural or Artificial Opening
	8 Via Natural or Artificial Opening
	    Endoscopic
		Z No Device	Z No Qualifier

N Pleura, Right P Pleura, Left T Diaphragm	Ø Open 3 Percutaneous 4 Percutaneous Endoscopic	Z No Device	Z No Qualifier

Respiratory System

Ø Medical and Surgical
B Respiratory System
P Removal

Definition: Taking out or off a device from a body part

Explanation: If a device is taken out and a similar device put in without cutting or puncturing the skin or mucous membrane, the procedure is coded to the root operation CHANGE. Otherwise, the procedure for taking out a device is coded to the root operation REMOVAL.

Body Part Character 4	Approach Character 5	Device Character 6	Qualifier Character 7
Ø Tracheobronchial Tree	Ø Open 3 Percutaneous 4 Percutaneous Endoscopic 7 Via Natural or Artificial Opening 8 Via Natural or Artificial Opening Endoscopic	Ø Drainage Device 1 Radioactive Element 2 Monitoring Device 3 Infusion Device 7 Autologous Tissue Substitute C Extraluminal Device D Intraluminal Device J Synthetic Substitute K Nonautologous Tissue Substitute Y Other Device	Z No Qualifier
Ø Tracheobronchial Tree	X External	Ø Drainage Device 1 Radioactive Element 2 Monitoring Device 3 Infusion Device D Intraluminal Device	Z No Qualifier
1 Trachea Cricoid cartilage	Ø Open 3 Percutaneous 4 Percutaneous Endoscopic 7 Via Natural or Artificial Opening 8 Via Natural or Artificial Opening Endoscopic	Ø Drainage Device 2 Monitoring Device 7 Autologous Tissue Substitute C Extraluminal Device D Intraluminal Device F Tracheostomy Device J Synthetic Substitute K Nonautologous Tissue Substitute	Z No Qualifier
1 Trachea Cricoid cartilage	X External	Ø Drainage Device 2 Monitoring Device D Intraluminal Device F Tracheostomy Device	Z No Qualifier
K Lung, Right L Lung, Left	Ø Open 3 Percutaneous 4 Percutaneous Endoscopic 7 Via Natural or Artificial Opening 8 Via Natural or Artificial Opening Endoscopic	Ø Drainage Device 1 Radioactive Element 2 Monitoring Device 3 Infusion Device Y Other Device	Z No Qualifier
K Lung, Right L Lung, Left	X External	Ø Drainage Device 1 Radioactive Element 2 Monitoring Device 3 Infusion Device	Z No Qualifier
Q Pleura	Ø Open 3 Percutaneous 4 Percutaneous Endoscopic 7 Via Natural or Artificial Opening 8 Via Natural or Artificial Opening Endoscopic	Ø Drainage Device 1 Radioactive Element 2 Monitoring Device Y Other Device	Z No Qualifier
Q Pleura	X External	Ø Drainage Device 1 Radioactive Element 2 Monitoring Device	Z No Qualifier
T Diaphragm	Ø Open 3 Percutaneous 4 Percutaneous Endoscopic 7 Via Natural or Artificial Opening 8 Via Natural or Artificial Opening Endoscopic	Ø Drainage Device 2 Monitoring Device 7 Autologous Tissue Substitute J Synthetic Substitute K Nonautologous Tissue Substitute M Diaphragmatic Pacemaker Lead Y Other Device	Z No Qualifier
T Diaphragm	X External	Ø Drainage Device 2 Monitoring Device M Diaphragmatic Pacemaker Lead	Z No Qualifier

Non-OR	ØBPØ[3,4]YZ	**Non-OR**	ØBPL7[Ø,2,3,Y]Z
Non-OR	ØBPØ[7,8][Ø,2,3,D,Y]Z	**Non-OR**	ØBPL8[Ø,2,3]Z
Non-OR	ØBPØX[Ø,1,2,3,D]Z	**Non-OR**	ØBP[K,L]X[Ø,1,2,3]Z
Non-OR	ØBP1[Ø,3,4]FZ	**Non-OR**	ØBPQ[Ø,3,4,7,8][Ø,1,2,]Z
Non-OR	ØBP1[7,8][Ø,2,D,F]Z	**Non-OR**	ØBPQ[3,7]YZ
Non-OR	ØBP1X[Ø,2,D,F]Z	**Non-OR**	ØBPQX[Ø,1,2]Z
Non-OR	ØBP[K,L]3YZ	**Non-OR**	ØBPT3YZ
Non-OR	ØBPK7[Ø,1,2,3,Y]Z	**Non-OR**	ØBPT[7,8][Ø,2,Y]Z
Non-OR	ØBPK8[Ø,1,2,3]Z	**Non-OR**	ØBPTX[Ø,2,M]Z

LC Limited Coverage   **NC** Noncovered   ⊞ Combination Member   HAC associated procedure   Combination Only   DRG Non-OR   Non-OR   New/Revised in GREEN

344   ICD-10-PCS 2021

Ø   **Medical and Surgical**
B   **Respiratory System**
Q   **Repair**   Definition: Restoring, to the extent possible, a body part to its normal anatomic structure and function

                                Explanation: Used only when the method to accomplish the repair is not one of the other root operations

Body Part Character 4	Approach Character 5	Device Character 6	Qualifier Character 7

1 Trachea
    Cricoid cartilage
2 Carina
3 Main Bronchus, Right
    Bronchus intermedius
    Intermediate bronchus
4 Upper Lobe Bronchus, Right
5 Middle Lobe Bronchus, Right
6 Lower Lobe Bronchus, Right
7 Main Bronchus, Left
8 Upper Lobe Bronchus, Left
9 Lingula Bronchus
B Lower Lobe Bronchus, Left
C Upper Lung Lobe, Right
D Middle Lung Lobe, Right
F Lower Lung Lobe, Right
G Upper Lung Lobe, Left
H Lung Lingula
J Lower Lung Lobe, Left
K Lung, Right
L Lung, Left
M Lungs, Bilateral
	Ø Open
	3 Percutaneous
	4 Percutaneous Endoscopic
	7 Via Natural or Artificial Opening
	8 Via Natural or Artificial Opening
	    Endoscopic
		Z No Device	**Z** No Qualifier

N Pleura, Right **P** Pleura, Left **T** Diaphragm	**Ø** Open **3** Percutaneous **4** Percutaneous Endoscopic	**Z** No Device	**Z** No Qualifier

Ø   Medical and Surgical
B   Respiratory System
R   Replacement   Definition: Putting in or on biological or synthetic material that physically takes the place and/or function of all or a portion of a body part
Explanation: The body part may have been taken out or replaced, or may be taken out, physically eradicated, or rendered nonfunctional during the REPLACEMENT procedure. A REMOVAL procedure is coded for taking out the device used in a previous replacement procedure.

Body Part Character 4	Approach Character 5	Device Character 6	Qualifier Character 7

1 Trachea
  Cricoid cartilage
2 Carina
3 Main Bronchus, Right
  Bronchus intermedius
  Intermediate bronchus
4 Upper Lobe Bronchus, Right
5 Middle Lobe Bronchus, Right
6 Lower Lobe Bronchus, Right
7 Main Bronchus, Left
8 Upper Lobe Bronchus, Left
9 Lingula Bronchus
B Lower Lobe Bronchus, Left
T Diaphragm
	Ø Open
	4 Percutaneous Endoscopic
		7 Autologous Tissue Substitute
		J Synthetic Substitute
		K Nonautologous Tissue Substitute
			Z No Qualifier

Ø   Medical and Surgical
B   Respiratory System
S   Reposition   Definition: Moving to its normal location, or other suitable location, all or a portion of a body part
Explanation: The body part is moved to a new location from an abnormal location, or from a normal location where it is not functioning correctly. The body part may or may not be cut out or off to be moved to the new location.

Body Part Character 4	Approach Character 5	Device Character 6	Qualifier Character 7

1 Trachea
  Cricoid cartilage
2 Carina
3 Main Bronchus, Right
  Bronchus intermedius
  Intermediate bronchus
4 Upper Lobe Bronchus, Right
5 Middle Lobe Bronchus, Right
6 Lower Lobe Bronchus, Right
7 Main Bronchus, Left
8 Upper Lobe Bronchus, Left
9 Lingula Bronchus
B Lower Lobe Bronchus, Left
C Upper Lung Lobe, Right
D Middle Lung Lobe, Right
F Lower Lung Lobe, Right
G Upper Lung Lobe, Left
H Lung Lingula
J Lower Lung Lobe, Left
K Lung, Right
L Lung, Left
T Diaphragm
	Ø Open	Z No Device	Z No Qualifier

Ø Medical and Surgical
B Respiratory System
T Resection　　Definition: Cutting out or off, without replacement, all of a body part
　　　　　　Explanation: None

Body Part Character 4	Approach Character 5	Device Character 6	Qualifier Character 7
1 Trachea 　Cricoid cartilage 2 Carina 3 Main Bronchus, Right 　Bronchus intermedius 　Intermediate bronchus 4 Upper Lobe Bronchus, Right 5 Middle Lobe Bronchus, Right 6 Lower Lobe Bronchus, Right 7 Main Bronchus, Left 8 Upper Lobe Bronchus, Left 9 Lingula Bronchus B Lower Lobe Bronchus, Left C Upper Lung Lobe, Right D Middle Lung Lobe, Right F Lower Lung Lobe, Right G Upper Lung Lobe, Left H Lung Lingula J Lower Lung Lobe, Left K Lung, Right L Lung, Left M Lungs, Bilateral T Diaphragm	Ø Open 4 Percutaneous Endoscopic	Z No Device	Z No Qualifier

Ø Medical and Surgical
B Respiratory System
U Supplement　　Definition: Putting in or on biological or synthetic material that physically reinforces and/or augments the function of a portion of a body part
　　　　　Explanation: The biological material is non-living, or is living and from the same individual. The body part may have been previously replaced, and the SUPPLEMENT procedure is performed to physically reinforce and/or augment the function of the replaced body part.

Body Part Character 4	Approach Character 5	Device Character 6	Qualifier Character 7
1 Trachea 　Cricoid cartilage 2 Carina 3 Main Bronchus, Right 　Bronchus intermedius 　Intermediate bronchus 4 Upper Lobe Bronchus, Right 5 Middle Lobe Bronchus, Right 6 Lower Lobe Bronchus, Right 7 Main Bronchus, Left 8 Upper Lobe Bronchus, Left 9 Lingula Bronchus B Lower Lobe Bronchus, Left	Ø Open 4 Percutaneous Endoscopic 8 Via Natural or Artificial Opening Endoscopic	7 Autologous Tissue Substitute J Synthetic Substitute K Nonautologous Tissue Substitute	Z No Qualifier
T Diaphragm	Ø Open 4 Percutaneous Endoscopic	7 Autologous Tissue Substitute J Synthetic Substitute K Nonautologous Tissue Substitute	Z No Qualifier

Respiratory System

Ø **Medical and Surgical**
B **Respiratory System**
V **Restriction**   Definition: Partially closing an orifice or the lumen of a tubular body part
                        Explanation: The orifice can be a natural orifice or an artificially created orifice

Body Part Character 4	Approach Character 5	Device Character 6	Qualifier Character 7

1 Trachea
   Cricoid cartilage
2 Carina
3 Main Bronchus, Right
   Bronchus intermedius
   Intermediate bronchus
4 Upper Lobe Bronchus, Right
5 Middle Lobe Bronchus, Right
6 Lower Lobe Bronchus, Right
7 Main Bronchus, Left
8 Upper Lobe Bronchus, Left
9 Lingula Bronchus
B Lower Lobe Bronchus, Left
	Ø Open
	3 Percutaneous
	4 Percutaneous Endoscopic
		C Extraluminal Device
		D Intraluminal Device
		Z No Device
			Z No Qualifier

1 Trachea
   Cricoid cartilage
2 Carina
3 Main Bronchus, Right
   Bronchus intermedius
   Intermediate bronchus
4 Upper Lobe Bronchus, Right
5 Middle Lobe Bronchus, Right
6 Lower Lobe Bronchus, Right
7 Main Bronchus, Left
8 Upper Lobe Bronchus, Left
9 Lingula Bronchus
B Lower Lobe Bronchus, Left
	7 Via Natural or Artificial Opening
	8 Via Natural or Artificial Opening Endoscopic
		D Intraluminal Device
		Z No Device
			Z No Qualifier

Ø   **Medical and Surgical**
B   **Respiratory System**
W   **Revision**   Definition: Correcting, to the extent possible, a portion of a malfunctioning device or the position of a displaced device

                            Explanation: Revision can include correcting a malfunctioning or displaced device by taking out or putting in components of the device such as a screw or pin

Body Part Character 4	Approach Character 5	Device Character 6	Qualifier Character 7
Ø Tracheobronchial Tree	**Ø** Open **3** Percutaneous **4** Percutaneous Endoscopic **7** Via Natural or Artificial Opening **8** Via Natural or Artificial Opening Endoscopic	**Ø** Drainage Device **2** Monitoring Device **3** Infusion Device **7** Autologous Tissue Substitute **C** Extraluminal Device **D** Intraluminal Device **J** Synthetic Substitute **K** Nonautologous Tissue Substitute **Y** Other Device	**Z** No Qualifier
Ø Tracheobronchial Tree	**X** External	**Ø** Drainage Device **2** Monitoring Device **3** Infusion Device **7** Autologous Tissue Substitute **C** Extraluminal Device **D** Intraluminal Device **J** Synthetic Substitute **K** Nonautologous Tissue Substitute	**Z** No Qualifier
1 Trachea Cricoid cartilage	**Ø** Open **3** Percutaneous **4** Percutaneous Endoscopic **7** Via Natural or Artificial Opening **8** Via Natural or Artificial Opening Endoscopic **X** External	**Ø** Drainage Device **2** Monitoring Device **7** Autologous Tissue Substitute **C** Extraluminal Device **D** Intraluminal Device **F** Tracheostomy Device **J** Synthetic Substitute **K** Nonautologous Tissue Substitute	**Z** No Qualifier
K Lung, Right **L Lung, Left**	**Ø** Open **3** Percutaneous **4** Percutaneous Endoscopic **7** Via Natural or Artificial Opening **8** Via Natural or Artificial Opening Endoscopic	**Ø** Drainage Device **2** Monitoring Device **3** Infusion Device **Y** Other Device	**Z** No Qualifier
K Lung, Right **L Lung, Left**	**X** External	**Ø** Drainage Device **2** Monitoring Device **3** Infusion Device	**Z** No Qualifier
Q Pleura	**Ø** Open **3** Percutaneous **4** Percutaneous Endoscopic **7** Via Natural or Artificial Opening **8** Via Natural or Artificial Opening Endoscopic	**Ø** Drainage Device **2** Monitoring Device **Y** Other Device	**Z** No Qualifier
Q Pleura	**X** External	**Ø** Drainage Device **2** Monitoring Device	**Z** No Qualifier
T Diaphragm	**Ø** Open **3** Percutaneous **4** Percutaneous Endoscopic **7** Via Natural or Artificial Opening **8** Via Natural or Artificial Opening Endoscopic	**Ø** Drainage Device **2** Monitoring Device **7** Autologous Tissue Substitute **J** Synthetic Substitute **K** Nonautologous Tissue Substitute **M** Diaphragmatic Pacemaker Lead **Y** Other Device	**Z** No Qualifier
T Diaphragm	**X** External	**Ø** Drainage Device **2** Monitoring Device **7** Autologous Tissue Substitute **J** Synthetic Substitute **K** Nonautologous Tissue Substitute **M** Diaphragmatic Pacemaker Lead	**Z** No Qualifier

Non-OR   ØBWØ[3,4]YZ
Non-OR   ØBWØ[7,8][2,3,D,Y]Z
Non-OR   ØBWØX[Ø,2,3,7,C,D,J,K]Z
Non-OR   ØBW1X[Ø,2,7,C,D,F,J,K]Z
Non-OR   ØBW[K,L]3YZ
Non-OR   ØBW[K,L]7[Ø,2,3,Y]Z
Non-OR   ØBW[K,L]8[Ø,2,3]Z
Non-OR   ØBW[K,L]X[Ø,2,3]Z
Non-OR   ØBWQ[Ø,3,4,7,8][Ø,2]Z
Non-OR   ØBWQ[Ø,3,7]YZ
Non-OR   ØBWQX[Ø,2]Z
Non-OR   ØBWT[3,7,8]YZ
Non-OR   ØBWTX[Ø,2,7,J,K,M]Z

IC Limited Coverage   NC Noncovered   ⊞ Combination Member   HAC associated procedure   Combination Only   DRG Non-OR   Non-OR   New/Revised in **GREEN**

ICD-10-PCS 2021   **349**

Ø   Medical and Surgical
B   Respiratory System
Y   Transplantation   Definition: Putting in or on all or a portion of a living body part taken from another individual or animal to physically take the place and/or function of all or a portion of a similar body part

Explanation: The native body part may or may not be taken out, and the transplanted body part may take over all or a portion of its function

Body Part Character 4	Approach Character 5	Device Character 6	Qualifier Character 7
C Upper Lung Lobe, Right LC D Middle Lung Lobe, Right LC F Lower Lung Lobe, Right LC G Upper Lung Lobe, Left LC H Lung Lingula LC J Lower Lung Lobe, Left LC K Lung, Right LC L Lung, Left LC M Lungs, Bilateral LC	Ø Open	Z No Device	Ø Allogeneic 1 Syngeneic 2 Zooplastic

LC   ØBY[C,D,F,G,H,J,K,L,M]ØZ[Ø,1,2]

Mouth and Throat ØCØ–ØCX

Character Meanings

This Character Meaning table is provided as a guide to assist the user in the identification of character members that may be found in this section of code tables. It **SHOULD NOT** be used to build a PCS code.

Operation–Character 3		Body Part–Character 4		Approach–Character 5		Device–Character 6		Qualifier–Character 7	
Ø	Alteration	Ø	Upper Lip	Ø	Open	Ø	Drainage Device	Ø	Single
2	Change	1	Lower Lip	3	Percutaneous	1	Radioactive Element	1	Multiple
5	Destruction	2	Hard Palate	4	Percutaneous Endoscopic	5	External Fixation Device	2	All
7	Dilation	3	Soft Palate	7	Via Natural or Artificial Opening	7	Autologous Tissue Substitute	X	Diagnostic
9	Drainage	4	Buccal Mucosa	8	Via Natural or Artificial Opening Endoscopic	B	Intraluminal Device, Airway	Z	No Qualifier
B	Excision	5	Upper Gingiva	X	External	C	Extraluminal Device		
C	Extirpation	6	Lower Gingiva			D	Intraluminal Device		
D	Extraction	7	Tongue			J	Synthetic Substitute		
F	Fragmentation	8	Parotid Gland, Right			K	Nonautologous Tissue Substitute		
H	Insertion	9	Parotid Gland, Left			Y	Other Device		
J	Inspection	A	Salivary Gland			Z	No Device		
L	Occlusion	B	Parotid Duct, Right						
M	Reattachment	C	Parotid Duct, Left						
N	Release	D	Sublingual Gland, Right						
P	Removal	F	Sublingual Gland, Left						
Q	Repair	G	Submaxillary Gland, Right						
R	Replacement	H	Submaxillary Gland, Left						
S	Reposition	J	Minor Salivary Gland						
T	Resection	M	Pharynx						
U	Supplement	N	Uvula						
V	Restriction	P	Tonsils						
W	Revision	Q	Adenoids						
X	Transfer	R	Epiglottis						
		S	Larynx						
		T	Vocal Cord, Right						
		V	Vocal Cord, Left						
		W	Upper Tooth						
		X	Lower Tooth						
		Y	Mouth and Throat						

AHA Coding Clinic for table ØC9
2017, 2Q, 16   Incision and drainage of floor of mouth

AHA Coding Clinic for table ØCB
2017, 2Q, 16   Excision of floor of mouth
2016, 3Q, 28   Lingual tonsillectomy, tongue base excision and epiglottopexy
2016, 2Q, 19   Biopsy of the base of tongue
2014, 3Q, 21   Superficial parotidectomy

AHA Coding Clinic for table ØCC
2016, 2Q, 20   Sialendoscopy with stone removal

AHA Coding Clinic for table ØCQ
2017, 1Q, 20   Preparatory nasal adhesion repair before definitive cleft palate repair

AHA Coding Clinic for table ØCR
2014, 3Q, 25   Excision of soft palate with placement of surgical obturator
2014, 2Q, 5   Oasis acellular matrix graft
2014, 2Q, 6   Composite grafting (synthetic versus nonautologous tissue substitute)

AHA Coding Clinic for table ØCS
2016, 3Q, 28   Lingual tonsillectomy, tongue base excision and epiglottopexy

AHA Coding Clinic for table ØCT
2016, 2Q, 12   Resection of malignant neoplasm of infratemporal fossa
2014, 3Q, 21   Superficial parotidectomy
2014, 3Q, 23   Le Fort I osteotomy

Mouth and Throat

Salivary Glands

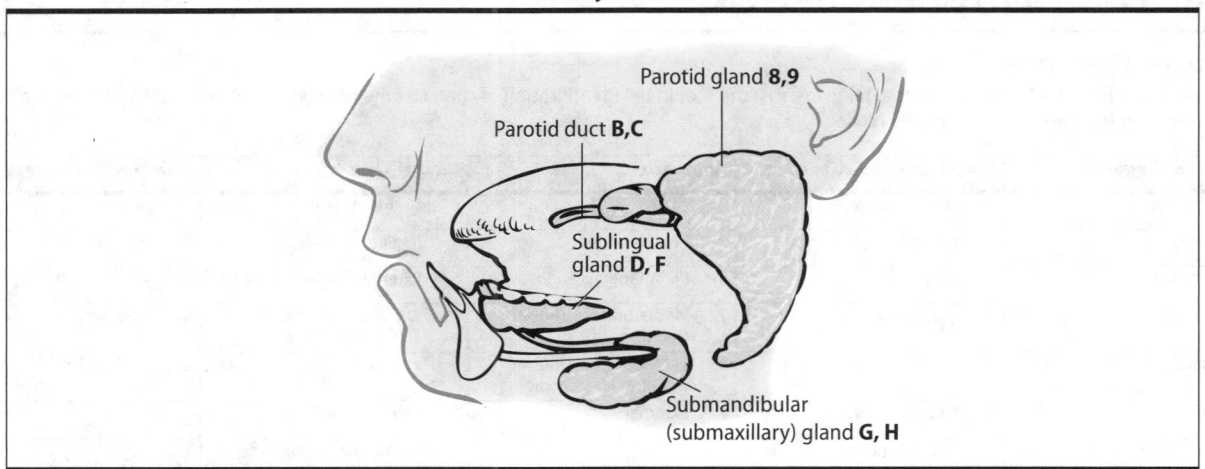

Parotid gland **8,9**

Parotid duct **B,C**

Sublingual gland **D, F**

Submandibular (submaxillary) gland **G, H**

Oral Anatomy

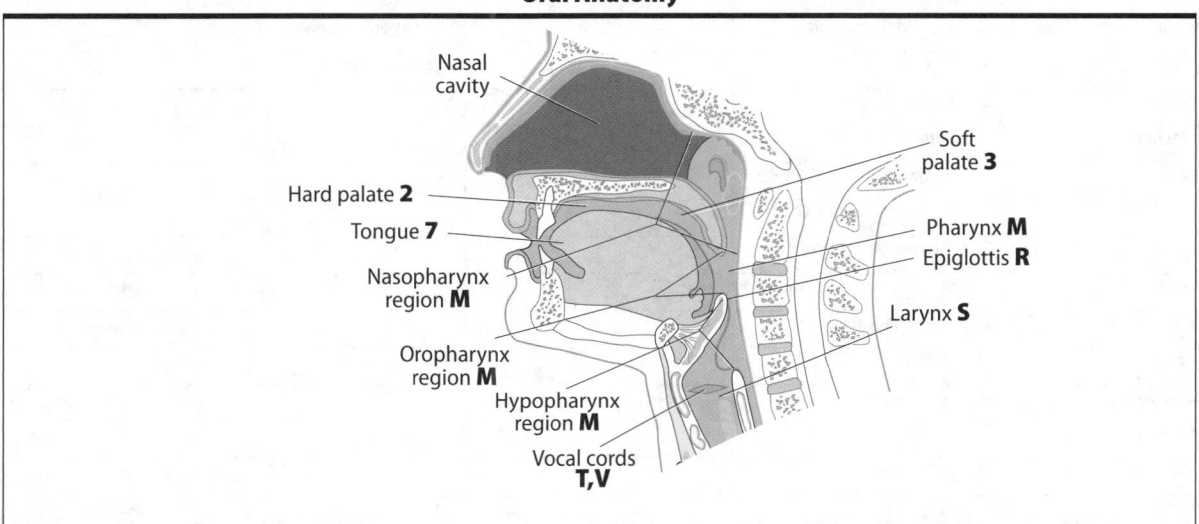

Nasal cavity

Soft palate **3**

Hard palate **2**

Tongue **7**

Pharynx **M**

Epiglottis **R**

Nasopharynx region **M**

Larynx **S**

Oropharynx region **M**

Hypopharynx region **M**

Vocal cords **T,V**

Mouth Frontal View (Upper)

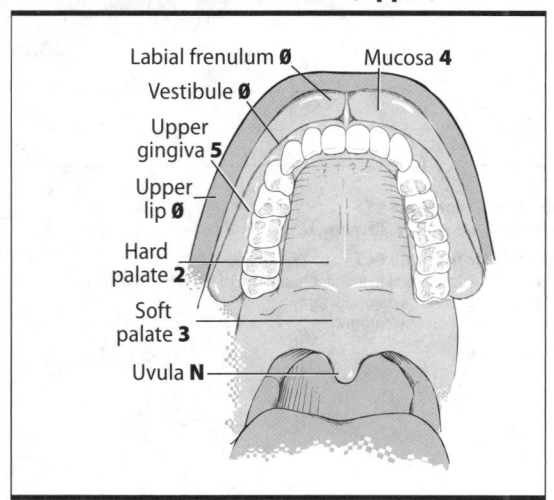

Labial frenulum **Ø**

Mucosa **4**

Vestibule **Ø**

Upper gingiva **5**

Upper lip **Ø**

Hard palate **2**

Soft palate **3**

Uvula **N**

Mouth Frontal View (Lower)

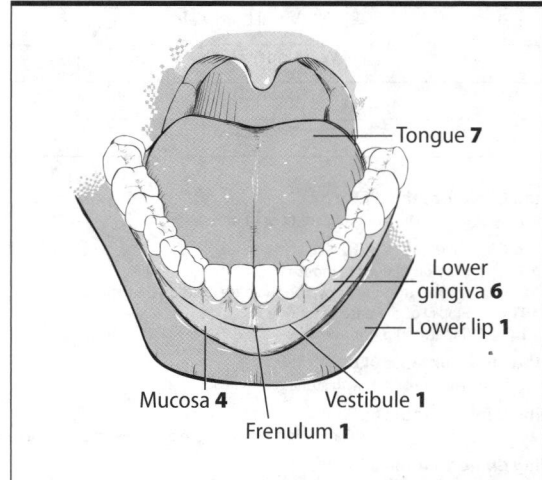

Tongue **7**

Lower gingiva **6**

Lower lip **1**

Mucosa **4**

Vestibule **1**

Frenulum **1**

0   Medical and Surgical
C   Mouth and Throat
0   Alteration   Definition: Modifying the anatomic structure of a body part without affecting the function of the body part
Explanation: Principal purpose is to improve appearance

Body Part Character 4	Approach Character 5	Device Character 6	Qualifier Character 7
0 Upper Lip Frenulum labii superioris Labial gland Vermilion border **1 Lower Lip** Frenulum labii inferioris Labial gland Vermilion border	**X External**	**7 Autologous Tissue Substitute** **J Synthetic Substitute** **K Nonautologous Tissue Substitute** **Z No Device**	**Z No Qualifier**

0   Medical and Surgical
C   Mouth and Throat
2   Change   Definition: Taking out or off a device from a body part and putting back an identical or similar device in or on the same body part without cutting or puncturing the skin or a mucous membrane
Explanation: All CHANGE procedures are coded using the approach EXTERNAL

Body Part Character 4	Approach Character 5	Device Character 6	Qualifier Character 7
A Salivary Gland **S Larynx** Aryepiglottic fold Arytenoid cartilage Corniculate cartilage Cuneiform cartilage False vocal cord Glottis Rima glottidis Thyroid cartilage Ventricular fold **Y Mouth and Throat**	**X External**	**0 Drainage Device** **Y Other Device**	**Z No Qualifier**

Non-OR   All body part, approach, device, and qualifier values

Mouth and Throat (side margin)

Ø **Medical and Surgical**
C **Mouth and Throat**
5 **Destruction**   Definition: Physical eradication of all or a portion of a body part by the direct use of energy, force, or a destructive agent
     Explanation: None of the body part is physically taken out

Body Part Character 4		Approach Character 5	Device Character 6	Qualifier Character 7
Ø Upper Lip Frenulum labii superioris Labial gland Vermilion border 1 Lower Lip Frenulum labii inferioris Labial gland Vermilion border 2 Hard Palate 3 Soft Palate 4 Buccal Mucosa Buccal gland Molar gland Palatine gland	5 Upper Gingiva 6 Lower Gingiva 7 Tongue Frenulum linguae N Uvula Palatine uvula P Tonsils Palatine tonsil Q Adenoids Pharyngeal tonsil	Ø Open 3 Percutaneous X External	Z No Device	Z No Qualifier
8 Parotid Gland, Right 9 Parotid Gland, Left B Parotid Duct, Right Stensen's duct C Parotid Duct, Left See B Parotid Duct, Right D Sublingual Gland, Right	F Sublingual Gland, Left G Submaxillary Gland, Right Submandibular gland H Submaxillary Gland, Left See G Submaxillary Gland, Right J Minor Salivary Gland Anterior lingual gland	Ø Open 3 Percutaneous	Z No Device	Z No Qualifier
M Pharynx Base of tongue Hypopharynx Laryngopharynx Lingual tonsil Oropharynx Piriform recess (sinus) Tongue, base of R Epiglottis Glossoepiglottic fold	S Larynx Aryepiglottic fold Arytenoid cartilage Corniculate cartilage Cuneiform cartilage False vocal cord Glottis Rima glottidis Thyroid cartilage Ventricular fold T Vocal Cord, Right Vocal fold V Vocal Cord, Left See T Vocal Cord, Right	Ø Open 3 Percutaneous 4 Percutaneous Endoscopic 7 Via Natural or Artificial Opening 8 Via Natural or Artificial Opening Endoscopic	Z No Device	Z No Qualifier
W Upper Tooth X Lower Tooth		Ø Open X External	Z No Device	Ø Single 1 Multiple 2 All

Non-OR   ØC5[5,6][Ø,3,X]ZZ
Non-OR   ØC5[W,X][Ø,X]Z[Ø,1,2]

Ø **Medical and Surgical**
C **Mouth and Throat**
7 **Dilation**   Definition: Expanding an orifice or the lumen of a tubular body part
     Explanation: The orifice can be a natural orifice or an artificially created orifice. Accomplished by stretching a tubular body part using intraluminal pressure or by cutting part of the orifice or wall of the tubular body part.

Body Part Character 4	Approach Character 5	Device Character 6	Qualifier Character 7
B Parotid Duct, Right Stensen's duct C Parotid Duct, Left See B Parotid Duct, Right	Ø Open 3 Percutaneous 7 Via Natural or Artificial Opening	D Intraluminal Device Z No Device	Z No Qualifier
M Pharynx Base of tongue Hypopharynx Laryngopharynx Lingual tonsil Oropharynx Piriform recess (sinus) Tongue, base of	7 Via Natural or Artificial Opening 8 Via Natural or Artificial Opening Endoscopic	D Intraluminal Device Z No Device	Z No Qualifier
S Larynx Aryepiglottic fold Arytenoid cartilage Corniculate cartilage Cuneiform cartilage False vocal cord Glottis Rima glottidis Thyroid cartilage Ventricular fold	Ø Open 3 Percutaneous 4 Percutaneous Endoscopic 7 Via Natural or Artificial Opening 8 Via Natural or Artificial Opening Endoscopic	D Intraluminal Device Z No Device	Z No Qualifier

Non-OR   ØC7[B,C][Ø,3,7][D,Z]Z
Non-OR   ØC7M[7,8][D,Z]Z

LC Limited Coverage   NC Noncovered   ⊞ Combination Member   HAC associated procedure   Combination Only   DRG Non-OR   Non-OR   New/Revised in GREEN

Ø　Medical and Surgical
C　Mouth and Throat
9　Drainage　　　Definition: Taking or letting out fluids and/or gases from a body part
　　　　　　　　　　 Explanation: The qualifier DIAGNOSTIC is used to identify drainage procedures that are biopsies

Body Part Character 4		Approach Character 5	Device Character 6	Qualifier Character 7
Ø　Upper Lip 　　Frenulum labii superioris 　　Labial gland 　　Vermilion border 1　Lower Lip 　　Frenulum labii inferioris 　　Labial gland 　　Vermilion border 2　Hard Palate 3　Soft Palate 4　Buccal Mucosa 　　Buccal gland 　　Molar gland 　　Palatine gland	5　Upper Gingiva 6　Lower Gingiva 7　Tongue 　　Frenulum linguae N　Uvula 　　Palatine uvula P　Tonsils 　　Palatine tonsil Q　Adenoids 　　Pharyngeal tonsil	Ø　Open 3　Percutaneous X　External	Ø　Drainage Device	Z　No Qualifier
Ø　Upper Lip 　　Frenulum labii superioris 　　Labial gland 　　Vermilion border 1　Lower Lip 　　Frenulum labii inferioris 　　Labial gland 　　Vermilion border 2　Hard Palate 3　Soft Palate 4　Buccal Mucosa 　　Buccal gland 　　Molar gland 　　Palatine gland	5　Upper Gingiva 6　Lower Gingiva 7　Tongue 　　Frenulum linguae N　Uvula 　　Palatine uvula P　Tonsils 　　Palatine tonsil Q　Adenoids 　　Pharyngeal tonsil	Ø　Open 3　Percutaneous X　External	Z　No Device	X　Diagnostic Z　No Qualifier
8　Parotid Gland, Right 9　Parotid Gland, Left B　Parotid Duct, Right 　　Stensen's duct C　Parotid Duct, Left 　　See B Parotid Duct, Right D　Sublingual Gland, Right	F　Sublingual Gland, Left G　Submaxillary Gland, Right 　　Submandibular gland H　Submaxillary Gland, Left 　　See G Submaxillary Gland, Right J　Minor Salivary Gland 　　Anterior lingual gland	Ø　Open 3　Percutaneous	Ø　Drainage Device	Z　No Qualifier
8　Parotid Gland, Right 9　Parotid Gland, Left B　Parotid Duct, Right 　　Stensen's duct C　Parotid Duct, Left 　　See B Parotid Duct, Right	D　Sublingual Gland, Right F　Sublingual Gland, Left G　Submaxillary Gland, Right 　　Submandibular gland H　Submaxillary Gland, Left 　　See G Submaxillary Gland, Right J　Minor Salivary Gland 　　Anterior lingual gland	Ø　Open 3　Percutaneous	Z　No Device	X　Diagnostic Z　No Qualifier
M　Pharynx 　　Base of tongue 　　Hypopharynx 　　Laryngopharynx 　　Lingual tonsil 　　Oropharynx 　　Piriform recess (sinus) 　　Tongue, base of R　Epiglottis 　　Glossoepiglottic fold	S　Larynx 　　Aryepiglottic fold 　　Arytenoid cartilage 　　Corniculate cartilage 　　Cuneiform cartilage 　　False vocal cord 　　Glottis 　　Rima glottidis 　　Thyroid cartilage 　　Ventricular fold T　Vocal Cord, Right 　　Vocal fold V　Vocal Cord, Left 　　See T Vocal Cord, Right	Ø　Open 3　Percutaneous 4　Percutaneous Endoscopic 7　Via Natural or Artificial 　　Opening 8　Via Natural or Artificial 　　Opening Endoscopic	Ø　Drainage Device	Z　No Qualifier

Non-OR　ØC9[Ø,1,2,3,4,7,N,P,Q]3ØZ
Non-OR　ØC9[5,6][Ø,3,X]ØZ
Non-OR　ØC9[Ø,1,4][Ø,3,X]ZX
Non-OR　ØC9[Ø,1,2,3,4,7,N,P,Q]3ZZ
Non-OR　ØC9[5,6][Ø,3,X]Z[X,Z]
Non-OR　ØC97[3,X]ZX
Non-OR　ØC9[8,9,B,C,D,F,G,H,J][Ø,3]ØZ
Non-OR　ØC9[8,9,B,C,D,F,G,H,J]3ZX
Non-OR　ØC9[8,9,G,H]3ZZ
Non-OR　ØC9[B,C,D, F,J][Ø,3]ZZ
Non-OR　ØC9[M,R,S,T,V]3ØZ

ØC9 Continued on next page

LC Limited Coverage　　NC Noncovered　　⊞ Combination Member　　HAC associated procedure　　Combination Only　　DRG Non-OR　　Non-OR　　New/Revised in GREEN

Mouth and Throat

0C9 Continued

0	Medical and Surgical
C	Mouth and Throat
9	Drainage

Definition: Taking or letting out fluids and/or gases from a body part

Explanation: The qualifier DIAGNOSTIC is used to identify drainage procedures that are biopsies

Body Part Character 4	Approach Character 5	Device Character 6	Qualifier Character 7

M Pharynx
  Base of tongue
  Hypopharynx
  Laryngopharynx
  Lingual tonsil
  Oropharynx
  Piriform recess (sinus)
  Tongue, base of
R Epiglottis
  Glossoepiglottic fold
 	
S Larynx
  Aryepiglottic fold
  Arytenoid cartilage
  Corniculate cartilage
  Cuneiform cartilage
  False vocal cord
  Glottis
  Rima glottidis
  Thyroid cartilage
  Ventricular fold
T Vocal Cord, Right
  Vocal fold
V Vocal Cord, Left
  See T Vocal Cord, Right
	0 Open
	3 Percutaneous
	4 Percutaneous Endoscopic
	7 Via Natural or Artificial Opening
	8 Via Natural or Artificial Opening Endoscopic
		Z No Device	X Diagnostic
			Z No Qualifier

W Upper Tooth X Lower Tooth	0 Open X External	0 Drainage Device Z No Device	0 Single 1 Multiple 2 All

Non-OR	0C9M[0,3,4,7,8]ZX
Non-OR	0C9[M,R,S,T,V]3ZZ
Non-OR	0C9[R,S,T,V][3,4,7,8]ZX
Non-OR	0C9[W,X][0,X][0,Z][0,1,2]

0	Medical and Surgical
C	Mouth and Throat
B	Excision

Definition: Cutting out or off, without replacement, a portion of a body part

Explanation: The qualifier DIAGNOSTIC is used to identify excision procedures that are biopsies

Body Part Character 4	Approach Character 5	Device Character 6	Qualifier Character 7

0 Upper Lip
  Frenulum labii superioris
  Labial gland
  Vermilion border
1 Lower Lip
  Frenulum labii inferioris
  Labial gland
  Vermilion border
2 Hard Palate
3 Soft Palate
4 Buccal Mucosa
  Buccal gland
  Molar gland
  Palatine gland
 	
5 Upper Gingiva
6 Lower Gingiva
7 Tongue
  Frenulum linguae
N Uvula
  Palatine uvula
P Tonsils
  Palatine tonsil
Q Adenoids
  Pharyngeal tonsil
	0 Open
	3 Percutaneous
	X External
		Z No Device	X Diagnostic
			Z No Qualifier

8 Parotid Gland, Right
9 Parotid Gland, Left
B Parotid Duct, Right
  Stensen's duct
C Parotid Duct, Left
  See B Parotid Duct, Right
D Sublingual Gland, Right
 	
F Sublingual Gland, Left
G Submaxillary Gland, Right
  Submandibular gland
H Submaxillary Gland, Left
  See G Submaxillary Gland, Right
J Minor Salivary Gland
  Anterior lingual gland
	0 Open
	3 Percutaneous
		Z No Device	X Diagnostic
			Z No Qualifier

M Pharynx
  Base of tongue
  Hypopharynx
  Laryngopharynx
  Lingual tonsil
  Oropharynx
  Piriform recess (sinus)
  Tongue, base of
R Epiglottis
  Glossoepiglottic fold
 	
S Larynx
  Aryepiglottic fold
  Arytenoid cartilage
  Corniculate cartilage
  Cuneiform cartilage
  False vocal cord
  Glottis
  Rima glottidis
  Thyroid cartilage
  Ventricular fold
T Vocal Cord, Right
  Vocal fold
V Vocal Cord, Left
  See T Vocal Cord, Right
	0 Open
	3 Percutaneous
	4 Percutaneous Endoscopic
	7 Via Natural or Artificial Opening
	8 Via Natural or Artificial Opening Endoscopic
		Z No Device	X Diagnostic
			Z No Qualifier

W Upper Tooth X Lower Tooth	0 Open X External	Z No Device	0 Single 1 Multiple 2 All

Non-OR	0CB[0,1,4][0,3,X]ZX	Non-OR	0CBM[0,3,4,7,8]ZX
Non-OR	0CB[5,6][0,3,X]Z[X,Z]	Non-OR	0CB[R,S,T,V][3,4,7,8]ZX
Non-OR	0CB7[3,X]ZX	Non-OR	0CB[W,X][0,X]Z[0,1,2]
Non-OR	0CB[8,9,B,C,D,F,G,H,J]3ZX		

LC Limited Coverage   NC Noncovered   ⊞ Combination Member   HAC associated procedure   Combination Only   DRG Non-OR   Non-OR   New/Revised in GREEN

356   ICD-10-PCS 2021

0   Medical and Surgical
C   Mouth and Throat
C   Extirpation   Definition: Taking or cutting out solid matter from a body part

Explanation: The solid matter may be an abnormal byproduct of a biological function or a foreign body; it may be imbedded in a body part or in the lumen of a tubular body part. The solid matter may or may not have been previously broken into pieces.

Body Part Character 4	Approach Character 5	Device Character 6	Qualifier Character 7
0 Upper Lip Frenulum labii superioris Labial gland Vermilion border **1 Lower Lip** Frenulum labii inferioris Labial gland Vermilion border **2 Hard Palate** **3 Soft Palate** **4 Buccal Mucosa** Buccal gland Molar gland Palatine gland **5 Upper Gingiva** **6 Lower Gingiva** **7 Tongue** Frenulum linguae **N Uvula** Palatine uvula **P Tonsils** Palatine tonsil **Q Adenoids** Pharyngeal tonsil	**0 Open** **3 Percutaneous** **X External**	**Z No Device**	**Z No Qualifier**
8 Parotid Gland, Right **9 Parotid Gland, Left** **B Parotid Duct, Right** Stensen's duct **C Parotid Duct, Left** *See B Parotid Duct, Right* **D Sublingual Gland, Right** **F Sublingual Gland, Left** **G Submaxillary Gland, Right** Submandibular gland **H Submaxillary Gland, Left** *See G Submaxillary Gland, Right* **J Minor Salivary Gland** Anterior lingual gland	**0 Open** **3 Percutaneous**	**Z No Device**	**Z No Qualifier**
M Pharynx Base of tongue Hypopharynx Laryngopharynx Lingual tonsil Oropharynx Piriform recess (sinus) Tongue, base of **R Epiglottis** Glossoepiglottic fold **S Larynx** Aryepiglottic fold Arytenoid cartilage Corniculate cartilage Cuneiform cartilage False vocal cord Glottis Rima glottidis Thyroid cartilage Ventricular fold **T Vocal Cord, Right** Vocal fold **V Vocal Cord, Left** *See T Vocal Cord, Right*	**0 Open** **3 Percutaneous** **4 Percutaneous Endoscopic** **7 Via Natural or Artificial Opening** **8 Via Natural or Artificial Opening Endoscopic**	**Z No Device**	**Z No Qualifier**
W Upper Tooth **X Lower Tooth**	**0 Open** **X External**	**Z No Device**	**0 Single** **1 Multiple** **2 All**

Non-OR	0CC[0,1,2,3,4,7,N,P,Q]XZZ
Non-OR	0CC[5,6][0,3,X]ZZ
Non-OR	0CC[8,9,G,H]3ZZ
Non-OR	0CC[B,C,D,F,J][0,3]ZZ
Non-OR	0CC[M,S][7,8]ZZ
Non-OR	0CC[W,X][0,X]Z[0,1,2]

0   Medical and Surgical
C   Mouth and Throat
D   Extraction   Definition: Pulling or stripping out or off all or a portion of a body part by the use of force

Explanation: The qualifier DIAGNOSTIC is used to identify extraction procedures that are biopsies

Body Part Character 4	Approach Character 5	Device Character 6	Qualifier Character 7
T Vocal Cord, Right Vocal fold **V Vocal Cord, Left** *See T Vocal Cord, Right*	**0 Open** **3 Percutaneous** **4 Percutaneous Endoscopic** **7 Via Natural or Artificial Opening** **8 Via Natural or Artificial Opening Endoscopic**	**Z No Device**	**Z No Qualifier**
W Upper Tooth **X Lower Tooth**	**X External**	**Z No Device**	**0 Single** **1 Multiple** **2 All**

Non-OR	0CD[W,X]XZ[0,1,2]

LC Limited Coverage   NC Noncovered   ⊞ Combination Member   HAC associated procedure   Combination Only   DRG Non-OR   Non-OR   New/Revised in GREEN

ICD-10-PCS 2021   357

0CC–0CD

Ø   Medical and Surgical
C   Mouth and Throat
F   Fragmentation   Definition: Breaking solid matter in a body part into pieces

Explanation: Physical force (e.g., manual, ultrasonic) applied directly or indirectly is used to break the solid matter into pieces. The solid matter may be an abnormal byproduct of a biological function or a foreign body. The pieces of solid matter are not taken out.

Body Part Character 4	Approach Character 5	Device Character 6	Qualifier Character 7

B   Parotid Duct, Right   NC
    Stensen's duct
C   Parotid Duct, Left   NC
    See B Parotid Duct, Right
	Ø Open
	3 Percutaneous
	7 Via Natural or Artificial Opening
	X External
		Z No Device	Z No Qualifier

Non-OR   All body part, approach, device, and qualifier values
NC   ØCF[B,C]XZZ

Ø   Medical and Surgical
C   Mouth and Throat
H   Insertion   Definition: Putting in a nonbiological appliance that monitors, assists, performs, or prevents a physiological function but does not physically take the place of a body part

Explanation: None

Body Part Character 4	Approach Character 5	Device Character 6	Qualifier Character 7
7 Tongue Frenulum linguae	Ø Open 3 Percutaneous X External	1 Radioactive Element	Z No Qualifier

A   Salivary Gland
S   Larynx
    Aryepiglottic fold
    Arytenoid cartilage
    Corniculate cartilage
    Cuneiform cartilage
    False vocal cord
    Glottis
    Rima glottidis
    Thyroid cartilage
    Ventricular fold
	Ø Open
	3 Percutaneous
	7 Via Natural or Artificial Opening
	8 Via Natural or Artificial Opening Endoscopic
		1 Radioactive Element
		Y Other Device
			Z No Qualifier

Y Mouth and Throat	Ø Open 3 Percutaneous	1 Radioactive Element Y Other Device	Z No Qualifier
Y Mouth and Throat	7 Via Natural or Artificial Opening 8 Via Natural or Artificial Opening Endoscopic	1 Radioactive Element B Intraluminal Device, Airway Y Other Device	Z No Qualifier

Non-OR   ØCH[A,S][3,7,8]YZ
Non-OR   ØCHSØYZ
Non-OR   ØCHY[Ø,3]YZ
Non-OR   ØCHY[7,8][B,Y]Z

Ø   Medical and Surgical
C   Mouth and Throat
J   Inspection   Definition: Visually and/or manually exploring a body part

Explanation: Visual exploration may be performed with or without optical instrumentation. Manual exploration may be performed directly or through intervening body layers.

Body Part Character 4	Approach Character 5	Device Character 6	Qualifier Character 7
A Salivary Gland	Ø Open 3 Percutaneous X External	Z No Device	Z No Qualifier

S   Larynx
    Aryepiglottic fold
    Arytenoid cartilage
    Corniculate cartilage
    Cuneiform cartilage
    False vocal cord
    Glottis
    Rima glottidis
    Thyroid cartilage
    Ventricular fold
Y   Mouth and Throat
	Ø Open
	3 Percutaneous
	4 Percutaneous Endoscopic
	7 Via Natural or Artificial Opening
	8 Via Natural or Artificial Opening Endoscopic
	X External
		Z No Device	Z No Qualifier

Non-OR   All body part, approach, device, and qualifier values

Ø   **Medical and Surgical**
C   **Mouth and Throat**
L   **Occlusion**   Definition: Completely closing an orifice or the lumen of a tubular body part
                      Explanation: The orifice can be a natural orifice or an artificially created orifice

Body Part Character 4	Approach Character 5	Device Character 6	Qualifier Character 7

B   **Parotid Duct, Right**
     Stensen's duct
C   **Parotid Duct, Left**
     See B Parotid Duct, Right
	Ø Open
	3 Percutaneous
	4 Percutaneous Endoscopic
		C Extraluminal Device
		D Intraluminal Device
		Z No Device
			Z No Qualifier

B   **Parotid Duct, Right**
     Stensen's duct
C   **Parotid Duct, Left**
     See B Parotid Duct, Right
	7 Via Natural or Artificial Opening
	8 Via Natural or Artificial Opening
	     Endoscopic
		D Intraluminal Device
		Z No Device
			Z No Qualifier

Ø   **Medical and Surgical**
C   **Mouth and Throat**
M   **Reattachment**   Definition: Putting back in or on all or a portion of a separated body part to its normal location or other suitable location
                    Explanation: Vascular circulation and nervous pathways may or may not be reestablished

Body Part Character 4	Approach Character 5	Device Character 6	Qualifier Character 7

Ø   **Upper Lip**
     Frenulum labii superioris
     Labial gland
     Vermilion border
1   **Lower Lip**
     Frenulum labii inferioris
     Labial gland
     Vermilion border
3   **Soft Palate**
7   **Tongue**
     Frenulum linguae
N   **Uvula**
     Palatine uvula
	Ø Open	**Z** No Device	**Z** No Qualifier

W **Upper Tooth** **X** **Lower Tooth**	**Ø** Open **X** External	**Z** No Device	**Ø** Single **1** Multiple **2** All

Non-OR   ØCM[W,X][Ø,X]Z[Ø,1,2]

Mouth and Throat (side tab)

Ø   **Medical and Surgical**
C   **Mouth and Throat**
N   **Release**   Definition: Freeing a body part from an abnormal physical constraint by cutting or by the use of force
                      Explanation: Some of the restraining tissue may be taken out but none of the body part is taken out

Body Part Character 4	Approach Character 5	Device Character 6	Qualifier Character 7
Ø **Upper Lip** Frenulum labii superioris Labial gland Vermilion border **1** **Lower Lip** Frenulum labii inferioris Labial gland Vermilion border **2** **Hard Palate** **3** **Soft Palate** **4** **Buccal Mucosa** Buccal gland Molar gland Palatine gland **5** **Upper Gingiva** **6** **Lower Gingiva** **7** **Tongue** Frenulum linguae **N** **Uvula** Palatine uvula **P** **Tonsils** Palatine tonsil **Q** **Adenoids** Pharyngeal tonsil	**Ø** Open **3** Percutaneous **X** External	**Z** No Device	**Z** No Qualifier
8 **Parotid Gland, Right** **9** **Parotid Gland, Left** **B** **Parotid Duct, Right** Stensen's duct **C** **Parotid Duct, Left** *See B Parotid Duct, Right* **D** **Sublingual Gland, Right** **F** **Sublingual Gland, Left** **G** **Submaxillary Gland, Right** Submandibular gland **H** **Submaxillary Gland, Left** *See G Submaxillary Gland, Right* **J** **Minor Salivary Gland** Anterior lingual gland	**Ø** Open **3** Percutaneous	**Z** No Device	**Z** No Qualifier
M **Pharynx** Base of tongue Hypopharynx Laryngopharynx Lingual tonsil Oropharynx Piriform recess (sinus) Tongue, base of **R** **Epiglottis** Glossoepiglottic fold **S** **Larynx** Aryepiglottic fold Arytenoid cartilage Corniculate cartilage Cuneiform cartilage False vocal cord Glottis Rima glottidis Thyroid cartilage Ventricular fold **T** **Vocal Cord, Right** Vocal fold **V** **Vocal Cord, Left** *See T Vocal Cord, Right*	**Ø** Open **3** Percutaneous **4** Percutaneous Endoscopic **7** Via Natural or Artificial Opening **8** Via Natural or Artificial Opening Endoscopic	**Z** No Device	**Z** No Qualifier
W **Upper Tooth** **X** **Lower Tooth**	**Ø** Open **X** External	**Z** No Device	**Ø** Single **1** Multiple **2** All

Non-OR   ØCN[Ø,1,5,6,7][Ø,3,X]ZZ
Non-OR   ØCN[W,X][Ø,X]Z[Ø,1,2]

LC Limited Coverage   **NC** Noncovered   ⊞ Combination Member   HAC associated procedure   Combination Only   DRG Non-OR   Non-OR   New/Revised in **GREEN**
360   ICD-10-PCS 2021

ØCN–ØCN (side tab)

Ø   Medical and Surgical
C   Mouth and Throat
P   Removal   Definition: Taking out or off a device from a body part

Explanation: If a device is taken out and a similar device put in without cutting or puncturing the skin or mucous membrane, the procedure is coded to the root operation CHANGE. Otherwise, the procedure for taking out a device is coded to the root operation REMOVAL.

Body Part Character 4	Approach Character 5	Device Character 6	Qualifier Character 7
A Salivary Gland	**Ø** Open **3** Percutaneous	**Ø** Drainage Device **C** Extraluminal Device **Y** Other Device	**Z** No Qualifier
A Salivary Gland	**7** Via Natural or Artificial Opening **8** Via Natural or Artificial Opening Endoscopic	**Y** Other Device	**Z** No Qualifier

S   Larynx
     Aryepiglottic fold
     Arytenoid cartilage
     Corniculate cartilage
     Cuneiform cartilage
     False vocal cord
     Glottis
     Rima glottidis
     Thyroid cartilage
     Ventricular fold
	Ø Open
	3 Percutaneous
	7 Via Natural or Artificial Opening
	8 Via Natural or Artificial Opening Endoscopic
		Ø Drainage Device
		7 Autologous Tissue Substitute
		D Intraluminal Device
		J Synthetic Substitute
		K Nonautologous Tissue Substitute
		Y Other Device
			Z No Qualifier

S   Larynx
     Aryepiglottic fold
     Arytenoid cartilage
     Corniculate cartilage
     Cuneiform cartilage
     False vocal cord
     Glottis
     Rima glottidis
     Thyroid cartilage
     Ventricular fold
	X External	**Ø** Drainage Device
		7 Autologous Tissue Substitute
		D Intraluminal Device
		J Synthetic Substitute
		K Nonautologous Tissue Substitute
			Z No Qualifier

Y Mouth and Throat	**Ø** Open **3** Percutaneous **7** Via Natural or Artificial Opening **8** Via Natural or Artificial Opening Endoscopic	**Ø** Drainage Device **1** Radioactive Element **7** Autologous Tissue Substitute **D** Intraluminal Device **J** Synthetic Substitute **K** Nonautologous Tissue Substitute **Y** Other Device	**Z** No Qualifier
Y Mouth and Throat	**X** External	**Ø** Drainage Device **1** Radioactive Element **7** Autologous Tissue Substitute **D** Intraluminal Device **J** Synthetic Substitute **K** Nonautologous Tissue Substitute	**Z** No Qualifier

Non-OR	ØCPA[Ø,3][Ø,C,Y]Z
Non-OR	ØCPA[7,8]YZ
Non-OR	ØCPS3YZ
Non-OR	ØCPS[7,8][Ø,D,Y]Z
Non-OR	ØCPSX[Ø,7,D,J,K]Z
Non-OR	ØCPY3YZ
Non-OR	ØCPY[7,8][Ø,D,Y]Z
Non-OR	ØCPYX[Ø,1,7,D,J,K]Z

LC Limited Coverage   **NC** Noncovered   ⊞ Combination Member   HAC associated procedure   Combination Only   DRG Non-OR   Non-OR   New/Revised in GREEN

ICD-10-PCS 2021   361

Mouth and Throat

Ø   **Medical and Surgical**
C   **Mouth and Throat**
Q   **Repair**   Definition: Restoring, to the extent possible, a body part to its normal anatomic structure and function
                     Explanation: Used only when the method to accomplish the repair is not one of the other root operations

Body Part Character 4	Approach Character 5	Device Character 6	Qualifier Character 7

Ø **Upper Lip**
    Frenulum labii superioris
    Labial gland
    Vermilion border
1 **Lower Lip**
    Frenulum labii inferioris
    Labial gland
    Vermilion border
2 **Hard Palate**
3 **Soft Palate**
4 **Buccal Mucosa**
    Buccal gland
    Molar gland
    Palatine gland
5 **Upper Gingiva**
6 **Lower Gingiva**
7 **Tongue**
    Frenulum linguae
N **Uvula**
    Palatine uvula
P **Tonsils**
    Palatine tonsil
Q **Adenoids**
    Pharyngeal tonsil
	Ø Open
	3 Percutaneous
	X External
		Z No Device	**Z** No Qualifier

8 **Parotid Gland, Right**
9 **Parotid Gland, Left**
B **Parotid Duct, Right**
    Stensen's duct
C **Parotid Duct, Left**
    See B Parotid Duct, Right
D **Sublingual Gland, Right**
F **Sublingual Gland, Left**
G **Submaxillary Gland, Right**
    Submandibular gland
H **Submaxillary Gland, Left**
    See G Submaxillary Gland, Right
J **Minor Salivary Gland**
    Anterior lingual gland
	Ø Open
	3 Percutaneous
		Z No Device	**Z** No Qualifier

M **Pharynx**
    Base of tongue
    Hypopharynx
    Laryngopharynx
    Lingual tonsil
    Oropharynx
    Piriform recess (sinus)
    Tongue, base of
R **Epiglottis**
    Glossoepiglottic fold
S **Larynx**
    Aryepiglottic fold
    Arytenoid cartilage
    Corniculate cartilage
    Cuneiform cartilage
    False vocal cord
    Glottis
    Rima glottidis
    Thyroid cartilage
    Ventricular fold
T **Vocal Cord, Right**
    Vocal fold
V **Vocal Cord, Left**
    See T Vocal Cord, Right
	Ø Open
	3 Percutaneous
	4 Percutaneous Endoscopic
	7 Via Natural or Artificial Opening
	8 Via Natural or Artificial Opening Endoscopic
		Z No Device	**Z** No Qualifier

W **Upper Tooth** **X** **Lower Tooth**	**Ø** Open **X** External	**Z** No Device	**Ø** Single **1** Multiple **2** All

Non-OR   ØCQ[Ø,1,4,7]XZZ
Non-OR   ØCQ[5,6][Ø,3,X]ZZ
Non-OR   ØCQ[W,X][Ø,X]Z[Ø,1,2]

Ø   Medical and Surgical
C   Mouth and Throat
R   Replacement   Definition: Putting in or on biological or synthetic material that physically takes the place and/or function of all or a portion of a body part

                             Explanation: The body part may have been taken out or replaced, or may be taken out, physically eradicated, or rendered nonfunctional during the REPLACEMENT procedure. A REMOVAL procedure is coded for taking out the device used in a previous replacement procedure.

Body Part Character 4	Approach Character 5	Device Character 6	Qualifier Character 7
Ø Upper Lip Frenulum labii superioris Labial gland Vermilion border **1 Lower Lip** Frenulum labii inferioris Labial gland Vermilion border **2 Hard Palate** **3 Soft Palate** **4 Buccal Mucosa** Buccal gland Molar gland Palatine gland **5 Upper Gingiva** **6 Lower Gingiva** **7 Tongue** Frenulum linguae **N Uvula** Palatine uvula	**Ø Open** **3 Percutaneous** **X External**	**7 Autologous Tissue Substitute** **J Synthetic Substitute** **K Nonautologous Tissue Substitute**	**Z No Qualifier**
B Parotid Duct, Right Stensen's duct **C Parotid Duct, Left** *See B Parotid Duct, Right*	**Ø Open** **3 Percutaneous**	**7 Autologous Tissue Substitute** **J Synthetic Substitute** **K Nonautologous Tissue Substitute**	**Z No Qualifier**
M Pharynx Base of tongue Hypopharynx Laryngopharynx Lingual tonsil Oropharynx Piriform recess (sinus) Tongue, base of **R Epiglottis** Glossoepiglottic fold **S Larynx** Aryepiglottic fold Arytenoid cartilage Corniculate cartilage Cuneiform cartilage False vocal cord Glottis Rima glottidis Thyroid cartilage Ventricular fold **T Vocal Cord, Right** Vocal fold **V Vocal Cord, Left** *See T Vocal Cord, Right*	**Ø Open** **7 Via Natural or Artificial Opening** **8 Via Natural or Artificial Opening Endoscopic**	**7 Autologous Tissue Substitute** **J Synthetic Substitute** **K Nonautologous Tissue Substitute**	**Z No Qualifier**
W Upper Tooth **X Lower Tooth**	**Ø Open** **X External**	**7 Autologous Tissue Substitute** **J Synthetic Substitute** **K Nonautologous Tissue Substitute**	**Ø Single** **1 Multiple** **2 All**

Non-OR   ØCR[W,X][Ø,X][7,J,K][Ø,1,2]

LC Limited Coverage   **NC** Noncovered   ⊞ Combination Member   HAC associated procedure   Combination Only   DRG Non-OR   Non-OR   New/Revised in **GREEN**

ICD-10-PCS 2021   **363**

Mouth and Throat

Ø **Medical and Surgical**
C **Mouth and Throat**
S **Reposition**　Definition: Moving to its normal location, or other suitable location, all or a portion of a body part

Explanation: The body part is moved to a new location from an abnormal location, or from a normal location where it is not functioning correctly. The body part may or may not be cut out or off to be moved to the new location.

Body Part Character 4	Approach Character 5	Device Character 6	Qualifier Character 7

Ø **Upper Lip**
  Frenulum labii superioris
  Labial gland
  Vermilion border
1 **Lower Lip**
  Frenulum labii inferioris
  Labial gland
  Vermilion border
2 **Hard Palate**
3 **Soft Palate**
7 **Tongue**
  Frenulum linguae
N **Uvula**
  Palatine uvula
	Ø Open
	X External
		Z No Device	**Z** No Qualifier

B **Parotid Duct, Right**
  Stensen's duct
C **Parotid Duct, Left**
  See B Parotid Duct, Right
	Ø Open
	3 Percutaneous
		Z No Device	**Z** No Qualifier

R **Epiglottis**
  Glossoepiglottic fold
T **Vocal Cord, Right**
  Vocal fold
V **Vocal Cord, Left**
  See T Vocal Cord, Right
	Ø Open
	7 Via Natural or Artificial Opening
	8 Via Natural or Artificial Opening
	  Endoscopic
		Z No Device	**Z** No Qualifier

W Upper Tooth **X** Lower Tooth	**Ø** Open **X** External	**5** External Fixation Device **Z** No Device	**Ø** Single **1** Multiple **2** All

Non-OR　ØCS[W,X][Ø,X][5,Z][Ø,1,2]

Ø   **Medical and Surgical**
C   **Mouth and Throat**
T   **Resection**   Definition: Cutting out or off, without replacement, all of a body part
                             Explanation: None

Body Part Character 4	Approach Character 5	Device Character 6	Qualifier Character 7

Ø **Upper Lip**
  Frenulum labii superioris
  Labial gland
  Vermilion border
1 **Lower Lip**
  Frenulum labii inferioris
  Labial gland
  Vermilion border
2 **Hard Palate**
3 **Soft Palate**
7 **Tongue**
  Frenulum linguae
N **Uvula**
  Palatine uvula
P **Tonsils**
  Palatine tonsil
Q **Adenoids**
  Pharyngeal tonsil
	Ø **Open**
	X **External**
		Z **No Device**	Z **No Qualifier**

8 **Parotid Gland, Right**
9 **Parotid Gland, Left**
B **Parotid Duct, Right**
  Stensen's duct
C **Parotid Duct, Left**
  See B Parotid Duct, Right
D **Sublingual Gland, Right**
F **Sublingual Gland, Left**
G **Submaxillary Gland, Right**
  Submandibular gland
H **Submaxillary Gland, Left**
  See G Submaxillary Gland, Right
J **Minor Salivary Gland**
  Anterior lingual gland
	Ø **Open**	Z **No Device**	Z **No Qualifier**

M **Pharynx**
  Base of tongue
  Hypopharynx
  Laryngopharynx
  Lingual tonsil
  Oropharynx
  Piriform recess (sinus)
  Tongue, base of
R **Epiglottis**
  Glossoepiglottic fold
S **Larynx**
  Aryepiglottic fold
  Arytenoid cartilage
  Corniculate cartilage
  Cuneiform cartilage
  False vocal cord
  Glottis
  Rima glottidis
  Thyroid cartilage
  Ventricular fold
T **Vocal Cord, Right**
  Vocal fold
V **Vocal Cord, Left**
  See T Vocal Cord, Right
	Ø **Open**
	4 **Percutaneous Endoscopic**
	7 **Via Natural or Artificial Opening**
	8 **Via Natural or Artificial Opening Endoscopic**
		Z **No Device**	Z **No Qualifier**

W **Upper Tooth** X **Lower Tooth**	Ø **Open**	Z **No Device**	Ø **Single** 1 **Multiple** 2 **All**

Non-OR   ØCT[W,X]ØZ[Ø,1,2]

LC Limited Coverage   **NC** Noncovered   ⊞ Combination Member   HAC associated procedure   Combination Only   DRG Non-OR   Non-OR   New/Revised in **GREEN**

ICD-10-PCS 2021   **365**

Mouth and Throat

Ø   **Medical and Surgical**
C   **Mouth and Throat**
U   **Supplement**   Definition: Putting in or on biological or synthetic material that physically reinforces and/or augments the function of a portion of a body part

Explanation: The biological material is non-living, or is living and from the same individual. The body part may have been previously replaced, and the SUPPLEMENT procedure is performed to physically reinforce and/or augment the function of the replaced body part.

Body Part Character 4	Approach Character 5	Device Character 6	Qualifier Character 7

Ø **Upper Lip**
  Frenulum labii superioris
  Labial gland
  Vermilion border
1 **Lower Lip**
  Frenulum labii inferioris
  Labial gland
  Vermilion border
2 **Hard Palate**
3 **Soft Palate**
4 **Buccal Mucosa**
  Buccal gland
  Molar gland
  Palatine gland
5 **Upper Gingiva**
6 **Lower Gingiva**
7 **Tongue**
  Frenulum linguae
N **Uvula**
  Palatine uvula
	Ø Open
	3 Percutaneous
	X External
		7 Autologous Tissue Substitute
		J Synthetic Substitute
		K Nonautologous Tissue Substitute
			Z No Qualifier

M **Pharynx**
  Base of tongue
  Hypopharynx
  Laryngopharynx
  Lingual tonsil
  Oropharynx
  Piriform recess (sinus)
  Tongue, base of
R **Epiglottis**
  Glossoepiglottic fold
S **Larynx**
  Aryepiglottic fold
  Arytenoid cartilage
  Corniculate cartilage
  Cuneiform cartilage
  False vocal cord
  Glottis
  Rima glottidis
  Thyroid cartilage
  Ventricular fold
T **Vocal Cord, Right**
  Vocal fold
V **Vocal Cord, Left**
  See T Vocal Cord, Right
	Ø Open
	7 Via Natural or Artificial Opening
	8 Via Natural or Artificial Opening Endoscopic
		7 Autologous Tissue Substitute
		J Synthetic Substitute
		K Nonautologous Tissue Substitute
			Z No Qualifier

Non-OR   ØCU2[Ø,3]JZ

Ø   **Medical and Surgical**
C   **Mouth and Throat**
V   **Restriction**   Definition: Partially closing an orifice or the lumen of a tubular body part

Explanation: The orifice can be a natural orifice or an artificially created orifice

Body Part Character 4	Approach Character 5	Device Character 6	Qualifier Character 7

B **Parotid Duct, Right**
  Stensen's duct
C **Parotid Duct, Left**
  See B Parotid Duct, Right
	Ø Open
	3 Percutaneous
		C Extraluminal Device
		D Intraluminal Device
		Z No Device
			Z No Qualifier

B **Parotid Duct, Right**
  Stensen's duct
C **Parotid Duct, Left**
  See B Parotid Duct, Right
	7 Via Natural or Artificial Opening
	8 Via Natural or Artificial Opening Endoscopic
		D Intraluminal Device
		Z No Device
			Z No Qualifier

LC Limited Coverage   NC Noncovered   ⊞ Combination Member   HAC associated procedure   Combination Only   DRG Non-OR   Non-OR   New/Revised in GREEN

366   ICD-10-PCS 2021

Ø   Medical and Surgical
C   Mouth and Throat
W   Revision   Definition: Correcting, to the extent possible, a portion of a malfunctioning device or the position of a displaced device

Explanation: Revision can include correcting a malfunctioning or displaced device by taking out or putting in components of the device such as a screw or pin

Body Part Character 4	Approach Character 5	Device Character 6	Qualifier Character 7
A Salivary Gland	**Ø Open** **3 Percutaneous**	**Ø Drainage Device** **C Extraluminal Device** **Y Other Device**	**Z No Qualifier**
A Salivary Gland	**7 Via Natural or Artificial Opening** **8 Via Natural or Artificial Opening Endoscopic**	**Y Other Device**	**Z No Qualifier**
A Salivary Gland	**X External**	**Ø Drainage Device** **C Extraluminal Device**	**Z No Qualifier**
S Larynx Aryepiglottic fold Arytenoid cartilage Corniculate cartilage Cuneiform cartilage False vocal cord Glottis Rima glottidis Thyroid cartilage Ventricular fold	**Ø Open** **3 Percutaneous** **7 Via Natural or Artificial Opening** **8 Via Natural or Artificial Opening Endoscopic**	**Ø Drainage Device** **7 Autologous Tissue Substitute** **D Intraluminal Device** **J Synthetic Substitute** **K Nonautologous Tissue Substitute** **Y Other Device**	**Z No Qualifier**
S Larynx Aryepiglottic fold Arytenoid cartilage Corniculate cartilage Cuneiform cartilage False vocal cord Glottis Rima glottidis Thyroid cartilage Ventricular fold	**X External**	**Ø Drainage Device** **7 Autologous Tissue Substitute** **D Intraluminal Device** **J Synthetic Substitute** **K Nonautologous Tissue Substitute**	**Z No Qualifier**
Y Mouth and Throat	**Ø Open** **3 Percutaneous** **7 Via Natural or Artificial Opening** **8 Via Natural or Artificial Opening Endoscopic**	**Ø Drainage Device** **1 Radioactive Element** **7 Autologous Tissue Substitute** **D Intraluminal Device** **J Synthetic Substitute** **K Nonautologous Tissue Substitute** **Y Other Device**	**Z No Qualifier**
Y Mouth and Throat	**X External**	**Ø Drainage Device** **1 Radioactive Element** **7 Autologous Tissue Substitute** **D Intraluminal Device** **J Synthetic Substitute** **K Nonautologous Tissue Substitute**	**Z No Qualifier**

Non-OR	ØCWA[Ø,3][Ø,C,Y]Z
Non-OR	ØCWA[7,8]YZ
Non-OR	ØCWAX[Ø,C]Z
Non-OR	ØCWS[3,7,8]YZ
Non-OR	ØCWSX[Ø,7,D,J,K]Z
Non-OR	ØCWYØ7Z
Non-OR	ØCWY[3,7,8]YZ
Non-OR	ØCWYX[Ø,1,7,D,J,K]Z

LC Limited Coverage   **NC** Noncovered   ⊞ Combination Member   HAC associated procedure   Combination Only   DRG Non-OR   Non-OR   New/Revised in **GREEN**

ICD-10-PCS 2021   **367**

Ø   **Medical and Surgical**
C   **Mouth and Throat**
X   **Transfer**   Definition: Moving, without taking out, all or a portion of a body part to another location to take over the function of all or a portion of a body part
                     Explanation: The body part transferred remains connected to its vascular and nervous supply

Body Part Character 4	Approach Character 5	Device Character 6	Qualifier Character 7

Ø Upper Lip
    Frenulum labii superioris
    Labial gland
    Vermilion border
1 Lower Lip
    Frenulum labii inferioris
    Labial gland
    Vermilion border
3 Soft Palate
4 Buccal Mucosa
    Buccal gland
    Molar gland
    Palatine gland
5 Upper Gingiva
6 Lower Gingiva
7 Tongue
    Frenulum linguae
	Ø Open
	X External
		Z No Device	**Z** No Qualifier

Gastrointestinal System ØD1–ØDY

Character Meanings

This Character Meaning table is provided as a guide to assist the user in the identification of character members that may be found in this section of code tables. It **SHOULD NOT** be used to build a PCS code.

Operation–Character 3		Body Part–Character 4		Approach–Character 5		Device–Character 6		Qualifier–Character 7	
1	Bypass	Ø	Upper Intestinal Tract	Ø	Open	Ø	Drainage Device	Ø	Allogeneic
2	Change	1	Esophagus, Upper	3	Percutaneous	1	Radioactive Element	1	Syngeneic
5	Destruction	2	Esophagus, Middle	4	Percutaneous Endoscopic	2	Monitoring Device	2	Zooplastic
7	Dilation	3	Esophagus, Lower	7	Via Natural or Artificial Opening	3	Infusion Device	3	Vertical
8	Division	4	Esophagogastric Junction	8	Via Natural or Artificial Opening Endoscopic	7	Autologous Tissue Substitute	4	Cutaneous
9	Drainage	5	Esophagus	F	Via Natural or Artificial Opening with Percutaneous Endoscopic Assistance	B	Intraluminal Device, Airway	5	Esophagus
B	Excision	6	Stomach	X	External	C	Extraluminal Device	6	Stomach
C	Extirpation	7	Stomach, Pylorus			D	Intraluminal Device	7	Vagina
D	Extraction	8	Small Intestine			J	Synthetic Substitute	8	Small Intestine
F	Fragmentation	9	Duodenum			K	Nonautologous Tissue Substitute	9	Duodenum
H	Insertion	A	Jejunum			L	Artificial Sphincter	A	Jejunum
J	Inspection	B	Ileum			M	Stimulator Lead	B	Ileum
L	Occlusion	C	Ileocecal Valve			U	Feeding Device	E	Large Intestine
M	Reattachment	D	Lower Intestinal Tract			Y	Other Device	H	Cecum
N	Release	E	Large Intestine			Z	No Device	K	Ascending Colon
P	Removal	F	Large Intestine, Right					L	Transverse Colon
Q	Repair	G	Large Intestine, Left					M	Descending Colon
R	Replacement	H	Cecum					N	Sigmoid Colon
S	Reposition	J	Appendix					P	Rectum
T	Resection	K	Ascending Colon					Q	Anus
U	Supplement	L	Transverse Colon					X	Diagnostic
V	Restriction	M	Descending Colon					Z	No Qualifier
W	Revision	N	Sigmoid Colon						
X	Transfer	P	Rectum						
Y	Transplantation	Q	Anus						
		R	Anal Sphincter						
		U	Omentum						
		V	Mesentery						
		W	Peritoneum						

AHA Coding Clinic for table ØD1

2019, 4Q, 29	Intestinal bypass
2017, 2Q, 17	Billroth II (distal gastrectomy and gastrojejunostomy)
2016, 2Q, 31	Laparoscopic biliopancreatic diversion with duodenal switch
2014, 4Q, 41	Abdominoperineal resection (APR) with flap closure of perineum and colostomy

AHA Coding Clinic for table ØD2

2019, 1Q, 26	Exchange of clogged gastrojejunostomy tube

AHA Coding Clinic for table ØD5

2017, 1Q, 34	Debulking of tumor and peritoneum ablation

AHA Coding Clinic for table ØD7

2017, 3Q, 23	Laparoscopic pyloromyotomy
2014, 4Q, 40	Dilation of gastrojejunostomy anastomosis stricture

AHA Coding Clinic for table ØD8

2019, 2Q, 15	Reversal of Roux-en-Y bypass
2017, 3Q, 22	Laparoscopic esophagomyotomy (Heller type) and Toupet fundoplication
2017, 3Q, 23	Laparoscopic pyloromyotomy

AHA Coding Clinic for table ØD9

2015, 2Q, 29	Insertion of nasogastric tube for drainage and feeding

AHA Coding Clinic for table ØDB

2019, 2Q, 15	Reversal of Roux-en-Y bypass
2019, 1Q, 3-8	Whipple procedure
2019, 1Q, 27	Excision of pelvic sidewall mass
2017, 2Q, 17	Billroth II (distal gastrectomy and gastrojejunostomy)
2017, 1Q, 16	Hepatic flexure versus transverse colon
2016, 3Q, 3-7	Stoma creation & takedown procedures
2016, 2Q, 31	Laparoscopic biliopancreatic diversion with duodenal switch
2016, 1Q, 22	Perineal proctectomy
2016, 1Q, 24	Endoscopic brush biopsy of esophagus
2014, 4Q, 40	Abdominoperineal resection (APR) with flap closure of perineum and colostomy
2014, 3Q, 28	Ileostomy takedown and parastomal hernia repair
2014, 3Q, 32	Pyloric-sparing Whipple procedure

AHA Coding Clinic for table ØDD

2017, 4Q, 41-42	Extraction procedures

AHA Coding Clinic for table ØDH

2019, 2Q, 18	Endoscopic wound VAC placement
2016, 3Q, 26	Insertion of gastrostomy tube
2013, 4Q, 117	Percutaneous endoscopic placement of gastrostomy tube

AHA Coding Clinic for table ØDJ

2019, 1Q, 25	Laparoscopic appendectomy converted to open procedure
2019, 1Q, 25	Milking of inspissated material from ileum to colon
2017, 2Q, 15	Low anterior resection with sigmoidoscopy
2016, 2Q, 20	Capsule endoscopy of small intestine
2015, 3Q, 24	Esophagogastroduodenoscopy with epinephrine injection for control of bleeding

AHA Coding Clinic for table ØDL

2013, 4Q, 112	Endoscopic banding of esophageal varices

AHA Coding Clinic for table ØDN

2017, 4Q, 49-50	New and revised body part values - Repositioning of the intestine
2017, 1Q, 35	Lysis of omental and peritoneal adhesions
2015, 3Q, 15	Vascular ring surgery with release of esophagus and trachea
2015, 3Q, 16	Vascular ring surgery and double aortic arch

AHA Coding Clinic for table ØDP

2019, 2Q, 18	Removal of wound VAC

AHA Coding Clinic for table ØDQ

2019, 2Q, 15	Reversal of Roux-en-Y bypass
2018, 2Q, 25	Third and fourth degree obstetric lacerations
2018, 1Q, 11	Repair of internal hernia at Petersen space
2017, 3Q, 17	Posterior sagittal anorectoplasty
2016, 3Q, 3-7	Stoma creation & takedown procedures
2016, 3Q, 26	Insertion of gastrostomy tube
2016, 1Q, 7	Obstetrical perineal laceration repair
2016, 1Q, 8	Obstetrical perineal laceration repair
2014, 4Q, 20	Control of bleeding duodenal ulcer

AHA Coding Clinic for table ØDS

2019, 1Q, 30	Laparoscopic-assisted rectopexy with manual reduction of prolapse
2017, 4Q, 49-50	New and revised body part values - Repositioning of the intestine
2017, 3Q, 9	Ileocolic intussusception reduction via air enema
2017, 3Q, 17	Posterior sagittal anorectoplasty
2016, 3Q, 3-5	Stoma creation & takedown procedures

AHA Coding Clinic for table ØDT

2019, 1Q, 3-8	Whipple procedure
2019, 1Q, 14	Esophagectomy with colon interposition
2017, 4Q, 49-50	New and revised body part values - Repositioning of the intestine
2014, 4Q, 40	Abdominoperineal resection (APR) with flap closure of perineum and colostomy
2014, 4Q, 42	Right colectomy with side-to-side functional end-to-end anastomosis
2014, 3Q, 6	Ileocecectomy including cecum, terminal ileum and appendix
2014, 3Q, 6	Right colectomy

AHA Coding Clinic for table ØDU

2019, 1Q, 30	Laparoscopic-assisted rectopexy with manual reduction of prolapse

AHA Coding Clinic for table ØDV

2017, 3Q, 22	Laparoscopic esophagomyotomy (Heller type) and Toupet fundoplication
2016, 2Q, 22	Esophageal lengthening Collis gastroplasty with Nissen fundoplication and hiatal hernia
2014, 3Q, 28	Laparoscopic Nissen fundoplication and diaphragmatic hernia repair

AHA Coding Clinic for table ØDW

2018, 1Q, 20	Adjustment of gastric band

AHA Coding Clinic for table ØDX

2019, 4Q, 29-30	Transfer large intestine to vagina
2019, 1Q, 14	Esophagectomy with colon interposition
2017, 2Q, 18	Esophagectomy and esophagogastrectomy with cervical esophagogastrostomy
2016, 2Q, 22	Esophageal lengthening Collis gastroplasty with Nissen fundoplication and hiatal hernia
2015, 1Q, 28	Repair of bronchopleural fistula using omental pedicle graft

Upper Intestinal Tract (Ø) and Lower Intestinal Tract (D)

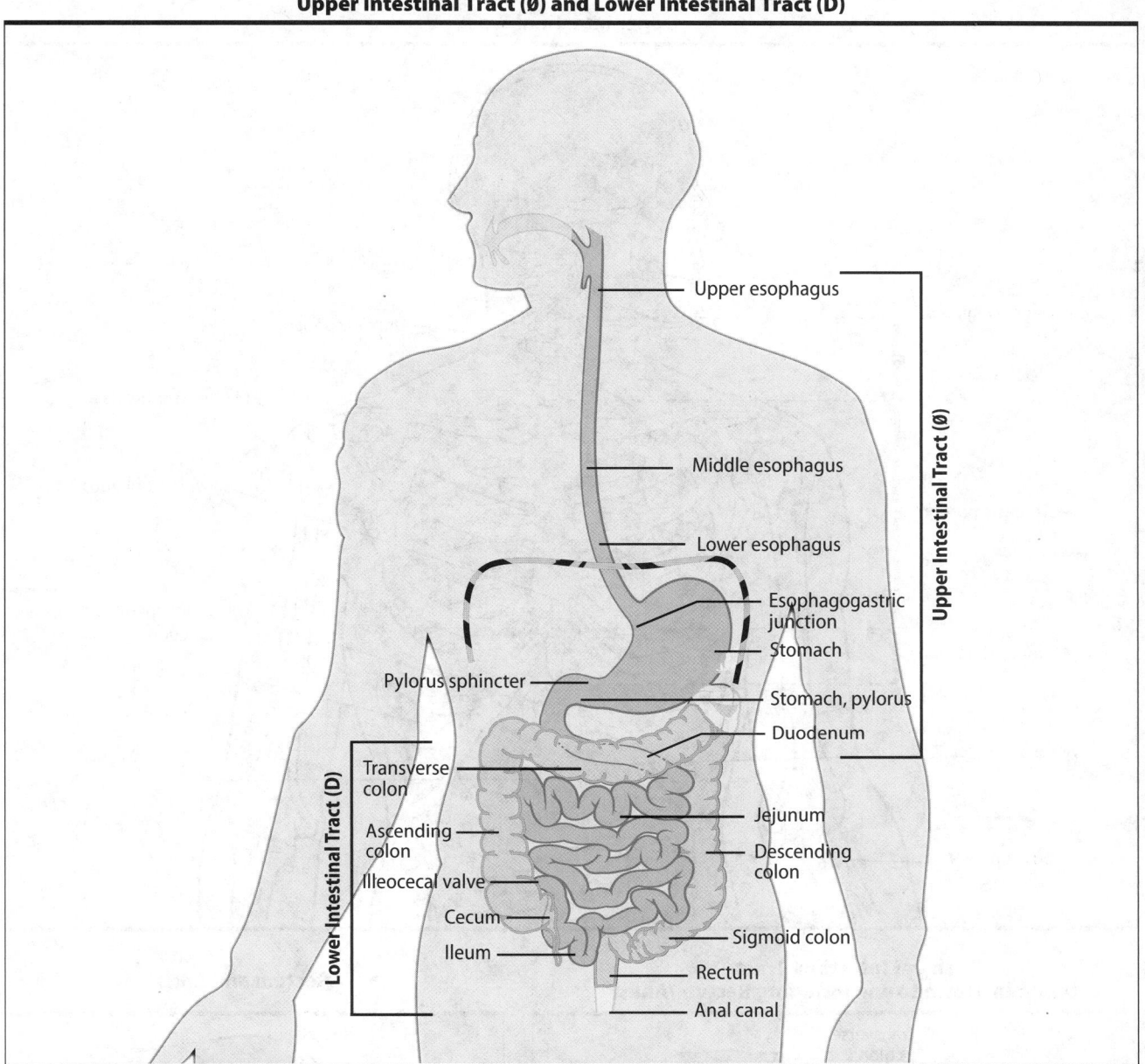

Upper Intestinal Tract

Esophageal region **5**:

Cervical portion

Thoracic portion

Abdominal portion

Pylorus sphincter **7**

Duodenum **9**

Upper esophagus **1**

Middle esophagus **2**

Lower esophagus **3**

Esophagogastric junction **4**

Stomach **6**

Stomach, pylorus **7**

Lower Intestinal Tract
(Jejunum Down to and Including Rectum/Anus)

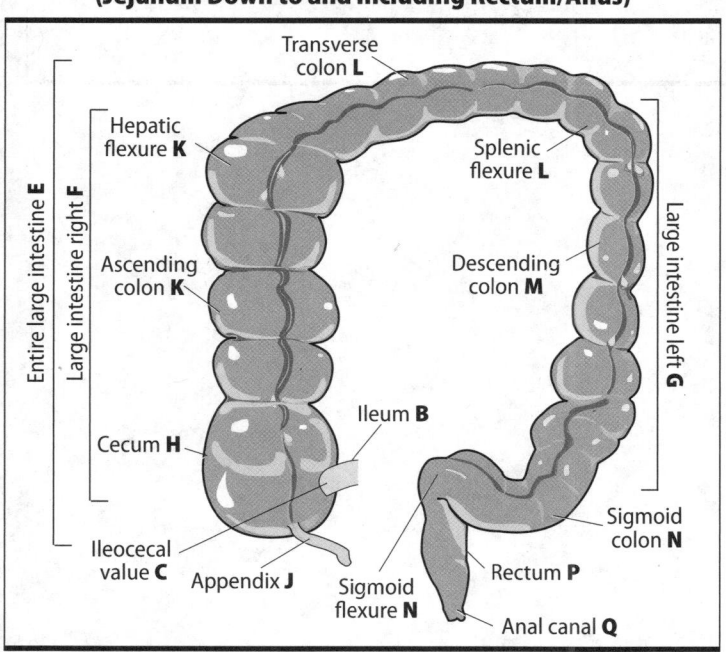

Transverse colon **L**

Hepatic flexure **K**

Splenic flexure **L**

Entire large intestine **E**

Large intestine right **F**

Ascending colon **K**

Descending colon **M**

Large intestine left **G**

Cecum **H**

Ileum **B**

Ileocecal value **C**

Appendix **J**

Sigmoid flexure **N**

Rectum **P**

Sigmoid colon **N**

Anal canal **Q**

Rectum and Anus

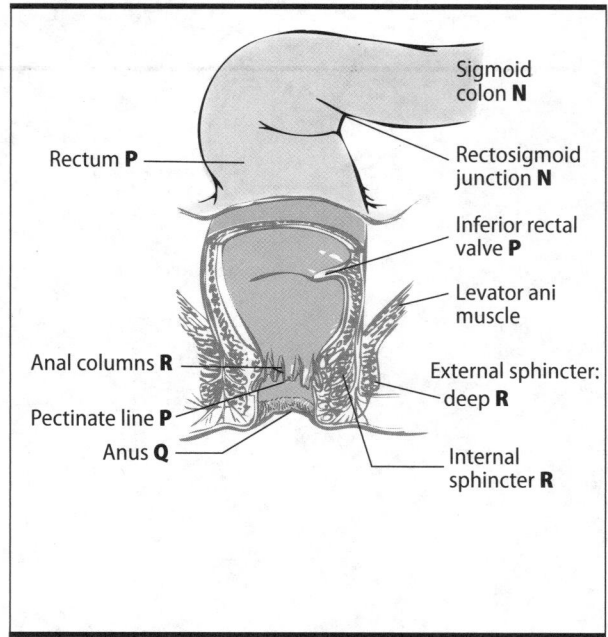

Sigmoid colon **N**

Rectum **P**

Rectosigmoid junction **N**

Inferior rectal valve **P**

Levator ani muscle

Anal columns **R**

Pectinate line **P**

Anus **Q**

External sphincter: deep **R**

Internal sphincter **R**

0   **Medical and Surgical**
D   **Gastrointestinal System**
1   **Bypass**   Definition: Altering the route of passage of the contents of a tubular body part

                Explanation: Rerouting contents of a body part to a downstream area of the normal route, to a similar route and body part, or to an abnormal route and dissimilar body part. Includes one or more anastomoses, with or without the use of a device.

Body Part Character 4	Approach Character 5	Device Character 6	Qualifier Character 7

1 Esophagus, Upper
   Cervical esophagus
2 Esophagus, Middle
   Thoracic esophagus
3 Esophagus, Lower
   Abdominal esophagus
5 Esophagus
	0 Open
	4 Percutaneous Endoscopic
	8 Via Natural or Artificial Opening Endoscopic
		7 Autologous Tissue Substitute
		J Synthetic Substitute
		K Nonautologous Tissue Substitute
		Z No Device
			4 Cutaneous
			6 Stomach
			9 Duodenum
			A Jejunum
			B Ileum

1 Esophagus, Upper
   Cervical esophagus
2 Esophagus, Middle
   Thoracic esophagus
3 Esophagus, Lower
   Abdominal esophagus
5 Esophagus
	3 Percutaneous	J Synthetic Substitute	4 Cutaneous

6 Stomach 9 Duodenum	0 Open 4 Percutaneous Endoscopic 8 Via Natural or Artificial Opening Endoscopic	7 Autologous Tissue Substitute J Synthetic Substitute K Nonautologous Tissue Substitute Z No Device	4 Cutaneous 9 Duodenum A Jejunum B Ileum L Transverse Colon
6 Stomach 9 Duodenum	3 Percutaneous	J Synthetic Substitute	4 Cutaneous
8 Small Intestine	0 Open 4 Percutaneous Endoscopic 8 Via Natural or Artificial Opening Endoscopic	7 Autologous Tissue Substitute J Synthetic Substitute K Nonautologous Tissue Substitute Z No Device	4 Cutaneous 8 Small Intestine H Cecum K Ascending Colon L Transverse Colon M Descending Colon N Sigmoid Colon P Rectum Q Anus
A Jejunum Duodenojejunal flexure	0 Open 4 Percutaneous Endoscopic 8 Via Natural or Artificial Opening Endoscopic	7 Autologous Tissue Substitute J Synthetic Substitute K Nonautologous Tissue Substitute Z No Device	4 Cutaneous A Jejunum B Ileum H Cecum K Ascending Colon L Transverse Colon M Descending Colon N Sigmoid Colon P Rectum Q Anus
A Jejunum Duodenojejunal flexure	3 Percutaneous	J Synthetic Substitute	4 Cutaneous
B Ileum	0 Open 4 Percutaneous Endoscopic 8 Via Natural or Artificial Opening Endoscopic	7 Autologous Tissue Substitute J Synthetic Substitute K Nonautologous Tissue Substitute Z No Device	4 Cutaneous B Ileum H Cecum K Ascending Colon L Transverse Colon M Descending Colon N Sigmoid Colon P Rectum Q Anus
B Ileum	3 Percutaneous	J Synthetic Substitute	4 Cutaneous
E Large Intestine	0 Open 4 Percutaneous Endoscopic 8 Via Natural or Artificial Opening Endoscopic	7 Autologous Tissue Substitute J Synthetic Substitute K Nonautologous Tissue Substitute Z No Device	4 Cutaneous E Large Intestine P Rectum
H Cecum	0 Open 4 Percutaneous Endoscopic 8 Via Natural or Artificial Opening Endoscopic	7 Autologous Tissue Substitute J Synthetic Substitute K Nonautologous Tissue Substitute Z No Device	4 Cutaneous H Cecum K Ascending Colon L Transverse Colon M Descending Colon N Sigmoid Colon P Rectum
H Cecum	3 Percutaneous	J Synthetic Substitute	4 Cutaneous

Non-OR   0D16[0,4,8][7,J,K,Z]4
Non-OR   0D163J4
HAC   0D16[0,4,8][7,J,K,Z][9,A,B,L] when reported with PDx E66.01 and SDx K68.11, K95.01, K95.81 or T81.40–T81.49 with7th character A

0D1 Continued on next page

LC Limited Coverage   NC Noncovered   ⊞ Combination Member   HAC associated procedure   Combination Only   DRG Non-OR   Non-OR   New/Revised in GREEN

Gastrointestinal System

Ø   **Medical and Surgical**
D   **Gastrointestinal System**
1   **Bypass**   Definition: Altering the route of passage of the contents of a tubular body part

                Explanation: Rerouting contents of a body part to a downstream area of the normal route, to a similar route and body part, or to an abnormal route and dissimilar body part. Includes one or more anastomoses, with or without the use of a device.

Body Part Character 4	Approach Character 5	Device Character 6	Qualifier Character 7
K Ascending Colon	Ø Open 4 Percutaneous Endoscopic 8 Via Natural or Artificial Opening Endoscopic	7 Autologous Tissue Substitute J Synthetic Substitute K Nonautologous Tissue Substitute Z No Device	4 Cutaneous K Ascending Colon L Transverse Colon M Descending Colon N Sigmoid Colon P Rectum
K Ascending Colon	3 Percutaneous	J Synthetic Substitute	4 Cutaneous

L   Transverse Colon
     Hepatic flexure
     Splenic flexure
	Ø Open
	4 Percutaneous Endoscopic
	8 Via Natural or Artificial Opening Endoscopic
		7 Autologous Tissue Substitute
		J Synthetic Substitute
		K Nonautologous Tissue Substitute
		Z No Device
			4 Cutaneous
			L Transverse Colon
			M Descending Colon
			N Sigmoid Colon
			P Rectum

L   Transverse Colon
     Hepatic flexure
     Splenic flexure
	3 Percutaneous	J Synthetic Substitute	4 Cutaneous

M Descending Colon	Ø Open 4 Percutaneous Endoscopic 8 Via Natural or Artificial Opening Endoscopic	7 Autologous Tissue Substitute J Synthetic Substitute K Nonautologous Tissue Substitute Z No Device	4 Cutaneous M Descending Colon N Sigmoid Colon P Rectum
M Descending Colon	3 Percutaneous	J Synthetic Substitute	4 Cutaneous

N   Sigmoid Colon
     Rectosigmoid junction
     Sigmoid flexure
	Ø Open
	4 Percutaneous Endoscopic
	8 Via Natural or Artificial Opening Endoscopic
		7 Autologous Tissue Substitute
		J Synthetic Substitute
		K Nonautologous Tissue Substitute
		Z No Device
			4 Cutaneous
			N Sigmoid Colon
			P Rectum

N   Sigmoid Colon
     Rectosigmoid junction
     Sigmoid flexure
	3 Percutaneous	J Synthetic Substitute	4 Cutaneous

Ø   **Medical and Surgical**
D   **Gastrointestinal System**
2   **Change**   Definition: Taking out or off a device from a body part and putting back an identical or similar device in or on the same body part without cutting or puncturing the skin or a mucous membrane

                Explanation: All CHANGE procedures are coded using the approach EXTERNAL

Body Part Character 4	Approach Character 5	Device Character 6	Qualifier Character 7
Ø Upper Intestinal Tract D Lower Intestinal Tract	X External	Ø Drainage Device U Feeding Device Y Other Device	Z No Qualifier

U   Omentum
     Gastrocolic ligament
     Gastrocolic omentum
     Gastrohepatic omentum
     Gastrophrenic ligament
     Gastrosplenic ligament
     Greater Omentum
     Hepatogastric ligament
     Lesser Omentum
V   Mesentery
     Mesoappendix
     Mesocolon
W   Peritoneum
     Epiploic foramen
	X External	Ø Drainage Device
		Y Other Device
			Z No Qualifier

Non-OR   All body part, approach, device, and qualifier values

LC Limited Coverage   NC Noncovered   ⊞ Combination Member   HAC associated procedure   Combination Only   DRG Non-OR   Non-OR   New/Revised in GREEN

374   ICD-10-PCS 2021

ØD1–ØD2

Ø   **Medical and Surgical**
D   **Gastrointestinal System**
5   **Destruction**   Definition: Physical eradication of all or a portion of a body part by the direct use of energy, force, or a destructive agent
                            Explanation: None of the body part is physically taken out

Body Part Character 4	Approach Character 5	Device Character 6	Qualifier Character 7

1 **Esophagus, Upper**
   Cervical esophagus
2 **Esophagus, Middle**
   Thoracic esophagus
3 **Esophagus, Lower**
   Abdominal esophagus
4 **Esophagogastric Junction**
   Cardia
   Cardioesophageal junction
   Gastroesophageal (GE) junction
5 **Esophagus**
6 **Stomach**
7 **Stomach, Pylorus**
   Pyloric antrum
   Pyloric canal
   Pyloric sphincter
8 **Small Intestine**
9 **Duodenum**
A **Jejunum**
   Duodenojejunal flexure
B **Ileum**
C **Ileocecal Valve**
E **Large Intestine**
F **Large Intestine, Right**
G **Large Intestine, Left**
H **Cecum**
J **Appendix**
   Vermiform appendix
K **Ascending Colon**
L **Transverse Colon**
   Hepatic flexure
   Splenic flexure
M **Descending Colon**
N **Sigmoid Colon**
   Rectosigmoid junction
   Sigmoid flexure
P **Rectum**
   Anorectal junction
	Ø **Open**
	3 **Percutaneous**
	4 **Percutaneous Endoscopic**
	7 **Via Natural or Artificial Opening**
	8 **Via Natural or Artificial Opening
	     Endoscopic**
		Z No Device	Z No Qualifier

Q **Anus**
   Anal orifice
	Ø **Open**
	3 **Percutaneous**
	4 **Percutaneous Endoscopic**
	7 **Via Natural or Artificial Opening**
	8 **Via Natural or Artificial Opening
	     Endoscopic**
	X **External**
		Z No Device	Z No Qualifier

R **Anal Sphincter**
   External anal sphincter
   Internal anal sphincter
U **Omentum**
   Gastrocolic ligament
   Gastrocolic omentum
   Gastrohepatic omentum
   Gastrophrenic ligament
   Gastrosplenic ligament
   Greater Omentum
   Hepatogastric ligament
   Lesser Omentum
V **Mesentery**
   Mesoappendix
   Mesocolon
W **Peritoneum**
   Epiploic foramen
	Ø **Open**
	3 **Percutaneous**
	4 **Percutaneous Endoscopic**
		Z No Device	Z No Qualifier

Non-OR   ØD5[1,2,3,4,5,6,7,9,E,F,G,H,K,L,M,N][4,8]ZZ
Non-OR   ØD5[8,A,B,C]8ZZ
Non-OR   ØD5P[Ø,3,4,7,8]ZZ
Non-OR   ØD5Q[4,8]ZZ
Non-OR   ØD5R4ZZ

Gastrointestinal System

Ø   Medical and Surgical
D   Gastrointestinal System
7   Dilation   Definition: Expanding an orifice or the lumen of a tubular body part

Explanation: The orifice can be a natural orifice or an artificially created orifice. Accomplished by stretching a tubular body part using intraluminal pressure or by cutting part of the orifice or wall of the tubular body part.

Body Part Character 4	Approach Character 5	Device Character 6	Qualifier Character 7

1   **Esophagus, Upper**
    Cervical esophagus
2   **Esophagus, Middle**
    Thoracic esophagus
3   **Esophagus, Lower**
    Abdominal esophagus
4   **Esophagogastric Junction**
    Cardia
    Cardioesophageal junction
    Gastroesophageal (GE) junction
5   **Esophagus**
6   **Stomach**
7   **Stomach, Pylorus**
    Pyloric antrum
    Pyloric canal
    Pyloric sphincter
8   **Small Intestine**
9   **Duodenum**
A   **Jejunum**
    Duodenojejunal flexure
B   **Ileum**
C   **Ileocecal Valve**
E   **Large Intestine**
F   **Large Intestine, Right**
G   **Large Intestine, Left**
H   **Cecum**
K   **Ascending Colon**
L   **Transverse Colon**
    Hepatic flexure
    Splenic flexure
M   **Descending Colon**
N   **Sigmoid Colon**
    Rectosigmoid junction
    Sigmoid flexure
P   **Rectum**
    Anorectal junction
Q   **Anus**
    Anal orifice
	Ø Open
	3 Percutaneous
	4 Percutaneous Endoscopic
	7 Via Natural or Artificial Opening
	8 Via Natural or Artificial Opening
	    Endoscopic
		D Intraluminal Device
		Z No Device
			Z No Qualifier

Non-OR	ØD7[1,2,3,4,5,6,8,9,A,B,C,E,F,G,H,K,L,M,N,P,Q][7,8][D,Z]Z
Non-OR	ØD77[4,8]DZ
Non-OR	ØD777[D,Z]Z
Non-OR	ØD7[8,9,A,B,C,E,F,G,H,K,L,M,N][Ø,3,4]DZ

Ø   Medical and Surgical
D   Gastrointestinal System
8   Division   Definition: Cutting into a body part, without draining fluids and/or gases from the body part, in order to separate or transect a body part

Explanation: All or a portion of the body part is separated into two or more portions

Body Part Character 4	Approach Character 5	Device Character 6	Qualifier Character 7

4   **Esophagogastric Junction**
    Cardia
    Cardioesophageal junction
    Gastroesophageal (GE) junction
7   **Stomach, Pylorus**
    Pyloric antrum
    Pyloric canal
    Pyloric sphincter
	Ø Open
	3 Percutaneous
	4 Percutaneous Endoscopic
	7 Via Natural or Artificial Opening
	8 Via Natural or Artificial Opening
	    Endoscopic
		Z No Device	Z No Qualifier

R   **Anal Sphincter**
    External anal sphincter
    Internal anal sphincter
	Ø Open
	3 Percutaneous
		Z No Device	Z No Qualifier

LC Limited Coverage   NC Noncovered   ⊞ Combination Member   HAC associated procedure   Combination Only   DRG Non-OR   Non-OR   New/Revised in GREEN

376   ICD-10-PCS 2021

0   **Medical and Surgical**
D   **Gastrointestinal System**
9   **Drainage**   Definition: Taking or letting out fluids and/or gases from a body part
                             Explanation: The qualifier DIAGNOSTIC is used to identify drainage procedures that are biopsies

Body Part Character 4		Approach Character 5	Device Character 6	Qualifier Character 7

1 Esophagus, Upper
  Cervical esophagus
2 Esophagus, Middle
  Thoracic esophagus
3 Esophagus, Lower
  Abdominal esophagus
4 Esophagogastric
  Junction
  Cardia
  Cardioesophageal
    junction
  Gastroesophageal (GE)
    junction
5 Esophagus
6 Stomach
7 Stomach, Pylorus
  Pyloric antrum
  Pyloric canal
  Pyloric sphincter
8 Small Intestine
9 Duodenum
	A Jejunum
	  Duodenojejunal flexure
	B Ileum
	C Ileocecal Valve
	E Large Intestine
	F Large Intestine, Right
	G Large Intestine, Left
	H Cecum
	J Appendix
	  Vermiform appendix
	K Ascending Colon
	L Transverse Colon
	  Hepatic flexure
	  Splenic flexure
	M Descending Colon
	N Sigmoid Colon
	  Rectosigmoid junction
	  Sigmoid flexure
	P Rectum
	  Anorectal junction
		0 Open
		3 Percutaneous
		4 Percutaneous Endoscopic
		7 Via Natural or Artificial
		  Opening
		8 Via Natural or Artificial
		  Opening Endoscopic
			0 Drainage Device	Z No Qualifier

1 Esophagus, Upper
  Cervical esophagus
2 Esophagus, Middle
  Thoracic esophagus
3 Esophagus, Lower
  Abdominal esophagus
4 Esophagogastric
  Junction
  Cardia
  Cardioesophageal
    junction
  Gastroesophageal (GE)
    junction
5 Esophagus
6 Stomach
7 Stomach, Pylorus
  Pyloric antrum
  Pyloric canal
  Pyloric sphincter
8 Small Intestine
9 Duodenum
	A Jejunum
	  Duodenojejunal flexure
	B Ileum
	C Ileocecal Valve
	E Large Intestine
	F Large Intestine, Right
	G Large Intestine, Left
	H Cecum
	J Appendix
	  Vermiform appendix
	K Ascending Colon
	L Transverse Colon
	  Hepatic flexure
	  Splenic flexure
	M Descending Colon
	N Sigmoid Colon
	  Rectosigmoid junction
	  Sigmoid flexure
	P Rectum
	  Anorectal junction
		0 Open
		3 Percutaneous
		4 Percutaneous Endoscopic
		7 Via Natural or Artificial
		  Opening
		8 Via Natural or Artificial
		  Opening Endoscopic
			Z No Device	X Diagnostic
				Z No Qualifier

Q Anus
  Anal orifice
		0 Open
		3 Percutaneous
		4 Percutaneous Endoscopic
		7 Via Natural or Artificial
		  Opening
		8 Via Natural or Artificial
		  Opening Endoscopic
		X External
			0 Drainage Device	Z No Qualifier

Q Anus
  Anal orifice
		0 Open
		3 Percutaneous
		4 Percutaneous Endoscopic
		7 Via Natural or Artificial
		  Opening
		8 Via Natural or Artificial
		  Opening Endoscopic
		X External
			Z No Device	X Diagnostic
				Z No Qualifier

Non-OR   0D9[1,2,3,4,5,C,J]30Z
Non-OR   0D9[6,7,8,9,A,B,E,F,G,H,K,L,M,N,P][3,7,8]0Z
Non-OR   0D9[1,2,3,4,5,6,7,8,9,A,B,C,E,F,G,H,K,L,M,N,P][3,4,7,8]ZX
Non-OR   0D9[1,2,3,4,5,6,7,8,9,A,B,C,E,F,G,H,J,K,L,M,N,P]3ZZ
Non-OR   0D9Q30Z
Non-OR   0D9Q[0,4,7,8,X]ZX
Non-OR   0D9Q3Z[X,Z]

0D9 Continued on next page

LC Limited Coverage   NC Noncovered   ⊞ Combination Member   HAC associated procedure   Combination Only   DRG Non-OR   Non-OR   New/Revised in GREEN

ICD-10-PCS 2021   377

0D9–0D9

ØD9 Continued

Ø Medical and Surgical
D Gastrointestinal System
9 Drainage   Definition: Taking or letting out fluids and/or gases from a body part
         Explanation: The qualifier DIAGNOSTIC is used to identify drainage procedures that are biopsies

Body Part Character 4	Approach Character 5	Device Character 6	Qualifier Character 7
R Anal Sphincter External anal sphincter Internal anal sphincter U Omentum Gastrocolic ligament Gastrocolic omentum Gastrohepatic omentum Gastrophrenic ligament Gastrosplenic ligament Greater Omentum Hepatogastric ligament Lesser Omentum V Mesentery Mesoappendix Mesocolon W Peritoneum Epiploic foramen	Ø Open 3 Percutaneous 4 Percutaneous Endoscopic	Ø Drainage Device	Z No Qualifier
R Anal Sphincter External anal sphincter Internal anal sphincter U Omentum Gastrocolic ligament Gastrocolic omentum Gastrohepatic omentum Gastrophrenic ligament Gastrosplenic ligament Greater Omentum Hepatogastric ligament Lesser Omentum V Mesentery Mesoappendix Mesocolon W Peritoneum Epiploic foramen	Ø Open 3 Percutaneous 4 Percutaneous Endoscopic	Z No Device	X Diagnostic Z No Qualifier

Non-OR   ØD9R3ØZ
Non-OR   ØD9[U,V,W][3,4]ØZ
Non-OR   ØD9R[Ø,4]ZX
Non-OR   ØD9[R,U,V,W]3Z[X,Z]
Non-OR   ØD9[U,V,W]4ZZ

Ø   **Medical and Surgical**
D   **Gastrointestinal System**
B   **Excision**   Definition: Cutting out or off, without replacement, a portion of a body part

              Explanation: The qualifier DIAGNOSTIC is used to identify excision procedures that are biopsies

Body Part — Character 4	Approach — Character 5	Device — Character 6	Qualifier — Character 7
1 Esophagus, Upper Cervical esophagus **2 Esophagus, Middle** Thoracic esophagus **3 Esophagus, Lower** Abdominal esophagus **4 Esophagogastric Junction** Cardia Cardioesophageal junction Gastroesophageal (GE) junction **5 Esophagus** **7 Stomach, Pylorus** Pyloric antrum Pyloric canal Pyloric sphincter **8 Small Intestine** **9 Duodenum** **A Jejunum** Duodenojejunal flexure **B Ileum** **C Ileocecal Valve** **E Large Intestine** **F Large Intestine, Right** **H Cecum** **J Appendix** Vermiform appendix **K Ascending Colon** **P Rectum** Anorectal junction	**Ø Open** **3 Percutaneous** **4 Percutaneous Endoscopic** **7 Via Natural or Artificial Opening** **8 Via Natural or Artificial Opening Endoscopic**	**Z No Device**	**X Diagnostic** **Z No Qualifier**
6 Stomach	**Ø Open** **3 Percutaneous** **4 Percutaneous Endoscopic** **7 Via Natural or Artificial Opening** **8 Via Natural or Artificial Opening Endoscopic**	**Z No Device**	**3 Vertical** **X Diagnostic** **Z No Qualifier**
G Large Intestine, Left **L Transverse Colon** Hepatic flexure Splenic flexure **M Descending Colon** **N Sigmoid Colon** Rectosigmoid junction Sigmoid flexure	**Ø Open** **3 Percutaneous** **4 Percutaneous Endoscopic** **7 Via Natural or Artificial Opening** **8 Via Natural or Artificial Opening Endoscopic**	**Z No Device**	**X Diagnostic** **Z No Qualifier**
G Large Intestine, Left **L Transverse Colon** Hepatic flexure Splenic flexure **M Descending Colon** **N Sigmoid Colon** Rectosigmoid junction Sigmoid flexure	**F Via Natural or Artificial Opening with Percutaneous Endoscopic Assistance**	**Z No Device**	**Z No Qualifier**
Q Anus Anal orifi	**Ø Open** **3 Percutaneous** **4 Percutaneous Endoscopic** **7 Via Natural or Artificial Opening** **8 Via Natural or Artificial Opening Endoscopic** **X External**	**Z No Device**	**X Diagnostic** **Z No Qualifier**
R Anal Sphincter External anal sphincter Internal anal sphincter **U Omentum** Gastrocolic ligament Gastrocolic omentum Gastrohepatic omentum Gastrophrenic ligament Gastrosplenic ligament Greater Omentum Hepatogastric ligament Lesser Omentum **V Mesentery** Mesoappendix Mesocolon **W Peritoneum** Epiploic foramen	**Ø Open** **3 Percutaneous** **4 Percutaneous Endoscopic**	**Z No Device**	**X Diagnostic** **Z No Qualifier**

Non-OR ØDB[1,2,3,4,5,7,8,9,A,B,C,E,F,H,K,P][3,4,7,8]ZX	**Non-OR** ØDB[G,L,M,N]8ZZ
Non-OR ØDB[1,2,3,5,7,9][4,8]ZZ	**Non-OR** ØDBQ[Ø,3,4,7,8,X]ZX
Non-OR ØDB[4,E,F,H,K,P]8ZZ	**Non-OR** ØDBQ8ZZ
Non-OR ØDB6[3,7,8]Z[3,X,Z]	**Non-OR** ØDBR[Ø,3,4]ZX
Non-OR ØDB[G,L,M,N][3,4,7,8]ZX	**Non-OR** ØDB[U,V,W][3,4]ZX

LC Limited Coverage   **NC** Noncovered   ⊞ Combination Member   HAC associated procedure   Combination Only   DRG Non-OR   Non-OR   New/Revised in GREEN

ICD-10-PCS 2021   **379**

ØDB–ØDB

Gastrointestinal System

Ø   **Medical and Surgical**
D   **Gastrointestinal System**
C   **Extirpation**   Definition: Taking or cutting out solid matter from a body part

Explanation: The solid matter may be an abnormal byproduct of a biological function or a foreign body; it may be imbedded in a body part or in the lumen of a tubular body part. The solid matter may or may not have been previously broken into pieces.

Body Part Character 4	Approach Character 5	Device Character 6	Qualifier Character 7

1 **Esophagus, Upper**
    Cervical esophagus
2 **Esophagus, Middle**
    Thoracic esophagus
3 **Esophagus, Lower**
    Abdominal esophagus
4 **Esophagogastric Junction**
    Cardia
    Cardioesophageal junction
    Gastroesophageal (GE) junction
5 **Esophagus**
6 **Stomach**
7 **Stomach, Pylorus**
    Pyloric antrum
    Pyloric canal
    Pyloric sphincter
8 **Small Intestine**
9 **Duodenum**
A **Jejunum**
    Duodenojejunal flexure
B **Ileum**
C **Ileocecal Valve**
E **Large Intestine**
F **Large Intestine, Right**
G **Large Intestine, Left**
H **Cecum**
J **Appendix**
    Vermiform appendix
K **Ascending Colon**
L **Transverse Colon**
    Hepatic flexure
    Splenic flexure
M **Descending Colon**
N **Sigmoid Colon**
    Rectosigmoid junction
    Sigmoid flexure
P **Rectum**
    Anorectal junction
	Ø **Open**
	3 **Percutaneous**
	4 **Percutaneous Endoscopic**
	7 **Via Natural or Artificial Opening**
	8 **Via Natural or Artificial Opening Endoscopic**
		Z **No Device**	**Z** **No Qualifier**

Q **Anus** Anal orifice	**Ø** **Open** **3** **Percutaneous** **4** **Percutaneous Endoscopic** **7** **Via Natural or Artificial Opening** **8** **Via Natural or Artificial Opening Endoscopic** **X** **External**	**Z** **No Device**	**Z** **No Qualifier**

R **Anal Sphincter**
    External anal sphincter
    Internal anal sphincter
U **Omentum**
    Gastrocolic ligament
    Gastrocolic omentum
    Gastrohepatic omentum
    Gastrophrenic ligament
    Gastrosplenic ligament
    Greater Omentum
    Hepatogastric ligament
    Lesser Omentum
V **Mesentery**
    Mesoappendix
    Mesocolon
W **Peritoneum**
    Epiploic foramen
	Ø **Open**
	3 **Percutaneous**
	4 **Percutaneous Endoscopic**
		Z **No Device**	**Z** **No Qualifier**

Non-OR   ØDC[1,2,3,4,5,6,7,8,9,A,B,C,E,F,G,H,K,L,M,N,P][7,8]ZZ
Non-OR   ØDCQ[7,8,X]ZZ

Ø   **Medical and Surgical**
D   **Gastrointestinal System**
D   **Extraction**   Definition: Pulling or stripping out or off all or a portion of a body part by the use of force
                                  Explanation: The qualifier DIAGNOSTIC is used to identify extraction procedures that are biopsies

Body Part Character 4	Approach Character 5	Device Character 6	Qualifier Character 7
1 Esophagus, Upper Cervical esophagus **2 Esophagus, Middle** Thoracic esophagus **3 Esophagus, Lower** Abdominal esophagus **4 Esophagogastric Junction** Cardia Cardioesophageal junction Gastroesophageal (GE) junction **5 Esophagus** **6 Stomach** **7 Stomach, Pylorus** Pyloric antrum Pyloric canal Pyloric sphincter **8 Small Intestine** **9 Duodenum** **A Jejunum** Duodenojejunal flexure **B Ileum** **C Ileocecal Valve** **E Large Intestine** **F Large Intestine, Right** **G Large Intestine, Left** **H Cecum** **J Appendix** Vermiform appendix **K Ascending Colon** **L Transverse Colon** Hepatic flexure Splenic flexure **M Descending Colon** **N Sigmoid Colon** Rectosigmoid junction Sigmoid flexure **P Rectum** Anorectal junction	**3 Percutaneous** **4 Percutaneous Endoscopic** **8 Via Natural or Artificial Opening Endoscopic**	**Z No Device**	**X Diagnostic**
Q Anus Anal orifice	**3 Percutaneous** **4 Percutaneous Endoscopic** **8 Via Natural or Artificial Opening Endoscopic** **X External**	**Z No Device**	**X Diagnostic**

Non-OR   ØDD[1,2,3,4,5,6,7,8,9,A,B,C,E,F,G,H,K,L,M,N,P][3,4,8]ZX
Non-OR   ØDDQ[3,4,8,X]ZX

Ø　Medical and Surgical
D　Gastrointestinal System
F　Fragmentation　　Definition: Breaking solid matter in a body part into pieces

　　　　　　　　　　　Explanation: Physical force (e.g., manual, ultrasonic) applied directly or indirectly is used to break the solid matter into pieces. The solid matter may be an abnormal byproduct of a biological function or a foreign body. The pieces of solid matter are not taken out.

Body Part Character 4	Approach Character 5	Device Character 6	Qualifier Character 7
5　Esophagus　　NC	Ø　Open	Z　No Device	Z　No Qualifier
6　Stomach　　NC	3　Percutaneous		
8　Small Intestine　　NC	4　Percutaneous Endoscopic		
9　Duodenum　　NC	7　Via Natural or Artificial Opening		
A　Jejunum　　NC 　　Duodenojejunal flexure	8　Via Natural or Artificial Opening 　　Endoscopic		
B　Ileum　　NC	X　External		
E　Large Intestine　　NC			
F　Large Intestine, Right　　NC			
G　Large Intestine, Left　　NC			
H　Cecum　　NC			
J　Appendix　　NC 　　Vermiform appendix			
K　Ascending Colon　　NC			
L　Transverse Colon　　NC 　　Hepatic flexure 　　Splenic flexure			
M　Descending Colon　　NC			
N　Sigmoid Colon　　NC 　　Rectosigmoid junction 　　Sigmoid flexure			
P　Rectum　　NC 　　Anorectal junction			
Q　Anus　　NC 　　Anal orifice			

Non-OR　　ØDF[5,6,8,9,A,B,E,F,G,H,J,K,L,M,N,P,Q]XZZ
NC　　　　ØDF[5,6,8,9,A,B,E,F,G,H,J,K,L,M,N,P,Q]XZZ

LC Limited Coverage　NC Noncovered　⊞ Combination Member　HAC associated procedure　Combination Only　DRG Non-OR　Non-OR　New/Revised in GREEN

382　　　　　　　　　　　　　　　　　　　　　　　　　　　　　　　　　　　　　　　ICD-10-PCS 2021

Ø   Medical and Surgical
D   Gastrointestinal System
H   Insertion   Definition: Putting in a nonbiological appliance that monitors, assists, performs, or prevents a physiological function but does not physically take the place of a body part
                  Explanation: None

Body Part Character 4	Approach Character 5	Device Character 6	Qualifier Character 7
Ø Upper Intestinal Tract D Lower Intestinal Tract	Ø Open 3 Percutaneous 4 Percutaneous Endoscopic 7 Via Natural or Artificial Opening 8 Via Natural or Artificial Opening Endoscopic	Y Other Device	Z No Qualifier
5 Esophagus	Ø Open 3 Percutaneous 4 Percutaneous Endoscopic	1 Radioactive Element 2 Monitoring Device 3 Infusion Device D Intraluminal Device U Feeding Device Y Other Device	Z No Qualifier
5 Esophagus	7 Via Natural or Artificial Opening 8 Via Natural or Artificial Opening Endoscopic	1 Radioactive Element 2 Monitoring Device 3 Infusion Device B Intraluminal Device, Airway D Intraluminal Device U Feeding Device Y Other Device	Z No Qualifier
6 Stomach ⊞	Ø Open 3 Percutaneous 4 Percutaneous Endoscopic	1 Radioactive Element 2 Monitoring Device 3 Infusion Device D Intraluminal Device M Stimulator Lead U Feeding Device Y Other Device	Z No Qualifier
6 Stomach	7 Via Natural or Artificial Opening 8 Via Natural or Artificial Opening Endoscopic	1 Radioactive Element 2 Monitoring Device 3 Infusion Device D Intraluminal Device U Feeding Device Y Other Device	Z No Qualifier
8 Small Intestine 9 Duodenum A Jejunum Duodenojejunal flexure B Ileum	Ø Open 3 Percutaneous 4 Percutaneous Endoscopic 7 Via Natural or Artificial Opening 8 Via Natural or Artificial Opening Endoscopic	1 Radioactive Element 2 Monitoring Device 3 Infusion Device D Intraluminal Device U Feeding Device	Z No Qualifier
E Large Intestine P Rectum Anorectal junction	Ø Open 3 Percutaneous 4 Percutaneous Endoscopic 7 Via Natural or Artificial Opening 8 Via Natural or Artificial Opening Endoscopic	1 Radioactive Element D Intraluminal Device	Z No Qualifier
Q Anus Anal orifice	Ø Open 3 Percutaneous 4 Percutaneous Endoscopic	D Intraluminal Device L Artificial Sphincter	Z No Qualifier
Q Anus Anal orifice	7 Via Natural or Artificial Opening 8 Via Natural or Artificial Opening Endoscopic	D Intraluminal Device	Z No Qualifier

R   Anal Sphincter
     External anal sphincter
     Internal anal sphincter
	Ø Open
	3 Percutaneous
	4 Percutaneous Endoscopic
		M Stimulator Lead	Z No Qualifier

Non-OR ØDH[Ø,D][Ø,3,4,7,8]YZ	**See Appendix L for Procedure Combinations**
Non-OR ØDH5[Ø,3,4][D,U]Z	⊞ ØDH6[Ø,3,4]MZ
Non-OR ØDH5[3,4]YZ	
Non-OR ØDH5[7,8][2,3,B,D,U,Y]Z	
Non-OR ØDH6[3,4][U,Y]Z	
Non-OR ØDH6[7,8][2,3,D,U,Y]Z	
Non-OR ØDH[8,9,A,B][Ø,3,4][D,U]Z	
Non-OR ØDH[8,9,A,B][7,8][2,3,D,U]Z	
Non-OR ØDH[E,P][Ø,3,4,7,8]DZ	

LC Limited Coverage   **NC** Noncovered   ⊞ Combination Member   HAC associated procedure   Combination Only   DRG Non-OR   Non-OR   New/Revised in GREEN

ICD-10-PCS 2021   **383**

Ø Medical and Surgical
D Gastrointestinal System
J Inspection   Definition: Visually and/or manually exploring a body part

Explanation: Visual exploration may be performed with or without optical instrumentation. Manual exploration may be performed directly or through intervening body layers.

Body Part Character 4	Approach Character 5	Device Character 6	Qualifier Character 7
Ø Upper Intestinal Tract 6 Stomach D Lower Intestinal Tract	Ø Open 3 Percutaneous 4 Percutaneous Endoscopic 7 Via Natural or Artificial Opening 8 Via Natural or Artificial Opening Endoscopic X External	Z No Device	Z No Qualifier

U Omentum
  Gastrocolic ligament
  Gastrocolic omentum
  Gastrohepatic omentum
  Gastrophrenic ligament
  Gastrosplenic ligament
  Greater Omentum
  Hepatogastric ligament
  Lesser Omentum
V Mesentery
  Mesoappendix
  Mesocolon
W Peritoneum
  Epiploic foramen
	Ø Open
	3 Percutaneous
	4 Percutaneous Endoscopic
	X External
		Z No Device	Z No Qualifier

Non-OR	ØDJ[Ø,6,D][3,7,8,X]ZZ
Non-OR	ØDJ[U,V,W][3,X]ZZ

Ø **Medical and Surgical**
D **Gastrointestinal System**
L **Occlusion**   Definition: Completely closing an orifice or the lumen of a tubular body part
                      Explanation: The orifice can be a natural orifice or an artificially created orifice

Body Part Character 4		Approach Character 5	Device Character 6	Qualifier Character 7
1 **Esophagus, Upper** Cervical esophagus **2** **Esophagus, Middle** Thoracic esophagus **3** **Esophagus, Lower** Abdominal esophagus **4** **Esophagogastric Junction** Cardia Cardioesophageal junction Gastroesophageal (GE) junction **5** **Esophagus** **6** Stomach **7** **Stomach, Pylorus** Pyloric antrum Pyloric canal Pyloric sphincter **8** **Small Intestine**	**9** Duodenum **A** Jejunum Duodenojejunal flexure **B** Ileum **C** Ileocecal Valve **E** Large Intestine **F** Large Intestine, Right **G** Large Intestine, Left **H** Cecum **K** Ascending Colon **L** Transverse Colon Hepatic flexure Splenic flexure **M** Descending Colon **N** Sigmoid Colon Rectosigmoid junction Sigmoid flexure **P** Rectum Anorectal junction	**Ø** Open **3** Percutaneous **4** Percutaneous Endoscopic	**C** Extraluminal Device **D** Intraluminal Device **Z** No Device	**Z** No Qualifier
1 **Esophagus, Upper** Cervical esophagus **2** **Esophagus, Middle** Thoracic esophagus **3** **Esophagus, Lower** Abdominal esophagus **4** **Esophagogastric Junction** Cardia Cardioesophageal junction Gastroesophageal (GE) junction **5** **Esophagus** **6** Stomach **7** **Stomach, Pylorus** Pyloric antrum Pyloric canal Pyloric sphincter **8** **Small Intestine**	**9** Duodenum **A** Jejunum Duodenojejunal flexure **B** Ileum **C** Ileocecal Valve **E** Large Intestine **F** Large Intestine, Right **G** Large Intestine, Left **H** Cecum **K** Ascending Colon **L** Transverse Colon Hepatic flexure Splenic flexure **M** Descending Colon **N** Sigmoid Colon Rectosigmoid junction Sigmoid flexure **P** Rectum Anorectal junction	**7** Via Natural or Artificial Opening **8** Via Natural or Artificial Opening Endoscopic	**D** Intraluminal Device **Z** No Device	**Z** No Qualifier
Q Anus Anal orifice		**Ø** Open **3** Percutaneous **4** Percutaneous Endoscopic **X** External	**C** Extraluminal Device **D** Intraluminal Device **Z** No Device	**Z** No Qualifier
Q Anus Anal orifice		**7** Via Natural or Artificial Opening **8** Via Natural or Artificial Opening Endoscopic	**D** Intraluminal Device **Z** No Device	**Z** No Qualifier

Non-OR ØDL[1,2,3,4,5][Ø,3,4][C,D,Z]Z
Non-OR ØDL[1,2,3,4,5][7,8][D,Z]Z

Gastrointestinal System

Ø   Medical and Surgical
D   Gastrointestinal System
M   Reattachment   Definition: Putting back in or on all or a portion of a separated body part to its normal location or other suitable location
                 Explanation: Vascular circulation and nervous pathways may or may not be reestablished

Body Part Character 4	Approach Character 5	Device Character 6	Qualifier Character 7

5   Esophagus
6   Stomach
8   Small Intestine
9   Duodenum
A   Jejunum
     Duodenojejunal flexure
B   Ileum
E   Large Intestine
F   Large Intestine, Right
G   Large Intestine, Left
H   Cecum
K   Ascending Colon
L   Transverse Colon
     Hepatic flexure
     Splenic flexure
M   Descending Colon
N   Sigmoid Colon
     Rectosigmoid junction
     Sigmoid flexure
P   Rectum
     Anorectal junction
	Ø Open
	4 Percutaneous Endoscopic
		Z No Device	Z No Qualifier

Ø   Medical and Surgical
D   Gastrointestinal System
N   Release   Definition: Freeing a body part from an abnormal physical constraint by cutting or by the use of force
                 Explanation: Some of the restraining tissue may be taken out but none of the body part is taken out

Body Part Character 4	Approach Character 5	Device Character 6	Qualifier Character 7

1   Esophagus, Upper
     Cervical esophagus
2   Esophagus, Middle
     Thoracic esophagus
3   Esophagus, Lower
     Abdominal esophagus
4   Esophagogastric
     Junction
     Cardia
     Cardioesophageal
     junction
     Gastroesophageal (GE)
     junction
5   Esophagus
6   Stomach
7   Stomach, Pylorus
     Pyloric antrum
     Pyloric canal
     Pyloric sphincter
8   Small Intestine
9   Duodenum
 	
A   Jejunum
     Duodenojejunal flexure
B   Ileum
C   Ileocecal Valve
E   Large Intestine
F   Large Intestine, Right
G   Large Intestine, Left
H   Cecum
J   Appendix
     Vermiform appendix
K   Ascending Colon
L   Transverse Colon
     Hepatic flexure
     Splenic flexure
M   Descending Colon
N   Sigmoid Colon
     Rectosigmoid junction
     Sigmoid flexure
P   Rectum
     Anorectal junction
	Ø Open
	3 Percutaneous
	4 Percutaneous Endoscopic
	7 Via Natural or Artificial
	     Opening
	8 Via Natural or Artificial
	     Opening Endoscopic
		Z No Device	Z No Qualifier

Q   Anus
     Anal orifice
	Ø Open
	3 Percutaneous
	4 Percutaneous Endoscopic
	7 Via Natural or Artificial
	     Opening
	8 Via Natural or Artificial
	     Opening Endoscopic
	X External
		Z No Device	Z No Qualifier

R   Anal Sphincter
     External anal sphincter
     Internal anal sphincter
U   Omentum
     Gastrocolic ligament
     Gastrocolic omentum
     Gastrohepatic omentum
     Gastrophrenic ligament
     Gastrosplenic ligament
     Greater Omentum
     Hepatogastric ligament
     Lesser Omentum
V   Mesentery
     Mesoappendix
     Mesocolon
W   Peritoneum
     Epiploic foramen
	Ø Open
	3 Percutaneous
	4 Percutaneous Endoscopic
		Z No Device	Z No Qualifier

Non-OR   ØDN[8,9,A,B,E,F,G,H,K,L,M,N][7,8]ZZ

LC Limited Coverage   NC Noncovered   ⊞ Combination Member   HAC associated procedure   Combination Only   DRG Non-OR   Non-OR   New/Revised in GREEN

386   ICD-10-PCS 2021

Ø   Medical and Surgical
D   Gastrointestinal System
P   Removal   Definition: Taking out or off a device from a body part

Explanation: If a device is taken out and a similar device put in without cutting or puncturing the skin or mucous membrane, the procedure is coded to the root operation CHANGE. Otherwise, the procedure for taking out a device is coded to the root operation REMOVAL.

Body Part Character 4	Approach Character 5	Device Character 6	Qualifier Character 7
Ø Upper Intestinal Tract D Lower Intestinal Tract	Ø Open 3 Percutaneous 4 Percutaneous Endoscopic 7 Via Natural or Artificial Opening 8 Via Natural or Artificial Opening Endoscopic	Ø Drainage Device 2 Monitoring Device 3 Infusion Device 7 Autologous Tissue Substitute C Extraluminal Device D Intraluminal Device J Synthetic Substitute K Nonautologous Tissue Substitute U Feeding Device Y Other Device	Z No Qualifier
Ø Upper Intestinal Tract D Lower Intestinal Tract	X External	Ø Drainage Device 2 Monitoring Device 3 Infusion Device D Intraluminal Device U Feeding Device	Z No Qualifier
5 Esophagus	Ø Open 3 Percutaneous 4 Percutaneous Endoscopic	1 Radioactive Element 2 Monitoring Device 3 Infusion Device U Feeding Device Y Other Device	Z No Qualifier
5 Esophagus	7 Via Natural or Artificial Opening 8 Via Natural or Artificial Opening Endoscopic	1 Radioactive Element D Intraluminal Device Y Other Device	Z No Qualifier
5 Esophagus	X External	1 Radioactive Element 2 Monitoring Device 3 Infusion Device D Intraluminal Device U Feeding Device	Z No Qualifier
6 Stomach	Ø Open 3 Percutaneous 4 Percutaneous Endoscopic	Ø Drainage Device 2 Monitoring Device 3 Infusion Device 7 Autologous Tissue Substitute C Extraluminal Device D Intraluminal Device J Synthetic Substitute K Nonautologous Tissue Substitute M Stimulator Lead U Feeding Device Y Other Device	Z No Qualifier
6 Stomach	7 Via Natural or Artificial Opening 8 Via Natural or Artificial Opening Endoscopic	Ø Drainage Device 2 Monitoring Device 3 Infusion Device 7 Autologous Tissue Substitute C Extraluminal Device D Intraluminal Device J Synthetic Substitute K Nonautologous Tissue Substitute U Feeding Device Y Other Device	Z No Qualifier
6 Stomach	X External	Ø Drainage Device 2 Monitoring Device 3 Infusion Device D Intraluminal Device U Feeding Device	Z No Qualifier

Non-OR   ØDP[Ø,D][3,4]YZ
Non-OR   ØDP[Ø,D][7,8][Ø,2,3,D,U,Y]Z
Non-OR   ØDP[Ø,D]X[Ø,2,3,D,U]Z
Non-OR   ØDP5[3,4]YZ
Non-OR   ØDP5[7,8][1,D,Y]Z
Non-OR   ØDP5X[1,2,3,D,U]Z
Non-OR   ØDP6[3,4]YZ
Non-OR   ØDP6[7,8][Ø,2,3,D,U,Y]Z
Non-OR   ØDP6X[Ø,2,3,D,U]Z

ØDP Continued on next page

LC Limited Coverage   NC Noncovered   ⊞ Combination Member   HAC associated procedure   Combination Only   DRG Non-OR   Non-OR   New/Revised in GREEN

Ø **Medical and Surgical**
D **Gastrointestinal System**
P **Removal**   Definition: Taking out or off a device from a body part

Explanation: If a device is taken out and a similar device put in without cutting or puncturing the skin or mucous membrane, the procedure is coded to the root operation CHANGE. Otherwise, the procedure for taking out a device is coded to the root operation REMOVAL.

Body Part Character 4	Approach Character 5	Device Character 6	Qualifier Character 7
P Rectum Anorectal junction	**Ø** Open **3** Percutaneous **4** Percutaneous Endoscopic **7** Via Natural or Artificial Opening **8** Via Natural or Artificial Opening Endoscopic **X** External	**1** Radioactive Element	**Z** No Qualifier
Q Anus Anal orifice	**Ø** Open **3** Percutaneous **4** Percutaneous Endoscopic **7** Via Natural or Artificial Opening **8** Via Natural or Artificial Opening Endoscopic	**L** Artificial Sphincter	**Z** No Qualifier
R Anal Sphincter External anal sphincter Internal anal sphincter	**Ø** Open **3** Percutaneous **4** Percutaneous Endoscopic	**M** Stimulator Lead	**Z** No Qualifier
U Omentum Gastrocolic ligament Gastrocolic omentum Gastrohepatic omentum Gastrophrenic ligament Gastrosplenic ligament Greater Omentum Hepatogastric ligament Lesser Omentum **V** Mesentery Mesoappendix Mesocolon **W** Peritoneum Epiploic foramen	**Ø** Open **3** Percutaneous **4** Percutaneous Endoscopic	**Ø** Drainage Device **1** Radioactive Element **7** Autologous Tissue Substitute **J** Synthetic Substitute **K** Nonautologous Tissue Substitute	**Z** No Qualifier

Non-OR   ØDPP[7,8,X]1Z

Gastrointestinal System

Ø   Medical and Surgical
D   Gastrointestinal System
Q   Repair   Definition: Restoring, to the extent possible, a body part to its normal anatomic structure and function
                     Explanation: Used only when the method to accomplish the repair is not one of the other root operations

Body Part Character 4	Approach Character 5	Device Character 6	Qualifier Character 7

1 Esophagus, Upper
   Cervical esophagus
2 Esophagus, Middle
   Thoracic esophagus
3 Esophagus, Lower
   Abdominal esophagus
4 Esophagogastric Junction
   Cardia
   Cardioesophageal junction
   Gastroesophageal (GE) junction
5 Esophagus
6 Stomach
7 Stomach, Pylorus
   Pyloric antrum
   Pyloric canal
   Pyloric sphincter
8 Small Intestine ⊞
9 Duodenum ⊞
A Jejunum ⊞
   Duodenojejunal flexure
B Ileum ⊞
C Ileocecal Valve
E Large Intestine ⊞
F Large Intestine, Right ⊞
G Large Intestine, Left ⊞
H Cecum ⊞
J Appendix
   Vermiform appendix
K Ascending Colon ⊞
L Transverse Colon ⊞
   Hepatic flexure
   Splenic flexure
M Descending Colon ⊞
N Sigmoid Colon ⊞
   Rectosigmoid junction
   Sigmoid flexure
P Rectum
   Anorectal junction
	Ø Open
	3 Percutaneous
	4 Percutaneous Endoscopic
	7 Via Natural or Artificial Opening
	8 Via Natural or Artificial Opening
	   Endoscopic
		Z No Device	Z No Qualifier

Q Anus
   Anal orifice
	Ø Open
	3 Percutaneous
	4 Percutaneous Endoscopic
	7 Via Natural or Artificial Opening
	8 Via Natural or Artificial Opening
	   Endoscopic
	X External
		Z No Device	Z No Qualifier

R Anal Sphincter
   External anal sphincter
   Internal anal sphincter
U Omentum
   Gastrocolic ligament
   Gastrocolic omentum
   Gastrohepatic omentum
   Gastrophrenic ligament
   Gastrosplenic ligament
   Greater Omentum
   Hepatogastric ligament
   Lesser Omentum
V Mesentery
   Mesoappendix
   Mesocolon
W Peritoneum
   Epiploic foramen
	Ø Open
	3 Percutaneous
	4 Percutaneous Endoscopic
		Z No Device	Z No Qualifier

Non-OR   ØDQU[Ø,3,4]ZZ

See Appendix L for Procedure Combinations
    ⊞   ØDQ[8,9,A,B,E,F,G,H,K,L,M,N]ØZZ

Ø   Medical and Surgical
D   Gastrointestinal System
R   Replacement   Definition: Putting in or on biological or synthetic material that physically takes the place and/or function of all or a portion of a body part

Explanation: The body part may have been taken out or replaced, or may be taken out, physically eradicated, or rendered nonfunctional during the REPLACEMENT procedure. A REMOVAL procedure is coded for taking out the device used in a previous replacement procedure.

Body Part Character 4	Approach Character 5	Device Character 6	Qualifier Character 7
5 Esophagus	Ø Open 4 Percutaneous Endoscopic 7 Via Natural or Artificial Opening 8 Via Natural or Artificial Opening Endoscopic	7 Autologous Tissue Substitute J Synthetic Substitute K Nonautologous Tissue Substitute	Z No Qualifier

R   Anal Sphincter
    External anal sphincter
    Internal anal sphincter
U   Omentum
    Gastrocolic ligament
    Gastrocolic omentum
    Gastrohepatic omentum
    Gastrophrenic ligament
    Gastrosplenic ligament
    Greater Omentum
    Hepatogastric ligament
    Lesser Omentum
V   Mesentery
    Mesoappendix
    Mesocolon
W   Peritoneum
    Epiploic foramen
	Ø Open
	4 Percutaneous Endoscopic
		7 Autologous Tissue Substitute
		J Synthetic Substitute
		K Nonautologous Tissue Substitute
			Z No Qualifier

Ø   Medical and Surgical
D   Gastrointestinal System
S   Reposition   Definition: Moving to its normal location, or other suitable location, all or a portion of a body part

Explanation: The body part is moved to a new location from an abnormal location, or from a normal location where it is not functioning correctly. The body part may or may not be cut out or off to be moved to the new location.

Body Part Character 4	Approach Character 5	Device Character 6	Qualifier Character 7

5   Esophagus
6   Stomach
9   Duodenum
A   Jejunum
    Duodenojejunal flexure
B   Ileum
H   Cecum
K   Ascending Colon
L   Transverse Colon
    Hepatic flexure
    Splenic flexure
M   Descending Colon
N   Sigmoid Colon
    Rectosigmoid junction
    Sigmoid flexure
P   Rectum
    Anorectal junction
Q   Anus
    Anal orifice
	Ø Open
	4 Percutaneous Endoscopic
	7 Via Natural or Artificial Opening
	8 Via Natural or Artificial Opening Endoscopic
	X External
		Z No Device	Z No Qualifier

8 Small Intestine E Large Intestine	Ø Open 4 Percutaneous Endoscopic 7 Via Natural or Artificial Opening 8 Via Natural or Artificial Opening Endoscopic	Z No Device	Z No Qualifier

Non-OR   ØDS[5,6,9,A,B,H,K,L,M,N,P,Q]XZZ

Ø **Medical and Surgical**
D **Gastrointestinal System**
T **Resection** 　　　Definition: Cutting out or off, without replacement, all of a body part
　　　　　　　　　　　Explanation: None

Body Part Character 4	Approach Character 5	Device Character 6	Qualifier Character 7
1 Esophagus, Upper 　Cervical esophagus **2 Esophagus, Middle** 　Thoracic esophagus **3 Esophagus, Lower** 　Abdominal esophagus **4 Esophagogastric Junction** 　Cardia 　Cardioesophageal junction 　Gastroesophageal (GE) junction **5 Esophagus** **6 Stomach** **7 Stomach, Pylorus** 　Pyloric antrum 　Pyloric canal 　Pyloric sphincter **8 Small Intestine** **9 Duodenum** ⊞ **A Jejunum** 　Duodenojejunal flexure **B Ileum** **C Ileocecal Valve** **E Large Intestine** **F Large Intestine, Right** **H Cecum** **J Appendix** 　Vermiform appendix **K Ascending Colon** **P Rectum** 　Anorectal junction **Q Anus** 　Anal orifice	**Ø Open** **4 Percutaneous Endoscopic** **7 Via Natural or Artificial Opening** **8 Via Natural or Artificial Opening Endoscopic**	**Z No Device**	**Z No Qualifier**
G Large Intestine, Left **L Transverse Colon** 　Hepatic flexure 　Splenic flexure **M Descending Colon** **N Sigmoid Colon** 　Rectosigmoid junction 　Sigmoid flexure	**Ø Open** **4 Percutaneous Endoscopic** **7 Via Natural or Artificial Opening** **8 Via Natural or Artificial Opening Endoscopic** **F Via Natural or Artificial Opening with Percutaneous Endoscopic Assistance**	**Z No Device**	**Z No Qualifier**
R Anal Sphincter 　External anal sphincter 　Internal anal sphincter **U Omentum** 　Gastrocolic ligament 　Gastrocolic omentum 　Gastrohepatic omentum 　Gastrophrenic ligament 　Gastrosplenic ligament 　Greater Omentum 　Hepatogastric ligament 　Lesser Omentum	**Ø Open** **4 Percutaneous Endoscopic**	**Z No Device**	**Z No Qualifier**

See Appendix L for Procedure Combinations
　⊞　　ØDT9ØZZ

LC Limited Coverage　NC Noncovered　⊞ Combination Member　HAC associated procedure　Combination Only　DRG Non-OR　Non-OR　New/Revised in GREEN

ICD-10-PCS 2021　　　　　　　　　　　　　　　　　　　　　　　　　　　　　　　391

Gastrointestinal System

Ø   Medical and Surgical
D   Gastrointestinal System
U   Supplement   Definition: Putting in or on biological or synthetic material that physically reinforces and/or augments the function of a portion of a body part

Explanation: The biological material is non-living, or is living and from the same individual. The body part may have been previously replaced, and the SUPPLEMENT procedure is performed to physically reinforce and/or augment the function of the replaced body part.

Body Part Character 4	Approach Character 5	Device Character 6	Qualifier Character 7

1   **Esophagus, Upper**
    Cervical esophagus
2   **Esophagus, Middle**
    Thoracic esophagus
3   **Esophagus, Lower**
    Abdominal esophagus
4   **Esophagogastric Junction**
    Cardia
    Cardioesophageal junction
    Gastroesophageal (GE) junction
5   **Esophagus**
6   **Stomach**
7   **Stomach, Pylorus**
    Pyloric antrum
    Pyloric canal
    Pyloric sphincter
8   **Small Intestine**
9   **Duodenum**
A   **Jejunum**
    Duodenojejunal flexure
B   **Ileum**
C   **Ileocecal Valve**
E   **Large Intestine**
F   **Large Intestine, Right**
G   **Large Intestine, Left**
H   **Cecum**
K   **Ascending Colon**
L   **Transverse Colon**
    Hepatic flexure
    Splenic flexure
M   **Descending Colon**
N   **Sigmoid Colon**
    Rectosigmoid junction
    Sigmoid flexure
P   **Rectum**
    Anorectal junction
	Ø **Open**
	4 **Percutaneous Endoscopic**
	7 **Via Natural or Artificial Opening**
	8 **Via Natural or Artificial Opening
	    Endoscopic**
		7 **Autologous Tissue Substitute**
		J **Synthetic Substitute**
		K **Nonautologous Tissue Substitute**
			Z **No Qualifier**

Q   **Anus**
    Anal orifice
	Ø **Open**
	4 **Percutaneous Endoscopic**
	7 **Via Natural or Artificial Opening**
	8 **Via Natural or Artificial Opening
	    Endoscopic**
	X **External**
		7 **Autologous Tissue Substitute**
		J **Synthetic Substitute**
		K **Nonautologous Tissue Substitute**
			Z **No Qualifier**

R   **Anal Sphincter**
    External anal sphincter
    Internal anal sphincter
U   **Omentum**
    Gastrocolic ligament
    Gastrocolic omentum
    Gastrohepatic omentum
    Gastrophrenic ligament
    Gastrosplenic ligament
    Greater Omentum
    Hepatogastric ligament
    Lesser Omentum
V   **Mesentery**
    Mesoappendix
    Mesocolon
W   **Peritoneum**
    Epiploic foramen
	Ø **Open**
	4 **Percutaneous Endoscopic**
		7 **Autologous Tissue Substitute**
		J **Synthetic Substitute**
		K **Nonautologous Tissue Substitute**
			Z **No Qualifier**

LC Limited Coverage   NC Noncovered   ⊞ Combination Member   HAC associated procedure   Combination Only   DRG Non-OR   Non-OR   New/Revised in GREEN

392   ICD-10-PCS 2021

Ø Medical and Surgical
D Gastrointestinal System
V Restriction   Definition: Partially closing an orifice or the lumen of a tubular body part
                Explanation: The orifice can be a natural orifice or an artificially created orifice

Body Part Character 4		Approach Character 5	Device Character 6	Qualifier Character 7

1 Esophagus, Upper
  Cervical esophagus
2 Esophagus, Middle
  Thoracic esophagus
3 Esophagus, Lower
  Abdominal esophagus
4 Esophagogastric
  Junction
  Cardia
  Cardioesophageal
    junction
  Gastroesophageal (GE)
    junction
5 Esophagus
6 Stomach
7 Stomach, Pylorus
  Pyloric antrum
  Pyloric canal
  Pyloric sphincter
8 Small Intestine
	9 Duodenum
	A Jejunum
	  Duodenojejunal flexure
	B Ileum
	C Ileocecal Valve
	E Large Intestine
	F Large Intestine, Right
	G Large Intestine, Left
	H Cecum
	K Ascending Colon
	L Transverse Colon
	  Hepatic flexure
	  Splenic flexure
	M Descending Colon
	N Sigmoid Colon
	  Rectosigmoid junction
	  Sigmoid flexure
	P Rectum
	  Anorectal junction
		Ø Open
		3 Percutaneous
		4 Percutaneous Endoscopic
			C Extraluminal Device
			D Intraluminal Device
			Z No Device
				Z No Qualifier

1 Esophagus, Upper
  Cervical esophagus
2 Esophagus, Middle
  Thoracic esophagus
3 Esophagus, Lower
  Abdominal esophagus
4 Esophagogastric
  Junction
  Cardia
  Cardioesophageal
    junction
  Gastroesophageal (GE)
    junction
5 Esophagus
6 Stomach NC
7 Stomach, Pylorus
  Pyloric antrum
  Pyloric canal
  Pyloric sphincter
8 Small Intestine
	9 Duodenum
	A Jejunum
	  Duodenojejunal flexure
	B Ileum
	C Ileocecal Valve
	E Large Intestine
	F Large Intestine, Right
	G Large Intestine, Left
	H Cecum
	K Ascending Colon
	L Transverse Colon
	  Hepatic flexure
	  Splenic flexure
	M Descending Colon
	N Sigmoid Colon
	  Rectosigmoid junction
	  Sigmoid flexure
	P Rectum
	  Anorectal junction
		7 Via Natural or Artificial
		  Opening
		8 Via Natural or Artificial
		  Opening Endoscopic
			D Intraluminal Device
			Z No Device
				Z No Qualifier

Q Anus Anal orifice		Ø Open 3 Percutaneous 4 Percutaneous Endoscopic X External	C Extraluminal Device D Intraluminal Device Z No Device	Z No Qualifier

Q Anus
  Anal orifice
		7 Via Natural or Artificial
		  Opening
		8 Via Natural or Artificial
		  Opening Endoscopic
			D Intraluminal Device
			Z No Device
				Z No Qualifier

Non-OR   ØDV6[7,8]DZ
HAC   ØDV64CZ when reported with PDx E66.Ø1 and SDx K68.11, K95.Ø1, K95.81, or T81.4Ø–T81.49 with 7th character A
NC   ØDV6[7,8]DZ

LC Limited Coverage   NC Noncovered   ⊞ Combination Member   HAC associated procedure   Combination Only   DRG Non-OR   Non-OR   New/Revised in GREEN
ICD-10-PCS 2021   393

ØDV–ØDV

Gastrointestinal System

Ø   **Medical and Surgical**
D   **Gastrointestinal System**
W   **Revision**   Definition: Correcting, to the extent possible, a portion of a malfunctioning device or the position of a displaced device

                  Explanation: Revision can include correcting a malfunctioning or displaced device by taking out or putting in components of the device such as a screw or pin

Body Part Character 4	Approach Character 5	Device Character 6	Qualifier Character 7
Ø Upper Intestinal Tract D Lower Intestinal Tract	Ø Open 3 Percutaneous 4 Percutaneous Endoscopic 7 Via Natural or Artificial Opening 8 Via Natural or Artificial Opening Endoscopic	Ø Drainage Device 2 Monitoring Device 3 Infusion Device 7 Autologous Tissue Substitute C Extraluminal Device D Intraluminal Device J Synthetic Substitute K Nonautologous Tissue Substitute U Feeding Device Y Other Device	Z No Qualifier
Ø Upper Intestinal Tract D Lower Intestinal Tract	X External	Ø Drainage Device 2 Monitoring Device 3 Infusion Device 7 Autologous Tissue Substitute C Extraluminal Device D Intraluminal Device J Synthetic Substitute K Nonautologous Tissue Substitute U Feeding Device	Z No Qualifier
5 Esophagus	Ø Open 3 Percutaneous 4 Percutaneous Endoscopic	Y Other Device	Z No Qualifier
5 Esophagus	7 Via Natural or Artificial Opening 8 Via Natural or Artificial Opening Endoscopic	D Intraluminal Device Y Other Device	Z No Qualifier
5 Esophagus	X External	D Intraluminal Device	Z No Qualifier
6 Stomach	Ø Open 3 Percutaneous 4 Percutaneous Endoscopic	Ø Drainage Device 2 Monitoring Device 3 Infusion Device 7 Autologous Tissue Substitute C Extraluminal Device D Intraluminal Device J Synthetic Substitute K Nonautologous Tissue Substitute M Stimulator Lead U Feeding Device Y Other Device	Z No Qualifier
6 Stomach	7 Via Natural or Artificial Opening 8 Via Natural or Artificial Opening Endoscopic	Ø Drainage Device 2 Monitoring Device 3 Infusion Device 7 Autologous Tissue Substitute C Extraluminal Device D Intraluminal Device J Synthetic Substitute K Nonautologous Tissue Substitute U Feeding Device Y Other Device	Z No Qualifier
6 Stomach	X External	Ø Drainage Device 2 Monitoring Device 3 Infusion Device 7 Autologous Tissue Substitute C Extraluminal Device D Intraluminal Device J Synthetic Substitute K Nonautologous Tissue Substitute U Feeding Device	Z No Qualifier

Non-OR   ØDW[Ø,D][3,4,7,8]YZ
Non-OR   ØDW[Ø,D]8UZ
Non-OR   ØDW[Ø,D]X[Ø,2,3,7,C,D,J,K,U]Z
Non-OR   ØDW5[Ø,3,4]YZ
Non-OR   ØDW5[7,8]YZ
Non-OR   ØDW5XDZ
Non-OR   ØDW6[3,4]YZ
Non-OR   ØDW68UZ
Non-OR   ØDW6[7,8]YZ
Non-OR   ØDW6X[Ø,2,3,7,C,D,J,K,U]Z

ØDW Continued on next page

LC Limited Coverage   NC Noncovered   ⊞ Combination Member   HAC associated procedure   Combination Only   DRG Non-OR   Non-OR   New/Revised in GREEN

Ø **Medical and Surgical**
D **Gastrointestinal System**
W **Revision**

ØDW Continued

Definition: Correcting, to the extent possible, a portion of a malfunctioning device or the position of a displaced device

Explanation: Revision can include correcting a malfunctioning or displaced device by taking out or putting in components of the device such as a screw or pin

Body Part Character 4	Approach Character 5	Device Character 6	Qualifier Character 7
8 Small Intestine E Large Intestine	Ø Open 4 Percutaneous Endoscopic 7 Via Natural or Artificial Opening 8 Via Natural or Artificial Opening Endoscopic	7 Autologous Tissue Substitute J Synthetic Substitute K Nonautologous Tissue Substitute	Z No Qualifier
Q Anus Anal orifice	Ø Open 3 Percutaneous 4 Percutaneous Endoscopic 7 Via Natural or Artificial Opening 8 Via Natural or Artificial Opening Endoscopic	L Artificial Sphincter	Z No Qualifier

R Anal Sphincter
  External anal sphincter
  Internal anal sphincter
	Ø Open
	3 Percutaneous
	4 Percutaneous Endoscopic
		M Stimulator Lead	Z No Qualifier

U Omentum
  Gastrocolic ligament
  Gastrocolic omentum
  Gastrohepatic omentum
  Gastrophrenic ligament
  Gastrosplenic ligament
  Greater Omentum
  Hepatogastric ligament
  Lesser Omentum
V Mesentery
  Mesoappendix
  Mesocolon
W Peritoneum
  Epiploic foramen
	Ø Open
	3 Percutaneous
	4 Percutaneous Endoscopic
		Ø Drainage Device
		7 Autologous Tissue Substitute
		J Synthetic Substitute
		K Nonautologous Tissue Substitute
			Z No Qualifier

Non-OR   ØDW[U,V,W][Ø,3,4]ØZ

Ø **Medical and Surgical**
D **Gastrointestinal System**
X **Transfer**

Definition: Moving, without taking out, all or a portion of a body part to another location to take over the function of all or a portion of a body part

Explanation: The body part transferred remains connected to its vascular and nervous supply

Body Part Character 4	Approach Character 5	Device Character 6	Qualifier Character 7
6 Stomach 8 Small Intestine	Ø Open 4 Percutaneous Endoscopic	Z No Device	5 Esophagus
E Large Intestine	Ø Open 4 Percutaneous Endoscopic	Z No Device	5 Esophagus 7 Vagina ♀

♀   ØDXE[Ø,4]Z7

Ø **Medical and Surgical**
D **Gastrointestinal System**
Y **Transplantation**

Definition: Putting in or on all or a portion of a living body part taken from another individual or animal to physically take the place and/or function of all or a portion of a similar body part

Explanation: The native body part may or may not be taken out, and the transplanted body part may take over all or a portion of its function

Body Part Character 4	Approach Character 5	Device Character 6	Qualifier Character 7
5 Esophagus 6 Stomach 8 Small Intestine **LC** E Large Intestine **LC**	Ø Open	Z No Device	Ø Allogeneic 1 Syngeneic 2 Zooplastic

Non-OR   ØDY5ØZ[Ø,1,2]
LC   ØDY[8,E]ØZ[Ø,1,2]

LC Limited Coverage   **NC** Noncovered   ⊞ Combination Member   HAC associated procedure   Combination Only   DRG Non-OR   Non-OR   New/Revised in GREEN

ICD-10-PCS 2021   395

ØDW–ØDY

Hepatobiliary System and Pancreas ØF1–ØFY

Character Meanings

This Character Meaning table is provided as a guide to assist the user in the identification of character members that may be found in this section of code tables. It **SHOULD NOT** be used to build a PCS code.

Operation–Character 3	Body Part–Character 4	Approach–Character 5	Device–Character 6	Qualifier–Character 7
1 Bypass	Ø Liver	Ø Open	Ø Drainage Device	Ø Allogeneic
2 Change	1 Liver, Right Lobe	3 Percutaneous	1 Radioactive Element	1 Syngeneic
5 Destruction	2 Liver, Left Lobe	4 Percutaneous Endoscopic	2 Monitoring Device	2 Zooplastic
7 Dilation	4 Gallbladder	7 Via Natural or Artificial Opening	3 Infusion Device	3 Duodenum
8 Division	5 Hepatic Duct, Right	8 Via Natural or Artificial Opening Endoscopic	7 Autologous Tissue Substitute	4 Stomach
9 Drainage	6 Hepatic Duct, Left	X External	C Extraluminal Device	5 Hepatic Duct, Right
B Excision	7 Hepatic Duct, Common		D Intraluminal Device	6 Hepatic Duct, Left
C Extirpation	8 Cystic Duct		J Synthetic Substitute	7 Hepatic Duct, Caudate
D Extraction	9 Common Bile Duct		K Nonautologous Tissue Substitute	8 Cystic Duct
F Fragmentation	B Hepatobiliary Duct		Y Other Device	9 Common Bile Duct
H Insertion	C Ampulla of Vater		Z No Device	B Small Intestine
J Inspection	D Pancreatic Duct			C Large Intestine
L Occlusion	F Pancreatic Duct, Accessory			F Irreversible Electroporation
M Reattachment	G Pancreas			X Diagnostic
N Release				Z No Qualifier
P Removal				
Q Repair				
R Replacement				
S Reposition				
T Resection				
U Supplement				
V Restriction				
W Revision				
Y Transplantation				

AHA Coding Clinic for table ØF5
2018, 4Q, 39   Irreversible electroporation

AHA Coding Clinic for table ØF7
2016, 3Q, 27   Endoscopic retrograde cholangiopancreatography with sphincterotomy and insertion of pancreatic stent
2016, 1Q, 25   Endoscopic retrograde cholangiopancreatography with brush biopsy of pancreatic and common bile ducts
2015, 1Q, 32   Percutaneous transhepatic biliary drainage catheter placement
2014, 3Q, 15   Drainage of pancreatic pseudocyst

AHA Coding Clinic for table ØF9
2015, 1Q, 32   Percutaneous transhepatic biliary drainage catheter placement
2014, 3Q, 15   Drainage of pancreatic pseudocyst

AHA Coding Clinic for table ØFB
2019, 1Q, 3-8   Whipple procedure
2016, 3Q, 41   Open cholecystectomy with needle biopsy of liver
2016, 1Q, 23   Endoscopic ultrasound with aspiration biopsy of common hepatic duct
2016, 1Q, 25   Endoscopic retrograde cholangiopancreatography with brush biopsy of pancreatic and common bile ducts
2014, 3Q, 32   Pyloric-sparing Whipple procedure

AHA Coding Clinic for table ØFC
2016, 3Q, 27   Endoscopic retrograde cholangiopancreatography with sphincterotomy and insertion of pancreatic stent

AHA Coding Clinic for table ØFQ
2016, 3Q, 27   Revision of common bile duct anastomosis
2013, 4Q, 109   Separating conjoined twins

AHA Coding Clinic for table ØFT
2019, 1Q, 3-8   Whipple Procedure
2012, 4Q, 99   Domino liver transplant

AHA Coding Clinic for table ØFY
2014, 3Q, 13   Orthotopic liver transplant with end to side cavoplasty
2012, 4Q, 99   Domino liver transplant

Liver

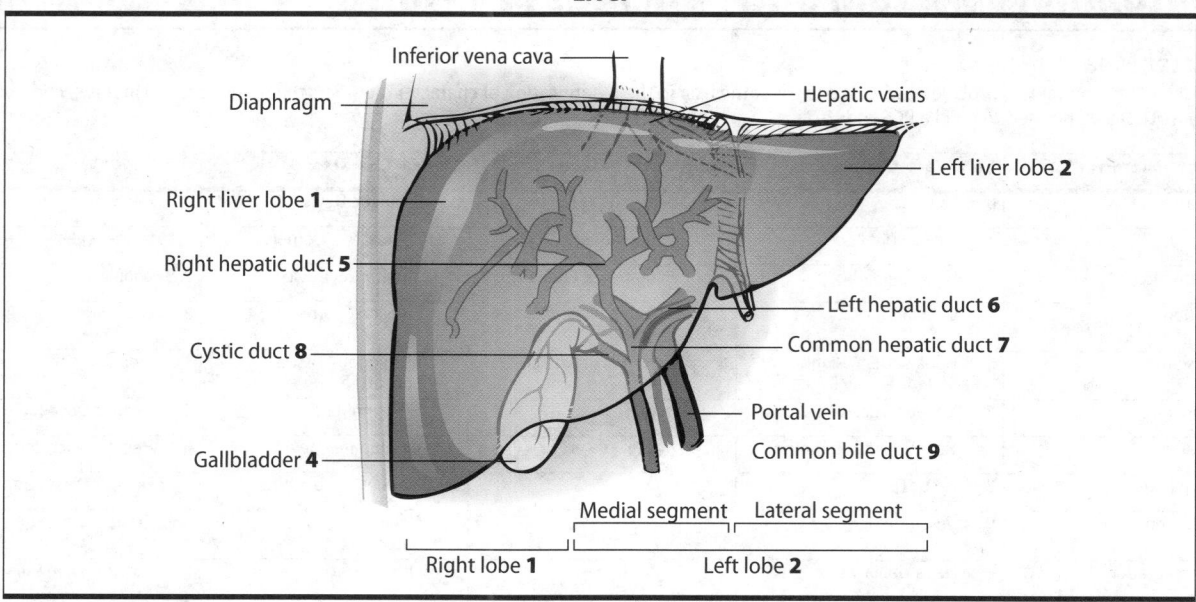

Inferior vena cava

Diaphragm

Hepatic veins

Left liver lobe **2**

Right liver lobe **1**

Right hepatic duct **5**

Left hepatic duct **6**

Common hepatic duct **7**

Cystic duct **8**

Portal vein

Gallbladder **4**

Common bile duct **9**

Medial segment | Lateral segment

Right lobe **1** | Left lobe **2**

Pancreas

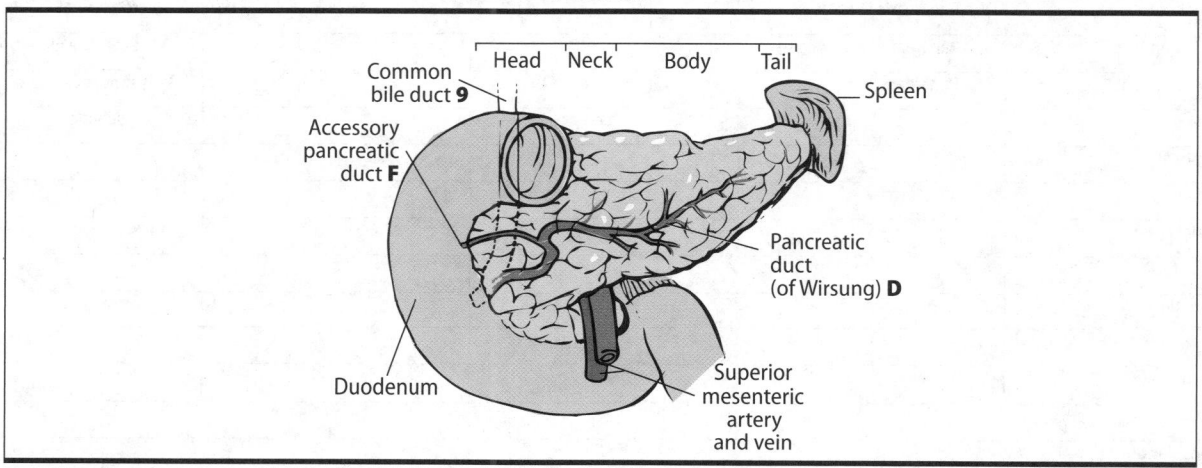

Head | Neck | Body | Tail

Common bile duct **9**

Spleen

Accessory pancreatic duct **F**

Pancreatic duct (of Wirsung) **D**

Duodenum

Superior mesenteric artery and vein

Gallbladder and Ducts

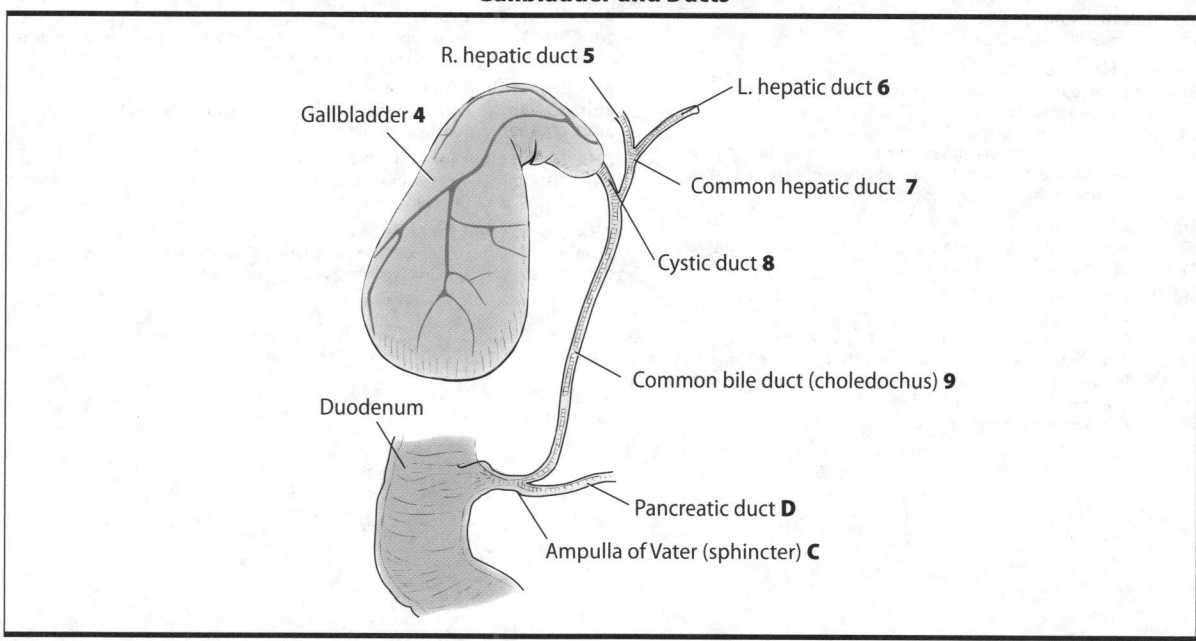

R. hepatic duct **5**

L. hepatic duct **6**

Gallbladder **4**

Common hepatic duct **7**

Cystic duct **8**

Common bile duct (choledochus) **9**

Duodenum

Pancreatic duct **D**

Ampulla of Vater (sphincter) **C**

Ø   Medical and Surgical
F   Hepatobiliary System and Pancreas
1   Bypass   Definition: Altering the route of passage of the contents of a tubular body part

Explanation: Rerouting contents of a body part to a downstream area of the normal route, to a similar route and body part, or to an abnormal route and dissimilar body part. Includes one or more anastomoses, with or without the use of a device.

Body Part Character 4	Approach Character 5	Device Character 6	Qualifier Character 7
4 Gallbladder 5 Hepatic Duct, Right 6 Hepatic Duct, Left 7 Hepatic Duct, Common 8 Cystic Duct 9 Common Bile Duct	Ø Open 4 Percutaneous Endoscopic	D Intraluminal Device Z No Device	3 Duodenum 4 Stomach 5 Hepatic Duct, Right 6 Hepatic Duct, Left 7 Hepatic Duct, Caudate 8 Cystic Duct 9 Common Bile Duct B Small Intestine
D Pancreatic Duct Duct of Wirsung	Ø Open 4 Percutaneous Endoscopic	D Intraluminal Device Z No Device	3 Duodenum 4 Stomach B Small Intestine C Large Intestine
F Pancreatic Duct, Accessory Duct of Santorini G Pancreas	Ø Open 4 Percutaneous Endoscopic	D Intraluminal Device Z No Device	3 Duodenum B Small Intestine C Large Intestine

Ø   Medical and Surgical
F   Hepatobiliary System and Pancreas
2   Change   Definition: Taking out or off a device from a body part and putting back an identical or similar device in or on the same body part without cutting or puncturing the skin or a mucous membrane

Explanation: All CHANGE procedures are coded using the approach EXTERNAL

Body Part Character 4	Approach Character 5	Device Character 6	Qualifier Character 7

Ø   Liver
     Quadrate lobe
4   Gallbladder
B   Hepatobiliary Duct
D   Pancreatic Duct
     Duct of Wirsung
G   Pancreas
	X External	Ø Drainage Device
		Y Other Device
			Z No Qualifier

Non-OR   All body part, approach, device, and qualifier values

Ø   Medical and Surgical
F   Hepatobiliary System and Pancreas
5   Destruction   Definition: Physical eradication of all or a portion of a body part by the direct use of energy, force, or a destructive agent

Explanation: None of the body part is physically taken out

Body Part Character 4	Approach Character 5	Device Character 6	Qualifier Character 7
Ø Liver Quadrate lobe 1 Liver, Right Lobe 2 Liver, Left Lobe	Ø Open 3 Percutaneous 4 Percutaneous Endoscopic	Z No Device	F Irreversible Electroporation Z No Qualifier
4 Gallbladder	Ø Open 3 Percutaneous 4 Percutaneous Endoscopic 8 Via Natural or Artificial Opening Endoscopic	Z No Device	Z No Qualifier

5   Hepatic Duct, Right
6   Hepatic Duct, Left
7   Hepatic Duct, Common
8   Cystic Duct
9   Common Bile Duct
C   Ampulla of Vater
     Duodenal ampulla
     Hepatopancreatic ampulla
D   Pancreatic Duct
     Duct of Wirsung
F   Pancreatic Duct, Accessory
     Duct of Santorini
	Ø Open
	3 Percutaneous
	4 Percutaneous Endoscopic
	7 Via Natural or Artificial Opening
	8 Via Natural or Artificial Opening Endoscopic
		Z No Device	Z No Qualifier

G Pancreas	Ø Open 3 Percutaneous 4 Percutaneous Endoscopic	Z No Device	F Irreversible Electroporation Z No Qualifier
G Pancreas	8 Via Natural or Artificial Opening Endoscopic	Z No Device	Z No Qualifier

Non-OR   ØF5[5,6,7,8,9,C,D,F][4,8]ZZ   Non-OR   ØF5G8ZZ
Non-OR   ØF5G4Z[F,Z]

LG Limited Coverage   NC Noncovered   ⊞ Combination Member   HAC associated procedure   Combination Only   DRG Non-OR   Non-OR   New/Revised in GREEN

Ø **Medical and Surgical**
F **Hepatobiliary System and Pancreas**
7 **Dilation** Definition: Expanding an orifice or the lumen of a tubular body part

Explanation: The orifice can be a natural orifice or an artificially created orifice. Accomplished by stretching a tubular body part using intraluminal pressure or by cutting part of the orifice or wall of the tubular body part.

Body Part Character 4	Approach Character 5	Device Character 6	Qualifier Character 7
5 Hepatic Duct, Right 6 Hepatic Duct, Left 7 Hepatic Duct, Common 8 Cystic Duct 9 Common Bile Duct C Ampulla of Vater 　Duodenal ampulla 　Hepatopancreatic ampulla D Pancreatic Duct 　Duct of Wirsung F Pancreatic Duct, Accessory 　Duct of Santorini	Ø Open 3 Percutaneous 4 Percutaneous Endoscopic 7 Via Natural or Artificial Opening 8 Via Natural or Artificial Opening 　Endoscopic	D Intraluminal Device Z No Device	Z No Qualifier

Non-OR　ØF7[5,6,7,8,9][3,4,8][D,Z]Z
Non-OR　ØF7[5,6,7,8,9,D]]7DZ
Non-OR　ØF7C8[D,Z]Z
Non-OR　ØF7[D,F][4,8][D,Z]Z

Ø **Medical and Surgical**
F **Hepatobiliary System and Pancreas**
8 **Division** Definition: Cutting into a body part, without draining fluids and/or gases from the body part, in order to separate or transect a body part

Explanation: All or a portion of the body part is separated into two or more portions

Body Part Character 4	Approach Character 5	Device Character 6	Qualifier Character 7
G Pancreas	Ø Open 3 Percutaneous 4 Percutaneous Endoscopic	Z No Device	Z No Qualifier

Ø Medical and Surgical
F Hepatobiliary System and Pancreas
9 Drainage　　Definition: Taking or letting out fluids and/or gases from a body part
　　　　Explanation: The qualifier DIAGNOSTIC is used to identify drainage procedures that are biopsies

Body Part Character 4	Approach Character 5	Device Character 6	Qualifier Character 7
Ø Liver 　Quadrate lobe 1 Liver, Right Lobe 2 Liver, Left Lobe	Ø Open 3 Percutaneous 4 Percutaneous Endoscopic	Ø Drainage Device	Z No Qualifier
Ø Liver 　Quadrate lobe 1 Liver, Right Lobe 2 Liver, Left Lobe	Ø Open 3 Percutaneous 4 Percutaneous Endoscopic	Z No Device	X Diagnostic Z No Qualifier
4 Gallbladder G Pancreas	Ø Open 3 Percutaneous 4 Percutaneous Endoscopic 8 Via Natural or Artificial Opening Endoscopic	Ø Drainage Device	Z No Qualifier
4 Gallbladder G Pancreas	Ø Open 3 Percutaneous 4 Percutaneous Endoscopic 8 Via Natural or Artificial Opening Endoscopic	Z No Device	X Diagnostic Z No Qualifier
5 Hepatic Duct, Right 6 Hepatic Duct, Left 7 Hepatic Duct, Common 8 Cystic Duct 9 Common Bile Duct C Ampulla of Vater 　Duodenal ampulla 　Hepatopancreatic ampulla D Pancreatic Duct 　Duct of Wirsung F Pancreatic Duct, Accessory 　Duct of Santorini	Ø Open 3 Percutaneous 4 Percutaneous Endoscopic 7 Via Natural or Artificial Opening 8 Via Natural or Artificial Opening Endoscopic	Ø Drainage Device	Z No Qualifier
5 Hepatic Duct, Right 6 Hepatic Duct, Left 7 Hepatic Duct, Common 8 Cystic Duct 9 Common Bile Duct C Ampulla of Vater 　Duodenal ampulla 　Hepatopancreatic ampulla D Pancreatic Duct 　Duct of Wirsung F Pancreatic Duct, Accessory 　Duct of Santorini	Ø Open 3 Percutaneous 4 Percutaneous Endoscopic 7 Via Natural or Artificial Opening 8 Via Natural or Artificial Opening Endoscopic	Z No Device	X Diagnostic Z No Qualifier

Non-OR ØF9[Ø,1,2][3,4]ØZ
Non-OR ØF9[Ø,1,2][3,4]Z[X,Z]
Non-OR ØF9[4,G]8ØZ
Non-OR ØF9G3ØZ
Non-OR ØF9[4,G]8Z[X,Z]
Non-OR ØF9G3Z[XZ]
Non-OR ØF9G4ZX
Non-OR ØF9[5,6,8][3,8]ØZ
Non-OR ØF97[3,4,7,8]ØZ

Non-OR ØF99[3,8]ØZ
Non-OR ØF9C[3,4,8]ØZ
Non-OR ØF9[D,F][3,8]ØZ
Non-OR ØF9[5,6,8,9,C,D,F]3Z[X,Z]
Non-OR ØF9[5,6,8,9,C,D,F][4,7,8]ZX
Non-OR ØF9[5,6,8,D,F]8ZZ
Non-OR ØF97[3,4,7,8]Z[X,Z]
Non-OR ØF99[4,7,8]ZZ
Non-OR ØF9C[4,8]ZZ

LC Limited Coverage　NC Noncovered　⊞ Combination Member　HAC associated procedure　Combination Only　DRG Non-OR　Non-OR　New/Revised in GREEN

Ø Medical and Surgical
F Hepatobiliary System and Pancreas
B Excision   Definition: Cutting out or off, without replacement, a portion of a body part
     Explanation: The qualifier DIAGNOSTIC is used to identify excision procedures that are biopsies

Body Part Character 4	Approach Character 5	Device Character 6	Qualifier Character 7
Ø Liver Quadrate lobe 1 Liver, Right Lobe 2 Liver, Left Lobe	Ø Open 3 Percutaneous 4 Percutaneous Endoscopic	Z No Device	X Diagnostic Z No Qualifier
4 Gallbladder G Pancreas	Ø Open 3 Percutaneous 4 Percutaneous Endoscopic 8 Via Natural or Artificial Opening Endoscopic	Z No Device	X Diagnostic Z No Qualifier

5 Hepatic Duct, Right
6 Hepatic Duct, Left
7 Hepatic Duct, Common
8 Cystic Duct
9 Common Bile Duct
C Ampulla of Vater
   Duodenal ampulla
   Hepatopancreatic ampulla
D Pancreatic Duct
   Duct of Wirsung
F Pancreatic Duct, Accessory
   Duct of Santorini
	Ø Open
	3 Percutaneous
	4 Percutaneous Endoscopic
	7 Via Natural or Artificial Opening
	8 Via Natural or Artificial Opening Endoscopic
		Z No Device	X Diagnostic
			Z No Qualifier

Non-OR   ØFB[Ø,1,2]3ZX
Non-OR   ØFB[4,G][3,4,8]ZX
Non-OR   ØFB[5,6,7,8,9,C,D,F][3,4,7,8]ZX
Non-OR   ØFB[5,6,7,8,9,C,D,F][4,8]ZZ

Ø Medical and Surgical
F Hepatobiliary System and Pancreas
C Extirpation   Definition: Taking or cutting out solid matter from a body part
     Explanation: The solid matter may be an abnormal byproduct of a biological function or a foreign body; it may be imbedded in a body part or in the lumen of a tubular body part. The solid matter may or may not have been previously broken into pieces.

Body Part Character 4	Approach Character 5	Device Character 6	Qualifier Character 7
Ø Liver Quadrate lobe 1 Liver, Right Lobe 2 Liver, Left Lobe	Ø Open 3 Percutaneous 4 Percutaneous Endoscopic	Z No Device	Z No Qualifier
4 Gallbladder G Pancreas	Ø Open 3 Percutaneous 4 Percutaneous Endoscopic 8 Via Natural or Artificial Opening Endoscopic	Z No Device	Z No Qualifier

5 Hepatic Duct, Right
6 Hepatic Duct, Left
7 Hepatic Duct, Common
8 Cystic Duct
9 Common Bile Duct
C Ampulla of Vater
   Duodenal ampulla
   Hepatopancreatic ampulla
D Pancreatic Duct
   Duct of Wirsung
F Pancreatic Duct, Accessory
   Duct of Santorini
	Ø Open
	3 Percutaneous
	4 Percutaneous Endoscopic
	7 Via Natural or Artificial Opening
	8 Via Natural or Artificial Opening Endoscopic
		Z No Device	Z No Qualifier

Non-OR   ØFC[5,6,7,8,9][3,4,7,8]ZZ
Non-OR   ØFCC[4,8]ZZ
Non-OR   ØFC[D,F][3,4,8]ZZ

Ø   Medical and Surgical
F   Hepatobiliary System and Pancreas
D   Extraction   Definition: Pulling or stripping out or off all or a portion of a body part by the use of force
                Explanation: The qualifier DIAGNOSTIC is used to identify extraction procedures that are biopsies

Body Part Character 4	Approach Character 5	Device Character 6	Qualifier Character 7
Ø Liver Quadrate lobe **1 Liver, Right Lobe** **2 Liver, Left Lobe**	**3** Percutaneous **4** Percutaneous Endoscopic	**Z** No Device	**X** Diagnostic

4 Gallbladder
5 Hepatic Duct, Right
6 Hepatic Duct, Left
7 Hepatic Duct, Common
8 Cystic Duct
9 Common Bile Duct
C Ampulla of Vater
   Duodenal ampulla
   Hepatopancreatic ampulla
D Pancreatic Duct
   Duct of Wirsung
F Pancreatic Duct, Accessory
   Duct of Santorini
G Pancreas
	3 Percutaneous
	4 Percutaneous Endoscopic
	8 Via Natural or Artificial Opening
	   Endoscopic
		Z No Device	**X** Diagnostic

Non-OR   ØFD[Ø,1,2]3ZX
Non-OR   ØFD[4,5,6,7,8,9,C,D,F,G][3,4,8]ZX

Ø   Medical and Surgical
F   Hepatobiliary System and Pancreas
F   Fragmentation   Definition: Breaking solid matter in a body part into pieces
                Explanation: Physical force (e.g., manual, ultrasonic) applied directly or indirectly is used to break the solid matter into pieces. The solid matter may be an abnormal byproduct of a biological function or a foreign body. The pieces of solid matter are not taken out.

Body Part Character 4	Approach Character 5	Device Character 6	Qualifier Character 7

4 Gallbladder   _{NC}
5 Hepatic Duct, Right   _{NC}
6 Hepatic Duct, Left   _{NC}
7 Hepatic Duct, Common
8 Cystic Duct   _{NC}
9 Common Bile Duct   _{NC}
C Ampulla of Vater   _{NC}
   Duodenal ampulla
   Hepatopancreatic ampulla
D Pancreatic Duct   _{NC}
   Duct of Wirsung
F Pancreatic Duct, Accessory   _{NC}
   Duct of Santorini
	Ø Open
	3 Percutaneous
	4 Percutaneous Endoscopic
	7 Via Natural or Artificial Opening
	8 Via Natural or Artificial Opening
	   Endoscopic
	X External
		Z No Device	**Z** No Qualifier

Non-OR   ØFF[4,5,6,7,8,9,C,D,F][8,X]ZZ
_{NC}   ØFF[4,5,6,8,9,C,D,F]XZZ

Ø   Medical and Surgical
F   Hepatobiliary System and Pancreas
H   Insertion   Definition: Putting in a nonbiological appliance that monitors, assists, performs, or prevents a physiological function but does not physically take the place of a body part
                Explanation: None

Body Part Character 4	Approach Character 5	Device Character 6	Qualifier Character 7
Ø Liver Quadrate lobe **4 Gallbladder** **G Pancreas**	**Ø** Open **3** Percutaneous **4** Percutaneous Endoscopic	**1** Radioactive Element **2** Monitoring Device **3** Infusion Device **Y** Other Device	**Z** No Qualifier
1 Liver, Right Lobe **2 Liver, Left Lobe**	**Ø** Open **3** Percutaneous **4** Percutaneous Endoscopic	**2** Monitoring Device **3** Infusion Device	**Z** No Qualifier

B Hepatobiliary Duct   ⊞
D Pancreatic Duct
   Duct of Wirsung
	Ø Open
	3 Percutaneous
	4 Percutaneous Endoscopic
	7 Via Natural or Artificial Opening
	8 Via Natural or Artificial Opening
	   Endoscopic
		1 Radioactive Element
		2 Monitoring Device
		3 Infusion Device
		D Intraluminal Device
		Y Other Device
			Z No Qualifier

Non-OR   ØFH[Ø,4,G][Ø,3,4]3Z   **Non-OR**   ØFH[B,D]4DZ   **See Appendix L for Procedure Combinations**
Non-OR   ØFH[Ø,4,G][3,4]YZ   **Non-OR**   ØFH[B,D][7,8][2,3]Z   ⊞   ØFHB7DZ
Non-OR   ØFH[1,2][Ø,3,4]3Z   **Non-OR**   ØFH[B,D]8DZ
Non-OR   ØFH[B,D][Ø,3,4]3Z   **Non-OR**   ØFH[B,D][3,4,7,8]YZ

_{LC} Limited Coverage   _{NC} Noncovered   ⊞ Combination Member   HAC associated procedure   Combination Only   DRG Non-OR   Non-OR   New/Revised in GREEN

Ø   Medical and Surgical
F   Hepatobiliary System and Pancreas
J   Inspection   Definition: Visually and/or manually exploring a body part

Explanation: Visual exploration may be performed with or without optical instrumentation. Manual exploration may be performed directly or through intervening body layers.

Body Part Character 4	Approach Character 5	Device Character 6	Qualifier Character 7
Ø Liver Quadrate lobe	Ø Open 3 Percutaneous 4 Percutaneous Endoscopic X External	Z No Device	Z No Qualifier
4 Gallbladder G Pancreas	Ø Open 3 Percutaneous 4 Percutaneous Endoscopic 8 Via Natural or Artificial Opening Endoscopic X External	Z No Device	Z No Qualifier
B Hepatobiliary Duct D Pancreatic Duct Duct of Wirsung	Ø Open 3 Percutaneous 4 Percutaneous Endoscopic 7 Via Natural or Artificial Opening 8 Via Natural or Artificial Opening Endoscopic	Z No Device	Z No Qualifier

Non-OR   ØFJØ[3,X]ZZ
Non-OR   ØFJ[4,G][3,8,X]ZZ
Non-OR   ØFJ[B,D][3,7,8]ZZ

Ø   Medical and Surgical
F   Hepatobiliary System and Pancreas
L   Occlusion   Definition: Completely closing an orifice or the lumen of a tubular body part

Explanation: The orifice can be a natural orifice or an artificially created orifice

Body Part Character 4	Approach Character 5	Device Character 6	Qualifier Character 7

5   Hepatic Duct, Right
6   Hepatic Duct, Left
7   Hepatic Duct, Common
8   Cystic Duct
9   Common Bile Duct
C   Ampulla of Vater
     Duodenal ampulla
     Hepatopancreatic ampulla
D   Pancreatic Duct
     Duct of Wirsung
F   Pancreatic Duct, Accessory
     Duct of Santorini
	Ø Open
	3 Percutaneous
	4 Percutaneous Endoscopic
		C Extraluminal Device
		D Intraluminal Device
		Z No Device
			Z No Qualifier

5   Hepatic Duct, Right
6   Hepatic Duct, Left
7   Hepatic Duct, Common
8   Cystic Duct
9   Common Bile Duct
C   Ampulla of Vater
     Duodenal ampulla
     Hepatopancreatic ampulla
D   Pancreatic Duct
     Duct of Wirsung
F   Pancreatic Duct, Accessory
     Duct of Santorini
	7 Via Natural or Artificial Opening
	8 Via Natural or Artificial Opening Endoscopic
		D Intraluminal Device
		Z No Device
			Z No Qualifier

Non-OR   ØFL[5,6,7,8,9][3,4][C,D,Z]Z
Non-OR   ØFL[5,6,7,8,9][7,8][D,Z]Z

Ø   Medical and Surgical
F   Hepatobiliary System and Pancreas
M   Reattachment   Definition: Putting back in or on all or a portion of a separated body part to its normal location or other suitable location
                        Explanation: Vascular circulation and nervous pathways may or may not be reestablished

Body Part Character 4	Approach Character 5	Device Character 6	Qualifier Character 7

Ø **Liver**
    Quadrate lobe
1 **Liver, Right Lobe**
2 **Liver, Left Lobe**
4 **Gallbladder**
5 **Hepatic Duct, Right**
6 **Hepatic Duct, Left**
7 **Hepatic Duct, Common**
8 **Cystic Duct**
9 **Common Bile Duct**
C **Ampulla of Vater**
    Duodenal ampulla
    Hepatopancreatic ampulla
D **Pancreatic Duct**
    Duct of Wirsung
F **Pancreatic Duct, Accessory**
    Duct of Santorini
G **Pancreas**
	Ø **Open**
	4 **Percutaneous Endoscopic**
		Z **No Device**	**Z** **No Qualifier**

Non-OR   ØFM[4,5,6,7,8,9]4ZZ

Ø   Medical and Surgical
F   Hepatobiliary System and Pancreas
N   Release   Definition: Freeing a body part from an abnormal physical constraint by cutting or by the use of force
                        Explanation: Some of the restraining tissue may be taken out but none of the body part is taken out

Body Part Character 4	Approach Character 5	Device Character 6	Qualifier Character 7
Ø **Liver** Quadrate lobe **1** **Liver, Right Lobe** **2** **Liver, Left Lobe**	**Ø** **Open** **3** **Percutaneous** **4** **Percutaneous Endoscopic**	**Z** **No Device**	**Z** **No Qualifier**
4 **Gallbladder** **G** **Pancreas**	**Ø** **Open** **3** **Percutaneous** **4** **Percutaneous Endoscopic** **8** **Via Natural or Artificial Opening Endoscopic**	**Z** **No Device**	**Z** **No Qualifier**

5 **Hepatic Duct, Right**
6 **Hepatic Duct, Left**
7 **Hepatic Duct, Common**
8 **Cystic Duct**
9 **Common Bile Duct**
C **Ampulla of Vater**
    Duodenal ampulla
    Hepatopancreatic ampulla
D **Pancreatic Duct**
    Duct of Wirsung
F **Pancreatic Duct, Accessory**
    Duct of Santorini
	Ø **Open**
	3 **Percutaneous**
	4 **Percutaneous Endoscopic**
	7 **Via Natural or Artificial Opening**
	8 **Via Natural or Artificial Opening Endoscopic**
		Z **No Device**	**Z** **No Qualifier**

LC Limited Coverage   **NC** Noncovered   ⊞ Combination Member   HAC associated procedure   Combination Only   DRG Non-OR   Non-OR   New/Revised in GREEN

ICD-10-PCS 2021   **405**

Ø **Medical and Surgical**
F **Hepatobiliary System and Pancreas**
P **Removal**   Definition: Taking out or off a device from a body part

Explanation: If a device is taken out and a similar device put in without cutting or puncturing the skin or mucous membrane, the procedure is coded to the root operation CHANGE. Otherwise, the procedure for taking out a device is coded to the root operation REMOVAL.

Body Part Character 4	Approach Character 5	Device Character 6	Qualifier Character 7
Ø Liver 　Quadrate lobe	Ø Open 3 Percutaneous 4 Percutaneous Endoscopic	Ø Drainage Device 2 Monitoring Device 3 Infusion Device Y Other Device	Z No Qualifier
Ø Liver 　Quadrate lobe	X External	Ø Drainage Device 2 Monitoring Device 3 Infusion Device	Z No Qualifier
4 Gallbladder G Pancreas	Ø Open 3 Percutaneous 4 Percutaneous Endoscopic	Ø Drainage Device 2 Monitoring Device 3 Infusion Device D Intraluminal Device Y Other Device	Z No Qualifier
4 Gallbladder G Pancreas	X External	Ø Drainage Device 2 Monitoring Device 3 Infusion Device D Intraluminal Device	Z No Qualifier
B Hepatobiliary Duct D Pancreatic Duct 　Duct of Wirsung	Ø Open 3 Percutaneous 4 Percutaneous Endoscopic 7 Via Natural or Artificial Opening 8 Via Natural or Artificial Opening 　Endoscopic	Ø Drainage Device 1 Radioactive Element 2 Monitoring Device 3 Infusion Device 7 Autologous Tissue Substitute C Extraluminal Device D Intraluminal Device J Synthetic Substitute K Nonautologous Tissue Substitute Y Other Device	Z No Qualifier
B Hepatobiliary Duct D Pancreatic Duct 　Duct of Wirsung	X External	Ø Drainage Device 1 Radioactive Element 2 Monitoring Device 3 Infusion Device D Intraluminal Device	Z No Qualifier

Non-OR ØFPØ[3,4]YZ		**See Appendix L for Procedure Combinations**
Non-OR ØFPØX[Ø,2,3]Z		**Combo-only** ØFP[B,D][7,8]DZ
Non-OR ØFPG3ØZ		**Combo-only** ØFP[B,D]XDZ
Non-OR ØFP[4,G][3,4]YZ		
Non-OR ØFP4X[Ø,2,3,D]Z		
Non-OR ØFPGX[Ø,2,3]Z		
Non-OR ØFP[B,D][3,4]YZ		
Non-OR ØFP[B,D][7,8][Ø,2,3,D,Y]Z		
Non-OR ØFP[B,D]X[Ø,1,2,3,D]Z		

Ø Medical and Surgical
F Hepatobiliary System and Pancreas
Q Repair   Definition: Restoring, to the extent possible, a body part to its normal anatomic structure and function

                Explanation: Used only when the method to accomplish the repair is not one of the other root operations

Body Part Character 4	Approach Character 5	Device Character 6	Qualifier Character 7
Ø Liver Quadrate lobe 1 Liver, Right Lobe 2 Liver, Left Lobe	Ø Open 3 Percutaneous 4 Percutaneous Endoscopic	Z No Device	Z No Qualifier
4 Gallbladder G Pancreas	Ø Open 3 Percutaneous 4 Percutaneous Endoscopic 8 Via Natural or Artificial Opening Endoscopic	Z No Device	Z No Qualifier

5 Hepatic Duct, Right
6 Hepatic Duct, Left
7 Hepatic Duct, Common
8 Cystic Duct
9 Common Bile Duct
C Ampulla of Vater
   Duodenal ampulla
   Hepatopancreatic ampulla
D Pancreatic Duct
   Duct of Wirsung
F Pancreatic Duct, Accessory
   Duct of Santorini
	Ø Open
	3 Percutaneous
	4 Percutaneous Endoscopic
	7 Via Natural or Artificial Opening
	8 Via Natural or Artificial Opening
	   Endoscopic
		Z No Device	Z No Qualifier

Ø Medical and Surgical
F Hepatobiliary System and Pancreas
R Replacement   Definition: Putting in or on biological or synthetic material that physically takes the place and/or function of all or a portion of a body part

                Explanation: The body part may have been taken out or replaced, or may be taken out, physically eradicated, or rendered nonfunctional during the REPLACEMENT procedure. A REMOVAL procedure is coded for taking out the device used in a previous replacement procedure.

Body Part Character 4	Approach Character 5	Device Character 6	Qualifier Character 7

5 Hepatic Duct, Right
6 Hepatic Duct, Left
7 Hepatic Duct, Common
8 Cystic Duct
9 Common Bile Duct
C Ampulla of Vater
   Duodenal ampulla
   Hepatopancreatic ampulla
D Pancreatic Duct
   Duct of Wirsung
F Pancreatic Duct, Accessory
   Duct of Santorini
	Ø Open
	4 Percutaneous Endoscopic
	8 Via Natural or Artificial Opening
	   Endoscopic
		7 Autologous Tissue Substitute
		J Synthetic Substitute
		K Nonautologous Tissue Substitute
			Z No Qualifier

Ø Medical and Surgical
F Hepatobiliary System and Pancreas
S Reposition   Definition: Moving to its normal location, or other suitable location, all or a portion of a body part

                Explanation: The body part is moved to a new location from an abnormal location, or from a normal location where it is not functioning correctly. The body part may or may not be cut out or off to be moved to the new location.

Body Part Character 4	Approach Character 5	Device Character 6	Qualifier Character 7

Ø Liver
   Quadrate lobe
4 Gallbladder
5 Hepatic Duct, Right
6 Hepatic Duct, Left
7 Hepatic Duct, Common
8 Cystic Duct
9 Common Bile Duct
C Ampulla of Vater
   Duodenal ampulla
   Hepatopancreatic ampulla
D Pancreatic Duct
   Duct of Wirsung
F Pancreatic Duct, Accessory
   Duct of Santorini
G Pancreas
	Ø Open
	4 Percutaneous Endoscopic
		Z No Device	Z No Qualifier

LC Limited Coverage   **NC** Noncovered   ⊞ Combination Member   HAC associated procedure   Combination Only   DRG Non-OR   Non-OR   New/Revised in GREEN

ICD-10-PCS 2021   407

Ø Medical and Surgical
F Hepatobiliary System and Pancreas
T Resection   Definition: Cutting out or off, without replacement, all of a body part
                   Explanation: None

Body Part Character 4	Approach Character 5	Device Character 6	Qualifier Character 7
Ø Liver Quadrate lobe 1 Liver, Right Lobe 2 Liver, Left Lobe 4 Gallbladder G Pancreas ⊞	Ø Open 4 Percutaneous Endoscopic	Z No Device	Z No Qualifier

5 Hepatic Duct, Right
6 Hepatic Duct, Left
7 Hepatic Duct, Common
8 Cystic Duct
9 Common Bile Duct
C Ampulla of Vater
    Duodenal ampulla
    Hepatopancreatic ampulla
D Pancreatic Duct
    Duct of Wirsung
F Pancreatic Duct, Accessory
    Duct of Santorini
	Ø Open
	4 Percutaneous Endoscopic
	7 Via Natural or Artificial Opening
	8 Via Natural or Artificial Opening
	    Endoscopic
		Z No Device	Z No Qualifier

Non-OR   ØFT[D,F][4,8]ZZ

See Appendix L for Procedure Combinations
  ⊞   ØFTGØZZ

Ø Medical and Surgical
F Hepatobiliary System and Pancreas
U Supplement   Definition: Putting in or on biological or synthetic material that physically reinforces and/or augments the function of a portion of a body part
                     Explanation: The biological material is non-living, or is living and from the same individual. The body part may have been previously replaced, and the SUPPLEMENT procedure is performed to physically reinforce and/or augment the function of the replaced body part.

Body Part Character 4	Approach Character 5	Device Character 6	Qualifier Character 7

5 Hepatic Duct, Right
6 Hepatic Duct, Left
7 Hepatic Duct, Common
8 Cystic Duct
9 Common Bile Duct
C Ampulla of Vater
    Duodenal ampulla
    Hepatopancreatic ampulla
D Pancreatic Duct
    Duct of Wirsung
F Pancreatic Duct, Accessory
    Duct of Santorini
	Ø Open
	3 Percutaneous
	4 Percutaneous Endoscopic
	8 Via Natural or Artificial Opening
	    Endoscopic
		7 Autologous Tissue Substitute
		J Synthetic Substitute
		K Nonautologous Tissue Substitute
			Z No Qualifier

Ø   **Medical and Surgical**
F   **Hepatobiliary System and Pancreas**
V   **Restriction**   Definition: Partially closing an orifice or the lumen of a tubular body part
                        Explanation: The orifice can be a natural orifice or an artificially created orifice

Body Part Character 4	Approach Character 5	Device Character 6	Qualifier Character 7

5 Hepatic Duct, Right
6 Hepatic Duct, Left
7 Hepatic Duct, Common
8 Cystic Duct
9 Common Bile Duct
C Ampulla of Vater
   Duodenal ampulla
   Hepatopancreatic ampulla
D Pancreatic Duct
   Duct of Wirsung
F Pancreatic Duct, Accessory
   Duct of Santorini
	Ø Open
	3 Percutaneous
	4 Percutaneous Endoscopic
		C Extraluminal Device
		D Intraluminal Device
		Z No Device
			Z No Qualifier

5 Hepatic Duct, Right
6 Hepatic Duct, Left
7 Hepatic Duct, Common
8 Cystic Duct
9 Common Bile Duct
C Ampulla of Vater
   Duodenal ampulla
   Hepatopancreatic ampulla
D Pancreatic Duct
   Duct of Wirsung
F Pancreatic Duct, Accessory
   Duct of Santorini
	7 Via Natural or Artificial Opening
	8 Via Natural or Artificial Opening Endoscopic
		D Intraluminal Device
		Z No Device
			Z No Qualifier

Non-OR   ØFV[5,6,7,8,9][3,4][C,D,Z]Z
Non-OR   ØFV[5,6,7,8,9][7,8][D,Z]Z

Ø   **Medical and Surgical**
F   **Hepatobiliary System and Pancreas**
W   **Revision**   Definition: Correcting, to the extent possible, a portion of a malfunctioning device or the position of a displaced device
                 Explanation: Revision can include correcting a malfunctioning or displaced device by taking out or putting in components of the device such as a screw or pin

Body Part Character 4	Approach Character 5	Device Character 6	Qualifier Character 7
Ø Liver Quadrate lobe	Ø Open 3 Percutaneous 4 Percutaneous Endoscopic	Ø Drainage Device 2 Monitoring Device 3 Infusion Device Y Other Device	Z No Qualifier
Ø Liver Quadrate lobe	X External	Ø Drainage Device 2 Monitoring Device 3 Infusion Device	Z No Qualifier
4 Gallbladder G Pancreas	Ø Open 3 Percutaneous 4 Percutaneous Endoscopic	Ø Drainage Device 2 Monitoring Device 3 Infusion Device D Intraluminal Device Y Other Device	Z No Qualifier
4 Gallbladder G Pancreas	X External	Ø Drainage Device 2 Monitoring Device 3 Infusion Device D Intraluminal Device	Z No Qualifier
B Hepatobiliary Duct D Pancreatic Duct Duct of Wirsung	Ø Open 3 Percutaneous 4 Percutaneous Endoscopic 7 Via Natural or Artificial Opening 8 Via Natural or Artificial Opening Endoscopic	Ø Drainage Device 2 Monitoring Device 3 Infusion Device 7 Autologous Tissue Substitute C Extraluminal Device D Intraluminal Device J Synthetic Substitute K Nonautologous Tissue Substitute Y Other Device	Z No Qualifier
B Hepatobiliary Duct D Pancreatic Duct Duct of Wirsung	X External	Ø Drainage Device 2 Monitoring Device 3 Infusion Device 7 Autologous Tissue Substitute C Extraluminal Device D Intraluminal Device J Synthetic Substitute K Nonautologous Tissue Substitute	Z No Qualifier

Non-OR   ØFWØ[3,4]YZ
Non-OR   ØFWØX[Ø,2,3]Z
Non-OR   ØFW[4,G][3,4]YZ
Non-OR   ØFW[4,G]X[Ø,2,3,D]Z
Non-OR   ØFW[B,D][3,4,7,8]YZ
Non-OR   ØFW[B,D]X[Ø,2,3,7,C,D,J,K]Z

Ø   **Medical and Surgical**
F   **Hepatobiliary System and Pancreas**
Y   **Transplantation**   Definition: Putting in or on all or a portion of a living body part taken from another individual or animal to physically take the place and/or function of all or a portion of a similar body part
                       Explanation: The native body part may or may not be taken out, and the transplanted body part may take over all or a portion of its function

Body Part Character 4	Approach Character 5	Device Character 6	Qualifier Character 7
Ø Liver LC Quadrate lobe G Pancreas LC NC ⊞	Ø Open	Z No Device	Ø Allogeneic 1 Syngeneic 2 Zooplastic

LC   ØFYØØZ[Ø,1,2]
LC   ØFYGØZ[Ø,1]
NC   ØFYGØZ2
NC   ØFYGØZ[Ø,1] If reported alone without one of the following procedures
        ØTYØØZ[Ø,1,2], ØTY1ØZ[Ø,1,2] and without one of the following
        diagnoses E1Ø.1Ø-E1Ø.9, E89.1

See Appendix L for Procedure Combinations
⊞   ØFYGØZ[Ø,1,2]

Endocrine System ØG2–ØGW

Character Meanings

This Character Meaning table is provided as a guide to assist the user in the identification of character members that may be found in this section of code tables. It **SHOULD NOT** be used to build a PCS code.

Operation–Character 3	Body Part–Character 4	Approach–Character 5	Device–Character 6	Qualifier–Character 7
2 Change	Ø Pituitary Gland	Ø Open	Ø Drainage Device	X Diagnostic
5 Destruction	1 Pineal Body	3 Percutaneous	1 Radioactive Element	Z No Qualifier
8 Division	2 Adrenal Gland, Left	4 Percutaneous Endoscopic	2 Monitoring Device	
9 Drainage	3 Adrenal Gland, Right	X External	3 Infusion Device	
B Excision	4 Adrenal Glands, Bilateral		Y Other Device	
C Extirpation	5 Adrenal Gland		Z No Device	
H Insertion	6 Carotid Body, Left			
J Inspection	7 Carotid Body, Right			
M Reattachment	8 Carotid Bodies, Bilateral			
N Release	9 Para-aortic Body			
P Removal	B Coccygeal Glomus			
Q Repair	C Glomus Jugulare			
S Reposition	D Aortic Body			
T Resection	F Paraganglion Extremity			
W Revision	G Thyroid Gland Lobe, Left			
	H Thyroid Gland Lobe, Right			
	J Thyroid Gland Isthmus			
	K Thyroid Gland			
	L Superior Parathyroid Gland, Right			
	M Superior Parathyroid Gland, Left			
	N Inferior Parathyroid Gland, Right			
	P Inferior Parathyroid Gland, Left			
	Q Parathyroid Glands, Multiple			
	R Parathyroid Gland			
	S Endocrine Gland			

AHA Coding Clinic for table ØGB

2017, 2Q, 20   Near total thyroidectomy
2014, 3Q, 22   Transsphenoidal removal of pituitary tumor and fat graft placement

AHA Coding Clinic for table ØGT

2017, 2Q, 20   Near total thyroidectomy

Endocrine System

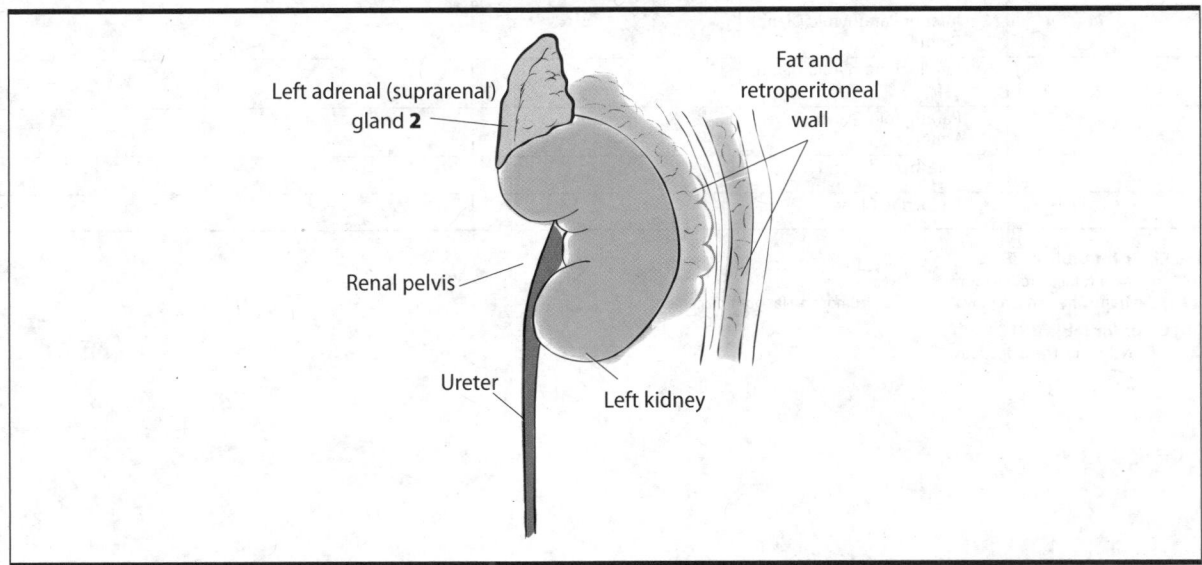

- Pineal gland **1**
- Pituitary **Ø**
- Parathyroid glands **L, M, N, P, Q, R**
- Thyroid gland **G, H, J, K**
- Thymus gland
- Thoracic duct
- Adrenals (suprarenal) gland **2, 3, 4, 5**
- Pancreas

Left Adrenal Gland

- Left adrenal (suprarenal) gland **2**
- Fat and retroperitoneal wall
- Renal pelvis
- Ureter
- Left kidney

Thyroid

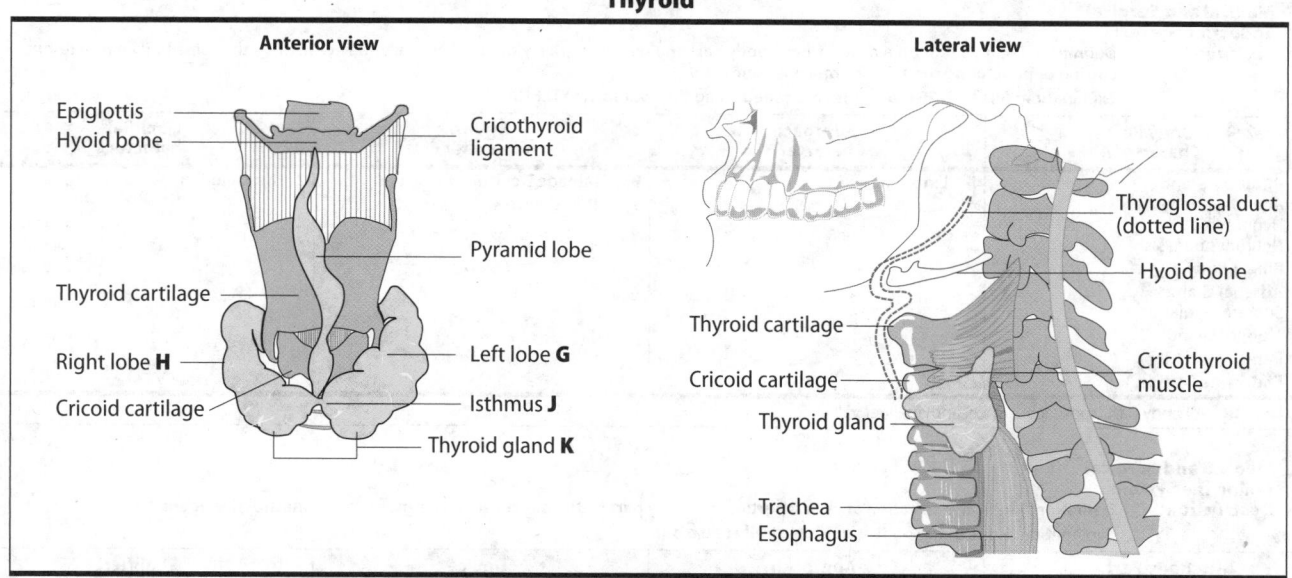

Anterior view

Epiglottis
Hyoid bone
Cricothyroid ligament
Pyramid lobe
Thyroid cartilage
Right lobe **H**
Left lobe **G**
Cricoid cartilage
Isthmus **J**
Thyroid gland **K**

Lateral view

Thyroglossal duct (dotted line)
Hyoid bone
Thyroid cartilage
Cricoid cartilage
Cricothyroid muscle
Thyroid gland
Trachea
Esophagus

Thyroid and Parathyroid Glands

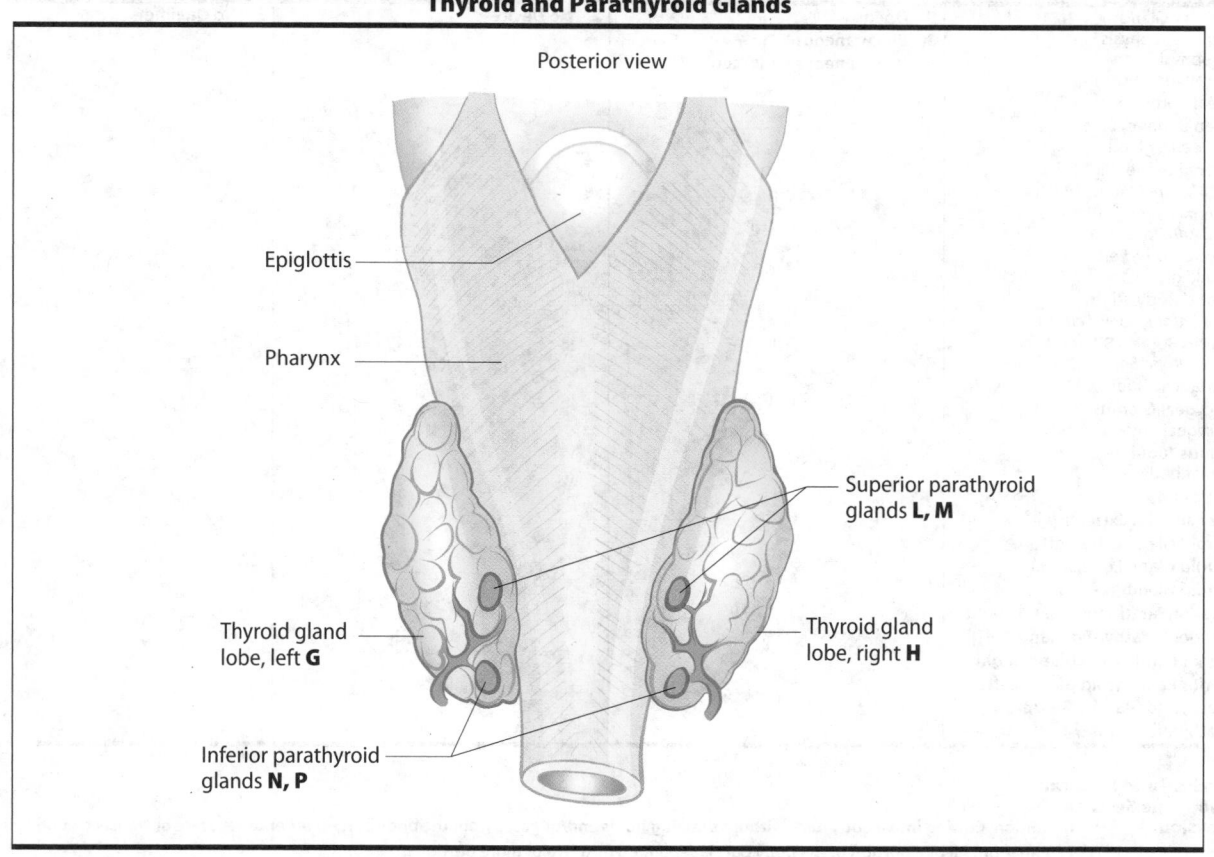

Posterior view

Epiglottis
Pharynx
Superior parathyroid glands **L, M**
Thyroid gland lobe, left **G**
Thyroid gland lobe, right **H**
Inferior parathyroid glands **N, P**

Ø　Medical and Surgical
G　Endocrine System
2　Change　　Definition: Taking out or off a device from a body part and putting back an identical or similar device in or on the same body part without cutting or puncturing the skin or a mucous membrane

Explanation: ALL CHANGE procedures are coded using the approach EXTERNAL

Body Part Character 4	Approach Character 5	Device Character 6	Qualifier Character 7
Ø Pituitary Gland 　Adenohypophysis 　Hypophysis 　Neurohypophysis 1 Pineal Body 5 Adrenal Gland 　Suprarenal gland K Thyroid Gland R Parathyroid Gland S Endocrine Gland	X External	Ø Drainage Device Y Other Device	Z No Qualifier

Non-OR　All body part, approach, device, and qualifier values

Ø　Medical and Surgical
G　Endocrine System
5　Destruction　　Definition: Physical eradication of all or a portion of a body part by the direct use of energy, force, or a destructive agent

Explanation: None of the body part is physically taken out

Body Part Character 4	Approach Character 5	Device Character 6	Qualifier Character 7
Ø Pituitary Gland 　Adenohypophysis 　Hypophysis 　Neurohypophysis 1 Pineal Body 2 Adrenal Gland, Left 　Suprarenal gland 3 Adrenal Gland, Right 　See 2 Adrenal Gland, Left 4 Adrenal Glands, Bilateral 　See 2 Adrenal Gland, Left 6 Carotid Body, Left 　Carotid glomus 7 Carotid Body, Right 　See 6 Carotid Body, Left 8 Carotid Bodies, Bilateral 　See 6 Carotid Body, Left 9 Para-aortic Body B Coccygeal Glomus 　Coccygeal body C Glomus Jugulare 　Jugular body D Aortic Body F Paraganglion Extremity G Thyroid Gland Lobe, Left H Thyroid Gland Lobe, Right K Thyroid Gland L Superior Parathyroid Gland, Right M Superior Parathyroid Gland, Left N Inferior Parathyroid Gland, Right P Inferior Parathyroid Gland, Left Q Parathyroid Glands, Multiple R Parathyroid Gland	Ø Open 3 Percutaneous 4 Percutaneous Endoscopic	Z No Device	Z No Qualifier

Ø　Medical and Surgical
G　Endocrine System
8　Division　　Definition: Cutting into a body part, without draining fluids and/or gases from the body part, in order to separate or transect a body part

Explanation: All or a portion of the body part is separated into two or more portions

Body Part Character 4	Approach Character 5	Device Character 6	Qualifier Character 7
Ø Pituitary Gland 　Adenohypophysis 　Hypophysis 　Neurohypophysis J Thyroid Gland Isthmus	Ø Open 3 Percutaneous 4 Percutaneous Endoscopic	Z No Device	Z No Qualifier

0   **Medical and Surgical**
G   **Endocrine System**
9   **Drainage**   Definition: Taking or letting out fluids and/or gases from a body part
                          Explanation: The qualifier DIAGNOSTIC is used to identify drainage procedures that are biopsies

Body Part Character 4	Approach Character 5	Device Character 6	Qualifier Character 7

0 **Pituitary Gland**
    Adenohypophysis
    Hypophysis
    Neurohypophysis
1 **Pineal Body**
2 **Adrenal Gland, Left**
    Suprarenal gland
3 **Adrenal Gland, Right**
    See 2 Adrenal Gland, Left
4 **Adrenal Glands, Bilateral**
    See 2 Adrenal Gland, Left
6 **Carotid Body, Left**
    Carotid glomus
7 **Carotid Body, Right**
    See 6 Carotid Body, Left
8 **Carotid Bodies, Bilateral**
    See 6 Carotid Body, Left
9 **Para-aortic Body**
B **Coccygeal Glomus**
    Coccygeal body
C **Glomus Jugulare**
    Jugular body
D **Aortic Body**
F **Paraganglion Extremity**
G **Thyroid Gland Lobe, Left**
H **Thyroid Gland Lobe, Right**
K **Thyroid Gland**
L **Superior Parathyroid Gland, Right**
M **Superior Parathyroid Gland, Left**
N **Inferior Parathyroid Gland, Right**
P **Inferior Parathyroid Gland, Left**
Q **Parathyroid Glands, Multiple**
R **Parathyroid Gland**
	0 Open
	3 Percutaneous
	4 Percutaneous Endoscopic
		0 Drainage Device	**Z** No Qualifier

0 **Pituitary Gland**
    Adenohypophysis
    Hypophysis
    Neurohypophysis
1 **Pineal Body**
2 **Adrenal Gland, Left**
    Suprarenal gland
3 **Adrenal Gland, Right**
    See 2 Adrenal Gland, Left
4 **Adrenal Glands, Bilateral**
    See 2 Adrenal Gland, Left
6 **Carotid Body, Left**
    Carotid glomus
7 **Carotid Body, Right**
    See 6 Carotid Body, Left
8 **Carotid Bodies, Bilateral**
    See 6 Carotid Body, Left
9 **Para-aortic Body**
B **Coccygeal Glomus**
    Coccygeal body
C **Glomus Jugulare**
    Jugular body
D **Aortic Body**
F **Paraganglion Extremity**
G **Thyroid Gland Lobe, Left**
H **Thyroid Gland Lobe, Right**
K **Thyroid Gland**
L **Superior Parathyroid Gland, Right**
M **Superior Parathyroid Gland, Left**
N **Inferior Parathyroid Gland, Right**
P **Inferior Parathyroid Gland, Left**
Q **Parathyroid Glands, Multiple**
R **Parathyroid Gland**
	0 Open
	3 Percutaneous
	4 Percutaneous Endoscopic
		Z No Device	**X** Diagnostic
			Z No Qualifier

Non-OR	0G9[0,1,2,3,4,6,7,8,9,B,C,D,F,G,H,K,L,M,N,P,Q,R]30Z
Non-OR	0G9[G,H,K,L,M,N,P,Q,R]40Z
Non-OR	0G9[2,3,4,G,H,K][3,4]ZX
Non-OR	0G9[0,1,2,3,4,6,7,8,9,B,C,D,F,G,H,K,L,M,N,P,Q,R]3ZZ
Non-OR	0G9[G,H,K,L,M,N,P,Q,R]4ZZ

[LC] Limited Coverage   [NC] Noncovered   ⊞ Combination Member   HAC associated procedure   Combination Only   DRG Non-OR   Non-OR   New/Revised in GREEN

ICD-10-PCS 2021   415

0G9–0G9

Endocrine System

Ø   **Medical and Surgical**
G   **Endocrine System**
B   **Excision**   Definition: Cutting out or off, without replacement, a portion of a body part
      Explanation: The qualifier DIAGNOSTIC is used to identify excision procedures that are biopsies

Body Part Character 4	Approach Character 5	Device Character 6	Qualifier Character 7

Ø Pituitary Gland
  Adenohypophysis
  Hypophysis
  Neurohypophysis
1 Pineal Body
2 Adrenal Gland, Left
  Suprarenal gland
3 Adrenal Gland, Right
  See 2 Adrenal Gland, Left
4 Adrenal Glands, Bilateral
  See 2 Adrenal Gland, Left
6 Carotid Body, Left
  Carotid glomus
7 Carotid Body, Right
  See 6 Carotid Body, Left
8 Carotid Bodies, Bilateral
  See 6 Carotid Body, Left
9 Para-aortic Body
B Coccygeal Glomus
  Coccygeal body
C Glomus Jugulare
  Jugular body
D Aortic Body
F Paraganglion Extremity
G Thyroid Gland Lobe, Left
H Thyroid Gland Lobe, Right
J Thyroid Gland Isthmus
L Superior Parathyroid Gland, Right
M Superior Parathyroid Gland, Left
N Inferior Parathyroid Gland, Right
P Inferior Parathyroid Gland, Left
Q Parathyroid Glands, Multiple
R Parathyroid Gland
	Ø Open
	3 Percutaneous
	4 Percutaneous Endoscopic
		Z No Device	X Diagnostic
			Z No Qualifier

Non-OR   ØGB[2,3,4,G,H,J][3,4]ZX

Ø   **Medical and Surgical**
G   **Endocrine System**
C   **Extirpation**   Definition: Taking or cutting out solid matter from a body part
      Explanation: The solid matter may be an abnormal byproduct of a biological function or a foreign body; it may be imbedded in a body part or in the lumen of a tubular body part. The solid matter may or may not have been previously broken into pieces.

Body Part Character 4	Approach Character 5	Device Character 6	Qualifier Character 7

Ø Pituitary Gland
  Adenohypophysis
  Hypophysis
  Neurohypophysis
1 Pineal Body
2 Adrenal Gland, Left
  Suprarenal gland
3 Adrenal Gland, Right
  See 2 Adrenal Gland, Left
4 Adrenal Glands, Bilateral
  See 2 Adrenal Gland, Left
6 Carotid Body, Left
  Carotid glomus
7 Carotid Body, Right
  See 6 Carotid Body, Left
8 Carotid Bodies, Bilateral
  See 6 Carotid Body, Left
9 Para-aortic Body
B Coccygeal Glomus
  Coccygeal body
C Glomus Jugulare
  Jugular body
D Aortic Body
F Paraganglion Extremity
G Thyroid Gland Lobe, Left
H Thyroid Gland Lobe, Right
K Thyroid Gland
L Superior Parathyroid Gland, Right
M Superior Parathyroid Gland, Left
N Inferior Parathyroid Gland, Right
P Inferior Parathyroid Gland, Left
Q Parathyroid Glands, Multiple
R Parathyroid Gland
	Ø Open
	3 Percutaneous
	4 Percutaneous Endoscopic
		Z No Device	Z No Qualifier

Ø   **Medical and Surgical**
G   **Endocrine System**
H   **Insertion**   Definition: Putting in a nonbiological appliance that monitors, assists, performs, or prevents a physiological function but does not physically take the place of a body part

Explanation: None

Body Part Character 4	Approach Character 5	Device Character 6	Qualifier Character 7
S Endocrine Gland	**Ø** Open **3** Percutaneous **4** Percutaneous Endoscopic	**1** Radioactive Element **2** Monitoring Device **3** Infusion Device **Y** Other Device	**Z** No Qualifier

Non-OR   ØGHS[3,4]YZ

Ø   **Medical and Surgical**
G   **Endocrine System**
J   **Inspection**   Definition: Visually and/or manually exploring a body part

Explanation: Visual exploration may be performed with or without optical instrumentation. Manual exploration may be performed directly or through intervening body layers.

Body Part Character 4	Approach Character 5	Device Character 6	Qualifier Character 7

Ø   Pituitary Gland
    Adenohypophysis
    Hypophysis
    Neurohypophysis
1   Pineal Body
5   Adrenal Gland
    Suprarenal gland
K   Thyroid Gland
R   Parathyroid Gland
S   Endocrine Gland
	Ø Open
	3 Percutaneous
	4 Percutaneous Endoscopic
		Z No Device	**Z** No Qualifier

Non-OR   ØGJ[Ø,1,5,K,R,S]3ZZ

Ø   **Medical and Surgical**
G   **Endocrine System**
M   **Reattachment**   Definition: Putting back in or on all or a portion of a separated body part to its normal location or other suitable location

Explanation: Vascular circulation and nervous pathways may or may not be reestablished

Body Part Character 4	Approach Character 5	Device Character 6	Qualifier Character 7

2   Adrenal Gland, Left
    Suprarenal gland
3   Adrenal Gland, Right
    See 2 Adrenal Gland, Left
G   Thyroid Gland Lobe, Left
H   Thyroid Gland Lobe, Right
L   Superior Parathyroid Gland, Right
M   Superior Parathyroid Gland, Left
N   Inferior Parathyroid Gland, Right
P   Inferior Parathyroid Gland, Left
Q   Parathyroid Glands, Multiple
R   Parathyroid Gland
	Ø Open
	4 Percutaneous Endoscopic
		Z No Device	**Z** No Qualifier

LC Limited Coverage   NC Noncovered   ⊞ Combination Member   HAC associated procedure   Combination Only   DRG Non-OR   Non-OR   New/Revised in **GREEN**

ICD-10-PCS 2021   **417**

ØGH–ØGM

Ø   Medical and Surgical
G   Endocrine System
N   Release   Definition: Freeing a body part from an abnormal physical constraint by cutting or by the use of force
                       Explanation: Some of the restraining tissue may be taken out but none of the body part is taken out

Body Part Character 4	Approach Character 5	Device Character 6	Qualifier Character 7

Ø Pituitary Gland
   Adenohypophysis
   Hypophysis
   Neurohypophysis
1 Pineal Body
2 Adrenal Gland, Left
   Suprarenal gland
3 Adrenal Gland, Right
   See 2 Adrenal Gland, Left
4 Adrenal Glands, Bilateral
   See 2 Adrenal Gland, Left
6 Carotid Body, Left
   Carotid glomus
7 Carotid Body, Right
   See 6 Carotid Body, Left
8 Carotid Bodies, Bilateral
   See 6 Carotid Body, Left
9 Para-aortic Body
B Coccygeal Glomus
   Coccygeal body
C Glomus Jugulare
   Jugular body
D Aortic Body
F Paraganglion Extremity
G Thyroid Gland Lobe, Left
H Thyroid Gland Lobe, Right
K Thyroid Gland
L Superior Parathyroid Gland, Right
M Superior Parathyroid Gland, Left
N Inferior Parathyroid Gland, Right
P Inferior Parathyroid Gland, Left
Q Parathyroid Glands, Multiple
R Parathyroid Gland
	Ø Open
	3 Percutaneous
	4 Percutaneous Endoscopic
		Z No Device	Z No Qualifier

Non-OR   ØGN[6,7,8,9,B,C,D,F][Ø,3,4]ZZ

Ø   Medical and Surgical
G   Endocrine System
P   Removal   Definition: Taking out or off a device from a body part
                       Explanation: If a device is taken out and a similar device put in without cutting or puncturing the skin or mucous membrane, the procedure is coded to the root operation CHANGE. Otherwise, the procedure for taking out a device is coded to the root operation REMOVAL.

Body Part Character 4	Approach Character 5	Device Character 6	Qualifier Character 7

Ø Pituitary Gland
   Adenohypophysis
   Hypophysis
   Neurohypophysis
1 Pineal Body
5 Adrenal Gland
   Suprarenal gland
K Thyroid Gland
R Parathyroid Gland
	Ø Open
	3 Percutaneous
	4 Percutaneous Endoscopic
	X External
		Ø Drainage Device	Z No Qualifier

S Endocrine Gland	Ø Open 3 Percutaneous 4 Percutaneous Endoscopic	Ø Drainage Device 2 Monitoring Device 3 Infusion Device Y Other Device	Z No Qualifier
S Endocrine Gland	X External	Ø Drainage Device 2 Monitoring Device 3 Infusion Device	Z No Qualifier

Non-OR   ØGP[Ø,1,5,K,R]XØZ
Non-OR   ØGPS[3,4]YZ
Non-OR   ØGPSX[Ø,2,3]Z

Ø   **Medical and Surgical**
G   **Endocrine System**
Q   **Repair**   Definition: Restoring, to the extent possible, a body part to its normal anatomic structure and function

                         Explanation: Used only when the method to accomplish the repair is not one of the other root operations

Body Part Character 4	Approach Character 5	Device Character 6	Qualifier Character 7

Ø Pituitary Gland
    Adenohypophysis
    Hypophysis
    Neurohypophysis
1 Pineal Body
2 Adrenal Gland, Left
    Suprarenal gland
3 Adrenal Gland, Right
    See 2 Adrenal Gland, Left
4 Adrenal Glands, Bilateral
    See 2 Adrenal Gland, Left
6 Carotid Body, Left
    Carotid glomus
7 Carotid Body, Right
    See 6 Carotid Body, Left
8 Carotid Bodies, Bilateral
    See 6 Carotid Body, Left
9 Para-aortic Body
B Coccygeal Glomus
    Coccygeal body
C Glomus Jugulare
    Jugular body
D Aortic Body
F Paraganglion Extremity
G Thyroid Gland Lobe, Left
H Thyroid Gland Lobe, Right
J Thyroid Gland Isthmus
K Thyroid Gland
L Superior Parathyroid Gland, Right
M Superior Parathyroid Gland, Left
N Inferior Parathyroid Gland, Right
P Inferior Parathyroid Gland, Left
Q Parathyroid Glands, Multiple
R Parathyroid Gland
	Ø Open
	3 Percutaneous
	4 Percutaneous Endoscopic
		Z No Device	Z No Qualifier

Ø   **Medical and Surgical**
G   **Endocrine System**
S   **Reposition**   Definition: Moving to its normal location, or other suitable location, all or a portion of a body part

                         Explanation: The body part is moved to a new location from an abnormal location, or from a normal location where it is not functioning correctly. The body part may or may not be cut out or off to be moved to the new location.

Body Part Character 4	Approach Character 5	Device Character 6	Qualifier Character 7

2 Adrenal Gland, Left
    Suprarenal gland
3 Adrenal Gland, Right
    See 2 Adrenal Gland, Left
G Thyroid Gland Lobe, Left
H Thyroid Gland Lobe, Right
L Superior Parathyroid Gland, Right
M Superior Parathyroid Gland, Left
N Inferior Parathyroid Gland, Right
P Inferior Parathyroid Gland, Left
Q Parathyroid Glands, Multiple
R Parathyroid Gland
	Ø Open
	4 Percutaneous Endoscopic
		Z No Device	Z No Qualifier

Endocrine System

Ø　**Medical and Surgical**
G　**Endocrine System**
T　**Resection**　　Definition: Cutting out or off, without replacement, all of a body part
　　　　　　　　　　Explanation: None

Body Part Character 4	Approach Character 5	Device Character 6	Qualifier Character 7
Ø　Pituitary Gland 　　Adenohypophysis 　　Hypophysis 　　Neurohypophysis 1　Pineal Body 2　Adrenal Gland, Left 　　Suprarenal gland 3　Adrenal Gland, Right 　　See 2 Adrenal Gland, Left 4　Adrenal Glands, Bilateral 　　See 2 Adrenal Gland, Left 6　Carotid Body, Left 　　Carotid glomus 7　Carotid Body, Right 　　See 6 Carotid Body, Left 8　Carotid Bodies, Bilateral 　　See 6 Carotid Body, Left 9　Para-aortic Body B　Coccygeal Glomus 　　Coccygeal body C　Glomus Jugulare 　　Jugular body D　Aortic Body F　Paraganglion Extremity G　Thyroid Gland Lobe, Left H　Thyroid Gland Lobe, Right J　Thyroid Gland Isthmus K　Thyroid Gland L　Superior Parathyroid Gland, Right M　Superior Parathyroid Gland, Left N　Inferior Parathyroid Gland, Right P　Inferior Parathyroid Gland, Left Q　Parathyroid Glands, Multiple R　Parathyroid Gland	Ø　Open 4　Percutaneous Endoscopic	Z　No Device	Z　No Qualifier

Non-OR　ØGT[6,7,8,9,B,C,D,F][Ø,4]ZZ

Ø　**Medical and Surgical**
G　**Endocrine System**
W　**Revision**　　Definition: Correcting, to the extent possible, a portion of a malfunctioning device or the position of a displaced device
　　　　　　　　　Explanation: Revision can include correcting a malfunctioning or displaced device by taking out or putting in components of the device such as a screw or pin

Body Part Character 4	Approach Character 5	Device Character 6	Qualifier Character 7
Ø　Pituitary Gland 　　Adenohypophysis 　　Hypophysis 　　Neurohypophysis 1　Pineal Body 5　Adrenal Gland 　　Suprarenal gland K　Thyroid Gland R　Parathyroid Gland	Ø　Open 3　Percutaneous 4　Percutaneous Endoscopic X　External	Ø　Drainage Device	Z　No Qualifier
S　Endocrine Gland	Ø　Open 3　Percutaneous 4　Percutaneous Endoscopic	Ø　Drainage Device 2　Monitoring Device 3　Infusion Device Y　Other Device	Z　No Qualifier
S　Endocrine Gland	X　External	Ø　Drainage Device 2　Monitoring Device 3　Infusion Device	Z　No Qualifier

Non-OR　ØGW[Ø,1,5,K,R]XØZ
Non-OR　ØGWS[3,4]YZ
Non-OR　ØGWSX[Ø,2,3]Z

Skin and Breast ØHØ–ØHX

Character Meanings*

This Character Meaning table is provided as a guide to assist the user in the identification of character members that may be found in this section of code tables. It **SHOULD NOT** be used to build a PCS code.

Operation–Character 3	Body Part–Character 4	Approach–Character 5	Device–Character 6	Qualifier–Character 7
Ø Alteration	Ø Skin, Scalp	Ø Open	Ø Drainage Device	2 Cell Suspension Technique
2 Change	1 Skin, Face	3 Percutaneous	1 Radioactive Element	3 Full Thickness
5 Destruction	2 Skin, Right Ear	7 Via Natural or Artificial Opening	7 Autologous Tissue Substitute	4 Partial Thickness
8 Division	3 Skin, Left Ear	8 Via Natural or Artificial Opening Endoscopic	J Synthetic Substitute	5 Latissimus Dorsi Myocutaneous Flap
9 Drainage	4 Skin, Neck	X External	K Nonautologous Tissue Substitute	6 Transverse Rectus Abdominis Myocutaneous Flap
B Excision	5 Skin, Chest		N Tissue Expander	7 Deep Inferior Epigastric Artery Perforator Flap
C Extirpation	6 Skin, Back		Y Other Device	8 Superficial Inferior Epigastric Artery Flap
D Extraction	7 Skin, Abdomen		Z No Device	9 Gluteal Artery Perforator Flap
H Insertion	8 Skin, Buttock			D Multiple
J Inspection	9 Skin, Perineum			X Diagnostic
M Reattachment	A Skin, Inguinal			Z No Qualifier
N Release	B Skin, Right Upper Arm			
P Removal	C Skin, Left Upper Arm			
Q Repair	D Skin, Right Lower Arm			
R Replacement	E Skin, Left Lower Arm			
S Reposition	F Skin, Right Hand			
T Resection	G Skin, Left Hand			
U Supplement	H Skin, Right Upper Leg			
W Revision	J Skin, Left Upper Leg			
X Transfer	K Skin, Right Lower Leg			
	L Skin, Left Lower Leg			
	M Skin, Right Foot			
	N Skin, Left Foot			
	P Skin			
	Q Finger Nail			
	R Toe Nail			
	S Hair			
	T Breast, Right			
	U Breast, Left			
	V Breast, Bilateral			
	W Nipple, Right			
	X Nipple, Left			
	Y Supernumerary Breast			

*   Includes skin and breast glands and ducts.

AHA Coding Clinic for table ØHØ

2019, 4Q, 30-31	Breast procedures

AHA Coding Clinic for table ØH5

2019, 4Q, 30-31	Breast procedures

AHA Coding Clinic for table ØH9

2019, 4Q, 30-31	Breast procedures

AHA Coding Clinic for table ØHB

2020, 1Q, 31	Repair of buried penis
2019, 4Q, 30-31	Breast procedures
2018, 1Q, 14	Excisional debridement of breast tissue and skin
2016, 3Q, 29	Closure of bilateral alveolar clefts
2015, 3Q, 3-8	Excisional and nonexcisional debridement

AHA Coding Clinic for table ØHC

2019, 4Q, 30-31	Breast procedures

AHA Coding Clinic for table ØHD

2019, 4Q, 30-31	Breast procedures
2016, 1Q, 40	Nonexcisional debridement of skin and subcutaneous tissue
2015, 3Q, 3-8	Excisional and nonexcisional debridement

AHA Coding Clinic for table ØHH

2019, 4Q, 30-31	Breast procedures
2017, 4Q, 67	New qualifier values - Pedicle flap procedures
2014, 2Q, 12	Pedicle latissimus myocutaneous flap with placement of breast tissue expanders
2013, 4Q, 107	Breast tissue expander placement using acellular dermal matrix

AHA Coding Clinic for table ØHJ

2019, 4Q, 30-31	Breast procedures

AHA Coding Clinic for table ØHN

2019, 4Q, 30-31	Breast procedures

AHA Coding Clinic for table ØHP

2019, 4Q, 30-31	Breast procedures
2018, 3Q, 13	Deep inferior epigastric artery perforator flap breast reconstruction
2016, 2Q, 27	Removal of nonviable transverse rectus abdominis myocutaneous (TRAM) flaps

AHA Coding Clinic for table ØHQ

2019, 4Q, 30-31	Breast procedures
2018, 2Q, 25	Third and fourth degree obstetric lacerations
2016, 1Q, 7	Obstetrical perineal laceration repair
2014, 4Q, 31	Delayed wound closure following fracture treatment

AHA Coding Clinic for table ØHR

2020, 1Q, 27	Delayed reconstruction following mastectomy using gracilis musculocutaneous free flap
2020, 1Q, 28	Free flap microvascular breast reconstruction
2020, 1Q, 30	Polarity Skin TE™ application
2019, 4Q, 30-31	Breast procedures
2019, 4Q, 32	Cell suspension epithelial autograft
2019, 3Q, 32	Breast reconstruction with neurotization
2018, 3Q, 13	Deep inferior epigastric artery perforator flap breast reconstruction
2017, 1Q, 35	Epifix® allograft
2014, 3Q, 14	Application of TheraSkin® and excisional debridement

AHA Coding Clinic for table ØHT

2018, 3Q, 13	Deep inferior epigastric artery perforator flap breast reconstruction
2014, 4Q, 34	Skin-sparing mastectomy

AHA Coding Clinic for table ØHU

2019, 4Q, 30-31	Breast procedures

AHA Coding Clinic for table ØHW

2019, 4Q, 30-31	Breast procedures

Integumentary Anatomy

Hair follicle **S**

Hair **S**

Sebaceous gland **Ø-9, A-P**

Arrector pili muscle

Epidermis

Thick-skin epidermis

Dermis

Hair shaft **S**

Pacinian corpuscle

Hair matrix **S**

Hypodermis (subcutaneous layer)

Sweat (eccrine gland) **Ø-9, A-P**

Sensory nerve

Bulb

Blood vessels

Nail Anatomy

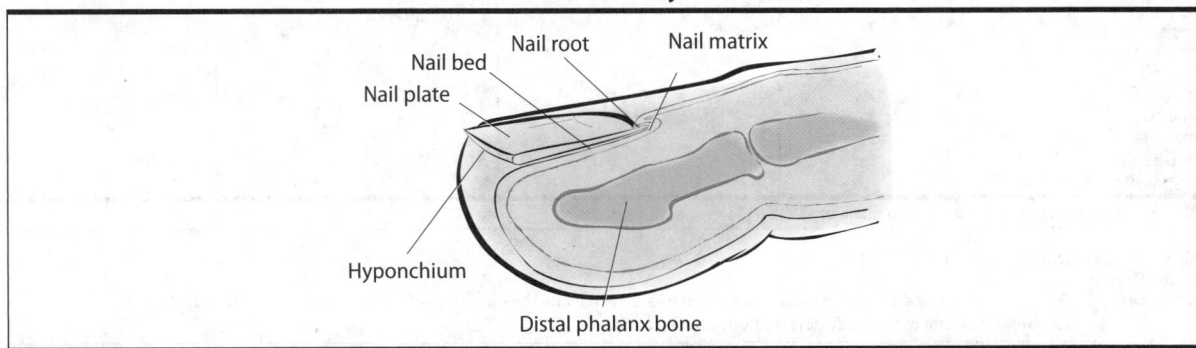

Nail bed

Nail root

Nail matrix

Nail plate

Hyponchium

Distal phalanx bone

Breast

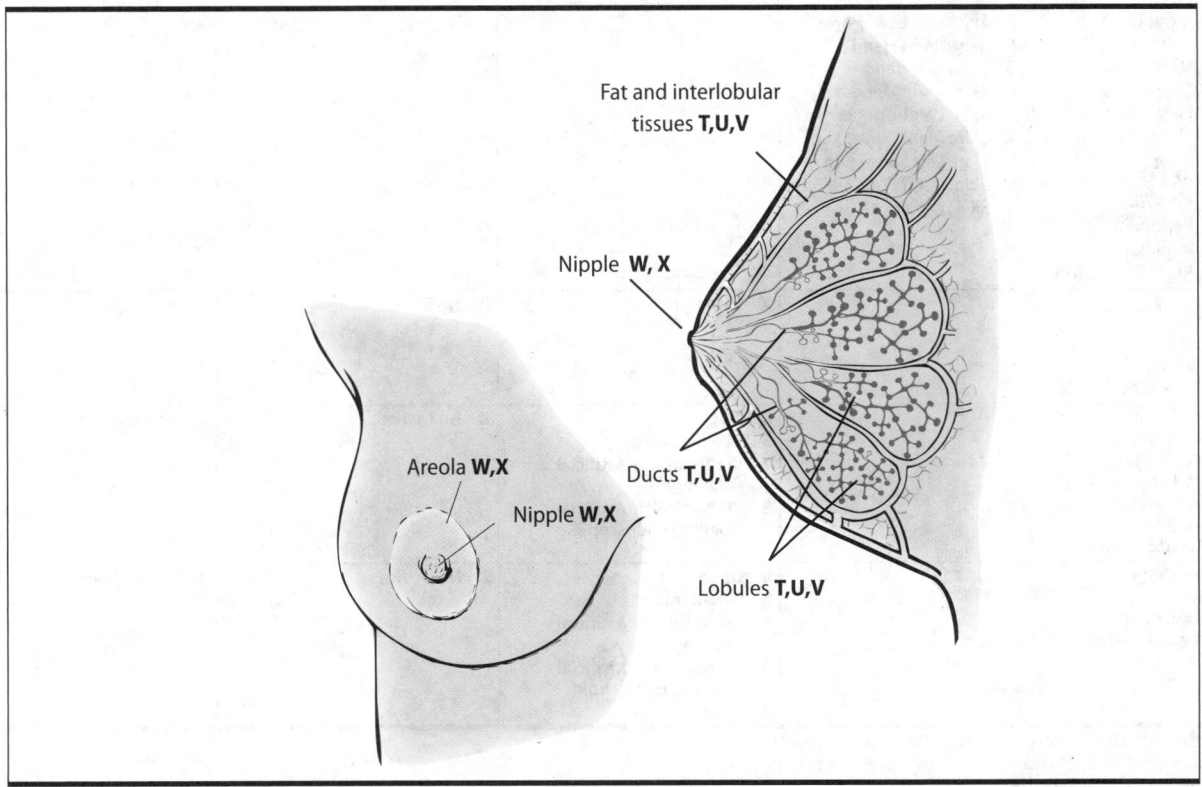

Fat and interlobular tissues **T,U,V**

Nipple **W, X**

Areola **W,X**

Nipple **W,X**

Ducts **T,U,V**

Lobules **T,U,V**

Ø　Medical and Surgical
H　Skin and Breast
Ø　Alteration　　Definition: Modifying the anatomic structure of a body part without affecting the function of the body part

Explanation: Principal purpose is to improve appearance

Body Part Character 4	Approach Character 5	Device Character 6	Qualifier Character 7
T　Breast, Right 　　Mammary duct 　　Mammary gland U　Breast, Left 　　*See T Breast, Right* V　Breast, Bilateral 　　*See T Breast, Right*	Ø　Open 3　Percutaneous	7　Autologous Tissue 　　Substitute J　Synthetic Substitute K　Nonautologous Tissue 　　Substitute Z　No Device	Z　No Qualifier

Non-OR　ØHØ[T,U,V]3JZ

Ø　Medical and Surgical
H　Skin and Breast
2　Change　　Definition: Taking out or off a device from a body part and putting back an identical or similar device in or on the same body part without cutting or puncturing the skin or a mucous membrane

Explanation: All CHANGE procedures are coded using the approach EXTERNAL

Body Part Character 4	Approach Character 5	Device Character 6	Qualifier Character 7
P　Skin 　　Dermis 　　Epidermis 　　Sebaceous gland 　　Sweat gland T　Breast, Right 　　Mammary duct 　　Mammary gland U　Breast, Left 　　*See T Breast, Right*	X　External	Ø　Drainage Device Y　Other Device	Z　No Qualifier

Non-OR　All body part, approach, device, and qualifier values

Ø　Medical and Surgical
H　Skin and Breast
5　Destruction　　Definition: Physical eradication of all or a portion of a body part by the direct use of energy, force, or a destructive agent

Explanation: None of the body part is physically taken out

Body Part Character 4	Approach Character 5	Device Character 6	Qualifier Character 7
Ø　Skin, Scalp 1　Skin, Face 2　Skin, Right Ear 3　Skin, Left Ear 4　Skin, Neck 5　Skin, Chest 　　Breast procedures, skin 　　only 6　Skin, Back 7　Skin, Abdomen 8　Skin, Buttock 9　Skin, Perineum A　Skin, Inguinal B　Skin, Right Upper Arm C　Skin, Left Upper Arm D　Skin, Right Lower Arm E　Skin, Left Lower Arm F　Skin, Right Hand G　Skin, Left Hand H　Skin, Right Upper Leg J　Skin, Left Upper Leg K　Skin, Right Lower Leg L　Skin, Left Lower Leg M　Skin, Right Foot N　Skin, Left Foot	X　External	Z　No Device	D　Multiple Z　No Qualifier
Q　Finger Nail 　　Nail bed 　　Nail plate R　Toe Nail 　　*See Q Finger Nail*	X　External	Z　No Device	Z　No Qualifier
T　Breast, Right 　　Mammary duct 　　Mammary gland U　Breast, Left 　　*See T Breast, Right* V　Breast, Bilateral 　　*See T Breast, Right*	Ø　Open 3　Percutaneous 7　Via Natural or Artificial 　　Opening 8　Via Natural or Artificial 　　Opening Endoscopic	Z　No Device	Z　No Qualifier
W　Nipple, Right 　　Areola X　Nipple, Left 　　*See W Nipple, Right*	Ø　Open 3　Percutaneous 7　Via Natural or Artificial 　　Opening 8　Via Natural or Artificial 　　Opening Endoscopic X　External	Z　No Device	Z　No Qualifier

DRG Non-OR　ØH5[Ø,1,4,5,6,7,8,9,A,B,C,D,E,F,G,H,J,K,L,M,N]XZ[D,Z]
DRG Non-OR　ØH5[Q,R]XZZ
Non-OR　　ØH5[2,3]XZ[D,Z]

LC Limited Coverage　　NC Noncovered　　⊞ Combination Member　　HAC associated procedure　　Combination Only　　DRG Non-OR　　Non-OR　　New/Revised in GREEN

Ø   **Medical and Surgical**
H   **Skin and Breast**
8   **Division**   Definition: Cutting into a body part, without draining fluids and/or gases from the body part, in order to separate or transect a body part
                              Explanation: All or a portion of the body part is separated into two or more portions

Body Part Character 4	Approach Character 5	Device Character 6	Qualifier Character 7
Ø Skin, Scalp	X External	Z No Device	Z No Qualifier
1 Skin, Face			
2 Skin, Right Ear			
3 Skin, Left Ear			
4 Skin, Neck			
5 Skin, Chest Breast procedures, skin only			
6 Skin, Back			
7 Skin, Abdomen			
8 Skin, Buttock			
9 Skin, Perineum			
A Skin, Inguinal			
B Skin, Right Upper Arm			
C Skin, Left Upper Arm			
D Skin, Right Lower Arm			
E Skin, Left Lower Arm			
F Skin, Right Hand			
G Skin, Left Hand			
H Skin, Right Upper Leg			
J Skin, Left Upper Leg			
K Skin, Right Lower Leg			
L Skin, Left Lower Leg			
M Skin, Right Foot			
N Skin, Left Foot			

Non-OR   All body part, approach, device, and qualifier values

Skin and Breast

Ø   **Medical and Surgical**
H   **Skin and Breast**
9   **Drainage**   Definition: Taking or letting out fluids and/or gases from a body part
                           Explanation: The qualifier DIAGNOSTIC is used to identify drainage procedures that are biopsies

Body Part Character 4		Approach Character 5	Device Character 6	Qualifier Character 7

Ø Skin, Scalp
1 Skin, Face
2 Skin, Right Ear
3 Skin, Left Ear
4 Skin, Neck
5 Skin, Chest
   Breast procedures, skin
     only
6 Skin, Back
7 Skin, Abdomen
8 Skin, Buttock
9 Skin, Perineum
A Skin, Inguinal
B Skin, Right Upper Arm
C Skin, Left Upper Arm
D Skin, Right Lower Arm
	E Skin, Left Lower Arm
	F Skin, Right Hand
	G Skin, Left Hand
	H Skin, Right Upper Leg
	J Skin, Left Upper Leg
	K Skin, Right Lower Leg
	L Skin, Left Lower Leg
	M Skin, Right Foot
	N Skin, Left Foot
	Q Finger Nail
	   Nail bed
	   Nail plate
	R Toe Nail
	   See Q Finger Nail
		X External	Ø Drainage Device	Z No Qualifier

Ø Skin, Scalp
1 Skin, Face
2 Skin, Right Ear
3 Skin, Left Ear
4 Skin, Neck
5 Skin, Chest
   Breast procedures, skin
     only
6 Skin, Back
7 Skin, Abdomen
8 Skin, Buttock
9 Skin, Perineum
A Skin, Inguinal
B Skin, Right Upper Arm
C Skin, Left Upper Arm
D Skin, Right Lower Arm
	E Skin, Left Lower Arm
	F Skin, Right Hand
	G Skin, Left Hand
	H Skin, Right Upper Leg
	J Skin, Left Upper Leg
	K Skin, Right Lower Leg
	L Skin, Left Lower Leg
	M Skin, Right Foot
	N Skin, Left Foot
	Q Finger Nail
	   Nail bed
	   Nail plate
	R Toe Nail
	   See Q Finger Nail
		X External	Z No Device	X Diagnostic
				Z No Qualifier

T Breast, Right
   Mammary duct
   Mammary gland
U Breast, Left
   See T Breast, Right
V Breast, Bilateral
   See T Breast, Right
		Ø Open
		3 Percutaneous
		7 Via Natural or Artificial
		   Opening
		8 Via Natural or Artificial
		   Opening Endoscopic
			Ø Drainage Device	Z No Qualifier

T Breast, Right
   Mammary duct
   Mammary gland
U Breast, Left
   See T Breast, Right
V Breast, Bilateral
   See T Breast, Right
		Ø Open
		3 Percutaneous
		7 Via Natural or Artificial
		   Opening
		8 Via Natural or Artificial
		   Opening Endoscopic
			Z No Device	X Diagnostic
				Z No Qualifier

W Nipple, Right
   Areola
X Nipple, Left
   See W Nipple, Right
		Ø Open
		3 Percutaneous
		7 Via Natural or Artificial
		   Opening
		8 Via Natural or Artificial
		   Opening Endoscopic
		X External
			Ø Drainage Device	Z No Qualifier

W Nipple, Right
   Areola
X Nipple, Left
   See W Nipple, Right
		Ø Open
		3 Percutaneous
		7 Via Natural or Artificial
		   Opening
		8 Via Natural or Artificial
		   Opening Endoscopic
		X External
			Z No Device	X Diagnostic
				Z No Qualifier

Non-OR   ØH9[Ø,1,2,3,4,5,6,7,8,A,B,C,D,E,F,G,H,J,K,L,M,N,Q,R]XØZ
Non-OR   ØH9[Ø,1,2,3,4,5,6,7,8,A,B,C,D,E,F,G,H,J,K,L,M,N,Q,R]XZ[X,Z]
Non-OR   ØH99XZX
Non-OR   ØH9[T,U,V][Ø,3,7,8]ØZ
Non-OR   ØH9[T,U,V][3,7,8]Z[X,Z]
Non-OR   ØH9[W,X][Ø,3,7,8,X]ØZ
Non-OR   ØH9[W,X][3,7,8,X]Z[X,Z]

Ø   **Medical and Surgical**
H   **Skin and Breast**
B   **Excision**   Definition: Cutting out or off, without replacement, a portion of a body part

                           Explanation: The qualifier DIAGNOSTIC is used to identify excision procedures that are biopsies

Body Part Character 4	Approach Character 5	Device Character 6	Qualifier Character 7

Ø Skin, Scalp
1 Skin, Face
2 Skin, Right Ear
3 Skin, Left Ear
4 Skin, Neck
5 Skin, Chest
     Breast procedures, skin only
6 Skin, Back
7 Skin, Abdomen
8 Skin, Buttock
9 Skin, Perineum
A Skin, Inguinal
B Skin, Right Upper Arm
C Skin, Left Upper Arm
D Skin, Right Lower Arm
E Skin, Left Lower Arm
F Skin, Right Hand
G Skin, Left Hand
H Skin, Right Upper Leg
J Skin, Left Upper Leg
K Skin, Right Lower Leg
L Skin, Left Lower Leg
M Skin, Right Foot
N Skin, Left Foot
Q Finger Nail
     Nail bed
     Nail plate
R Toe Nail
     See Q Finger Nail
	X External	**Z** No Device	**X** Diagnostic
			Z No Qualifier

T Breast, Right
     Mammary duct
     Mammary gland
U Breast, Left
     See T Breast, Right
V Breast, Bilateral
     See T Breast, Right
Y Supernumerary Breast
	Ø Open
	3 Percutaneous
	7 Via Natural or Artificial Opening
	8 Via Natural or Artificial Opening
	     Endoscopic
		Z No Device	**X** Diagnostic
			Z No Qualifier

W Nipple, Right
     Areola
X Nipple, Left
     See W Nipple, Right
	Ø Open
	3 Percutaneous
	7 Via Natural or Artificial Opening
	8 Via Natural or Artificial Opening
	     Endoscopic
	X External
		Z No Device	**X** Diagnostic
			Z No Qualifier

DRG Non-OR	ØHB9XZZ
Non-OR	ØHB[Ø,1,2,3,4,5,6,7,8,A,B,C,D,E,F,G,H,J,K,L,M,N,Q,R]XZ[X,Z]
Non-OR	ØHB9XZX
Non-OR	ØHB[T,U,V,Y][3,7,8]ZX
Non-OR	ØHB[W,X][3,7,8,X]ZX

Ø   **Medical and Surgical**
H   **Skin and Breast**
C   **Extirpation**   Definition: Taking or cutting out solid matter from a body part

Explanation: The solid matter may be an abnormal byproduct of a biological function or a foreign body; it may be imbedded in a body part or in the lumen of a tubular body part. The solid matter may or may not have been previously broken into pieces.

Body Part Character 4	Approach Character 5	Device Character 6	Qualifier Character 7
Ø Skin, Scalp	**X** External	**Z** No Device	**Z** No Qualifier
1 Skin, Face			
2 Skin, Right Ear			
3 Skin, Left Ear			
4 Skin, Neck			
5 Skin, Chest Breast procedures, skin only			
6 Skin, Back			
7 Skin, Abdomen			
8 Skin, Buttock			
9 Skin, Perineum			
A Skin, Inguinal			
B Skin, Right Upper Arm			
C Skin, Left Upper Arm			
D Skin, Right Lower Arm			
E Skin, Left Lower Arm			
F Skin, Right Hand			
G Skin, Left Hand			
H Skin, Right Upper Leg			
J Skin, Left Upper Leg			
K Skin, Right Lower Leg			
L Skin, Left Lower Leg			
M Skin, Right Foot			
N Skin, Left Foot			

Q Finger Nail
   Nail bed
   Nail plate			

R Toe Nail *See Q Finger Nail*			

T Breast, Right
   Mammary duct
   Mammary gland
	Ø Open
	3 Percutaneous
	7 Via Natural or Artificial Opening
	8 Via Natural or Artificial Opening Endoscopic
		Z No Device	**Z** No Qualifier

U Breast, Left *See T Breast, Right*			
V Breast, Bilateral *See T Breast, Right*			
W Nipple, Right Areola	**Ø** Open **3** Percutaneous **7** Via Natural or Artificial Opening **8** Via Natural or Artificial Opening Endoscopic **X** External	**Z** No Device	**Z** No Qualifier
X Nipple, Left *See W Nipple, Right*			

Non-OR   ØHC[Ø,1,2,3,4,5,6,7,8,9,A,B,C,D,E,F,G,H,J,K,L,M,N,Q,R]XZZ
Non-OR   ØHC[T,U,V][3,7,8]ZZ
Non-OR   ØHC[W,X][3,7,8,X]ZZ

Ø   Medical and Surgical
H   Skin and Breast
D   Extraction   Definition: Pulling or stripping out or off all or a portion of a body part by the use of force
                                Explanation: The qualifier DIAGNOSTIC is used to identify extraction procedures that are biopsies

Body Part Character 4	Approach Character 5	Device Character 6	Qualifier Character 7

Ø Skin, Scalp
1 Skin, Face
2 Skin, Right Ear
3 Skin, Left Ear
4 Skin, Neck
5 Skin, Chest
     Breast procedures, skin only
6 Skin, Back
7 Skin, Abdomen
8 Skin, Buttock
9 Skin, Perineum
A Skin, Inguinal
B Skin, Right Upper Arm
C Skin, Left Upper Arm
D Skin, Right Lower Arm
E Skin, Left Lower Arm
F Skin, Right Hand
G Skin, Left Hand
H Skin, Right Upper Leg
J Skin, Left Upper Leg
K Skin, Right Lower Leg
L Skin, Left Lower Leg
M Skin, Right Foot
N Skin, Left Foot
Q Finger Nail
     Nail bed
     Nail plate
R Toe Nail
     See Q Finger Nail
S Hair
	X External	**Z** No Device	**Z** No Qualifier

T Breast, Right
     Mammary duct
     Mammary gland
U Breast, Left
     See T Breast, Right
V Breast, Bilateral
     See T Breast, Right
Y Supernumerary Breast
	Ø Open	**Z** No Device	**Z** No Qualifier

Non-OR   All body part, approach, device, and qualifier values

---

LC Limited Coverage   NC Noncovered   ⊞ Combination Member   HAC associated procedure   Combination Only   DRG Non-OR   Non-OR   New/Revised in GREEN

Ø Medical and Surgical
H Skin and Breast
H Insertion   Definition: Putting in a nonbiological appliance that monitors, assists, performs, or prevents a physiological function but does not physically take the place of a body part
                 Explanation: None

Body Part Character 4	Approach Character 5	Device Character 6	Qualifier Character 7
P Skin	**X** External	**Y** Other Device	**Z** No Qualifier
T Breast, Right Mammary duct Mammary gland **U Breast, Left** *See T Breast, Right*	**Ø** Open **3** Percutaneous **7** Via Natural or Artificial Opening **8** Via Natural or Artificial Opening Endoscopic	**1** Radioactive Element **N** Tissue Expander **Y** Other Device	**Z** No Qualifier
V Breast, Bilateral Mammary duct Mammary gland	**Ø** Open **3** Percutaneous **7** Via Natural or Artificial Opening **8** Via Natural or Artificial Opening Endoscopic	**1** Radioactive Element **N** Tissue Expander	**Z** No Qualifier
W Nipple, Right Areola **X Nipple, Left** *See W Nipple, Right*	**Ø** Open **3** Percutaneous **7** Via Natural or Artificial Opening **8** Via Natural or Artificial Opening Endoscopic	**1** Radioactive Element **N** Tissue Expander	**Z** No Qualifier
W Nipple, Right Areola **X Nipple, Left** *See W Nipple, Right*	**X** External	**1** Radioactive Element	**Z** No Qualifier

Non-OR   ØHHPXYZ
Non-OR   ØHH[T,U][3,7,8]YZ

Ø Medical and Surgical
H Skin and Breast
J Inspection   Definition: Visually and/or manually exploring a body part
                 Explanation: Visual exploration may be performed with or without optical instrumentation. Manual exploration may be performed directly or through intervening body layers.

Body Part Character 4	Approach Character 5	Device Character 6	Qualifier Character 7
P Skin Dermis Epidermis Sebaceous gland Sweat gland **Q Finger Nail** Nail bed Nail plate **R Toe Nail** *See Q Finger Nail*	**X** External	**Z** No Device	**Z** No Qualifier
T Breast, Right Mammary duct Mammary gland **U Breast, Left** *See T Breast, Right*	**Ø** Open **3** Percutaneous **7** Via Natural or Artificial Opening **8** Via Natural or Artificial Opening Endoscopic	**Z** No Device	**Z** No Qualifier

Non-OR   All body part, approach, device and qualifier values

Ø   **Medical and Surgical**
H   **Skin and Breast**
M   **Reattachment**   Definition: Putting back in or on all or a portion of a separated body part to its normal location or other suitable location
                               Explanation: Vascular circulation and nervous pathways may or may not be reestablished

Body Part Character 4	Approach Character 5	Device Character 6	Qualifier Character 7
Ø Skin, Scalp	**X** External	**Z** No Device	**Z** No Qualifier
1 Skin, Face			
2 Skin, Right Ear			
3 Skin, Left Ear			
4 Skin, Neck			
5 Skin, Chest Breast procedures, skin only			
6 Skin, Back			
7 Skin, Abdomen			
8 Skin, Buttock			
9 Skin, Perineum			
A Skin, Inguinal			
B Skin, Right Upper Arm			
C Skin, Left Upper Arm			
D Skin, Right Lower Arm			
E Skin, Left Lower Arm			
F Skin, Right Hand			
G Skin, Left Hand			
H Skin, Right Upper Leg			
J Skin, Left Upper Leg			
K Skin, Right Lower Leg			
L Skin, Left Lower Leg			
M Skin, Right Foot			
N Skin, Left Foot			

T Breast, Right
    Mammary duct
    Mammary gland			

U Breast, Left *See T Breast, Right*			
V Breast, Bilateral *See T Breast, Right*			
W Nipple, Right Areola			
X Nipple, Left *See W Nipple, Right*			

Non-OR   ØHMØXZZ

Skin and Breast

Ø   **Medical and Surgical**
H   **Skin and Breast**
N   **Release**   Definition: Freeing a body part from an abnormal physical constraint by cutting or by the use of force
                            Explanation: Some of the restraining tissue may be taken out but none of the body part is taken out

Body Part Character 4	Approach Character 5	Device Character 6	Qualifier Character 7

Ø   Skin, Scalp
1   Skin, Face
2   Skin, Right Ear
3   Skin, Left Ear
4   Skin, Neck
5   Skin, Chest
     Breast procedures, skin only
6   Skin, Back
7   Skin, Abdomen
8   Skin, Buttock
9   Skin, Perineum
A   Skin, Inguinal
B   Skin, Right Upper Arm
C   Skin, Left Upper Arm
D   Skin, Right Lower Arm
E   Skin, Left Lower Arm
F   Skin, Right Hand
G   Skin, Left Hand
H   Skin, Right Upper Leg
J   Skin, Left Upper Leg
K   Skin, Right Lower Leg
L   Skin, Left Lower Leg
M   Skin, Right Foot
N   Skin, Left Foot
Q   Finger Nail
     Nail bed
     Nail plate
R   Toe Nail
     See Q Finger Nail
	X External	Z No Device	Z No Qualifier

T   Breast, Right
     Mammary duct
     Mammary gland
U   Breast, Left
     See T Breast, Right
V   Breast, Bilateral
     See T Breast, Right
	Ø Open
	3 Percutaneous
	7 Via Natural or Artificial Opening
	8 Via Natural or Artificial Opening
	     Endoscopic
		Z No Device	Z No Qualifier

W   Nipple, Right
     Areola
X   Nipple, Left
     See W Nipple, Right
	Ø Open
	3 Percutaneous
	7 Via Natural or Artificial Opening
	8 Via Natural or Artificial Opening
	     Endoscopic
	X External
		Z No Device	Z No Qualifier

Ø   **Medical and Surgical**
H   **Skin and Breast**
P   **Removal**   Definition: Taking out or off a device from a body part

Explanation: If a device is taken out and a similar device put in without cutting or puncturing the skin or mucous membrane, the procedure is coded to the root operation CHANGE. Otherwise, the procedure for taking out a device is coded to the root operation REMOVAL.

Body Part Character 4	Approach Character 5	Device Character 6	Qualifier Character 7

P   **Skin**
   Dermis
   Epidermis
   Sebaceous gland
   Sweat gland
	X External	**Ø** Drainage Device
		7 Autologous Tissue Substitute
		J Synthetic Substitute
		K Nonautologous Tissue Substitute
		Y Other Device
			Z No Qualifier

Q   **Finger Nail**
   Nail bed
   Nail plate
R   **Toe Nail**
   See Q Finger Nail
	X External	**Ø** Drainage Device
		7 Autologous Tissue Substitute
		J Synthetic Substitute
		K Nonautologous Tissue Substitute
			Z No Qualifier

S **Hair**	**X** External	**7** Autologous Tissue Substitute **J** Synthetic Substitute **K** Nonautologous Tissue Substitute	**Z** No Qualifier

T   **Breast, Right**
   Mammary duct
   Mammary gland
U   **Breast, Left**
   See T Breast, Right
	Ø Open
	3 Percutaneous
	7 Via Natural or Artificial Opening
	8 Via Natural or Artificial Opening Endoscopic
		Ø Drainage Device
		1 Radioactive Element
		7 Autologous Tissue Substitute
		J Synthetic Substitute
		K Nonautologous Tissue Substitute
		N Tissue Expander
		Y Other Device
			Z No Qualifier

Non-OR   ØHPPX[Ø,7,J,K,Y]Z
Non-OR   ØHP[Q,R]X[Ø,7,J,K]Z
Non-OR   ØHPSX[7,J,K]Z
Non-OR   ØHP[T,U]Ø[Ø,1,7,K]Z
Non-OR   ØHP[T,U]3[Ø,1,7,K,Y]Z
Non-OR   ØHP[T,U][7,8][Ø,1,7,J,K,N,Y]Z

LC Limited Coverage   **NC** Noncovered   ⊞ Combination Member   HAC associated procedure   Combination Only   DRG Non-OR   Non-OR   New/Revised in GREEN

ICD-10-PCS 2021   **433**

ØHP–ØHP

Ø   Medical and Surgical
H   Skin and Breast
Q   Repair   Definition: Restoring, to the extent possible, a body part to its normal anatomic structure and function
                    Explanation: Used only when the method to accomplish the repair is not one of the other root operations

Body Part Character 4	Approach Character 5	Device Character 6	Qualifier Character 7

Ø Skin, Scalp
1 Skin, Face
2 Skin, Right Ear
3 Skin, Left Ear
4 Skin, Neck
5 Skin, Chest
    Breast procedures, skin only
6 Skin, Back
7 Skin, Abdomen
8 Skin, Buttock
9 Skin, Perineum
A Skin, Inguinal
B Skin, Right Upper Arm
C Skin, Left Upper Arm
D Skin, Right Lower Arm
E Skin, Left Lower Arm
F Skin, Right Hand
G Skin, Left Hand
H Skin, Right Upper Leg
J Skin, Left Upper Leg
K Skin, Right Lower Leg
L Skin, Left Lower Leg
M Skin, Right Foot
N Skin, Left Foot
Q Finger Nail
    Nail bed
    Nail plate
R Toe Nail
    See Q Finger Nail
	X External	**Z** No Device	**Z** No Qualifier

T Breast, Right
    Mammary duct
    Mammary gland
U Breast, Left
    See T Breast, Right
V Breast, Bilateral
    See T Breast, Right
Y Supernumerary Breast
	Ø Open
	3 Percutaneous
	7 Via Natural or Artificial Opening
	8 Via Natural or Artificial Opening
	    Endoscopic
		Z No Device	**Z** No Qualifier

W Nipple, Right
    Areola
X Nipple, Left
    See W Nipple, Right
	Ø Open
	3 Percutaneous
	7 Via Natural or Artificial Opening
	8 Via Natural or Artificial Opening
	    Endoscopic
	X External
		Z No Device	**Z** No Qualifier

DRG Non-OR   ØHQ9XZZ
Non-OR   ØHQ[Ø,1,2,3,4,5,6,7,8,A,B,C,D,E,F,G,H,J,K,L,M,N]XZZ

Ø   Medical and Surgical
H   Skin and Breast
R   Replacement   Definition: Putting in or on biological or synthetic material that physically takes the place and/or function of all or a portion of a body part
                           Explanation: The body part may have been taken out or replaced, or may be taken out, physically eradicated, or rendered nonfunctional during the REPLACEMENT procedure. A REMOVAL procedure is coded for taking out the device used in a previous replacement procedure.

Body Part Character 4		Approach Character 5	Device Character 6	Qualifier Character 7
Ø Skin, Scalp 1 Skin, Face 2 Skin, Right Ear 3 Skin, Left Ear 4 Skin, Neck 5 Skin, Chest Breast procedures, skin only 6 Skin, Back 7 Skin, Abdomen 8 Skin, Buttock 9 Skin, Perineum A Skin, Inguinal	B Skin, Right Upper Arm C Skin, Left Upper Arm D Skin, Right Lower Arm E Skin, Left Lower Arm F Skin, Right Hand G Skin, Left Hand H Skin, Right Upper Leg J Skin, Left Upper Leg K Skin, Right Lower Leg L Skin, Left Lower Leg M Skin, Right Foot N Skin, Left Foot	X External	7 Autologous Tissue Substitute	2 Cell Suspension Technique 3 Full Thickness 4 Partial Thickness
Ø Skin, Scalp 1 Skin, Face 2 Skin, Right Ear 3 Skin, Left Ear 4 Skin, Neck 5 Skin, Chest Breast procedures, skin only 6 Skin, Back 7 Skin, Abdomen 8 Skin, Buttock 9 Skin, Perineum A Skin, Inguinal	B Skin, Right Upper Arm C Skin, Left Upper Arm D Skin, Right Lower Arm E Skin, Left Lower Arm F Skin, Right Hand G Skin, Left Hand H Skin, Right Upper Leg J Skin, Left Upper Leg K Skin, Right Lower Leg L Skin, Left Lower Leg M Skin, Right Foot N Skin, Left Foot	X External	J Synthetic Substitute	3 Full Thickness 4 Partial Thickness Z No Qualifier
Ø Skin, Scalp 1 Skin, Face 2 Skin, Right Ear 3 Skin, Left Ear 4 Skin, Neck 5 Skin, Chest Breast procedures, skin only 6 Skin, Back 7 Skin, Abdomen 8 Skin Buttock 9 Skin, Perineum A Skin, Inguinal	B Skin, Right Upper Arm C Skin, Left Upper Arm D Skin, Right Lower Arm E Skin, Left Lower Arm F Skin, Right Hand G Skin, Left Hand H Skin, Right Upper Leg J Skin, Left Upper Leg K Skin, Right Lower Leg L Skin, Left Lower Leg M Skin, Right Foot N Skin, Left Foot	X External	K Nonautologous Tissue Substitute	3 Full Thickness 4 Partial Thickness

Q Finger Nail
    Nail bed
    Nail plate
	R Toe Nail
	    See Q Finger Nail
	S Hair
		X External	7 Autologous Tissue Substitute
			J Synthetic Substitute
			K Nonautologous Tissue Substitute
				Z No Qualifier

T Breast, Right
    Mammary duct
    Mammary gland
	U Breast, Left
	    See T Breast, Right
	V Breast, Bilateral
	    See T Breast, Right
		Ø Open	7 Autologous Tissue Substitute	5 Latissimus Dorsi Myocutaneous Flap
				6 Transverse Rectus Abdominis Myocutaneous Flap
				7 Deep Inferior Epigastric Artery Perforator Flap
				8 Superficial Inferior Epigastric Artery Flap
				9 Gluteal Artery Perforator Flap
				Z No Qualifier

T Breast, Right
    Mammary duct
    Mammary gland
	U Breast, Left
	    See T Breast, Right
	V Breast, Bilateral
	    See T Breast, Right
		Ø Open	J Synthetic Substitute
			K Nonautologous Tissue Substitute
				Z No Qualifier

T Breast, Right ⊞
    Mammary duct
    Mammary gland
U Breast, Left ⊞
    See T Breast, Right
	V Breast, Bilateral ⊞
	    See T Breast, Right
		3 Percutaneous	7 Autologous Tissue Substitute
			J Synthetic Substitute
			K Nonautologous Tissue Substitute
				Z No Qualifier

W Nipple, Right
    Areola
	X Nipple, Left
	    See W Nipple, Right
		Ø Open
		3 Percutaneous
		X External
			7 Autologous Tissue Substitute
			J Synthetic Substitute
			K Nonautologous Tissue Substitute
				Z No Qualifier

Non-OR   ØHRSX7Z   **See Appendix L for Procedure Combinations**
                                          ⊞   ØHR[T,U,V]37Z

ⒾⒸ Limited Coverage   ⓃⒸ Noncovered   ⊞ Combination Member   HAC associated procedure   Combination Only   DRG Non-OR   Non-OR   New/Revised in GREEN

ICD-10-PCS 2021   435

ØHR–ØHR

Ø Medical and Surgical
H Skin and Breast
S Reposition

Definition: Moving to its normal location, or other suitable location, all or a portion of a body part

Explanation: The body part is moved to a new location from an abnormal location, or from a normal location where it is not functioning correctly. The body part may or may not be cut out or off to be moved to the new location.

Body Part Character 4	Approach Character 5	Device Character 6	Qualifier Character 7

S Hair
W Nipple, Right
   Areola
X Nipple, Left
   See W Nipple, Right
	X External	Z No Device	Z No Qualifier

T Breast, Right
   Mammary duct
   Mammary gland
U Breast, Left
   See T Breast, Right
V Breast, Bilateral
   See T Breast, Right
	Ø Open	Z No Device	Z No Qualifier

Non-OR ØHSSXZZ

Ø Medical and Surgical
H Skin and Breast
T Resection

Definition: Cutting out or off, without replacement, all of a body part

Explanation: None

Body Part Character 4	Approach Character 5	Device Character 6	Qualifier Character 7

Q Finger Nail
   Nail bed
   Nail plate
R Toe Nail
   See Q Finger Nail
W Nipple, Right
   Areola
X Nipple, Left
   See W Nipple, Right
	X External	Z No Device	Z No Qualifier

⊞ T Breast, Right
   Mammary duct
   Mammary gland
⊞ U Breast, Left
   See T Breast, Right
⊞ V Breast, Bilateral
   See T Breast, Right
Y Supernumerary Breast
	Ø Open	Z No Device	Z No Qualifier

Non-OR ØHT[Q,R]XZZ

See Appendix L for Procedure Combinations
⊞   ØHT[T,U,V]ØZZ

Ø Medical and Surgical
H Skin and Breast
U Supplement

Definition: Putting in or on biological or synthetic material that physically reinforces and/or augments the function of a portion of a body part

Explanation: The biological material is non-living, or is living and from the same individual. The body part may have been previously replaced, and the SUPPLEMENT procedure is performed to physically reinforce and/or augment the function of the replaced body part.

Body Part Character 4	Approach Character 5	Device Character 6	Qualifier Character 7

T Breast, Right
   Mammary duct
   Mammary gland
U Breast, Left
   See T Breast, Right
V Breast, Bilateral
   See T Breast, Right
	Ø Open
	3 Percutaneous
	7 Via Natural or Artificial Opening
	8 Via Natural or Artificial Opening Endoscopic
		7 Autologous Tissue Substitute
		J Synthetic Substitute
		K Nonautologous Tissue Substitute
			Z No Qualifier

W Nipple, Right
   Areola
X Nipple, Left
   See W Nipple, Right
	Ø Open
	3 Percutaneous
	7 Via Natural or Artificial Opening
	8 Via Natural or Artificial Opening Endoscopic
	X External
		7 Autologous Tissue Substitute
		J Synthetic Substitute
		K Nonautologous Tissue Substitute
			Z No Qualifier

Non-OR ØHU[T,U,V]3JZ

⟦LC⟧ Limited Coverage   ⟦NC⟧ Noncovered   ⊞ Combination Member   HAC associated procedure   Combination Only   DRG Non-OR   Non-OR   New/Revised in **GREEN**

436   ICD-10-PCS 2021

Ø   Medical and Surgical
H   Skin and Breast
W   Revision   Definition: Correcting, to the extent possible, a portion of a malfunctioning device or the position of a displaced device
                    Explanation: Revision can include correcting a malfunctioning or displaced device by taking out or putting in components of the device such as a screw or pin

Body Part Character 4	Approach Character 5	Device Character 6	Qualifier Character 7

P **Skin**
    Dermis
    Epidermis
    Sebaceous gland
    Sweat gland
	X External	**Ø** Drainage Device
		7 Autologous Tissue Substitute
		J Synthetic Substitute
		K Nonautologous Tissue Substitute
		Y Other Device
			Z No Qualifier

Q **Finger Nail**
    Nail bed
    Nail plate
R **Toe Nail**
    See Q Finger Nail
	X External	**Ø** Drainage Device
		7 Autologous Tissue Substitute
		J Synthetic Substitute
		K Nonautologous Tissue Substitute
			Z No Qualifier

S **Hair**	**X** External	**7** Autologous Tissue Substitute **J** Synthetic Substitute **K** Nonautologous Tissue Substitute	**Z** No Qualifier

T **Breast, Right**
    Mammary duct
    Mammary gland
U **Breast, Left**
    See T Breast, Right
	Ø Open
	3 Percutaneous
	7 Via Natural or Artificial Opening
	8 Via Natural or Artificial Opening Endoscopic
		Ø Drainage Device
		7 Autologous Tissue Substitute
		J Synthetic Substitute
		K Nonautologous Tissue Substitute
		N Tissue Expander
		Y Other Device
			Z No Qualifier

Non-OR	ØHWPX[Ø,7,J,K,Y]Z
Non-OR	ØHW[Q,R]X[Ø,7,J,K]Z
Non-OR	ØHWSX[7,J,K]Z
Non-OR	ØHW[T,U]Ø[Ø,7,K,N]Z
Non-OR	ØHW[T,U]3[Ø,7,K,N,Y]Z
Non-OR	ØHW[T,U][7,8][Ø,7,J,K,N,Y]Z

Ø   Medical and Surgical
H   Skin and Breast
X   Transfer   Definition: Moving, without taking out, all or a portion of a body part to another location to take over the function of all or a portion of a body part
                    Explanation: The body part transferred remains connected to its vascular and nervous supply

Body Part Character 4	Approach Character 5	Device Character 6	Qualifier Character 7
Ø Skin, Scalp **1** Skin, Face **2** Skin, Right Ear **3** Skin, Left Ear **4** Skin, Neck **5** Skin, Chest Breast procedures, skin only **6** Skin, Back **7** Skin, Abdomen **8** Skin, Buttock **9** Skin, Perineum **A** Skin, Inguinal **B** Skin, Right Upper Arm **C** Skin, Left Upper Arm **D** Skin, Right Lower Arm **E** Skin, Left Lower Arm **F** Skin, Right Hand **G** Skin, Left Hand **H** Skin, Right Upper Leg **J** Skin, Left Upper Leg **K** Skin, Right Lower Leg **L** Skin, Left Lower Leg **M** Skin, Right Foot **N** Skin, Left Foot	**X** External	**Z** No Device	**Z** No Qualifier

LC Limited Coverage   **NC** Noncovered   ⊞ Combination Member   HAC associated procedure   Combination Only   DRG Non-OR   Non-OR   New/Revised in GREEN

ICD-10-PCS 2021   437

ØHW–ØHX

Subcutaneous Tissue and Fascia ØJØ–ØJX

Character Meanings

This Character Meaning table is provided as a guide to assist the user in the identification of character members that may be found in this section of code tables. It **SHOULD NOT** be used to build a PCS code.

Operation–Character 3		Body Part–Character 4		Approach–Character 5		Device–Character 6		Qualifier–Character 7	
Ø	Alteration	Ø	Subcutaneous Tissue and Fascia, Scalp	Ø	Open	Ø	Drainage Device OR Monitoring Device, Hemodynamic	B	Skin and Subcutaneous Tissue
2	Change	1	Subcutaneous Tissue and Fascia, Face	3	Percutaneous	1	Radioactive Element	C	Skin, Subcutaneous Tissue and Fascia
5	Destruction	4	Subcutaneous Tissue and Fascia, Right Neck	X	External	2	Monitoring Device	X	Diagnostic
8	Division	5	Subcutaneous Tissue and Fascia, Left Neck			3	Infusion Device	Z	No Qualifier
9	Drainage	6	Subcutaneous Tissue and Fascia, Chest			4	Pacemaker, Single Chamber		
B	Excision	7	Subcutaneous Tissue and Fascia, Back			5	Pacemaker, Single Chamber Rate Responsive		
C	Extirpation	8	Subcutaneous Tissue and Fascia, Abdomen			6	Pacemaker, Dual Chamber		
D	Extraction	9	Subcutaneous Tissue and Fascia, Buttock			7	Autologous Tissue Substitute OR Cardiac Resynchronization Pacemaker Pulse Generator		
H	Insertion	B	Subcutaneous Tissue and Fascia, Perineum			8	Defibrillator Generator		
J	Inspection	C	Subcutaneous Tissue and Fascia, Pelvic Region			9	Cardiac Resynchronization Defibrillator Pulse Generator		
N	Release	D	Subcutaneous Tissue and Fascia, Right Upper Arm			A	Contractility Modulation Device		
P	Removal	F	Subcutaneous Tissue and Fascia, Left Upper Arm			B	Stimulator Generator, Single Array		
Q	Repair	G	Subcutaneous Tissue and Fascia, Right Lower Arm			C	Stimulator Generator, Single Array Rechargeable		
R	Replacement	H	Subcutaneous Tissue and Fascia, Left Lower Arm			D	Stimulator Generator, Multiple Array		
U	Supplement	J	Subcutaneous Tissue and Fascia, Right Hand			E	Stimulator Generator, Multiple Array Rechargeable		
W	Revision	K	Subcutaneous Tissue and Fascia, Left Hand			F	Subcutaneous Defibrillator Lead		
X	Transfer	L	Subcutaneous Tissue and Fascia, Right Upper Leg			H	Contraceptive Device		
		M	Subcutaneous Tissue and Fascia, Left Upper Leg			J	Synthetic Substitute		
		N	Subcutaneous Tissue and Fascia, Right Lower Leg			K	Nonautologous Tissue Substitute		
		P	Subcutaneous Tissue and Fascia, Left Lower Leg			M	Stimulator Generator		
		Q	Subcutaneous Tissue and Fascia, Right Foot			N	Tissue Expander		
		R	Subcutaneous Tissue and Fascia, Left Foot			P	Cardiac Rhythm Related Device		
		S	Subcutaneous Tissue and Fascia, Head and Neck			V	Infusion Device, Pump		
		T	Subcutaneous Tissue and Fascia, Trunk			W	Vascular Access Device, Totally Implantable		
		V	Subcutaneous Tissue and Fascia, Upper Extremity			X	Vascular Access Device, Tunneled		
		W	Subcutaneous Tissue and Fascia, Lower Extremity			Y	Other Device		
						Z	No Device		

AHA Coding Clinic for table ØJ2

2018, 3Q, 10	Disruption of perma-catheter fibrin sheath via angioplasty of superior vena cava
2017, 2Q, 26	Exchange of tunneled catheter

AHA Coding Clinic for table ØJ5

2019, 3Q, 25	Endoscopic removal of pilonidal sinus and cyst

AHA Coding Clinic for table ØJ8

2017, 3Q, 11	Bilateral escharotomy of leg, thigh and foot

AHA Coding Clinic for table ØJ9

2018, 3Q, 16	Incision and drainage of submandibular space
2018, 3Q, 16	Incision and drainage of neck abscess
2015, 3Q, 23	Incision and drainage of multiple abscess cavities using vessel loop

AHA Coding Clinic for table ØJB

2020, 1Q, 31	Repair of buried penis
2019, 3Q, 25	Endoscopic removal of pilonidal sinus and cyst
2018, 3Q, 17	Excisional debridement of periosteum
2018, 1Q, 7	Placement of fat graft following lumbar decompression surgery
2015, 3Q, 3-8	Excisional and nonexcisional debridement
2015, 2Q, 13	Transfer of free flap to reconstruct orbital defect
2015, 1Q, 29	Fistulectomy with placement of seton
2014, 4Q, 38	Abdominoplasty and abdominal wall plication for hernia repair
2014, 3Q, 22	Transsphenoidal removal of pituitary tumor and fat graft placement

AHA Coding Clinic for table ØJC

2017, 3Q, 22	Replacement of native skull bone flap

AHA Coding Clinic for table ØJD

2016, 3Q, 20	VersaJet™ nonexcisional debridement of leg muscle
2016, 3Q, 21	Nonexcisional debridement of infected lumbar wound
2016, 3Q, 21	Nonexcisional pulsed lavage debridement
2016, 3Q, 22	Debridement of bone and tendon using Tenex ultrasound device
2016, 1Q, 40	Nonexcisional debridement of skin and subcutaneous tissue
2015, 3Q, 3-8	Excisional and nonexcisional debridement
2015, 1Q, 23	Non-Excisional debridement with lavage of wound

AHA Coding Clinic for table ØJH

2020, 2Q, 15	Ommaya Reservoir with Ventricular Catheter Placement
2020, 2Q, 16	Ommaya Reservoir Placement for Cerebrospinal Fluid Infusion Therapy
2019, 4Q, 33	Subcutaneous implantable cardioverter defibrillator lead
2017, 4Q, 63-64	Added and revised device values - Vascular access reservoir
2017, 2Q, 24	Tunneled catheter versus totally implantable catheter
2017, 2Q, 26	Exchange of tunneled catheter
2016, 4Q, 97-98	Phrenic neurostimulator
2016, 2Q, 14	Insertion of peritoneal totally implantable venous access device
2016, 2Q, 15	Removal and replacement of tunneled internal jugular catheter
2015, 4Q, 14	New Section X codes—New Technology procedures
2015, 4Q, 30-31	Vascular access devices
2015, 2Q, 33	Totally implantable central venous access device (Port-a-Cath)
2014, 3Q, 19	End of life replacement of Baclofen pump
2013, 4Q, 116	Device character for Port-A-Cath placement
2012, 4Q, 104	Placement of subcutaneous implantable cardioverter defibrillator

AHA Coding Clinic for table ØJN

2017, 3Q, 11	Bilateral escharotomy of leg, thigh and foot

AHA Coding Clinic for table ØJP

2019, 4Q, 33	Subcutaneous implantable cardioverter defibrillator lead
2018, 4Q, 86	Placement of lumboatrial shunt
2018, 3Q, 29	Decommissioning of left ventricular assist device with exploration of mediastinum
2016, 2Q, 15	Removal and replacement of tunneled internal jugular catheter
2015, 4Q, 31	Vascular access devices
2014, 3Q, 19	End of life replacement of Baclofen pump
2013, 4Q, 109	Separating conjoined twins
2012, 4Q, 104	Placement of subcutaneous implantable cardioverter defibrillator

AHA Coding Clinic for table ØJQ

2017, 3Q, 19	Anterior repair of cystocele
2014, 4Q, 44	Posterior colporrhaphy/rectocele repair

AHA Coding Clinic for table ØJR

2015, 2Q, 13	Transfer of free flap to reconstruct orbital defect

AHA Coding Clinic for table ØJU

2018, 2Q, 20	Prelaminated free flap graft using Alloderm™
2018, 1Q, 7	Placement of fat graft following lumbar decompression surgery

AHA Coding Clinic for table ØJW

2019, 4Q, 33	Subcutaneous implantable cardioverter defibrillator lead
2018, 1Q, 8	Ventricular peritoneal shunt ligation
2015, 4Q, 33	Externalization of peritoneal dialysis catheter
2015, 2Q, 9	Revision of ventriculoperitoneal (VP) shunt
2012, 4Q, 104	Placement of subcutaneous implantable cardioverter defibrillator

AHA Coding Clinic for table ØJX

2018, 1Q, 10	Complex wound closure using pericranial flap
2014, 3Q, 18	Placement of reverse sural fasciocutaneous pedicle flap
2013, 4Q, 109	Separating conjoined twins

Ø Medical and Surgical
J Subcutaneous Tissue and Fascia
Ø Alteration   Definition: Modifying the anatomic structure of a body part without affecting the function of the body part
            Explanation: Principal purpose is to improve appearance

Body Part Character 4		Approach Character 5	Device Character 6	Qualifier Character 7

1 Subcutaneous Tissue and Fascia, Face
  Masseteric fascia
  Orbital fascia
  Submandibular space
	F Subcutaneous Tissue and Fascia, Left Upper Arm
	  See D Subcutaneous Tissue and Fascia, Right Upper Arm
		Ø Open
		3 Percutaneous
			Z No Device	Z No Qualifier

4 Subcutaneous Tissue and Fascia, Right Neck
  Deep cervical fascia
  Pretracheal fascia
  Prevertebral fascia
	G Subcutaneous Tissue and Fascia, Right Lower Arm
	  Antebrachial fascia
	  Bicipital aponeurosis			

5 Subcutaneous Tissue and Fascia, Left Neck
  See 4 Subcutaneous Tissue and Fascia, Right Neck
	H Subcutaneous Tissue and Fascia, Left Lower Arm
	  See G Subcutaneous Tissue and Fascia, Right Lower Arm			

6 Subcutaneous Tissue and Fascia, Chest
  Pectoral fascia
	L Subcutaneous Tissue and Fascia, Right Upper Leg
	  Crural fascia
	  Fascia lata
	  Iliac fascia
	  Iliotibial tract (band)			

7 Subcutaneous Tissue and Fascia, Back	M Subcutaneous Tissue and Fascia, Left Upper Leg *See L Subcutaneous Tissue and Fascia, Right Upper Leg*			
8 Subcutaneous Tissue and Fascia, Abdomen				
9 Subcutaneous Tissue and Fascia, Buttock	N Subcutaneous Tissue and Fascia, Right Lower Leg			

D Subcutaneous Tissue and Fascia, Right Upper Arm
  Axillary fascia
  Deltoid fascia
  Infraspinatus fascia
  Subscapular aponeurosis
  Supraspinatus fascia
	P Subcutaneous Tissue and Fascia, Left Lower Leg			

Ø Medical and Surgical
J Subcutaneous Tissue and Fascia
2 Change   Definition: Taking out or off a device from a body part and putting back an identical or similar device in or on the same body part without cutting or puncturing the skin or a mucous membrane
            Explanation: All CHANGE procedures are coded using the approach EXTERNAL

Body Part Character 4	Approach Character 5	Device Character 6	Qualifier Character 7
S Subcutaneous Tissue and Fascia, Head and Neck	X External	Ø Drainage Device	Z No Qualifier

T Subcutaneous Tissue and Fascia, Trunk
  External oblique aponeurosis
  Transversalis fascia
		Y Other Device	

V Subcutaneous Tissue and Fascia, Upper Extremity			
W Subcutaneous Tissue and Fascia, Lower Extremity			

   Non-OR   All body part, approach, device, and qualifier values

---

Ø   Medical and Surgical
J   Subcutaneous Tissue and Fascia
5   Destruction   Definition: Physical eradication of all or a portion of a body part by the direct use of energy, force, or a destructive agent
                       Explanation: None of the body part is physically taken out

Body Part Character 4		Approach Character 5	Device Character 6	Qualifier Character 7
Ø Subcutaneous Tissue and Fascia, Scalp Galea aponeurotica **1 Subcutaneous Tissue and Fascia, Face** Masseteric fascia Orbital fascia Submandibular space **4 Subcutaneous Tissue and Fascia, Right Neck** Deep cervical fascia Pretracheal fascia Prevertebral fascia **5 Subcutaneous Tissue and Fascia, Left Neck** *See 4 Subcutaneous Tissue and Fascia, Right Neck* **6 Subcutaneous Tissue and Fascia, Chest** Pectoral fascia **7 Subcutaneous Tissue and Fascia, Back** **8 Subcutaneous Tissue and Fascia, Abdomen** **9 Subcutaneous Tissue and Fascia, Buttock** **B Subcutaneous Tissue and Fascia, Perineum** **C Subcutaneous Tissue and Fascia, Pelvic Region** **D Subcutaneous Tissue and Fascia, Right Upper Arm** Axillary fascia Deltoid fascia Infraspinatus fascia Subscapular aponeurosis Supraspinatus fascia **F Subcutaneous Tissue and Fascia, Left Upper Arm** *See D Subcutaneous Tissue and Fascia, Right Upper Arm*	**G Subcutaneous Tissue and Fascia, Right Lower Arm** Antebrachial fascia Bicipital aponeurosis **H Subcutaneous Tissue and Fascia, Left Lower Arm** *See G Subcutaneous Tissue and Fascia, Right Lower Arm* **J Subcutaneous Tissue and Fascia, Right Hand** Palmar fascia (aponeurosis) **K Subcutaneous Tissue and Fascia, Left Hand** *See J Subcutaneous Tissue and Fascia, Right Hand* **L Subcutaneous Tissue and Fascia, Right Upper Leg** Crural fascia Fascia lata Iliac fascia Iliotibial tract (band) **M Subcutaneous Tissue and Fascia, Left Upper Leg** *See L Subcutaneous Tissue and Fascia, Right Upper Leg* **N Subcutaneous Tissue and Fascia, Right Lower Leg** **P Subcutaneous Tissue and Fascia, Left Lower Leg** **Q Subcutaneous Tissue and Fascia, Right Foot** Plantar fascia (aponeurosis) **R Subcutaneous Tissue and Fascia, Left Foot** *See Q Subcutaneous Tissue and Fascia, Right Foot*	**Ø Open** **3 Percutaneous**	**Z No Device**	**Z No Qualifier**

DRG Non-OR   All body part, approach, device, and qualifier values

Ø   **Medical and Surgical**
J   **Subcutaneous Tissue and Fascia**
8   **Division**   Definition: Cutting into a body part, without draining fluids and/or gases from the body part, in order to separate or transect a body part
                             Explanation: All or a portion of the body part is separated into two or more portions

Body Part Character 4		Approach Character 5	Device Character 6	Qualifier Character 7
Ø **Subcutaneous Tissue and Fascia, Scalp** Galea aponeurotica **1** **Subcutaneous Tissue and Fascia, Face** Masseteric fascia Orbital fascia Submandibular space **4** **Subcutaneous Tissue and Fascia, Right Neck** Deep cervical fascia Pretracheal fascia Prevertebral fascia **5** **Subcutaneous Tissue and Fascia, Left Neck** *See 4 Subcutaneous Tissue and Fascia, Right Neck* **6** **Subcutaneous Tissue and Fascia, Chest** Pectoral fascia **7** **Subcutaneous Tissue and Fascia, Back** **8** **Subcutaneous Tissue and Fascia, Abdomen** **9** **Subcutaneous Tissue and Fascia, Buttock** **B** **Subcutaneous Tissue and Fascia, Perineum** **C** **Subcutaneous Tissue and Fascia, Pelvic Region** **D** **Subcutaneous Tissue and Fascia, Right Upper Arm** Axillary fascia Deltoid fascia Infraspinatus fascia Subscapular aponeurosis Supraspinatus fascia **F** **Subcutaneous Tissue and Fascia, Left Upper Arm** *See D Subcutaneous Tissue and Fascia, Right Upper Arm* **G** **Subcutaneous Tissue and Fascia, Right Lower Arm** Antebrachial fascia Bicipital aponeurosis	**H** **Subcutaneous Tissue and Fascia, Left Lower Arm** *See G Subcutaneous Tissue and Fascia, Right Lower Arm* **J** **Subcutaneous Tissue and Fascia, Right Hand** Palmar fascia (aponeurosis) **K** **Subcutaneous Tissue and Fascia, Left Hand** *See J Subcutaneous Tissue and Fascia, Right Hand* **L** **Subcutaneous Tissue and Fascia, Right Upper Leg** Crural fascia Fascia lata Iliac fascia Iliotibial tract (band) **M** **Subcutaneous Tissue and Fascia, Left Upper Leg** *See L Subcutaneous Tissue and Fascia, Right Upper Leg* **N** **Subcutaneous Tissue and Fascia, Right Lower Leg** **P** **Subcutaneous Tissue and Fascia, Left Lower Leg** **Q** **Subcutaneous Tissue and Fascia, Right Foot** Plantar fascia (aponeurosis) **R** **Subcutaneous Tissue and Fascia, Left Foot** *See Q Subcutaneous Tissue and Fascia, Right Foot* **S** **Subcutaneous Tissue and Fascia, Head and Neck** **T** **Subcutaneous Tissue and Fascia, Trunk** External oblique aponeurosis Transversalis fascia **V** **Subcutaneous Tissue and Fascia, Upper Extremity** **W** **Subcutaneous Tissue and Fascia, Lower Extremity**	**Ø** Open **3** Percutaneous	**Z** No Device	**Z** No Qualifier

LC Limited Coverage   **NC** Noncovered   ⊞ Combination Member   HAC associated procedure   Combination Only   DRG Non-OR   Non-OR   New/Revised in GREEN

ICD-10-PCS 2021   **443**

Ø   Medical and Surgical
J   Subcutaneous Tissue and Fascia
9   Drainage   Definition: Taking or letting out fluids and/or gases from a body part
                       Explanation: The qualifier DIAGNOSTIC is used to identify drainage procedures that are biopsies

Body Part Character 4		Approach Character 5	Device Character 6	Qualifier Character 7
Ø Subcutaneous Tissue and Fascia, Scalp Galea aponeurotica **1 Subcutaneous Tissue and Fascia, Face** Masseteric fascia Orbital fascia Submandibular space **4 Subcutaneous Tissue and Fascia, Right Neck** Deep cervical fascia Pretracheal fascia Prevertebral fascia **5 Subcutaneous Tissue and Fascia, Left Neck** *See 4 Subcutaneous Tissue and Fascia, Right Neck* **6 Subcutaneous Tissue and Fascia, Chest** Pectoral fascia **7 Subcutaneous Tissue and Fascia, Back** **8 Subcutaneous Tissue and Fascia, Abdomen** **9 Subcutaneous Tissue and Fascia, Buttock** **B Subcutaneous Tissue and Fascia, Perineum** **C Subcutaneous Tissue and Fascia, Pelvic Region** **D Subcutaneous Tissue and Fascia, Right Upper Arm** Axillary fascia Deltoid fascia Infraspinatus fascia Subscapular aponeurosis Supraspinatus fascia **F Subcutaneous Tissue and Fascia, Left Upper Arm** *See D Subcutaneous Tissue and Fascia, Right Upper Arm*	**G Subcutaneous Tissue and Fascia, Right Lower Arm** Antebrachial fascia Bicipital aponeurosis **H Subcutaneous Tissue and Fascia, Left Lower Arm** *See G Subcutaneous Tissue and Fascia, Right Lower Arm* **J Subcutaneous Tissue and Fascia, Right Hand** Palmar fascia (aponeurosis) **K Subcutaneous Tissue and Fascia, Left Hand** *See J Subcutaneous Tissue and Fascia, Right Hand* **L Subcutaneous Tissue and Fascia, Right Upper Leg** Crural fascia Fascia lata Iliac fascia Iliotibial tract (band) **M Subcutaneous Tissue and Fascia, Left Upper Leg** *See L Subcutaneous Tissue and Fascia, Right Upper Leg* **N Subcutaneous Tissue and Fascia, Right Lower Leg** **P Subcutaneous Tissue and Fascia, Left Lower Leg** **Q Subcutaneous Tissue and Fascia, Right Foot** Plantar fascia (aponeurosis) **R Subcutaneous Tissue and Fascia, Left Foot** *See Q Subcutaneous Tissue and Fascia, Right Foot*	**Ø Open** **3 Percutaneous**	**Ø Drainage Device**	**Z No Qualifier**

Non-OR   0J9[0,1,4,5,6,7,8,9,B,C,D,F,G,H,J,K,L,M,N,P,Q,R][0,3]0Z

0J9 Continued on next page

LG Limited Coverage   **NC** Noncovered   ⊞ Combination Member   HAC associated procedure   Combination Only   DRG Non-OR   Non-OR   New/Revised in **GREEN**

444   ICD-10-PCS 2021

Ø   Medical and Surgical
J   Subcutaneous Tissue and Fascia
9   Drainage   Definition: Taking or letting out fluids and/or gases from a body part

ØJ9 Continued

                           Explanation: The qualifier DIAGNOSTIC is used to identify drainage procedures that are biopsies

Body Part Character 4		Approach Character 5	Device Character 6	Qualifier Character 7
Ø Subcutaneous Tissue and Fascia, Scalp Galea aponeurotica **1 Subcutaneous Tissue and Fascia, Face** Masseteric fascia Orbital fascia Submandibular space **4 Subcutaneous Tissue and Fascia, Right Neck** Deep cervical fascia Pretracheal fascia Prevertebral fascia **5 Subcutaneous Tissue and Fascia, Left Neck** *See 4 Subcutaneous Tissue and Fascia, Right Neck* **6 Subcutaneous Tissue and Fascia, Chest** Pectoral fascia **7 Subcutaneous Tissue and Fascia, Back** **8 Subcutaneous Tissue and Fascia, Abdomen** **9 Subcutaneous Tissue and Fascia, Buttock** **B Subcutaneous Tissue and Fascia, Perineum** **C Subcutaneous Tissue and Fascia, Pelvic Region** **D Subcutaneous Tissue and Fascia, Right Upper Arm** Axillary fascia Deltoid fascia Infraspinatus fascia Subscapular aponeurosis Supraspinatus fascia **F Subcutaneous Tissue and Fascia, Left Upper Arm** *See D Subcutaneous Tissue and Fascia, Right Upper Arm*	**G Subcutaneous Tissue and Fascia, Right Lower Arm** Antebrachial fascia Bicipital aponeurosis **H Subcutaneous Tissue and Fascia, Left Lower Arm** *See G Subcutaneous Tissue and Fascia, Right Lower Arm* **J Subcutaneous Tissue and Fascia, Right Hand** Palmar fascia (aponeurosis) **K Subcutaenous Tissue and Fascia, Left Hand** *See J Subcutaneous Tissue and Fascia, Right Hand* **L Subcutaneous Tissue and Fascia, Right Upper Leg** Crural fascia Fascia lata Iliac fascia Iliotibial tract (band) **M Subcutaneous Tissue and Fascia, Left Upper Leg** *See L Subcutaneous Tissue and Fascia, Right Upper Leg* **N Subcutaneous Tissue and Fascia, Right Lower Leg** **P Subcutaneous Tissue and Fascia, Left Lower Leg** **Q Subcutaneous Tissue and Fascia, Right Foot** Plantar fascia (aponeurosis) **R Subcutaneous Tissue and Fascia, Left Foot** *See Q Subcutaneous Tissue and Fascia, Right Foot*	**Ø Open** **3 Percutaneous**	**Z No Device**	**X Diagnostic** **Z No Qualifier**

Non-OR   ØJ9[Ø,1,4,5,6,7,8,9,B,C,D,F,G,H,J,K,L,M,N,P,Q,R][Ø,3]ZX
Non-OR   ØJ9[Ø,1,4,5,6,7,8,9,B,C,D,F,G,H,J,K,L,M,N,P,Q,R]3ZZ

LC Limited Coverage   NC Noncovered   ⊞ Combination Member   HAC associated procedure   Combination Only   DRG Non-OR   Non-OR   New/Revised in GREEN

ICD-10-PCS 2021   445

Ø   **Medical and Surgical**
J   **Subcutaneous Tissue and Fascia**
B   **Excision**   Definition: Cutting out or off, without replacement, a portion of a body part
                       Explanation: The qualifier DIAGNOSTIC is used to identify excision procedures that are biopsies

Body Part Character 4		Approach Character 5	Device Character 6	Qualifier Character 7
Ø Subcutaneous Tissue and Fascia, Scalp Galea aponeurotica **1 Subcutaneous Tissue and Fascia, Face** Masseteric fascia Orbital fascia Submandibular space **4 Subcutaneous Tissue and Fascia, Right Neck** Deep cervical fascia Pretracheal fascia Prevertebral fascia **5 Subcutaneous Tissue and Fascia, Left Neck** *See 4 Subcutaneous Tissue and Fascia, Right Neck* **6 Subcutaneous Tissue and Fascia, Chest** Pectoral fascia **7 Subcutaneous Tissue and Fascia, Back** **8 Subcutaneous Tissue and Fascia, Abdomen** **9 Subcutaneous Tissue and Fascia, Buttock** **B Subcutaneous Tissue and Fascia, Perineum** **C Subcutaneous Tissue and Fascia, Pelvic Region** **D Subcutaneous Tissue and Fascia, Right Upper Arm** Axillary fascia Deltoid fascia Infraspinatus fascia Subscapular aponeurosis Supraspinatus fascia **F Subcutaneous Tissue and Fascia, Left Upper Arm** *See D Subcutaneous Tissue and Fascia, Right Upper Arm*	**G Subcutaneous Tissue and Fascia, Right Lower Arm** Antebrachial fascia Bicipital aponeurosis **H Subcutaneous Tissue and Fascia, Left Lower Arm** *See G Subcutaneous Tissue and Fascia, Right Lower Arm* **J Subcutaneous Tissue and Fascia, Right Hand** Palmar fascia (aponeurosis) **K Subcutaneous Tissue and Fascia, Left Hand** *See J Subcutaneous Tissue and Fascia, Right Hand* **L Subcutaneous Tissue and Fascia, Right Upper Leg** Crural fascia Fascia lata Iliac fascia Iliotibial tract (band) **M Subcutaneous Tissue and Fascia, Left Upper Leg** *See L Subcutaneous Tissue and Fascia, Right Upper Leg* **N Subcutaneous Tissue and Fascia, Right Lower Leg** **P Subcutaneous Tissue and Fascia, Left Lower Leg** **Q Subcutaneous Tissue and Fascia, Right Foot** Plantar fascia (aponeurosis) **R Subcutaneous Tissue and Fascia, Left Foot** *See Q Subcutaneous Tissue and Fascia, Right Foot*	**Ø** Open **3** Percutaneous	**Z** No Device	**X** Diagnostic **Z** No Qualifier

DRG Non-OR   ØJB[Ø,4,5,6,7,8,9,B,C,D,F,G,H,L,M,N,P,Q,R]3ZZ
Non-OR   ØJB[Ø,1,4,5,6,7,8,9,B,C,D,F,G,H,J,K,L,M,N,P,Q,R][Ø,3]ZX

LC Limited Coverage   NC Noncovered   ⊞ Combination Member   HAC associated procedure   Combination Only   DRG Non-OR   Non-OR   New/Revised in GREEN

446   ICD-10-PCS 2021

Ø   Medical and Surgical
J   Subcutaneous Tissue and Fascia
C   Extirpation   Definition: Taking or cutting out solid matter from a body part

Explanation: The solid matter may be an abnormal byproduct of a biological function or a foreign body; it may be imbedded in a body part or in the lumen of a tubular body part. The solid matter may or may not have been previously broken into pieces.

Body Part Character 4		Approach Character 5	Device Character 6	Qualifier Character 7
Ø Subcutaneous Tissue and Fascia, Scalp Galea aponeurotica	**G Subcutaneous Tissue and Fascia, Right Lower Arm** Antebrachial fascia Bicipital aponeurosis	**Ø Open** **3 Percutaneous**	**Z No Device**	**Z No Qualifier**
1 Subcutaneous Tissue and Fascia, Face Masseteric fascia Orbital fascia Submandibular space	**H Subcutaneous Tissue and Fascia, Left Lower Arm** *See* G Subcutaneous Tissue and Fascia, Right Lower Arm			
4 Subcutaneous Tissue and Fascia, Right Neck Deep cervical fascia Pretracheal fascia Prevertebral fascia	**J Subcutaneous Tissue and Fascia, Right Hand** Palmar fascia (aponeurosis)			
5 Subcutaneous Tissue and Fascia, Left Neck *See* 4 Subcutaneous Tissue and Fascia, Right Neck	**K Subcutaneous Tissue and Fascia, Left Hand** *See* J Subcutaneous Tissue and Fascia, Right Hand			
6 Subcutaneous Tissue and Fascia, Chest Pectoral fascia	**L Subcutaneous Tissue and Fascia, Right Upper Leg** Crural fascia Fascia lata Iliac fascia Iliotibial tract (band)			
7 Subcutaneous Tissue and Fascia, Back	**M Subcutaneous Tissue and Fascia, Left Upper Leg** *See* L Subcutaneous Tissue and Fascia, Right Upper Leg			
8 Subcutaneous Tissue and Fascia, Abdomen	**N Subcutaneous Tissue and Fascia, Right Lower Leg**			
9 Subcutaneous Tissue and Fascia, Buttock	**P Subcutaneous Tissue and Fascia, Left Lower Leg**			
B Subcutaneous Tissue and Fascia, Perineum	**Q Subcutaneous Tissue and Fascia, Right Foot** Plantar fascia (aponeurosis)			
C Subcutaneous Tissue and Fascia, Pelvic Region	**R Subcutaneous Tissue and Fascia, Left Foot** *See* Q Subcutaneous Tissue and Fascia, Right Foot			
D Subcutaneous Tissue and Fascia, Right Upper Arm Axillary fascia Deltoid fascia Infraspinatus fascia Subscapular aponeurosis Supraspinatus fascia				
F Subcutaneous Tissue and Fascia, Left Upper Arm *See* D Subcutaneous Tissue and Fascia, Right Upper Arm				

Non-OR   All body part, approach, device, and qualifier values

Ø   Medical and Surgical
J   Subcutaneous Tissue and Fascia
D   Extraction   Definition: Pulling or stripping out or off all or a portion of a body part by the use of force
                       Explanation: The qualifier DIAGNOSTIC is used to identify extraction procedures that are biopsies

Body Part Character 4		Approach Character 5	Device Character 6	Qualifier Character 7

Ø   Subcutaneous Tissue and Fascia, Scalp
     Galea aponeurotica
 1   Subcutaneous Tissue and Fascia, Face
     Masseteric fascia
     Orbital fascia
     Submandibular space
 4   Subcutaneous Tissue and Fascia, Right Neck
     Deep cervical fascia
     Pretracheal fascia
     Prevertebral fascia
 5   Subcutaneous Tissue and Fascia, Left Neck
     See 4 *Subcutaneous Tissue and Fascia, Right Neck*
 6   Subcutaneous Tissue and Fascia, Chest
     Pectoral fascia
 7   Subcutaneous Tissue and Fascia, Back
 8   Subcutaneous Tissue and Fascia, Abdomen
 9   Subcutaneous Tissue and Fascia, Buttock
 B   Subcutaneous Tissue and Fascia, Perineum
 C   Subcutaneous Tissue and Fascia, Pelvic Region
 D   Subcutaneous Tissue and Fascia, Right Upper Arm
     Axillary fascia
     Deltoid fascia
     Infraspinatus fascia
     Subscapular aponeurosis
     Supraspinatus fascia
 F   Subcutaneous Tissue and Fascia, Left Upper Arm
     See D *Subcutaneous Tissue and Fascia, Right Upper Arm*
	G Subcutaneous Tissue and Fascia, Right Lower Arm
	     Antebrachial fascia
	     Bicipital aponeurosis
	 H Subcutaneous Tissue and Fascia, Left Lower Arm
	     See G *Subcutaneous Tissue and Fascia, Right Lower Arm*
	 J Subcutaneous Tissue and Fascia, Right Hand
	     Palmar fascia (aponeurosis)
	 K Subcutaneous Tissue and Fascia, Left Hand
	     See J *Subcutaneous Tissue and Fascia, Right Hand*
	 L Subcutaneous Tissue and Fascia, Right Upper Leg
	     Crural fascia
	     Fascia lata
	     Iliac fascia
	     Iliotibial tract (band)
	 M Subcutaneous Tissue and Fascia, Left Upper Leg
	     See L *Subcutaneous Tissue and Fascia, Right Upper Leg*
	 N Subcutaneous Tissue and Fascia, Right Lower Leg
	 P Subcutaneous Tissue and Fascia, Left Lower Leg
	 Q Subcutaneous Tissue and Fascia, Right Foot
	     Plantar fascia (aponeurosis)
	 R Subcutaneous Tissue and Fascia, Left Foot
	     See Q *Subcutaneous Tissue and Fascia, Right Foot*
		Ø Open
		 3 Percutaneous
			Z No Device	Z No Qualifier

Non-OR   ØJD[Ø,1,4,5,B,C,D,F,G,H,J,K,N,P,Q,R]3ZZ

See Appendix L for Procedure Combinations
Combo-only   ØJD[6,7,8,9,L,M]3ZZ

Ø   Medical and Surgical
J   Subcutaneous Tissue and Fascia
H   Insertion   Definition: Putting in a nonbiological appliance that monitors, assists, performs, or prevents a physiological function but does not physically take the place of a body part
                    Explanation: None

Body Part Character 4	Approach Character 5	Device Character 6	Qualifier Character 7

Ø Subcutaneous Tissue and Fascia, Scalp
  Galea aponeurotica
1 Subcutaneous Tissue and Fascia, Face
  Masseteric fascia
  Orbital fascia
  Submandibular space
4 Subcutaneous Tissue and Fascia, Right Neck
  Deep cervical fascia
  Pretracheal fascia
  Prevertebral fascia
5 Subcutaneous Tissue and Fascia, Left Neck
  See 4 Subcutaneous Tissue and Fascia, Right Neck
9 Subcutaneous Tissue and Fascia, Buttock
B Subcutaneous Tissue and Fascia, Perineum
	C Subcutaneous Tissue and Fascia, Pelvic Region
	J Subcutaneous Tissue and Fascia, Right Hand
	  Palmar fascia (aponeurosis)
	K Subcutaneous Tissue and Fascia, Left Hand
	  See J Subcutaneous Tissue and Fascia, Right Hand
	Q Subcutaneous Tissue and Fascia, Right Foot
	  Plantar fascia (aponeurosis)
	R Subcutaneous Tissue and Fascia, Left Foot
	  See Q Subcutaneous Tissue and Fascia, Right Foot
		Ø Open
		3 Percutaneous
			N Tissue Expander	**Z** No Qualifier

6 Subcutaneous Tissue and Fascia, Chest ⊞ Pectoral fascia	**Ø** Open **3** Percutaneous	**Ø** Monitoring Device, Hemodynamic **2** Monitoring Device **4** Pacemaker, Single Chamber **5** Pacemaker, Single Chamber Rate Responsive **6** Pacemaker, Dual Chamber **7** Cardiac Resynchronization Pacemaker Pulse Generator **8** Defibrillator Generator **9** Cardiac Resynchronization Defibrillator Pulse Generator **A** Contractility Modulation Device **B** Stimulator Generator, Single Array **C** Stimulator Generator, Single Array Rechargeable **D** Stimulator Generator, Multiple Array **E** Stimulator Generator, Multiple Array Rechargeable **F** Subcutaneous Defibrillator Lead **H** Contraceptive Device **M** Stimulator Generator **N** Tissue Expander **P** Cardiac Rhythm Related Device **V** Infusion Device, Pump **W** Vascular Access Device, Totally Implantable **X** Vascular Access Device, Tunneled **Y** Other Device	**Z** No Qualifier
7 Subcutaneous Tissue and Fascia, Back NC ⊞	**Ø** Open **3** Percutaneous	**B** Stimulator Generator, Single Array **C** Stimulator Generator, Single Array Rechargeable **D** Stimulator Generator, Multiple Array **E** Stimulator Generator, Multiple Array Rechargeable **M** Stimulator Generator **N** Tissue Expander **V** Infusion Device, Pump **Y** Other Device	**Z** No Qualifier

DRG Non-OR   ØJH6[Ø,3][4,5,6,7,H,P,X]Z
DRG Non-OR   ØJH63WX
HAC   ØJH6[Ø,3][4,5,6,7,8,9,P]Z when reported with SDx K68.11 or T81.4Ø-T81.49, T82.6-T82.7 with 7th character A
HAC   ØJH63XZ when reported with SDx J95.811
NC   ØJH7[Ø,3]MZ

See Appendix L for Procedure Combinations
⊞   ØJH6[Ø,3][4,5,6,7,8,9,A,B,C,D,E,F,P]Z
⊞   ØJH7[Ø,3][B,C,D,E]Z

ØJH Continued on next page

Subcutaneous Tissue and Fascia *(left margin)*

Ø **Medical and Surgical**
J   **Subcutaneous Tissue and Fascia**
H **Insertion**

ØJH Continued

Definition: Putting in a nonbiological appliance that monitors, assists, performs, or prevents a physiological function but does not physically take the place of a body part

Explanation: None

Body Part Character 4		Approach Character 5	Device Character 6	Qualifier Character 7
8 Subcutaneous Tissue and Fascia, Abdomen NC ⊞		Ø Open 3 Percutaneous	Ø Monitoring Device, Hemodynamic 2 Monitoring Device 4 Pacemaker, Single Chamber 5 Pacemaker, Single Chamber Rate Responsive 6 Pacemaker, Dual Chamber 7 Cardiac Resynchronization Pacemaker Pulse Generator 8 Defibrillator Generator 9 Cardiac Resynchronization Defibrillator Pulse Generator A Contractility Modulation Device B Stimulator Generator, Single Array C Stimulator Generator, Single Array Rechargeable D Stimulator Generator, Multiple Array E Stimulator Generator, Multiple Array Rechargeable H Contraceptive Device M Stimulator Generator N Tissue Expander P Cardiac Rhythm Related Device V Infusion Device, Pump W Vascular Access Device, Totally Implantable X Vascular Access Device, Tunneled Y Other Device	Z No Qualifier

D Subcutaneous Tissue and Fascia, Right Upper Arm
  Axillary fascia
  Deltoid fascia
  Infraspinatus fascia
  Subscapular aponeurosis
  Supraspinatus fascia
F Subcutaneous Tissue and Fascia, Left Upper Arm
  See D Subcutaneous Tissue and Fascia, Right Upper Arm
G Subcutaneous Tissue and Fascia, Right Lower Arm
  Antebrachial fascia
  Bicipital aponeurosis
H Subcutaneous Tissue and Fascia, Left Lower Arm
  See G Subcutaneous Tissue and Fascia, Right Lower Arm
	L Subcutaneous Tissue and Fascia, Right Upper Leg
	  Crural fascia
	  Fascia lata
	  Iliac fascia
	  Iliotibial tract (band)
	M Subcutaneous Tissue and Fascia, Left Upper Leg
	  See L Subcutaneous Tissue and Fascia, Right Upper Leg
	N Subcutaneous Tissue and Fascia, Right Lower Leg
	P Subcutaneous Tissue and Fascia, Left Lower Leg
		Ø Open
		3 Percutaneous
			H Contraceptive Device
			N Tissue Expander
			V Infusion Device, Pump
			W Vascular Access Device, Totally Implantable
			X Vascular Access Device, Tunneled
				Z No Qualifier

S Subcutaneous Tissue and Fascia, Head and Neck V Subcutaneous Tissue and Fascia, Upper Extremity W Subcutaneous Tissue and Fascia, Lower Extremity		Ø Open 3 Percutaneous	1 Radioactive Element 3 Infusion Device Y Other Device	Z No Qualifier

T Subcutaneous Tissue and Fascia, Trunk
  External oblique aponeurosis
  Transversalis fascia
		Ø Open
		3 Percutaneous
			1 Radioactive Element
			3 Infusion Device
			V Infusion Device, Pump
			Y Other Device
				Z No Qualifier

DRG Non-OR	ØJH8[Ø,3][2,4,5,6,7,H,P,X]Z	**Non-OR**	ØJH[D,F,G,H,L,M][Ø,3]HZ	**HAC** ØJH8[Ø,3][4,5,6,7,8,9,P]Z when reported with SDx K68.11 or T81.4Ø-T81.49, T82.6-T82.7 with 7th character A
DRG Non-OR	ØJH83WX	**Non-OR**	ØJHNØHZ	
DRG Non-OR	ØJH[D,F,G,H,L,M,N,P]ØXZ	**Non-OR**	ØJH[S,V,W]Ø3Z	NC ØJH8[Ø,3]MZ
DRG Non-OR	ØJH[D,F,G,H,L,M,N,P]3[W,X]Z	**Non-OR**	ØJH[S,V,W]3[3,Y]Z	**See Appendix L for Procedure Combinations**
DRG Non-OR	ØJHN3HZ	**Non-OR**	ØJHTØ3Z	⊞ ØJH8[Ø,3][4,5,6,7,8,9,A,B,C,D,E,P]Z
DRG Non-OR	ØJHP[Ø,3]HZ	**Non-OR**	ØJHT3[3,Y]Z	

LC Limited Coverage   NC Noncovered   ⊞ Combination Member   HAC associated procedure   Combination Only   DRG Non-OR   Non-OR   New/Revised in GREEN

450   ICD-10-PCS 2021

ØJH–ØJH *(left margin bottom)*

Ø **Medical and Surgical**
J **Subcutaneous Tissue and Fascia**
J **Inspection**　　Definition: Visually and/or manually exploring a body part

Explanation: Visual exploration may be performed with or without optical instrumentation. Manual exploration may be performed directly or through intervening body layers.

Body Part Character 4	Approach Character 5	Device Character 6	Qualifier Character 7
S　Subcutaneous Tissue and Fascia, Head and Neck T　Subcutaneous Tissue and Fascia, Trunk 　External oblique aponeurosis 　Transversalis fascia V　Subcutaneous Tissue and Fascia, Upper Extremity W　Subcutaneous Tissue and Fascia, Lower Extremity	Ø　Open 3　Percutaneous X　External	Z　No Device	Z　No Qualifier

Non-OR　All body part, approach, device, and qualifier values

Ø **Medical and Surgical**
J **Subcutaneous Tissue and Fascia**
N **Release**　　Definition: Freeing a body part from an abnormal physical constraint by cutting or by the use of force

Explanation: Some of the restraining tissue may be taken out but none of the body part is taken out

Body Part Character 4	Approach Character 5	Device Character 6	Qualifier Character 7
Ø　Subcutaneous Tissue and Fascia, Scalp 　Galea aponeurotica 1　Subcutaneous Tissue and Fascia, Face 　Masseteric fascia 　Orbital fascia 　Submandibular space 4　Subcutaneous Tissue and Fascia, Right Neck 　Deep cervical fascia 　Pretracheal fascia 　Prevertebral fascia 5　Subcutaneous Tissue and Fascia, Left Neck 　*See 4 Subcutaneous Tissue and Fascia, Right Neck* 6　Subcutaneous Tissue and Fascia, Chest 　Pectoral fascia 7　Subcutaneous Tissue and Fascia, Back 8　Subcutaneous Tissue and Fascia, Abdomen 9　Subcutaneous Tissue and Fascia, Buttock B　Subcutaneous Tissue and Fascia, Perineum C　Subcutaneous Tissue and Fascia, Pelvic Region D　Subcutaneous Tissue and Fascia, Right Upper Arm 　Axillary fascia 　Deltoid fascia 　Infraspinatus fascia 　Subscapular aponeurosis 　Supraspinatus fascia F　Subcutaneous Tissue and Fascia, Left Upper Arm 　*See D Subcutaneous Tissue and Fascia, Right Upper Arm* G　Subcutaneous Tissue and Fascia, Right Lower Arm 　Antebrachial fascia 　Bicipital aponeurosis H　Subcutaneous Tissue and Fascia, Left Lower Arm 　*See G Subcutaneous Tissue and Fascia, Right Lower Arm* J　Subcutaneous Tissue and Fascia, Right Hand 　Palmar fascia (aponeurosis) K　Subcutaneous Tissue and Fascia, Left Hand 　*See J Subcutaneous Tissue and Fascia, Right Hand* L　Subcutaneous Tissue and Fascia, Right Upper Leg 　Crural fascia 　Fascia lata 　Iliac fascia 　Iliotibial tract (band) M　Subcutaneous Tissue and Fascia, Left Upper Leg 　*See L Subcutaneous Tissue and Fascia, Right Upper Leg* N　Subcutaneous Tissue and Fascia, Right Lower Leg P　Subcutaneous Tissue and Fascia, Left Lower Leg Q　Subcutaneous Tissue and Fascia, Right Foot 　Plantar fascia (aponeurosis) R　Subcutaneous Tissue and Fascia, Left Foot 　*See Q Subcutaneous Tissue and Fascia, Right Foot*	Ø　Open 3　Percutaneous X　External	Z　No Device	Z　No Qualifier

Non-OR　ØJN[Ø,1,4,5,6,7,8,9,B,C,D,F,G,H,J,K,L,M,N,P,Q,R]XZZ

LC Limited Coverage　**NC** Noncovered　⊞ Combination Member　HAC associated procedure　Combination Only　DRG Non-OR　Non-OR　New/Revised in GREEN

Ø **Medical and Surgical**
J **Subcutaneous Tissue and Fascia**
P **Removal**   Definition: Taking out or off a device from a body part

Explanation: If a device is taken out and a similar device put in without cutting or puncturing the skin or mucous membrane, the procedure is coded to the root operation CHANGE. Otherwise, the procedure for taking out a device is coded to the root operation REMOVAL.

Body Part Character 4	Approach Character 5	Device Character 6	Qualifier Character 7
S Subcutaneous Tissue and Fascia, Head and Neck	**Ø** Open **3** Percutaneous	**Ø** Drainage Device **1** Radioactive Element **3** Infusion Device **7** Autologous Tissue Substitute **J** Synthetic Substitute **K** Nonautologous Tissue Substitute **N** Tissue Expander **Y** Other Device	**Z** No Qualifier
S Subcutaneous Tissue and Fascia, Head and Neck	**X** External	**Ø** Drainage Device **1** Radioactive Element **3** Infusion Device	**Z** No Qualifier
T Subcutaneous Tissue and Fascia, Trunk External oblique aponeurosis Transversalis fascia	**Ø** Open **3** Percutaneous	**Ø** Drainage Device **1** Radioactive Element **2** Monitoring Device **3** Infusion Device **7** Autologous Tissue Substitute **F** Subcutaneous Defibrillator Lead **H** Contraceptive Device **J** Synthetic Substitute **K** Nonautologous Tissue Substitute **M** Stimulator Generator **N** Tissue Expander **P** Cardiac Rhythm Related Device **V** Infusion Device, Pump **W** Vascular Access Device, Totally Implantable **X** Vascular Access Device, Tunneled **Y** Other Device	**Z** No Qualifier
T Subcutaneous Tissue and Fascia, Trunk External oblique aponeurosis Transversalis fascia	**X** External	**Ø** Drainage Device **1** Radioactive Element **2** Monitoring Device **3** Infusion Device **H** Contraceptive Device **V** Infusion Device, Pump **X** Vascular Access Device, Tunneled	**Z** No Qualifier
V Subcutaneous Tissue and Fascia, Upper Extremity **W** Subcutaneous Tissue and Fascia, Lower Extremity	**Ø** Open **3** Percutaneous	**Ø** Drainage Device **1** Radioactive Element **3** Infusion Device **7** Autologous Tissue Substitute **H** Contraceptive Device **J** Synthetic Substitute **K** Nonautologous Tissue Substitute **N** Tissue Expander **V** Infusion Device, Pump **W** Vascular Access Device, Totally Implantable **X** Vascular Access Device, Tunneled **Y** Other Device	**Z** No Qualifier
V Subcutaneous Tissue and Fascia, Upper Extremity **W** Subcutaneous Tissue and Fascia, Lower Extremity	**X** External	**Ø** Drainage Device **1** Radioactive Element **3** Infusion Device **H** Contraceptive Device **V** Infusion Device, Pump **X** Vascular Access Device, Tunneled	**Z** No Qualifier

Non-OR	ØJPS[Ø,3][Ø,1,3,7,J,K,N,Y]Z
Non-OR	ØJPSX[Ø,1,3]Z
Non-OR	ØJPT[Ø,3][Ø,1,2,3,7,H,J,K,M,N,V,W,X,Y]Z
Non-OR	ØJPTX[Ø,1,2,3,H,V,X]Z
Non-OR	ØJP[V,W][Ø,3][Ø,1,3,7,H,J,K,N,V,W,X,Y]Z
Non-OR	ØJP[V,W]X[Ø,1,3,H,V,X]Z
HAC	ØJPT[Ø,3][F,P]Z when reported with SDx K68.11 or T81.4Ø-T81.49, T82.6-T82.7 with 7th character A

Ø Medical and Surgical
J Subcutaneous Tissue and Fascia
Q Repair   Definition: Restoring, to the extent possible, a body part to its normal anatomic structure and function

Explanation: Used only when the method to accomplish the repair is not one of the other root operations

Body Part Character 4	Approach Character 5	Device Character 6	Qualifier Character 7
Ø Subcutaneous Tissue and Fascia, Scalp Galea aponeurotica **1 Subcutaneous Tissue and Fascia, Face** Masseteric fascia Orbital fascia Submandibular space **4 Subcutaneous Tissue and Fascia, Right Neck** Deep cervical fascia Pretracheal fascia Prevertebral fascia **5 Subcutaneous Tissue and Fascia, Left Neck** See 4 Subcutaneous Tissue and Fascia, Right Neck **6 Subcutaneous Tissue and Fascia, Chest** Pectoral fascia **7 Subcutaneous Tissue and Fascia, Back** **8 Subcutaneous Tissue and Fascia, Abdomen** **9 Subcutaneous Tissue and Fascia, Buttock** **B Subcutaneous Tissue and Fascia, Perineum** **C Subcutaneous Tissue and Fascia, Pelvic Region** **D Subcutaneous Tissue and Fascia, Right Upper Arm** Axillary fascia Deltoid fascia Infraspinatus fascia Subscapular aponeurosis Supraspinatus fascia **F Subcutaneous Tissue and Fascia, Left Upper Arm** See D Subcutaneous Tissue and Fascia, Right Upper Arm **G Subcutaneous Tissue and Fascia, Right Lower Arm** Antebrachial fascia Bicipital aponeurosis **H Subcutaneous Tissue and Fascia, Left Lower Arm** See G Subcutaneous Tissue and Fascia, Right Lower Arm **J Subcutaneous Tissue and Fascia, Right Hand** Palmar fascia (aponeurosis) **K Subcutaneous Tissue and Fascia, Left Hand** See J Subcutaneous Tissue and Fascia, Right Hand **L Subcutaneous Tissue and Fascia, Right Upper Leg** Crural fascia Fascia lata Iliac fascia Iliotibial tract (band) **M Subcutaneous Tissue and Fascia, Left Upper Leg** See L Subcutaneous Tissue and Fascia, Right Upper Leg **N Subcutaneous Tissue and Fascia, Right Lower Leg** **P Subcutaneous Tissue and Fascia, Left Lower Leg** **Q Subcutaneous Tissue and Fascia, Right Foot** Plantar fascia (aponeurosis) **R Subcutaneous Tissue and Fascia, Left Foot** See Q Subcutaneous Tissue and Fascia, Right Foot	Ø Open 3 Percutaneous	Z No Device	Z No Qualifier

Non-OR ØJQ[Ø,1,4,5,6,7,8,9,B,C,D,F,G,H,J,K,L,M,N,P,Q,R]3ZZ

Subcutaneous Tissue and Fascia *(side tab, left margin)*

Ø   **Medical and Surgical**
J   **Subcutaneous Tissue and Fascia**
R   **Replacement**   Definition: Putting in or on biological or synthetic material that physically takes the place and/or function of all or a portion of a body part

Explanation: The body part may have been taken out or replaced, or may be taken out, physically eradicated, or rendered nonfunctional during the REPLACEMENT procedure. A REMOVAL procedure is coded for taking out the device used in a previous replacement procedure.

Body Part Character 4		Approach Character 5	Device Character 6	Qualifier Character 7

Ø   **Subcutaneous Tissue and Fascia, Scalp**
    Galea aponeurotica
1   **Subcutaneous Tissue and Fascia, Face**
    Masseteric fascia
    Orbital fascia
    Submandibular space
4   **Subcutaneous Tissue and Fascia, Right Neck**
    Deep cervical fascia
    Pretracheal fascia
    Prevertebral fascia
5   **Subcutaneous Tissue and Fascia, Left Neck**
    See 4 *Subcutaneous Tissue and Fascia, Right Neck*
6   **Subcutaneous Tissue and Fascia, Chest**
    Pectoral fascia
7   **Subcutaneous Tissue and Fascia, Back**
8   **Subcutaneous Tissue and Fascia, Abdomen**
9   **Subcutaneous Tissue and Fascia, Buttock**
B   **Subcutaneous Tissue and Fascia, Perineum**
C   **Subcutaneous Tissue and Fascia, Pelvic Region**
D   **Subcutaneous Tissue and Fascia, Right Upper Arm**
    Axillary fascia
    Deltoid fascia
    Infraspinatus fascia
    Subscapular aponeurosis
    Supraspinatus fascia
F   **Subcutaneous Tissue and Fascia, Left Upper Arm**
    See D *Subcutaneous Tissue and Fascia, Right Upper Arm*
	G **Subcutaneous Tissue and Fascia, Right Lower Arm**
	    Antebrachial fascia
	    Bicipital aponeurosis
	H **Subcutaneous Tissue and Fascia, Left Lower Arm**
	    See G *Subcutaneous Tissue and Fascia, Right Lower Arm*
	J **Subcutaneous Tissue and Fascia, Right Hand**
	    Palmar fascia (aponeurosis)
	K **Subcutaneous Tissue and Fascia, Left Hand**
	    See J *Subcutaneous Tissue and Fascia, Right Hand*
	L **Subcutaneous Tissue and Fascia, Right Upper Leg**
	    Crural fascia
	    Fascia lata
	    Iliac fascia
	    Iliotibial tract (band)
	M **Subcutaneous Tissue and Fascia, Left Upper Leg**
	    See L *Subcutaneous Tissue and Fascia, Right Upper Leg*
	N **Subcutaneous Tissue and Fascia, Right Lower Leg**
	P **Subcutaneous Tissue and Fascia, Left Lower Leg**
	Q **Subcutaneous Tissue and Fascia, Right Foot**
	    Plantar fascia (aponeurosis)
	R **Subcutaneous Tissue and Fascia, Left Foot**
	    See Q *Subcutaneous Tissue and Fascia, Right Foot*
		Ø Open
		3 Percutaneous
			7 Autologous Tissue Substitute
			J Synthetic Substitute
			K Nonautologous Tissue Substitute
				Z No Qualifier

LC Limited Coverage   NC Noncovered   ⊞ Combination Member   HAC associated procedure   Combination Only   DRG Non-OR   Non-OR   New/Revised in GREEN

454   ICD-10-PCS 2021

Ø   Medical and Surgical
J   Subcutaneous Tissue and Fascia
U   Supplement: Definition: Putting in or on biological or synthetic material that physically reinforces and/or augments the function of a portion of a body part

Explanation: The biological material is non-living, or is living and from the same individual. The body part may have been previously replaced, and the SUPPLEMENT procedure is performed to physically reinforce and/or augment the function of the replaced body part.

Body Part Character 4		Approach Character 5	Device Character 6	Qualifier Character 7
Ø Subcutaneous Tissue and Fascia, Scalp Galea aponeurotica	**G Subcutaneous Tissue and Fascia, Right Lower Arm** Antebrachial fascia Bicipital aponeurosis	**Ø Open** **3 Percutaneous**	**7 Autologous Tissue Substitute** **J Synthetic Substitute** **K Nonautologous Tissue Substitute**	**Z No Qualifier**
1 Subcutaneous Tissue and Fascia, Face Masseteric fascia Orbital fascia Submandibular space	**H Subcutaneous Tissue and Fascia, Left Lower Arm** *See G Subcutaneous Tissue and Fascia, Right Lower Arm*			
4 Subcutaneous Tissue and Fascia, Right Neck Deep cervical fascia Pretracheal fascia Prevertebral fascia	**J Subcutaneous Tissue and Fascia, Right Hand** Palmar fascia (aponeurosis)			
5 Subcutaneous Tissue and Fascia, Left Neck *See 4 Subcutaneous Tissue and Fascia, Right Neck*	**K Subcutaneous Tissue and Fascia, Left Hand** *See J Subcutaneous Tissue and Fascia, Right Hand*			
6 Subcutaneous Tissue and Fascia, Chest Pectoral fascia	**L Subcutaneous Tissue and Fascia, Right Upper Leg** Crural fascia Fascia lata Iliac fascia Iliotibial tract (band)			
7 Subcutaneous Tissue and Fascia, Back	**M Subcutaneous Tissue and Fascia, Left Upper Leg** *See L Subcutaneous Tissue and Fascia, Right Upper Leg*			
8 Subcutaneous Tissue and Fascia, Abdomen	**N Subcutaneous Tissue and Fascia, Right Lower Leg**			
9 Subcutaneous Tissue and Fascia, Buttock	**P Subcutaneous Tissue and Fascia, Left Lower Leg**			
B Subcutaneous Tissue and Fascia, Perineum	**Q Subcutaneous Tissue and Fascia, Right Foot** Plantar fascia (aponeurosis)			
C Subcutaneous Tissue and Fascia, Pelvic Region	**R Subcutaneous Tissue and Fascia, Left Foot** *See Q Subcutaneous Tissue and Fascia, Right Foot*			
D Subcutaneous Tissue and Fascia, Right Upper Arm Axillary fascia Deltoid fascia Infraspinatus fascia Subscapular aponeurosis Supraspinatus fascia				
F Subcutaneous Tissue and Fascia, Left Upper Arm *See D Subcutaneous Tissue and Fascia, Right Upper Arm*				

LC Limited Coverage   **NC** Noncovered   ⊞ Combination Member   HAC associated procedure   Combination Only   DRG Non-OR   Non-OR   New/Revised in GREEN

ICD-10-PCS 2021   455

Ø Medical and Surgical
J Subcutaneous Tissue and Fascia
W Revision   Definition: Correcting, to the extent possible, a portion of a malfunctioning device or the position of a displaced device

                    Explanation: Revision can include correcting a malfunctioning or displaced device by taking out or putting in components of the device such as a screw or pin

Body Part Character 4	Approach Character 5	Device Character 6	Qualifier Character 7
S Subcutaneous Tissue and Fascia, Head and Neck	**Ø** Open **3** Percutaneous	**Ø** Drainage Device **3** Infusion Device **7** Autologous Tissue Substitute **J** Synthetic Substitute **K** Nonautologous Tissue Substitute **N** Tissue Expander **Y** Other Device	**Z** No Qualifier
S Subcutaneous Tissue and Fascia, Head and Neck	**X** External	**Ø** Drainage Device **3** Infusion Device **7** Autologous Tissue Substitute **J** Synthetic Substitute **K** Nonautologous Tissue Substitute **N** Tissue Expander	**Z** No Qualifier
T Subcutaneous Tissue and Fascia, Trunk External oblique aponeurosis Transversalis fascia	**Ø** Open **3** Percutaneous	**Ø** Drainage Device **2** Monitoring Device **3** Infusion Device **7** Autologous Tissue Substitute **F** Subcutaneous Defibrillator Lead **H** Contraceptive Device **J** Synthetic Substitute **K** Nonautologous Tissue Substitute **M** Stimulator Generator **N** Tissue Expander **P** Cardiac Rhythm Related Device **V** Infusion Device, Pump **W** Vascular Access Device, Totally Implantable **X** Vascular Access Device, Tunneled **Y** Other Device	**Z** No Qualifier
T Subcutaneous Tissue and Fascia, Trunk External oblique aponeurosis Transversalis fascia	**X** External	**Ø** Drainage Device **2** Monitoring Device **3** Infusion Device **7** Autologous Tissue Substitute **F** Subcutaneous Defibrillator Lead **H** Contraceptive Device **J** Synthetic Substitute **K** Nonautologous Tissue Substitute **M** Stimulator Generator **N** Tissue Expander **P** Cardiac Rhythm Related Device **V** Infusion Device, Pump **W** Vascular Access Device, Totally Implantable **X** Vascular Access Device, Tunneled	**Z** No Qualifier
V Subcutaneous Tissue and Fascia, Upper Extremity **W** Subcutaneous Tissue and Fascia, Lower Extremity	**Ø** Open **3** Percutaneous	**Ø** Drainage Device **3** Infusion Device **7** Autologous Tissue Substitute **H** Contraceptive Device **J** Synthetic Substitute **K** Nonautologous Tissue Substitute **N** Tissue Expander **V** Infusion Device, Pump **W** Vascular Access Device, Totally Implantable **X** Vascular Access Device, Tunneled **Y** Other Device	**Z** No Qualifier
V Subcutaneous Tissue and Fascia, Upper Extremity **W** Subcutaneous Tissue and Fascia, Lower Extremity	**X** External	**Ø** Drainage Device **3** Infusion Device **7** Autologous Tissue Substitute **H** Contraceptive Device **J** Synthetic Substitute **K** Nonautologous Tissue Substitute **N** Tissue Expander **V** Infusion Device, Pump **W** Vascular Access Device, Totally Implantable **X** Vascular Access Device, Tunneled	**Z** No Qualifier

DRG Non-OR ØJWS[Ø,3][Ø,3,7,J,K,N,Y]Z	**HAC** ØJWT[Ø,3][F,P]Z when reported with SDx K68.11 or T81.4Ø-T81.49, T82.6-T82.7
DRG Non-OR ØJWT[Ø,3][Ø,3,7,H,J,K,M,N,V,W,X]Z	with 7th character A
DRG Non-OR ØJWTXMZ	
DRG Non-OR ØJW[V,W][Ø,3][Ø,3,7,H,J,K,N,V,W,X,Y]Z	
Non-OR ØJWSX[Ø,3,7,J,K,N]Z	
Non-OR ØJWT3YZ	
Non-OR ØJWTX[Ø,2,3,7,F,H,J,K,N,P,V,W,X]Z	
Non-OR ØJW[V,W]X[Ø,3,7,H,J,K,N,V,W,X]Z	

LC Limited Coverage   **NC** Noncovered   ⊞ Combination Member   HAC associated procedure   Combination Only   DRG Non-OR   Non-OR   New/Revised in GREEN

456   ICD-10-PCS 2021

Ø   Medical and Surgical
J   Subcutaneous Tissue and Fascia
X   Transfer   Definition: Moving, without taking out, all or a portion of a body part to another location to take over the function of all or a portion of a body part

                       Explanation: The body part transferred remains connected to its vascular and nervous supply

Body Part Character 4		Approach Character 5	Device Character 6	Qualifier Character 7
Ø Subcutaneous Tissue and Fascia, Scalp Galea aponeurotica **1 Subcutaneous Tissue and Fascia, Face** Masseteric fascia Orbital fascia Submandibular space **4 Subcutaneous Tissue and Fascia, Right Neck** Deep cervical fascia Pretracheal fascia Prevertebral fascia **5 Subcutaneous Tissue and Fascia, Left Neck** *See 4 Subcutaneous Tissue and Fascia, Right Neck* **6 Subcutaneous Tissue and Fascia, Chest** Pectoral fascia **7 Subcutaneous Tissue and Fascia, Back** **8 Subcutaneous Tissue and Fascia, Abdomen** **9 Subcutaneous Tissue and Fascia, Buttock** **B Subcutaneous Tissue and Fascia, Perineum** **C Subcutaneous Tissue and Fascia, Pelvic Region** **D Subcutaneous Tissue and Fascia, Right Upper Arm** Axillary fascia Deltoid fascia Infraspinatus fascia Subscapular aponeurosis Supraspinatus fascia **F Subcutaneous Tissue and Fascia, Left Upper Arm** *See D Subcutaneous Tissue and Fascia, Right Upper Arm*	**G Subcutaneous Tissue and Fascia, Right Lower Arm** Antebrachial fascia Bicipital aponeurosis **H Subcutaneous Tissue and Fascia, Left Lower Arm** *See G Subcutaneous Tissue and Fascia, Right Lower Arm* **J Subcutaneous Tissue and Fascia, Right Hand** Palmar fascia (aponeurosis) **K Subcutaneous Tissue and Fascia, Left Hand** *See J Subcutaneous Tissue and Fascia, Right Hand* **L Subcutaneous Tissue and Fascia, Right Upper Leg** Crural fascia Fascia lata Iliac fascia Iliotibial tract (band) **M Subcutaneous Tissue and Fascia, Left Upper Leg** *See L Subcutaneous Tissue and Fascia, Right Upper Leg* **N Subcutaneous Tissue and Fascia, Right Lower Leg** **P Subcutaneous Tissue and Fascia, Left Lower Leg** **Q Subcutaneous Tissue and Fascia, Right Foot** Plantar fascia (aponeurosis) **R Subcutaneous Tissue and Fascia, Left Foot** *See Q Subcutaneous Tissue and Fascia, Right Foot*	**Ø Open** **3 Percutaneous**	**Z No Device**	**B Skin and Subcutaneous Tissue** **C Skin, Subcutaneous Tissue and Fascia** **Z No Qualifier**

Muscles ØK2–ØKX

Character Meanings

This Character Meaning table is provided as a guide to assist the user in the identification of character members that may be found in this section of code tables. It **SHOULD NOT** be used to build a PCS code.

Operation–Character 3	Body Part–Character 4	Approach–Character 5	Device–Character 6	Qualifier–Character 7
2 Change	Ø Head Muscle	Ø Open	Ø Drainage Device	Ø Skin
5 Destruction	1 Facial Muscle	3 Percutaneous	7 Autologous Tissue Substitute	1 Subcutaneous Tissue
8 Division	2 Neck Muscle, Right	4 Percutaneous Endoscopic	J Synthetic Substitute	2 Skin and Subcutaneous Tissue
9 Drainage	3 Neck Muscle, Left	X External	K Nonautologous Tissue Substitute	5 Latissimus Dorsi Myocutaneous Flap
B Excision	4 Tongue, Palate, Pharynx Muscle		M Stimulator Lead	6 Transverse Rectus Abdominis Myocutaneous Flap
C Extirpation	5 Shoulder Muscle, Right		Y Other Device	7 Deep Inferior Epigastric Artery Perforator Flap
D Extraction	6 Shoulder Muscle, Left		Z No Device	8 Superficial Inferior Epigastric Artery Flap
H Insertion	7 Upper Arm Muscle, Right			9 Gluteal Artery Perforator Flap
J Inspection	8 Upper Arm Muscle, Left			X Diagnostic
M Reattachment	9 Lower Arm and Wrist Muscle, Right			Z No Qualifier
N Release	B Lower Arm and Wrist Muscle, Left			
P Removal	C Hand Muscle, Right			
Q Repair	D Hand Muscle, Left			
R Replacement	F Trunk Muscle, Right			
S Reposition	G Trunk Muscle, Left			
T Resection	H Thorax Muscle, Right			
U Supplement	J Thorax Muscle, Left			
W Revision	K Abdomen Muscle, Right			
X Transfer	L Abdomen Muscle, Left			
	M Perineum Muscle			
	N Hip Muscle, Right			
	P Hip Muscle, Left			
	Q Upper Leg Muscle, Right			
	R Upper Leg Muscle, Left			
	S Lower Leg Muscle, Right			
	T Lower Leg Muscle, Left			
	V Foot Muscle, Right			
	W Foot Muscle, Left			
	X Upper Muscle			
	Y Lower Muscle			

AHA Coding Clinic for table ØK8
2020, 2Q, 25   Endoscopic Stapling of Zenker's Diverticulum

AHA Coding Clinic for table ØKB
2020, 1Q, 27   Delayed reconstruction following mastectomy using gracilis musculocutaneous free flap
2016, 3Q, 20   Excisional debridement of sacrum
2015, 3Q, 3-8   Excisional and nonexcisional debridement

AHA Coding Clinic for table ØKD
2017, 4Q, 41-42   Extraction procedures

AHA Coding Clinic for table ØKN
2017, 2Q, 12   Compartment syndrome and fasciotomy of foot
2017, 2Q, 13   Compartment syndrome and fasciotomy of leg
2015, 2Q, 22   Arthroscopic subacromial decompression
2014, 4Q, 39   Abdominal component release with placement of mesh for hernia repair

AHA Coding Clinic for table ØKQ
2018, 2Q, 25   Third and fourth degree obstetric lacerations
2016, 2Q, 34   Assisted vaginal delivery
2016, 1Q, 7   Obstetrical perineal laceration repair
2014, 4Q, 43   Second degree obstetric perineal laceration
2013, 4Q, 120   Repair of second degree perineum obstetric laceration

AHA Coding Clinic for table ØKS
2017, 1Q, 41   Manual reduction of hernia

AHA Coding Clinic for table ØKT
2016, 2Q, 12   Resection of malignant neoplasm of infratemporal fossa
2015, 1Q, 38   Abdominoperineal resection with flap closure of the perineum and colostomy

AHA Coding Clinic for table ØKX
2018, 2Q, 18   Transverse rectus abdominis myocutaneous (TRAM) delay
2017, 4Q, 67   New qualifier values – Pedicle flap procedures
2016, 3Q, 30   Resection of femur with interposition arthroplasty
2015, 3Q, 33   Cleft lip repair using Millard rotation advancement
2015, 2Q, 26   Pharyngeal flap to soft palate
2014, 4Q, 41   Abdominoperineal resection (APR) with flap closure of perineum and colostomy
2014, 2Q, 10   Transverse abdominomyocutaneous (TRAM) breast reconstruction
2014, 2Q, 12   Pedicle latissimus myocutaneous flap with placement of breast tissue expanders

Muscles

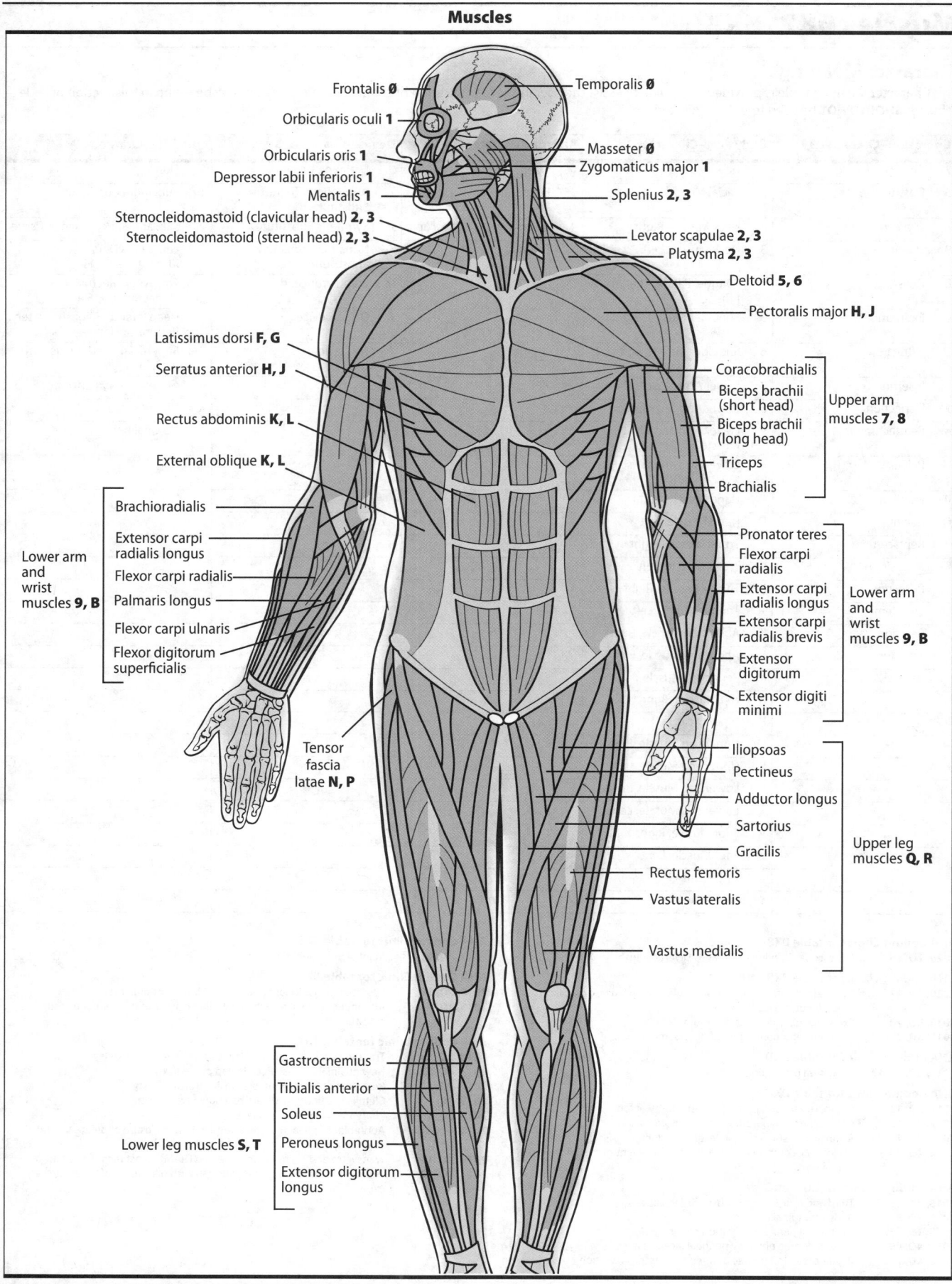

Frontalis **Ø**

Temporalis **Ø**

Orbicularis oculi **1**

Orbicularis oris **1**

Masseter **Ø**

Zygomaticus major **1**

Depressor labii inferioris **1**

Mentalis **1**

Splenius **2, 3**

Sternocleidomastoid (clavicular head) **2, 3**

Sternocleidomastoid (sternal head) **2, 3**

Levator scapulae **2, 3**

Platysma **2, 3**

Deltoid **5, 6**

Pectoralis major **H, J**

Latissimus dorsi **F, G**

Coracobrachialis

Serratus anterior **H, J**

Biceps brachii (short head)

Upper arm muscles **7, 8**

Rectus abdominis **K, L**

Biceps brachii (long head)

External oblique **K, L**

Triceps

Brachialis

Brachioradialis

Pronator teres

Extensor carpi radialis longus

Flexor carpi radialis

Flexor carpi radialis

Extensor carpi radialis longus

Lower arm and wrist muscles **9, B**

Lower arm and wrist muscles **9, B**

Palmaris longus

Extensor carpi radialis brevis

Flexor carpi ulnaris

Extensor digitorum

Flexor digitorum superficialis

Extensor digiti minimi

Iliopsoas

Pectineus

Tensor fascia latae **N, P**

Adductor longus

Sartorius

Gracilis

Upper leg muscles **Q, R**

Rectus femoris

Vastus lateralis

Vastus medialis

Gastrocnemius

Tibialis anterior

Soleus

Lower leg muscles **S, T**

Peroneus longus

Extensor digitorum longus

0   Medical and Surgical
K   Muscles
2   Change   Definition: Taking out or off a device from a body part and putting back an identical or similar device in or on the same body part without cutting or puncturing the skin or a mucous membrane

Explanation: All CHANGE procedures are coded using the approach EXTERNAL

Body Part Character 4	Approach Character 5	Device Character 6	Qualifier Character 7
X Upper Muscle Y Lower Muscle	X External	0 Drainage Device Y Other Device	Z No Qualifier

Non-OR	All body part, approach, device, and qualifier values

0   Medical and Surgical
K   Muscles
5   Destruction   Definition: Physical eradication of all or a portion of a body part by the direct use of energy, force, or a destructive agent

Explanation: None of the body part is physically taken out

Body Part Character 4		Approach Character 5	Device Character 6	Qualifier Character 7
0 Head Muscle Auricularis muscle Masseter muscle Pterygoid muscle Splenius capitis muscle Temporalis muscle Temporoparietalis muscle **1 Facial Muscle** Buccinator muscle Corrugator supercilii muscle Depressor anguli oris muscle Depressor labii inferioris muscle Depressor septi nasi muscle Depressor supercilii muscle Levator anguli oris muscle Levator labii superioris alaeque nasi muscle Levator labii superioris muscle Mentalis muscle Nasalis muscle Occipitofrontalis muscle Orbicularis oris muscle Procerus muscle Risorius muscle Zygomaticus muscle **2 Neck Muscle, Right** Anterior vertebral muscle Arytenoid muscle Cricothyroid muscle Infrahyoid muscle Levator scapulae muscle Platysma muscle Scalene muscle Splenius cervicis muscle Sternocleidomastoid muscle Suprahyoid muscle Thyroarytenoid muscle **3 Neck Muscle, Left** *See 2 Neck Muscle, Right* **4 Tongue, Palate, Pharynx Muscle** Chondroglossus muscle Genioglossus muscle Hyoglossus muscle Inferior longitudinal muscle Levator veli palatini muscle Palatoglossal muscle Palatopharyngeal muscle Pharyngeal constrictor muscle Salpingopharyngeus muscle Styloglossus muscle Stylopharyngeus muscle Superior longitudinal muscle Tensor veli palatini muscle **5 Shoulder Muscle, Right** Deltoid muscle Infraspinatus muscle Subscapularis muscle Supraspinatus muscle Teres major muscle Teres minor muscle **6 Shoulder Muscle, Left** *See 5 Shoulder Muscle, Right*	**7 Upper Arm Muscle, Right** Biceps brachii muscle Brachialis muscle Coracobrachialis muscle Triceps brachii muscle **8 Upper Arm Muscle, Left** *See 7 Upper Arm Muscle, Right* **9 Lower Arm and Wrist Muscle, Right** Anatomical snuffbox Brachioradialis muscle Extensor carpi radialis muscle Extensor carpi ulnaris muscle Flexor carpi radialis muscle Flexor carpi ulnaris muscle Flexor pollicis longus muscle Palmaris longus muscle Pronator quadratus muscle Pronator teres muscle **B Lower Arm and Wrist Muscle, Left** *See 9 Lower Arm and Wrist Muscle, Right* **C Hand Muscle, Right** Hypothenar muscle Palmar interosseous muscle Thenar muscle **D Hand Muscle, Left** *See C Hand Muscle, Right* **F Trunk Muscle, Right** Coccygeus muscle Erector spinae muscle Interspinalis muscle Intertransversarius muscle Latissimus dorsi muscle Quadratus lumborum muscle Rhomboid major muscle Rhomboid minor muscle Serratus posterior muscle Transversospinalis muscle Trapezius muscle **G Trunk Muscle, Left** *See F Trunk Muscle, Right* **H Thorax Muscle, Right** Intercostal muscle Levatores costarum muscle Pectoralis major muscle Pectoralis minor muscle Serratus anterior muscle Subclavius muscle Subcostal muscle Transverse thoracis muscle **J Thorax Muscle, Left** *See H Thorax Muscle, Right* **K Abdomen Muscle, Right** External oblique muscle Internal oblique muscle Pyramidalis muscle Rectus abdominis muscle Transversus abdominis muscle **L Abdomen Muscle, Left** *See K Abdomen Muscle, Right*	**M Perineum Muscle** Bulbospongiosus muscle Cremaster muscle Deep transverse perineal muscle Ischiocavernosus muscle Levator ani muscle Superficial transverse perineal muscle **N Hip Muscle, Right** Gemellus muscle Gluteus maximus muscle Gluteus medius muscle Gluteus minimus muscle Iliacus muscle Obturator muscle Piriformis muscle Psoas muscle Quadratus femoris muscle Tensor fasciae latae muscle **P Hip Muscle, Left** *See N Hip Muscle, Right* **Q Upper Leg Muscle, Right** Adductor brevis muscle Adductor longus muscle Adductor magnus muscle Biceps femoris muscle Gracilis muscle Pectineus muscle Quadriceps (femoris) Rectus femoris muscle Sartorius muscle Semimembranosus muscle Semitendinosus muscle Vastus intermedius muscle Vastus lateralis muscle Vastus medialis muscle **R Upper Leg Muscle, Left** *See Q Upper Leg Muscle, Right* **S Lower Leg Muscle, Right** Extensor digitorum longus muscle Extensor hallucis longus muscle Fibularis brevis muscle Fibularis longus muscle Flexor digitorum longus muscle Flexor hallucis longus muscle Gastrocnemius muscle Peroneus brevis muscle Peroneus longus muscle Popliteus muscle Soleus muscle Tibialis anterior muscle Tibialis posterior muscle **T Lower Leg Muscle, Left** *See S Lower Leg Muscle, Right* **V Foot Muscle, Right** Abductor hallucis muscle Adductor hallucis muscle Extensor digitorum brevis muscle Extensor hallucis brevis muscle Flexor digitorum brevis muscle Flexor hallucis brevis muscle Quadratus plantae muscle **W Foot Muscle, Left** *See V Foot Muscle, Right*	0 Open 3 Percutaneous 4 Percutaneous Endoscopic	Z No Device	Z No Qualifier

LC Limited Coverage   **NC** Noncovered   ⊞ Combination Member   HAC associated procedure   Combination Only   DRG Non-OR   Non-OR   New/Revised in GREEN

Ø   Medical and Surgical
K   Muscles
8   Division   Definition: Cutting into a body part, without draining fluids and/or gases from the body part, in order to separate or transect a body part
                     Explanation: All or a portion of the body part is separated into two or more portions

Body Part Character 4			Approach Character 5	Device Character 6	Qualifier Character 7

Ø Head Muscle
Auricularis muscle
Masseter muscle
Pterygoid muscle
Splenius capitis muscle
Temporalis muscle
Temporoparietalis muscle
1 Facial Muscle
Buccinator muscle
Corrugator supercilii
  muscle
Depressor anguli oris
  muscle
Depressor labii inferioris
  muscle
Depressor septi nasi
  muscle
Depressor supercilii
  muscle
Levator anguli oris muscle
Levator labii superioris
  alaeque nasi muscle
Levator labii superioris
  muscle
Mentalis muscle
Nasalis muscle
Occipitofrontalis muscle
Orbicularis oris muscle
Procerus muscle
Risorius muscle
Zygomaticus muscle
2 Neck Muscle, Right
Anterior vertebral muscle
Arytenoid muscle
Cricothyroid muscle
Infrahyoid muscle
Levator scapulae muscle
Platysma muscle
Scalene muscle
Splenius cervicis muscle
Sternocleidomastoid
  muscle
Suprahyoid muscle
Thyroarytenoid muscle
3 Neck Muscle, Left
See 2 Neck Muscle, Right
4 Tongue, Palate, Pharynx
Muscle
Chondroglossus muscle
Genioglossus muscle
Hyoglossus muscle
Inferior longitudinal
  muscle
Levator veli palatini
  muscle
Palatoglossal muscle
Palatopharyngeal muscle
Pharyngeal constrictor
  muscle
Salpingopharyngeus
  muscle
Styloglossus muscle
Stylopharyngeus muscle
Superior longitudinal
  muscle
Tensor veli palatini muscle
5 Shoulder Muscle, Right
Deltoid muscle
Infraspinatus muscle
Subscapularis muscle
Supraspinatus muscle
Teres major muscle
Teres minor muscle
6 Shoulder Muscle, Left
See 5 Shoulder Muscle,
  Right
	7 Upper Arm Muscle, Right
	Biceps brachii muscle
	Brachialis muscle
	Coracobrachialis muscle
	Triceps brachii muscle
	8 Upper Arm Muscle, Left
	See 7 Upper Arm Muscle,
	  Right
	9 Lower Arm and Wrist
	Muscle, Right
	Anatomical snuffbox
	Brachioradialis muscle
	Extensor carpi radialis
	  muscle
	Extensor carpi ulnaris
	  muscle
	Flexor carpi radialis muscle
	Flexor carpi ulnaris muscle
	Flexor pollicis longus
	  muscle
	Palmaris longus muscle
	Pronator quadratus
	  muscle
	Pronator teres muscle
	B Lower Arm and Wrist
	Muscle, Left
	See 9 Lower Arm and Wrist
	  Muscle, Right
	C Hand Muscle, Right
	Hypothenar muscle
	Palmar interosseous
	  muscle
	Thenar muscle
	D Hand Muscle, Left
	See C Hand Muscle, Right
	F Trunk Muscle, Right
	Coccygeus muscle
	Erector spinae muscle
	Interspinalis muscle
	Intertransversarius muscle
	Latissimus dorsi muscle
	Quadratus lumborum
	  muscle
	Rhomboid major muscle
	Rhomboid minor muscle
	Serratus posterior muscle
	Transversospinalis muscle
	Trapezius muscle
	G Trunk Muscle, Left
	See F Trunk Muscle, Right
	H Thorax Muscle, Right
	Intercostal muscle
	Levatores costarum
	  muscle
	Pectoralis major muscle
	Pectoralis minor muscle
	Serratus anterior muscle
	Subclavius muscle
	Subcostal muscle
	Transverse thoracis muscle
	J Thorax Muscle, Left
	See H Thorax Muscle, Right
	K Abdomen Muscle, Right
	External oblique muscle
	Internal oblique muscle
	Pyramidalis muscle
	Rectus abdominis muscle
	Transversus abdominis
	  muscle
	L Abdomen Muscle, Left
	See K Abdomen Muscle,
	  Right
		M Perineum Muscle
		Bulbospongiosus muscle
		Cremaster muscle
		Deep transverse perineal
		  muscle
		Ischiocavernosus muscle
		Levator ani muscle
		Superficial transverse
		  perineal muscle
		N Hip Muscle, Right
		Gemellus muscle
		Gluteus maximus muscle
		Gluteus medius muscle
		Gluteus minimus muscle
		Iliacus muscle
		Obturator muscle
		Piriformis muscle
		Psoas muscle
		Quadratus femoris muscle
		Tensor fasciae latae
		  muscle
		P Hip Muscle, Left
		See N Hip Muscle, Right
		Q Upper Leg Muscle, Right
		Adductor brevis muscle
		Adductor longus muscle
		Adductor magnus muscle
		Biceps femoris muscle
		Gracilis muscle
		Pectineus muscle
		Quadriceps (femoris)
		Rectus femoris muscle
		Sartorius muscle
		Semimembranosus
		  muscle
		Semitendinosus muscle
		Vastus intermedius muscle
		Vastus lateralis muscle
		Vastus medialis muscle
		R Upper Leg Muscle, Left
		See Q Upper Leg Muscle,
		  Right
		S Lower Leg Muscle, Right
		Extensor digitorum longus
		  muscle
		Extensor hallucis longus
		  muscle
		Fibularis brevis muscle
		Fibularis longus muscle
		Flexor digitorum longus
		  muscle
		Flexor hallucis longus
		  muscle
		Gastrocnemius muscle
		Peroneus brevis muscle
		Peroneus longus muscle
		Popliteus muscle
		Soleus muscle
		Tibialis anterior muscle
		Tibialis posterior muscle
		T Lower Leg Muscle, Left
		See S Lower Leg Muscle,
		  Right
		V Foot Muscle, Right
		Abductor hallucis muscle
		Adductor hallucis muscle
		Extensor digitorum brevis
		  muscle
		Extensor hallucis brevis
		  muscle
		Flexor digitorum brevis
		  muscle
		Flexor hallucis brevis
		  muscle
		Quadratus plantae muscle
		W Foot Muscle, Left
		See V Foot Muscle, Right
			Ø Open
			3 Percutaneous
			4 Percutaneous
			  Endoscopic
				Z No Device	**Z** No Qualifier

LC Limited Coverage   **NC** Noncovered   ⊞ Combination Member   HAC associated procedure   Combination Only   DRG Non-OR   Non-OR   New/Revised in GREEN

462   ICD-10-PCS 2021

ØK8–ØK8

Ø   **Medical and Surgical**
K   **Muscles**
9   **Drainage**   Definition: Taking or letting out fluids and/or gases from a body part

Explanation: The qualifier DIAGNOSTIC is used to identify drainage procedures that are biopsies

Body Part Character 4			Approach Character 5	Device Character 6	Qualifier Character 7
Ø Head Muscle	**7 Upper Arm Muscle, Right**	**M Perineum Muscle**	**Ø Open**	**Ø Drainage Device**	**Z No Qualifier**
Auricularis muscle	Biceps brachii muscle	Bulbospongiosus muscle	**3 Percutaneous**		
Masseter muscle	Brachialis muscle	Cremaster muscle	**4 Percutaneous Endoscopic**		
Pterygoid muscle	Coracobrachialis muscle	Deep transverse perineal muscle			
Splenius capitis muscle	Triceps brachii muscle	Ischiocavernosus muscle			
Temporalis muscle	**8 Upper Arm Muscle, Left**	Levator ani muscle			
Temporoparietalis muscle	*See 7 Upper Arm Muscle, Right*	Superficial transverse perineal muscle			
1 Facial Muscle	**9 Lower Arm and Wrist Muscle, Right**	**N Hip Muscle, Right**			
Buccinator muscle	Anatomical snuffbox	Gemellus muscle			
Corrugator supercilii muscle	Brachioradialis muscle	Gluteus maximus muscle			
Depressor anguli oris muscle	Extensor carpi radialis muscle	Gluteus medius muscle			
Depressor labii inferioris muscle	Extensor carpi ulnaris muscle	Gluteus minimus muscle			
Depressor septi nasi muscle	Flexor carpi radialis muscle	Iliacus muscle			
Depressor supercilii muscle	Flexor carpi ulnaris muscle	Obturator muscle			
Levator anguli oris muscle	Flexor pollicis longus muscle	Piriformis muscle			
Levator labii superioris alaeque nasi muscle	Palmaris longus muscle	Psoas muscle			
Levator labii superioris muscle	Pronator quadratus muscle	Quadratus femoris muscle			
Mentalis muscle	Pronator teres muscle	Tensor fasciae latae muscle			
Nasalis muscle	**B Lower Arm and Wrist Muscle, Left**	**P Hip Muscle, Left**			
Occipitofrontalis muscle	*See 9 Lower Arm and Wrist Muscle, Right*	*See N Hip Muscle, Right*			
Orbicularis oris muscle	**C Hand Muscle, Right**	**Q Upper Leg Muscle, Right**			
Procerus muscle	Hypothenar muscle	Adductor brevis muscle			
Risorius muscle	Palmar interosseous muscle	Adductor longus muscle			
Zygomaticus muscle	Thenar muscle	Adductor magnus muscle			
2 Neck Muscle, Right	**D Hand Muscle, Left**	Biceps femoris muscle			
Anterior vertebral muscle	*See C Hand Muscle, Right*	Gracilis muscle			
Arytenoid muscle	**F Trunk Muscle, Right**	Pectineus muscle			
Cricothyroid muscle	Coccygeus muscle	Quadriceps (femoris)			
Infrahyoid muscle	Erector spinae muscle	Rectus femoris muscle			
Levator scapulae muscle	Interspinalis muscle	Sartorius muscle			
Platysma muscle	Intertransversarius muscle	Semimembranosus muscle			
Scalene muscle	Latissimus dorsi muscle	Semitendinosus muscle			
Splenius cervicis muscle	Quadratus lumborum muscle	Vastus intermedius muscle			
Sternocleidomastoid muscle	Rhomboid major muscle	Vastus lateralis muscle			
Suprahyoid muscle	Rhomboid minor muscle	Vastus medialis muscle			
Thyroarytenoid muscle	Serratus posterior muscle	**R Upper Leg Muscle, Left**			
3 Neck Muscle, Left	Transversospinalis muscle	*See Q Upper Leg Muscle, Right*			
See 2 Neck Muscle, Right	Trapezius muscle	**S Lower Leg Muscle, Right**			
4 Tongue, Palate, Pharynx Muscle	**G Trunk Muscle, Left**	Extensor digitorum longus muscle			
Chondroglossus muscle	*See F Trunk Muscle, Right*	Extensor hallucis longus muscle			
Genioglossus muscle	**H Thorax Muscle, Right**	Fibularis brevis muscle			
Hyoglossus muscle	Intercostal muscle	Fibularis longus muscle			
Inferior longitudinal muscle	Levatores costarum muscle	Flexor digitorum longus muscle			
Levator veli palatini muscle	Pectoralis major muscle	Flexor hallucis longus muscle			
Palatoglossal muscle	Pectoralis minor muscle	Gastrocnemius muscle			
Palatopharyngeal muscle	Serratus anterior muscle	Peroneus brevis muscle			
Pharyngeal constrictor muscle	Subclavius muscle	Peroneus longus muscle			
Salpingopharyngeus muscle	Subcostal muscle	Popliteus muscle			
Styloglossus muscle	Transverse thoracis muscle	Soleus muscle			
Stylopharyngeus muscle	**J Thorax Muscle, Left**	Tibialis anterior muscle			
Superior longitudinal muscle	*See H Thorax Muscle, Right*	Tibialis posterior muscle			
Tensor veli palatini muscle	**K Abdomen Muscle, Right**	**T Lower Leg Muscle, Left**			
5 Shoulder Muscle, Right	External oblique muscle	*See S Lower Leg Muscle, Right*			
Deltoid muscle	Internal oblique muscle	**V Foot Muscle, Right**			
Infraspinatus muscle	Pyramidalis muscle	Abductor hallucis muscle			
Subscapularis muscle	Rectus abdominis muscle	Adductor hallucis muscle			
Supraspinatus muscle	Transversus abdominis muscle	Extensor digitorum brevis muscle			
Teres major muscle	**L Abdomen Muscle, Left**	Extensor hallucis brevis muscle			
Teres minor muscle	*See K Abdomen Muscle, Right*	Flexor digitorum brevis muscle			
6 Shoulder Muscle, Left		Flexor hallucis brevis muscle			
See 5 Shoulder Muscle, Right		Quadratus plantae muscle			
		W Foot Muscle, Left			
		See V Foot Muscle, Right			

Non-OR   ØK9[Ø,1,2,3,4,5,6,7,8,9,B,C,D,F,G,H,J,K,L,M,N,P,Q,R,S,T,V,W]3ØZ

ØK9 Continued on next page

LC Limited Coverage   **NC** Noncovered   ⊞ Combination Member   HAC associated procedure   Combination Only   DRG Non-OR   Non-OR   New/Revised in GREEN

Ø **Medical and Surgical**   *ØK9 Continued*
K **Muscles**
9 **Drainage**

Definition: Taking or letting out fluids and/or gases from a body part

Explanation: The qualifier DIAGNOSTIC is used to identify drainage procedures that are biopsies

Body Part Character 4			Approach Character 5	Device Character 6	Qualifier Character 7
Ø Head Muscle Auricularis muscle Masseter muscle Pterygoid muscle Splenius capitis muscle Temporalis muscle Temporoparietalis muscle **1 Facial Muscle** Buccinator muscle Corrugator supercilii muscle Depressor anguli oris muscle Depressor labii inferioris muscle Depressor septi nasi muscle Depressor supercilii muscle Levator anguli oris muscle Levator labii superioris alaeque nasi muscle Levator labii superioris muscle Mentalis muscle Nasalis muscle Occipitofrontalis muscle Orbicularis oris muscle Procerus muscle Risorius muscle Zygomaticus muscle **2 Neck Muscle, Right** Anterior vertebral muscle Arytenoid muscle Cricothyroid muscle Infrahyoid muscle Levator scapulae muscle Platysma muscle Scalene muscle Splenius cervicis muscle Sternocleidomastoid muscle Suprahyoid muscle Thyroarytenoid muscle **3 Neck Muscle, Left** *See 2 Neck Muscle, Right* **4 Tongue, Palate, Pharynx Muscle** Chondroglossus muscle Genioglossus muscle Hyoglossus muscle Inferior longitudinal muscle Levator veli palatini muscle Palatoglossal muscle Palatopharyngeal muscle Pharyngeal constrictor muscle Salpingopharyngeus muscle Styloglossus muscle Stylopharyngeus muscle Superior longitudinal muscle Tensor veli palatini muscle **5 Shoulder Muscle, Right** Deltoid muscle Infraspinatus muscle Subscapularis muscle Supraspinatus muscle Teres major muscle Teres minor muscle **6 Shoulder Muscle, Left** *See 5 Shoulder Muscle, Right*	**7 Upper Arm Muscle, Right** Biceps brachii muscle Brachialis muscle Coracobrachialis muscle Triceps brachii muscle **8 Upper Arm Muscle, Left** *See 7 Upper Arm Muscle, Right* **9 Lower Arm and Wrist Muscle, Right** Anatomical snuffbox Brachioradialis muscle Extensor carpi radialis muscle Extensor carpi ulnaris muscle Flexor carpi radialis muscle Flexor carpi ulnaris muscle Flexor pollicis longus muscle Palmaris longus muscle Pronator quadratus muscle Pronator teres muscle **B Lower Arm and Wrist Muscle, Left** *See 9 Lower Arm and Wrist Muscle, Right* **C Hand Muscle, Right** Hypothenar muscle Palmar interosseous muscle Thenar muscle **D Hand Muscle, Left** *See C Hand Muscle, Right* **F Trunk Muscle, Right** Coccygeus muscle Erector spinae muscle Interspinalis muscle Intertransversarius muscle Latissimus dorsi muscle Quadratus lumborum muscle Rhomboid major muscle Rhomboid minor muscle Serratus posterior muscle Transversospinalis muscle Trapezius muscle **G Trunk Muscle, Left** *See F Trunk Muscle, Right* **H Thorax Muscle, Right** Intercostal muscle Levatores costarum muscle Pectoralis major muscle Pectoralis minor muscle Serratus anterior muscle Subclavius muscle Subcostal muscle Transverse thoracis muscle **J Thorax Muscle, Left** *See H Thorax Muscle, Right* **K Abdomen Muscle, Right** External oblique muscle Internal oblique muscle Pyramidalis muscle Rectus abdominis muscle Transversus abdominis muscle **L Abdomen Muscle, Left** *See K Abdomen Muscle, Right*	**M Perineum Muscle** Bulbospongiosus muscle Cremaster muscle Deep transverse perineal muscle Ischiocavernosus muscle Levator ani muscle Superficial transverse perineal muscle **N Hip Muscle, Right** Gemellus muscle Gluteus maximus muscle Gluteus medius muscle Gluteus minimus muscle Iliacus muscle Obturator muscle Piriformis muscle Psoas muscle Quadratus femoris muscle Tensor fasciae latae muscle **P Hip Muscle, Left** *See N Hip Muscle, Right* **Q Upper Leg Muscle, Right** Adductor brevis muscle Adductor longus muscle Adductor magnus muscle Biceps femoris muscle Gracilis muscle Pectineus muscle Quadriceps (femoris) Rectus femoris muscle Sartorius muscle Semimembranosus muscle Semitendinosus muscle Vastus intermedius muscle Vastus lateralis muscle Vastus medialis muscle **R Upper Leg Muscle, Left** *See Q Upper Leg Muscle, Right* **S Lower Leg Muscle, Right** Extensor digitorum longus muscle Extensor hallucis longus muscle Fibularis brevis muscle Fibularis longus muscle Flexor digitorum longus muscle Flexor hallucis longus muscle Gastrocnemius muscle Peroneus brevis muscle Peroneus longus muscle Popliteus muscle Soleus muscle Tibialis anterior muscle Tibialis posterior muscle **T Lower Leg Muscle, Left** *See S Lower Leg Muscle, Right* **V Foot Muscle, Right** Abductor hallucis muscle Adductor hallucis muscle Extensor digitorum brevis muscle Extensor hallucis brevis muscle Flexor digitorum brevis muscle Flexor hallucis brevis muscle Quadratus plantae muscle **W Foot Muscle, Left** *See V Foot Muscle, Right*	**Ø Open** **3 Percutaneous** **4 Percutaneous Endoscopic**	**Z No Device**	**X Diagnostic** **Z No Qualifier**

Non-OR	ØK9[Ø,1,2,3,4,5,6,7,8,9,B,F,G,H,J,K,L,M,N,P,Q,R,S,T,V,W]3ZZ
Non-OR	ØK9[C,D][3,4]ZZ

■ Limited Coverage   ■ Noncovered   ⊞ Combination Member   HAC associated procedure   Combination Only   DRG Non-OR   Non-OR   New/Revised in GREEN

464   ICD-10-PCS 2021

Ø   **Medical and Surgical**
K   **Muscles**
B   **Excision**   **Definition:** Cutting out or off, without replacement, a portion of a body part

                  Explanation: The qualifier DIAGNOSTIC is used to identify excision procedures that are biopsies

Body Part Character 4			Approach Character 5	Device Character 6	Qualifier Character 7

Ø Head Muscle
Auricularis muscle
Masseter muscle
Pterygoid muscle
Splenius capitis muscle
Temporalis muscle
Temporoparietalis muscle
1 Facial Muscle
Buccinator muscle
Corrugator supercilii
  muscle
Depressor anguli oris
  muscle
Depressor labii inferioris
  muscle
Depressor septi nasi
  muscle
Depressor supercilii
  muscle
Levator anguli oris muscle
Levator labii superioris
  alaeque nasi muscle
Levator labii superioris
  muscle
Mentalis muscle
Nasalis muscle
Occipitofrontalis muscle
Orbicularis oris muscle
Procerus muscle
Risorius muscle
Zygomaticus muscle
2 Neck Muscle, Right
Anterior vertebral muscle
Arytenoid muscle
Cricothyroid muscle
Infrahyoid muscle
Levator scapulae muscle
Platysma muscle
Scalene muscle
Splenius cervicis muscle
Sternocleidomastoid
  muscle
Suprahyoid muscle
Thyroarytenoid muscle
3 Neck Muscle, Left
See 2 Neck Muscle, Right
**4 Tongue, Palate, Pharynx
  Muscle**
Chondroglossus muscle
Genioglossus muscle
Hyoglossus muscle
Inferior longitudinal
  muscle
Levator veli palatini
  muscle
Palatoglossal muscle
Palatopharyngeal muscle
Pharyngeal constrictor
  muscle
Salpingopharyngeus
  muscle
Styloglossus muscle
Stylopharyngeus muscle
Superior longitudinal
  muscle
Tensor veli palatini muscle
5 Shoulder Muscle, Right
Deltoid muscle
Infraspinatus muscle
Subscapularis muscle
Supraspinatus muscle
Teres major muscle
Teres minor muscle
6 Shoulder Muscle, Left
*See 5 Shoulder Muscle,
  Right*
	7 Upper Arm Muscle, Right
	Biceps brachii muscle
	Brachialis muscle
	Coracobrachialis muscle
	Triceps brachii muscle
	8 Upper Arm Muscle, Left
	*See 7 Upper Arm Muscle,
	  Right*
	**9 Lower Arm and Wrist
	  Muscle, Right**
	Anatomical snuffbox
	Brachioradialis muscle
	Extensor carpi radialis
	  muscle
	Extensor carpi ulnaris
	  muscle
	Flexor carpi radialis muscle
	Flexor carpi ulnaris muscle
	Flexor pollicis longus
	  muscle
	Palmaris longus muscle
	Pronator quadratus
	  muscle
	Pronator teres muscle
	**B Lower Arm and Wrist
	  Muscle, Left**
	*See 9 Lower Arm and Wrist
	  Muscle, Right*
	C Hand Muscle, Right
	Hypothenar muscle
	Palmar interosseous
	  muscle
	Thenar muscle
	D Hand Muscle, Left
	See C Hand Muscle, Right
	F Trunk Muscle, Right
	Coccygeus muscle
	Erector spinae muscle
	Interspinalis muscle
	Intertransversarius muscle
	Latissimus dorsi muscle
	Quadratus lumborum
	  muscle
	Rhomboid major muscle
	Rhomboid minor muscle
	Serratus posterior muscle
	Transversospinalis muscle
	Trapezius muscle
	G Trunk Muscle, Left
	See F Trunk Muscle, Right
	H Thorax Muscle, Right
	Intercostal muscle
	Levatores costarum
	  muscle
	Pectoralis major muscle
	Pectoralis minor muscle
	Serratus anterior muscle
	Subclavius muscle
	Subcostal muscle
	Transverse thoracis muscle
	J Thorax Muscle, Left
	See H Thorax Muscle, Right
	K Abdomen Muscle, Right
	External oblique muscle
	Internal oblique muscle
	Pyramidalis muscle
	Rectus abdominis muscle
	Transversus abdominis
	  muscle
	L Abdomen Muscle, Left
	*See K Abdomen Muscle,
	  Right*
		M Perineum Muscle
		Bulbospongiosus muscle
		Cremaster muscle
		Deep transverse perineal
		  muscle
		Ischiocavernosus muscle
		Levator ani muscle
		Superficial transverse
		  perineal muscle
		N Hip Muscle, Right
		Gemellus muscle
		Gluteus maximus muscle
		Gluteus medius muscle
		Gluteus minimus muscle
		Iliacus muscle
		Obturator muscle
		Piriformis muscle
		Psoas muscle
		Quadratus femoris muscle
		Tensor fasciae latae
		  muscle
		P Hip Muscle, Left
		See N Hip Muscle, Right
		Q Upper Leg Muscle, Right
		Adductor brevis muscle
		Adductor longus muscle
		Adductor magnus muscle
		Biceps femoris muscle
		Gracilis muscle
		Pectineus muscle
		Quadriceps (femoris)
		Rectus femoris muscle
		Sartorius muscle
		Semimembranosus
		  muscle
		Semitendinosus muscle
		Vastus intermedius muscle
		Vastus lateralis muscle
		Vastus medialis muscle
		R Upper Leg Muscle, Left
		*See Q Upper Leg Muscle,
		  Right*
		S Lower Leg Muscle, Right
		Extensor digitorum longus
		  muscle
		Extensor hallucis longus
		  muscle
		Fibularis brevis muscle
		Fibularis longus muscle
		Flexor digitorum longus
		  muscle
		Flexor hallucis longus
		  muscle
		Gastrocnemius muscle
		Peroneus brevis muscle
		Peroneus longus muscle
		Popliteus muscle
		Soleus muscle
		Tibialis anterior muscle
		Tibialis posterior muscle
		T Lower Leg Muscle, Left
		*See S Lower Leg Muscle,
		  Right*
		V Foot Muscle, Right
		Abductor hallucis muscle
		Adductor hallucis muscle
		Extensor digitorum brevis
		  muscle
		Extensor hallucis brevis
		  muscle
		Flexor digitorum brevis
		  muscle
		Flexor hallucis brevis
		  muscle
		Quadratus plantae muscle
		W Foot Muscle, Left
		See V Foot Muscle, Right
			Ø Open
			3 Percutaneous
			4 Percutaneous
			  Endoscopic
				Z No Device	**X** Diagnostic
					Z No Qualifier

LC Limited Coverage   **NC** Noncovered   ⊞ Combination Member   HAC associated procedure   Combination Only   DRG Non-OR   Non-OR   New/Revised in **GREEN**

ICD-10-PCS 2021   465

ØKB–ØKB

Ø   **Medical and Surgical**
K   **Muscles**
C   **Extirpation**   Definition: Taking or cutting out solid matter from a body part

Explanation: The solid matter may be an abnormal byproduct of a biological function or a foreign body; it may be imbedded in a body part or in the lumen of a tubular body part. The solid matter may or may not have been previously broken into pieces.

Body Part Character 4			Approach Character 5	Device Character 6	Qualifier Character 7
Ø Head Muscle Auricularis muscle Masseter muscle Pterygoid muscle Splenius capitis muscle Temporalis muscle Temporoparietalis muscle **1 Facial Muscle** Buccinator muscle Corrugator supercilii muscle Depressor anguli oris muscle Depressor labii inferioris muscle Depressor septi nasi muscle Depressor supercilii muscle Levator anguli oris muscle Levator labii superioris alaeque nasi muscle Levator labii superioris muscle Mentalis muscle Nasalis muscle Occipitofrontalis muscle Orbicularis oris muscle Procerus muscle Risorius muscle Zygomaticus muscle **2 Neck Muscle, Right** Anterior vertebral muscle Arytenoid muscle Cricothyroid muscle Infrahyoid muscle Levator scapulae muscle Platysma muscle Scalene muscle Splenius cervicis muscle Sternocleidomastoid muscle Suprahyoid muscle Thyroarytenoid muscle **3 Neck Muscle, Left** *See 2 Neck Muscle, Right* **4 Tongue, Palate, Pharynx Muscle** Chondroglossus muscle Genioglossus muscle Hyoglossus muscle Inferior longitudinal muscle Levator veli palatini muscle Palatoglossal muscle Palatopharyngeal muscle Pharyngeal constrictor muscle Salpingopharyngeus muscle Styloglossus muscle Stylopharyngeus muscle Superior longitudinal muscle Tensor veli palatini muscle **5 Shoulder Muscle, Right** Deltoid muscle Infraspinatus muscle Subscapularis muscle Supraspinatus muscle Teres major muscle Teres minor muscle **6 Shoulder Muscle, Left** *See 5 Shoulder Muscle, Right*	**7 Upper Arm Muscle, Right** Biceps brachii muscle Brachialis muscle Coracobrachialis muscle Triceps brachii muscle **8 Upper Arm Muscle, Left** *See 7 Upper Arm Muscle, Right* **9 Lower Arm and Wrist Muscle, Right** Anatomical snuffbox Brachioradialis muscle Extensor carpi radialis muscle Extensor carpi ulnaris muscle Flexor carpi radialis muscle Flexor carpi ulnaris muscle Flexor pollicis longus muscle Palmaris longus muscle Pronator quadratus muscle Pronator teres muscle **B Lower Arm and Wrist Muscle, Left** *See 9 Lower Arm and Wrist Muscle, Right* **C Hand Muscle, Right** Hypothenar muscle Palmar interosseous muscle Thenar muscle **D Hand Muscle, Left** *See C Hand Muscle, Right* **F Trunk Muscle, Right** Coccygeus muscle Erector spinae muscle Interspinalis muscle Intertransversarius muscle Latissimus dorsi muscle Quadratus lumborum muscle Rhomboid major muscle Rhomboid minor muscle Serratus posterior muscle Transversospinalis muscle Trapezius muscle **G Trunk Muscle, Left** *See F Trunk Muscle, Right* **H Thorax Muscle, Right** Intercostal muscle Levatores costarum muscle Pectoralis major muscle Pectoralis minor muscle Serratus anterior muscle Subclavius muscle Subcostal muscle Transverse thoracis muscle **J Thorax Muscle, Left** *See H Thorax Muscle, Right* **K Abdomen Muscle, Right** External oblique muscle Internal oblique muscle Pyramidalis muscle Rectus abdominis muscle Transversus abdominis muscle **L Abdomen Muscle, Left** *See K Abdomen Muscle, Right*	**M Perineum Muscle** Bulbospongiosus muscle Cremaster muscle Deep transverse perineal muscle Ischiocavernosus muscle Levator ani muscle Superficial transverse perineal muscle **N Hip Muscle, Right** Gemellus muscle Gluteus maximus muscle Gluteus medius muscle Gluteus minimus muscle Iliacus muscle Obturator muscle Piriformis muscle Psoas muscle Quadratus femoris muscle Tensor fasciae latae muscle **P Hip Muscle, Left** *See N Hip Muscle, Right* **Q Upper Leg Muscle, Right** Adductor brevis muscle Adductor longus muscle Adductor magnus muscle Biceps femoris muscle Gracilis muscle Pectineus muscle Quadriceps (femoris) Rectus femoris muscle Sartorius muscle Semimembranosus muscle Semitendinosus muscle Vastus intermedius muscle Vastus lateralis muscle Vastus medialis muscle **R Upper Leg Muscle, Left** *See Q Upper Leg Muscle, Right* **S Lower Leg Muscle, Right** Extensor digitorum longus muscle Extensor hallucis longus muscle Fibularis brevis muscle Fibularis longus muscle Flexor digitorum longus muscle Flexor hallucis longus muscle Gastrocnemius muscle Peroneus brevis muscle Peroneus longus muscle Popliteus muscle Soleus muscle Tibialis anterior muscle Tibialis posterior muscle **T Lower Leg Muscle, Left** *See S Lower Leg Muscle, Right* **V Foot Muscle, Right** Abductor hallucis muscle Adductor hallucis muscle Extensor digitorum brevis muscle Extensor hallucis brevis muscle Flexor digitorum brevis muscle Flexor hallucis brevis muscle Quadratus plantae muscle **W Foot Muscle, Left** *See V Foot Muscle, Right*	**Ø Open** **3 Percutaneous** **4 Percutaneous Endoscopic**	**Z No Device**	**Z No Qualifier**

LC Limited Coverage   **NC** Noncovered   ⊞ Combination Member   HAC associated procedure   Combination Only   DRG Non-OR   Non-OR   New/Revised in GREEN

466   ICD-10-PCS 2021

ØKC–ØKC

Muscles

Ø Medical and Surgical
K Muscles
D Extraction

Definition: Pulling or stripping out or off all or a portion of a body part by the use of force
Explanation: The qualifier DIAGNOSTIC is used to identify extraction procedures that are biopsies

Body Part Character 4			Approach Character 5	Device Character 6	Qualifier Character 7

Ø Head Muscle
Auricularis muscle
Masseter muscle
Pterygoid muscle
Splenius capitis muscle
Temporalis muscle
Temporoparietalis muscle
1 Facial Muscle
Buccinator muscle
Corrugator supercilii
  muscle
Depressor anguli oris
  muscle
Depressor labii inferioris
  muscle
Depressor septi nasi
  muscle
Depressor supercilii
  muscle
Levator anguli oris muscle
Levator labii superioris
  alaeque nasi muscle
Levator labii superioris
  muscle
Mentalis muscle
Nasalis muscle
Occipitofrontalis muscle
Orbicularis oris muscle
Procerus muscle
Risorius muscle
Zygomaticus muscle
2 Neck Muscle, Right
Anterior vertebral muscle
Arytenoid muscle
Cricothyroid muscle
Infrahyoid muscle
Levator scapulae muscle
Platysma muscle
Scalene muscle
Splenius cervicis muscle
Sternocleidomastoid
  muscle
Suprahyoid muscle
Thyroarytenoid muscle
3 Neck Muscle, Left
See 2 Neck Muscle, Right
4 Tongue, Palate, Pharynx
Muscle
Chondroglossus muscle
Genioglossus muscle
Hyoglossus muscle
Inferior longitudinal
  muscle
Levator veli palatini
  muscle
Palatoglossal muscle
Palatopharyngeal muscle
Pharyngeal constrictor
  muscle
Salpingopharyngeus
  muscle
Styloglossus muscle
Stylopharyngeus muscle
Superior longitudinal
  muscle
Tensor veli palatini muscle
5 Shoulder Muscle, Right
Deltoid muscle
Infraspinatus muscle
Subscapularis muscle
Supraspinatus muscle
Teres major muscle
Teres minor muscle
6 Shoulder Muscle, Left
See 5 Shoulder Muscle,
Right
	7 Upper Arm Muscle, Right
	Biceps brachii muscle
	Brachialis muscle
	Coracobrachialis muscle
	Triceps brachii muscle
	8 Upper Arm Muscle, Left
	See 7 Upper Arm Muscle,
	Right
	9 Lower Arm and Wrist
	Muscle, Right
	Anatomical snuffbox
	Brachioradialis muscle
	Extensor carpi radialis
	  muscle
	Extensor carpi ulnaris
	  muscle
	Flexor carpi radialis muscle
	Flexor carpi ulnaris muscle
	Flexor pollicis longus
	  muscle
	Palmaris longus muscle
	Pronator quadratus
	  muscle
	Pronator teres muscle
	B Lower Arm and Wrist
	Muscle, Left
	See 9 Lower Arm and Wrist
	Muscle, Right
	C Hand Muscle, Right
	Hypothenar muscle
	Palmar interosseous
	  muscle
	Thenar muscle
	D Hand Muscle, Left
	See C Hand Muscle, Right
	F Trunk Muscle, Right
	Coccygeus muscle
	Erector spinae muscle
	Interspinalis muscle
	Intertransversarius muscle
	Latissimus dorsi muscle
	Quadratus lumborum
	  muscle
	Rhomboid major muscle
	Rhomboid minor muscle
	Serratus posterior muscle
	Transversospinalis muscle
	Trapezius muscle
	G Trunk Muscle, Left
	See F Trunk Muscle, Right
	H Thorax Muscle, Right
	Intercostal muscle
	Levatores costarum
	  muscle
	Pectoralis major muscle
	Pectoralis minor muscle
	Serratus anterior muscle
	Subclavius muscle
	Subcostal muscle
	Transverse thoracis muscle
	J Thorax Muscle, Left
	See H Thorax Muscle, Right
	K Abdomen Muscle, Right
	External oblique muscle
	Internal oblique muscle
	Pyramidalis muscle
	Rectus abdominis muscle
	Transversus abdominis
	  muscle
	L Abdomen Muscle, Left
	See K Abdomen Muscle,
	Right
		M Perineum Muscle
		Bulbospongiosus muscle
		Cremaster muscle
		Deep transverse perineal
		  muscle
		Ischiocavernosus muscle
		Levator ani muscle
		Superficial transverse
		  perineal muscle
		N Hip Muscle, Right
		Gemellus muscle
		Gluteus maximus muscle
		Gluteus medius muscle
		Gluteus minimus muscle
		Iliacus muscle
		Obturator muscle
		Piriformis muscle
		Psoas muscle
		Quadratus femoris muscle
		Tensor fasciae latae
		  muscle
		P Hip Muscle, Left
		See N Hip Muscle, Right
		Q Upper Leg Muscle, Right
		Adductor brevis muscle
		Adductor longus muscle
		Adductor magnus muscle
		Biceps femoris muscle
		Gracilis muscle
		Pectineus muscle
		Quadriceps (femoris)
		Rectus femoris muscle
		Sartorius muscle
		Semimembranosus
		  muscle
		Semitendinosus muscle
		Vastus intermedius muscle
		Vastus lateralis muscle
		Vastus medialis muscle
		R Upper Leg Muscle, Left
		See Q Upper Leg Muscle,
		Right
		S Lower Leg Muscle, Right
		Extensor digitorum longus
		  muscle
		Extensor hallucis longus
		  muscle
		Fibularis brevis muscle
		Fibularis longus muscle
		Flexor digitorum longus
		  muscle
		Flexor hallucis longus
		  muscle
		Gastrocnemius muscle
		Peroneus brevis muscle
		Peroneus longus muscle
		Popliteus muscle
		Soleus muscle
		Tibialis anterior muscle
		Tibialis posterior muscle
		T Lower Leg Muscle, Left
		See S Lower Leg Muscle,
		Right
		V Foot Muscle, Right
		Abductor hallucis muscle
		Adductor hallucis muscle
		Extensor digitorum brevis
		  muscle
		Extensor hallucis brevis
		  muscle
		Flexor digitorum brevis
		  muscle
		Flexor hallucis brevis
		  muscle
		Quadratus plantae muscle
		W Foot Muscle, Left
		See V Foot Muscle, Right
			Ø Open	**Z No Device**	**Z No Qualifier**

LC Limited Coverage   **NC** Noncovered   ⊞ Combination Member   HAC associated procedure   Combination Only   DRG Non-OR   Non-OR   New/Revised in **GREEN**

ICD-10-PCS 2021   467

Ø   Medical and Surgical
K   Muscles
H   Insertion   Definition: Putting in a nonbiological appliance that monitors, assists, performs, or prevents a physiological function but does not physically take the place of a body part

                 Explanation: None

Body Part Character 4	Approach Character 5	Device Character 6	Qualifier Character 7
X Upper Muscle Y Lower Muscle	Ø Open 3 Percutaneous 4 Percutaneous Endoscopic	M Stimulator Lead Y Other Device	Z No Qualifier

Non-OR   ØKH[X,Y][3,4]YZ

Ø   Medical and Surgical
K   Muscles
J   Inspection   Definition: Visually and/or manually exploring a body part

                 Explanation: Visual exploration may be performed with or without optical instrumentation. Manual exploration may be performed directly or through intervening body layers.

Body Part Character 4	Approach Character 5	Device Character 6	Qualifier Character 7
X Upper Muscle Y Lower Muscle	Ø Open 3 Percutaneous 4 Percutaneous Endoscopic X External	Z No Device	Z No Qualifier

Non-OR   ØKJ[X,Y][3,X]ZZ

LC Limited Coverage   **NC** Noncovered   ⊞ Combination Member   HAC associated procedure   Combination Only   DRG Non-OR   Non-OR   New/Revised in GREEN

468   ICD-10-PCS 2021

Ø Medical and Surgical
K Muscles
M Reattachment   Definition: Putting back in or on all or a portion of a separated body part to its normal location or other suitable location
                 Explanation: Vascular circulation and nervous pathways may or may not be reestablished

Body Part Character 4			Approach Character 5	Device Character 6	Qualifier Character 7
Ø Head Muscle Auricularis muscle Masseter muscle Pterygoid muscle Splenius capitis muscle Temporalis muscle Temporoparietalis muscle **1 Facial Muscle** Buccinator muscle Corrugator supercilii muscle Depressor anguli oris muscle Depressor labii inferioris muscle Depressor septi nasi muscle Depressor supercilii muscle Levator anguli oris muscle Levator labii superioris alaeque nasi muscle Levator labii superioris muscle Mentalis muscle Nasalis muscle Occipitofrontalis muscle Orbicularis oris muscle Procerus muscle Risorius muscle Zygomaticus muscle **2 Neck Muscle, Right** Anterior vertebral muscle Arytenoid muscle Cricothyroid muscle Infrahyoid muscle Levator scapulae muscle Platysma muscle Scalene muscle Splenius cervicis muscle Sternocleidomastoid muscle Suprahyoid muscle Thyroarytenoid muscle **3 Neck Muscle, Left** *See 2 Neck Muscle, Right* **4 Tongue, Palate, Pharynx Muscle** Chondroglossus muscle Genioglossus muscle Hyoglossus muscle Inferior longitudinal muscle Levator veli palatini muscle Palatoglossal muscle Palatopharyngeal muscle Pharyngeal constrictor muscle Salpingopharyngeus muscle Styloglossus muscle Stylopharyngeus muscle Superior longitudinal muscle Tensor veli palatini muscle **5 Shoulder Muscle, Right** Deltoid muscle Infraspinatus muscle Subscapularis muscle Supraspinatus muscle Teres major muscle Teres minor muscle **6 Shoulder Muscle, Left** *See 5 Shoulder Muscle, Right*	**7 Upper Arm Muscle, Right** Biceps brachii muscle Brachialis muscle Coracobrachialis muscle Triceps brachii muscle **8 Upper Arm Muscle, Left** *See 7 Upper Arm Muscle, Right* **9 Lower Arm and Wrist Muscle, Right** Anatomical snuffbox Brachioradialis muscle Extensor carpi radialis muscle Extensor carpi ulnaris muscle Flexor carpi radialis muscle Flexor carpi ulnaris muscle Flexor pollicis longus muscle Palmaris longus muscle Pronator quadratus muscle Pronator teres muscle **B Lower Arm and Wrist Muscle, Left** *See 9 Lower Arm and Wrist Muscle, Right* **C Hand Muscle, Right** Hypothenar muscle Palmar interosseous muscle Thenar muscle **D Hand Muscle, Left** *See C Hand Muscle, Right* **F Trunk Muscle, Right** Coccygeus muscle Erector spinae muscle Interspinalis muscle Intertransversarius muscle Latissimus dorsi muscle Quadratus lumborum muscle Rhomboid major muscle Rhomboid minor muscle Serratus posterior muscle Transversospinalis muscle Trapezius muscle **G Trunk Muscle, Left** *See F Trunk Muscle, Right* **H Thorax Muscle, Right** Intercostal muscle Levatores costarum muscle Pectoralis major muscle Pectoralis minor muscle Serratus anterior muscle Subclavius muscle Subcostal muscle Transverse thoracis muscle **J Thorax Muscle, Left** *See H Thorax Muscle, Right* **K Abdomen Muscle, Right** External oblique muscle Internal oblique muscle Pyramidalis muscle Rectus abdominis muscle Transversus abdominis muscle **L Abdomen Muscle, Left** *See K Abdomen Muscle, Right*	**M Perineum Muscle** Bulbospongiosus muscle Cremaster muscle Deep transverse perineal muscle Ischiocavernosus muscle Levator ani muscle Superficial transverse perineal muscle **N Hip Muscle, Right** Gemellus muscle Gluteus maximus muscle Gluteus medius muscle Gluteus minimus muscle Iliacus muscle Obturator muscle Piriformis muscle Psoas muscle Quadratus femoris muscle Tensor fasciae latae muscle **P Hip Muscle, Left** *See N Hip Muscle, Right* **Q Upper Leg Muscle, Right** Adductor brevis muscle Adductor longus muscle Adductor magnus muscle Biceps femoris muscle Gracilis muscle Pectineus muscle Quadriceps (femoris) Rectus femoris muscle Sartorius muscle Semimembranosus muscle Semitendinosus muscle Vastus intermedius muscle Vastus lateralis muscle Vastus medialis muscle **R Upper Leg Muscle, Left** *See Q Upper Leg Muscle, Right* **S Lower Leg Muscle, Right** Extensor digitorum longus muscle Extensor hallucis longus muscle Fibularis brevis muscle Fibularis longus muscle Flexor digitorum longus muscle Flexor hallucis longus muscle Gastrocnemius muscle Peroneus brevis muscle Peroneus longus muscle Popliteus muscle Soleus muscle Tibialis anterior muscle Tibialis posterior muscle **T Lower Leg Muscle, Left** *See S Lower Leg Muscle, Right* **V Foot Muscle, Right** Abductor hallucis muscle Adductor hallucis muscle Extensor digitorum brevis muscle Extensor hallucis brevis muscle Flexor digitorum brevis muscle Flexor hallucis brevis muscle Quadratus plantae muscle **W Foot Muscle, Left** *See V Foot Muscle, Right*	**Ø Open** **4 Percutaneous Endoscopic**	**Z No Device**	**Z No Qualifier**

LC Limited Coverage   NC Noncovered   ⊞ Combination Member   HAC associated procedure   Combination Only   DRG Non-OR   Non-OR   New/Revised in GREEN

ICD-10-PCS 2021   469

ØKM–ØKM

Ø   **Medical and Surgical**
K   **Muscles**
N   **Release**

Definition: Freeing a body part from an abnormal physical constraint by cutting or by the use of force
Explanation: Some of the restraining tissue may be taken out but none of the body part is taken out

Body Part Character 4			Approach Character 5	Device Character 6	Qualifier Character 7

Ø Head Muscle
Auricularis muscle
Masseter muscle
Pterygoid muscle
Splenius capitis muscle
Temporalis muscle
Temporoparietalis muscle
1 Facial Muscle
Buccinator muscle
Corrugator supercilii
  muscle
Depressor anguli oris
  muscle
Depressor labii inferioris
  muscle
Depressor septi nasi
  muscle
Depressor supercilii
  muscle
Levator anguli oris muscle
Levator labii superioris
  alaeque nasi muscle
Levator labii superioris
  muscle
Mentalis muscle
Nasalis muscle
Occipitofrontalis muscle
Orbicularis oris muscle
Procerus muscle
Risorius muscle
Zygomaticus muscle
2 Neck Muscle, Right
Anterior vertebral muscle
Arytenoid muscle
Cricothyroid muscle
Infrahyoid muscle
Levator scapulae muscle
Platysma muscle
Scalene muscle
Splenius cervicis muscle
Sternocleidomastoid
  muscle
Suprahyoid muscle
Thyroarytenoid muscle
3 Neck Muscle, Left
See 2 Neck Muscle, Right
4 Tongue, Palate, Pharynx
Muscle
Chondroglossus muscle
Genioglossus muscle
Hyoglossus muscle
Inferior longitudinal
  muscle
Levator veli palatini
  muscle
Palatoglossal muscle
Palatopharyngeal muscle
Pharyngeal constrictor
  muscle
Salpingopharyngeus
  muscle
Styloglossus muscle
Stylopharyngeus muscle
Superior longitudinal
  muscle
Tensor veli palatini muscle
5 Shoulder Muscle, Right
Deltoid muscle
Infraspinatus muscle
Subscapularis muscle
Supraspinatus muscle
Teres major muscle
Teres minor muscle
6 Shoulder Muscle, Left
See 5 Shoulder Muscle,
Right
	7 Upper Arm Muscle, Right
	Biceps brachii muscle
	Brachialis muscle
	Coracobrachialis muscle
	Triceps brachii muscle
	8 Upper Arm Muscle, Left
	See 7 Upper Arm Muscle,
	Right
	9 Lower Arm and Wrist
	Muscle, Right
	Anatomical snuffbox
	Brachioradialis muscle
	Extensor carpi radialis
	  muscle
	Extensor carpi ulnaris
	  muscle
	Flexor carpi radialis muscle
	Flexor carpi ulnaris muscle
	Flexor pollicis longus
	  muscle
	Palmaris longus muscle
	Pronator quadratus
	  muscle
	Pronator teres muscle
	B Lower Arm and Wrist
	Muscle, Left
	See 9 Lower Arm and Wrist
	Muscle, Right
	C Hand Muscle, Right
	Hypothenar muscle
	Palmar interosseous
	  muscle
	Thenar muscle
	D Hand Muscle, Left
	See C Hand Muscle, Right
	F Trunk Muscle, Right
	Coccygeus muscle
	Erector spinae muscle
	Interspinalis muscle
	Intertransversarius muscle
	Latissimus dorsi muscle
	Quadratus lumborum
	  muscle
	Rhomboid major muscle
	Rhomboid minor muscle
	Serratus posterior muscle
	Transversospinalis muscle
	Trapezius muscle
	G Trunk Muscle, Left
	See F Trunk Muscle, Right
	H Thorax Muscle, Right
	Intercostal muscle
	Levatores costarum
	  muscle
	Pectoralis major muscle
	Pectoralis minor muscle
	Serratus anterior muscle
	Subclavius muscle
	Subcostal muscle
	Transverse thoracis muscle
	J Thorax Muscle, Left
	See H Thorax Muscle, Right
	K Abdomen Muscle, Right
	External oblique muscle
	Internal oblique muscle
	Pyramidalis muscle
	Rectus abdominis muscle
	Transversus abdominis
	  muscle
	L Abdomen Muscle, Left
	See K Abdomen Muscle,
	Right
		M Perineum Muscle
		Bulbospongiosus muscle
		Cremaster muscle
		Deep transverse perineal
		  muscle
		Ischiocavernosus muscle
		Levator ani muscle
		Superficial transverse
		  perineal muscle
		N Hip Muscle, Right
		Gemellus muscle
		Gluteus maximus muscle
		Gluteus medius muscle
		Gluteus minimus muscle
		Iliacus muscle
		Obturator muscle
		Piriformis muscle
		Psoas muscle
		Quadratus femoris muscle
		Tensor fasciae latae
		  muscle
		P Hip Muscle, Left
		See N Hip Muscle, Right
		Q Upper Leg Muscle, Right
		Adductor brevis muscle
		Adductor longus muscle
		Adductor magnus muscle
		Biceps femoris muscle
		Gracilis muscle
		Pectineus muscle
		Quadriceps (femoris)
		Rectus femoris muscle
		Sartorius muscle
		Semimembranosus
		  muscle
		Semitendinosus muscle
		Vastus intermedius muscle
		Vastus lateralis muscle
		Vastus medialis muscle
		R Upper Leg Muscle, Left
		See Q Upper Leg Muscle,
		Right
		S Lower Leg Muscle, Right
		Extensor digitorum longus
		  muscle
		Extensor hallucis longus
		  muscle
		Fibularis brevis muscle
		Fibularis longus muscle
		Flexor digitorum longus
		  muscle
		Flexor hallucis longus
		  muscle
		Gastrocnemius muscle
		Peroneus brevis muscle
		Peroneus longus muscle
		Popliteus muscle
		Soleus muscle
		Tibialis anterior muscle
		Tibialis posterior muscle
		T Lower Leg Muscle, Left
		See S Lower Leg Muscle,
		Right
		V Foot Muscle, Right
		Abductor hallucis muscle
		Adductor hallucis muscle
		Extensor digitorum brevis
		  muscle
		Extensor hallucis brevis
		  muscle
		Flexor digitorum brevis
		  muscle
		Flexor hallucis brevis
		  muscle
		Quadratus plantae muscle
		W Foot Muscle, Left
		See V Foot Muscle, Right
			Ø Open
			3 Percutaneous
			4 Percutaneous
			  Endoscopic
			X External
				Z No Device	**Z** No Qualifier

Non-OR   ØKN[Ø,1,2,3,4,5,6,7,8,9,B,C,D,F,G,H,J,K,L,M,N,P,Q,R,S,T,V,W]XZZ

LC Limited Coverage   **NC** Noncovered   ⊞ Combination Member   HAC associated procedure   Combination Only   DRG Non-OR   Non-OR   New/Revised in **GREEN**

470   ICD-10-PCS 2021

Ø   Medical and Surgical
K   Muscles
P   Removal

Definition: Taking out or off a device from a body part

Explanation: If a device is taken out and a similar device put in without cutting or puncturing the skin or mucous membrane, the procedure is coded to the root operation CHANGE. Otherwise, the procedure for taking out a device is coded to the root operation REMOVAL.

Body Part Character 4	Approach Character 5	Device Character 6	Qualifier Character 7
X Upper Muscle **Y** Lower Muscle	**Ø** Open **3** Percutaneous **4** Percutaneous Endoscopic	**Ø** Drainage Device **7** Autologous Tissue Substitute **J** Synthetic Substitute **K** Nonautologous Tissue Substitute **M** Stimulator Lead **Y** Other Device	**Z** No Qualifier
X Upper Muscle **Y** Lower Muscle	**X** External	**Ø** Drainage Device **M** Stimulator Lead	**Z** No Qualifier

Non-OR   ØKP[X,Y][3,4]YZ
Non-OR   ØKP[X,Y]X[Ø,M]Z

LC Limited Coverage   **NC** Noncovered   ⊞ Combination Member   HAC associated procedure   Combination Only   DRG Non-OR   Non-OR   New/Revised in GREEN

ICD-10-PCS 2021   471

ØKP–ØKP

Ø Medical and Surgical
K Muscles
Q Repair

Definition: Restoring, to the extent possible, a body part to its normal anatomic structure and function

Explanation: Used only when the method to accomplish the repair is not one of the other root operations

Body Part Character 4			Approach Character 5	Device Character 6	Qualifier Character 7

Ø Head Muscle
Auricularis muscle
Masseter muscle
Pterygoid muscle
Splenius capitis muscle
Temporalis muscle
Temporoparietalis muscle

1 Facial Muscle
Buccinator muscle
Corrugator supercilii muscle
Depressor anguli oris muscle
Depressor labii inferioris muscle
Depressor septi nasi muscle
Depressor supercilii muscle
Levator anguli oris muscle
Levator labii superioris alaeque nasi muscle
Levator labii superioris muscle
Mentalis muscle
Nasalis muscle
Occipitofrontalis muscle
Orbicularis oris muscle
Procerus muscle
Risorius muscle
Zygomaticus muscle

2 Neck Muscle, Right
Anterior vertebral muscle
Arytenoid muscle
Cricothyroid muscle
Infrahyoid muscle
Levator scapulae muscle
Platysma muscle
Scalene muscle
Splenius cervicis muscle
Sternocleidomastoid muscle
Suprahyoid muscle
Thyroarytenoid muscle

3 Neck Muscle, Left
See 2 Neck Muscle, Right

4 Tongue, Palate, Pharynx Muscle
Chondroglossus muscle
Genioglossus muscle
Hyoglossus muscle
Inferior longitudinal muscle
Levator veli palatini muscle
Palatoglossal muscle
Palatopharyngeal muscle
Pharyngeal constrictor muscle
Salpingopharyngeus muscle
Styloglossus muscle
Stylopharyngeus muscle
Superior longitudinal muscle
Tensor veli palatini muscle

5 Shoulder Muscle, Right
Deltoid muscle
Infraspinatus muscle
Subscapularis muscle
Supraspinatus muscle
Teres major muscle
Teres minor muscle

6 Shoulder Muscle, Left
See 5 Shoulder Muscle, Right

7 Upper Arm Muscle, Right
Biceps brachii muscle
Brachialis muscle
Coracobrachialis muscle
Triceps brachii muscle

8 Upper Arm Muscle, Left
See 7 Upper Arm Muscle, Right

9 Lower Arm and Wrist Muscle, Right
Anatomical snuffbox
Brachioradialis muscle
Extensor carpi radialis muscle
Extensor carpi ulnaris muscle
Flexor carpi radialis muscle
Flexor carpi ulnaris muscle
Flexor pollicis longus muscle
Palmaris longus muscle
Pronator quadratus muscle
Pronator teres muscle

B Lower Arm and Wrist Muscle, Left
See 9 Lower Arm and Wrist Muscle, Right

C Hand Muscle, Right
Hypothenar muscle
Palmar interosseous muscle
Thenar muscle

D Hand Muscle, Left
See C Hand Muscle, Right

F Trunk Muscle, Right
Coccygeus muscle
Erector spinae muscle
Interspinalis muscle
Intertransversarius muscle
Latissimus dorsi muscle
Quadratus lumborum muscle
Rhomboid major muscle
Rhomboid minor muscle
Serratus posterior muscle
Transversospinalis muscle
Trapezius muscle

G Trunk Muscle, Left
See F Trunk Muscle, Right

H Thorax Muscle, Right
Intercostal muscle
Levatores costarum muscle
Pectoralis major muscle
Pectoralis minor muscle
Serratus anterior muscle
Subclavius muscle
Subcostal muscle
Transverse thoracis muscle

J Thorax Muscle, Left
See H Thorax Muscle, Right

K Abdomen Muscle, Right
External oblique muscle
Internal oblique muscle
Pyramidalis muscle
Rectus abdominis muscle
Transversus abdominis muscle

L Abdomen Muscle, Left
See K Abdomen Muscle, Right

M Perineum Muscle
Bulbospongiosus muscle
Cremaster muscle
Deep transverse perineal muscle
Ischiocavernosus muscle
Levator ani muscle
Superficial transverse perineal muscle

N Hip Muscle, Right
Gemellus muscle
Gluteus maximus muscle
Gluteus medius muscle
Gluteus minimus muscle
Iliacus muscle
Obturator muscle
Piriformis muscle
Psoas muscle
Quadratus femoris muscle
Tensor fasciae latae muscle

P Hip Muscle, Left
See N Hip Muscle, Right

Q Upper Leg Muscle, Right
Adductor brevis muscle
Adductor longus muscle
Adductor magnus muscle
Biceps femoris muscle
Gracilis muscle
Pectineus muscle
Quadriceps (femoris)
Rectus femoris muscle
Sartorius muscle
Semimembranosus muscle
Semitendinosus muscle
Vastus intermedius muscle
Vastus lateralis muscle
Vastus medialis muscle

R Upper Leg Muscle, Left
See Q Upper Leg Muscle, Right

S Lower Leg Muscle, Right
Extensor digitorum longus muscle
Extensor hallucis longus muscle
Fibularis brevis muscle
Fibularis longus muscle
Flexor digitorum longus muscle
Flexor hallucis longus muscle
Gastrocnemius muscle
Peroneus brevis muscle
Peroneus longus muscle
Popliteus muscle
Soleus muscle
Tibialis anterior muscle
Tibialis posterior muscle

T Lower Leg Muscle, Left
See S Lower Leg Muscle, Right

V Foot Muscle, Right
Abductor hallucis muscle
Adductor hallucis muscle
Extensor digitorum brevis muscle
Extensor hallucis brevis muscle
Flexor digitorum brevis muscle
Flexor hallucis brevis muscle
Quadratus plantae muscle

W Foot Muscle, Left
See V Foot Muscle, Right

Approach Character 5
Ø Open
3 Percutaneous
4 Percutaneous Endoscopic

Device Character 6
Z No Device

Qualifier Character 7
Z No Qualifier

LC Limited Coverage   NC Noncovered   ⊞ Combination Member   HAC associated procedure   Combination Only   DRG Non-OR   Non-OR   New/Revised in GREEN

472   ICD-10-PCS 2021

Ø   Medical and Surgical
K   Muscles
R   Replacement   Definition: Putting in or on biological or synthetic material that physically takes the place and/or function of all or a portion of a body part

Explanation: The body part may have been taken out or replaced, or may be taken out, physically eradicated, or rendered nonfunctional during the REPLACEMENT procedure. A REMOVAL procedure is coded for taking out the device used in a previous replacement procedure.

Body Part Character 4		Approach Character 5	Device Character 6	Qualifier Character 7
Ø Head Muscle Auricularis muscle Masseter muscle Pterygoid muscle Splenius capitis muscle Temporalis muscle Temporoparietalis muscle **1 Facial Muscle** Buccinator muscle Corrugator supercilii muscle Depressor anguli oris muscle Depressor labii inferioris muscle Depressor septi nasi muscle Depressor supercilii muscle Levator anguli oris muscle Levator labii superioris alaeque nasi muscle Levator labii superioris muscle Mentalis muscle Nasalis muscle Occipitofrontalis muscle Orbicularis oris muscle Procerus muscle Risorius muscle Zygomaticus muscle **2 Neck Muscle, Right** Anterior vertebral muscle Arytenoid muscle Cricothyroid muscle Infrahyoid muscle Levator scapulae muscle Platysma muscle Scalene muscle Splenius cervicis muscle Sternocleidomastoid muscle Suprahyoid muscle Thyroarytenoid muscle **3 Neck Muscle, Left** *See 2 Neck Muscle, Right* **4 Tongue, Palate, Pharynx Muscle** Chondroglossus muscle Genioglossus muscle Hyoglossus muscle Inferior longitudinal muscle Levator veli palatini muscle Palatoglossal muscle Palatopharyngeal muscle Pharyngeal constrictor muscle Salpingopharyngeus muscle Styloglossus muscle Stylopharyngeus muscle Superior longitudinal muscle Tensor veli palatini muscle **5 Shoulder Muscle, Right** Deltoid muscle Infraspinatus muscle Subscapularis muscle Supraspinatus muscle Teres major muscle Teres minor muscle **6 Shoulder Muscle, Left** *See 5 Shoulder Muscle, Right*	**7 Upper Arm Muscle, Right** Biceps brachii muscle Brachialis muscle Coracobrachialis muscle Triceps brachii muscle **8 Upper Arm Muscle, Left** *See 7 Upper Arm Muscle, Right* **9 Lower Arm and Wrist Muscle, Right** Anatomical snuffbox Brachioradialis muscle Extensor carpi radialis muscle Extensor carpi ulnaris muscle Flexor carpi radialis muscle Flexor carpi ulnaris muscle Flexor pollicis longus muscle Palmaris longus muscle Pronator quadratus muscle Pronator teres muscle **B Lower Arm and Wrist Muscle, Left** *See 9 Lower Arm and Wrist Muscle, Right* **C Hand Muscle, Right** Hypothenar muscle Palmar interosseous muscle Thenar muscle **D Hand Muscle, Left** *See C Hand Muscle, Right* **F Trunk Muscle, Right** Coccygeus muscle Erector spinae muscle Interspinalis muscle Intertransversarius muscle Latissimus dorsi muscle Quadratus lumborum muscle Rhomboid major muscle Rhomboid minor muscle Serratus posterior muscle Transversospinalis muscle Trapezius muscle **G Trunk Muscle, Left** *See F Trunk Muscle, Right* **H Thorax Muscle, Right** Intercostal muscle Levatores costarum muscle Pectoralis major muscle Pectoralis minor muscle Serratus anterior muscle Subclavius muscle Subcostal muscle Transverse thoracis muscle **J Thorax Muscle, Left** *See H Thorax Muscle, Right* **K Abdomen Muscle, Right** External oblique muscle Internal oblique muscle Pyramidalis muscle Rectus abdominis muscle Transversus abdominis muscle **L Abdomen Muscle, Left** *See K Abdomen Muscle, Right*	**M Perineum Muscle** Bulbospongiosus muscle Cremaster muscle Deep transverse perineal muscle Ischiocavernosus muscle Levator ani muscle Superficial transverse perineal muscle **N Hip Muscle, Right** Gemellus muscle Gluteus maximus muscle Gluteus medius muscle Gluteus minimus muscle Iliacus muscle Obturator muscle Piriformis muscle Psoas muscle Quadratus femoris muscle Tensor fasciae latae muscle **P Hip Muscle, Left** *See N Hip Muscle, Right* **Q Upper Leg Muscle, Right** Adductor brevis muscle Adductor longus muscle Adductor magnus muscle Biceps femoris muscle Gracilis muscle Pectineus muscle Quadriceps (femoris) Rectus femoris muscle Sartorius muscle Semimembranosus muscle Semitendinosus muscle Vastus intermedius muscle Vastus lateralis muscle Vastus medialis muscle **R Upper Leg Muscle, Left** *See Q Upper Leg Muscle, Right* **S Lower Leg Muscle, Right** Extensor digitorum longus muscle Extensor hallucis longus muscle Fibularis brevis muscle Fibularis longus muscle Flexor digitorum longus muscle Flexor hallucis longus muscle Gastrocnemius muscle Peroneus brevis muscle Peroneus longus muscle Popliteus muscle Soleus muscle Tibialis anterior muscle Tibialis posterior muscle **T Lower Leg Muscle, Left** *See S Lower Leg Muscle, Right* **V Foot Muscle, Right** Abductor hallucis muscle Adductor hallucis muscle Extensor digitorum brevis muscle Extensor hallucis brevis muscle Flexor digitorum brevis muscle Flexor hallucis brevis muscle Quadratus plantae muscle **W Foot Muscle, Left** *See V Foot Muscle, Right*	**Ø Open** **4 Percutaneous Endoscopic**	**7 Autologous Tissue Substitute** **J Synthetic Substitute** **K Nonautologous Tissue Substitute**	**Z No Qualifier**

LC Limited Coverage   NC Noncovered   ⊞ Combination Member   HAC associated procedure   Combination Only   DRG Non-OR   Non-OR   New/Revised in GREEN

ICD-10-PCS 2021   473

Muscles

Ø Medical and Surgical
K Muscles
S Reposition

Definition: Moving to its normal location, or other suitable location, all or a portion of a body part

Explanation: The body part is moved to a new location from an abnormal location, or from a normal location where it is not functioning correctly. The body part may or may not be cut out or off to be moved to the new location.

Body Part Character 4		Approach Character 5	Device Character 6	Qualifier Character 7
Ø Head Muscle	M Perineum Muscle	Ø Open	Z No Device	Z No Qualifier

Ø Head Muscle
Auricularis muscle
Masseter muscle
Pterygoid muscle
Splenius capitis muscle
Temporalis muscle
Temporoparietalis muscle

1 Facial Muscle
Buccinator muscle
Corrugator supercilii muscle
Depressor anguli oris muscle
Depressor labii inferioris muscle
Depressor septi nasi muscle
Depressor supercilii muscle
Levator anguli oris muscle
Levator labii superioris alaeque nasi muscle
Levator labii superioris muscle
Mentalis muscle
Nasalis muscle
Occipitofrontalis muscle
Orbicularis oris muscle
Procerus muscle
Risorius muscle
Zygomaticus muscle

2 Neck Muscle, Right
Anterior vertebral muscle
Arytenoid muscle
Cricothyroid muscle
Infrahyoid muscle
Levator scapulae muscle
Platysma muscle
Scalene muscle
Splenius cervicis muscle
Sternocleidomastoid muscle
Suprahyoid muscle
Thyroarytenoid muscle

3 Neck Muscle, Left
See 2 Neck Muscle, Right

4 Tongue, Palate, Pharynx Muscle
Chondroglossus muscle
Genioglossus muscle
Hyoglossus muscle
Inferior longitudinal muscle
Levator veli palatini muscle
Palatoglossal muscle
Palatopharyngeal muscle
Pharyngeal constrictor muscle
Salpingopharyngeus muscle
Styloglossus muscle
Stylopharyngeus muscle
Superior longitudinal muscle
Tensor veli palatini muscle

5 Shoulder Muscle, Right
Deltoid muscle
Infraspinatus muscle
Subscapularis muscle
Supraspinatus muscle
Teres major muscle
Teres minor muscle

6 Shoulder Muscle, Left
See 5 Shoulder Muscle, Right

7 Upper Arm Muscle, Right
Biceps brachii muscle
Brachialis muscle
Coracobrachialis muscle
Triceps brachii muscle

8 Upper Arm Muscle, Left
See 7 Upper Arm Muscle, Right

9 Lower Arm and Wrist Muscle, Right
Anatomical snuffbox
Brachioradialis muscle
Extensor carpi radialis muscle
Extensor carpi ulnaris muscle
Flexor carpi radialis muscle
Flexor carpi ulnaris muscle
Flexor pollicis longus muscle
Palmaris longus muscle
Pronator quadratus muscle
Pronator teres muscle

B Lower Arm and Wrist Muscle, Left
See 9 Lower Arm and Wrist Muscle, Right

C Hand Muscle, Right
Hypothenar muscle
Palmar interosseous muscle
Thenar muscle

D Hand Muscle, Left
See C Hand Muscle, Right

F Trunk Muscle, Right
Coccygeus muscle
Erector spinae muscle
Interspinalis muscle
Intertransversarius muscle
Latissimus dorsi muscle
Quadratus lumborum muscle
Rhomboid major muscle
Rhomboid minor muscle
Serratus posterior muscle
Transversospinalis muscle
Trapezius muscle

G Trunk Muscle, Left
See F Trunk Muscle, Right

H Thorax Muscle, Right
Intercostal muscle
Levatores costarum muscle
Pectoralis major muscle
Pectoralis minor muscle
Serratus anterior muscle
Subclavius muscle
Subcostal muscle
Transverse thoracis muscle

J Thorax Muscle, Left
See H Thorax Muscle, Right

K Abdomen Muscle, Right
External oblique muscle
Internal oblique muscle
Pyramidalis muscle
Rectus abdominis muscle
Transversus abdominis muscle

L Abdomen Muscle, Left
See K Abdomen Muscle, Right

M Perineum Muscle
Bulbospongiosus muscle
Cremaster muscle
Deep transverse perineal muscle
Ischiocavernosus muscle
Levator ani muscle
Superficial transverse perineal muscle

N Hip Muscle, Right
Gemellus muscle
Gluteus maximus muscle
Gluteus medius muscle
Gluteus minimus muscle
Iliacus muscle
Obturator muscle
Piriformis muscle
Psoas muscle
Quadratus femoris muscle
Tensor fasciae latae muscle

P Hip Muscle, Left
See N Hip Muscle, Right

Q Upper Leg Muscle, Right
Adductor brevis muscle
Adductor longus muscle
Adductor magnus muscle
Biceps femoris muscle
Gracilis muscle
Pectineus muscle
Quadriceps (femoris)
Rectus femoris muscle
Sartorius muscle
Semimembranosus muscle
Semitendinosus muscle
Vastus intermedius muscle
Vastus lateralis muscle
Vastus medialis muscle

R Upper Leg Muscle, Left
See Q Upper Leg Muscle, Right

S Lower Leg Muscle, Right
Extensor digitorum longus muscle
Extensor hallucis longus muscle
Fibularis brevis muscle
Fibularis longus muscle
Flexor digitorum longus muscle
Flexor hallucis longus muscle
Gastrocnemius muscle
Peroneus brevis muscle
Peroneus longus muscle
Popliteus muscle
Soleus muscle
Tibialis anterior muscle
Tibialis posterior muscle

T Lower Leg Muscle, Left
See S Lower Leg Muscle, Right

V Foot Muscle, Right
Abductor hallucis muscle
Adductor hallucis muscle
Extensor digitorum brevis muscle
Extensor hallucis brevis muscle
Flexor digitorum brevis muscle
Flexor hallucis brevis muscle
Quadratus plantae muscle

W Foot Muscle, Left
See V Foot Muscle, Right

Approach
Ø Open
4 Percutaneous Endoscopic

Device
Z No Device

Qualifier
Z No Qualifier

Ø   **Medical and Surgical**
K   **Muscles**
T   **Resection**   Definition: Cutting out or off, without replacement, all of a body part
                   Explanation: None

Body Part Character 4			Approach Character 5	Device Character 6	Qualifier Character 7
Ø Head Muscle Auricularis muscle Masseter muscle Pterygoid muscle Splenius capitis muscle Temporalis muscle Temporoparietalis muscle **1 Facial Muscle** Buccinator muscle Corrugator supercilii muscle Depressor anguli oris muscle Depressor labii inferioris muscle Depressor septi nasi muscle Depressor supercilii muscle Levator anguli oris muscle Levator labii superioris alaeque nasi muscle Levator labii superioris muscle Mentalis muscle Nasalis muscle Occipitofrontalis muscle Orbicularis oris muscle Procerus muscle Risorius muscle Zygomaticus muscle **2 Neck Muscle, Right** Anterior vertebral muscle Arytenoid muscle Cricothyroid muscle Infrahyoid muscle Levator scapulae muscle Platysma muscle Scalene muscle Splenius cervicis muscle Sternocleidomastoid muscle Suprahyoid muscle Thyroarytenoid muscle **3 Neck Muscle, Left** *See 2 Neck Muscle, Right* **4 Tongue, Palate, Pharynx Muscle** Chondroglossus muscle Genioglossus muscle Hyoglossus muscle Inferior longitudinal muscle Levator veli palatini muscle Palatoglossal muscle Palatopharyngeal muscle Pharyngeal constrictor muscle Salpingopharyngeus muscle Styloglossus muscle Stylopharyngeus muscle Superior longitudinal muscle Tensor veli palatini muscle **5 Shoulder Muscle, Right** Deltoid muscle Infraspinatus muscle Subscapularis muscle Supraspinatus muscle Teres major muscle Teres minor muscle **6 Shoulder Muscle, Left** *See 5 Shoulder Muscle, Right*	**7 Upper Arm Muscle, Right** Biceps brachii muscle Brachialis muscle Coracobrachialis muscle Triceps brachii muscle **8 Upper Arm Muscle, Left** *See 7 Upper Arm Muscle, Right* **9 Lower Arm and Wrist Muscle, Right** Anatomical snuffbox Brachioradialis muscle Extensor carpi radialis muscle Extensor carpi ulnaris muscle Flexor carpi radialis muscle Flexor carpi ulnaris muscle Flexor pollicis longus muscle Palmaris longus muscle Pronator quadratus muscle Pronator teres muscle **B Lower Arm and Wrist Muscle, Left** *See 9 Lower Arm and Wrist Muscle, Right* **C Hand Muscle, Right** Hypothenar muscle Palmar interosseous muscle Thenar muscle **D Hand Muscle, Left** *See C Hand Muscle, Right* **F Trunk Muscle, Right** Coccygeus muscle Erector spinae muscle Interspinalis muscle Intertransversarius muscle Latissimus dorsi muscle Quadratus lumborum muscle Rhomboid major muscle Rhomboid minor muscle Serratus posterior muscle Transversospinalis muscle Trapezius muscle **G Trunk Muscle, Left** *See F Trunk Muscle, Right* **H Thorax Muscle, Right** ⊞ Intercostal muscle Levatores costarum muscle Pectoralis major muscle Pectoralis minor muscle Serratus anterior muscle Subclavius muscle Subcostal muscle Transverse thoracis muscle **J Thorax Muscle, Left** ⊞ *See H Thorax Muscle, Right* **K Abdomen Muscle, Right** External oblique muscle Internal oblique muscle Pyramidalis muscle Rectus abdominis muscle Transversus abdominis muscle **L Abdomen Muscle, Left** *See K Abdomen Muscle, Right*	**M Perineum Muscle** Bulbospongiosus muscle Cremaster muscle Deep transverse perineal muscle Ischiocavernosus muscle Levator ani muscle Superficial transverse perineal muscle **N Hip Muscle, Right** Gemellus muscle Gluteus maximus muscle Gluteus medius muscle Gluteus minimus muscle Iliacus muscle Obturator muscle Piriformis muscle Psoas muscle Quadratus femoris muscle Tensor fasciae latae muscle **P Hip Muscle, Left** *See N Hip Muscle, Right* **Q Upper Leg Muscle, Right** Adductor brevis muscle Adductor longus muscle Adductor magnus muscle Biceps femoris muscle Gracilis muscle Pectineus muscle Quadriceps (femoris) Rectus femoris muscle Sartorius muscle Semimembranosus muscle Semitendinosus muscle Vastus intermedius muscle Vastus lateralis muscle Vastus medialis muscle **R Upper Leg Muscle, Left** *See Q Upper Leg Muscle, Right* **S Lower Leg Muscle, Right** Extensor digitorum longus muscle Extensor hallucis longus muscle Fibularis brevis muscle Fibularis longus muscle Flexor digitorum longus muscle Flexor hallucis longus muscle Gastrocnemius muscle Peroneus brevis muscle Peroneus longus muscle Popliteus muscle Soleus muscle Tibialis anterior muscle Tibialis posterior muscle **T Lower Leg Muscle, Left** *See S Lower Leg Muscle, Right* **V Foot Muscle, Right** Abductor hallucis muscle Adductor hallucis muscle Extensor digitorum brevis muscle Extensor hallucis brevis muscle Flexor digitorum brevis muscle Flexor hallucis brevis muscle Quadratus plantae muscle **W Foot Muscle, Left** *See V Foot Muscle, Right*	**Ø Open** **4 Percutaneous Endoscopic**	**Z No Device**	**Z No Qualifier**

See Appendix L for Procedure Combinations
    ⊞   ØKT[H,J]ØZZ

🆛 Limited Coverage   🅝🅒 Noncovered   ⊞ Combination Member   HAC associated procedure   Combination Only   DRG Non-OR   Non-OR   New/Revised in GREEN

ICD-10-PCS 2021   475

ØKT–ØKT

Ø Medical and Surgical
K Muscles
U Supplement

Definition: Putting in or on biological or synthetic material that physically reinforces and/or augments the function of a portion of a body part

Explanation: The biological material is non-living, or is living and from the same individual. The body part may have been previously replaced, and the SUPPLEMENT procedure is performed to physically reinforce and/or augment the function of the replaced body part.

Body Part Character 4		Approach Character 5	Device Character 6	Qualifier Character 7
Ø Head Muscle Auricularis muscle Masseter muscle Pterygoid muscle Splenius capitis muscle Temporalis muscle Temporoparietalis muscle **1 Facial Muscle** Buccinator muscle Corrugator supercilii muscle Depressor anguli oris muscle Depressor labii inferioris muscle Depressor septi nasi muscle Depressor supercilii muscle Levator anguli oris muscle Levator labii superioris alaeque nasi muscle Levator labii superioris muscle Mentalis muscle Nasalis muscle Occipitofrontalis muscle Orbicularis oris muscle Procerus muscle Risorius muscle Zygomaticus muscle **2 Neck Muscle, Right** Anterior vertebral muscle Arytenoid muscle Cricothyroid muscle Infrahyoid muscle Levator scapulae muscle Platysma muscle Scalene muscle Splenius cervicis muscle Sternocleidomastoid muscle Suprahyoid muscle Thyroarytenoid muscle **3 Neck Muscle, Left** *See 2 Neck Muscle, Right* **4 Tongue, Palate, Pharynx Muscle** Chondroglossus muscle Genioglossus muscle Hyoglossus muscle Inferior longitudinal muscle Levator veli palatini muscle Palatoglossal muscle Palatopharyngeal muscle Pharyngeal constrictor muscle Salpingopharyngeus muscle Styloglossus muscle Stylopharyngeus muscle Superior longitudinal muscle Tensor veli palatini muscle **5 Shoulder Muscle, Right** Deltoid muscle Infraspinatus muscle Subscapularis muscle Supraspinatus muscle Teres major muscle Teres minor muscle **6 Shoulder Muscle, Left** *See 5 Shoulder Muscle, Right*	**7 Upper Arm Muscle, Right** Biceps brachii muscle Brachialis muscle Coracobrachialis muscle Triceps brachii muscle **8 Upper Arm Muscle, Left** *See 7 Upper Arm Muscle, Right* **9 Lower Arm and Wrist Muscle, Right** Anatomical snuffbox Brachioradialis muscle Extensor carpi radialis muscle Extensor carpi ulnaris muscle Flexor carpi radialis muscle Flexor carpi ulnaris muscle Flexor pollicis longus muscle Palmaris longus muscle Pronator quadratus muscle Pronator teres muscle **B Lower Arm and Wrist Muscle, Left** *See 9 Lower Arm and Wrist Muscle, Right* **C Hand Muscle, Right** Hypothenar muscle Palmar interosseous muscle Thenar muscle **D Hand Muscle, Left** *See C Hand Muscle, Right* **F Trunk Muscle, Right** Coccygeus muscle Erector spinae muscle Interspinalis muscle Intertransversarius muscle Latissimus dorsi muscle Quadratus lumborum muscle Rhomboid major muscle Rhomboid minor muscle Serratus posterior muscle Transversospinalis muscle Trapezius muscle **G Trunk Muscle, Left** *See F Trunk Muscle, Right* **H Thorax Muscle, Right** Intercostal muscle Levatores costarum muscle Pectoralis major muscle Pectoralis minor muscle Serratus anterior muscle Subclavius muscle Subcostal muscle Transverse thoracis muscle **J Thorax Muscle, Left** *See H Thorax Muscle, Right* **K Abdomen Muscle, Right** External oblique muscle Internal oblique muscle Pyramidalis muscle Rectus abdominis muscle Transversus abdominis muscle **L Abdomen Muscle, Left** *See K Abdomen Muscle, Right*	**M Perineum Muscle** Bulbospongiosus muscle Cremaster muscle Deep transverse perineal muscle Ischiocavernosus muscle Levator ani muscle Superficial transverse perineal muscle **N Hip Muscle, Right** Gemellus muscle Gluteus maximus muscle Gluteus medius muscle Gluteus minimus muscle Iliacus muscle Obturator muscle Piriformis muscle Psoas muscle Quadratus femoris muscle Tensor fasciae latae muscle **P Hip Muscle, Left** *See N Hip Muscle, Right* **Q Upper Leg Muscle, Right** Adductor brevis muscle Adductor longus muscle Adductor magnus muscle Biceps femoris muscle Gracilis muscle Pectineus muscle Quadriceps (femoris) Rectus femoris muscle Sartorius muscle Semimembranosus muscle Semitendinosus muscle Vastus intermedius muscle Vastus lateralis muscle Vastus medialis muscle **R Upper Leg Muscle, Left** *See Q Upper Leg Muscle, Right* **S Lower Leg Muscle, Right** Extensor digitorum longus muscle Extensor hallucis longus muscle Fibularis brevis muscle Fibularis longus muscle Flexor digitorum longus muscle Flexor hallucis longus muscle Gastrocnemius muscle Peroneus brevis muscle Peroneus longus muscle Popliteus muscle Soleus muscle Tibialis anterior muscle Tibialis posterior muscle **T Lower Leg Muscle, Left** *See S Lower Leg Muscle, Right* **V Foot Muscle, Right** Abductor hallucis muscle Adductor hallucis muscle Extensor digitorum brevis muscle Extensor hallucis brevis muscle Flexor digitorum brevis muscle Flexor hallucis brevis muscle Quadratus plantae muscle **W Foot Muscle, Left** *See V Foot Muscle, Right*	**Ø Open** **4 Percutaneous Endoscopic**	**7 Autologous Tissue Substitute** **J Synthetic Substitute** **K Nonautologous Tissue Substitute**	**Z No Qualifier**

LC Limited Coverage   NC Noncovered   ⊞ Combination Member   HAC associated procedure   Combination Only   DRG Non-OR   Non-OR   New/Revised in GREEN

476   ICD-10-PCS 2021

ØKU–ØKU

Ø   Medical and Surgical
K   Muscles
W   Revision   Definition: Correcting, to the extent possible, a portion of a malfunctioning device or the position of a displaced device

                     Explanation: Revision can include correcting a malfunctioning or displaced device by taking out or putting in components of the device such as a screw or pin

Body Part Character 4	Approach Character 5	Device Character 6	Qualifier Character 7
X Upper Muscle Y Lower Muscle	Ø Open 3 Percutaneous 4 Percutaneous Endoscopic	Ø Drainage Device 7 Autologous Tissue Substitute J Synthetic Substitute K Nonautologous Tissue Substitute M Stimulator Lead Y Other Device	Z No Qualifier
X Upper Muscle Y Lower Muscle	X External	Ø Drainage Device 7 Autologous Tissue Substitute J Synthetic Substitute K Nonautologous Tissue Substitute M Stimulator Lead	Z No Qualifier

Non-OR   ØKW[X,Y][3,4]YZ
Non-OR   ØKW[X,Y]X[Ø,7,J,K,M]Z

LC Limited Coverage   NC Noncovered   ⊞ Combination Member   HAC associated procedure   Combination Only   DRG Non-OR   Non-OR   New/Revised in GREEN

ICD-10-PCS 2021   477

ØKW–ØKW

Muscles

Ø Medical and Surgical
K Muscles
X Transfer

Definition: Moving, without taking out, all or a portion of a body part to another location to take over the function of all or a portion of a body part
Explanation: The body part transferred remains connected to its vascular and nervous supply

Body Part — Character 4		Approach Character 5	Device Character 6	Qualifier Character 7
Ø Head Muscle Auricularis muscle Masseter muscle Pterygoid muscle Splenius capitis muscle Temporalis muscle Temporoparietalis muscle **1 Facial Muscle** Buccinator muscle Corrugator supercilii muscle Depressor anguli oris muscle Depressor labii inferioris muscle Depressor septi nasi muscle Depressor supercilii muscle Levator anguli oris muscle Levator labii superioris alaeque nasi muscle Levator labii superioris muscle Mentalis muscle Nasalis muscle Occipitofrontalis muscle Orbicularis oris muscle Procerus muscle Risorius muscle Zygomaticus muscle **2 Neck Muscle, Right** Anterior vertebral muscle Arytenoid muscle Cricothyroid muscle Infrahyoid muscle Levator scapulae muscle Platysma muscle Scalene muscle Splenius cervicis muscle Sternocleidomastoid muscle Suprahyoid muscle Thyroarytenoid muscle **3 Neck Muscle, Left** *See 2 Neck Muscle, Right* **4 Tongue, Palate, Pharynx Muscle** Chondroglossus muscle Genioglossus muscle Hyoglossus muscle Inferior longitudinal muscle Levator veli palatini muscle Palatoglossal muscle Palatopharyngeal muscle Pharyngeal constrictor muscle Salpingopharyngeus muscle Styloglossus muscle Stylopharyngeus muscle Superior longitudinal muscle Tensor veli palatini muscle **5 Shoulder Muscle, Right** Deltoid muscle Infraspinatus muscle Subscapularis muscle Supraspinatus muscle Teres major muscle Teres minor muscle	**6 Shoulder Muscle, Left** *See 5 Shoulder Muscle, Right* **7 Upper Arm Muscle, Right** Biceps brachii muscle Brachialis muscle Coracobrachialis muscle Triceps brachii muscle **8 Upper Arm Muscle, Left** *See 7 Upper Arm Muscle, Right* **9 Lower Arm and Wrist Muscle, Right** Anatomical snuffbox Brachioradialis muscle Extensor carpi radialis muscle Extensor carpi ulnaris muscle Flexor carpi radialis muscle Flexor carpi ulnaris muscle Flexor pollicis longus muscle Palmaris longus muscle Pronator quadratus muscle Pronator teres muscle **B Lower Arm and Wrist Muscle, Left** *See 9 Lower Arm and Wrist Muscle, Right* **C Hand Muscle, Right** Hypothenar muscle Palmar interosseous muscle Thenar muscle **D Hand Muscle, Left** *See C Hand Muscle, Right* **H Thorax Muscle, Right** Intercostal muscle Levatores costarum muscle Pectoralis major muscle Pectoralis minor muscle Serratus anterior muscle Subclavius muscle Subcostal muscle Transverse thoracis muscle **J Thorax Muscle, Left** *See H Thorax Muscle, Right* **M Perineum Muscle** Bulbospongiosus muscle Cremaster muscle Deep transverse perineal muscle Ischiocavernosus muscle Levator ani muscle Superficial transverse perineal muscle **N Hip Muscle, Right** Gemellus muscle Gluteus maximus muscle Gluteus medius muscle Gluteus minimus muscle Iliacus muscle Obturator muscle Piriformis muscle Psoas muscle Quadratus femoris muscle Tensor fasciae latae muscle	**P Hip Muscle, Left** *See N Hip Muscle, Right* **Q Upper Leg Muscle, Right** Adductor brevis muscle Adductor longus muscle Adductor magnus muscle Biceps femoris muscle Gracilis muscle Pectineus muscle Quadriceps (femoris) Rectus femoris muscle Sartorius muscle Semimembranosus muscle Semitendinosus muscle Vastus intermedius muscle Vastus lateralis muscle Vastus medialis muscle **R Upper Leg Muscle, Left** *See Q Upper Leg Muscle, Right* **S Lower Leg Muscle, Right** Extensor digitorum longus muscle Extensor hallucis longus muscle Fibularis brevis muscle Fibularis longus muscle Flexor digitorum longus muscle Flexor hallucis longus muscle Gastrocnemius muscle Peroneus brevis muscle Peroneus longus muscle Popliteus muscle Soleus muscle Tibialis anterior muscle Tibialis posterior muscle **T Lower Leg Muscle, Left** *See S Lower Leg Muscle, Right* **V Foot Muscle, Right** Abductor hallucis muscle Adductor hallucis muscle Extensor digitorum brevis muscle Extensor hallucis brevis muscle Flexor digitorum brevis muscle Flexor hallucis brevis muscle Quadratus plantae muscle **W Foot Muscle, Left** *See V Foot Muscle, Right*	**Ø** Open **4** Percutaneous Endoscopic	**Z** No Device	**Ø** Skin **1** Subcutaneous Tissue **2** Skin and Subcutaneous Tissue **Z** No Qualifier

ØKX Continued on next page

Muscles

Ø   Medical and Surgical
K   Muscles
X   Transfer

ØKX Continued

Definition: Moving, without taking out, all or a portion of a body part to another location to take over the function of all or a portion of a body part
Explanation: The body part transferred remains connected to its vascular and nervous supply

Body Part Character 4	Approach Character 5	Device Character 6	Qualifier Character 7

F **Trunk Muscle, Right**
   Coccygeus muscle
   Erector spinae muscle
   Interspinalis muscle
   Intertransversarius muscle
   Latissimus dorsi muscle
   Quadratus lumborum muscle
   Rhomboid major muscle
   Rhomboid minor muscle
   Serratus posterior muscle
   Transversospinalis muscle
   Trapezius muscle
G **Trunk Muscle, Left**
   See F Trunk Muscle, Right
	Ø Open
	4 Percutaneous Endoscopic
		Z No Device	**Ø** Skin
			1 Subcutaneous Tissue
			2 Skin and Subcutaneous Tissue
			5 Latissimus Dorsi Myocutaneous Flap
			7 Deep Inferior Epigastric Artery Perforator Flap
			8 Superficial Inferior Epigastric Artery Flap
			9 Gluteal Artery Perforator Flap
			Z No Qualifier

K **Abdomen Muscle, Right**
   External oblique muscle
   Internal oblique muscle
   Pyramidalis muscle
   Rectus abdominis muscle
   Transversus abdominis muscle
L **Abdomen Muscle, Left**
   See K Abdomen Muscle, Right
	Ø Open
	4 Percutaneous Endoscopic
		Z No Device	**Ø** Skin
			1 Subcutaneous Tissue
			2 Skin and Subcutaneous Tissue
			6 Transverse Rectus Abdominis Myocutaneous Flap
			Z No Qualifier

Tendons ØL2–ØLX

Character Meanings*

This Character Meaning table is provided as a guide to assist the user in the identification of character members that may be found in this section of code tables. It **SHOULD NOT** be used to build a PCS code.

Operation–Character 3	Body Part–Character 4	Approach–Character 5	Device–Character 6	Qualifier–Character 7
2 Change	Ø Head and Neck Tendon	Ø Open	Ø Drainage Device	X Diagnostic
5 Destruction	1 Shoulder Tendon, Right	3 Percutaneous	7 Autologous Tissue Substitute	Z No Qualifier
8 Division	2 Shoulder Tendon, Left	4 Percutaneous Endoscopic	J Synthetic Substitute	
9 Drainage	3 Upper Arm Tendon, Right	X External	K Nonautologous Tissue Substitute	
B Excision	4 Upper Arm Tendon, Left		Y Other Device	
C Extirpation	5 Lower Arm and Wrist Tendon, Right		Z No Device	
D Extraction	6 Lower Arm and Wrist Tendon, Left			
H Insertion	7 Hand Tendon, Right			
J Inspection	8 Hand Tendon, Left			
M Reattachment	9 Trunk Tendon, Right			
N Release	B Trunk Tendon, Left			
P Removal	C Thorax Tendon, Right			
Q Repair	D Thorax Tendon, Left			
R Replacement	F Abdomen Tendon, Right			
S Reposition	G Abdomen Tendon, Left			
T Resection	H Perineum Tendon			
U Supplement	J Hip Tendon, Right			
W Revision	K Hip Tendon, Left			
X Transfer	L Upper Leg Tendon, Right			
	M Upper Leg Tendon, Left			
	N Lower Leg Tendon, Right			
	P Lower Leg Tendon, Left			
	Q Knee Tendon, Right			
	R Knee Tendon, Left			
	S Ankle Tendon, Right			
	T Ankle Tendon, Left			
	V Foot Tendon, Right			
	W Foot Tendon, Left			
	X Upper Tendon			
	Y Lower Tendon			

* Includes synovial membrane.

AHA Coding Clinic for table ØL8
2016, 3Q, 30   Resection of femur with interposition arthroplasty

AHA Coding Clinic for table ØLB
2017, 2Q, 21   Arthroscopic anterior cruciate ligament revision using autograft with anterolateral ligament reconstruction
2015, 3Q, 26   Thumb arthroplasty with resection of trapezium
2014, 3Q, 14   Application of TheraSkin® and excisional debridement
2014, 3Q, 18   Placement of reverse sural fasciocutaneous pedicle flap

AHA Coding Clinic for table ØLD
2017, 4Q, 41   Extraction procedures

AHA Coding Clinic for table ØLQ
2016, 3Q, 32   Rotator cuff repair, tenodesis, decompression, acromioplasty and coracoplasty
2015, 2Q, 11   Repair of patellar and quadriceps tendons with allograft
2013, 3Q, 20   Superior labrum anterior posterior (SLAP) repair and subacromial decompression

AHA Coding Clinic for table ØLS
2016, 3Q, 32   Rotator cuff repair, tenodesis, decompression, acromioplasty and coracoplasty
2015, 3Q, 14   Endoprosthetic replacement of humerus and tendon reattachment

AHA Coding Clinic for table ØLU
2015, 2Q, 11   Repair of patellar and quadriceps tendons with allograft

Foot Tendons

Lateral malleolus of fibula

Medial malleolus of tibia

Peroneus brevis **N, P**

Extensor hallucis longus **N, P**

Extensor digitorum longus **N, P**

Select extensors of the foot

Shoulder Tendons

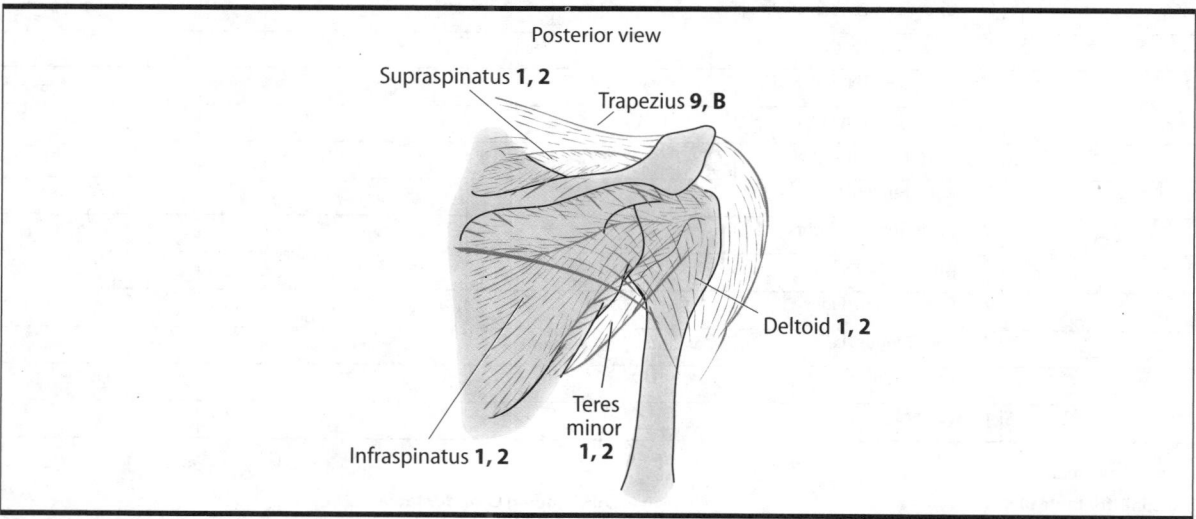

Posterior view

Supraspinatus **1, 2**

Trapezius **9, B**

Deltoid **1, 2**

Infraspinatus **1, 2**

Teres minor **1, 2**

Tendons of Wrist and Hand

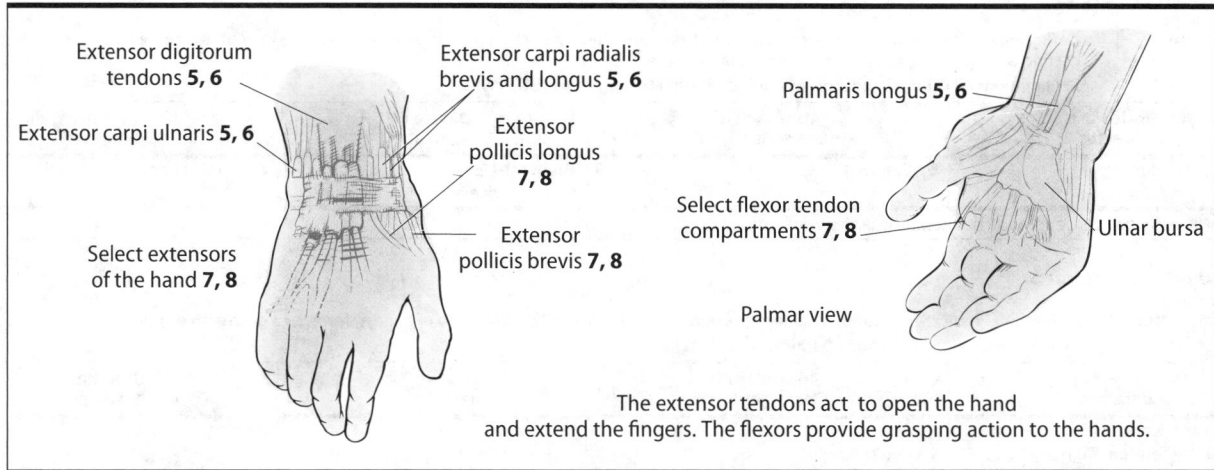

Extensor digitorum tendons **5, 6**

Extensor carpi ulnaris **5, 6**

Extensor carpi radialis brevis and longus **5, 6**

Extensor pollicis longus **7, 8**

Select extensors of the hand **7, 8**

Extensor pollicis brevis **7, 8**

Palmaris longus **5, 6**

Select flexor tendon compartments **7, 8**

Ulnar bursa

Palmar view

The extensor tendons act to open the hand and extend the fingers. The flexors provide grasping action to the hands.

Leg Muscles and Tendons

Head of fibula

Patella

Soleus **N, P**

Anterior tibialis **N, P**

Gastrocnemius **N, P**

Extensor longus **N, P**

Peroneus longus **N, P**

Peroneus brevis **N, P**

Head of femur

Rectus femoris **L, M**

Adductor longus **L, M**

Sartorius **L, M**

Vastus lateralis **L, M**

Patella

Fibula

Tendons

Ø **Medical and Surgical**
L **Tendons**
2 **Change**　Definition: Taking out or off a device from a body part and putting back an identical or similar device in or on the same body part without cutting or puncturing the skin or a mucous membrane
Explanation: All CHANGE procedures are coded using the approach EXTERNAL

Body Part Character 4	Approach Character 5	Device Character 6	Qualifier Character 7
X Upper Tendon Y Lower Tendon	X External	Ø Drainage Device Y Other Device	Z No Qualifier

Non-OR　All body part, approach, device, and qualifier values

Ø **Medical and Surgical**
L **Tendons**
5 **Destruction**　Definition: Physical eradication of all or a portion of a body part by the direct use of energy, force, or a destructive agent
Explanation: None of the body part is physically taken out

Body Part Character 4	Approach Character 5	Device Character 6	Qualifier Character 7
Ø Head and Neck Tendon 1 Shoulder Tendon, Right 2 Shoulder Tendon, Left 3 Upper Arm Tendon, Right 4 Upper Arm Tendon, Left 5 Lower Arm and Wrist Tendon, Right 6 Lower Arm and Wrist Tendon, Left 7 Hand Tendon, Right 8 Hand Tendon, Left 9 Trunk Tendon, Right B Trunk Tendon, Left C Thorax Tendon, Right D Thorax Tendon, Left F Abdomen Tendon, Right G Abdomen Tendon, Left H Perineum Tendon J Hip Tendon, Right K Hip Tendon, Left L Upper Leg Tendon, Right M Upper Leg Tendon, Left N Lower Leg Tendon, Right 　　Achilles tendon P Lower Leg Tendon, Left 　　*See* N Lower Leg Tendon, Right Q Knee Tendon, Right 　　Patellar tendon R Knee Tendon, Left 　　*See* Q Knee Tendon, Right S Ankle Tendon, Right T Ankle Tendon, Left V Foot Tendon, Right W Foot Tendon, Left	Ø Open 3 Percutaneous 4 Percutaneous Endoscopic	Z No Device	Z No Qualifier

Ø **Medical and Surgical**
L **Tendons**
8 **Division**   Definition: Cutting into a body part, without draining fluids and/or gases from the body part, in order to separate or transect a body part
Explanation: All or a portion of the body part is separated into two or more portions

Body Part Character 4	Approach Character 5	Device Character 6	Qualifier Character 7
Ø Head and Neck Tendon	**Ø** Open	**Z** No Device	**Z** No Qualifier
1 Shoulder Tendon, Right	**3** Percutaneous		
2 Shoulder Tendon, Left	**4** Percutaneous Endoscopic		
3 Upper Arm Tendon, Right			
4 Upper Arm Tendon, Left			
5 Lower Arm and Wrist Tendon, Right			
6 Lower Arm and Wrist Tendon, Left			
7 Hand Tendon, Right			
8 Hand Tendon, Left			
9 Trunk Tendon, Right			
B Trunk Tendon, Left			
C Thorax Tendon, Right			
D Thorax Tendon, Left			
F Abdomen Tendon, Right			
G Abdomen Tendon, Left			
H Perineum Tendon			
J Hip Tendon, Right			
K Hip Tendon, Left			
L Upper Leg Tendon, Right			
M Upper Leg Tendon, Left			
N Lower Leg Tendon, Right Achilles tendon			
P Lower Leg Tendon, Left *See N Lower Leg Tendon, Right*			
Q Knee Tendon, Right Patellar tendon			
R Knee Tendon, Left *See Q Knee Tendon, Right*			
S Ankle Tendon, Right			
T Ankle Tendon, Left			
V Foot Tendon, Right			
W Foot Tendon, Left			

Ø   Medical and Surgical
L   Tendons
9   Drainage   Definition: Taking or letting out fluids and/or gases from a body part

                     Explanation: The qualifier DIAGNOSTIC is used to identify drainage procedures that are biopsies

Body Part Character 4	Approach Character 5	Device Character 6	Qualifier Character 7

Ø   Head and Neck Tendon
1   Shoulder Tendon, Right
2   Shoulder Tendon, Left
3   Upper Arm Tendon, Right
4   Upper Arm Tendon, Left
5   Lower Arm and Wrist Tendon, Right
6   Lower Arm and Wrist Tendon, Left
7   Hand Tendon, Right
8   Hand Tendon, Left
9   Trunk Tendon, Right
B   Trunk Tendon, Left
C   Thorax Tendon, Right
D   Thorax Tendon, Left
F   Abdomen Tendon, Right
G   Abdomen Tendon, Left
H   Perineum Tendon
J   Hip Tendon, Right
K   Hip Tendon, Left
L   Upper Leg Tendon, Right
M   Upper Leg Tendon, Left
N   Lower Leg Tendon, Right
     Achilles tendon
P   Lower Leg Tendon, Left
     See N Lower Leg Tendon, Right
Q   Knee Tendon, Right
     Patellar tendon
R   Knee Tendon, Left
     See Q Knee Tendon, Right
S   Ankle Tendon, Right
T   Ankle Tendon, Left
V   Foot Tendon, Right
W   Foot Tendon, Left
	Ø Open
	3 Percutaneous
	4 Percutaneous Endoscopic
		Ø Drainage Device	Z No Qualifier

Ø   Head and Neck Tendon
1   Shoulder Tendon, Right
2   Shoulder Tendon, Left
3   Upper Arm Tendon, Right
4   Upper Arm Tendon, Left
5   Lower Arm and Wrist Tendon, Right
6   Lower Arm and Wrist Tendon, Left
7   Hand Tendon, Right
8   Hand Tendon, Left
9   Trunk Tendon, Right
B   Trunk Tendon, Left
C   Thorax Tendon, Right
D   Thorax Tendon, Left
F   Abdomen Tendon, Right
G   Abdomen Tendon, Left
H   Perineum Tendon
J   Hip Tendon, Right
K   Hip Tendon, Left
L   Upper Leg Tendon, Right
M   Upper Leg Tendon, Left
N   Lower Leg Tendon, Right
     Achilles tendon
P   Lower Leg Tendon, Left
     See N Lower Leg Tendon, Right
Q   Knee Tendon, Right
     Patellar tendon
R   Knee Tendon, Left
     See Q Knee Tendon, Right
S   Ankle Tendon, Right
T   Ankle Tendon, Left
V   Foot Tendon, Right
W   Foot Tendon, Left
	Ø Open
	3 Percutaneous
	4 Percutaneous Endoscopic
		Z No Device	X Diagnostic
			Z No Qualifier

Non-OR   ØL9[Ø,1,2,3,4,5,6,7,8,9,B,C,D,F,G,H,J,K,L,M,N,P,Q,R,S,T,V,W]3ØZ   **Non-OR**   ØL9[7,8]4ZZ
Non-OR   ØL9[Ø,1,2,3,4,5,6,7,8,9,B,C,D,F,G,H,J,K,L,M,N,P,Q,R,S,T,V,W]3ZZ

LC Limited Coverage   NC Noncovered   ⊞ Combination Member   HAC associated procedure   Combination Only   DRG Non-OR   Non-OR   New/Revised in GREEN

486   ICD-10-PCS 2021

ØL9–ØL9

Ø   **Medical and Surgical**
L   **Tendons**
B   **Excision**   Definition: Cutting out or off, without replacement, a portion of a body part

                       Explanation: The qualifier DIAGNOSTIC is used to identify excision procedures that are biopsies

Body Part Character 4	Approach Character 5	Device Character 6	Qualifier Character 7

Ø   Head and Neck Tendon
1   Shoulder Tendon, Right
2   Shoulder Tendon, Left
3   Upper Arm Tendon, Right
4   Upper Arm Tendon, Left
5   Lower Arm and Wrist Tendon, Right
6   Lower Arm and Wrist Tendon, Left
7   Hand Tendon, Right
8   Hand Tendon, Left
9   Trunk Tendon, Right
B   Trunk Tendon, Left
C   Thorax Tendon, Right
D   Thorax Tendon, Left
F   Abdomen Tendon, Right
G   Abdomen Tendon, Left
H   Perineum Tendon
J   Hip Tendon, Right
K   Hip Tendon, Left
L   Upper Leg Tendon, Right
M   Upper Leg Tendon, Left
N   Lower Leg Tendon, Right
     Achilles tendon
P   Lower Leg Tendon, Left
     See N Lower Leg Tendon, Right
Q   Knee Tendon, Right
     Patellar tendon
R   Knee Tendon, Left
     See Q Knee Tendon, Right
S   Ankle Tendon, Right
T   Ankle Tendon, Left
V   Foot Tendon, Right
W   Foot Tendon, Left
	Ø Open
	3 Percutaneous
	4 Percutaneous Endoscopic
		Z No Device	X Diagnostic
			Z No Qualifier

LC Limited Coverage   NC Noncovered   ⊞ Combination Member   HAC associated procedure   Combination Only   DRG Non-OR   Non-OR   New/Revised in GREEN

ICD-10-PCS 2021   487

Ø   Medical and Surgical
L   Tendons
C   Extirpation   Definition: Taking or cutting out solid matter from a body part

Explanation: The solid matter may be an abnormal byproduct of a biological function or a foreign body; it may be imbedded in a body part or in the lumen of a tubular body part. The solid matter may or may not have been previously broken into pieces.

Body Part Character 4	Approach Character 5	Device Character 6	Qualifier Character 7

Ø Head and Neck Tendon
1 Shoulder Tendon, Right
2 Shoulder Tendon, Left
3 Upper Arm Tendon, Right
4 Upper Arm Tendon, Left
5 Lower Arm and Wrist Tendon, Right
6 Lower Arm and Wrist Tendon, Left
7 Hand Tendon, Right
8 Hand Tendon, Left
9 Trunk Tendon, Right
B Trunk Tendon, Left
C Thorax Tendon, Right
D Thorax Tendon, Left
F Abdomen Tendon, Right
G Abdomen Tendon, Left
H Perineum Tendon
J Hip Tendon, Right
K Hip Tendon, Left
L Upper Leg Tendon, Right
M Upper Leg Tendon, Left
N Lower Leg Tendon, Right
    Achilles tendon
P Lower Leg Tendon, Left
    See N Lower Leg Tendon, Right
Q Knee Tendon, Right
    Patellar tendon
R Knee Tendon, Left
    See Q Knee Tendon, Right
S Ankle Tendon, Right
T Ankle Tendon, Left
V Foot Tendon, Right
W Foot Tendon, Left
	Ø Open
	3 Percutaneous
	4 Percutaneous Endoscopic
		Z No Device	Z No Qualifier

LC Limited Coverage   NC Noncovered   ⊞ Combination Member   HAC associated procedure   Combination Only   DRG Non-OR   Non-OR   New/Revised in GREEN

488   ICD-10-PCS 2021

Ø   Medical and Surgical
L   Tendons
D   Extraction   Definition: Pulling or stripping out or off all or a portion of a body part by the use of force

                    Explanation: The qualifier DIAGNOSTIC is used to identify extraction procedures that are biopsies

Body Part Character 4	Approach Character 5	Device Character 6	Qualifier Character 7

Ø Head and Neck Tendon
1 Shoulder Tendon, Right
2 Shoulder Tendon, Left
3 Upper Arm Tendon, Right
4 Upper Arm Tendon, Left
5 Lower Arm and Wrist Tendon, Right
6 Lower Arm and Wrist Tendon, Left
7 Hand Tendon, Right
8 Hand Tendon, Left
9 Trunk Tendon, Right
B Trunk Tendon, Left
C Thorax Tendon, Right
D Thorax Tendon, Left
F Abdomen Tendon, Right
G Abdomen Tendon, Left
H Perineum Tendon
J Hip Tendon, Right
K Hip Tendon, Left
L Upper Leg Tendon, Right
M Upper Leg Tendon, Left
N Lower Leg Tendon, Right
    Achilles tendon
P Lower Leg Tendon, Left
    See N Lower Leg Tendon, Right
Q Knee Tendon, Right
    Patellar tendon
R Knee Tendon, Left
    See Q Knee Tendon, Right
S Ankle Tendon, Right
T Ankle Tendon, Left
V Foot Tendon, Right
W Foot Tendon, Left
	Ø Open	**Z** No Device	**Z** No Qualifier

Ø   Medical and Surgical
L   Tendons
H   Insertion   Definition: Putting in a nonbiological appliance that monitors, assists, performs, or prevents a physiological function but does not physically take the place of a body part

                    Explanation: None

Body Part Character 4	Approach Character 5	Device Character 6	Qualifier Character 7
X Upper Tendon **Y** Lower Tendon	**Ø** Open **3** Percutaneous **4** Percutaneous Endoscopic	**Y** Other Device	**Z** No Qualifier

Non-OR   ØLH[X,Y][3,4]YZ

Ø   Medical and Surgical
L   Tendons
J   Inspection   Definition: Visually and/or manually exploring a body part

                    Explanation: Visual exploration may be performed with or without optical instrumentation. Manual exploration may be performed directly or through intervening body layers.

Body Part Character 4	Approach Character 5	Device Character 6	Qualifier Character 7
X Upper Tendon **Y** Lower Tendon	**Ø** Open **3** Percutaneous **4** Percutaneous Endoscopic **X** External	**Z** No Device	**Z** No Qualifier

Non-OR   ØLJ[X,Y][3,X]ZZ

LC Limited Coverage   NC Noncovered   ⊞ Combination Member   HAC associated procedure   Combination Only   DRG Non-OR   Non-OR   New/Revised in GREEN

ICD-10-PCS 2021   489

Ø   **Medical and Surgical**
L   **Tendons**
M   **Reattachment**   Definition: Putting back in or on all or a portion of a separated body part to its normal location or other suitable location
           Explanation: Vascular circulation and nervous pathways may or may not be reestablished

Body Part Character 4	Approach Character 5	Device Character 6	Qualifier Character 7

Ø   Head and Neck Tendon
1   Shoulder Tendon, Right
2   Shoulder Tendon, Left
3   Upper Arm Tendon, Right
4   Upper Arm Tendon, Left
5   Lower Arm and Wrist Tendon, Right
6   Lower Arm and Wrist Tendon, Left
7   Hand Tendon, Right
8   Hand Tendon, Left
9   Trunk Tendon, Right
B   Trunk Tendon, Left
C   Thorax Tendon, Right
D   Thorax Tendon, Left
F   Abdomen Tendon, Right
G   Abdomen Tendon, Left
H   Perineum Tendon
J   Hip Tendon, Right
K   Hip Tendon, Left
L   Upper Leg Tendon, Right
M   Upper Leg Tendon, Left
N   Lower Leg Tendon, Right
     Achilles tendon
P   Lower Leg Tendon, Left
     See N Lower Leg Tendon, Right
Q   Knee Tendon, Right
     Patellar tendon
R   Knee Tendon, Left
     See Q Knee Tendon, Right
S   Ankle Tendon, Right
T   Ankle Tendon, Left
V   Foot Tendon, Right
W   Foot Tendon, Left
	Ø Open
	4 Percutaneous Endoscopic
		Z No Device	Z No Qualifier

Ø   **Medical and Surgical**
L   **Tendons**
N   **Release**   Definition: Freeing a body part from an abnormal physical constraint by cutting or by the use of force
           Explanation: Some of the restraining tissue may be taken out but none of the body part is taken out

Body Part Character 4	Approach Character 5	Device Character 6	Qualifier Character 7

Ø   Head and Neck Tendon
1   Shoulder Tendon, Right
2   Shoulder Tendon, Left
3   Upper Arm Tendon, Right
4   Upper Arm Tendon, Left
5   Lower Arm and Wrist Tendon, Right
6   Lower Arm and Wrist Tendon, Left
7   Hand Tendon, Right
8   Hand Tendon, Left
9   Trunk Tendon, Right
B   Trunk Tendon, Left
C   Thorax Tendon, Right
D   Thorax Tendon, Left
F   Abdomen Tendon, Right
G   Abdomen Tendon, Left
H   Perineum Tendon
J   Hip Tendon, Right
K   Hip Tendon, Left
L   Upper Leg Tendon, Right
M   Upper Leg Tendon, Left
N   Lower Leg Tendon, Right
     Achilles tendon
P   Lower Leg Tendon, Left
     See N Lower Leg Tendon, Right
Q   Knee Tendon, Right
     Patellar tendon
R   Knee Tendon, Left
     See Q Knee Tendon, Right
S   Ankle Tendon, Right
T   Ankle Tendon, Left
V   Foot Tendon, Right
W   Foot Tendon, Left
	Ø Open
	3 Percutaneous
	4 Percutaneous Endoscopic
	X External
		Z No Device	Z No Qualifier

Non-OR   ØLN[Ø,1,2,3,4,5,6,7,8,9,B,C,D,F,G,H,J,K,L,M,N,P,Q,R,S,T,V,W]XZZ

LC Limited Coverage   NC Noncovered   ⊞ Combination Member   HAC associated procedure   Combination Only   DRG Non-OR   Non-OR   New/Revised in GREEN

Ø   **Medical and Surgical**
L   **Tendons**
P   **Removal**   Definition: Taking out or off a device from a body part

                       Explanation: If a device is taken out and a similar device put in without cutting or puncturing the skin or mucous membrane, the procedure is coded to the root operation CHANGE. Otherwise, the procedure for taking out a device is coded to the root operation REMOVAL.

Body Part Character 4	Approach Character 5	Device Character 6	Qualifier Character 7
X Upper Tendon Y Lower Tendon	Ø Open 3 Percutaneous 4 Percutaneous Endoscopic	Ø Drainage Device 7 Autologous Tissue Substitute J Synthetic Substitute K Nonautologous Tissue Substitute Y Other Device	Z No Qualifier
X Upper Tendon Y Lower Tendon	X External	Ø Drainage Device	Z No Qualifier

Non-OR	ØLP[X,Y]3ØZ
Non-OR	ØLP[X,Y][3,4]YZ
Non-OR	ØLP[X,Y]XØZ

Ø   **Medical and Surgical**
L   **Tendons**
Q   **Repair**   Definition: Restoring, to the extent possible, a body part to its normal anatomic structure and function

                       Explanation: Used only when the method to accomplish the repair is not one of the other root operations

Body Part Character 4	Approach Character 5	Device Character 6	Qualifier Character 7

Ø   Head and Neck Tendon
1   Shoulder Tendon, Right
2   Shoulder Tendon, Left
3   Upper Arm Tendon, Right
4   Upper Arm Tendon, Left
5   Lower Arm and Wrist Tendon, Right
6   Lower Arm and Wrist Tendon, Left
7   Hand Tendon, Right
8   Hand Tendon, Left
9   Trunk Tendon, Right
B   Trunk Tendon, Left
C   Thorax Tendon, Right
D   Thorax Tendon, Left
F   Abdomen Tendon, Right
G   Abdomen Tendon, Left
H   Perineum Tendon
J   Hip Tendon, Right
K   Hip Tendon, Left
L   Upper Leg Tendon, Right
M   Upper Leg Tendon, Left
N   Lower Leg Tendon, Right
     Achilles tendon
P   Lower Leg Tendon, Left
     See N Lower Leg Tendon, Right
Q   Knee Tendon, Right
     Patellar tendon
R   Knee Tendon, Left
     See Q Knee Tendon, Right
S   Ankle Tendon, Right
T   Ankle Tendon, Left
V   Foot Tendon, Right
W   Foot Tendon, Left
	Ø Open
	3 Percutaneous
	4 Percutaneous Endoscopic
		Z No Device	Z No Qualifier

LC Limited Coverage   **NC** Noncovered   ⊞ Combination Member   HAC associated procedure   Combination Only   DRG Non-OR   Non-OR   New/Revised in GREEN

ICD-10-PCS 2021   **491**

ØLP–ØLQ

Tendons (side tab)

ØLR–ØLS (side tab)

Ø **Medical and Surgical**
L **Tendons**
R **Replacement**   Definition: Putting in or on biological or synthetic material that physically takes the place and/or function of all or a portion of a body part

        Explanation: The body part may have been taken out or replaced, or may be taken out, physically eradicated, or rendered nonfunctional during the REPLACEMENT procedure. A REMOVAL procedure is coded for taking out the device used in a previous replacement procedure.

Body Part Character 4	Approach Character 5	Device Character 6	Qualifier Character 7

Ø Head and Neck Tendon
1 Shoulder Tendon, Right
2 Shoulder Tendon, Left
3 Upper Arm Tendon, Right
4 Upper Arm Tendon, Left
5 Lower Arm and Wrist Tendon, Right
6 Lower Arm and Wrist Tendon, Left
7 Hand Tendon, Right
8 Hand Tendon, Left
9 Trunk Tendon, Right
B Trunk Tendon, Left
C Thorax Tendon, Right
D Thorax Tendon, Left
F Abdomen Tendon, Right
G Abdomen Tendon, Left
H Perineum Tendon
J Hip Tendon, Right
K Hip Tendon, Left
L Upper Leg Tendon, Right
M Upper Leg Tendon, Left
N Lower Leg Tendon, Right
    Achilles tendon
P Lower Leg Tendon, Left
    See N Lower Leg Tendon, Right
Q Knee Tendon, Right
    Patellar tendon
R Knee Tendon, Left
    See Q Knee Tendon, Right
S Ankle Tendon, Right
T Ankle Tendon, Left
V Foot Tendon, Right
W Foot Tendon, Left
	Ø Open
	4 Percutaneous Endoscopic
		7 Autologous Tissue Substitute
		J Synthetic Substitute
		K Nonautologous Tissue Substitute
			Z No Qualifier

Ø **Medical and Surgical**
L **Tendons**
S **Reposition**   Definition: Moving to its normal location, or other suitable location, all or a portion of a body part

        Explanation: The body part is moved to a new location from an abnormal location, or from a normal location where it is not functioning correctly. The body part may or may not be cut out or off to be moved to the new location.

Body Part Character 4	Approach Character 5	Device Character 6	Qualifier Character 7

Ø Head and Neck Tendon
1 Shoulder Tendon, Right
2 Shoulder Tendon, Left
3 Upper Arm Tendon, Right
4 Upper Arm Tendon, Left
5 Lower Arm and Wrist Tendon, Right
6 Lower Arm and Wrist Tendon, Left
7 Hand Tendon, Right
8 Hand Tendon, Left
9 Trunk Tendon, Right
B Trunk Tendon, Left
C Thorax Tendon, Right
D Thorax Tendon, Left
F Abdomen Tendon, Right
G Abdomen Tendon, Left
H Perineum Tendon
J Hip Tendon, Right
K Hip Tendon, Left
L Upper Leg Tendon, Right
M Upper Leg Tendon, Left
N Lower Leg Tendon, Right
    Achilles tendon
P Lower Leg Tendon, Left
    See N Lower Leg Tendon, Right
Q Knee Tendon, Right
    Patellar tendon
R Knee Tendon, Left
    See Q Knee Tendon, Right
S Ankle Tendon, Right
T Ankle Tendon, Left
V Foot Tendon, Right
W Foot Tendon, Left
	Ø Open
	4 Percutaneous Endoscopic
		Z No Device	**Z** No Qualifier

Ø   Medical and Surgical
L   Tendons
T   Resection   Definition: Cutting out or off, without replacement, all of a body part
                            Explanation: None

Body Part Character 4	Approach Character 5	Device Character 6	Qualifier Character 7

Ø Head and Neck Tendon
1 Shoulder Tendon, Right
2 Shoulder Tendon, Left
3 Upper Arm Tendon, Right
4 Upper Arm Tendon, Left
5 Lower Arm and Wrist Tendon, Right
6 Lower Arm and Wrist Tendon, Left
7 Hand Tendon, Right
8 Hand Tendon, Left
9 Trunk Tendon, Right
B Trunk Tendon, Left
C Thorax Tendon, Right
D Thorax Tendon, Left
F Abdomen Tendon, Right
G Abdomen Tendon, Left
H Perineum Tendon
J Hip Tendon, Right
K Hip Tendon, Left
L Upper Leg Tendon, Right
M Upper Leg Tendon, Left
N Lower Leg Tendon, Right
    Achilles tendon
P Lower Leg Tendon, Left
    See N Lower Leg Tendon, Right
Q Knee Tendon, Right
    Patellar tendon
R Knee Tendon, Left
    See Q Knee Tendon, Right
S Ankle Tendon, Right
T Ankle Tendon, Left
V Foot Tendon, Right
W Foot Tendon, Left
	Ø Open
	4 Percutaneous Endoscopic
		Z No Device	Z No Qualifier

Ø   Medical and Surgical
L   Tendons
U   Supplement   Definition: Putting in or on biological or synthetic material that physically reinforces and/or augments the function of a portion of a body part
                            Explanation: The biological material is non-living, or is living and from the same individual. The body part may have been previously replaced, and the SUPPLEMENT procedure is performed to physically reinforce and/or augment the function of the replaced body part.

Body Part Character 4	Approach Character 5	Device Character 6	Qualifier Character 7

Ø Head and Neck Tendon
1 Shoulder Tendon, Right
2 Shoulder Tendon, Left
3 Upper Arm Tendon, Right
4 Upper Arm Tendon, Left
5 Lower Arm and Wrist Tendon, Right
6 Lower Arm and Wrist Tendon, Left
7 Hand Tendon, Right
8 Hand Tendon, Left
9 Trunk Tendon, Right
B Trunk Tendon, Left
C Thorax Tendon, Right
D Thorax Tendon, Left
F Abdomen Tendon, Right
G Abdomen Tendon, Left
H Perineum Tendon
J Hip Tendon, Right
K Hip Tendon, Left
L Upper Leg Tendon, Right
M Upper Leg Tendon, Left
N Lower Leg Tendon, Right
    Achilles tendon
P Lower Leg Tendon, Left
    See N Lower Leg Tendon, Right
Q Knee Tendon, Right
    Patellar tendon
R Knee Tendon, Left
    See Q Knee Tendon, Right
S Ankle Tendon, Right
T Ankle Tendon, Left
V Foot Tendon, Right
W Foot Tendon, Left
	Ø Open
	4 Percutaneous Endoscopic
		7 Autologous Tissue Substitute
		J Synthetic Substitute
		K Nonautologous Tissue Substitute
			Z No Qualifier

LC Limited Coverage   NC Noncovered   ⊞ Combination Member   HAC associated procedure   Combination Only   DRG Non-OR   Non-OR   New/Revised in GREEN

ICD-10-PCS 2021   **493**

ØLT–ØLU

Ø **Medical and Surgical**
L **Tendons**
W **Revision**   Definition: Correcting, to the extent possible, a portion of a malfunctioning device or the position of a displaced device

Explanation: Revision can include correcting a malfunctioning or displaced device by taking out or putting in components of the device such as a screw or pin

Body Part Character 4	Approach Character 5	Device Character 6	Qualifier Character 7
X Upper Tendon **Y** Lower Tendon	**Ø** Open **3** Percutaneous **4** Percutaneous Endoscopic	**Ø** Drainage Device **7** Autologous Tissue Substitute **J** Synthetic Substitute **K** Nonautologous Tissue Substitute **Y** Other Device	**Z** No Qualifier
X Upper Tendon **Y** Lower Tendon	**X** External	**Ø** Drainage Device **7** Autologous Tissue Substitute **J** Synthetic Substitute **K** Nonautologous Tissue Substitute	**Z** No Qualifier

Non-OR ØLW[X,Y][3,4]YZ
Non-OR ØLW[X,Y]X[Ø,7,J,K]Z

Ø **Medical and Surgical**
L **Tendons**
X **Transfer**   Definition: Moving, without taking out, all or a portion of a body part to another location to take over the function of all or a portion of a body part

Explanation: The body part transferred remains connected to its vascular and nervous supply

Body Part Character 4	Approach Character 5	Device Character 6	Qualifier Character 7

Ø Head and Neck Tendon
1 Shoulder Tendon, Right
2 Shoulder Tendon, Left
3 Upper Arm Tendon, Right
4 Upper Arm Tendon, Left
5 Lower Arm and Wrist Tendon, Right
6 Lower Arm and Wrist Tendon, Left
7 Hand Tendon, Right
8 Hand Tendon, Left
9 Trunk Tendon, Right
B Trunk Tendon, Left
C Thorax Tendon, Right
D Thorax Tendon, Left
F Abdomen Tendon, Right
G Abdomen Tendon, Left
H Perineum Tendon
J Hip Tendon, Right
K Hip Tendon, Left
L Upper Leg Tendon, Right
M Upper Leg Tendon, Left
N Lower Leg Tendon, Right
    Achilles tendon
P Lower Leg Tendon, Left
    See N Lower Leg Tendon, Right
Q Knee Tendon, Right
    Patellar tendon
R Knee Tendon, Left
    See Q Knee Tendon, Right
S Ankle Tendon, Right
T Ankle Tendon, Left
V Foot Tendon, Right
W Foot Tendon, Left
	Ø Open
	4 Percutaneous Endoscopic
		Z No Device	**Z** No Qualifier

Bursae and Ligaments ØM2–ØMX

Character Meanings*

This Character Meaning table is provided as a guide to assist the user in the identification of character members that may be found in this section of code tables. It **SHOULD NOT** be used to build a PCS code.

Operation–Character 3	Body Part–Character 4	Approach–Character 5	Device–Character 6	Qualifier–Character 7
2 Change	Ø Head and Neck Bursa and Ligament	Ø Open	Ø Drainage Device	X Diagnostic
5 Destruction	1 Shoulder Bursa and Ligament, Right	3 Percutaneous	7 Autologous Tissue Substitute	Z No Qualifier
8 Division	2 Shoulder Bursa and Ligament, Left	4 Percutaneous Endoscopic	J Synthetic Substitute	
9 Drainage	3 Elbow Bursa and Ligament, Right	X External	K Nonautologous Tissue Substitute	
B Excision	4 Elbow Bursa and Ligament, Left		Y Other Device	
C Extirpation	5 Wrist Bursa and Ligament, Right		Z No Device	
D Extraction	6 Wrist Bursa and Ligament, Left			
H Insertion	7 Hand Bursa and Ligament, Right			
J Inspection	8 Hand Bursa and Ligament, Left			
M Reattachment	9 Upper Extremity Bursa and Ligament, Right			
N Release	B Upper Extremity Bursa and Ligament, Left			
P Removal	C Upper Spine Bursa and Ligament			
Q Repair	D Lower Spine Bursa and Ligament			
R Replacement	F Sternum Bursa and Ligament			
S Reposition	G Rib(s) Bursa and Ligament			
T Resection	H Abdomen Bursa and Ligament, Right			
U Supplement	J Abdomen Bursa and Ligament, Left			
W Revision	K Perineum Bursa and Ligament			
X Transfer	L Hip Bursa and Ligament, Right			
	M Hip Bursa and Ligament, Left			
	N Knee Bursa and Ligament, Right			
	P Knee Bursa and Ligament, Left			
	Q Ankle Bursa and Ligament, Right			
	R Ankle Bursa and Ligament, Left			
	S Foot Bursa and Ligament, Right			
	T Foot Bursa and Ligament, Left			
	V Lower Extremity Bursa and Ligament, Right			
	W Lower Extremity Bursa and Ligament, Left			
	X Upper Bursa and Ligament			
	Y Lower Bursa and Ligament			

* Includes synovial membrane.

AHA Coding Clinic for table ØMB
2018, 3Q, 17   Excisional debridement of periosteum

AHA Coding Clinic for table ØMM
2013, 3Q, 20   Superior labrum anterior posterior (SLAP) repair and subacromial decompression

AHA Coding Clinic for table ØMQ
2014, 3Q, 9   Interspinous ligamentoplasty

AHA Coding Clinic for table ØMT
2017, 2Q, 21   Arthroscopic anterior cruciate ligament revision using autograft with anterolateral ligament reconstruction

AHA Coding Clinic for table ØMU
2017, 2Q, 21   Arthroscopic anterior cruciate ligament revision using autograft with anterolateral ligament reconstruction

Shoulder Ligaments

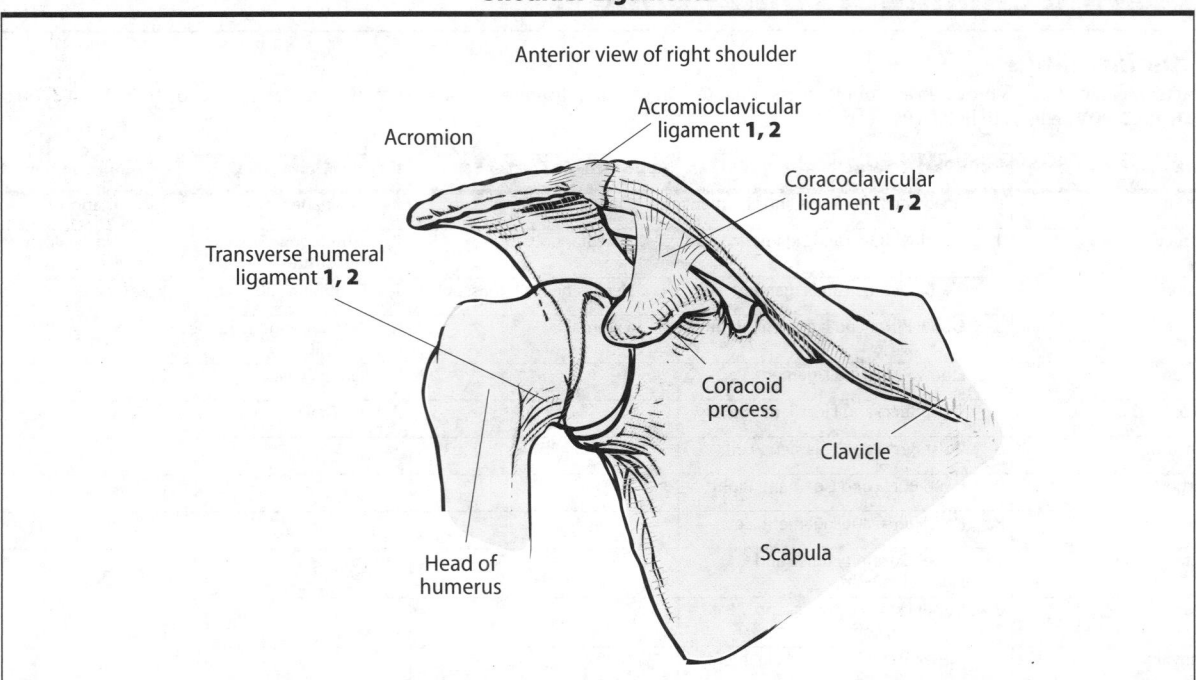

Anterior view of right shoulder

Acromioclavicular ligament **1, 2**

Coracoclavicular ligament **1, 2**

Acromion

Transverse humeral ligament **1, 2**

Coracoid process

Clavicle

Head of humerus

Scapula

Knee Bursae

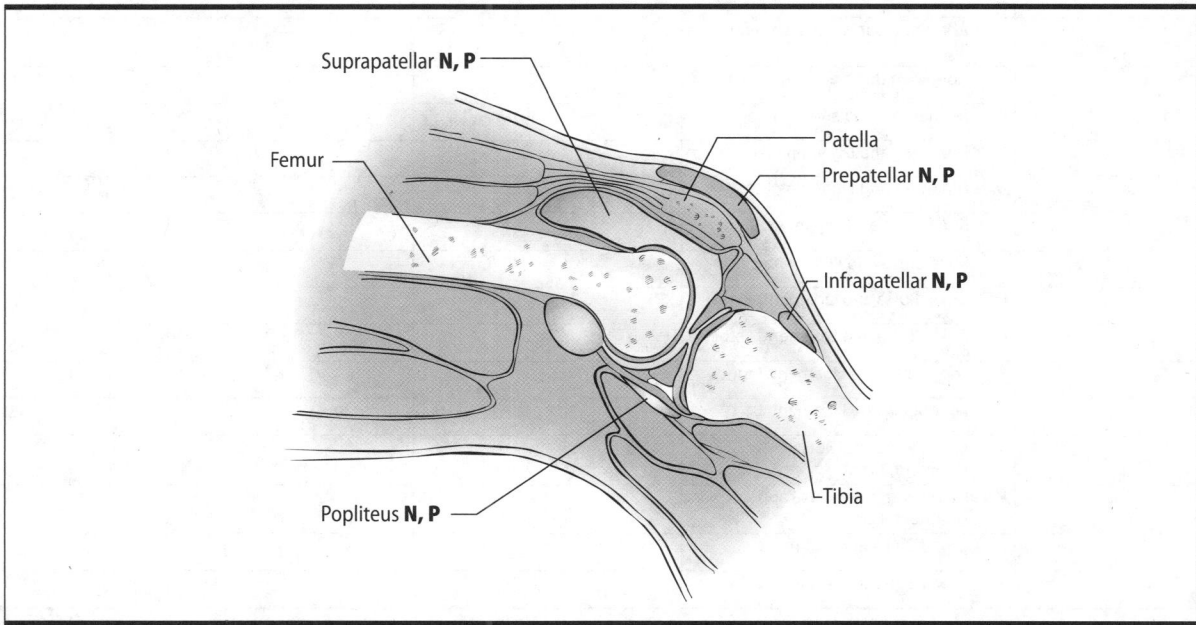

Suprapatellar **N, P**

Femur

Patella

Prepatellar **N, P**

Infrapatellar **N, P**

Popliteus **N, P**

Tibia

Knee Ligaments

Anterior view

Lateral collateral ligament **N, P**

Medial collateral ligament **N, P**

Patella

Posterior cruciate ligament **N, P**
(Behind the Anterior cruciate)

Anterior cruciate ligament **N, P**

Fibula

Tibia

Posterior cruciate ligament **N, P**

Anterior cruciate ligament **N, P**

Wrist Ligaments

Palmar view

5 4 3 2 1

Flexor carpi ulnaris **5, 6**

Radial collateral carpal **5, 6**

Ulnar collateral carpal **5, 6**

Palmar radiocarpal **5, 6**

Dorsal view

1 2 3 4 5

Radial collateral carpal **5, 6**

Ulnar collateral carpal **5, 6**

Dorsal radiocarpal **5, 6**

Ulnocarpal **5, 6**

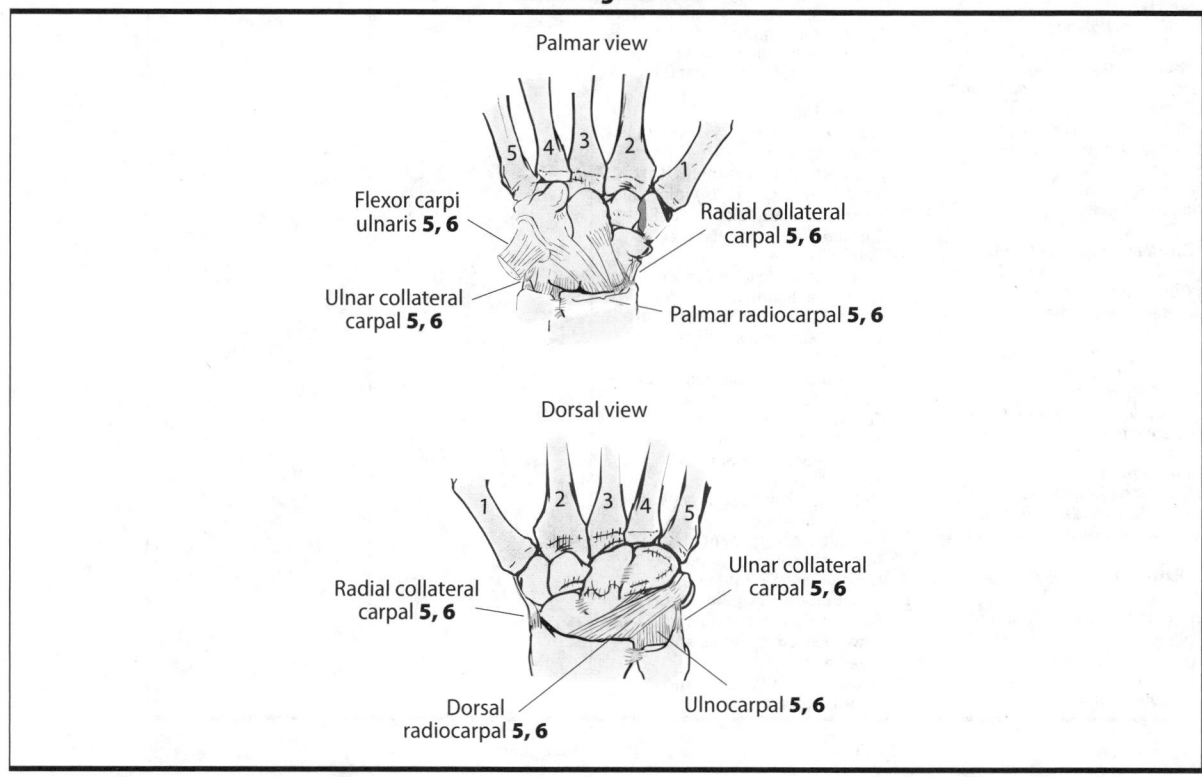

Bursae and Ligaments

Ø   **Medical and Surgical**
M   **Bursae and Ligaments**
2   **Change**   Definition: Taking out or off a device from a body part and putting back an identical or similar device in or on the same body part without cutting or puncturing the skin or a mucous membrane

                    Explanation: All CHANGE procedures are coded using the approach EXTERNAL

Body Part Character 4	Approach Character 5	Device Character 6	Qualifier Character 7
X Upper Bursa and Ligament Y Lower Bursa and Ligament	X External	Ø Drainage Device Y Other Device	Z No Qualifier

Non-OR   All body part, approach, device, and qualifier values

---

Ø   **Medical and Surgical**
M   **Bursae and Ligaments**
5   **Destruction**   Definition: Physical eradication of all or a portion of a body part by the direct use of energy, force, or a destructive agent

                       Explanation: None of the body part is physically taken out

Body Part Character 4	Approach Character 5	Device Character 6	Qualifier Character 7

Ø   **Head and Neck Bursa and Ligament**
    Alar ligament of axis
    Cervical interspinous ligament
    Cervical intertransverse ligament
    Cervical ligamentum flavum
    Interspinous ligament, cervical
    Intertransverse ligament, cervical
    Lateral temporomandibular ligament
    Ligamentum flavum, cervical
    Sphenomandibular ligament
    Stylomandibular ligament
    Transverse ligament of atlas
1   **Shoulder Bursa and Ligament, Right**
    Acromioclavicular ligament
    Coracoacromial ligament
    Coracoclavicular ligament
    Coracohumeral ligament
    Costoclavicular ligament
    Glenohumeral ligament
    Interclavicular ligament
    Sternoclavicular ligament
    Subacromial bursa
    Transverse humeral ligament
    Transverse scapular ligament
2   **Shoulder Bursa and Ligament, Left**
    See 1 Shoulder Bursa and Ligament, Right
3   **Elbow Bursa and Ligfament, Right**
    Annular ligament
    Olecranon bursa
    Radial collateral ligament
    Ulnar collateral ligament
4   **Elbow Bursa and Ligament, Left**
    See 3 Elbow Bursa and Ligament, Right
5   **Wrist Bursa and Ligament, Right**
    Palmar ulnocarpal ligament
    Radial collateral carpal ligament
    Radiocarpal ligament
    Radioulnar ligament
    Scapholunate ligament
    Ulnar collateral carpal ligament
6   **Wrist Bursa and Ligament, Left**
    See 5 Wrist Bursa and Ligament, Right
7   **Hand Bursa and Ligament, Right**
    Carpometacarpal ligament
    Intercarpal ligament
    Interphalangeal ligament
    Lunotriquetral ligament
    Metacarpal ligament
    Metacarpophalangeal ligament
    Pisohamate ligament
    Pisometacarpal ligament
    Scaphotrapezium ligament
8   **Hand Bursa and Ligament, Left**
    See 7 Hand Bursa and Ligament, Right
9   **Upper Extremity Bursa and Ligament, Right**
B   **Upper Extremity Bursa and Ligament, Left**
C   **Upper Spine Bursa and Ligament**
    Interspinous ligament, thoracic
    Intertransverse ligament, thoracic
    Ligamentum flavum, thoracic
    Supraspinous ligament
 	
D   **Lower Spine Bursa and Ligament**
    Iliolumbar ligament
    Interspinous ligament, lumbar
    Intertransverse ligament, lumbar
    Ligamentum flavum, lumbar
    Sacrococcygeal ligament
    Sacroiliac ligament
    Sacrospinous ligament
    Sacrotuberous ligament
    Supraspinous ligament
F   **Sternum Bursa and Ligament**
    Costoxiphoid ligament
    Sternocostal ligament
G   **Rib(s) Bursa and Ligament**
    Costotransverse ligament
H   **Abdomen Bursa and Ligament, Right**
J   **Abdomen Bursa and Ligament, Left**
K   **Perineum Bursa and Ligament**
L   **Hip Bursa and Ligament, Right**
    Iliofemoral ligament
    Ischiofemoral ligament
    Pubofemoral ligament
    Transverse acetabular ligament
    Trochanteric bursa
M   **Hip Bursa and Ligament, Left**
    See L Hip Bursa and Ligament, Right
N   **Knee Bursa and Ligament, Right**
    Anterior cruciate ligament (ACL)
    Lateral collateral ligament (LCL)
    Ligament of head of fibula
    Medial collateral ligament (MCL)
    Patellar ligament
    Popliteal ligament
    Posterior cruciate ligament (PCL)
    Prepatellar bursa
P   **Knee Bursa and Ligament, Left**
    See N Knee Bursa and Ligament, Right
Q   **Ankle Bursa and Ligament, Right**
    Calcaneofibular ligament
    Deltoid ligament
    Ligament of the lateral malleolus
    Talofibular ligament
R   **Ankle Bursa and Ligament, Left**
    See Q Ankle Bursa and Ligament, Right
S   **Foot Bursa and Ligament, Right**
    Calcaneocuboid ligament
    Cuneonavicular ligament
    Intercuneiform ligament
    Interphalangeal ligament
    Metatarsal ligament
    Metatarsophalangeal ligament
    Subtalar ligament
    Talocalcaneal ligament
    Talocalcaneonavicular ligament
    Tarsometatarsal ligament
T   **Foot Bursa and Ligament, Left**
    See S Foot Bursa and Ligament, Right
V   **Lower Extremity Bursa and Ligament, Right**
W   **Lower Extremity Bursa and Ligament, Left**
	Ø Open
	3 Percutaneous
	4 Percutaneous Endoscopic
		Z No Device	Z No Qualifier

LC Limited Coverage   NC Noncovered   ⊞ Combination Member   HAC associated procedure   Combination Only   DRG Non-OR   Non-OR   New/Revised in GREEN

498   ICD-10-PCS 2021

Ø   **Medical and Surgical**
M   **Bursae and Ligaments**
8   **Division**   Definition: Cutting into a body part, without draining fluids and/or gases from the body part, in order to separate or transect a body part
                           Explanation: All or a portion of the body part is separated into two or more portions

Body Part Character 4		Approach Character 5	Device Character 6	Qualifier Character 7
Ø Head and Neck Bursa and Ligament Alar ligament of axis Cervical interspinous ligament Cervical intertransverse ligament Cervical ligamentum flavum Interspinous ligament, cervical Intertransverse ligament, cervical Lateral temporomandibular ligament Ligamentum flavum, cervical Sphenomandibular ligament Stylomandibular ligament Transverse ligament of atlas **1 Shoulder Bursa and Ligament, Right** Acromioclavicular ligament Coracoacromial ligament Coracoclavicular ligament Coracohumeral ligament Costoclavicular ligament Glenohumeral ligament Interclavicular ligament Sternoclavicular ligament Subacromial bursa Transverse humeral ligament Transverse scapular ligament **2 Shoulder Bursa and Ligament, Left** *See 1 Shoulder Bursa and Ligament, Right* **3 Elbow Bursa and Ligament, Right** Annular ligament Olecranon bursa Radial collateral ligament Ulnar collateral ligament **4 Elbow Bursa and Ligament, Left** *See 3 Elbow Bursa and Ligament, Right* **5 Wrist Bursa and Ligament, Right** Palmar ulnocarpal ligament Radial collateral carpal ligament Radiocarpal ligament Radioulnar ligament Scapholunate ligament Ulnar collateral carpal ligament **6 Wrist Bursa and Ligament, Left** *See 5 Wrist Bursa and Ligament, Right* **7 Hand Bursa and Ligament, Right** Carpometacarpal ligament Intercarpal ligament Interphalangeal ligament Lunotriquetral ligament Metacarpal ligament Metacarpophalangeal ligament Pisohamate ligament Pisometacarpal ligament Scaphotrapezium ligament **8 Hand Bursa and Ligament, Left** *See 7 Hand Bursa and Ligament, Right* **9 Upper Extremity Bursa and Ligament, Right** **B Upper Extremity Bursa and Ligament, Left** **C Upper Spine Bursa and Ligament** Interspinous ligament, thoracic Intertransverse ligament, thoracic Ligamentum flavum, thoracic Supraspinous ligament	**D Lower Spine Bursa and Ligament** Iliolumbar ligament Interspinous ligament, lumbar Intertransverse ligament, lumbar Ligamentum flavum, lumbar Sacrococcygeal ligament Sacroiliac ligament Sacrospinous ligament Sacrotuberous ligament Supraspinous ligament **F Sternum Bursa and Ligament** Costoxiphoid ligament Sternocostal ligament **G Rib(s) Bursa and Ligament** Costotransverse ligament **H Abdomen Bursa and Ligament, Right** **J Abdomen Bursa and Ligament, Left** **K Perineum Bursa and Ligament** **L Hip Bursa and Ligament, Right** Iliofemoral ligament Ischiofemoral ligament Pubofemoral ligament Transverse acetabular ligament Trochanteric bursa **M Hip Bursa and Ligament, Left** *See L Hip Bursa and Ligament, Right* **N Knee Bursa and Ligament, Right** Anterior cruciate ligament (ACL) Lateral collateral ligament (LCL) Ligament of head of fibula Medial collateral ligament (MCL) Patellar ligament Popliteal ligament Posterior cruciate ligament (PCL) Prepatellar bursa **P Knee Bursa and Ligament, Left** *See N Knee Bursa and Ligament, Right* **Q Ankle Bursa and Ligament, Right** Calcaneofibular ligament Deltoid ligament Ligament of the lateral malleolus Talofibular ligament **R Ankle Bursa and Ligament, Left** *See Q Ankle Bursa and Ligament, Right* **S Foot Bursa and Ligament, Right** Calcaneocuboid ligament Cuneonavicular ligament Intercuneiform ligament Interphalangeal ligament Metatarsal ligament Metatarsophalangeal ligament Subtalar ligament Talocalcaneal ligament Talocalcaneonavicular ligament Tarsometatarsal ligament **T Foot Bursa and Ligament, Left** *See S Foot Bursa and Ligament, Right* **V Lower Extremity Bursa and Ligament, Right** **W Lower Extremity Bursa and Ligament, Left**	**Ø Open** **3 Percutaneous** **4 Percutaneous Endoscopic**	**Z No Device**	**Z No Qualifier**

Bursae and Ligaments

Ø   Medical and Surgical
M   Bursae and Ligaments
9   Drainage   Definition: Taking or letting out fluids and/or gases from a body part
                        Explanation: The qualifier DIAGNOSTIC is used to identify drainage procedures that are biopsies

Body Part Character 4		Approach Character 5	Device Character 6	Qualifier Character 7

Ø Head and Neck Bursa and Ligament
Alar ligament of axis
Cervical interspinous ligament
Cervical intertransverse ligament
Cervical ligamentum flavum
Interspinous ligament, cervical
Intertransverse ligament, cervical
Lateral temporomandibular
   ligament
Ligamentum flavum, cervical
Sphenomandibular ligament
Stylomandibular ligament
Transverse ligament of atlas
1 Shoulder Bursa and Ligament, Right
Acromioclavicular ligament
Coracoacromial ligament
Coracoclavicular ligament
Coracohumeral ligament
Costoclavicular ligament
Glenohumeral ligament
Interclavicular ligament
Sternoclavicular ligament
Subacromial bursa
Transverse humeral ligament
Transverse scapular ligament
2 Shoulder Bursa and Ligament, Left
See 1 Shoulder Bursa and
   Ligament, Right
3 Elbow Bursa and Ligament, Right
Annular ligament
Olecranon bursa
Radial collateral ligament
Ulnar collateral ligament
4 Elbow Bursa and Ligament, Left
See 3 Elbow Bursa and Ligament,
   Right
5 Wrist Bursa and Ligament, Right
Palmar ulnocarpal ligament
Radial collateral carpal ligament
Radiocarpal ligament
Radioulnar ligament
Scapholunate ligament
Ulnar collateral carpal ligament
6 Wrist Bursa and Ligament, Left
See 5 Wrist Bursa and Ligament,
   Right
7 Hand Bursa and Ligament, Right
Carpometacarpal ligament
Intercarpal ligament
Interphalangeal ligament
Lunotriquetral ligament
Metacarpal ligament
Metacarpophalangeal ligament
Pisohamate ligament
Pisometacarpal ligament
Scaphotrapezium ligament
8 Hand Bursa and Ligament, Left
See 7 Hand Bursa and Ligament,
   Right
9 Upper Extremity Bursa and Ligament, Right
B Upper Extremity Bursa and Ligament, Left
C Upper Spine Bursa and Ligament
Interspinous ligament, thoracic
Intertransverse ligament, thoracic
Ligamentum flavum, thoracic
Supraspinous ligament
	D Lower Spine Bursa and Ligament
	Iliolumbar ligament
	Interspinous ligament, lumbar
	Intertransverse ligament, lumbar
	Ligamentum flavum, lumbar
	Sacrococcygeal ligament
	Sacroiliac ligament
	Sacrospinous ligament
	Sacrotuberous ligament
	Supraspinous ligament
	F Sternum Bursa and Ligament
	Costoxiphoid ligament
	Sternocostal ligament
	G Rib(s) Bursa and Ligament
	Costotransverse ligament
	H Abdomen Bursa and Ligament, Right
	J Abdomen Bursa and Ligament, Left
	K Perineum Bursa and Ligament
	L Hip Bursa and Ligament, Right
	Iliofemoral ligament
	Ischiofemoral ligament
	Pubofemoral ligament
	Transverse acetabular ligament
	Trochanteric bursa
	M Hip Bursa and Ligament, Left
	See L Hip Bursa and Ligament,
	   Right
	N Knee Bursa and Ligament, Right
	Anterior cruciate ligament (ACL)
	Lateral collateral ligament (LCL)
	Ligament of head of fibula
	Medial collateral ligament (MCL)
	Patellar ligament
	Popliteal ligament
	Posterior cruciate ligament (PCL)
	Prepatellar bursa
	P Knee Bursa and Ligament, Left
	See N Knee Bursa and Ligament,
	   Right
	Q Ankle Bursa and Ligament, Right
	Calcaneofibular ligament
	Deltoid ligament
	Ligament of the lateral malleolus
	Talofibular ligament
	R Ankle Bursa and Ligament, Left
	See Q Ankle Bursa and Ligament,
	   Right
	S Foot Bursa and Ligament, Right
	Calcaneocuboid ligament
	Cuneonavicular ligament
	Intercuneiform ligament
	Interphalangeal ligament
	Metatarsal ligament
	Metatarsophalangeal ligament
	Subtalar ligament
	Talocalcaneal ligament
	Talocalcaneonavicular ligament
	Tarsometatarsal ligament
	T Foot Bursa and Ligament, Left
	See S Foot Bursa and Ligament,
	   Right
	V Lower Extremity Bursa and Ligament, Right
	W Lower Extremity Bursa and Ligament, Left
		Ø Open
		3 Percutaneous
		4 Percutaneous Endoscopic
			Ø Drainage Device	**Z No Qualifier**

Non-OR   ØM9[Ø,1,2,3,4,5,6,7,8,9,B,C,D,F,G,H,J,K,L,M,N,P,Q,R,S,T,V,W]3ØZ
Non-OR   ØM9[1,2,3,4,7,8,9,B,C,D,F,G,H,J,K,L,M,V,W]4ØZ

ØM9 Continued on next page

Ø   **Medical and Surgical**
M **Bursae and Ligaments**
9   **Drainage**

ØM9 Continued

Definition: Taking or letting out fluids and/or gases from a body part
Explanation: The qualifier DIAGNOSTIC is used to identify drainage procedures that are biopsies

Body Part Character 4		Approach Character 5	Device Character 6	Qualifier Character 7
Ø Head and Neck Bursa and Ligament Alar ligament of axis Cervical interspinous ligament Cervical intertransverse ligament Cervical ligamentum flavum Interspinous ligament, cervical Intertransverse ligament, cervical Lateral temporomandibular ligament Ligamentum flavum, cervical Sphenomandibular ligament Stylomandibular ligament Transverse ligament of atlas	**D Lower Spine Bursa and Ligament** Iliolumbar ligament Interspinous ligament, lumbar Intertransverse ligament, lumbar Ligamentum flavum, lumbar Sacrococcygeal ligament Sacroiliac ligament Sacrospinous ligament Sacrotuberous ligament Supraspinous ligament	**Ø Open** **3 Percutaneous** **4 Percutaneous Endoscopic**	**Z No Device**	**X Diagnostic** **Z No Qualifier**
1 Shoulder Bursa and Ligament, Right Acromioclavicular ligament Coracoacromial ligament Coracoclavicular ligament Coracohumeral ligament Costoclavicular ligament Glenohumeral ligament Interclavicular ligament Sternoclavicular ligament Subacromial bursa Transverse humeral ligament Transverse scapular ligament	**F Sternum Bursa and Ligament** Costoxiphoid ligament Sternocostal ligament **G Rib(s) Bursa and Ligament** Costotransverse ligament **H Abdomen Bursa and Ligament, Right** **J Abdomen Bursa and Ligament, Left** **K Perineum Bursa and Ligament** **L Hip Bursa and Ligament, Right** Iliofemoral ligament Ischiofemoral ligament Pubofemoral ligament Transverse acetabular ligament Trochanteric bursa			
2 Shoulder Bursa and Ligament, Left *See 1 Shoulder Bursa and Ligament, Right*	**M Hip Bursa and Ligament, Left** *See L Hip Bursa and Ligament, Right*			
3 Elbow Bursa and Ligament, Right Annular ligament Olecranon bursa Radial collateral ligament Ulnar collateral ligament	**N Knee Bursa and Ligament, Right** Anterior cruciate ligament (ACL) Lateral collateral ligament (LCL) Ligament of head of fibula Medial collateral ligament (MCL) Patellar ligament Popliteal ligament Posterior cruciate ligament (PCL) Prepatellar bursa			
4 Elbow Bursa and Ligament, Left *See 3 Elbow Bursa and Ligament, Right*	**P Knee Bursa and Ligament, Left** *See N Knee Bursa and Ligament, Right*			
5 Wrist Bursa and Ligament, Right Palmar ulnocarpal ligament Radial collateral carpal ligament Radiocarpal ligament Radioulnar ligament Scapholunate ligament Ulnar collateral carpal ligament	**Q Ankle Bursa and Ligament, Right** Calcaneofibular ligament Deltoid ligament Ligament of the lateral malleolus Talofibular ligament			
6 Wrist Bursa and Ligament, Left *See 5 Wrist Bursa and Ligament, Right*	**R Ankle Bursa and Ligament, Left** *See Q Ankle Bursa and Ligament, Right*			
7 Hand Bursa and Ligament, Right Carpometacarpal ligament Intercarpal ligament Interphalangeal ligament Lunotriquetral ligament Metacarpal ligament Metacarpophalangeal ligament Pisohamate ligament Pisometacarpal ligament Scaphotrapezium ligament	**S Foot Bursa and Ligament, Right** Calcaneocuboid ligament Cuneonavicular ligament Intercuneiform ligament Interphalangeal ligament Metatarsal ligament Metatarsophalangeal ligament Subtalar ligament Talocalcaneal ligament Talocalcaneonavicular ligament Tarsometatarsal ligament			
8 Hand Bursa and Ligament, Left *See 7 Hand Bursa and Ligament, Right*	**T Foot Bursa and Ligament, Left** *See S Foot Bursa and Ligament, Right*			
9 Upper Extremity Bursa and Ligament, Right **B Upper Extremity Bursa and Ligament, Left** **C Upper Spine Bursa and Ligament** Interspinous ligament, thoracic Intertransverse ligament, thoracic Ligamentum flavum, thoracic Supraspinous ligament	**V Lower Extremity Bursa and Ligament, Right** **W Lower Extremity Bursa and Ligament, Left**			

Non-OR	ØM9[Ø,1,2,3,4,5,6,7,8,C,D,F,G,L,M,N,P,Q,R,S,T][Ø,3,4]ZX
Non-OR	ØM9[Ø,1,2,3,4,5,6,7,8,9,B,C,D,F,G,H,J,K,L,M,N,P,Q,R,S,T,V,W]3ZZ
Non-OR	ØM9[Ø,5,6,7,8,9,B,C,D,F,G,H,J,K,N,P,Q,R,S,T,V,W]4ZZ

Bursae and Ligaments

Ø   Medical and Surgical
M   Bursae and Ligaments
B   Excision   Definition: Cutting out or off, without replacement, a portion of a body part
                       Explanation: The qualifier DIAGNOSTIC is used to identify excision procedures that are biopsies

Body Part – Character 4		Approach – Character 5	Device – Character 6	Qualifier – Character 7
Ø Head and Neck Bursa and Ligament Alar ligament of axis Cervical interspinous ligament Cervical intertransverse ligament Cervical ligamentum flavum Interspinous ligament, cervical Intertransverse ligament, cervical Lateral temporomandibular ligament Ligamentum flavum, cervical Sphenomandibular ligament Stylomandibular ligament Transverse ligament of atlas **1 Shoulder Bursa and Ligament, Right** Acromioclavicular ligament Coracoacromial ligament Coracoclavicular ligament Coracohumeral ligament Costoclavicular ligament Glenohumeral ligament Interclavicular ligament Sternoclavicular ligament Subacromial bursa Transverse humeral ligament Transverse scapular ligament **2 Shoulder Bursa and Ligament, Left** *See 1 Shoulder Bursa and Ligament, Right* **3 Elbow Bursa and Ligament, Right** Annular ligament Olecranon bursa Radial collateral ligament Ulnar collateral ligament **4 Elbow Bursa and Ligament, Left** *See 3 Elbow Bursa and Ligament, Right* **5 Wrist Bursa and Ligament, Right** Palmar ulnocarpal ligament Radial collateral carpal ligament Radiocarpal ligament Radioulnar ligament Scapholunate ligament Ulnar collateral carpal ligament **6 Wrist Bursa and Ligament, Left** *See 5 Wrist Bursa and Ligament, Right* **7 Hand Bursa and Ligament, Right** Carpometacarpal ligament Intercarpal ligament Interphalangeal ligament Lunotriquetral ligament Metacarpal ligament Metacarpophalangeal ligament Pisohamate ligament Pisometacarpal ligament Scaphotrapezium ligament **8 Hand Bursa and Ligament, Left** *See 7 Hand Bursa and Ligament, Right* **9 Upper Extremity Bursa and Ligament, Right** **B Upper Extremity Bursa and Ligament, Left** **C Upper Spine Bursa and Ligament** Interspinous ligament, thoracic Intertransverse ligament, thoracic Ligamentum flavum, thoracic Supraspinous ligament	**D Lower Spine Bursa and Ligament** Iliolumbar ligament Interspinous ligament, lumbar Intertransverse ligament, lumbar Ligamentum flavum, lumbar Sacrococcygeal ligament Sacroiliac ligament Sacrospinous ligament Sacrotuberous ligament Supraspinous ligament **F Sternum Bursa and Ligament** Costoxiphoid ligament Sternocostal ligament **G Rib(s) Bursa and Ligament** Costotransverse ligament **H Abdomen Bursa and Ligament, Right** **J Abdomen Bursa and Ligament, Left** **K Perineum Bursa and Ligament** **L Hip Bursa and Ligament, Right** Iliofemoral ligament Ischiofemoral ligament Pubofemoral ligament Transverse acetabular ligament Trochanteric bursa **M Hip Bursa and Ligament, Left** *See L Hip Bursa and Ligament, Right* **N Knee Bursa and Ligament, Right** Anterior cruciate ligament (ACL) Lateral collateral ligament (LCL) Ligament of head of fibula Medial collateral ligament (MCL) Patellar ligament Popliteal ligament Posterior cruciate ligament (PCL) Prepatellar bursa **P Knee Bursa and Ligament, Left** *See N Knee Bursa and Ligament, Right* **Q Ankle Bursa and Ligament, Right** Calcaneofibular ligament Deltoid ligament Ligament of the lateral malleolus Talofibular ligament **R Ankle Bursa and Ligament, Left** *See Q Ankle Bursa and Ligament, Right* **S Foot Bursa and Ligament, Right** Calcaneocuboid ligament Cuneonavicular ligament Intercuneiform ligament Interphalangeal ligament Metatarsal ligament Metatarsophalangeal ligament Subtalar ligament Talocalcaneal ligament Talocalcaneonavicular ligament Tarsometatarsal ligament **T Foot Bursa and Ligament, Left** *See S Foot Bursa and Ligament, Right* **V Lower Extremity Bursa and Ligament, Right** **W Lower Extremity Bursa and Ligament, Left**	**Ø Open** **3 Percutaneous** **4 Percutaneous Endoscopic**	**Z No Device**	**X Diagnostic** **Z No Qualifier**

Non-OR   ØMB[Ø,1,2,3,4,5,6,7,8,B,C,D,F,G,L,M,N,P,Q,R,S,T][Ø,3,4]ZX
Non-OR   ØMB94ZX

Ø   Medical and Surgical
M   Bursae and Ligaments
C   Extirpation   Definition: Taking or cutting out solid matter from a body part

Explanation: The solid matter may be an abnormal byproduct of a biological function or a foreign body; it may be imbedded in a body part or in the lumen of a tubular body part. The solid matter may or may not have been previously broken into pieces.

Body Part Character 4		Approach Character 5	Device Character 6	Qualifier Character 7
Ø Head and Neck Bursa and Ligament Alar ligament of axis Cervical interspinous ligament Cervical intertransverse ligament Cervical ligamentum flavum Interspinous ligament, cervical Intertransverse ligament, cervical Lateral temporomandibular ligament Ligamentum flavum, cervical Sphenomandibular ligament Stylomandibular ligament Transverse ligament of atlas **1 Shoulder Bursa and Ligament, Right** Acromioclavicular ligament Coracoacromial ligament Coracoclavicular ligament Coracohumeral ligament Costoclavicular ligament Glenohumeral ligament Interclavicular ligament Sternoclavicular ligament Subacromial bursa Transverse humeral ligament Transverse scapular ligament **2 Shoulder Bursa and Ligament, Left** *See 1 Shoulder Bursa and Ligament, Right* **3 Elbow Bursa and Ligament, Right** Annular ligament Olecranon bursa Radial collateral ligament Ulnar collateral ligament **4 Elbow Bursa and Ligament, Left** *See 3 Elbow Bursa and Ligament, Right* **5 Wrist Bursa and Ligament, Right** Palmar ulnocarpal ligament Radial collateral carpal ligament Radiocarpal ligament Radioulnar ligament Scapholunate ligament Ulnar collateral carpal ligament **6 Wrist Bursa and Ligament, Left** *See 5 Wrist Bursa and Ligament, Right* **7 Hand Bursa and Ligament, Right** Carpometacarpal ligament Intercarpal ligament Interphalangeal ligament Lunotriquetral ligament Metacarpal ligament Metacarpophalangeal ligament Pisohamate ligament Pisometacarpal ligament Scaphotrapezium ligament **8 Hand Bursa and Ligament, Left** *See 7 Hand Bursa and Ligament, Right* **9 Upper Extremity Bursa and Ligament, Right** **B Upper Extremity Bursa and Ligament, Left** **C Upper Spine Bursa and Ligament** Interspinous ligament, thoracic Intertransverse ligament, thoracic Ligamentum flavum, thoracic Supraspinous ligament	**D Lower Spine Bursa and Ligament** Iliolumbar ligament Interspinous ligament, lumbar Intertransverse ligament, lumbar Ligamentum flavum, lumbar Sacrococcygeal ligament Sacroiliac ligament Sacrospinous ligament Sacrotuberous ligament Supraspinous ligament **F Sternum Bursa and Ligament** Costoxiphoid ligament Sternocostal ligament **G Rib(s) Bursa and Ligament** Costotransverse ligament **H Abdomen Bursa and Ligament, Right** **J Abdomen Bursa and Ligament, Left** **K Perineum Bursa and Ligament** **L Hip Bursa and Ligament, Right** Iliofemoral ligament Ischiofemoral ligament Pubofemoral ligament Transverse acetabular ligament Trochanteric bursa **M Hip Bursa and Ligament, Left** *See L Hip Bursa and Ligament, Right* **N Knee Bursa and Ligament, Right** Anterior cruciate ligament (ACL) Lateral collateral ligament (LCL) Ligament of head of fibula Medial collateral ligament (MCL) Patellar ligament Popliteal ligament Posterior cruciate ligament (PCL) Prepatellar bursa **P Knee Bursa and Ligament, Left** *See N Knee Bursa and Ligament, Right* **Q Ankle Bursa and Ligament, Right** Calcaneofibular ligament Deltoid ligament Ligament of the lateral malleolus Talofibular ligament **R Ankle Bursa and Ligament, Left** *See Q Ankle Bursa and Ligament, Right* **S Foot Bursa and Ligament, Right** Calcaneocuboid ligament Cuneonavicular ligament Intercuneiform ligament Interphalangeal ligament Metatarsal ligament Metatarsophalangeal ligament Subtalar ligament Talocalcaneal ligament Talocalcaneonavicular ligament Tarsometatarsal ligament **T Foot Bursa and Ligament, Left** *See S Foot Bursa and Ligament, Right* **V Lower Extremity Bursa and Ligament, Right** **W Lower Extremity Bursa and Ligament, Left**	**Ø Open** **3 Percutaneous** **4 Percutaneous Endoscopic**	**Z No Device**	**Z No Qualifier**

Bursae and Ligaments

Ø Medical and Surgical
M Bursae and Ligaments
D Extraction Definition: Pulling or stripping out or off all or a portion of a body part by the use of force
Explanation: The qualifier DIAGNOSTIC is used to identify extraction procedures that are biopsies

Body Part Character 4		Approach Character 5	Device Character 6	Qualifier Character 7
Ø Head and Neck Bursa and Ligament Alar ligament of axis Cervical interspinous ligament Cervical intertransverse ligament Cervical ligamentum flavum Interspinous ligament, cervical Intertransverse ligament, cervical Lateral temporomandibular ligament Ligamentum flavum, cervical Sphenomandibular ligament Stylomandibular ligament Transverse ligament of atlas **1 Shoulder Bursa and Ligament, Right** Acromioclavicular ligament Coracoacromial ligament Coracoclavicular ligament Coracohumeral ligament Costoclavicular ligament Glenohumeral ligament Interclavicular ligament Sternoclavicular ligament Subacromial bursa Transverse humeral ligament Transverse scapular ligament **2 Shoulder Bursa and Ligament, Left** *See 1 Shoulder Bursa and Ligament, Right* **3 Elbow Bursa and Ligament, Right** Annular ligament Olecranon bursa Radial collateral ligament Ulnar collateral ligament **4 Elbow Bursa and Ligament, Left** *See 3 Elbow Bursa and Ligament, Right* **5 Wrist Bursa and Ligament, Right** Palmar ulnocarpal ligament Radial collateral carpal ligament Radiocarpal ligament Radioulnar ligament Scapholunate ligament Ulnar collateral carpal ligament **6 Wrist Bursa and Ligament, Left** *See 5 Wrist Bursa and Ligament, Right* **7 Hand Bursa and Ligament, Right** Carpometacarpal ligament Intercarpal ligament Interphalangeal ligament Lunotriquetral ligament Metacarpal ligament Metacarpophalangeal ligament Pisohamate ligament Pisometacarpal ligament Scaphotrapezium ligament **8 Hand Bursa and Ligament, Left** *See 7 Hand Bursa and Ligament, Right* **9 Upper Extremity Bursa and Ligament, Right** **B Upper Extremity Bursa and Ligament, Left** **C Upper Spine Bursa and Ligament** Interspinous ligament, thoracic Intertransverse ligament, thoracic Ligamentum flavum, thoracic Supraspinous ligament	**D Lower Spine Bursa and Ligament** Iliolumbar ligament Interspinous ligament, lumbar Intertransverse ligament, lumbar Ligamentum flavum, lumbar Sacrococcygeal ligament Sacroiliac ligament Sacrospinous ligament Sacrotuberous ligament Supraspinous ligament **F Sternum Bursa and Ligament** Costoxiphoid ligament Sternocostal ligament **G Rib(s) Bursa and Ligament** Costotransverse ligament **H Abdomen Bursa and Ligament, Right** **J Abdomen Bursa and Ligament, Left** **K Perineum Bursa and Ligament** **L Hip Bursa and Ligament, Right** Iliofemoral ligament Ischiofemoral ligament Pubofemoral ligament Transverse acetabular ligament Trochanteric bursa **M Hip Bursa and Ligament, Left** *See L Hip Bursa and Ligament, Right* **N Knee Bursa and Ligament, Right** Anterior cruciate ligament (ACL) Lateral collateral ligament (LCL) Ligament of head of fibula Medial collateral ligament (MCL) Patellar ligament Popliteal ligament Posterior cruciate ligament (PCL) Prepatellar bursa **P Knee Bursa and Ligament, Left** *See N Knee Bursa and Ligament, Right* **Q Ankle Bursa and Ligament, Right** Calcaneofibular ligament Deltoid ligament Ligament of the lateral malleolus Talofibular ligament **R Ankle Bursa and Ligament, Left** *See Q Ankle Bursa and Ligament, Right* **S Foot Bursa and Ligament, Right** Calcaneocuboid ligament Cuneonavicular ligament Intercuneiform ligament Interphalangeal ligament Metatarsal ligament Metatarsophalangeal ligament Subtalar ligament Talocalcaneal ligament Talocalcaneonavicular ligament Tarsometatarsal ligament **T Foot Bursa and Ligament, Left** *See S Foot Bursa and Ligament, Right* **V Lower Extremity Bursa and Ligament, Right** **W Lower Extremity Bursa and Ligament, Left**	**Ø Open** **3 Percutaneous** **4 Percutaneous Endoscopic**	**Z No Device**	**Z No Qualifier**

Ø   Medical and Surgical
M   Bursae and Ligaments
H   Insertion   Definition: Putting in a nonbiological appliance that monitors, assists, performs, or prevents a physiological function but does not physically take the place of a body part

                      Explanation: None

Body Part Character 4	Approach Character 5	Device Character 6	Qualifier Character 7
X Upper Bursa and Ligament Y Lower Bursa and Ligament	Ø Open 3 Percutaneous 4 Percutaneous Endoscopic	Y Other Device	Z No Qualifier

Non-OR   ØMH[X,Y][3,4]YZ

Ø   Medical and Surgical
M   Bursae and Ligaments
J   Inspection   Definition: Visually and/or manually exploring a body part

                      Explanation: Visual exploration may be performed with or without optical instrumentation. Manual exploration may be performed directly or through intervening body layers.

Body Part Character 4	Approach Character 5	Device Character 6	Qualifier Character 7
X Upper Bursa and Ligament Y Lower Bursa and Ligament	Ø Open 3 Percutaneous 4 Percutaneous Endoscopic X External	Z No Device	Z No Qualifier

Non-OR   ØMJ[X,Y][3,X]ZZ

Bursae and Ligaments

Ø   **Medical and Surgical**
M   **Bursae and Ligaments**
M   **Reattachment**   Definition: Putting back in or on all or a portion of a separated body part to its normal location or other suitable location
                        Explanation: Vascular circulation and nervous pathways may or may not be reestablished

Body Part Character 4		Approach Character 5	Device Character 6	Qualifier Character 7
Ø **Head and Neck Bursa and Ligament** Alar ligament of axis Cervical interspinous ligament Cervical intertransverse ligament Cervical ligamentum flavum Interspinous ligament, cervical Intertransverse ligament, cervical Lateral temporomandibular ligament Ligamentum flavum, cervical Sphenomandibular ligament Stylomandibular ligament Transverse ligament of atlas **1** **Shoulder Bursa and Ligament, Right** Acromioclavicular ligament Coracoacromial ligament Coracoclavicular ligament Coracohumeral ligament Costoclavicular ligament Glenohumeral ligament Interclavicular ligament Sternoclavicular ligament Subacromial bursa Transverse humeral ligament Transverse scapular ligament **2** **Shoulder Bursa and Ligament, Left** *See 1 Shoulder Bursa and Ligament, Right* **3** **Elbow Bursa and Ligament, Right** Annular ligament Olecranon bursa Radial collateral ligament Ulnar collateral ligament **4** **Elbow Bursa and Ligament, Left** *See 3 Elbow Bursa and Ligament, Right* **5** **Wrist Bursa and Ligament, Right** Palmar ulnocarpal ligament Radial collateral carpal ligament Radiocarpal ligament Radioulnar ligament Scapholunate ligament Ulnar collateral carpal ligament **6** **Wrist Bursa and Ligament, Left** *See 5 Wrist Bursa and Ligament, Right* **7** **Hand Bursa and Ligament, Right** Carpometacarpal ligament Intercarpal ligament Interphalangeal ligament Lunotriquetral ligament Metacarpal ligament Metacarpophalangeal ligament Pisohamate ligament Pisometacarpal ligament Scaphotrapezium ligament **8** **Hand Bursa and Ligament, Left** *See 7 Hand Bursa and Ligament, Right* **9** **Upper Extremity Bursa and Ligament, Right** **B** **Upper Extremity Bursa and Ligament, Left** **C** **Upper Spine Bursa and Ligament** Interspinous ligament, thoracic Intertransverse ligament, thoracic Ligamentum flavum, thoracic Supraspinous ligament	**D** **Lower Spine Bursa and Ligament** Iliolumbar ligament Interspinous ligament, lumbar Intertransverse ligament, lumbar Ligamentum flavum, lumbar Sacrococcygeal ligament Sacroiliac ligament Sacrospinous ligament Sacrotuberous ligament Supraspinous ligament **F** **Sternum Bursa and Ligament** Costoxiphoid ligament Sternocostal ligament **G** **Rib(s) Bursa and Ligament** Costotransverse ligament **H** **Abdomen Bursa and Ligament, Right** **J** **Abdomen Bursa and Ligament, Left** **K** **Perineum Bursa and Ligament** **L** **Hip Bursa and Ligament, Right** Iliofemoral ligament Ischiofemoral ligament Pubofemoral ligament Transverse acetabular ligament Trochanteric bursa **M** **Hip Bursa and Ligament, Left** *See L Hip Bursa and Ligament, Right* **N** **Knee Bursa and Ligament, Right** Anterior cruciate ligament (ACL) Lateral collateral ligament (LCL) Ligament of head of fibula Medial collateral ligament (MCL) Patellar ligament Popliteal ligament Posterior cruciate ligament (PCL) Prepatellar bursa **P** **Knee Bursa and Ligament, Left** *See N Knee Bursa and Ligament, Right* **Q** **Ankle Bursa and Ligament, Right** Calcaneofibular ligament Deltoid ligament Ligament of the lateral malleolus Talofibular ligament **R** **Ankle Bursa and Ligament, Left** *See Q Ankle Bursa and Ligament, Right* **S** **Foot Bursa and Ligament, Right** Calcaneocuboid ligament Cuneonavicular ligament Intercuneiform ligament Interphalangeal ligament Metatarsal ligament Metatarsophalangeal ligament Subtalar ligament Talocalcaneal ligament Talocalcaneonavicular ligament Tarsometatarsal ligament **T** **Foot Bursa and Ligament, Left** *See S Foot Bursa and Ligament, Right* **V** **Lower Extremity Bursa and Ligament, Right** **W** **Lower Extremity Bursa and Ligament, Left**	**Ø** Open **4** Percutaneous Endoscopic	**Z** No Device	**Z** No Qualifier

LC Limited Coverage   **NC** Noncovered   ⊞ Combination Member   HAC associated procedure   Combination Only   DRG Non-OR   Non-OR   New/Revised in GREEN

506   ICD-10-PCS 2021

Ø   Medical and Surgical
M   Bursae and Ligaments
N   Release   Definition: Freeing a body part from an abnormal physical constraint by cutting or by the use of force
                     Explanation: Some of the restraining tissue may be taken out but none of the body part is taken out

Body Part Character 4		Approach Character 5	Device Character 6	Qualifier Character 7
Ø Head and Neck Bursa and Ligament Alar ligament of axis Cervical interspinous ligament Cervical intertransverse ligament Cervical ligamentum flavum Interspinous ligament, cervical Intertransverse ligament, cervical Lateral temporomandibular ligament Ligamentum flavum, cervical Sphenomandibular ligament Stylomandibular ligament Transverse ligament of atlas **1 Shoulder Bursa and Ligament, Right** Acromioclavicular ligament Coracoacromial ligament Coracoclavicular ligament Coracohumeral ligament Costoclavicular ligament Glenohumeral ligament Interclavicular ligament Sternoclavicular ligament Subacromial bursa Transverse humeral ligament Transverse scapular ligament **2 Shoulder Bursa and Ligament, Left** *See 1 Shoulder Bursa and Ligament, Right* **3 Elbow Bursa and Ligament, Right** Annular ligament Olecranon bursa Radial collateral ligament Ulnar collateral ligament **4 Elbow Bursa and Ligament, Left** *See 3 Elbow Bursa and Ligament, Right* **5 Wrist Bursa and Ligament, Right** Palmar ulnocarpal ligament Radial collateral carpal ligament Radiocarpal ligament Radioulnar ligament Scapholunate ligament Ulnar collateral carpal ligament **6 Wrist Bursa and Ligament, Left** *See 5 Wrist Bursa and Ligament, Right* **7 Hand Bursa and Ligament, Right** Carpometacarpal ligament Intercarpal ligament Interphalangeal ligament Lunotriquetral ligament Metacarpal ligament Metacarpophalangeal ligament Pisohamate ligament Pisometacarpal ligament Scaphotrapezium ligament **8 Hand Bursa and Ligament, Left** *See 7 Hand Bursa and Ligament, Right* **9 Upper Extremity Bursa and Ligament, Right** **B Upper Extremity Bursa and Ligament, Left** **C Upper Spine Bursa and Ligament** Interspinous ligament, thoracic Intertransverse ligament, thoracic Ligamentum flavum, thoracic Supraspinous ligament	**D Lower Spine Bursa and Ligament** Iliolumbar ligament Interspinous ligament, lumbar Intertransverse ligament, lumbar Ligamentum flavum, lumbar Sacrococcygeal ligament Sacroiliac ligament Sacrospinous ligament Sacrotuberous ligament Supraspinous ligament **F Sternum Bursa and Ligament** Costoxiphoid ligament Sternocostal ligament **G Rib(s) Bursa and Ligament** Costotransverse ligament **H Abdomen Bursa and Ligament, Right** **J Abdomen Bursa and Ligament, Left** **K Perineum Bursa and Ligament** **L Hip Bursa and Ligament, Right** Iliofemoral ligament Ischiofemoral ligament Pubofemoral ligament Transverse acetabular ligament Trochanteric bursa **M Hip Bursa and Ligament, Left** *See L Hip Bursa and Ligament, Right* **N Knee Bursa and Ligament, Right** Anterior cruciate ligament (ACL) Lateral collateral ligament (LCL) Ligament of head of fibula Medial collateral ligament (MCL) Patellar ligament Popliteal ligament Posterior cruciate ligament (PCL) Prepatellar bursa **P Knee Bursa and Ligament, Left** *See N Knee Bursa and Ligament, Right* **Q Ankle Bursa and Ligament, Right** Calcaneofibular ligament Deltoid ligament Ligament of the lateral malleolus Talofibular ligament **R Ankle Bursa and Ligament, Left** *See Q Ankle Bursa and Ligament, Right* **S Foot Bursa and Ligament, Right** Calcaneocuboid ligament Cuneonavicular ligament Intercuneiform ligament Interphalangeal ligament Metatarsal ligament Metatarsophalangeal ligament Subtalar ligament Talocalcaneal ligament Talocalcaneonavicular ligament Tarsometatarsal ligament **T Foot Bursa and Ligament, Left** *See S Foot Bursa and Ligament, Right* **V Lower Extremity Bursa and Ligament, Right** **W Lower Extremity Bursa and Ligament, Left**	**Ø Open** **3 Percutaneous** **4 Percutaneous Endoscopic** **X External**	**Z No Device**	**Z No Qualifier**

Non-OR   ØMN[Ø,1,2,3,4,5,6,7,8,9,B,C,D,F,G,H,J,K,L,M,N,P,Q,R,S,T,V,W]XZZ

LC Limited Coverage   **NC** Noncovered   ⊞ Combination Member   HAC associated procedure   Combination Only   DRG Non-OR   Non-OR   New/Revised in GREEN

ICD-10-PCS 2021   507

Ø   **Medical and Surgical**
M   **Bursae and Ligaments**
P   **Removal**   Definition: Taking out or off a device from a body part

                         Explanation: If a device is taken out and a similar device put in without cutting or puncturing the skin or mucous membrane, the procedure is coded to the root operation CHANGE. Otherwise, the procedure for taking out a device is coded to the root operation REMOVAL.

Body Part Character 4	Approach Character 5	Device Character 6	Qualifier Character 7
X Upper Bursa and Ligament **Y** Lower Bursa and Ligament	**Ø** Open **3** Percutaneous **4** Percutaneous Endoscopic	**Ø** Drainage Device **7** Autologous Tissue Substitute **J** Synthetic Substitute **K** Nonautologous Tissue Substitute **Y** Other Device	**Z** No Qualifier
X Upper Bursa and Ligament **Y** Lower Bursa and Ligament	**X** External	**Ø** Drainage Device	**Z** No Qualifier

Non-OR   ØMP[X,Y]3ØZ
Non-OR   ØMP[X,Y][3,4]YZ
Non-OR   ØMP[X,Y]XØZ

Ø   Medical and Surgical
M Bursae and Ligaments
Q Repair   Definition: Restoring, to the extent possible, a body part to its normal anatomic structure and function
                     Explanation: Used only when the method to accomplish the repair is not one of the other root operations

Body Part Character 4		Approach Character 5	Device Character 6	Qualifier Character 7
Ø Head and Neck Bursa and Ligament Alar ligament of axis Cervical interspinous ligament Cervical intertransverse ligament Cervical ligamentum flavum Interspinous ligament, cervical Intertransverse ligament, cervical Lateral temporomandibular ligament Ligamentum flavum, cervical Sphenomandibular ligament Stylomandibular ligament Transverse ligament of atlas **1 Shoulder Bursa and Ligament, Right** Acromioclavicular ligament Coracoacromial ligament Coracoclavicular ligament Coracohumeral ligament Costoclavicular ligament Glenohumeral ligament Interclavicular ligament Sternoclavicular ligament Subacromial bursa Transverse humeral ligament Transverse scapular ligament **2 Shoulder Bursa and Ligament, Left** *See 1 Shoulder Bursa and Ligament, Right* **3 Elbow Bursa and Ligament, Right** Annular ligament Olecranon bursa Radial collateral ligament Ulnar collateral ligament **4 Elbow Bursa and Ligament, Left** *See 3 Elbow Bursa and Ligament, Right* **5 Wrist Bursa and Ligament, Right** Palmar ulnocarpal ligament Radial collateral carpal ligament Radiocarpal ligament Radioulnar ligament Scapholunate ligament Ulnar collateral carpal ligament **6 Wrist Bursa and Ligament, Left** *See 5 Wrist Bursa and Ligament, Right* **7 Hand Bursa and Ligament, Right** Carpometacarpal ligament Intercarpal ligament Interphalangeal ligament Lunotriquetral ligament Metacarpal ligament Metacarpophalangeal ligament Pisohamate ligament Pisometacarpal ligament Scaphotrapezium ligament **8 Hand Bursa and Ligament, Left** *See 7 Hand Bursa and Ligament, Right* **9 Upper Extremity Bursa and Ligament, Right** **B Upper Extremity Bursa and Ligament, Left** **C Upper Spine Bursa and Ligament** Interspinous ligament, thoracic Intertransverse ligament, thoracic Ligamentum flavum, thoracic Supraspinous ligament	**D Lower Spine Bursa and Ligament** Iliolumbar ligament Interspinous ligament, lumbar Intertransverse ligament, lumbar Ligamentum flavum, lumbar Sacrococcygeal ligament Sacroiliac ligament Sacrospinous ligament Sacrotuberous ligament Supraspinous ligament **F Sternum Bursa and Ligament** Costoxiphoid ligament Sternocostal ligament **G Rib(s) Bursa and Ligament** Costotransverse ligament **H Abdomen Bursa and Ligament, Right** **J Abdomen Bursa and Ligament, Left** **K Perineum Bursa and Ligament** **L Hip Bursa and Ligament, Right** Iliofemoral ligament Ischiofemoral ligament Pubofemoral ligament Transverse acetabular ligament Trochanteric bursa **M Hip Bursa and Ligament, Left** *See L Hip Bursa and Ligament, Right* **N Knee Bursa and Ligament, Right** Anterior cruciate ligament (ACL) Lateral collateral ligament (LCL) Ligament of head of fibula Medial collateral ligament (MCL) Patellar ligament Popliteal ligament Posterior cruciate ligament (PCL) Prepatellar bursa **P Knee Bursa and Ligament, Left** *See N Knee Bursa and Ligament, Right* **Q Ankle Bursa and Ligament, Right** Calcaneofibular ligament Deltoid ligament Ligament of the lateral malleolus Talofibular ligament **R Ankle Bursa and Ligament, Left** *See Q Ankle Bursa and Ligament, Right* **S Foot Bursa and Ligament, Right** Calcaneocuboid ligament Cuneonavicular ligament Intercuneiform ligament Interphalangeal ligament Metatarsal ligament Metatarsophalangeal ligament Subtalar ligament Talocalcaneal ligament Talocalcaneonavicular ligament Tarsometatarsal ligament **T Foot Bursa and Ligament, Left** *See S Foot Bursa and Ligament, Right* **V Lower Extremity Bursa and Ligament, Right** **W Lower Extremity Bursa and Ligament, Left**	**Ø Open** **3 Percutaneous** **4 Percutaneous Endoscopic**	**Z No Device**	**Z No Qualifier**

LC Limited Coverage   NC Noncovered   ⊞ Combination Member   HAC associated procedure   Combination Only   DRG Non-OR   Non-OR   New/Revised in GREEN

Bursae and Ligaments *(side tab)*

Ø   **Medical and Surgical**
M   **Bursae and Ligaments**
R   **Replacement**   Definition: Putting in or on biological or synthetic material that physically takes the place and/or function of all or a portion of a body part
           Explanation: The body part may have been taken out or replaced, or may be taken out, physically eradicated, or rendered nonfunctional during the REPLACEMENT procedure. A REMOVAL procedure is coded for taking out the device used in a previous replacement procedure.

Body Part Character 4		Approach Character 5	Device Character 6	Qualifier Character 7
Ø Head and Neck Bursa and Ligament Alar ligament of axis Cervical interspinous ligament Cervical intertransverse ligament Cervical ligamentum flavum Interspinous ligament, cervical Intertransverse ligament, cervical Lateral temporomandibular ligament Ligamentum flavum, cervical Sphenomandibular ligament Stylomandibular ligament Transverse ligament of atlas **1 Shoulder Bursa and Ligament, Right** Acromioclavicular ligament Coracoacromial ligament Coracoclavicular ligament Coracohumeral ligament Costoclavicular ligament Glenohumeral ligament Interclavicular ligament Sternoclavicular ligament Subacromial bursa Transverse humeral ligament Transverse scapular ligament **2 Shoulder Bursa and Ligament, Left** *See 1 Shoulder Bursa and Ligament, Right* **3 Elbow Bursa and Ligament, Right** Annular ligament Olecranon bursa Radial collateral ligament Ulnar collateral ligament **4 Elbow Bursa and Ligament, Left** *See 3 Elbow Bursa and Ligament, Right* **5 Wrist Bursa and Ligament, Right** Palmar ulnocarpal ligament Radial collateral carpal ligament Radiocarpal ligament Radioulnar ligament Scapholunate ligament Ulnar collateral carpal ligament **6 Wrist Bursa and Ligament, Left** *See 5 Wrist Bursa and Ligament, Right* **7 Hand Bursa and Ligament, Right** Carpometacarpal ligament Intercarpal ligament Interphalangeal ligament Lunotriquetral ligament Metacarpal ligament Metacarpophalangeal ligament Pisohamate ligament Pisometacarpal ligament Scaphotrapezium ligament **8 Hand Bursa and Ligament, Left** *See 7 Hand Bursa and Ligament, Right* **9 Upper Extremity Bursa and Ligament, Right** **B Upper Extremity Bursa and Ligament, Left** **C Upper Spine Bursa and Ligament** Interspinous ligament, thoracic Intertransverse ligament, thoracic Ligamentum flavum, thoracic Supraspinous ligament	**D Lower Spine Bursa and Ligament** Iliolumbar ligament Interspinous ligament, lumbar Intertransverse ligament, lumbar Ligamentum flavum, lumbar Sacrococcygeal ligament Sacroiliac ligament Sacrospinous ligament Sacrotuberous ligament Supraspinous ligament **F Sternum Bursa and Ligament** Costoxiphoid ligament Sternocostal ligament **G Rib(s) Bursa and Ligament** Costotransverse ligament **H Abdomen Bursa and Ligament, Right** **J Abdomen Bursa and Ligament, Left** **K Perineum Bursa and Ligament** **L Hip Bursa and Ligament, Right** Iliofemoral ligament Ischiofemoral ligament Pubofemoral ligament Transverse acetabular ligament Trochanteric bursa **M Hip Bursa and Ligament, Left** *See L Hip Bursa and Ligament, Right* **N Knee Bursa and Ligament, Right** Anterior cruciate ligament (ACL) Lateral collateral ligament (LCL) Ligament of head of fibula Medial collateral ligament (MCL) Patellar ligament Popliteal ligament Posterior cruciate ligament (PCL) Prepatellar bursa **P Knee Bursa and Ligament, Left** *See N Knee Bursa and Ligament, Right* **Q Ankle Bursa and Ligament, Right** Calcaneofibular ligament Deltoid ligament Ligament of the lateral malleolus Talofibular ligament **R Ankle Bursa and Ligament, Left** *See Q Ankle Bursa and Ligament, Right* **S Foot Bursa and Ligament, Right** Calcaneocuboid ligament Cuneonavicular ligament Intercuneiform ligament Interphalangeal ligament Metatarsal ligament Metatarsophalangeal ligament Subtalar ligament Talocalcaneal ligament Talocalcaneonavicular ligament Tarsometatarsal ligament **T Foot Bursa and Ligament, Left** *See S Foot Bursa and Ligament, Right* **V Lower Extremity Bursa and Ligament, Right** **W Lower Extremity Bursa and Ligament, Left**	**Ø Open** **4 Percutaneous Endoscopic**	**7 Autologous Tissue Substitute** **J Synthetic Substitute** **K Nonautologous Tissue Substitute**	**Z No Qualifier**

LG Limited Coverage   NC Noncovered   ⊞ Combination Member   HAC associated procedure   Combination Only   DRG Non-OR   Non-OR   New/Revised in GREEN
510   ICD-10-PCS 2021

ØMR–ØMR *(side tab)*

Ø　Medical and Surgical
M　Bursae and Ligaments
S　Reposition　Definition: Moving to its normal location, or other suitable location, all or a portion of a body part

Explanation: The body part is moved to a new location from an abnormal location, or from a normal location where it is not functioning correctly. The body part may or may not be cut out or off to be moved to the new location.

Body Part Character 4		Approach Character 5	Device Character 6	Qualifier Character 7
Ø　Head and Neck Bursa and Ligament Alar ligament of axis Cervical interspinous ligament Cervical intertransverse ligament Cervical ligamentum flavum Interspinous ligament, cervical Intertransverse ligament, cervical Lateral temporomandibular ligament Ligamentum flavum, cervical Sphenomandibular ligament Stylomandibular ligament Transverse ligament of atlas **1　Shoulder Bursa and Ligament, Right** Acromioclavicular ligament Coracoacromial ligament Coracoclavicular ligament Coracohumeral ligament Costoclavicular ligament Glenohumeral ligament Interclavicular ligament Sternoclavicular ligament Subacromial bursa Transverse humeral ligament Transverse scapular ligament **2　Shoulder Bursa and Ligament, Left** *See 1 Shoulder Bursa and Ligament, Right* **3　Elbow Bursa and Ligament, Right** Annular ligament Olecranon bursa Radial collateral ligament Ulnar collateral ligament **4　Elbow Bursa and Ligament, Left** *See 3 Elbow Bursa and Ligament, Right* **5　Wrist Bursa and Ligament, Right** Palmar ulnocarpal ligament Radial collateral carpal ligament Radiocarpal ligament Radioulnar ligament Scapholunate ligament Ulnar collateral carpal ligament **6　Wrist Bursa and Ligament, Left** *See 5 Wrist Bursa and Ligament, Right* **7　Hand Bursa and Ligament, Right** Carpometacarpal ligament Intercarpal ligament Interphalangeal ligament Lunotriquetral ligament Metacarpal ligament Metacarpophalangeal ligament Pisohamate ligament Pisometacarpal ligament Scaphotrapezium ligament **8　Hand Bursa and Ligament, Left** *See 7 Hand Bursa and Ligament, Right* **9　Upper Extremity Bursa and Ligament, Right** **B　Upper Extremity Bursa and Ligament, Left** **C　Upper Spine Bursa and Ligament** Interspinous ligament, thoracic Intertransverse ligament, thoracic Ligamentum flavum, thoracic Supraspinous ligament	**D　Lower Spine Bursa and Ligament** Iliolumbar ligament Interspinous ligament, lumbar Intertransverse ligament, lumbar Ligamentum flavum, lumbar Sacrococcygeal ligament Sacroiliac ligament Sacrospinous ligament Sacrotuberous ligament Supraspinous ligament **F　Sternum Bursa and Ligament** Costoxiphoid ligament Sternocostal ligament **G　Rib(s) Bursa and Ligament** Costotransverse ligament **H　Abdomen Bursa and Ligament, Right** **J　Abdomen Bursa and Ligament, Left** **K　Perineum Bursa and Ligament** **L　Hip Bursa and Ligament, Right** Iliofemoral ligament Ischiofemoral ligament Pubofemoral ligament Transverse acetabular ligament Trochanteric bursa **M　Hip Bursa and Ligament, Left** *See L Hip Bursa and Ligament, Right* **N　Knee Bursa and Ligament, Right** Anterior cruciate ligament (ACL) Lateral collateral ligament (LCL) Ligament of head of fibula Medial collateral ligament (MCL) Patellar ligament Popliteal ligament Posterior cruciate ligament (PCL) Prepatellar bursa **P　Knee Bursa and Ligament, Left** *See N Knee Bursa and Ligament, Right* **Q　Ankle Bursa and Ligament, Right** Calcaneofibular ligament Deltoid ligament Ligament of the lateral malleolus Talofibular ligament **R　Ankle Bursa and Ligament, Left** *See Q Ankle Bursa and Ligament, Right* **S　Foot Bursa and Ligament, Right** Calcaneocuboid ligament Cuneonavicular ligament Intercuneiform ligament Interphalangeal ligament Metatarsal ligament Metatarsophalangeal ligament Subtalar ligament Talocalcaneal ligament Talocalcaneonavicular ligament Tarsometatarsal ligament **T　Foot Bursa and Ligament, Left** *See S Foot Bursa and Ligament, Right* **V　Lower Extremity Bursa and Ligament, Right** **W　Lower Extremity Bursa and Ligament, Left**	**Ø　Open** **4　Percutaneous Endoscopic**	**Z　No Device**	**Z　No Qualifier**

Bursae and Ligaments

Ø   **Medical and Surgical**
M   **Bursae and Ligaments**
T   **Resection**   Definition: Cutting out or off, without replacement, all of a body part
                   Explanation: None

Body Part Character 4		Approach Character 5	Device Character 6	Qualifier Character 7
Ø **Head and Neck Bursa and Ligament** Alar ligament of axis Cervical interspinous ligament Cervical intertransverse ligament Cervical ligamentum flavum Interspinous ligament, cervical Intertransverse ligament, cervical Lateral temporomandibular ligament Ligamentum flavum, cervical Sphenomandibular ligament Stylomandibular ligament Transverse ligament of atlas **1** **Shoulder Bursa and Ligament, Right** Acromioclavicular ligament Coracoacromial ligament Coracoclavicular ligament Coracohumeral ligament Costoclavicular ligament Glenohumeral ligament Interclavicular ligament Sternoclavicular ligament Subacromial bursa Transverse humeral ligament Transverse scapular ligament **2** **Shoulder Bursa and Ligament, Left** *See 1 Shoulder Bursa and Ligament, Right* **3** **Elbow Bursa and Ligament, Right** Annular ligament Olecranon bursa Radial collateral ligament Ulnar collateral ligament **4** **Elbow Bursa and Ligament, Left** *See 3 Elbow Bursa and Ligament, Right* **5** **Wrist Bursa and Ligament, Right** Palmar ulnocarpal ligament Radial collateral carpal ligament Radiocarpal ligament Radioulnar ligament Scapholunate ligament Ulnar collateral carpal ligament **6** **Wrist Bursa and Ligament, Left** *See 5 Wrist Bursa and Ligament, Right* **7** **Hand Bursa and Ligament, Right** Carpometacarpal ligament Intercarpal ligament Interphalangeal ligament Lunotriquetral ligament Metacarpal ligament Metacarpophalangeal ligament Pisohamate ligament Pisometacarpal ligament Scaphotrapezium ligament **8** **Hand Bursa and Ligament, Left** *See 7 Hand Bursa and Ligament, Right* **9** **Upper Extremity Bursa and Ligament, Right** **B** **Upper Extremity Bursa and Ligament, Left** **C** **Upper Spine Bursa and Ligament** Interspinous ligament, thoracic Intertransverse ligament, thoracic Ligamentum flavum, thoracic Supraspinous ligament	**D** **Lower Spine Bursa and Ligament** Iliolumbar ligament Interspinous ligament, lumbar Intertransverse ligament, lumbar Ligamentum flavum, lumbar Sacrococcygeal ligament Sacroiliac ligament Sacrospinous ligament Sacrotuberous ligament Supraspinous ligament **F** **Sternum Bursa and Ligament** Costoxiphoid ligament Sternocostal ligament **G** **Rib(s) Bursa and Ligament** Costotransverse ligament **H** **Abdomen Bursa and Ligament, Right** **J** **Abdomen Bursa and Ligament, Left** **K** **Perineum Bursa and Ligament** **L** **Hip Bursa and Ligament, Right** Iliofemoral ligament Ischiofemoral ligament Pubofemoral ligament Transverse acetabular ligament Trochanteric bursa **M** **Hip Bursa and Ligament, Left** *See L Hip Bursa and Ligament, Right* **N** **Knee Bursa and Ligament, Right** Anterior cruciate ligament (ACL) Lateral collateral ligament (LCL) Ligament of head of fibula Medial collateral ligament (MCL) Patellar ligament Popliteal ligament Posterior cruciate ligament (PCL) Prepatellar bursa **P** **Knee Bursa and Ligament, Left** *See N Knee Bursa and Ligament, Right* **Q** **Ankle Bursa and Ligament, Right** Calcaneofibular ligament Deltoid ligament Ligament of the lateral malleolus Talofibular ligament **R** **Ankle Bursa and Ligament, Left** *See Q Ankle Bursa and Ligament, Right* **S** **Foot Bursa and Ligament, Right** Calcaneocuboid ligament Cuneonavicular ligament Intercuneiform ligament Interphalangeal ligament Metatarsal ligament Metatarsophalangeal ligament Subtalar ligament Talocalcaneal ligament Talocalcaneonavicular ligament Tarsometatarsal ligament **T** **Foot Bursa and Ligament, Left** *See S Foot Bursa and Ligament, Right* **V** **Lower Extremity Bursa and Ligament, Right** **W** **Lower Extremity Bursa and Ligament, Left**	**Ø** Open **4** Percutaneous Endoscopic	**Z** No Device	**Z** No Qualifier

LC Limited Coverage   NC Noncovered   ⊞ Combination Member   HAC associated procedure   Combination Only   DRG Non-OR   Non-OR   New/Revised in GREEN

512   ICD-10-PCS 2021

Ø   Medical and Surgical
M   Bursae and Ligaments
U   Supplement   Definition: Putting in or on biological or synthetic material that physically reinforces and/or augments the function of a portion of a body part
                          Explanation: The biological material is non-living, or is living and from the same individual. The body part may have been previously replaced, and the SUPPLEMENT procedure is performed to physically reinforce and/or augment the function of the replaced body part.

Body Part Character 4		Approach Character 5	Device Character 6	Qualifier Character 7
Ø Head and Neck Bursa and Ligament Alar ligament of axis Cervical interspinous ligament Cervical intertransverse ligament Cervical ligamentum flavum Interspinous ligament, cervical Intertransverse ligament, cervical Lateral temporomandibular ligament Ligamentum flavum, cervical Sphenomandibular ligament Stylomandibular ligament Transverse ligament of atlas **1 Shoulder Bursa and Ligament, Right** Acromioclavicular ligament Coracoacromial ligament Coracoclavicular ligament Coracohumeral ligament Costoclavicular ligament Glenohumeral ligament Interclavicular ligament Sternoclavicular ligament Subacromial bursa Transverse humeral ligament Transverse scapular ligament **2 Shoulder Bursa and Ligament, Left** *See 1 Shoulder Bursa and Ligament, Right* **3 Elbow Bursa and Ligament, Right** Annular ligament Olecranon bursa Radial collateral ligament Ulnar collateral ligament **4 Elbow Bursa and Ligament, Left** *See 3 Elbow Bursa and Ligament, Right* **5 Wrist Bursa and Ligament, Right** Palmar ulnocarpal ligament Radial collateral carpal ligament Radiocarpal ligament Radioulnar ligament Scapholunate ligament Ulnar collateral carpal ligament **6 Wrist Bursa and Ligament, Left** *See 5 Wrist Bursa and Ligament, Right* **7 Hand Bursa and Ligament, Right** Carpometacarpal ligament Intercarpal ligament Interphalangeal ligament Lunotriquetral ligament Metacarpal ligament Metacarpophalangeal ligament Pisohamate ligament Pisometacarpal ligament Scaphotrapezium ligament **8 Hand Bursa and Ligament, Left** *See 7 Hand Bursa and Ligament, Right* **9 Upper Extremity Bursa and Ligament, Right** **B Upper Extremity Bursa and Ligament, Left** **C Upper Spine Bursa and Ligament** Interspinous ligament, thoracic Intertransverse ligament, thoracic Ligamentum flavum, thoracic Supraspinous ligament	**D Lower Spine Bursa and Ligament** Iliolumbar ligament Interspinous ligament, lumbar Intertransverse ligament, lumbar Ligamentum flavum, lumbar Sacrococcygeal ligament Sacroiliac ligament Sacrospinous ligament Sacrotuberous ligament Supraspinous ligament **F Sternum Bursa and Ligament** Costoxiphoid ligament Sternocostal ligament **G Rib(s) Bursa and Ligament** Costotransverse ligament **H Abdomen Bursa and Ligament, Right** **J Abdomen Bursa and Ligament, Left** **K Perineum Bursa and Ligament** **L Hip Bursa and Ligament, Right** Iliofemoral ligament Ischiofemoral ligament Pubofemoral ligament Transverse acetabular ligament Trochanteric bursa **M Hip Bursa and Ligament, Left** *See L Hip Bursa and Ligament, Right* **N Knee Bursa and Ligament, Right** Anterior cruciate ligament (ACL) Lateral collateral ligament (LCL) Ligament of head of fibula Medial collateral ligament (MCL) Patellar ligament Popliteal ligament Posterior cruciate ligament (PCL) Prepatellar bursa **P Knee Bursa and Ligament, Left** *See N Knee Bursa and Ligament, Right* **Q Ankle Bursa and Ligament, Right** Calcaneofibular ligament Deltoid ligament Ligament of the lateral malleolus Talofibular ligament **R Ankle Bursa and Ligament, Left** *See Q Ankle Bursa and Ligament, Right* **S Foot Bursa and Ligament, Right** Calcaneocuboid ligament Cuneonavicular ligament Intercuneiform ligament Interphalangeal ligament Metatarsal ligament Metatarsophalangeal ligament Subtalar ligament Talocalcaneal ligament Talocalcaneonavicular ligament Tarsometatarsal ligament **T Foot Bursa and Ligament, Left** *See S Foot Bursa and Ligament, Right* **V Lower Extremity Bursa and Ligament, Right** **W Lower Extremity Bursa and Ligament, Left**	**Ø Open** **4 Percutaneous Endoscopic**	**7 Autologous Tissue Substitute** **J Synthetic Substitute** **K Nonautologous Tissue Substitute**	**Z No Qualifier**

LC Limited Coverage   **NC** Noncovered   ⊞ Combination Member   HAC associated procedure   Combination Only   DRG Non-OR   Non-OR   New/Revised in GREEN

ICD-10-PCS 2021   513

Ø   Medical and Surgical
M   Bursae and Ligaments
W   Revision   Definition: Correcting, to the extent possible, a portion of a malfunctioning device or the position of a displaced device
                          Explanation: Revision can include correcting a malfunctioning or displaced device by taking out or putting in components of the device such as a screw or pin

Body Part Character 4	Approach Character 5	Device Character 6	Qualifier Character 7
X Upper Bursa and Ligament Y Lower Bursa and Ligament	Ø Open 3 Percutaneous 4 Percutaneous Endoscopic	Ø Drainage Device 7 Autologous Tissue Substitute J Synthetic Substitute K Nonautologous Tissue Substitute Y Other Device	Z No Qualifier
X Upper Bursa and Ligament Y Lower Bursa and Ligament	X External	Ø Drainage Device 7 Autologous Tissue Substitute J Synthetic Substitute K Nonautologous Tissue Substitute	Z No Qualifier

Non-OR	ØMW[X,Y][3,4]YZ
Non-OR	ØMW[X,Y]X[Ø,7,J,K]Z

Ø   **Medical and Surgical**
M   **Bursae and Ligaments**
X   **Transfer**   Definition: Moving, without taking out, all or a portion of a body part to another location to take over the function of all or a portion of a body part
                           Explanation: The body part transferred remains connected to its vascular and nervous supply

Body Part Character 4		Approach Character 5	Device Character 6	Qualifier Character 7
Ø Head and Neck Bursa and Ligament Alar ligament of axis Cervical interspinous ligament Cervical intertransverse ligament Cervical ligamentum flavum Interspinous ligament, cervical Intertransverse ligament, cervical Lateral temporomandibular ligament Ligamentum flavum, cervical Sphenomandibular ligament Stylomandibular ligament Transverse ligament of atlas **1 Shoulder Bursa and Ligament, Right** Acromioclavicular ligament Coracoacromial ligament Coracoclavicular ligament Coracohumeral ligament Costoclavicular ligament Glenohumeral ligament Interclavicular ligament Sternoclavicular ligament Subacromial bursa Transverse humeral ligament Transverse scapular ligament **2 Shoulder Bursa and Ligament, Left** *See 1 Shoulder Bursa and Ligament, Right* **3 Elbow Bursa and Ligament, Right** Annular ligament Olecranon bursa Radial collateral ligament Ulnar collateral ligament **4 Elbow Bursa and Ligament, Left** *See 3 Elbow Bursa and Ligament, Right* **5 Wrist Bursa and Ligament, Right** Palmar ulnocarpal ligament Radial collateral carpal ligament Radiocarpal ligament Radioulnar ligament Scapholunate ligament Ulnar collateral carpal ligament **6 Wrist Bursa and Ligament, Left** *See 5 Wrist Bursa and Ligament, Right* **7 Hand Bursa and Ligament, Right** Carpometacarpal ligament Intercarpal ligament Interphalangeal ligament Lunotriquetral ligament Metacarpal ligament Metacarpophalangeal ligament Pisohamate ligament Pisometacarpal ligament Scaphotrapezium ligament **8 Hand Bursa and Ligament, Left** *See 7 Hand Bursa and Ligament, Right* **9 Upper Extremity Bursa and Ligament, Right** **B Upper Extremity Bursa and Ligament, Left** **C Upper Spine Bursa and Ligament** Interspinous ligament, thoracic Intertransverse ligament, thoracic Ligamentum flavum, thoracic Supraspinous ligament	**D Lower Spine Bursa and Ligament** Iliolumbar ligament Interspinous ligament, lumbar Intertransverse ligament, lumbar Ligamentum flavum, lumbar Sacrococcygeal ligament Sacroiliac ligament Sacrospinous ligament Sacrotuberous ligament Supraspinous ligament **F Sternum Bursa and Ligament** Costoxiphoid ligament Sternocostal ligament **G Rib(s) Bursa and Ligament** Costotransverse ligament **H Abdomen Bursa and Ligament, Right** **J Abdomen Bursa and Ligament, Left** **K Perineum Bursa and Ligament** **L Hip Bursa and Ligament, Right** Iliofemoral ligament Ischiofemoral ligament Pubofemoral ligament Transverse acetabular ligament Trochanteric bursa **M Hip Bursa and Ligament, Left** *See L Hip Bursa and Ligament, Right* **N Knee Bursa and Ligament, Right** Anterior cruciate ligament (ACL) Lateral collateral ligament (LCL) Ligament of head of fibula Medial collateral ligament (MCL) Patellar ligament Popliteal ligament Posterior cruciate ligament (PCL) Prepatellar bursa **P Knee Bursa and Ligament, Left** *See N Knee Bursa and Ligament, Right* **Q Ankle Bursa and Ligament, Right** Calcaneofibular ligament Deltoid ligament Ligament of the lateral malleolus Talofibular ligament **R Ankle Bursa and Ligament, Left** *See Q Ankle Bursa and Ligament, Right* **S Foot Bursa and Ligament, Right** Calcaneocuboid ligament Cuneonavicular ligament Intercuneiform ligament Interphalangeal ligament Metatarsal ligament Metatarsophalangeal ligament Subtalar ligament Talocalcaneal ligament Talocalcaneonavicular ligament Tarsometatarsal ligament **T Foot Bursa and Ligament, Left** *See S Foot Bursa and Ligament, Right* **V Lower Extremity Bursa and Ligament, Right** **W Lower Extremity Bursa and Ligament, Left**	**Ø** Open **4** Percutaneous Endoscopic	**Z** No Device	**Z** No Qualifier

Head and Facial Bones ØN2–ØNW

Character Meanings

This Character Meaning table is provided as a guide to assist the user in the identification of character members that may be found in this section of code tables. It **SHOULD NOT** be used to build a PCS code.

Operation–Character 3	Body Part–Character 4	Approach–Character 5	Device–Character 6	Qualifier–Character 7
2 Change	Ø Skull	Ø Open	Ø Drainage Device	X Diagnostic
5 Destruction	1 Frontal Bone	3 Percutaneous	4 Internal Fixation Device	Z No Qualifier
8 Division	3 Parietal Bone, Right	4 Percutaneous Endoscopic	5 External Fixation Device	
9 Drainage	4 Parietal Bone, Left	X External	7 Autologous Tissue Substitute	
B Excision	5 Temporal Bone, Right		J Synthetic Substitute	
C Extirpation	6 Temporal Bone, Left		K Nonautologous Tissue Substitute	
D Extraction	7 Occipital Bone		M Bone Growth Stimulator	
H Insertion	B Nasal Bone		N Neurostimulator Generator	
J Inspection	C Sphenoid Bone		S Hearing Device	
N Release	F Ethmoid Bone, Right		Y Other Device	
P Removal	G Ethmoid Bone, Left		Z No Device	
Q Repair	H Lacrimal Bone, Right			
R Replacement	J Lacrimal Bone, Left			
S Reposition	K Palatine Bone, Right			
T Resection	L Palatine Bone, Left			
U Supplement	M Zygomatic Bone, Right			
W Revision	N Zygomatic Bone, Left			
	P Orbit, Right			
	Q Orbit, Left			
	R Maxilla			
	T Mandible, Right			
	V Mandible, Left			
	W Facial Bone			
	X Hyoid Bone			

AHA Coding Clinic for table ØNB
2017, 1Q, 20   Preparatory nasal adhesion repair before definitive cleft palate repair
2015, 3Q, 3-8   Excisional and nonexcisional debridement
2015, 2Q, 12   Orbital exenteration

AHA Coding Clinic for table ØND
2017, 4Q, 41   Extraction procedures

AHA Coding Clinic for table ØNH
2015, 3Q, 13   Nonexcisional debridement of cranial wound with removal and replacement of hardware

AHA Coding Clinic for table ØNP
2015, 3Q, 13   Nonexcisional debridement of cranial wound with removal and replacement of hardware

AHA Coding Clinic for table ØNQ
2016, 3Q, 29   Closure of bilateral alveolar clefts

AHA Coding Clinic for table ØNR
2017, 3Q, 17   Resection of schwannoma and placement of DuraGen and Lorenz cranial plating system
2017, 3Q, 22   Replacement of native skull bone flap
2017, 1Q, 23   Reconstruction of mandible using titanium and bone
2014, 3Q, 7   Hemi-cranioplasty for repair of cranial defect

AHA Coding Clinic for table ØNS
2017, 3Q, 22   Replacement of native skull bone flap
2017, 1Q, 20   Preparatory nasal adhesion repair before definitive cleft palate repair
2016, 2Q, 30   Clipping (occlusion) of cerebral artery, decompressive craniectomy and storage of bone flap in abdominal wall
2015, 3Q, 17   Craniosynostosis with cranial vault reconstruction
2015, 3Q, 27   Moyamoya disease and hemispheric pial synagiosis with craniotomy
2014, 3Q, 23   Le Fort I osteotomy
2013, 3Q, 24   Distraction osteogenesis
2013, 3Q, 25   Fracture of frontal bone with repair and coagulation for hemostasis

AHA Coding Clinic for table ØNU
2016, 3Q, 29   Closure of bilateral alveolar clefts
2013, 3Q, 24   Distraction osteogenesis

Head and Facial Bones

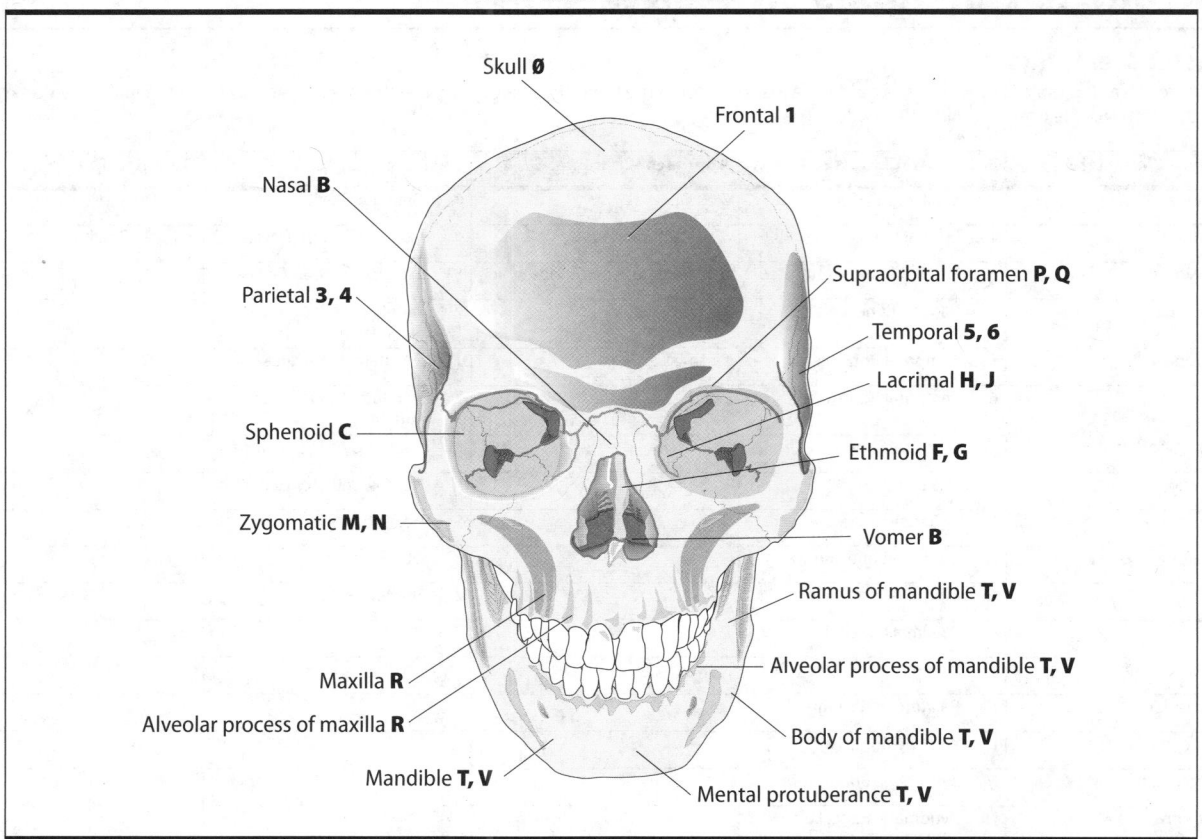

Skull **Ø**
Frontal **1**
Nasal **B**
Supraorbital foramen **P, Q**
Parietal **3, 4**
Temporal **5, 6**
Lacrimal **H, J**
Sphenoid **C**
Ethmoid **F, G**
Zygomatic **M, N**
Vomer **B**
Ramus of mandible **T, V**
Alveolar process of mandible **T, V**
Maxilla **R**
Body of mandible **T, V**
Alveolar process of maxilla **R**
Mandible **T, V**
Mental protuberance **T, V**

Skull Bones

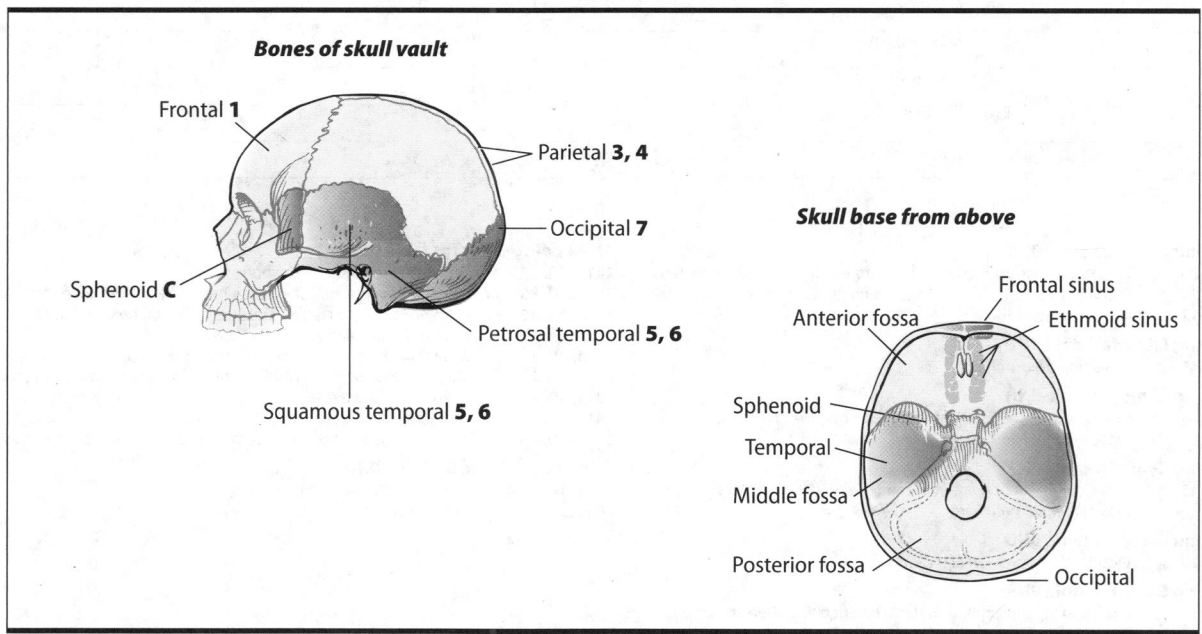

Bones of skull vault

Frontal **1**
Parietal **3, 4**
Occipital **7**
Sphenoid **C**
Petrosal temporal **5, 6**
Squamous temporal **5, 6**

Skull base from above

Frontal sinus
Anterior fossa
Ethmoid sinus
Sphenoid
Temporal
Middle fossa
Posterior fossa
Occipital

Ø   Medical and Surgical
N   Head and Facial Bones
2   Change   Definition: Taking out or off a device from a body part and putting back an identical or similar device in or on the same body part without cutting or puncturing the skin or a mucous membrane
                         Explanation: All CHANGE procedures are coded using the approach EXTERNAL

Body Part Character 4	Approach Character 5	Device Character 6	Qualifier Character 7
Ø Skull B Nasal Bone Vomer of nasal septum W Facial Bone	X External	Ø Drainage Device Y Other Device	Z No Qualifier

Non-OR   All body part, approach, device, and qualifier values

Ø   Medical and Surgical
N   Head and Facial Bones
5   Destruction   Definition: Physical eradication of all or a portion of a body part by the direct use of energy, force, or a destructive agent
                        Explanation: None of the body part is physically taken out

Body Part Character 4	Approach Character 5	Device Character 6	Qualifier Character 7

Ø Skull
1 Frontal Bone
   Zygomatic process of frontal bone
3 Parietal Bone, Right
4 Parietal Bone, Left
5 Temporal Bone, Right
   Mastoid process
   Petrous part of temporal bone
   Tympanic part of temporal bone
   Zygomatic process of temporal bone
6 Temporal Bone, Left
   See 5 Temporal Bone, Right
7 Occipital Bone
   Foramen magnum
B Nasal Bone
   Vomer of nasal septum
C Sphenoid Bone
   Greater wing
   Lesser wing
   Optic foramen
   Pterygoid process
   Sella turcica
F Ethmoid Bone, Right
   Cribriform plate
G Ethmoid Bone, Left
   See F Ethmoid Bone, Right
H Lacrimal Bone, Right
J Lacrimal Bone, Left
K Palatine Bone, Right
L Palatine Bone, Left
M Zygomatic Bone, Right
N Zygomatic Bone, Left
P Orbit, Right
   Bony orbit
   Orbital portion of ethmoid bone
   Orbital portion of frontal bone
   Orbital portion of lacrimal bone
   Orbital portion of maxilla
   Orbital portion of palatine bone
   Orbital portion of sphenoid bone
   Orbital portion of zygomatic bone
Q Orbit, Left
   See P Orbit, Right
R Maxilla
   Alveolar process of maxilla
T Mandible, Right
   Alveolar process of mandible
   Condyloid process
   Mandibular notch
   Mental foramen
V Mandible, Left
   See T Mandible, Right
X Hyoid Bone
	Ø Open
	3 Percutaneous
	4 Percutaneous Endoscopic
		Z No Device	Z No Qualifier

LC Limited Coverage   **NC** Noncovered   ⊞ Combination Member   HAC associated procedure   Combination Only   DRG Non-OR   Non-OR   New/Revised in GREEN

ICD-10-PCS 2021   519

Head and Facial Bones (side tab)

Ø Medical and Surgical
N Head and Facial Bones
8 Division

Definition: Cutting into a body part, without draining fluids and/or gases from the body part, in order to separate or transect a body part
Explanation: All or a portion of the body part is separated into two or more portions

Body Part Character 4	Approach Character 5	Device Character 6	Qualifier Character 7
Ø Skull	**Ø Open**	**Z No Device**	**Z No Qualifier**
1 Frontal Bone	**3 Percutaneous**		
Zygomatic process of frontal bone	**4 Percutaneous Endoscopic**		
3 Parietal Bone, Right			
4 Parietal Bone, Left			
5 Temporal Bone, Right			
Mastoid process			
Petrous part of temporal bone			
Tympanic part of temporal bone			
Zygomatic process of temporal bone			
6 Temporal Bone, Left			
See 5 Temporal Bone, Right			
7 Occipital Bone			
Foramen magnum			
B Nasal Bone			
Vomer of nasal septum			
C Sphenoid Bone			
Greater wing			
Lesser wing			
Optic foramen			
Pterygoid process			
Sella turcica			
F Ethmoid Bone, Right			
Cribriform plate			
G Ethmoid Bone, Left			
See F Ethmoid Bone, Right			
H Lacrimal Bone, Right			
J Lacrimal Bone, Left			
K Palatine Bone, Right			
L Palatine Bone, Left			
M Zygomatic Bone, Right			
N Zygomatic Bone, Left			
P Orbit, Right			
Bony orbit			
Orbital portion of ethmoid bone			
Orbital portion of frontal bone			
Orbital portion of lacrimal bone			
Orbital portion of maxilla			
Orbital portion of palatine bone			
Orbital portion of sphenoid bone			
Orbital portion of zygomatic bone			
Q Orbit, Left			
See P Orbit, Right			
R Maxilla			
Alveolar process of maxilla			
T Mandible, Right			
Alveolar process of mandible			
Condyloid process			
Mandibular notch			
Mental foramen			
V Mandible, Left			
See T Mandible, Right			
X Hyoid Bone			

Non-OR   ØN8B[Ø,3,4]ZZ

LC Limited Coverage   **NC** Noncovered   ⊞ Combination Member   HAC associated procedure   Combination Only   DRG Non-OR   Non-OR   New/Revised in GREEN

520   ICD-10-PCS 2021

Ø   **Medical and Surgical**
N   **Head and Facial Bones**
9   **Drainage**   Definition: Taking or letting out fluids and/or gases from a body part
                       Explanation: The qualifier DIAGNOSTIC is used to identify drainage procedures that are biopsies

Body Part Character 4	Approach Character 5	Device Character 6	Qualifier Character 7
Ø Skull	**Ø** Open	**Ø** Drainage Device	**Z** No Qualifier
1 **Frontal Bone** Zygomatic process of frontal bone	**3** Percutaneous **4** Percutaneous Endoscopic		
3 **Parietal Bone, Right**			
4 **Parietal Bone, Left**			

5 **Temporal Bone, Right**
   Mastoid process
   Petrous part of temporal bone
   Tympanic part of temporal bone
   Zygomatic process of temporal bone			

6 **Temporal Bone, Left** *See 5 Temporal Bone, Right*			
7 **Occipital Bone** Foramen magnum			
B **Nasal Bone** Vomer of nasal septum			

C **Sphenoid Bone**
   Greater wing
   Lesser wing
   Optic foramen
   Pterygoid process
   Sella turcica			

F **Ethmoid Bone, Right** Cribriform plate			
G **Ethmoid Bone, Left** *See F Ethmoid Bone, Right*			
H **Lacrimal Bone, Right**			
J **Lacrimal Bone, Left**			
K **Palatine Bone, Right**			
L **Palatine Bone, Left**			
M **Zygomatic Bone, Right**			
N **Zygomatic Bone, Left**			

P **Orbit, Right**
   Bony orbit
   Orbital portion of ethmoid bone
   Orbital portion of frontal bone
   Orbital portion of lacrimal bone
   Orbital portion of maxilla
   Orbital portion of palatine bone
   Orbital portion of sphenoid bone
   Orbital portion of zygomatic bone			

Q **Orbit, Left** *See P Orbit, Right*			
R **Maxilla** Alveolar process of maxilla			

T **Mandible, Right**
   Alveolar process of mandible
   Condyloid process
   Mandibular notch
   Mental foramen			

V **Mandible, Left** *See T Mandible, Right*			
X **Hyoid Bone**			

Non-OR   ØN9[Ø,1,3,4,5,6,7,C,F,G,H,J,K,L,M,N,P,Q,X]3ØZ
Non-OR   ØN9[B,R,T,V][Ø,3,4]ØZ

ØN9 Continued on next page

LC Limited Coverage   **NC** Noncovered   ⊞ Combination Member   HAC associated procedure   Combination Only   DRG Non-OR   Non-OR   New/Revised in **GREEN**

ICD-10-PCS 2021   **521**

Head and Facial Bones

Ø **Medical and Surgical**   *ØN9 Continued*
N **Head and Facial Bones**
9 **Drainage**   Definition: Taking or letting out fluids and/or gases from a body part
                         Explanation: The qualifier DIAGNOSTIC is used to identify drainage procedures that are biopsies

Body Part Character 4	Approach Character 5	Device Character 6	Qualifier Character 7
Ø Skull	**Ø** Open	**Z** No Device	**X** Diagnostic
1 Frontal Bone Zygomatic process of frontal bone	**3** Percutaneous		**Z** No Qualifier
3 Parietal Bone, Right	**4** Percutaneous Endoscopic		
4 Parietal Bone, Left			

5 Temporal Bone, Right
    Mastoid process
    Petrous part of temporal bone
    Tympanic part of temporal bone
    Zygomatic process of temporal bone			

6 Temporal Bone, Left *See 5 Temporal Bone, Right*			
7 Occipital Bone Foramen magnum			
B Nasal Bone Vomer of nasal septum			

C Sphenoid Bone
    Greater wing
    Lesser wing
    Optic foramen
    Pterygoid process
    Sella turcica			

F Ethmoid Bone, Right Cribriform plate			
G Ethmoid Bone, Left *See F Ethmoid Bone, Right*			
H Lacrimal Bone, Right			
J Lacrimal Bone, Left			
K Palatine Bone, Right			
L Palatine Bone, Left			
M Zygomatic Bone, Right			
N Zygomatic Bone, Left			

P Orbit, Right
    Bony orbit
    Orbital portion of ethmoid bone
    Orbital portion of frontal bone
    Orbital portion of lacrimal bone
    Orbital portion of maxilla
    Orbital portion of palatine bone
    Orbital portion of sphenoid bone
    Orbital portion of zygomatic bone			

Q Orbit, Left *See P Orbit, Right*			
R Maxilla Alveolar process of maxilla			

T Mandible, Right
    Alveolar process of mandible
    Condyloid process
    Mandibular notch
    Mental foramen			

V Mandible, Left *See T Mandible, Right*			
X Hyoid Bone			

Non-OR   ØN9[Ø,1,3,4,5,6,7,C,F,G,H,J,K,L,M,N,P,Q,X]3ZZ
Non-OR   ØN9B[Ø,3,4]Z[X,Z]
Non-OR   ØN9[R,T,V][Ø,3,4]ZZ

Ø   **Medical and Surgical**
N   **Head and Facial Bones**
B   **Excision**   Definition: Cutting out or off, without replacement, a portion of a body part
                               Explanation: The qualifier DIAGNOSTIC is used to identify excision procedures that are biopsies

Body Part Character 4	Approach Character 5	Device Character 6	Qualifier Character 7
Ø Skull	**Ø** Open	**Z** No Device	**X** Diagnostic
1 **Frontal Bone**	**3** Percutaneous		**Z** No Qualifier
Zygomatic process of frontal bone	**4** Percutaneous Endoscopic		
3 **Parietal Bone, Right**			
4 **Parietal Bone, Left**			
5 **Temporal Bone, Right**			
Mastoid process			
Petrous part of temporal bone			
Tympanic part of temporal bone			
Zygomatic process of temporal bone			
6 **Temporal Bone, Left**			
See 5 Temporal Bone, Right			
7 **Occipital Bone**			
Foramen magnum			
B Nasal Bone			
Vomer of nasal septum			
C **Sphenoid Bone**			
Greater wing			
Lesser wing			
Optic foramen			
Pterygoid process			
Sella turcica			
F **Ethmoid Bone, Right**			
Cribriform plate			
G **Ethmoid Bone, Left**			
See F Ethmoid Bone, Right			
H **Lacrimal Bone, Right**			
J **Lacrimal Bone, Left**			
K **Palatine Bone, Right**			
L **Palatine Bone, Left**			
M **Zygomatic Bone, Right**			
N **Zygomatic Bone, Left**			
P **Orbit, Right**			
Bony orbit			
Orbital portion of ethmoid bone			
Orbital portion of frontal bone			
Orbital portion of lacrimal bone			
Orbital portion of maxilla			
Orbital portion of palatine bone			
Orbital portion of sphenoid bone			
Orbital portion of zygomatic bone			
Q **Orbit, Left**			
See P Orbit, Right			
R Maxilla			
Alveolar process of maxilla			
T Mandible, Right			
Alveolar process of mandible			
Condyloid process			
Mandibular notch			
Mental foramen			
V Mandible, Left			
See T Mandible, Right			
X **Hyoid Bone**			

Non-OR   ØNB[B,R,T,V][Ø,3,4]ZX

LC Limited Coverage   **NC** Noncovered   ⊞ Combination Member   HAC associated procedure   Combination Only   DRG Non-OR   Non-OR   New/Revised in GREEN

ICD-10-PCS 2021   **523**

ØNB–ØNB

Head and Facial Bones

Ø   **Medical and Surgical**
N   **Head and Facial Bones**
C   **Extirpation**   Definition: Taking or cutting out solid matter from a body part

                        Explanation: The solid matter may be an abnormal byproduct of a biological function or a foreign body; it may be imbedded in a body part or in the lumen of a tubular body part. The solid matter may or may not have been previously broken into pieces.

Body Part Character 4	Approach Character 5	Device Character 6	Qualifier Character 7

1 **Frontal Bone**
    Zygomatic process of frontal bone
3 **Parietal Bone, Right**
4 **Parietal Bone, Left**
5 **Temporal Bone, Right**
    Mastoid process
    Petrous part of temporal bone
    Tympanic part of temporal bone
    Zygomatic process of temporal bone
6 **Temporal Bone, Left**
    See 5 Temporal Bone, Right
7 **Occipital Bone**
    Foramen magnum
B **Nasal Bone**
    Vomer of nasal septum
C **Sphenoid Bone**
    Greater wing
    Lesser wing
    Optic foramen
    Pterygoid process
    Sella turcica
F **Ethmoid Bone, Right**
    Cribriform plate
G **Ethmoid Bone, Left**
    See F Ethmoid Bone, Right
H **Lacrimal Bone, Right**
J **Lacrimal Bone, Left**
K **Palatine Bone, Right**
L **Palatine Bone, Left**
M **Zygomatic Bone, Right**
N **Zygomatic Bone, Left**
P **Orbit, Right**
    Bony orbit
    Orbital portion of ethmoid bone
    Orbital portion of frontal bone
    Orbital portion of lacrimal bone
    Orbital portion of maxilla
    Orbital portion of palatine bone
    Orbital portion of sphenoid bone
    Orbital portion of zygomatic bone
Q **Orbit, Left**
    See P Orbit, Right
R **Maxilla**
    Alveolar process of maxilla
T **Mandible, Right**
    Alveolar process of mandible
    Condyloid process
    Mandibular notch
    Mental foramen
V **Mandible, Left**
    See T Mandible, Right
X **Hyoid Bone**
	Ø **Open**
	3 **Percutaneous**
	4 **Percutaneous Endoscopic**
		Z **No Device**	**Z** **No Qualifier**

Non-OR   ØNC[B,R,T,V][Ø,3,4]ZZ

Ø   Medical and Surgical
N   Head and Facial Bones
D   Extraction   Definition: Pulling or stripping out or off all or a portion of a body part by the use of force
                       Explanation: The qualifier DIAGNOSTIC is used to identify extraction procedures that are biopsies

Body Part Character 4	Approach Character 5	Device Character 6	Qualifier Character 7
Ø Skull	**Ø Open**	**Z No Device**	**Z No Qualifier**
1 Frontal Bone Zygomatic process of frontal bone			
3 Parietal Bone, Right			
4 Parietal Bone, Left			

5   Temporal Bone, Right
      Mastoid process
      Petrous part of temporal bone
      Tympanic part of temporal bone
      Zygomatic process of temporal bone			

6 Temporal Bone, Left *See 5 Temporal Bone, Right*			
7 Occipital Bone Foramen magnum			
B Nasal Bone Vomer of nasal septum			

C   Sphenoid Bone
      Greater wing
      Lesser wing
      Optic foramen
      Pterygoid process
      Sella turcica			

F Ethmoid Bone, Right Cribriform plate			
G Ethmoid Bone, Left *See F Ethmoid Bone, Right*			
H Lacrimal Bone, Right			
J Lacrimal Bone, Left			
K Palatine Bone, Right			
L Palatine Bone, Left			
M Zygomatic Bone, Right			
N Zygomatic Bone, Left			

P   Orbit, Right
      Bony orbit
      Orbital portion of ethmoid bone
      Orbital portion of frontal bone
      Orbital portion of lacrimal bone
      Orbital portion of maxilla
      Orbital portion of palatine bone
      Orbital portion of sphenoid bone
      Orbital portion of zygomatic bone			

Q Orbit, Left *See P Orbit, Right*			
R Maxilla Alveolar process of maxilla			

T   Mandible, Right
      Alveolar process of mandible
      Condyloid process
      Mandibular notch
      Mental foramen			

V Mandible, Left *See T Mandible, Right*			
X Hyoid Bone			

LC Limited Coverage   NC Noncovered   ⊞ Combination Member   HAC associated procedure   Combination Only   DRG Non-OR   Non-OR   New/Revised in GREEN

ICD-10-PCS 2021   **525**

Head and Facial Bones

Ø   **Medical and Surgical**
N   **Head and Facial Bones**
H   **Insertion**   Definition: Putting in a nonbiological appliance that monitors, assists, performs, or prevents a physiological function but does not physically take the place of a body part
                    Explanation: None

Body Part Character 4	Approach Character 5	Device Character 6	Qualifier Character 7
Ø Skull ⊞	**Ø** Open	**4** Internal Fixation Device **5** External Fixation Device **M** Bone Growth Stimulator **N** Neurostimulator Generator	**Z** No Qualifier
Ø Skull	**3** Percutaneous **4** Percutaneous Endoscopic	**4** Internal Fixation Device **5** External Fixation Device **M** Bone Growth Stimulator	**Z** No Qualifier

1 **Frontal Bone**
    Zygomatic process of frontal bone
3 **Parietal Bone, Right**
4 **Parietal Bone, Left**
7 **Occipital Bone**
    Foramen magnum
C **Sphenoid Bone**
    Greater wing
    Lesser wing
    Optic foramen
    Pterygoid process
    Sella turcica
F **Ethmoid Bone, Right**
    Cribriform plate
G **Ethmoid Bone, Left**
    See F Ethmoid Bone, Right
H **Lacrimal Bone, Right**
J **Lacrimal Bone, Left**
K **Palatine Bone, Right**
L **Palatine Bone, Left**
M **Zygomatic Bone, Right**
N **Zygomatic Bone, Left**
P **Orbit, Right**
    Bony orbit
    Orbital portion of ethmoid bone
    Orbital portion of frontal bone
    Orbital portion of lacrimal bone
    Orbital portion of maxilla
    Orbital portion of palatine bone
    Orbital portion of sphenoid bone
    Orbital portion of zygomatic bone
Q **Orbit, Left**
    See P Orbit, Right
X **Hyoid Bone**
	Ø Open
	3 Percutaneous
	4 Percutaneous Endoscopic
		4 Internal Fixation Device	**Z** No Qualifier

5 **Temporal Bone, Right**
    Mastoid process
    Petrous part of temporal bone
    Tympanic part of temporal bone
    Zygomatic process of temporal bone
6 **Temporal Bone, Left**
    See 5 Temporal Bone, Right
	Ø Open
	3 Percutaneous
	4 Percutaneous Endoscopic
		4 Internal Fixation Device
		S Hearing Device
			Z No Qualifier

B **Nasal Bone** Vomer of nasal septum	**Ø** Open **3** Percutaneous **4** Percutaneous Endoscopic	**4** Internal Fixation Device **M** Bone Growth Stimulator	**Z** No Qualifier

R **Maxilla**
    Alveolar process of maxilla
T **Mandible, Right**
    Alveolar process of mandible
    Condyloid process
    Mandibular notch
    Mental foramen
V **Mandible, Left**
    See T Mandible, Right
	Ø Open
	3 Percutaneous
	4 Percutaneous Endoscopic
		4 Internal Fixation Device
		5 External Fixation Device
			Z No Qualifier

W Facial Bone	**Ø** Open **3** Percutaneous **4** Percutaneous Endoscopic	**M** Bone Growth Stimulator	**Z** No Qualifier

Non-OR   ØNHØØ5Z
Non-OR   ØNHØ[3,4]5Z
Non-OR   ØNHB[Ø,3,4][4,M]Z

See Appendix L for Procedure Combinations
  ⊞   ØNHØØNZ

Ø   Medical and Surgical
N   Head and Facial Bones
J   Inspection   Definition: Visually and/or manually exploring a body part

                  Explanation: Visual exploration may be performed with or without optical instrumentation. Manual exploration may be performed directly or through intervening body layers.

Body Part Character 4	Approach Character 5	Device Character 6	Qualifier Character 7
Ø **Skull**	**Ø** Open	**Z** No Device	**Z** No Qualifier
B Nasal Bone	**3** Percutaneous		
Vomer of nasal septum	**4** Percutaneous Endoscopic		
W **Facial Bone**	**X** External		

    Non-OR   ØNJ[Ø,B,W][3,X]ZZ

Ø   Medical and Surgical
N   Head and Facial Bones
N   Release   Definition: Freeing a body part from an abnormal physical constraint by cutting or by the use of force

                  Explanation: Some of the restraining tissue may be taken out but none of the body part is taken out

Body Part Character 4	Approach Character 5	Device Character 6	Qualifier Character 7
1 **Frontal Bone**	**Ø** Open	**Z** No Device	**Z** No Qualifier
Zygomatic process of frontal bone	**3** Percutaneous		
3 **Parietal Bone, Right**	**4** Percutaneous Endoscopic		
4 **Parietal Bone, Left**			
5 **Temporal Bone, Right**			
Mastoid process			
Petrous part of temporal bone			
Tympanic part of temporal bone			
Zygomatic process of temporal bone			
6 **Temporal Bone, Left**			
See 5 Temporal Bone, Right			
7 **Occipital Bone**			
Foramen magnum			
B Nasal Bone			
Vomer of nasal septum			
C **Sphenoid Bone**			
Greater wing			
Lesser wing			
Optic foramen			
Pterygoid process			
Sella turcica			
F **Ethmoid Bone, Right**			
Cribriform plate			
G **Ethmoid Bone, Left**			
See F Ethmoid Bone, Right			
H **Lacrimal Bone, Right**			
J **Lacrimal Bone, Left**			
K **Palatine Bone, Right**			
L **Palatine Bone, Left**			
M **Zygomatic Bone, Right**			
N **Zygomatic Bone, Left**			
P **Orbit, Right**			
Bony orbit			
Orbital portion of ethmoid bone			
Orbital portion of frontal bone			
Orbital portion of lacrimal bone			
Orbital portion of maxilla			
Orbital portion of palatine bone			
Orbital portion of sphenoid bone			
Orbital portion of zygomatic bone			
Q **Orbit, Left**			
See P Orbit, Right			
R **Maxilla**			
Alveolar process of maxilla			
T **Mandible, Right**			
Alveolar process of mandible			
Condyloid process			
Mandibular notch			
Mental foramen			
V **Mandible, Left**			
See T Mandible, Right			
X **Hyoid Bone**			

    Non-OR   ØNNB[Ø,3,4]ZZ

Ø **Medical and Surgical**
N **Head and Facial Bones**
P **Removal**   Definition: Taking out or off a device from a body part

Explanation: If a device is taken out and a similar device put in without cutting or puncturing the skin or mucous membrane, the procedure is coded to the root operation CHANGE. Otherwise, the procedure for taking out a device is coded to the root operation REMOVAL.

Body Part Character 4	Approach Character 5	Device Character 6	Qualifier Character 7
Ø Skull	Ø Open	Ø Drainage Device 4 Internal Fixation Device 5 External Fixation Device 7 Autologous Tissue Substitute J Synthetic Substitute K Nonautologous Tissue Substitute M Bone Growth Stimulator N Neurostimulator Generator S Hearing Device	Z No Qualifier
Ø Skull	3 Percutaneous 4 Percutaneous Endoscopic	Ø Drainage Device 4 Internal Fixation Device 5 External Fixation Device 7 Autologous Tissue Substitute J Synthetic Substitute K Nonautologous Tissue Substitute M Bone Growth Stimulator S Hearing Device	Z No Qualifier
Ø Skull	X External	Ø Drainage Device 4 Internal Fixation Device 5 External Fixation Device M Bone Growth Stimulator S Hearing Device	Z No Qualifier
B Nasal Bone Vomer of nasal septum W Facial Bone	Ø Open 3 Percutaneous 4 Percutaneous Endoscopic	Ø Drainage Device 4 Internal Fixation Device 7 Autologous Tissue Substitute J Synthetic Substitute K Nonautologous Tissue Substitute M Bone Growth Stimulator	Z No Qualifier
B Nasal Bone Vomer of nasal septum W Facial Bone	X External	Ø Drainage Device 4 Internal Fixation Device M Bone Growth Stimulator	Z No Qualifier

Non-OR   ØNPØ[3,4]5Z
Non-OR   ØNPØX[Ø,5]Z
Non-OR   ØNPB[Ø,3,4][Ø,4,7,J,K,M]Z
Non-OR   ØNPBX[Ø,4,M]Z
Non-OR   ØNPWX[Ø,M]Z

Ø   Medical and Surgical
N   Head and Facial Bones
Q   Repair   Definition: Restoring, to the extent possible, a body part to its normal anatomic structure and function
                    Explanation: Used only when the method to accomplish the repair is not one of the other root operations

Body Part Character 4	Approach Character 5	Device Character 6	Qualifier Character 7
Ø Skull	**Ø** Open	**Z** No Device	**Z** No Qualifier
1 Frontal Bone	**3** Percutaneous		
Zygomatic process of frontal bone	**4** Percutaneous Endoscopic		
3 Parietal Bone, Right	**X** External		
4 Parietal Bone, Left			
5 Temporal Bone, Right			
Mastoid process			
Petrous part of temporal bone			
Tympanic part of temporal bone			
Zygomatic process of temporal bone			
6 Temporal Bone, Left			
See 5 Temporal Bone, Right			
7 Occipital Bone			
Foramen magnum			
B Nasal Bone			
Vomer of nasal septum			
C Sphenoid Bone			
Greater wing			
Lesser wing			
Optic foramen			
Pterygoid process			
Sella turcica			
F Ethmoid Bone, Right			
Cribriform plate			
G Ethmoid Bone, Left			
See F Ethmoid Bone, Right			
H Lacrimal Bone, Right			
J Lacrimal Bone, Left			
K Palatine Bone, Right			
L Palatine Bone, Left			
M Zygomatic Bone, Right			
N Zygomatic Bone, Left			
P Orbit, Right			
Bony orbit			
Orbital portion of ethmoid bone			
Orbital portion of frontal bone			
Orbital portion of lacrimal bone			
Orbital portion of maxilla			
Orbital portion of palatine bone			
Orbital portion of sphenoid bone			
Orbital portion of zygomatic bone			
Q Orbit, Left			
See P Orbit, Right			
R Maxilla			
Alveolar process of maxilla			
T Mandible, Right			
Alveolar process of mandible			
Condyloid process			
Mandibular notch			
Mental foramen			
V Mandible, Left			
See T Mandible, Right			
X Hyoid Bone			

Non-OR   ØNQ[Ø,1,3,4,5,6,7,B,C,F,G,H,J,K,L,M,N,P,Q,R,T,V,X]XZZ

Head and Facial Bones

Ø **Medical and Surgical**
N **Head and Facial Bones**
R **Replacement**   Definition: Putting in or on biological or synthetic material that physically takes the place and/or function of all or a portion of a body part
Explanation: The body part may have been taken out or replaced, or may be taken out, physically eradicated, or rendered nonfunctional during the REPLACEMENT procedure. A REMOVAL procedure is coded for taking out the device used in a previous replacement procedure.

Body Part Character 4	Approach Character 5	Device Character 6	Qualifier Character 7
Ø **Skull**	**Ø** **Open**	**7** **Autologous Tissue Substitute**	**Z** **No Qualifier**
1 **Frontal Bone**	**3** **Percutaneous**	**J** **Synthetic Substitute**	
Zygomatic process of frontal bone	**4** **Percutaneous Endoscopic**	**K** **Nonautologous Tissue Substitute**	
3 **Parietal Bone, Right**			
4 **Parietal Bone, Left**			
5 **Temporal Bone, Right**			
Mastoid process			
Petrous part of temporal bone			
Tympanic part of temporal bone			
Zygomatic process of temporal bone			
6 **Temporal Bone, Left**			
See 5 Temporal Bone, Right			
7 **Occipital Bone**			
Foramen magnum			
B **Nasal Bone**			
Vomer of nasal septum			
C **Sphenoid Bone**			
Greater wing			
Lesser wing			
Optic foramen			
Pterygoid process			
Sella turcica			
F **Ethmoid Bone, Right**			
Cribriform plate			
G **Ethmoid Bone, Left**			
See F Ethmoid Bone, Right			
H **Lacrimal Bone, Right**			
J **Lacrimal Bone, Left**			
K **Palatine Bone, Right**			
L **Palatine Bone, Left**			
M **Zygomatic Bone, Right**			
N **Zygomatic Bone, Left**			
P **Orbit, Right**			
Bony orbit			
Orbital portion of ethmoid bone			
Orbital portion of frontal bone			
Orbital portion of lacrimal bone			
Orbital portion of maxilla			
Orbital portion of palatine bone			
Orbital portion of sphenoid bone			
Orbital portion of zygomatic bone			
Q **Orbit, Left**			
See P Orbit, Right			
R **Maxilla**			
Alveolar process of maxilla			
T **Mandible, Right**			
Alveolar process of mandible			
Condyloid process			
Mandibular notch			
Mental foramen			
V **Mandible, Left**			
See T Mandible, Right			
X **Hyoid Bone**			

LC Limited Coverage **NC** Noncovered ⊞ Combination Member HAC associated procedure Combination Only DRG Non-OR Non-OR New/Revised in GREEN

530 ICD-10-PCS 2021

Ø **Medical and Surgical**
N **Head and Facial Bones**
S **Reposition**   Definition: Moving to its normal location, or other suitable location, all or a portion of a body part

Explanation: The body part is moved to a new location from an abnormal location, or from a normal location where it is not functioning correctly. The body part may or may not be cut out or off to be moved to the new location.

Body Part Character 4	Approach Character 5	Device Character 6	Qualifier Character 7

Ø Skull
R Maxilla
   Alveolar process of maxilla
T Mandible, Right
   Alveolar process of mandible
   Condyloid process
   Mandibular notch
   Mental foramen
V Mandible, Left
   See T Mandible, Right
	Ø Open
	3 Percutaneous
	4 Percutaneous Endoscopic
		4 Internal Fixation Device
		5 External Fixation Device
		Z No Device
			Z No Qualifier

Ø Skull
R Maxilla
   Alveolar process of maxilla
T Mandible, Right
   Alveolar process of mandible
   Condyloid process
   Mandibular notch
   Mental foramen
V Mandible, Left
   See T Mandible, Right
	X External	Z No Device	Z No Qualifier

1 Frontal Bone
   Zygomatic process of frontal bone
3 Parietal Bone, Right
4 Parietal Bone, Left
5 Temporal Bone, Right
   Mastoid process
   Petrous part of temporal bone
   Tympanic part of temporal bone
   Zygomatic process of temporal bone
6 Temporal Bone, Left
   See 5 Temporal Bone, Right
7 Occipital Bone
   Foramen magnum
B Nasal Bone
   Vomer of nasal septum
C Sphenoid Bone
   Greater wing
   Lesser wing
   Optic foramen
   Pterygoid process
   Sella turcica
F Ethmoid Bone, Right
   Cribriform plate
G Ethmoid Bone, Left
   See F Ethmoid Bone, Right
H Lacrimal Bone, Right
J Lacrimal Bone, Left
K Palatine Bone, Right
L Palatine Bone, Left
M Zygomatic Bone, Right
N Zygomatic Bone, Left
P Orbit, Right
   Bony orbit
   Orbital portion of ethmoid bone
   Orbital portion of frontal bone
   Orbital portion of lacrimal bone
   Orbital portion of maxilla
   Orbital portion of palatine bone
   Orbital portion of sphenoid bone
   Orbital portion of zygomatic bone
Q Orbit, Left
   See P Orbit, Right
X Hyoid Bone
	Ø Open
	3 Percutaneous
	4 Percutaneous Endoscopic
		4 Internal Fixation Device
		Z No Device
			Z No Qualifier

Non-OR ØNS[R,T,V][3,4][4,5,Z]Z
Non-OR ØNS[Ø,R,T,V]XZZ
Non-OR ØNS[B,C,F,G,H,J,K,L,M,N,P,Q,X][3,4][4,Z]Z

ØNS Continued on next page

LC Limited Coverage NC Noncovered ⊞ Combination Member HAC associated procedure Combination Only DRG Non-OR Non-OR New/Revised in GREEN

ICD-10-PCS 2021 531

ØNS–ØNS

Head and Facial Bones

ØNS Continued

Ø   Medical and Surgical
N   Head and Facial Bones
S   Reposition   Definition: Moving to its normal location, or other suitable location, all or a portion of a body part

                     Explanation: The body part is moved to a new location from an abnormal location, or from a normal location where it is not functioning correctly. The body part may or may not be cut out or off to be moved to the new location.

Body Part Character 4	Approach Character 5	Device Character 6	Qualifier Character 7

1 **Frontal Bone**
   Zygomatic process of frontal bone
3 **Parietal Bone, Right**
4 **Parietal Bone, Left**
5 **Temporal Bone, Right**
   Mastoid process
   Petrous part of temporal bone
   Tympanic part of temporal bone
   Zygomatic process of temporal bone
6 **Temporal Bone, Left**
   See 5 Temporal Bone, Right
7 **Occipital Bone**
   Foramen magnum
B **Nasal Bone**
   Vomer of nasal septum
C **Sphenoid Bone**
   Greater wing
   Lesser wing
   Optic foramen
   Pterygoid process
   Sella turcica
F **Ethmoid Bone, Right**
   Cribriform plate
G **Ethmoid Bone, Left**
   See F Ethmoid Bone, Right
H **Lacrimal Bone, Right**
J **Lacrimal Bone, Left**
K **Palatine Bone, Right**
L **Palatine Bone, Left**
M **Zygomatic Bone, Right**
N **Zygomatic Bone, Left**
P **Orbit, Right**
   Bony orbit
   Orbital portion of ethmoid bone
   Orbital portion of frontal bone
   Orbital portion of lacrimal bone
   Orbital portion of maxilla
   Orbital portion of palatine bone
   Orbital portion of sphenoid bone
   Orbital portion of zygomatic bone
Q **Orbit, Left**
   See P Orbit, Right
X **Hyoid Bone**
	X External	Z No Device	Z No Qualifier

Non-OR   ØNS[1,3,4,5,6,7,B,C,F,G,H,J,K,L,M,N,P,Q,X]XZZ

Ø   Medical and Surgical
N   Head and Facial Bones
T   Resection   Definition: Cutting out or off, without replacement, all of a body part
                       Explanation: None

Body Part Character 4	Approach Character 5	Device Character 6	Qualifier Character 7

1 Frontal Bone
   Zygomatic process of frontal bone
3 Parietal Bone, Right
4 Parietal Bone, Left
5 Temporal Bone, Right
   Mastoid process
   Petrous part of temporal bone
   Tympanic part of temporal bone
   Zygomatic process of temporal bone
6 Temporal Bone, Left
   See 5 Temporal Bone, Right
7 Occipital Bone
   Foramen magnum
B Nasal Bone
   Vomer of nasal septum
C Sphenoid Bone
   Greater wing
   Lesser wing
   Optic foramen
   Pterygoid process
   Sella turcica
F Ethmoid Bone, Right
   Cribriform plate
G Ethmoid Bone, Left
   See F Ethmoid Bone, Right
H Lacrimal Bone, Right
J Lacrimal Bone, Left
K Palatine Bone, Right
L Palatine Bone, Left
M Zygomatic Bone, Right
N Zygomatic Bone, Left
P Orbit, Right
   Bony orbit
   Orbital portion of ethmoid bone
   Orbital portion of frontal bone
   Orbital portion of lacrimal bone
   Orbital portion of maxilla
   Orbital portion of palatine bone
   Orbital portion of sphenoid bone
   Orbital portion of zygomatic bone
Q Orbit, Left
   See P Orbit, Right
R Maxilla
   Alveolar process of maxilla
T Mandible, Right
   Alveolar process of mandible
   Condyloid process
   Mandibular notch
   Mental foramen
V Mandible, Left
   See T Mandible, Right
X Hyoid Bone
	Ø Open	**Z No Device**	**Z No Qualifier**

Head and Facial Bones

Ø   Medical and Surgical
N   Head and Facial Bones
U   Supplement   Definition: Putting in or on biological or synthetic material that physically reinforces and/or augments the function of a portion of a body part

     Explanation: The biological material is non-living, or is living and from the same individual. The body part may have been previously replaced, and the SUPPLEMENT procedure is performed to physically reinforce and/or augment the function of the replaced body part.

Body Part Character 4	Approach Character 5	Device Character 6	Qualifier Character 7
Ø Skull	**Ø** Open	**7** Autologous Tissue Substitute	**Z** No Qualifier
1 Frontal Bone	**3** Percutaneous	**J** Synthetic Substitute	
Zygomatic process of frontal bone	**4** Percutaneous Endoscopic	**K** Nonautologous Tissue Substitute	
3 Parietal Bone, Right			
4 Parietal Bone, Left			
5 Temporal Bone, Right			
Mastoid process			
Petrous part of temporal bone			
Tympanic part of temporal bone			
Zygomatic process of temporal bone			
6 Temporal Bone, Left			
See 5 Temporal Bone, Right			
7 Occipital Bone			
Foramen magnum			
B Nasal Bone			
Vomer of nasal septum			
C Sphenoid Bone			
Greater wing			
Lesser wing			
Optic foramen			
Pterygoid process			
Sella turcica			
F Ethmoid Bone, Right			
Cribriform plate			
G Ethmoid Bone, Left			
See F Ethmoid Bone, Right			
H Lacrimal Bone, Right			
J Lacrimal Bone, Left			
K Palatine Bone, Right			
L Palatine Bone, Left			
M Zygomatic Bone, Right			
N Zygomatic Bone, Left			
P Orbit, Right			
Bony orbit			
Orbital portion of ethmoid bone			
Orbital portion of frontal bone			
Orbital portion of lacrimal bone			
Orbital portion of maxilla			
Orbital portion of palatine bone			
Orbital portion of sphenoid bone			
Orbital portion of zygomatic bone			
Q Orbit, Left			
See P Orbit, Right			
R Maxilla			
Alveolar process of maxilla			
T Mandible, Right			
Alveolar process of mandible			
Condyloid process			
Mandibular notch			
Mental foramen			
V Mandible, Left			
See T Mandible, Right			
X Hyoid Bone			

LC Limited Coverage   **NC** Noncovered   ⊞ Combination Member   HAC associated procedure   Combination Only   DRG Non-OR   Non-OR   New/Revised in GREEN

534   ICD-10-PCS 2021

Ø   **Medical and Surgical**
N   **Head and Facial Bones**
W   **Revision**   Definition: Correcting, to the extent possible, a portion of a malfunctioning device or the position of a displaced device

                           Explanation: Revision can include correcting a malfunctioning or displaced device by taking out or putting in components of the device such as a screw or pin

Body Part Character 4	Approach Character 5	Device Character 6	Qualifier Character 7
Ø Skull	**Ø** Open	**Ø** Drainage Device **4** Internal Fixation Device **5** External Fixation Device **7** Autologous Tissue Substitute **J** Synthetic Substitute **K** Nonautologous Tissue Substitute **M** Bone Growth Stimulator **N** Neurostimulator Generator **S** Hearing Device	**Z** No Qualifier
Ø Skull	**3** Percutaneous **4** Percutaneous Endoscopic **X** External	**Ø** Drainage Device **4** Internal Fixation Device **5** External Fixation Device **7** Autologous Tissue Substitute **J** Synthetic Substitute **K** Nonautologous Tissue Substitute **M** Bone Growth Stimulator **S** Hearing Device	**Z** No Qualifier
B Nasal Bone Vomer of nasal septum **W** Facial Bone	**Ø** Open **3** Percutaneous **4** Percutaneous Endoscopic **X** External	**Ø** Drainage Device **4** Internal Fixation Device **7** Autologous Tissue Substitute **J** Synthetic Substitute **K** Nonautologous Tissue Substitute **M** Bone Growth Stimulator	**Z** No Qualifier

Non-OR   ØNWØX[Ø,4,5,7,J,K,M,S]Z
Non-OR   ØNWB[Ø,3,4,X][Ø,4,7,J,K,M]Z
Non-OR   ØNWWX[Ø,4,7,J,K,M]Z

Upper Bones ØP2–ØPW

Character Meanings

This Character Meaning table is provided as a guide to assist the user in the identification of character members that may be found in this section of code tables. It **SHOULD NOT** be used to build a PCS code.

Operation–Character 3	Body Part–Character 4	Approach–Character 5	Device–Character 6	Qualifier–Character 7
2 Change	Ø Sternum	Ø Open	Ø Drainage Device OR Internal Fixation Device, Rigid Plate	X Diagnostic
5 Destruction	1 Ribs, 1 to 2	3 Percutaneous	4 Internal Fixation Device	Z No Qualifier
8 Division	2 Ribs, 3 or more	4 Percutaneous Endoscopic	5 External Fixation Device	
9 Drainage	3 Cervical Vertebra	X External	6 Internal Fixation Device, Intramedullary	
B Excision	4 Thoracic Vertebra		7 Autologous Tissue Substitute OR Internal Fixation Device, Intramedullary Limb Lengthening	
C Extirpation	5 Scapula, Right		8 External Fixation Device, Limb Lengthening	
D Extraction	6 Scapula, Left		B External Fixation Device, Monoplanar	
H Insertion	7 Glenoid Cavity, Right		C External Fixation Device, Ring	
J Inspection	8 Glenoid Cavity, Left		D External Fixation Device, Hybrid	
N Release	9 Clavicle, Right		J Synthetic Substitute	
P Removal	B Clavicle, Left		K Nonautologous Tissue Substitute	
Q Repair	C Humeral Head, Right		M Bone Growth Stimulator	
R Replacement	D Humeral Head, Left		Y Other Device	
S Reposition	F Humeral Shaft, Right		Z No Device	
T Resection	G Humeral Shaft, Left			
U Supplement	H Radius, Right			
W Revision	J Radius, Left			
	K Ulna, Right			
	L Ulna, Left			
	M Carpal, Right			
	N Carpal, Left			
	P Metacarpal, Right			
	Q Metacarpal, Left			
	R Thumb Phalanx, Right			
	S Thumb Phalanx, Left			
	T Finger Phalanx, Right			
	V Finger Phalanx, Left			
	Y Upper Bone			

AHA Coding Clinic for table ØPB

2015, 3Q, 3-8   Excisional and nonexcisional debridement
2015, 2Q, 34   Decompressive laminectomy
2013, 4Q, 109   Separating conjoined twins
2013, 4Q, 116   Spinal decompression
2013, 3Q, 20   Superior labrum anterior posterior (SLAP) repair and subacromialdecompression
2012, 4Q, 101   Rib resection with reconstruction of anterior chest wall
2012, 2Q, 19   Multiple decompressive cervical laminectomies

AHA Coding Clinic for table ØPC

2019, 3Q, 19   Removal of sternal wire

AHA Coding Clinic for table ØPD

2017, 4Q, 41   Extraction procedures

AHA Coding Clinic for table ØPH

2020, 1Q, 29   Repair of sternal dehiscence using Sternal Talon® device
2019, 4Q, 34   Intramedullary limb lengthening internal fixation device
2019, 2Q, 40   Decompression of spinal cord and placement of instrumentation
2018, 3Q, 26   Anterior vertebral tethering using Dynesys Tethering System
2017, 2Q, 20   Exchange of intramedullary antibiotic impregnated spacer
2016, 4Q, 117 Placement of magnetic growth rods
2014, 4Q, 28   Removal and replacement of displaced growing rods

AHA Coding Clinic for table ØPP

2019, 3Q, 19   Removal of sternal wire
2017, 2Q, 20   Exchange of intramedullary antibiotic impregnated spacer
2016, 4Q, 117 Placement of magnetic growth rods
2014, 4Q, 28   Removal and replacement of displaced growing rods

AHA Coding Clinic for table ØPR

2018, 4Q, 92   Radial head arthroplasty

AHA Coding Clinic for table ØPS

2020, 1Q, 33   Spinal fusion without use of bone graft
2018, 3Q, 26   Anterior vertebral tethering using Dynesys Tethering System
2017, 4Q, 53   New and revised body part values - Ribs
2016, 1Q, 21   Elongation derotation flexion casting
2015, 4Q, 33   Ravitch operation
2015, 2Q, 35   Application of tongs to reduce and stabilize cervical fracture
2014, 4Q, 26   Placement of vertical expandable prosthetic titanium rib (VEPTR)
2014, 4Q, 32   Open reduction internal fixation of fracture with debridement
2014, 3Q, 33   Radial fracture treatment with open reduction internal fixation, and release of carpal ligament

AHA Coding Clinic for table ØPT

2015, 3Q, 26   Thumb arthroplasty with resection of trapezium

AHA Coding Clinic for table ØPU

2015, 2Q, 20   Cervical laminoplasty
2013, 4Q, 109   Separating conjoined twins

AHA Coding Clinic for table ØPW

2014, 4Q, 26   Adjustment of VEPTR lengthening mechanism
2014, 4Q, 27   Bilateral lengthening of growing rods

Upper Bones

Cervical vertebra **3**

Clavicle **9, B**

Sternum **Ø**

Rib **1, 2**

Thoracic vertebra **4**

Scapula **5, 6**

Humerus **C, D, F, G**

Ulna **K, L**

Radius **H, J**

Carpal **M, N**

Metacarpal **P, Q**

Thumb phalanx **R, S**

Finger phalanx **T, V**

Humerus and Scapula

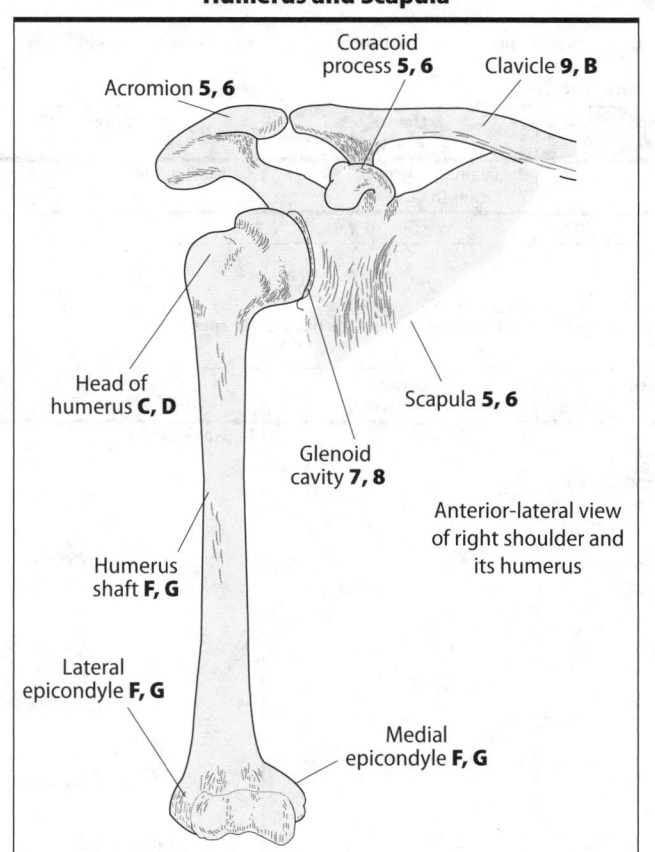

Coracoid process **5, 6**

Clavicle **9, B**

Acromion **5, 6**

Head of humerus **C, D**

Scapula **5, 6**

Glenoid cavity **7, 8**

Anterior-lateral view of right shoulder and its humerus

Humerus shaft **F, G**

Lateral epicondyle **F, G**

Medial epicondyle **F, G**

Radius and Ulna

Olecranon process **K, L**

Radius **H, J**

Coronoid process **K, L**

Ulna **K, L**

Shaft **H, J**

Shaft **K, L**

Radial styloid process **H, J**

Ulnar styloid process **K, L**

Carpal **M, N**

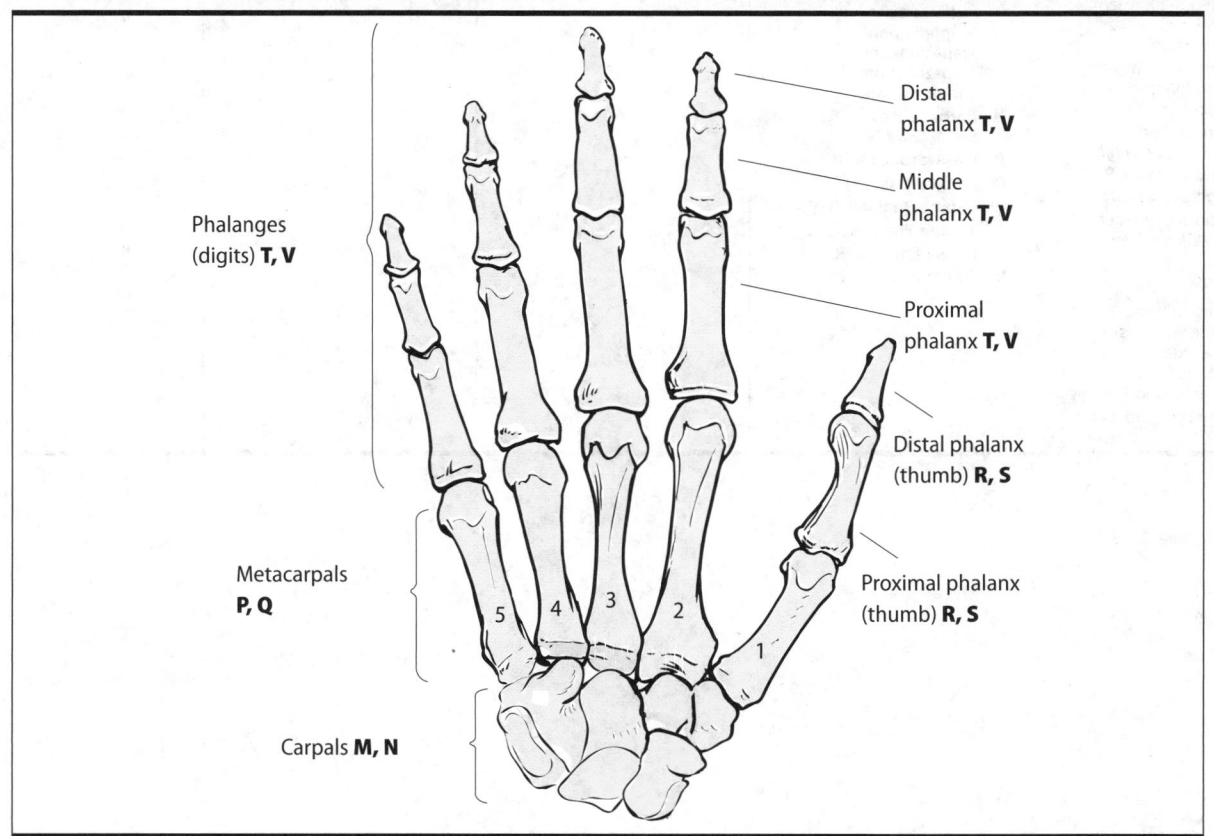

Distal phalanx **T, V**

Middle phalanx **T, V**

Phalanges (digits) **T, V**

Proximal phalanx **T, V**

Distal phalanx (thumb) **R, S**

Metacarpals **P, Q**

Proximal phalanx (thumb) **R, S**

Carpals **M, N**

Upper Bones

Ø   Medical and Surgical
P   Upper Bones
2   Change   Definition: Taking out or off a device from a body part and putting back an identical or similar device in or on the same body part without cutting or puncturing the skin or a mucous membrane

Explanation: All CHANGE procedures are coded using the approach EXTERNAL

Body Part Character 4	Approach Character 5	Device Character 6	Qualifier Character 7
Y Upper Bone	X External	Ø Drainage Device Y Other Device	Z No Qualifier

Non-OR   All body part, approach, device, and qualifier values

Ø   Medical and Surgical
P   Upper Bones
5   Destruction   Definition: Physical eradication of all or a portion of a body part by the direct use of energy, force, or a destructive agent

Explanation: None of the body part is physically taken out

Body Part Character 4	Approach Character 5	Device Character 6	Qualifier Character 7

0 Sternum
   Manubrium
   Suprasternal notch
   Xiphoid process
1 Ribs, 1 to 2
2 Ribs, 3 or More
3 Cervical Vertebra
   Dens
   Odontoid process
   Spinous process
   Transverse foramen
   Transverse process
   Vertebral arch
   Vertebral body
   Vertebral foramen
   Vertebral lamina
   Vertebral pedicle
4 Thoracic Vertebra
   Spinous process
   Transverse process
   Vertebral arch
   Vertebral body
   Vertebral foramen
   Vertebral lamina
   Vertebral pedicle
5 Scapula, Right
   Acromion (process)
   Coracoid process
6 Scapula, Left
   See 5 Scapula, Right
7 Glenoid Cavity, Right
   Glenoid fossa (of scapula)
8 Glenoid Cavity, Left
   See 7 Glenoid Cavity, Right
9 Clavicle, Right
B Clavicle, Left
C Humeral Head, Right
   Greater tuberosity
   Lesser tuberosity
   Neck of humerus
     (anatomical)(surgical)
D Humeral Head, Left
   See C Humeral Head, Right
 	
F Humeral Shaft, Right
   Distal humerus
   Humerus, distal
   Lateral epicondyle of
     humerus
   Medial epicondyle of
     humerus
G Humeral Shaft, Left
   See F Humeral Shaft, Right
H Radius, Right
   Ulnar notch
J Radius, Left
   See H Radius, Right
K Ulna, Right
   Olecranon process
   Radial notch
L Ulna, Left
   See K Ulna, Right
M Carpal, Right
   Capitate bone
   Hamate bone
   Lunate bone
   Pisiform bone
   Scaphoid bone
   Trapezium bone
   Trapezoid bone
   Triquetral bone
N Carpal, Left
   See M Carpal, Right
P Metacarpal, Right
Q Metacarpal, Left
R Thumb Phalanx, Right
S Thumb Phalanx, Left
T Finger Phalanx, Right
V Finger Phalanx, Left
	0 Open
	3 Percutaneous
	4 Percutaneous Endoscopic
		Z No Device	**Z** No Qualifier

Ø　Medical and Surgical
P　Upper Bones
8　Division　　　Definition: Cutting into a body part, without draining fluids and/or gases from the body part, in order to separate or transect a body part
　　　　　　　　　　　Explanation: All or a portion of the body part is separated into two or more portions

Body Part Character 4		Approach Character 5	Device Character 6	Qualifier Character 7
Ø　Sternum 　　Manubrium 　　Suprasternal notch 　　Xiphoid process **1　Ribs, 1 to 2** **2　Ribs, 3 or More** **3　Cervical Vertebra** 　　Dens 　　Odontoid process 　　Spinous process 　　Transverse foramen 　　Transverse process 　　Vertebral arch 　　Vertebral body 　　Vertebral foramen 　　Vertebral lamina 　　Vertebral pedicle **4　Thoracic Vertebra** 　　Spinous process 　　Transverse process 　　Vertebral arch 　　Vertebral body 　　Vertebral foramen 　　Vertebral lamina 　　Vertebral pedicle **5　Scapula, Right** 　　Acromion (process) 　　Coracoid process **6　Scapula, Left** 　　*See 5 Scapula, Right* **7　Glenoid Cavity, Right** 　　Glenoid fossa (of scapula) **8　Glenoid Cavity, Left** 　　*See 7 Glenoid Cavity, Right* **9　Clavicle, Right** **B　Clavicle, Left** **C　Humeral Head, Right** 　　Greater tuberosity 　　Lesser tuberosity 　　Neck of humerus 　　　(anatomical)(surgical) **D　Humeral Head, Left** 　　*See C Humeral Head, Right*	**F　Humeral Shaft, Right** 　　Distal humerus 　　Humerus, distal 　　Lateral epicondyle of 　　　humerus 　　Medial epicondyle of 　　　humerus **G　Humeral Shaft, Left** 　　*See F Humeral Shaft, Right* **H　Radius, Right** 　　Ulnar notch **J　Radius, Left** 　　*See H Radius, Right* **K　Ulna, Right** 　　Olecranon process 　　Radial notch **L　Ulna, Left** 　　*See K Ulna, Right* **M　Carpal, Right** 　　Capitate bone 　　Hamate bone 　　Lunate bone 　　Pisiform bone 　　Scaphoid bone 　　Trapezium bone 　　Trapezoid bone 　　Triquetral bone **N　Carpal, Left** 　　*See M Carpal, Right* **P　Metacarpal, Right** **Q　Metacarpal, Left** **R　Thumb Phalanx, Right** **S　Thumb Phalanx, Left** **T　Finger Phalanx, Right** **V　Finger Phalanx, Left**	**Ø　Open** **3　Percutaneous** **4　Percutaneous Endoscopic**	**Z　No Device**	**Z　No Qualifier**

Upper Bones

Ø　Medical and Surgical
P　Upper Bones
9　Drainage　　Definition: Taking or letting out fluids and/or gases from a body part

Explanation: The qualifier DIAGNOSTIC is used to identify drainage procedures that are biopsies

Body Part Character 4		Approach Character 5	Device Character 6	Qualifier Character 7
Ø Sternum Manubrium Suprasternal notch Xiphoid process **1 Ribs, 1 to 2** **2 Ribs, 3 or More** **3 Cervical Vertebra** Dens Odontoid process Spinous process Transverse foramen Transverse process Vertebral arch Vertebral body Vertebral foramen Vertebral lamina Vertebral pedicle **4 Thoracic Vertebra** Spinous process Transverse process Vertebral arch Vertebral body Vertebral foramen Vertebral lamina Vertebral pedicle **5 Scapula, Right** Acromion (process) Coracoid process **6 Scapula, Left** *See 5 Scapula, Right* **7 Glenoid Cavity, Right** Glenoid fossa (of scapula) **8 Glenoid Cavity, Left** *See 7 Glenoid Cavity, Right* **9 Clavicle, Right** **B Clavicle, Left** **C Humeral Head, Right** Greater tuberosity Lesser tuberosity Neck of humerus 　(anatomical)(surgical)	**D Humeral Head, Left** *See C Humeral Head, Right* **F Humeral Shaft, Right** Distal humerus Humerus, distal Lateral epicondyle of 　humerus Medial epicondyle of 　humerus **G Humeral Shaft, Left** *See F Humeral Shaft, Right* **H Radius, Right** Ulnar notch **J Radius, Left** *See H Radius, Right* **K Ulna, Right** Olecranon process Radial notch **L Ulna, Left** *See K Ulna, Right* **M Carpal, Right** Capitate bone Hamate bone Lunate bone Pisiform bone Scaphoid bone Trapezium bone Trapezoid bone Triquetral bone **N Carpal, Left** *See M Carpal, Right* **P Metacarpal, Right** **Q Metacarpal, Left** **R Thumb Phalanx, Right** **S Thumb Phalanx, Left** **T Finger Phalanx, Right** **V Finger Phalanx, Left**	**Ø Open** **3 Percutaneous** **4 Percutaneous Endoscopic**	**Ø Drainage Device**	**Z No Qualifier**

Non-OR　ØP9[Ø,1,2,3,4,5,6,7,8,9,B,C,D,F,G,H,J,K,L,M,N,P,Q,R,S,T,V]3ØZ

ØP9 Continued on next page

LC Limited Coverage　**NC** Noncovered　⊞ Combination Member　HAC associated procedure　Combination Only　DRG Non-OR　Non-OR　New/Revised in GREEN

542　　　　　　　　　　　　　　　　　　　　　　　　　　　　　　　　　　　ICD-10-PCS 2021

Ø　Medical and Surgical
P　Upper Bones
9　Drainage

Definition: Taking or letting out fluids and/or gases from a body part

Explanation: The qualifier DIAGNOSTIC is used to identify drainage procedures that are biopsies

Body Part Character 4		Approach Character 5	Device Character 6	Qualifier Character 7
Ø Sternum 　Manubrium 　Suprasternal notch 　Xiphoid process **1 Ribs, 1 to 2** **2 Ribs, 3 or More** **3 Cervical Vertebra** 　Dens 　Odontoid process 　Spinous process 　Transverse foramen 　Transverse process 　Vertebral arch 　Vertebral body 　Vertebral foramen 　Vertebral lamina 　Vertebral pedicle **4 Thoracic Vertebra** 　Spinous process 　Transverse process 　Vertebral arch 　Vertebral body 　Vertebral foramen 　Vertebral lamina 　Vertebral pedicle **5 Scapula, Right** 　Acromion (process) 　Coracoid process **6 Scapula, Left** 　*See 5 Scapula, Right* **7 Glenoid Cavity, Right** 　Glenoid fossa (of scapula) **8 Glenoid Cavity, Left** 　*See 7 Glenoid Cavity, Right* **9 Clavicle, Right** **B Clavicle, Left** **C Humeral Head, Right** 　Greater tuberosity 　Lesser tuberosity 　Neck of humerus 　　(anatomical)(surgical)	**D Humeral Head, Left** 　*See C Humeral Head, Right* **F Humeral Shaft, Right** 　Distal humerus 　Humerus, distal 　Lateral epicondyle of 　　humerus 　Medial epicondyle of 　　humerus **G Humeral Shaft, Left** 　*See F Humeral Shaft, Right* **H Radius, Right** 　Ulnar notch **J Radius, Left** 　*See H Radius, Right* **K Ulna, Right** 　Olecranon process 　Radial notch **L Ulna, Left** 　*See K Ulna, Right* **M Carpal, Right** 　Capitate bone 　Hamate bone 　Lunate bone 　Pisiform bone 　Scaphoid bone 　Trapezium bone 　Trapezoid bone 　Triquetral bone **N Carpal, Left** 　*See M Carpal, Right* **P Metacarpal, Right** **Q Metacarpal, Left** **R Thumb Phalanx, Right** **S Thumb Phalanx, Left** **T Finger Phalanx, Right** **V Finger Phalanx, Left**	**Ø Open** **3 Percutaneous** **4 Percutaneous Endoscopic**	**Z No Device**	**X Diagnostic** **Z No Qualifier**

Non-OR　ØP9[Ø,1,2,3,4,5,6,7,8,9,B,C,D,F,G,H,J,K,L,M,N,P,Q,R,S,T,V]3ZZ

Ø   Medical and Surgical
P   Upper Bones
B   Excision

Definition: Cutting out or off, without replacement, a portion of a body part

Explanation: The qualifier DIAGNOSTIC is used to identify excision procedures that are biopsies

Body Part Character 4		Approach Character 5	Device Character 6	Qualifier Character 7

Ø Sternum
  Manubrium
  Suprasternal notch
  Xiphoid process
1 Ribs, 1 to 2
2 Ribs, 3 or More
3 Cervical Vertebra
  Dens
  Odontoid process
  Spinous process
  Transverse foramen
  Transverse process
  Vertebral arch
  Vertebral body
  Vertebral foramen
  Vertebral lamina
  Vertebral pedicle
4 Thoracic Vertebra
  Spinous process
  Transverse process
  Vertebral arch
  Vertebral body
  Vertebral foramen
  Vertebral lamina
  Vertebral pedicle
5 Scapula, Right
  Acromion (process)
  Coracoid process
6 Scapula, Left
  See 5 Scapula, Right
7 Glenoid Cavity, Right
  Glenoid fossa (of scapula)
8 Glenoid Cavity, Left
  See 7 Glenoid Cavity, Right
9 Clavicle, Right
B Clavicle, Left
C Humeral Head, Right
  Greater tuberosity
  Lesser tuberosity
  Neck of humerus
    (anatomical)(surgical)
D Humeral Head, Left
  See C Humeral Head, Right
	F Humeral Shaft, Right
	  Distal humerus
	  Humerus, distal
	  Lateral epicondyle of
	    humerus
	  Medial epicondyle of
	    humerus
	G Humeral Shaft, Left
	  See F Humeral Shaft, Right
	H Radius, Right
	  Ulnar notch
	J Radius, Left
	  See H Radius, Right
	K Ulna, Right
	  Olecranon process
	  Radial notch
	L Ulna, Left
	  See K Ulna, Right
	M Carpal, Right
	  Capitate bone
	  Hamate bone
	  Lunate bone
	  Pisiform bone
	  Scaphoid bone
	  Trapezium bone
	  Trapezoid bone
	  Triquetral bone
	N Carpal, Left
	  See M Carpal, Right
	P Metacarpal, Right
	Q Metacarpal, Left
	R Thumb Phalanx, Right
	S Thumb Phalanx, Left
	T Finger Phalanx, Right
	V Finger Phalanx, Left
		Ø Open
		3 Percutaneous
		4 Percutaneous Endoscopic
			Z No Device	**X** Diagnostic
				Z No Qualifier

LC Limited Coverage   **NC** Noncovered   ⊞ Combination Member   HAC associated procedure   Combination Only   DRG Non-OR   Non-OR   New/Revised in GREEN

544

ICD-10-PCS 2021

ØPB–ØPB

Ø   Medical and Surgical
P   Upper Bones
C   Extirpation

Definition: Taking or cutting out solid matter from a body part

Explanation: The solid matter may be an abnormal byproduct of a biological function or a foreign body; it may be imbedded in a body part or in the lumen of a tubular body part. The solid matter may or may not have been previously broken into pieces.

Body Part Character 4		Approach Character 5	Device Character 6	Qualifier Character 7

Ø Sternum
   Manubrium
   Suprasternal notch
   Xiphoid process
 1 Ribs, 1 to 2
 2 Ribs, 3 or More
 3 Cervical Vertebra
   Dens
   Odontoid process
   Spinous process
   Transverse foramen
   Transverse process
   Vertebral arch
   Vertebral body
   Vertebral foramen
   Vertebral lamina
   Vertebral pedicle
 4 Thoracic Vertebra
   Spinous process
   Transverse process
   Vertebral arch
   Vertebral body
   Vertebral foramen
   Vertebral lamina
   Vertebral pedicle
 5 Scapula, Right
   Acromion (process)
   Coracoid process
 6 Scapula, Left
   See 5 Scapula, Right
 7 Glenoid Cavity, Right
   Glenoid fossa (of scapula)
 8 Glenoid Cavity, Left
   See 7 Glenoid Cavity, Right
 9 Clavicle, Right
 B Clavicle, Left
 C Humeral Head, Right
   Greater tuberosity
   Lesser tuberosity
   Neck of humerus
     (anatomical)(surgical)
 D Humeral Head, Left
   See C Humeral Head, Right
	F Humeral Shaft, Right
	   Distal humerus
	   Humerus, distal
	   Lateral epicondyle of
	     humerus
	   Medial epicondyle of
	     humerus
	 G Humeral Shaft, Left
	   See F Humeral Shaft, Right
	 H Radius, Right
	   Ulnar notch
	 J Radius, Left
	   See H Radius, Right
	 K Ulna, Right
	   Olecranon process
	   Radial notch
	 L Ulna, Left
	   See K Ulna, Right
	 M Carpal, Right
	   Capitate bone
	   Hamate bone
	   Lunate bone
	   Pisiform bone
	   Scaphoid bone
	   Trapezium bone
	   Trapezoid bone
	   Triquetral bone
	 N Carpal, Left
	   See M Carpal, Right
	 P Metacarpal, Right
	 Q Metacarpal, Left
	 R Thumb Phalanx, Right
	 S Thumb Phalanx, Left
	 T Finger Phalanx, Right
	 V Finger Phalanx, Left
		Ø Open
		 3 Percutaneous
		 4 Percutaneous Endoscopic
			Z No Device	**Z No Qualifier**

LC Limited Coverage   **NC** Noncovered   ⊞ Combination Member   HAC associated procedure   Combination Only   DRG Non-OR   Non-OR   New/Revised in **GREEN**

ICD-10-PCS 2021

545

ØPC–ØPC

Ø Medical and Surgical
P Upper Bones
D Extraction   Definition: Pulling or stripping out or off all or a portion of a body part by the use of force
                 Explanation: The qualifier DIAGNOSTIC is used to identify extraction procedures that are biopsies

Body Part Character 4		Approach Character 5	Device Character 6	Qualifier Character 7

Ø Sternum
  Manubrium
  Suprasternal notch
  Xiphoid process
1 Ribs, 1 to 2
2 Ribs, 3 or More
3 Cervical Vertebra
  Dens
  Odontoid process
  Spinous process
  Transverse foramen
  Transverse process
  Vertebral arch
  Vertebral body
  Vertebral foramen
  Vertebral lamina
  Vertebral pedicle
4 Thoracic Vertebra
  Spinous process
  Transverse process
  Vertebral arch
  Vertebral body
  Vertebral foramen
  Vertebral lamina
  Vertebral pedicle
5 Scapula, Right
  Acromion (process)
  Coracoid process
6 Scapula, Left
  See 5 Scapula, Right
7 Glenoid Cavity, Right
  Glenoid fossa (of scapula)
8 Glenoid Cavity, Left
  See 7 Glenoid Cavity, Right
9 Clavicle, Right
B Clavicle, Left
C Humeral Head, Right
  Greater tuberosity
  Lesser tuberosity
  Neck of humerus
    (anatomical)(surgical)
D Humeral Head, Left
  See C Humeral Head, Right
	F Humeral Shaft, Right
	  Distal humerus
	  Humerus, distal
	  Lateral epicondyle of
	    humerus
	  Medial epicondyle of
	    humerus
	G Humeral Shaft, Left
	  See F Humeral Shaft, Right
	H Radius, Right
	  Ulnar notch
	J Radius, Left
	  See H Radius, Right
	K Ulna, Right
	  Olecranon process
	  Radial notch
	L Ulna, Left
	  See K Ulna, Right
	M Carpal, Right
	  Capitate bone
	  Hamate bone
	  Lunate bone
	  Pisiform bone
	  Scaphoid bone
	  Trapezium bone
	  Trapezoid bone
	  Triquetral bone
	N Carpal, Left
	  See M Carpal, Right
	P Metacarpal, Right
	Q Metacarpal, Left
	R Thumb Phalanx, Right
	S Thumb Phalanx, Left
	T Finger Phalanx, Right
	V Finger Phalanx, Left
		Ø Open	**Z No Device**	**Z No Qualifier**

Upper Bones

Ø   Medical and Surgical
P   Upper Bones
H   Insertion   Definition: Putting in a nonbiological appliance that monitors, assists, performs, or prevents a physiological function but does not physically take the place of a body part
                  Explanation: None

Body Part Character 4		Approach Character 5	Device Character 6	Qualifier Character 7
Ø Sternum Manubrium Suprasternal notch Xiphoid process		**Ø Open** **3 Percutaneous** **4 Percutaneous Endoscopic**	**Ø Internal Fixation Device, Rigid Plate** **4 Internal Fixation Device**	**Z No Qualifier**
1 Ribs, 1 to 2 **2 Ribs, 3 or More** **3 Cervical Vertebra** Dens Odontoid process Spinous process Transverse foramen Transverse process Vertebral arch Vertebral body Vertebral foramen Vertebral lamina Vertebral pedicle **4 Thoracic Vertebra** Spinous process Transverse process Vertebral arch Vertebral body Vertebral foramen Vertebral lamina Vertebral pedicle	**5 Scapula, Right** Acromion (process) Coracoid process **6 Scapula, Left** *See 5 Scapula, Right* **7 Glenoid Cavity, Right** Glenoid fossa (of scapula) **8 Glenoid Cavity, Left** *See 7 Glenoid Cavity, Right* **9 Clavicle, Right** **B Clavicle, Left**	**Ø Open** **3 Percutaneous** **4 Percutaneous Endoscopic**	**4 Internal Fixation Device**	**Z No Qualifier**

C   Humeral Head, Right
Greater tuberosity
Lesser tuberosity
Neck of humerus
     (anatomical)(surgical)
D   Humeral Head, Left
See C Humeral Head, Right
	H Radius, Right
	Ulnar notch
	J Radius, Left
	See H Radius, Right
	K Ulna, Right
	Olecranon process
	Radial notch
	L Ulna, Left
	See K Ulna, Right
		Ø Open
		3 Percutaneous
		4 Percutaneous Endoscopic
			4 Internal Fixation Device
			5 External Fixation Device
			**6 Internal Fixation Device,
			     Intramedullary**
			**8 External Fixation Device,
			     Limb Lengthening**
			**B External Fixation Device,
			     Monoplanar**
			C External Fixation Device, Ring
			**D External Fixation Device,
			     Hybrid**
				Z No Qualifier

F   Humeral Shaft, Right
Distal humerus
Humerus, distal
Lateral epicondyle of
     humerus
Medial epicondyle of
     humerus
	G Humeral Shaft, Left
	See F Humeral Shaft, Right
		Ø Open
		3 Percutaneous
		4 Percutaneous Endoscopic
			4 Internal Fixation Device
			5 External Fixation Device
			**6 Internal Fixation Device,
			     Intramedullary**
			**7 Internal Fixation Device,
			     Intramedullary Limb
			     Lengthening**
			**8 External Fixation Device,
			     Limb Lengthening**
			**B External Fixation Device,
			     Monoplanar**
			C External Fixation Device, Ring
			**D External Fixation Device,
			     Hybrid**
				Z No Qualifier

M Carpal, Right Capitate bone Hamate bone Lunate bone Pisiform bone Scaphoid bone Trapezium bone Trapezoid bone Triquetral bone **N Carpal, Left** *See M Carpal, Right*	**P Metacarpal, Right** **Q Metacarpal, Left** **R Thumb Phalanx, Right** **S Thumb Phalanx, Left** **T Finger Phalanx, Right** **V Finger Phalanx, Left**	**Ø Open** **3 Percutaneous** **4 Percutaneous Endoscopic**	**4 Internal Fixation Device** **5 External Fixation Device**	**Z No Qualifier**
Y Upper Bone		**Ø Open** **3 Percutaneous** **4 Percutaneous Endoscopic**	**M Bone Growth Stimulator**	**Z No Qualifier**

Non-OR   ØPH[C,D,H,J,K,L][Ø,3,4]8Z
Non-OR   ØPH[F,G][Ø,3,4]8Z

LC Limited Coverage   **NC** Noncovered   ⊞ Combination Member   HAC associated procedure   Combination Only   DRG Non-OR   Non-OR   New/Revised in GREEN

Ø   **Medical and Surgical**
P   **Upper Bones**
J   **Inspection**   Definition: Visually and/or manually exploring a body part

Explanation: Visual exploration may be performed with or without optical instrumentation. Manual exploration may be performed directly or through intervening body layers.

Body Part Character 4	Approach Character 5	Device Character 6	Qualifier Character 7
Y Upper Bone	**Ø** Open **3** Percutaneous **4** Percutaneous Endoscopic **X** External	**Z** No Device	**Z** No Qualifier

Non-OR   ØPJY[3,X]ZZ

Ø   **Medical and Surgical**
P   **Upper Bones**
N   **Release**   Definition: Freeing a body part from an abnormal physical constraint by cutting or by the use of force

Explanation: Some of the restraining tissue may be taken out but none of the body part is taken out

Body Part Character 4	Approach Character 5	Device Character 6	Qualifier Character 7

Ø   Sternum
     Manubrium
     Suprasternal notch
     Xiphoid process
1   Ribs, 1 to 2
2   Ribs, 3 or More
3   Cervical Vertebra
     Dens
     Odontoid process
     Spinous process
     Transverse foramen
     Transverse process
     Vertebral arch
     Vertebral body
     Vertebral foramen
     Vertebral lamina
     Vertebral pedicle
4   Thoracic Vertebra
     Spinous process
     Transverse process
     Vertebral arch
     Vertebral body
     Vertebral foramen
     Vertebral lamina
     Vertebral pedicle
5   Scapula, Right
     Acromion (process)
     Coracoid process
6   Scapula, Left
     See 5 Scapula, Right
7   Glenoid Cavity, Right
     Glenoid fossa (of scapula)
8   Glenoid Cavity, Left
     See 7 Glenoid Cavity, Right
9   Clavicle, Right
B   Clavicle, Left
C   Humeral Head, Right
     Greater tuberosity
     Lesser tuberosity
     Neck of humerus
       (anatomical) (surgical)
D   Humeral Head, Left
     See C Humeral Head, Right
	F Humeral Shaft, Right
	     Distal humerus
	     Humerus, distal
	     Lateral epicondyle of
	       humerus
	     Medial epicondyle of
	       humerus
	G Humeral Shaft, Left
	     See F Humeral Shaft, Right
	H Radius, Right
	     Ulnar notch
	J Radius, Left
	     See H Radius, Right
	K Ulna, Right
	     Olecranon process
	     Radial notch
	L Ulna, Left
	     See K Ulna, Right
	M Carpal, Right
	     Capitate bone
	     Hamate bone
	     Lunate bone
	     Pisiform bone
	     Scaphoid bone
	     Trapezium bone
	     Trapezoid bone
	     Triquetral bone
	N Carpal, Left
	     See M Carpal, Right
	P Metacarpal, Right
	Q Metacarpal, Left
	R Thumb Phalanx, Right
	S Thumb Phalanx, Left
	T Finger Phalanx, Right
	V Finger Phalanx, Left
		Ø Open
		3 Percutaneous
		4 Percutaneous Endoscopic
			Z No Device	**Z** No Qualifier

Ø **Medical and Surgical**
P **Upper Bones**
P **Removal** 　　Definition: Taking out or off a device from a body part

Explanation: If a device is taken out and a similar device put in without cutting or puncturing the skin or mucous membrane, the procedure is coded to the root operation CHANGE. Otherwise, the procedure for taking out a device is coded to the root operation REMOVAL.

Body Part Character 4		Approach Character 5	Device Character 6	Qualifier Character 7
Ø Sternum Manubrium Suprasternal notch Xiphoid process **1 Ribs, 1 to 2** **2 Ribs, 3 or More** **3 Cervical Vertebra** Dens Odontoid process Spinous process Transverse foramen Transverse process Vertebral arch Vertebral body Vertebral foramen Vertebral lamina Vertebral pedicle	**4 Thoracic Vertebra** Spinous process Transverse process Vertebral arch Vertebral body Vertebral foramen Vertebral lamina Vertebral pedicle **5 Scapula, Right** Acromion (process) Coracoid process **6 Scapula, Left** *See 5 Scapula, Right* **7 Glenoid Cavity, Right** Glenoid fossa (of scapula) **8 Glenoid Cavity, Left** *See 7 Glenoid Cavity, Right* **9 Clavicle, Right** **B Clavicle, Left**	**Ø Open** **3 Percutaneous** **4 Percutaneous Endoscopic**	**4 Internal Fixation Device** **7 Autologous Tissue Substitute** **J Synthetic Substitute** **K Nonautologous Tissue Substitute**	**Z No Qualifier**
Ø Sternum Manubrium Suprasternal notch Xiphoid process **1 Ribs, 1 to 2** **2 Ribs, 3 or More** **3 Cervical Vertebra** Dens Odontoid process Spinous process Transverse foramen Transverse process Vertebral arch Vertebral body Vertebral foramen Vertebral lamina Vertebral pedicle	**4 Thoracic Vertebra** Spinous process Transverse process Vertebral arch Vertebral body Vertebral foramen Vertebral lamina Vertebral pedicle **5 Scapula, Right** Acromion (process) Coracoid process **6 Scapula, Left** *See 5 Scapula, Right* **7 Glenoid Cavity, Right** Glenoid fossa (of scapula) **8 Glenoid Cavity, Left** *See 7 Glenoid Cavity, Right* **9 Clavicle, Right** **B Clavicle, Left**	**X External**	**4 Internal Fixation Device**	**Z No Qualifier**
C Humeral Head, Right Greater tuberosity Lesser tuberosity Neck of humerus (anatomical) (surgical) **D Humeral Head, Left** *See C Humeral Head, Right* **F Humeral Shaft, Right** Distal humerus Humerus, distal Lateral epicondyle of humerus Medial epicondyle of humerus **G Humeral Shaft, Left** *See F Humeral Shaft, Right* **H Radius, Right** Ulnar notch **J Radius, Left** *See H Radius, Right* **K Ulna, Right** Olecranon process Radial notch	**L Ulna, Left** *See K Ulna, Right* **M Carpal, Right** Capitate bone Hamate bone Lunate bone Pisiform bone Scaphoid bone Trapezium bone Trapezoid bone Triquetral bone **N Carpal, Left** *See M Carpal, Right* **P Metacarpal, Right** **Q Metacarpal, Left** **R Thumb Phalanx, Right** **S Thumb Phalanx, Left** **T Finger Phalanx, Right** **V Finger Phalanx, Left**	**Ø Open** **3 Percutaneous** **4 Percutaneous Endoscopic**	**4 Internal Fixation Device** **5 External Fixation Device** **7 Autologous Tissue Substitute** **J Synthetic Substitute** **K Nonautologous Tissue Substitute**	**Z No Qualifier**

Non-OR 　ØPP[Ø,1,2,3,4,5,6,7,8,9,B]X4Z

ØPP Continued on next page

LC Limited Coverage　NC Noncovered　⊞ Combination Member　HAC associated procedure　Combination Only　DRG Non-OR　Non-OR　New/Revised in GREEN

ICD-10-PCS 2021　　　　　　　　　　　　　　　　　　　　　　　　　　　　　　　549

ØPP–ØPP

Ø   **Medical and Surgical**   *ØPP Continued*
P   **Upper Bones**
P   **Removal**   Definition: Taking out or off a device from a body part

Explanation: If a device is taken out and a similar device put in without cutting or puncturing the skin or mucous membrane, the procedure is coded to the root operation CHANGE. Otherwise, the procedure for taking out a device is coded to the root operation REMOVAL.

Body Part Character 4		Approach Character 5	Device Character 6	Qualifier Character 7

C **Humeral Head, Right**
 Greater tuberosity
 Lesser tuberosity
 Neck of humerus
   (anatomical) (surgical)
 D **Humeral Head, Left**
 See C Humeral Head, Right
 F **Humeral Shaft, Right**
 Distal humerus
 Humerus, distal
 Lateral epicondyle of
   humerus
 Medial epicondyle of
   humerus
 G **Humeral Shaft, Left**
 See F Humeral Shaft, Right
 H **Radius, Right**
 Ulnar notch
 J **Radius, Left**
 See H Radius, Right
 K **Ulna, Right**
 Olecranon process
 Radial notch
	L **Ulna, Left**
	 See K Ulna, Right
	 M **Carpal, Right**
	 Capitate bone
	 Hamate bone
	 Lunate bone
	 Pisiform bone
	 Scaphoid bone
	 Trapezium bone
	 Trapezoid bone
	 Triquetral bone
	 N **Carpal, Left**
	 See M Carpal, Right
	 P **Metacarpal, Right**
	 Q **Metacarpal, Left**
	 R **Thumb Phalanx, Right**
	 S **Thumb Phalanx, Left**
	 T **Finger Phalanx, Right**
	 V **Finger Phalanx, Left**
		X External	**4** Internal Fixation Device
			 5 External Fixation Device
				Z No Qualifier

Y **Upper Bone**		**Ø** Open **3** Percutaneous **4** Percutaneous Endoscopic **X** External	**Ø** Drainage Device **M** Bone Growth Stimulator	**Z** No Qualifier

Non-OR   ØPP[C,D,F,G,H,J,K,L,M,N,P,Q,R,S,T,V]X[4,5]Z
Non-OR   ØPPY3ØZ
Non-OR   ØPPYX[Ø,M]Z

LC Limited Coverage   NC Noncovered   ⊞ Combination Member   HAC associated procedure   Combination Only   DRG Non-OR   Non-OR   New/Revised in GREEN

550   ICD-10-PCS 2021

ØPP–ØPP

Ø   **Medical and Surgical**
P   **Upper Bones**
Q   **Repair**   Definition: Restoring, to the extent possible, a body part to its normal anatomic structure and function
                  Explanation: Used only when the method to accomplish the repair is not one of the other root operations

Body Part Character 4		Approach Character 5	Device Character 6	Qualifier Character 7

Ø **Sternum**
  Manubrium
  Suprasternal notch
  Xiphoid process
1 **Ribs, 1 to 2**
2 **Ribs, 3 or More**
3 **Cervical Vertebra**
  Dens
  Odontoid process
  Spinous process
  Transverse foramen
  Transverse process
  Vertebral arch
  Vertebral body
  Vertebral foramen
  Vertebral lamina
  Vertebral pedicle
4 **Thoracic Vertebra**
  Spinous process
  Transverse process
  Vertebral arch
  Vertebral body
  Vertebral foramen
  Vertebral lamina
  Vertebral pedicle
5 **Scapula, Right**
  Acromion (process)
  Coracoid process
6 **Scapula, Left**
  See 5 Scapula, Right
7 **Glenoid Cavity, Right**
  Glenoid fossa (of scapula)
8 **Glenoid Cavity, Left**
  See 7 Glenoid Cavity, Right
9 **Clavicle, Right**
B **Clavicle, Left**
C **Humeral Head, Right**
  Greater tuberosity
  Lesser tuberosity
  Neck of humerus
    (anatomical)(surgical)
D **Humeral Head, Left**
  See C Humeral Head, Right
	F **Humeral Shaft, Right**
	  Distal humerus
	  Humerus, distal
	  Lateral epicondyle of
	    humerus
	  Medial epicondyle of
	    humerus
	G **Humeral Shaft, Left**
	  See F Humeral Shaft, Right
	H **Radius, Right**
	  Ulnar notch
	J **Radius, Left**
	  See H Radius, Right
	K **Ulna, Right**
	  Olecranon process
	  Radial notch
	L **Ulna, Left**
	  See K Ulna, Right
	M **Carpal, Right**
	  Capitate bone
	  Hamate bone
	  Lunate bone
	  Pisiform bone
	  Scaphoid bone
	  Trapezium bone
	  Trapezoid bone
	  Triquetral bone
	N **Carpal, Left**
	  See M Carpal, Right
	P **Metacarpal, Right**
	Q **Metacarpal, Left**
	R **Thumb Phalanx, Right**
	S **Thumb Phalanx, Left**
	T **Finger Phalanx, Right**
	V **Finger Phalanx, Left**
		Ø Open
		3 Percutaneous
		4 Percutaneous Endoscopic
		X External
			Z No Device	Z No Qualifier

Non-OR   ØPQ[Ø,1,2,3,4,5,6,7,8,9,B,C,D,F,G,H,J,K,L,M,N,P,Q,R,S,T,V]XZZ

LC Limited Coverage   **NC** Noncovered   ⊞ Combination Member   HAC associated procedure   Combination Only   DRG Non-OR   Non-OR   New/Revised in **GREEN**

ICD-10-PCS 2021   **551**

ØPQ–ØPQ

Upper Bones

Ø   **Medical and Surgical**
P   **Upper Bones**
R   **Replacement**

Definition: Putting in or on biological or synthetic material that physically takes the place and/or function of all or a portion of a body part

Explanation: The body part may have been taken out or replaced, or may be taken out, physically eradicated, or rendered nonfunctional during the REPLACEMENT procedure. A REMOVAL procedure is coded for taking out the device used in a previous replacement procedure.

Body Part Character 4		Approach Character 5	Device Character 6	Qualifier Character 7

Ø **Sternum**
  Manubrium
  Suprasternal notch
  Xiphoid process
1 **Ribs, 1 to 2**
2 **Ribs, 3 or More**
3 **Cervical Vertebra**
  Dens
  Odontoid process
  Spinous process
  Transverse foramen
  Transverse process
  Vertebral arch
  Vertebral body
  Vertebral foramen
  Vertebral lamina
  Vertebral pedicle
4 **Thoracic Vertebra**
  Spinous process
  Transverse process
  Vertebral arch
  Vertebral body
  Vertebral foramen
  Vertebral lamina
  Vertebral pedicle
5 **Scapula, Right**
  Acromion (process)
  Coracoid process
6 **Scapula, Left**
  See 5 Scapula, Right
7 **Glenoid Cavity, Right**
  Glenoid fossa (of scapula)
8 **Glenoid Cavity, Left**
  See 7 Glenoid Cavity, Right
9 **Clavicle, Right**
B **Clavicle, Left**
C **Humeral Head, Right**
  Greater tuberosity
  Lesser tuberosity
  Neck of humerus
    (anatomical)(surgical)
D **Humeral Head, Left**
  See C Humeral Head, Right
	F **Humeral Shaft, Right**
	  Distal humerus
	  Humerus, distal
	  Lateral epicondyle of
	    humerus
	  Medial epicondyle of
	    humerus
	G **Humeral Shaft, Left**
	  See F Humeral Shaft, Right
	H **Radius, Right**
	  Ulnar notch
	J **Radius, Left**
	  See H Radius, Right
	K **Ulna, Right**
	  Olecranon process
	  Radial notch
	L **Ulna, Left**
	  See K Ulna, Right
	M **Carpal, Right**
	  Capitate bone
	  Hamate bone
	  Lunate bone
	  Pisiform bone
	  Scaphoid bone
	  Trapezium bone
	  Trapezoid bone
	  Triquetral bone
	N **Carpal, Left**
	  See M Carpal, Right
	P **Metacarpal, Right**
	Q **Metacarpal, Left**
	R **Thumb Phalanx, Right**
	S **Thumb Phalanx, Left**
	T **Finger Phalanx, Right**
	V **Finger Phalanx, Left**
		Ø Open
		3 Percutaneous
		4 Percutaneous Endoscopic
			7 Autologous Tissue
			  Substitute
			J Synthetic Substitute
			K Nonautologous Tissue
			  Substitute
				Z No Qualifier

LC Limited Coverage   NC Noncovered   ⊞ Combination Member   HAC associated procedure   Combination Only   DRG Non-OR   Non-OR   New/Revised in GREEN

552   ICD-10-PCS 2021

Ø   **Medical and Surgical**
P   **Upper Bones**
S   **Reposition**   Definition: Moving to its normal location, or other suitable location, all or a portion of a body part

Explanation: The body part is moved to a new location from an abnormal location, or from a normal location where it is not functioning correctly. The body part may or may not be cut out or off to be moved to the new location.

Body Part Character 4		Approach Character 5	Device Character 6	Qualifier Character 7
Ø **Sternum** Manubrium Suprasternal notch Xiphoid process		**Ø** Open **3** Percutaneous **4** Percutaneous Endoscopic	**Ø** Internal Fixation Device, Rigid Plate **4** Internal Fixation Device **Z** No Device	**Z** No Qualifier
Ø **Sternum** Manubrium Suprasternal notch Xiphoid process		**X** External	**Z** No Device	**Z** No Qualifier
1 **Ribs, 1 to 2** **2** **Ribs, 3 or More** **3** **Cervical Vertebra** ⊞ Dens Odontoid process Spinous process Transverse foramen Transverse process Vertebral arch Vertebral body Vertebral foramen Vertebral lamina Vertebral pedicle **4** **Thoracic Vertebra** ⊞ Spinous process Transverse process Vertebral arch Vertebral body Vertebral foramen Vertebral lamina Vertebral pedicle	**5** **Scapula, Right** Acromion (process) Coracoid process **6** **Scapula, Left** *See 5 Scapula, Right* **7** **Glenoid Cavity, Right** Glenoid fossa (of scapula) **8** **Glenoid Cavity, Left** *See 7 Glenoid Cavity, Right* **9** **Clavicle, Right** **B** **Clavicle, Left**	**Ø** Open **3** Percutaneous **4** Percutaneous Endoscopic	**4** Internal Fixation Device **Z** No Device	**Z** No Qualifier
1 **Ribs, 1 to 2** **2** **Ribs, 3 or More** **3** **Cervical Vertebra** Dens Odontoid process Spinous process Transverse foramen Transverse process Vertebral arch Vertebral body Vertebral foramen Vertebral lamina Vertebral pedicle **4** **Thoracic Vertebra** Spinous process Transverse process Vertebral arch Vertebral body Vertebral foramen Vertebral lamina Vertebral pedicle	**5** **Scapula, Right** Acromion (process) Coracoid process **6** **Scapula, Left** *See 5 Scapula, Right* **7** **Glenoid Cavity, Right** Glenoid fossa (of scapula) **8** **Glenoid Cavity, Left** *See 7 Glenoid Cavity, Right* **9** **Clavicle, Right** **B** **Clavicle, Left**	**X** External	**Z** No Device	**Z** No Qualifier
C **Humeral Head, Right** Greater tuberosity Lesser tuberosity Neck of humerus (anatomical)(surgical) **D** **Humeral Head, Left** *See C Humeral Head, Right* **F** **Humeral Shaft, Right** Distal humerus Humerus, distal Lateral epicondyle of humerus Medial epicondyle of humerus	**G** **Humeral Shaft, Left** *See F Humeral Shaft, Right* **H** **Radius, Right** Ulnar notch **J** **Radius, Left** *See H Radius, Right* **K** **Ulna, Right** Olecranon process Radial notch **L** **Ulna, Left** *See K Ulna, Right*	**Ø** Open **3** Percutaneous **4** Percutaneous Endoscopic	**4** Internal Fixation Device **5** External Fixation Device **6** Internal Fixation Device, Intramedullary **B** External Fixation Device, Monoplanar **C** External Fixation Device, Ring **D** External Fixation Device, Hybrid **Z** No Device	**Z** No Qualifier

Non-OR ØPSØ[3,4]ZZ		
Non-OR ØPSØXZZ		
Non-OR ØPS[1,2,5,6,7,8,9,B][3,4]ZZ	**See Appendix L for Procedure Combinations**	
Non-OR ØPS[1,2,3,4,5,6,7,8,9,B]XZZ	⊞ ØPS[3,4]3ZZ	
Non-OR ØPS[C,D,F,G,H,J,K,L][3,4]ZZ		

ØPS Continued on next page

LC Limited Coverage   **NC** Noncovered   ⊞ Combination Member   HAC associated procedure   Combination Only   DRG Non-OR   Non-OR   New/Revised in GREEN

ICD-10-PCS 2021   553

ØPS–ØPS

Ø   **Medical and Surgical**
P   **Upper Bones**
S   **Reposition**

Definition: Moving to its normal location, or other suitable location, all or a portion of a body part

Explanation: The body part is moved to a new location from an abnormal location, or from a normal location where it is not functioning correctly. The body part may or may not be cut out or off to be moved to the new location.

Body Part — Character 4		Approach — Character 5	Device — Character 6	Qualifier — Character 7

C Humeral Head, Right
  Greater tuberosity
  Lesser tuberosity
  Neck of humerus
    (anatomical)(surgical)
D Humeral Head, Left
  See C Humeral Head, Right
F Humeral Shaft, Right
  Distal humerus
  Humerus, distal
  Lateral epicondyle of
    humerus
  Medial epicondyle of
    humerus
	G Humeral Shaft, Left
	  See F Humeral Shaft, Right
	H Radius, Right
	  Ulnar notch
	J Radius, Left
	  See H Radius, Right
	K Ulna, Right
	  Olecranon process
	  Radial notch
	L Ulna, Left
	  See K Ulna, Right
		X External	**Z** No Device	**Z** No Qualifier

M Carpal, Right
  Capitate bone
  Hamate bone
  Lunate bone
  Pisiform bone
  Scaphoid bone
  Trapezium bone
  Trapezoid bone
  Triquetral bone
	N Carpal, Left
	  See M Carpal, Right
	P Metacarpal, Right
	Q Metacarpal, Left
	R Thumb Phalanx, Right
	S Thumb Phalanx, Left
	T Finger Phalanx, Right
	V Finger Phalanx, Left
		Ø Open
		3 Percutaneous
		4 Percutaneous Endoscopic
			4 Internal Fixation Device
			5 External Fixation Device
			Z No Device
				Z No Qualifier

M Carpal, Right
  Capitate bone
  Hamate bone
  Lunate bone
  Pisiform bone
  Scaphoid bone
  Trapezium bone
  Trapezoid bone
  Triquetral bone
	N Carpal, Left
	  See M Carpal, Right
	P Metacarpal, Right
	Q Metacarpal, Left
	R Thumb Phalanx, Right
	S Thumb Phalanx, Left
	T Finger Phalanx, Right
	V Finger Phalanx, Left
		X External	**Z** No Device	**Z** No Qualifier

Non-OR   ØPS[C,D,F,G,H,J,K,L]XZZ
Non-OR   ØPS[M,N,P,Q,R,S,T,V][3,4]ZZ
Non-OR   ØPS[M,N,P,Q,R,S,T,V]XZZ

Ø   **Medical and Surgical**
P   **Upper Bones**
T   **Resection**

Definition: Cutting out or off, without replacement, all of a body part

Explanation: None

Body Part — Character 4		Approach — Character 5	Device — Character 6	Qualifier — Character 7

Ø Sternum
  Manubrium
  Suprasternal notch
  Xiphoid process
1 Ribs, 1 to 2
2 Ribs, 3 or More
5 Scapula, Right
  Acromion (process)
  Coracoid process
6 Scapula, Left
  See 5 Scapula, Right
7 Glenoid Cavity, Right
  Glenoid fossa (of scapula)
8 Glenoid Cavity, Left
  See 7 Glenoid Cavity, Right
9 Clavicle, Right
B Clavicle, Left
C Humeral Head, Right
  Greater tuberosity
  Lesser tuberosity
  Neck of humerus
    (anatomical) (surgical)
D Humeral Head, Left
  See C Humeral Head, Right
F Humeral Shaft, Right
  Distal humerus
  Humerus, distal
  Lateral epicondyle of humerus
  Medial epicondyle of humerus
	G Humeral Shaft, Left
	  See F Humeral Shaft, Right
	H Radius, Right
	  Ulnar notch
	J Radius, Left
	  See H Radius, Right
	K Ulna, Right
	  Olecranon process
	  Radial notch
	L Ulna, Left
	  See K Ulna, Right
	M Carpal, Right
	  Capitate bone
	  Hamate bone
	  Lunate bone
	  Pisiform bone
	  Scaphoid bone
	  Trapezium bone
	  Trapezoid bone
	  Triquetral bone
	N Carpal, Left
	  See M Carpal, Right
	P Metacarpal, Right
	Q Metacarpal, Left
	R Thumb Phalanx, Right
	S Thumb Phalanx, Left
	T Finger Phalanx, Right
	V Finger Phalanx, Left
		Ø Open	**Z** No Device	**Z** No Qualifier

LC Limited Coverage   NC Noncovered   ⊞ Combination Member   HAC associated procedure   Combination Only   DRG Non-OR   Non-OR   New/Revised in GREEN

554   ICD-10-PCS 2021

ØPS–ØPT

Ø   Medical and Surgical
P   Upper Bones
U   Supplement

Definition: Putting in or on biological or synthetic material that physically reinforces and/or augments the function of a portion of a body part
Explanation: The biological material is non-living, or is living and from the same individual. The body part may have been previously replaced, and the SUPPLEMENT procedure is performed to physically reinforce and/or augment the function of the replaced body part.

Body Part Character 4		Approach Character 5	Device Character 6	Qualifier Character 7
Ø Sternum	**D Humeral Head, Left**	**Ø Open**	**7 Autologous Tissue**	**Z No Qualifier**
Manubrium	*See C Humeral Head, Right*	**3 Percutaneous**	**Substitute**	
Suprasternal notch	**F Humeral Shaft, Right**	**4 Percutaneous Endoscopic**	**J Synthetic Substitute**	
Xiphoid process	Distal humerus		**K Nonautologous Tissue**	
1 Ribs, 1 to 2	Humerus, distal		**Substitute**	
2 Ribs, 3 or More	Lateral epicondyle of			
3 Cervical Vertebra ⊞	humerus			
Dens	Medial epicondyle of			
Odontoid process	humerus			
Spinous process	**G Humeral Shaft, Left**			
Transverse foramen	*See F Humeral Shaft, Right*			
Transverse process	**H Radius, Right**			
Vertebral arch	Ulnar notch			
Vertebral body	**J Radius, Left**			
Vertebral foramen	*See H Radius, Right*			
Vertebral lamina	**K Ulna, Right**			
Vertebral pedicle	Olecranon process			
4 Thoracic Vertebra ⊞	Radial notch			
Spinous process	**L Ulna, Left**			
Transverse process	*See K Ulna, Right*			
Vertebral arch	**M Carpal, Right**			
Vertebral body	Capitate bone			
Vertebral foramen	Hamate bone			
Vertebral lamina	Lunate bone			
Vertebral pedicle	Pisiform bone			
5 Scapula, Right	Scaphoid bone			
Acromion (process)	Trapezium bone			
Coracoid process	Trapezoid bone			
6 Scapula, Left	Triquetral bone			
See 5 Scapula, Right	**N Carpal, Left**			
7 Glenoid Cavity, Right	*See M Carpal, Right*			
Glenoid fossa (of scapula)	**P Metacarpal, Right**			
8 Glenoid Cavity, Left	**Q Metacarpal, Left**			
See 7 Glenoid Cavity, Right	**R Thumb Phalanx, Right**			
9 Clavicle, Right	**S Thumb Phalanx, Left**			
B Clavicle, Left	**T Finger Phalanx, Right**			
C Humeral Head, Right	**V Finger Phalanx, Left**			
Greater tuberosity				
Lesser tuberosity				
Neck of humerus (anatomical) (surgical)				

See Appendix L for Procedure Combinations
⊞   ØPU[3,4]3JZ

Upper Bones

Ø **Medical and Surgical**
P **Upper Bones**
W **Revision**   Definition: Correcting, to the extent possible, a portion of a malfunctioning device or the position of a displaced device

Explanation: Revision can include correcting a malfunctioning or displaced device by taking out or putting in components of the device such as a screw or pin

Body Part Character 4		Approach Character 5	Device Character 6	Qualifier Character 7
Ø Sternum Manubrium Suprasternal notch Xiphoid process **1** Ribs, 1 to 2 **2** Ribs, 3 or More **3** Cervical Vertebra Dens Odontoid process Spinous process Transverse foramen Transverse process Vertebral arch Vertebral body Vertebral foramen Vertebral lamina Vertebral pedicle **4** Thoracic Vertebra Spinous process Transverse process Vertebral arch Vertebral body Vertebral foramen Vertebral lamina Vertebral pedicle	**5** Scapula, Right Acromion (process) Coracoid process **6** Scapula, Left *See 5 Scapula, Right* **7** Glenoid Cavity, Right Glenoid fossa (of scapula) **8** Glenoid Cavity, Left *See 7 Glenoid Cavity, Right* **9** Clavicle, Right **B** Clavicle, Left	**Ø** Open **3** Percutaneous **4** Percutaneous Endoscopic **X** External	**4** Internal Fixation Device **7** Autologous Tissue Substitute **J** Synthetic Substitute **K** Nonautologous Tissue Substitute	**Z** No Qualifier
C Humeral Head, Right Greater tuberosity Lesser tuberosity Neck of humerus (anatomical)(surgical) **D** Humeral Head, Left *See C Humeral Head, Right* **F** Humeral Shaft, Right Distal humerus Humerus, distal Lateral epicondyle of humerus Medial epicondyle of humerus **G** Humeral Shaft, Left *See F Humeral Shaft, Right* **H** Radius, Right Ulnar notch **J** Radius, Left *See H Radius, Right* **K** Ulna, Right Olecranon process Radial notch	**L** Ulna, Left *See K Ulna, Right* **M** Carpal, Right Capitate bone Hamate bone Lunate bone Pisiform bone Scaphoid bone Trapezium bone Trapezoid bone Triquetral bone **N** Carpal, Left *See M Carpal, Right* **P** Metacarpal, Right **Q** Metacarpal, Left **R** Thumb Phalanx, Right **S** Thumb Phalanx, Left **T** Finger Phalanx, Right **V** Finger Phalanx, Left	**Ø** Open **3** Percutaneous **4** Percutaneous Endoscopic **X** External	**4** Internal Fixation Device **5** External Fixation Device **7** Autologous Tissue Substitute **J** Synthetic Substitute **K** Nonautologous Tissue Substitute	**Z** No Qualifier
Y Upper Bone		**Ø** Open **3** Percutaneous **4** Percutaneous Endoscopic **X** External	**Ø** Drainage Device **M** Bone Growth Stimulator	**Z** No Qualifier

Non-OR   ØPW[Ø,1,2,3,4,5,6,7,8,9,B]X[4,7,J,K]Z
Non-OR   ØPW[C,D,F,G,H,J,K,L,M,N,P,Q,R,S,T,V]X[4,5,7,J,K]Z
Non-OR   ØPWYX[Ø,M]Z

Lower Bones ØQ2–ØQW

Character Meanings

This Character Meaning table is provided as a guide to assist the user in the identification of character members that may be found in this section of code tables. It **SHOULD NOT** be used to build a PCS code.

Operation–Character 3		Body Part–Character 4		Approach–Character 5		Device–Character 6		Qualifier–Character 7	
2	Change	Ø	Lumbar Vertebra	Ø	Open	Ø	Drainage Device	2	Sesamoid Bone(s) 1st Toe
5	Destruction	1	Sacrum	3	Percutaneous	4	Internal Fixation Device	X	Diagnostic
8	Division	2	Pelvic Bone, Right	4	Percutaneous Endoscopic	5	External Fixation Device	Z	No Qualifier
9	Drainage	3	Pelvic Bone, Left	X	External	6	Internal Fixation Device, Intramedullary		
B	Excision	4	Acetabulum, Right			7	Autologous Tissue Substitute OR Internal Fixation Device, Intramedullary Limb Lengthening		
C	Extirpation	5	Acetabulum, Left			8	External Fixation Device, Limb Lengthening		
D	Extraction	6	Upper Femur, Right			B	External Fixation Device, Monoplanar		
H	Insertion	7	Upper Femur, Left			C	External Fixation Device, Ring		
J	Inspection	8	Femoral Shaft, Right			D	External Fixation Device, Hybrid		
N	Release	9	Femoral Shaft, Left			J	Synthetic Substitute		
P	Removal	B	Lower Femur, Right			K	Nonautologous Tissue Substitute		
Q	Repair	C	Lower Femur, Left			M	Bone Growth Stimulator		
R	Replacement	D	Patella, Right			Y	Other Device		
S	Reposition	F	Patella, Left			Z	No Device		
T	Resection	G	Tibia, Right						
U	Supplement	H	Tibia, Left						
W	Revision	J	Fibula, Right						
		K	Fibula, Left						
		L	Tarsal, Right						
		M	Tarsal, Left						
		N	Metatarsal, Right						
		P	Metatarsal, Left						
		Q	Toe Phalanx, Right						
		R	Toe Phalanx, Left						
		S	Coccyx						
		Y	Lower Bone						

AHA Coding Clinic for table 0Q8

2018, 1Q, 25	Periacetabular osteotomy for repair of congenital hip dysplasia
2016, 2Q, 31	Periacetabular ostectomy for repair of congenital hip dysplasia

AHA Coding Clinic for table 0QB

2020, 2Q, 26	Sacral Pressure Ulcer with Excisional and Nonexcisional Debridement of Same Site
2019, 2Q, 19	Cervical spinal fusion, decompression and placement of interfacet stabilization device
2018, 3Q, 17	Excisional debridement of periosteum
2017, 1Q, 23	Reconstruction of mandible using titanium and bone
2016, 3Q, 30	Resection of femur with interposition arthroplasty
2015, 3Q, 3-8	Excisional and nonexcisional debridement
2015, 3Q, 26	Femoral head resection
2015, 2Q, 34	Decompressive laminectomy
2014, 4Q, 25	Femoroacetabular impingement and labral tear with repair
2014, 2Q, 6	Posterior lumbar fusion with discectomy
2013, 4Q, 116	Spinal decompression
2013, 2Q, 39	Ankle fusion, osteotomy, and removal of hardware
2012, 2Q, 19	Multiple decompressive cervical laminectomies

AHA Coding Clinic for table 0QD

2017, 4Q, 41	Extraction procedures

AHA Coding Clinic for table 0QH

2019, 4Q, 34	Intramedullary limb lengthening internal fixation device
2017, 1Q, 21	Staged scoliosis surgery with iliac fixation and spinal fusion
2016, 3Q, 34	Tibial/fibula epiphysiodesis

AHA Coding Clinic for table 0QP

2017, 4Q, 74-75	Magnetic growth rods
2015, 2Q, 6	Planned implant break

AHA Coding Clinic for table 0QQ

2018, 1Q, 15	Pubic symphysis fusion
2014, 3Q, 24	Repair of lipomyelomeningocele and tethered cord

AHA Coding Clinic for table 0QR

2017, 1Q, 22	Total knee replacement and patellar component
2016, 3Q, 30	Resection of femur with interposition arthroplasty

AHA Coding Clinic for table 0QS

2020, 1Q, 33	Spinal fusion without use of bone graft
2019, 3Q, 26	Open reduction with internal fixation and placement of strut allograft
2018, 1Q, 13	Bilateral cuboid osteotomy for repair of congenital talipes equinovarus
2018, 1Q, 25	Periacetabular osteotomy for repair of congenital hip dysplasia
2016, 3Q, 34	Tibial/fibula epiphysiodesis
2014, 4Q, 29	Rotational osteosynthesis
2014, 4Q, 29	Reposition of femur for correction of valgus and recurvatum deformities

AHA Coding Clinic for table 0QT

2017, 1Q, 22	Chopart amputation of foot
2016, 3Q, 30	Resection of femur with interposition arthroplasty
2015, 3Q, 26	Femoral head resection
2014, 4Q, 29	Rotational osteosynthesis

AHA Coding Clinic for table 0QU

2019, 3Q, 26	Open reduction with internal fixation and placement of strut allograft
2019, 2Q, 35	Kiva® kyphoplasty
2015, 3Q, 18	Total hip replacement with acetabular reconstruction
2014, 4Q, 31	Reposition of femur for correction of valgus and recurvatum deformities
2014, 2Q, 12	Percutaneous vertebroplasty using cement
2013, 2Q, 35	Use of bone void filler in grafting

AHA Coding Clinic for table 0QW

2017, 4Q, 74-75	Magnetic growth rods

Lower Bones

Lumbar vertebra **Ø**

Pelvic **2, 3**

Sacrum **1**

Coccyx **S**

Acetabulum **4, 5**

Femur **6, 7, 8, 9, B, C**

Patella **D, F**

Tibia **G, H**

Fibula **J, K**

Metatarsal **N, P**

Tarsal **L, M**

Toe phalanx **Q, R**

Hip Bone Anatomy

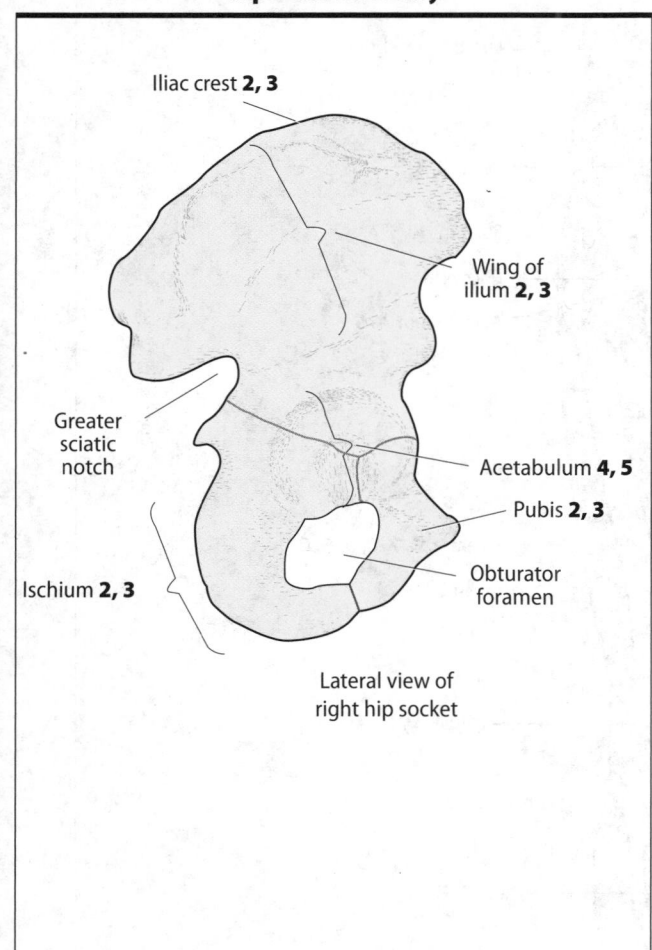

Iliac crest **2, 3**

Wing of ilium **2, 3**

Acetabulum **4, 5**

Greater sciatic notch

Pubis **2, 3**

Obturator foramen

Ischium **2, 3**

Lateral view of right hip socket

Pelvic and Lower Extremity Bones

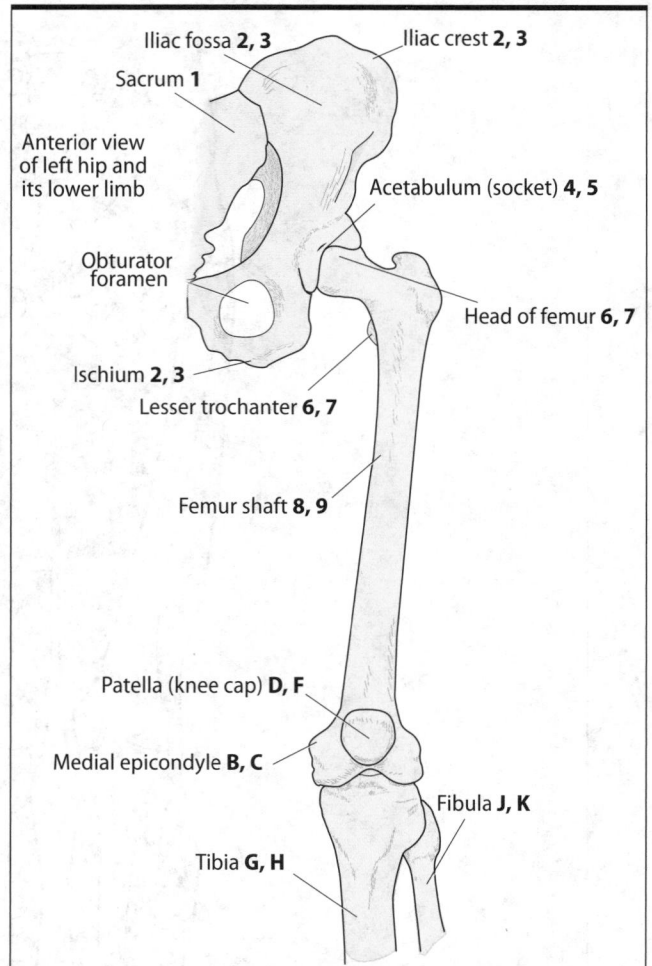

Iliac fossa **2, 3**

Sacrum **1**

Iliac crest **2, 3**

Anterior view of left hip and its lower limb

Acetabulum (socket) **4, 5**

Obturator foramen

Head of femur **6, 7**

Ischium **2, 3**

Lesser trochanter **6, 7**

Femur shaft **8, 9**

Patella (knee cap) **D, F**

Medial epicondyle **B, C**

Fibula **J, K**

Tibia **G, H**

Foot Bones

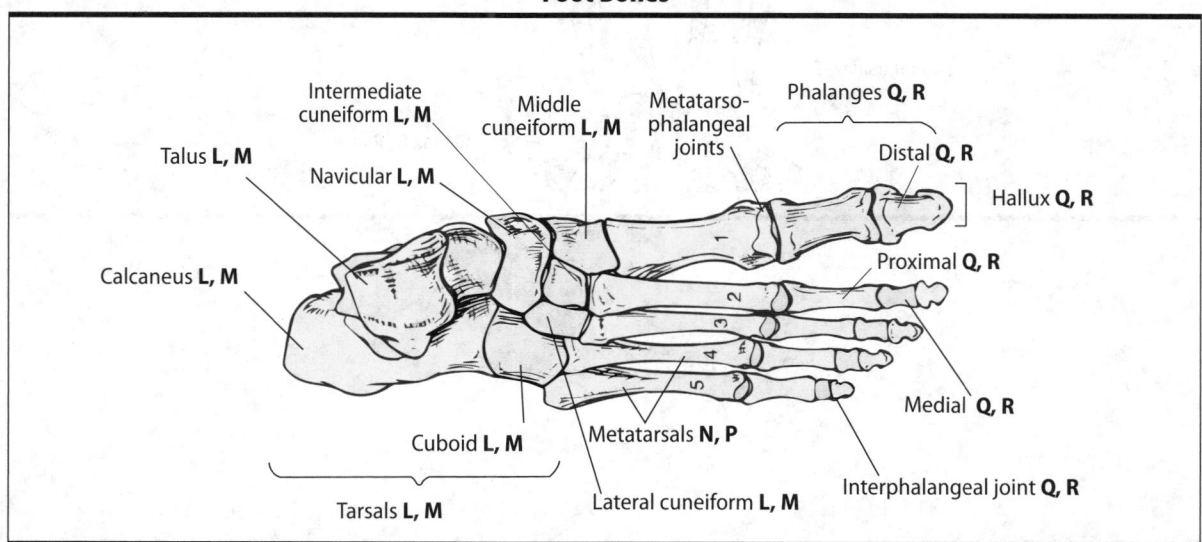

Intermediate cuneiform **L, M**

Middle cuneiform **L, M**

Metatarso-phalangeal joints

Phalanges **Q, R**

Talus **L, M**

Navicular **L, M**

Distal **Q, R**

Hallux **Q, R**

Calcaneus **L, M**

Proximal **Q, R**

Medial **Q, R**

Cuboid **L, M**

Metatarsals **N, P**

Tarsals **L, M**

Lateral cuneiform **L, M**

Interphalangeal joint **Q, R**

Ø   Medical and Surgical
Q   Lower Bones
2   Change   Definition: Taking out or off a device from a body part and putting back an identical or similar device in or on the same body part without cutting or puncturing the skin or a mucous membrane

Explanation: All CHANGE procedures are coded using the approach EXTERNAL

Body Part Character 4	Approach Character 5	Device Character 6	Qualifier Character 7
Y Lower Bone	X External	Ø Drainage Device Y Other Device	Z No Qualifier

Non-OR	All body part, approach, device, and qualifier values

Ø   Medical and Surgical
Q   Lower Bones
5   Destruction   Definition: Physical eradication of all or a portion of a body part by the direct use of energy, force, or a destructive agent

Explanation: None of the body part is physically taken out

Body Part Character 4		Approach Character 5	Device Character 6	Qualifier Character 7

Ø   Lumbar Vertebra
    Spinous process
    Transverse process
    Vertebral arch
    Vertebral body
    Vertebral foramen
    Vertebral lamina
    Vertebral pedicle
1   Sacrum
2   Pelvic Bone, Right
    Iliac crest
    Ilium
    Ischium
    Pubis
3   Pelvic Bone, Left
    See 2 Pelvic Bone, Right
4   Acetabulum, Right
5   Acetabulum, Left
6   Upper Femur, Right
    Femoral head
    Greater trochanter
    Lesser trochanter
    Neck of femur
7   Upper Femur, Left
    See 6 Upper Femur, Right
8   Femoral Shaft, Right
    Body of femur
9   Femoral Shaft, Left
    See 8 Femoral Shaft, Right
B   Lower Femur, Right
    Lateral condyle of femur
    Lateral epicondyle of femur
    Medial condyle of femur
    Medial epicondyle of femur
C   Lower Femur, Left
    See B Lower Femur, Right
	D Patella, Right
	F Patella, Left
	G Tibia, Right
	    Lateral condyle of tibia
	    Medial condyle of tibia
	    Medial malleolus
	H Tibia, Left
	    See G Tibia, Right
	J Fibula, Right
	    Body of fibula
	    Head of fibula
	    Lateral malleolus
	K Fibula, Left
	    See J Fibula, Right
	L Tarsal, Right
	    Calcaneus
	    Cuboid bone
	    Intermediate cuneiform
	       bone
	    Lateral cuneiform bone
	    Medial cuneiform bone
	    Navicular bone
	    Talus bone
	M Tarsal, Left
	    See L Tarsal, Right
	N Metatarsal, Right
	P Metatarsal, Left
	Q Toe Phalanx, Right
	R Toe Phalanx, Left
	S Coccyx
		Ø Open
		3 Percutaneous
		4 Percutaneous Endoscopic
			Z No Device	Z No Qualifier

LC Limited Coverage **NC** Noncovered ⊞ Combination Member HAC associated procedure Combination Only DRG Non-OR Non-OR New/Revised in GREEN

ICD-10-PCS 2021   561

Lower Bones

Ø   **Medical and Surgical**
Q   **Lower Bones**
8   **Division**   Definition: Cutting into a body part, without draining fluids and/or gases from the body part, in order to separate or transect a body part
                     Explanation: All or a portion of the body part is separated into two or more portions

Body Part Character 4	Approach Character 5	Device Character 6	Qualifier Character 7

Ø **Lumbar Vertebra**
    Spinous process
    Transverse process
    Vertebral arch
    Vertebral body
    Vertebral foramen
    Vertebral lamina
    Vertebral pedicle
1 **Sacrum**
2 **Pelvic Bone, Right**
    Iliac crest
    Ilium
    Ischium
    Pubis
3 **Pelvic Bone, Left**
    See 2 Pelvic Bone, Right
4 **Acetabulum, Right**
5 **Acetabulum, Left**
6 **Upper Femur, Right**
    Femoral head
    Greater trochanter
    Lesser trochanter
    Neck of femur
7 **Upper Femur, Left**
    See 6 Upper Femur, Right
8 **Femoral Shaft, Right**
    Body of femur
9 **Femoral Shaft, Left**
    See 8 Femoral Shaft, Right
B **Lower Femur, Right**
    Lateral condyle of femur
    Lateral epicondyle of femur
    Medial condyle of femur
    Medial epicondyle of femur
C **Lower Femur, Left**
    See B Lower Femur, Right
D **Patella, Right**
F **Patella, Left**
G **Tibia, Right**
    Lateral condyle of tibia
    Medial condyle of tibia
    Medial malleolus
H **Tibia, Left**
    See G Tibia, Right
J **Fibula, Right**
    Body of fibula
    Head of fibula
    Lateral malleolus
K **Fibula, Left**
    See J Fibula, Right
L **Tarsal, Right**
    Calcaneus
    Cuboid bone
    Intermediate cuneiform bone
    Lateral cuneiform bone
    Medial cuneiform bone
    Navicular bone
    Talus bone
M **Tarsal, Left**
    See L Tarsal, Right
N **Metatarsal, Right**
P **Metatarsal, Left**
Q **Toe Phalanx, Right**
R **Toe Phalanx, Left**
S **Coccyx**
	Ø Open
	3 Percutaneous
	4 Percutaneous Endoscopic
		Z No Device	Z No Qualifier

LC Limited Coverage   **NC** Noncovered   ⊞ Combination Member   HAC associated procedure   Combination Only   DRG Non-OR   Non-OR   New/Revised in GREEN

562   ICD-10-PCS 2021

0 **Medical and Surgical**
Q **Lower Bones**
9 **Drainage** Definition: Taking or letting out fluids and/or gases from a body part

Explanation: The qualifier DIAGNOSTIC is used to identify drainage procedures that are biopsies

Body Part Character 4		Approach Character 5	Device Character 6	Qualifier Character 7
0 **Lumbar Vertebra** Spinous process Transverse process Vertebral arch Vertebral body Vertebral foramen Vertebral lamina Vertebral pedicle **1** **Sacrum** **2** **Pelvic Bone, Right** Iliac crest Ilium Ischium Pubis **3** **Pelvic Bone, Left** *See 2 Pelvic Bone, Right* **4** **Acetabulum, Right** **5** **Acetabulum, Left** **6** **Upper Femur, Right** Femoral head Greater trochanter Lesser trochanter Neck of femur **7** **Upper Femur, Left** *See 6 Upper Femur, Right* **8** **Femoral Shaft, Right** Body of femur **9** **Femoral Shaft, Left** *See 8 Femoral Shaft, Right* **B** **Lower Femur, Right** Lateral condyle of femur Lateral epicondyle of femur Medial condyle of femur Medial epicondyle of femur	**C** **Lower Femur, Left** *See B Lower Femur, Right* **D** **Patella, Right** **F** **Patella, Left** **G** **Tibia, Right** Lateral condyle of tibia Medial condyle of tibia Medial malleolus **H** **Tibia, Left** *See G Tibia, Right* **J** **Fibula, Right** Body of fibula Head of fibula Lateral malleolus **K** **Fibula, Left** *See J Fibula, Right* **L** **Tarsal, Right** Calcaneus Cuboid bone Intermediate cuneiform bone Lateral cuneiform bone Medial cuneiform bone Navicular bone Talus bone **M** **Tarsal, Left** *See L Tarsal, Right* **N** **Metatarsal, Right** **P** **Metatarsal, Left** **Q** **Toe Phalanx, Right** **R** **Toe Phalanx, Left** **S** **Coccyx**	**0** Open **3** Percutaneous **4** Percutaneous Endoscopic	**0** Drainage Device	**Z** No Qualifier
0 **Lumbar Vertebra** Spinous process Transverse process Vertebral arch Vertebral body Vertebral foramen Vertebral lamina Vertebral pedicle **1** **Sacrum** **2** **Pelvic Bone, Right** Iliac crest Ilium Ischium Pubis **3** **Pelvic Bone, Left** *See 2 Pelvic Bone, Right* **4** **Acetabulum, Right** **5** **Acetabulum, Left** **6** **Upper Femur, Right** Femoral head Greater trochanter Lesser trochanter Neck of femur **7** **Upper Femur, Left** *See 6 Upper Femur, Right* **8** **Femoral Shaft, Right** Body of femur **9** **Femoral Shaft, Left** *See 8 Femoral Shaft, Right* **B** **Lower Femur, Right** Lateral condyle of femur Lateral epicondyle of femur Medial condyle of femur Medial epicondyle of femur	**C** **Lower Femur, Left** *See B Lower Femur, Right* **D** **Patella, Right** **F** **Patella, Left** **G** **Tibia, Right** Lateral condyle of tibia Medial condyle of tibia Medial malleolus **H** **Tibia, Left** *See G Tibia, Right* **J** **Fibula, Right** Body of fibula Head of fibula Lateral malleolus **K** **Fibula, Left** *See J Fibula, Right* **L** **Tarsal, Right** Calcaneus Cuboid bone Intermediate cuneiform bone Lateral cuneiform bone Medial cuneiform bone Navicular bone Talus bone **M** **Tarsal, Left** *See L Tarsal, Right* **N** **Metatarsal, Right** **P** **Metatarsal, Left** **Q** **Toe Phalanx, Right** **R** **Toe Phalanx, Left** **S** **Coccyx**	**0** Open **3** Percutaneous **4** Percutaneous Endoscopic	**Z** No Device	**X** Diagnostic **Z** No Qualifier

Non-OR 0Q9[0,1,2,3,4,5,6,7,8,9,B,C,D,F,G,H,J,K,L,M,P,Q,R,S]30Z
Non-OR 0Q9[0,1,2,3,4,5,6,7,8,9,B,C,D,F,G,H,J,K,L,M,P,Q,R,S]3ZZ

LC Limited Coverage **NC** Noncovered ⊞ Combination Member HAC associated procedure Combination Only DRG Non-OR Non-OR New/Revised in GREEN

ICD-10-PCS 2021 563

Ø Medical and Surgical
Q Lower Bones
B Excision

Definition: Cutting out or off, without replacement, a portion of a body part

Explanation: The qualifier DIAGNOSTIC is used to identify excision procedures that are biopsies

Body Part Character 4	Approach Character 5	Device Character 6	Qualifier Character 7
Ø Lumbar Vertebra Spinous process Transverse process Vertebral arch Vertebral body Vertebral foramen Vertebral lamina Vertebral pedicle **1 Sacrum** **2 Pelvic Bone, Right** Iliac crest Ilium Ischium Pubis **3 Pelvic Bone, Left** *See 2 Pelvic Bone, Right* **4 Acetabulum, Right** **5 Acetabulum, Left** **6 Upper Femur, Right** Femoral head Greater trochanter Lesser trochanter Neck of femur **7 Upper Femur, Left** *See 6 Upper Femur, Right* **8 Femoral Shaft, Right** Body of femur **9 Femoral Shaft, Left** *See 8 Femoral Shaft, Right* **B Lower Femur, Right** Lateral condyle of femur Lateral epicondyle of femur Medial condyle of femur Medial epicondyle of femur **C Lower Femur, Left** *See B Lower Femur, Right* **D Patella, Right** **F Patella, Left** **G Tibia, Right** Lateral condyle of tibia Medial condyle of tibia Medial malleolus **H Tibia, Left** *See G Tibia, Right* **J Fibula, Right** Body of fibula Head of fibula Lateral malleolus **K Fibula, Left** *See J Fibula, Right* **L Tarsal, Right** Calcaneus Cuboid bone Intermediate cuneiform bone Lateral cuneiform bone Medial cuneiform bone Navicular bone Talus bone **M Tarsal, Left** *See L Tarsal, Right* **N Metatarsal, Right** **P Metatarsal, Left** **Q Toe Phalanx, Right** **R Toe Phalanx, Left** **S Coccyx**	**Ø Open** **3 Percutaneous** **4 Percutaneous Endoscopic**	**Z No Device**	**X Diagnostic** **Z No Qualifier**

LC Limited Coverage   NC Noncovered   ⊞ Combination Member   HAC associated procedure   Combination Only   DRG Non-OR   Non-OR   New/Revised in GREEN

564   ICD-10-PCS 2021

Ø **Medical and Surgical**
Q **Lower Bones**
C **Extirpation**   Definition: Taking or cutting out solid matter from a body part

Explanation: The solid matter may be an abnormal byproduct of a biological function or a foreign body; it may be imbedded in a body part or in the lumen of a tubular body part. The solid matter may or may not have been previously broken into pieces.

Body Part Character 4		Approach Character 5	Device Character 6	Qualifier Character 7
Ø Lumbar Vertebra Spinous process Transverse process Vertebral arch Vertebral body Vertebral foramen Vertebral lamina Vertebral pedicle **1 Sacrum** **2 Pelvic Bone, Right** Iliac crest Ilium Ischium Pubis **3 Pelvic Bone, Left** *See 2 Pelvic Bone, Right* **4 Acetabulum, Right** **5 Acetabulum, Left** **6 Upper Femur, Right** Femoral head Greater trochanter Lesser trochanter Neck of femur **7 Upper Femur, Left** *See 6 Upper Femur, Right* **8 Femoral Shaft, Right** Body of femur **9 Femoral Shaft, Left** *See 8 Femoral Shaft, Right* **B Lower Femur, Right** Lateral condyle of femur Lateral epicondyle of femur Medial condyle of femur Medial epicondyle of femur	**C Lower Femur, Left** *See B Lower Femur, Right* **D Patella, Right** **F Patella, Left** **G Tibia, Right** Lateral condyle of tibia Medial condyle of tibia Medial malleolus **H Tibia, Left** *See G Tibia, Right* **J Fibula, Right** Body of fibula Head of fibula Lateral malleolus **K Fibula, Left** *See J Fibula, Right* **L Tarsal, Right** Calcaneus Cuboid bone Intermediate cuneiform bone Lateral cuneiform bone Medial cuneiform bone Navicular bone Talus bone **M Tarsal, Left** *See L Tarsal, Right* **N Metatarsal, Right** **P Metatarsal, Left** **Q Toe Phalanx, Right** **R Toe Phalanx, Left** **S Coccyx**	**Ø Open** **3 Percutaneous** **4 Percutaneous Endoscopic**	**Z No Device**	**Z No Qualifier**

Ø **Medical and Surgical**
Q **Lower Bones**
D **Extraction**   Definition: Pulling or stripping out or off all or a portion of a body part by the use of force

Explanation: The qualifier DIAGNOSTIC is used to identify extraction procedures that are biopsies

Body Part Character 4		Approach Character 5	Device Character 6	Qualifier Character 7
Ø Lumbar Vertebra Spinous process Transverse process Vertebral arch Vertebral body Vertebral foramen Vertebral lamina Vertebral pedicle **1 Sacrum** **2 Pelvic Bone, Right** Iliac crest Ilium Ischium Pubis **3 Pelvic Bone, Left** *See 2 Pelvic Bone, Right* **4 Acetabulum, Right** **5 Acetabulum, Left** **6 Upper Femur, Right** Femoral head Greater trochanter Lesser trochanter Neck of femur **7 Upper Femur, Left** *See 6 Upper Femur, Right* **8 Femoral Shaft, Right** Body of femur **9 Femoral Shaft, Left** *See 8 Femoral Shaft, Right* **B Lower Femur, Right** Lateral condyle of femur Lateral epicondyle of femur Medial condyle of femur Medial epicondyle of femur	**C Lower Femur, Left** *See B Lower Femur, Right* **D Patella, Right** **F Patella, Left** **G Tibia, Right** Lateral condyle of tibia Medial condyle of tibia Medial malleolus **H Tibia, Left** *See G Tibia, Right* **J Fibula, Right** Body of fibula Head of fibula Lateral malleolus **K Fibula, Left** *See J Fibula, Right* **L Tarsal, Right** Calcaneus Cuboid bone Intermediate cuneiform bone Lateral cuneiform bone Medial cuneiform bone Navicular bone Talus bone **M Tarsal, Left** *See L Tarsal, Right* **N Metatarsal, Right** **P Metatarsal, Left** **Q Toe Phalanx, Right** **R Toe Phalanx, Left** **S Coccyx**	**Ø Open**	**Z No Device**	**Z No Qualifier**

[LC] Limited Coverage   [NC] Noncovered   ⊞ Combination Member   HAC associated procedure   Combination Only   DRG Non-OR   Non-OR   New/Revised in GREEN

ICD-10-PCS 2021   **565**

Ø **Medical and Surgical**
Q **Lower Bones**
H **Insertion** Definition: Putting in a nonbiological appliance that monitors, assists, performs, or prevents a physiological function but does not physically take the place of a body part

Explanation: None

Body Part Character 4		Approach Character 5	Device Character 6	Qualifier Character 7
Ø **Lumbar Vertebra** Spinous process Transverse process Vertebral arch Vertebral body Vertebral foramen Vertebral lamina Vertebral pedicle **1** **Sacrum** **2** **Pelvic Bone, Right** Iliac crest Ilium Ischium Pubis **3** **Pelvic Bone, Left** *See* 2 Pelvic Bone, Right **4** **Acetabulum, Right** **5** **Acetabulum, Left**	**D** **Patella, Right** **F** **Patella, Left** **L** **Tarsal, Right** Calcaneus Cuboid bone Intermediate cuneiform bone Lateral cuneiform bone Medial cuneiform bone Navicular bone Talus bone **M** **Tarsal, Left** *See* L Tarsal, Right **N** **Metatarsal, Right** **P** **Metatarsal, Left** **Q** **Toe Phalanx, Right** **R** **Toe Phalanx, Left** **S** **Coccyx**	**Ø** **Open** **3** **Percutaneous** **4** **Percutaneous Endoscopic**	**4** **Internal Fixation Device** **5** **External Fixation Device**	**Z** **No Qualifier**
6 **Upper Femur, Right** Femoral head Greater trochanter Lesser trochanter Neck of femur **7** **Upper Femur, Left** *See* 6 Upper Femur, Right **B** **Lower Femur, Right** Lateral condyle of femur Lateral epicondyle of femur Medial condyle of femur Medial epicondyle of femur	**C** **Lower Femur, Left** *See* B Lower Femur, Right **J** **Fibula, Right** Body of fibula Head of fibula Lateral malleolus **K** **Fibula, Left** *See* J Fibula, Right	**Ø** **Open** **3** **Percutaneous** **4** **Percutaneous Endoscopic**	**4** **Internal Fixation Device** **5** **External Fixation Device** **6** **Internal Fixation Device, Intramedullary** **8** **External Fixation Device, Limb Lengthening** **B** **External Fixation Device, Monoplanar** **C** **External Fixation Device, Ring** **D** **External Fixation Device, Hybrid**	**Z** **No Qualifier**
8 **Femoral Shaft, Right** Body of femur **9** **Femoral Shaft, Left** *See* 8 Femoral Shaft, Right	**G** **Tibia, Right** Lateral condyle of tibia Medial condyle of tibia Medial malleolus **H** **Tibia, Left** *See* G Tibia, Right	**Ø** **Open** **3** **Percutaneous** **4** **Percutaneous Endoscopic**	**4** **Internal Fixation Device** **5** **External Fixation Device** **6** **Internal Fixation Device, Intramedullary** **7** **Internal Fixation Device, Intramedullary Limb Lengthening** **8** **External Fixation Device, Limb Lengthening** **B** **External Fixation Device, Monoplanar** **C** **External Fixation Device, Ring** **D** **External Fixation Device, Hybrid**	**Z** **No Qualifier**
Y **Lower Bone**		**Ø** **Open** **3** **Percutaneous** **4** **Percutaneous Endoscopic**	**M** **Bone Growth Stimulator**	**Z** **No Qualifier**

Non-OR ØQH[6,7,B,C,J,K][Ø,3,4]8Z
Non-OR ØQH[8,9,G,H][Ø,3,4]8Z

Ø **Medical and Surgical**
Q **Lower Bones**
J **Inspection** Definition: Visually and/or manually exploring a body part

Explanation: Visual exploration may be performed with or without optical instrumentation. Manual exploration may be performed directly or through intervening body layers.

Body Part Character 4	Approach Character 5	Device Character 6	Qualifier Character 7
Y **Lower Bone**	**Ø** **Open** **3** **Percutaneous** **4** **Percutaneous Endoscopic** **X** **External**	**Z** **No Device**	**Z** **No Qualifier**

Non-OR ØQJY[3,X]ZZ

LC Limited Coverage   NC Noncovered   ⊞ Combination Member   HAC associated procedure   Combination Only   DRG Non-OR   Non-OR   New/Revised in GREEN

566

ICD-10-PCS 2021

ØQH–ØQJ

Ø   Medical and Surgical
Q   Lower Bones
N   Release   Definition: Freeing a body part from an abnormal physical constraint by cutting or by the use of force
               Explanation: Some of the restraining tissue may be taken out but none of the body part is taken out

Body Part — Character 4		Approach — Character 5	Device — Character 6	Qualifier — Character 7
Ø **Lumbar Vertebra** Spinous process Transverse process Vertebral arch Vertebral body Vertebral foramen Vertebral lamina Vertebral pedicle **1** **Sacrum** **2** **Pelvic Bone, Right** Iliac crest Ilium Ischium Pubis **3** **Pelvic Bone, Left** *See 2 Pelvic Bone, Right* **4** **Acetabulum, Right** **5** **Acetabulum, Left** **6** **Upper Femur, Right** Femoral head Greater trochanter Lesser trochanter Neck of femur **7** **Upper Femur, Left** *See 6 Upper Femur, Right* **8** **Femoral Shaft, Right** Body of femur **9** **Femoral Shaft, Left** *See 8 Femoral Shaft, Right* **B** **Lower Femur, Right** Lateral condyle of femur Lateral epicondyle of femur Medial condyle of femur Medial epicondyle of femur	**C** **Lower Femur, Left** *See B Lower Femur, Right* **D** **Patella, Right** **F** **Patella, Left** **G** **Tibia, Right** Lateral condyle of tibia Medial condyle of tibia Medial malleolus **H** **Tibia, Left** *See G Tibia, Right* **J** **Fibula, Right** Body of fibula Head of fibula Lateral malleolus **K** **Fibula, Left** *See J Fibula, Right* **L** **Tarsal, Right** Calcaneus Cuboid bone Intermediate cuneiform bone Lateral cuneiform bone Medial cuneiform bone Navicular bone Talus bone **M** **Tarsal, Left** *See L Tarsal, Right* **N** **Metatarsal, Right** **P** **Metatarsal, Left** **Q** **Toe Phalanx, Right** **R** **Toe Phalanx, Left** **S** **Coccyx**	**Ø** **Open** **3** **Percutaneous** **4** **Percutaneous Endoscopic**	**Z** **No Device**	**Z** **No Qualifier**

Lower Bones *(side margin)*

Ø   Medical and Surgical
Q   Lower Bones
P   Removal

Definition: Taking out or off a device from a body part

Explanation: If a device is taken out and a similar device put in without cutting or puncturing the skin or mucous membrane, the procedure is coded to the root operation CHANGE. Otherwise, the procedure for taking out a device is coded to the root operation REMOVAL.

Body Part Character 4		Approach Character 5	Device Character 6	Qualifier Character 7
Ø Lumbar Vertebra Spinous process Transverse process Vertebral arch Vertebral body Vertebral foramen Vertebral lamina Vertebral pedicle **1 Sacrum** **2 Pelvic Bone, Right** Iliac crest Ilium Ischium Pubis **3 Pelvic Bone, Left** *See 2 Pelvic Bone, Right* **4 Acetabulum, Right** **5 Acetabulum, Left** **6 Upper Femur, Right** Femoral head Greater trochanter Lesser trochanter Neck of femur **7 Upper Femur, Left** *See 6 Upper Femur, Right* **8 Femoral Shaft, Right** Body of femur **9 Femoral Shaft, Left** *See 8 Femoral Shaft, Right* **B Lower Femur, Right** Lateral condyle of femur Lateral epicondyle of femur Medial condyle of femur Medial epicondyle of femur	**C Lower Femur, Left** *See B Lower Femur, Right* **D Patella, Right** **F Patella, Left** **G Tibia, Right** Lateral condyle of tibia Medial condyle of tibia Medial malleolus **H Tibia, Left** *See G Tibia, Right* **J Fibula, Right** Body of fibula Head of fibula Lateral malleolus **K Fibula, Left** *See J Fibula, Right* **L Tarsal, Right** Calcaneus Cuboid bone Intermediate cuneiform bone Lateral cuneiform bone Medial cuneiform bone Navicular bone Talus bone **M Tarsal, Left** *See L Tarsal, Right* **N Metatarsal, Right** **P Metatarsal, Left** **Q Toe Phalanx, Right** **R Toe Phalanx, Left** **S Coccyx**	**Ø Open** **3 Percutaneous** **4 Percutaneous Endoscopic**	**4 Internal Fixation Device** **5 External Fixation Device** **7 Autologous Tissue Substitute** **J Synthetic Substitute** **K Nonautologous Tissue Substitute**	**Z No Qualifier**
Ø Lumbar Vertebra Spinous process Transverse process Vertebral arch Vertebral body Vertebral foramen Vertebral lamina Vertebral pedicle **1 Sacrum** **2 Pelvic Bone, Right** Iliac crest Ilium Ischium Pubis **3 Pelvic Bone, Left** *See 2 Pelvic Bone, Right* **4 Acetabulum, Right** **5 Acetabulum, Left** **6 Upper Femur, Right** Femoral head Greater trochanter Lesser trochanter Neck of femur **7 Upper Femur, Left** *See 6 Upper Femur, Right* **8 Femoral Shaft, Right** Body of femur **9 Femoral Shaft, Left** *See 8 Femoral Shaft, Right* **B Lower Femur, Right** Lateral condyle of femur Lateral epicondyle of femur Medial condyle of femur Medial epicondyle of femur	**C Lower Femur, Left** *See B Lower Femur, Right* **D Patella, Right** **F Patella, Left** **G Tibia, Right** Lateral condyle of tibia Medial condyle of tibia Medial malleolus **H Tibia, Left** *See G Tibia, Right* **J Fibula, Right** Body of fibula Head of fibula Lateral malleolus **K Fibula, Left** *See J Fibula, Right* **L Tarsal, Right** Calcaneus Cuboid bone Intermediate cuneiform bone Lateral cuneiform bone Medial cuneiform bone Navicular bone Talus bone **M Tarsal, Left** *See L Tarsal, Right* **N Metatarsal, Right** **P Metatarsal, Left** **Q Toe Phalanx, Right** **R Toe Phalanx, Left** **S Coccyx**	**X External**	**4 Internal Fixation Device** **5 External Fixation Device**	**Z No Qualifier**
Y Lower Bone		**Ø Open** **3 Percutaneous** **4 Percutaneous Endoscopic** **X External**	**Ø Drainage Device** **M Bone Growth Stimulator**	**Z No Qualifier**

Non-OR	ØQP[Ø,1,4,5,S]X4Z	Non-OR	ØQPY3ØZ
Non-OR	ØQP[2,3,6,7,8,9,B,C,D,F,G,H,J,K,L,M,N,P,Q,R]X[4,5]Z	Non-OR	ØQPYX[Ø,M]Z

Ø   **Medical and Surgical**
Q   **Lower Bones**
Q   **Repair**   Definition: Restoring, to the extent possible, a body part to its normal anatomic structure and function
                   Explanation: Used only when the method to accomplish the repair is not one of the other root operations

Body Part Character 4	Approach Character 5	Device Character 6	Qualifier Character 7

Ø Lumbar Vertebra
  Spinous process
  Transverse process
  Vertebral arch
  Vertebral body
  Vertebral foramen
  Vertebral lamina
  Vertebral pedicle
1 Sacrum
2 Pelvic Bone, Right
  Iliac crest
  Ilium
  Ischium
  Pubis
3 Pelvic Bone, Left
  See 2 Pelvic Bone, Right
4 Acetabulum, Right
5 Acetabulum, Left
6 Upper Femur, Right
  Femoral head
  Greater trochanter
  Lesser trochanter
  Neck of femur
7 Upper Femur, Left
  See 6 Upper Femur, Right
8 Femoral Shaft, Right
  Body of femur
9 Femoral Shaft, Left
  See 8 Femoral Shaft, Right
B Lower Femur, Right
  Lateral condyle of femur
  Lateral epicondyle of femur
  Medial condyle of femur
  Medial epicondyle of femur
C Lower Femur, Left
  See B Lower Femur, Right
D Patella, Right
F Patella, Left
G Tibia, Right
  Lateral condyle of tibia
  Medial condyle of tibia
  Medial malleolus
H Tibia, Left
  See G Tibia, Right
J Fibula, Right
  Body of fibula
  Head of fibula
  Lateral malleolus
K Fibula, Left
  See J Fibula, Right
L Tarsal, Right
  Calcaneus
  Cuboid bone
  Intermediate cuneiform bone
  Lateral cuneiform bone
  Medial cuneiform bone
  Navicular bone
  Talus bone
M Tarsal, Left
  See L Tarsal, Right
N Metatarsal, Right
P Metatarsal, Left
Q Toe Phalanx, Right
R Toe Phalanx, Left
S Coccyx
	Ø Open
	3 Percutaneous
	4 Percutaneous Endoscopic
	X External
		Z No Device	**Z No Qualifier**

Non-OR   ØQQ[Ø,1,2,3,4,5,6,7,8,9,B,C,D,F,G,H,J,K,L,M,N,P,Q,R,S]XZZ

Lower Bones

Ø   **Medical and Surgical**
Q   **Lower Bones**
R   **Replacement**   Definition: Putting in or on biological or synthetic material that physically takes the place and/or function of all or a portion of a body part

                           Explanation: The body part may have been taken out or replaced, or may be taken out, physically eradicated, or rendered nonfunctional during the REPLACEMENT procedure. A REMOVAL procedure is coded for taking out the device used in a previous replacement procedure.

Body Part Character 4	Approach Character 5	Device Character 6	Qualifier Character 7

Ø Lumbar Vertebra
   Spinous process
   Transverse process
   Vertebral arch
   Vertebral body
   Vertebral foramen
   Vertebral lamina
   Vertebral pedicle
1 Sacrum
2 Pelvic Bone, Right
   Iliac crest
   Ilium
   Ischium
   Pubis
3 Pelvic Bone, Left
   See 2 Pelvic Bone, Right
4 Acetabulum, Right
5 Acetabulum, Left
6 Upper Femur, Right
   Femoral head
   Greater trochanter
   Lesser trochanter
   Neck of femur
7 Upper Femur, Left
   See 6 Upper Femur, Right
8 Femoral Shaft, Right
   Body of femur
9 Femoral Shaft, Left
   See 8 Femoral Shaft, Right
B Lower Femur, Right
   Lateral condyle of femur
   Lateral epicondyle of femur
   Medial condyle of femur
   Medial epicondyle of femur
C Lower Femur, Left
   See B Lower Femur, Right
D Patella, Right
F Patella, Left
G Tibia, Right
   Lateral condyle of tibia
   Medial condyle of tibia
   Medial malleolus
H Tibia, Left
   See G Tibia, Right
J Fibula, Right
   Body of fibula
   Head of fibula
   Lateral malleolus
K Fibula, Left
   See J Fibula, Right
L Tarsal, Right
   Calcaneus
   Cuboid bone
   Intermediate cuneiform bone
   Lateral cuneiform bone
   Medial cuneiform bone
   Navicular bone
   Talus bone
M Tarsal, Left
   See L Tarsal, Right
N Metatarsal, Right
P Metatarsal, Left
Q Toe Phalanx, Right
R Toe Phalanx, Left
S Coccyx
	Ø Open
	3 Percutaneous
	4 Percutaneous Endoscopic
		7 Autologous Tissue Substitute
		J Synthetic Substitute
		K Nonautologous Tissue Substitute
			Z No Qualifier

Lower Bones

Ø　**Medical and Surgical**
Q　**Lower Bones**
S　**Reposition**　　Definition: Moving to its normal location, or other suitable location, all or a portion of a body part

Explanation: The body part is moved to a new location from an abnormal location, or from a normal location where it is not functioning correctly. The body part may or may not be cut out or off to be moved to the new location.

Body Part Character 4	Approach Character 5	Device Character 6	Qualifier Character 7
Ø　Lumbar Vertebra ⊞ 　　Spinous process 　　Transverse process 　　Vertebral arch 　　Vertebral body 　　Vertebral foramen 　　Vertebral lamina 　　Vertebral pedicle **1　Sacrum** ⊞ **4　Acetabulum, Right** **5　Acetabulum, Left** **S　Coccyx** ⊞	**Ø　Open** **3　Percutaneous** **4　Percutaneous Endoscopic**	**4　Internal Fixation Device** **Z　No Device**	**Z　No Qualifier**
Ø　Lumbar Vertebra 　　Spinous process 　　Transverse process 　　Vertebral arch 　　Vertebral body 　　Vertebral foramen 　　Vertebral lamina 　　Vertebral pedicle **1　Sacrum** **4　Acetabulum, Right** **5　Acetabulum, Left** **S　Coccyx**	**X　External**	**Z　No Device**	**Z　No Qualifier**
2　Pelvic Bone, Right 　　Iliac crest 　　Ilium 　　Ischium 　　Pubis **3　Pelvic Bone, Left** 　　*See 2 Pelvic Bone, Right* **D　Patella, Right** **F　Patella, Left** **L　Tarsal, Right** 　　Calcaneus 　　Cuboid bone 　　Intermediate cuneiform bone 　　Lateral cuneiform bone 　　Medial cuneiform bone 　　Navicular bone 　　Talus bone **M　Tarsal, Left** 　　*See L Tarsal, Right* **Q　Toe Phalanx, Right** **R　Toe Phalanx, Left**	**Ø　Open** **3　Percutaneous** **4　Percutaneous Endoscopic**	**4　Internal Fixation Device** **5　External Fixation Device** **Z　No Device**	**Z　No Qualifier**
2　Pelvic Bone, Right 　　Iliac crest 　　Ilium 　　Ischium 　　Pubis **3　Pelvic Bone, Left** 　　*See 2 Pelvic Bone, Right* **D　Patella, Right** **F　Patella, Left** **L　Tarsal, Right** 　　Calcaneus 　　Cuboid bone 　　Intermediate cuneiform bone 　　Lateral cuneiform bone 　　Medial cuneiform bone 　　Navicular bone 　　Talus bone **M　Tarsal, Left** 　　*See L Tarsal, Right* **Q　Toe Phalanx, Right** **R　Toe Phalanx, Left**	**X　External**	**Z　No Device**	**Z　No Qualifier**

Non-OR	ØQS[4,5][3,4]ZZ
Non-OR	ØQS[Ø,1,4,5,S]XZZ
Non-OR	ØQS[2,3,D,F,L,M,Q,R][3,4]ZZ
Non-OR	ØQS[2,3,D,F,L,M,Q,R]XZZ

See Appendix L for Procedure Combinations
　⊞　　ØQS[Ø,1,S]3ZZ

ØQS Continued on next page

ØQS–ØQS

Ø   Medical and Surgical
Q   Lower Bones
S   Reposition

Definition: Moving to its normal location, or other suitable location, all or a portion of a body part

Explanation: The body part is moved to a new location from an abnormal location, or from a normal location where it is not functioning correctly. The body part may or may not be cut out or off to be moved to the new location.

Body Part Character 4	Approach Character 5	Device Character 6	Qualifier Character 7

6 Upper Femur, Right
Femoral head
Greater trochanter
Lesser trochanter
Neck of femur
7 Upper Femur, Left
See 6 Upper Femur, Right
8 Femoral Shaft, Right
Body of femur
9 Femoral Shaft, Left
See 8 Femoral Shaft, Right
B Lower Femur, Right
Lateral condyle of femur
Lateral epicondyle of femur
Medial condyle of femur
Medial epicondyle of femur
C Lower Femur, Left
See B Lower Femur, Right
G Tibia, Right
Lateral condyle of tibia
Medial condyle of tibia
Medial malleolus
H Tibia, Left
See G Tibia, Right
J Fibula, Right
Body of fibula
Head of fibula
Lateral malleolus
K Fibula, Left
See J Fibula, Right
	Ø Open
	3 Percutaneous
	4 Percutaneous Endoscopic
		4 Internal Fixation Device
		5 External Fixation Device
		**6 Internal Fixation Device,
		    Intramedullary**
		**B External Fixation Device,
		    Monoplanar**
		C External Fixation Device, Ring
		D External Fixation Device, Hybrid
		Z No Device
			Z No Qualifier

6 Upper Femur, Right Femoral head Greater trochanter Lesser trochanter Neck of femur **7 Upper Femur, Left** *See 6 Upper Femur, Right* **8 Femoral Shaft, Right** Body of femur **9 Femoral Shaft, Left** *See 8 Femoral Shaft, Right* **B Lower Femur, Right** Lateral condyle of femur Lateral epicondyle of femur Medial condyle of femur Medial epicondyle of femur **C Lower Femur, Left** *See B Lower Femur, Right* **G Tibia, Right** Lateral condyle of tibia Medial condyle of tibia Medial malleolus **H Tibia, Left** *See G Tibia, Right* **J Fibula, Right** Body of fibula Head of fibula Lateral malleolus **K Fibula, Left** *See J Fibula, Right*	**X External**	**Z No Device**	**Z No Qualifier**
N Metatarsal, Right **P Metatarsal, Left**	**Ø Open** **3 Percutaneous** **4 Percutaneous Endoscopic**	**4 Internal Fixation Device** **5 External Fixation Device** **Z No Device**	**2 Sesamoid Bone(s) 1st Toe** **Z No Qualifier**
N Metatarsal, Right **P Metatarsal, Left**	**X External**	**Z No Device**	**2 Sesamoid Bone(s) 1st Toe** **Z No Qualifier**

Non-OR   ØQS[6,7,8,9,B,C,G,H,J,K][3,4]ZZ
Non-OR   ØQS[6,7,8,9,B,C,G,H,J,K]XZZ
Non-OR   ØQS[N,P][3,4]Z[2,Z]
Non-OR   ØQS[N,P]XZ[2,Z]

LC Limited Coverage NC Noncovered ⊞ Combination Member HAC associated procedure Combination Only DRG Non-OR Non-OR New/Revised in GREEN

572   ICD-10-PCS 2021

Ø   **Medical and Surgical**
Q   **Lower Bones**
T   **Resection**   Definition: Cutting out or off, without replacement, all of a body part
                  Explanation: None

Body Part Character 4		Approach Character 5	Device Character 6	Qualifier Character 7
2 Pelvic Bone, Right Iliac crest Ilium Ischium Pubis **3 Pelvic Bone, Left** *See 2 Pelvic Bone, Right* **4 Acetabulum, Right** **5 Acetabulum, Left** **6 Upper Femur, Right** Femoral head Greater trochanter Lesser trochanter Neck of femur **7 Upper Femur, Left** *See 6 Upper Femur, Right* **8 Femoral Shaft, Right** Body of femur **9 Femoral Shaft, Left** *See 8 Femoral Shaft, Right* **B Lower Femur, Right** Lateral condyle of femur Lateral epicondyle of femur Medial condyle of femur Medial epicondyle of femur **C Lower Femur, Left** *See B Lower Femur, Right* **D Patella, Right**	**F Patella, Left** **G Tibia, Right** Lateral condyle of tibia Medial condyle of tibia Medial malleolus **H Tibia, Left** *See G Tibia, Right* **J Fibula, Right** Body of fibula Head of fibula Lateral malleolus **K Fibula, Left** *See J Fibula, Right* **L Tarsal, Right** Calcaneus Cuboid bone Intermediate cuneiform bone Lateral cuneiform bone Medial cuneiform bone Navicular bone Talus bone **M Tarsal, Left** *See L Tarsal, Right* **N Metatarsal, Right** **P Metatarsal, Left** **Q Toe Phalanx, Right** **R Toe Phalanx, Left** **S Coccyx**	**Ø Open**	**Z No Device**	**Z No Qualifier**

Ø   **Medical and Surgical**
Q   **Lower Bones**
U   **Supplement**   Definition: Putting in or on biological or synthetic material that physically reinforces and/or augments the function of a portion of a body part
                  Explanation: The biological material is non-living, or is living and from the same individual. The body part may have been previously replaced, and the SUPPLEMENT procedure is performed to physically reinforce and/or augment the function of the replaced body part.

Body Part Character 4		Approach Character 5	Device Character 6	Qualifier Character 7
Ø Lumbar Vertebra ⊞ Spinous process Transverse process Vertebral arch Vertebral body Vertebral foramen Vertebral lamina Vertebral pedicle **1 Sacrum** ⊞ **2 Pelvic Bone, Right** Iliac crest Ilium Ischium Pubis **3 Pelvic Bone, Left** *See 2 Pelvic Bone, Right* **4 Acetabulum, Right** **5 Acetabulum, Left** **6 Upper Femur, Right** Femoral head Greater trochanter Lesser trochanter Neck of femur **7 Upper Femur, Left** *See 6 Upper Femur, Right* **8 Femoral Shaft, Right** Body of femur **9 Femoral Shaft, Left** *See 8 Femoral Shaft, Right* **B Lower Femur, Right** Lateral condyle of femur Lateral epicondyle of femur Medial condyle of femur Medial epicondyle of femur	**C Lower Femur, Left** *See B Lower Femur, Right* **D Patella, Right** **F Patella, Left** **G Tibia, Right** Lateral condyle of tibia Medial condyle of tibia Medial malleolus **H Tibia, Left** *See G Tibia, Right* **J Fibula, Right** Body of fibula Head of fibula Lateral malleolus **K Fibula, Left** *See J Fibula, Right* **L Tarsal, Right** Calcaneus Cuboid bone Intermediate cuneiform bone Lateral cuneiform bone Medial cuneiform bone Navicular bone Talus bone **M Tarsal, Left** *See L Tarsal, Right* **N Metatarsal, Right** **P Metatarsal, Left** **Q Toe Phalanx, Right** **R Toe Phalanx, Left** **S Coccyx** ⊞	**Ø Open** **3 Percutaneous** **4 Percutaneous Endoscopic**	**7 Autologous Tissue Substitute** **J Synthetic Substitute** **K Nonautologous Tissue Substitute**	**Z No Qualifier**

See Appendix L for Procedure Combinations
⊞   ØQU[Ø,1,S]3JZ

LC Limited Coverage   **NC** Noncovered   ⊞ Combination Member   HAC associated procedure   Combination Only   DRG Non-OR   Non-OR   New/Revised in GREEN

ICD-10-PCS 2021   573

ØQT–ØQU

Lower Bones

ØQW–ØQW

Ø **Medical and Surgical**
Q **Lower Bones**
W **Revision**

Definition: Correcting, to the extent possible, a portion of a malfunctioning device or the position of a displaced device

Explanation: Revision can include correcting a malfunctioning or displaced device by taking out or putting in components of the device such as a screw or pin

Body Part Character 4	Approach Character 5	Device Character 6	Qualifier Character 7

Ø **Lumbar Vertebra**
  Spinous process
  Transverse process
  Vertebral arch
  Vertebral body
  Vertebral foramen
  Vertebral lamina
  Vertebral pedicle
1 **Sacrum**
4 **Acetabulum, Right**
5 **Acetabulum, Left**
S **Coccyx**
	Ø Open
	3 Percutaneous
	4 Percutaneous Endoscopic
	X External
		4 Internal Fixation Device
		7 Autologous Tissue Substitute
		J Synthetic Substitute
		K Nonautologous Tissue Substitute
			Z No Qualifier

2 **Pelvic Bone, Right**
  Iliac crest
  Ilium
  Ischium
  Pubis
3 **Pelvic Bone, Left**
  See 2 Pelvic Bone, Right
6 **Upper Femur, Right**
  Femoral head
  Greater trochanter
  Lesser trochanter
  Neck of femur
7 **Upper Femur, Left**
  See 6 Upper Femur, Right
8 **Femoral Shaft, Right**
  Body of femur
9 **Femoral Shaft, Left**
  See 8 Femoral Shaft, Right
B **Lower Femur, Right**
  Lateral condyle of femur
  Lateral epicondyle of femur
  Medial condyle of femur
  Medial epicondyle of femur
C **Lower Femur, Left**
  See B Lower Femur, Right
D **Patella, Right**
F **Patella, Left**
G **Tibia, Right**
  Lateral condyle of tibia
  Medial condyle of tibia
  Medial malleolus
H **Tibia, Left**
  See G Tibia, Right
J **Fibula, Right**
  Body of fibula
  Head of fibula
  Lateral malleolus
K **Fibula, Left**
  See J Fibula, Right
L **Tarsal, Right**
  Calcaneus
  Cuboid bone
  Intermediate cuneiform bone
  Lateral cuneiform bone
  Medial cuneiform bone
  Navicular bone
  Talus bone
M **Tarsal, Left**
  See L Tarsal, Right
N **Metatarsal, Right**
P **Metatarsal, Left**
Q **Toe Phalanx, Right**
R **Toe Phalanx, Left**
	Ø Open
	3 Percutaneous
	4 Percutaneous Endoscopic
	X External
		4 Internal Fixation Device
		5 External Fixation Device
		7 Autologous Tissue Substitute
		J Synthetic Substitute
		K Nonautologous Tissue Substitute
			Z No Qualifier

Y **Lower Bone**	Ø Open 3 Percutaneous 4 Percutaneous Endoscopic X External	Ø Drainage Device M Bone Growth Stimulator	Z No Qualifier

Non-OR   ØQW[Ø,1,4,5,S]X[4,7,J,K]Z
Non-OR   ØQW[2,3,6,7,8,9,B,C,D,F,G,H,J,K,L,M,N,P,Q,R]X[4,5,7,J,K]Z
Non-OR   ØQWYX[Ø,M]Z

LC Limited Coverage   **NC** Noncovered   ⊞ Combination Member   HAC associated procedure   Combination Only   DRG Non-OR   Non-OR   New/Revised in GREEN

Upper Joints ØR2–ØRW

Character Meanings*

This Character Meaning table is provided as a guide to assist the user in the identification of character members that may be found in this section of code tables. It **SHOULD NOT** be used to build a PCS code.

Operation–Character 3	Body Part–Character 4	Approach–Character 5	Device–Character 6	Qualifier–Character 7
2 Change	Ø Occipital-cervical Joint	Ø Open	Ø Drainage Device OR Synthetic Substitute, Reverse Ball and Socket	Ø Anterior Approach, Anterior Column
5 Destruction	1 Cervical Vertebral Joint	3 Percutaneous	3 Infusion Device OR Internal Fixation Device, Sustained Compression	1 Posterior Approach, Posterior Column
9 Drainage	2 Cervical Vertebral Joint, 2 or more	4 Percutaneous Endoscopic	4 Internal Fixation Device	6 Humeral Surface
B Excision	3 Cervical Vertebral Disc	X External	5 External Fixation Device	7 Glenoid Surface
C Extirpation	4 Cervicothoracic Vertebral Joint		7 Autologous Tissue Substitute	J Posterior Approach, Anterior Column
G Fusion	5 Cervicothoracic Vertebral Disc		8 Spacer	X Diagnostic
H Insertion	6 Thoracic Vertebral Joint		A Interbody Fusion Device	Z No Qualifier
J Inspection	7 Thoracic Vertebral Joint, 2 to 7		B Spinal Stabilization Device, Interspinous Process	
N Release	8 Thoracic Vertebral Joint, 8 or more		C Spinal Stabilization Device, Pedicle-Based	
P Removal	9 Thoracic Vertebral Disc		D Spinal Stabilization Device, Facet Replacement	
Q Repair	A Thoracolumbar Vertebral Joint		J Synthetic Substitute	
R Replacement	B Thoracolumbar Vertebral Disc		K Nonautologous Tissue Substitute	
S Reposition	C Temporomandibular Joint, Right		Y Other Device	
T Resection	D Temporomandibular Joint, Left		Z No Device	
U Supplement	E Sternoclavicular Joint, Right			
W Revision	F Sternoclavicular Joint, Left			
	G Acromioclavicular Joint, Right			
	H Acromioclavicular Joint, Left			
	J Shoulder Joint, Right			
	K Shoulder Joint, Left			
	L Elbow Joint, Right			
	M Elbow Joint, Left			
	N Wrist Joint, Right			
	P Wrist Joint, Left			
	Q Carpal Joint, Right			
	R Carpal Joint, Left			
	S Carpometacarpal Joint, Right			
	T Carpometacarpal Joint, Left			
	U Metacarpophalangeal Joint, Right			
	V Metacarpophalangeal Joint, Left			
	W Finger Phalangeal Joint, Right			
	X Finger Phalangeal Joint, Left			
	Y Upper Joint			

* Includes synovial membrane.

AHA Coding Clinic for table ØRB

2019, 3Q, 26	Acromioclavicular joint reconstruction using allograft

AHA Coding Clinic for table ØRG

2020, 2Q, 27	Spinal Fusion with NuVasive® VersaTie®
2020, 1Q, 33	Spinal fusion without use of bone graft
2019, 3Q, 28	Use of VERTE-STACK™ implant with fusion
2019, 3Q, 35	Fusion procedures of the spine (guideline B3.1Øc)
2019, 2Q, 19	Cervical spinal fusion, decompression and placement of interfacet stabilization device
2019, 1Q, 30	Spinal fusion performed at same level as decompressive laminectomy
2018, 4Q, 43	Joint fusion device value
2018, 1Q, 22	Spinal fusion procedures without bone graft
2017, 4Q, 62	Added and revised device values - Nerve substitutes
2017, 4Q, 76	Radiolucent porous interbody fusion device
2017, 2Q, 23	Decompression of spinal cord and placement of instrumentation
2014, 3Q, 30	Spinal fusion and fixation instrumentation
2014, 2Q, 7	Anterior cervical thoracic fusion with total discectomy
2013, 1Q, 21-23	Spinal fusion of thoracic and lumbar vertebrae
2013, 1Q, 29	Cervical and thoracic spinal fusion

AHA Coding Clinic for table ØRH

2019, 2Q, 40	Decompression of spinal cord and placement of instrumentation
2018, 3Q, 26	Anterior vertebral tethering using Dynesys Tethering System
2017, 2Q, 23	Decompression of spinal cord and placement of instrumentation
2016, 3Q, 32	Rotator cuff repair, tenodesis, decompression, acromioplasty and coracoplasty

AHA Coding Clinic for table ØRN

2019, 1Q, 30	Spinal fusion performed at same level as decompressive laminectomy
2016, 3Q, 32	Rotator cuff repair, tenodesis, decompression, acromioplasty and coracoplasty
2015, 2Q, 22	Arthroscopic subacromial decompression
2015, 2Q, 23	Arthroscopic release of shoulder joint

AHA Coding Clinic for table ØRP

2017, 4Q, 107	Total ankle replacement versus revision

AHA Coding Clinic for table ØRQ

2016, 1Q, 30	Thermal capsulorrhapy of shoulder

AHA Coding Clinic for table ØRR

2018, 4Q, 92	Radial head arthroplasty
2017, 4Q, 107	Total ankle replacement versus revision
2015, 3Q, 14	Endoprosthetic replacement of humerus and tendon reattachment
2015, 1Q, 27	Reverse total shoulder arthroplasty

AHA Coding Clinic for table ØRS

2019, 3Q, 26	Acromioclavicular joint reconstruction using allograft
2018, 3Q, 26	Anterior vertebral tethering using Dynesys Tethering System
2015, 2Q, 35	Application of tongs to reduce and stabilize cervical fracture
2014, 4Q, 32	Open reduction internal fixation of fracture with debridement
2014, 3Q, 33	Radial fracture treatment with open reduction internal fixation, and release of carpal ligament
2013, 2Q, 39	Application of cervical tongs for reduction of cervical fracture

AHA Coding Clinic for table ØRT

2019, 3Q, 26	Acromioclavicular joint reconstruction using allograft
2014, 2Q, 7	Anterior cervical thoracic fusion with total discectomy

AHA Coding Clinic for table ØRU

2019, 3Q, 26	Acromioclavicular joint reconstruction using allograft
2015, 3Q, 26	Thumb arthroplasty with resection of trapezium

AHA Coding Clinic for table ØRW

2017, 4Q, 107	Total ankle replacement versus revision

Upper Joints

Temporomandibular **C, D**

Acromioclavicular **G, H**

Sternoclavicular **E, F**

Shoulder **J, K**

Elbow **L, M**

Wrist: Radiocarpal **N, P**

Wrist: Midcarpal **N, P**

Carpometacarpal **S, T**

Metacarpophalangeal **U, V**

Hand Joints

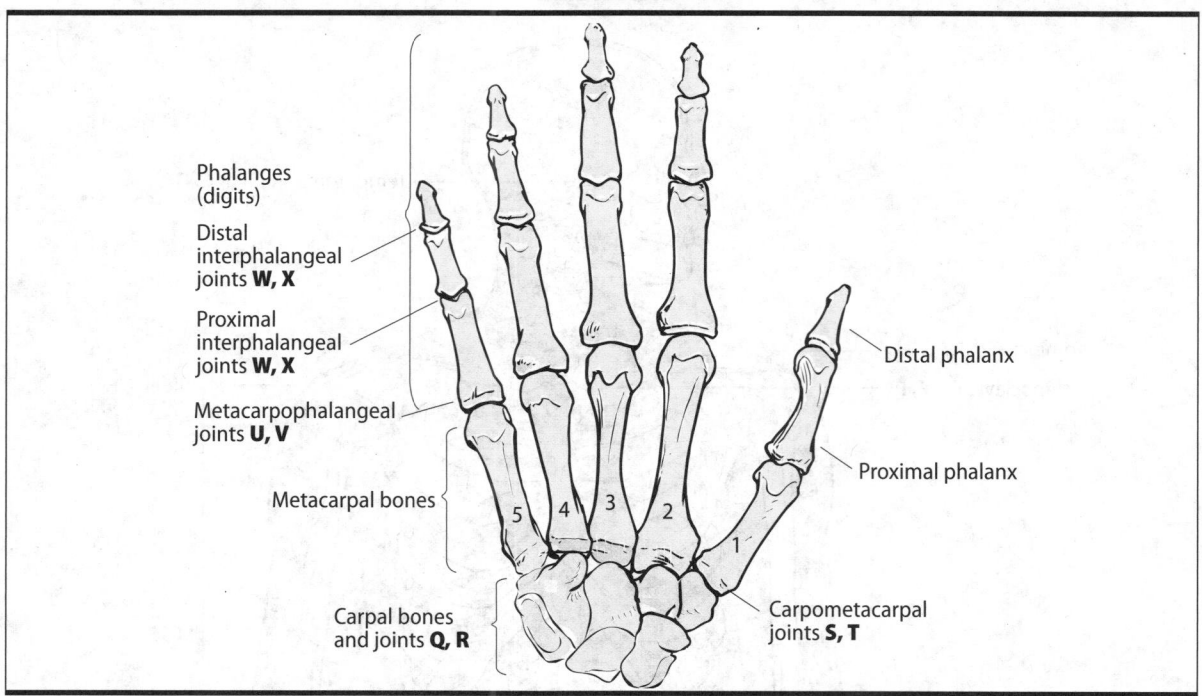

Phalanges (digits)

Distal interphalangeal joints **W, X**

Proximal interphalangeal joints **W, X**

Metacarpophalangeal joints **U, V**

Metacarpal bones

Carpal bones and joints **Q, R**

Distal phalanx

Proximal phalanx

Carpometacarpal joints **S, T**

Shoulder Joints

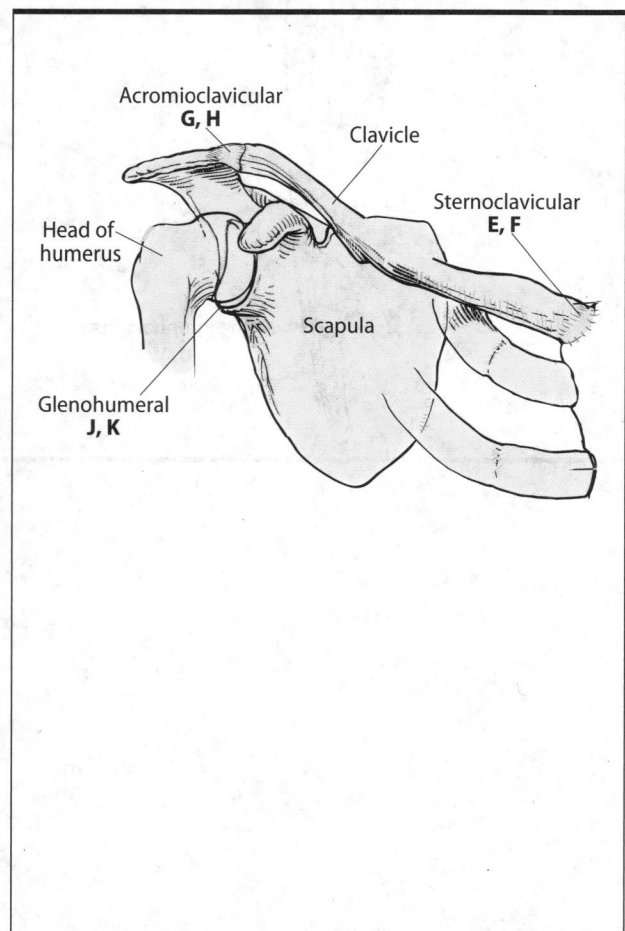

Acromioclavicular **G, H**

Clavicle

Head of humerus

Sternoclavicular **E, F**

Scapula

Glenohumeral **J, K**

Upper Vertebral Joints

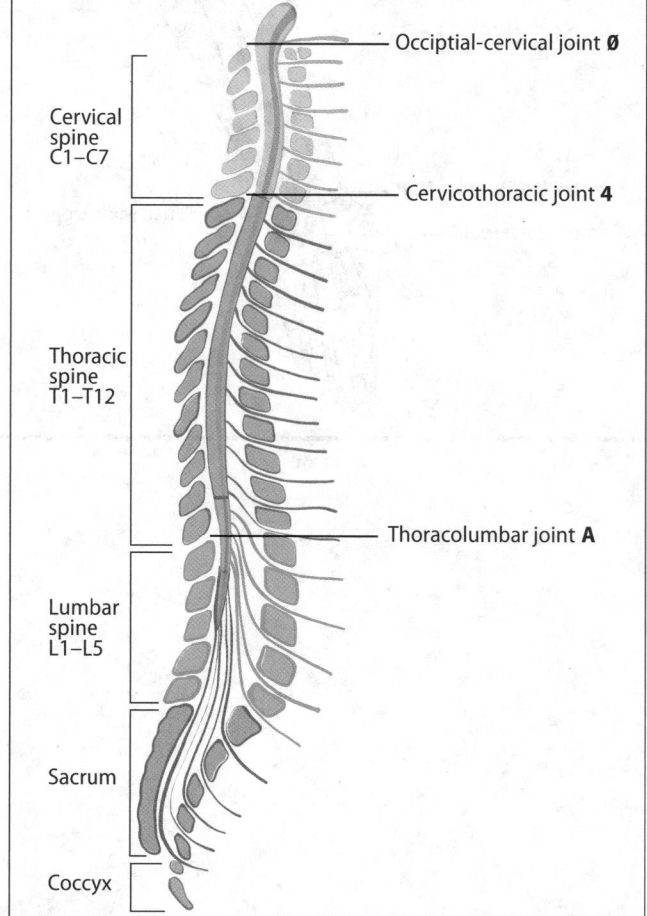

Occiptial-cervical joint **Ø**

Cervical spine C1–C7

Cervicothoracic joint **4**

Thoracic spine T1–T12

Thoracolumbar joint **A**

Lumbar spine L1–L5

Sacrum

Coccyx

Ø   Medical and Surgical
R   Upper Joints
2   Change   Definition: Taking out or off a device from a body part and putting back an identical or similar device in or on the same body part without cutting or puncturing the skin or a mucous membrane

Explanation: All CHANGE procedures are coded using the approach EXTERNAL

Body Part Character 4	Approach Character 5	Device Character 6	Qualifier Character 7
Y Upper Joint	X External	Ø Drainage Device Y Other Device	Z No Qualifier

Non-OR   All body part, approach, device, and qualifier values

Ø   Medical and Surgical
R   Upper Joints
5   Destruction   Definition: Physical eradication of all or a portion of a body part by the direct use of energy, force, or a destructive agent

Explanation: None of the body part is physically taken out

Body Part Character 4	Approach Character 5	Device Character 6	Qualifier Character 7

Ø   Occipital-cervical Joint
1   Cervical Vertebral Joint
    Atlantoaxial joint
    Cervical facet joint
3   Cervical Vertebral Disc
4   Cervicothoracic Vertebral Joint
    Cervicothoracic facet joint
5   Cervicothoracic Vertebral Disc
6   Thoracic Vertebral Joint
    Costotransverse joint
    Costovertebral joint
    Thoracic facet joint
9   Thoracic Vertebral Disc
A   Thoracolumbar Vertebral Joint
    Thoracolumbar facet joint
B   Thoracolumbar Vertebral Disc
C   Temporomandibular Joint, Right
D   Temporomandibular Joint, Left
E   Sternoclavicular Joint, Right
F   Sternoclavicular Joint, Left
G   Acromioclavicular Joint, Right
H   Acromioclavicular Joint, Left
J   Shoulder Joint, Right
    Glenohumeral joint
    Glenoid ligament (labrum)
K   Shoulder Joint, Left
    See J Shoulder Joint, Right
L   Elbow Joint, Right
    Distal humerus, involving joint
    Humeroradial joint
    Humeroulnar joint
    Proximal radioulnar joint
M   Elbow Joint, Left
    See L Elbow Joint, Right
N   Wrist Joint, Right
    Distal radioulnar joint
    Radiocarpal joint
P   Wrist Joint, Left
    See N Wrist Joint, Right
Q   Carpal Joint, Right
    Intercarpal joint
    Midcarpal joint
R   Carpal Joint, Left
    See Q Carpal Joint, Right
S   Carpometacarpal Joint, Right
T   Carpometacarpal Joint, Left
U   Metacarpophalangeal Joint, Right
V   Metacarpophalangeal Joint, Left
W   Finger Phalangeal Joint, Right
    Interphalangeal (IP) joint
X   Finger Phalangeal Joint, Left
    See W Finger Phalangeal Joint, Right
	Ø Open
	3 Percutaneous
	4 Percutaneous Endoscopic
		Z No Device	Z No Qualifier

Non-OR   ØR5[3,5,9,B][3,4]ZZ

LC Limited Coverage   NC Noncovered   ⊞ Combination Member   HAC associated procedure   Combination Only   DRG Non-OR   Non-OR   New/Revised in GREEN

ICD-10-PCS 2021   579

ØR2–ØR5

Ø   **Medical and Surgical**
R   **Upper Joints**
9   **Drainage**

Definition: Taking or letting out fluids and/or gases from a body part

Explanation: The qualifier DIAGNOSTIC is used to identify drainage procedures that are biopsies

Body Part		Approach	Device	Qualifier
Character 4		**Character 5**	**Character 6**	**Character 7**
Ø Occipital-cervical Joint	L Elbow Joint, Right	Ø Open	Ø Drainage Device	Z No Qualifier
1 Cervical Vertebral Joint	Distal humerus, involving	3 Percutaneous		
Atlantoaxial joint	joint	4 Percutaneous Endoscopic		
Cervical facet joint	Humeroradial joint			
3 Cervical Vertebral Disc	Humeroulnar joint			
4 Cervicothoracic Vertebral	Proximal radioulnar joint			
Joint	M Elbow Joint, Left			
Cervicothoracic facet joint	*See L Elbow Joint, Right*			
5 Cervicothoracic Vertebral	N Wrist Joint, Right			
Disc	Distal radioulnar joint			
6 Thoracic Vertebral Joint	Radiocarpal joint			
Costotransverse joint	P Wrist Joint, Left			
Costovertebral joint	*See N Wrist Joint, Right*			
Thoracic facet joint	Q Carpal Joint, Right			
9 Thoracic Vertebral Disc	Intercarpal joint			
A Thoracolumbar Vertebral	Midcarpal joint			
Joint	R Carpal Joint, Left			
Thoracolumbar facet joint	*See Q Carpal Joint, Right*			
B Thoracolumbar Vertebral	S Carpometacarpal Joint,			
Disc	Right			
C Temporomandibular Joint,	T Carpometacarpal Joint, Left			
Right	U Metacarpophalangeal Joint,			
D Temporomandibular Joint,	Right			
Left	V Metacarpophalangeal Joint,			
E Sternoclavicular Joint, Right	Left			
F Sternoclavicular Joint, Left	W Finger Phalangeal Joint,			
G Acromioclavicular Joint,	Right			
Right	Interphalangeal (IP) joint			
H Acromioclavicular Joint, Left	X Finger Phalangeal Joint, Left			
J Shoulder Joint, Right	*See W Finger Phalangeal Joint,*			
Glenohumeral joint	*Right*			
Glenoid ligament (labrum)				
K Shoulder Joint, Left				
See J Shoulder Joint, Right				
Ø Occipital-cervical Joint	L Elbow Joint, Right	Ø Open	Z No Device	X Diagnostic
1 Cervical Vertebral Joint	Distal humerus, involving	3 Percutaneous		Z No Qualifier
Atlantoaxial joint	joint	4 Percutaneous Endoscopic		
Cervical facet joint	Humeroradial joint			
3 Cervical Vertebral Disc	Humeroulnar joint			
4 Cervicothoracic Vertebral	Proximal radioulnar joint			
Joint	M Elbow Joint, Left			
Cervicothoracic facet joint	*See L Elbow Joint, Right*			
5 Cervicothoracic Vertebral	N Wrist Joint, Right			
Disc	Distal radioulnar joint			
6 Thoracic Vertebral Joint	Radiocarpal joint			
Costotransverse joint	P Wrist Joint, Left			
Costovertebral joint	*See N Wrist Joint, Right*			
Thoracic facet joint	Q Carpal Joint, Right			
9 Thoracic Vertebral Disc	Intercarpal joint			
A Thoracolumbar Vertebral	Midcarpal joint			
Joint	R Carpal Joint, Left			
Thoracolumbar facet joint	*See Q Carpal Joint, Right*			
B Thoracolumbar Vertebral	S Carpometacarpal Joint,			
Disc	Right			
C Temporomandibular Joint,	T Carpometacarpal Joint, Left			
Right	U Metacarpophalangeal Joint,			
D Temporomandibular Joint,	Right			
Left	V Metacarpophalangeal Joint,			
E Sternoclavicular Joint, Right	Left			
F Sternoclavicular Joint, Left	W Finger Phalangeal Joint,			
G Acromioclavicular Joint,	Right			
Right	Interphalangeal (IP) joint			
H Acromioclavicular Joint, Left	X Finger Phalangeal Joint, Left			
J Shoulder Joint, Right	*See W Finger Phalangeal Joint,*			
Glenohumeral joint	*Right*			
Glenoid ligament (labrum)				
K Shoulder Joint, Left				
See J Shoulder Joint, Right				

Non-OR	ØR9[Ø,1,3,4,5,6,9,A,B,E,F,G,H,J,K,L,M,N,P,Q,R,S,T,U,V,W,X][3,4]ØZ
Non-OR	ØR9[C,D]3ØZ
Non-OR	ØR9[Ø,1,3,4,5,6,9,A,B,E,F,G,H,J,K,L,M,N,P,Q,R,S,T,U,V,W,X][Ø,3,4]ZX
Non-OR	ØR9[Ø,1,3,4,5,6,9,A,B,E,F,G,H,J,K,L,M,N,P,Q,R,S,T,U,V,W,X][3,4]ZZ
Non-OR	ØR9[C,D]3ZZ

LC Limited Coverage   **NC** Noncovered   ⊞ Combination Member   HAC associated procedure   Combination Only   DRG Non-OR   Non-OR   New/Revised in **GREEN**

580   ICD-10-PCS 2021

ØR9–ØR9

Ø   Medical and Surgical
R   Upper Joints
B   Excision   Definition: Cutting out or off, without replacement, a portion of a body part
                       Explanation: The qualifier DIAGNOSTIC is used to identify excision procedures that are biopsies

Body Part Character 4	Approach Character 5	Device Character 6	Qualifier Character 7
Ø **Occipital-cervical Joint**	**Ø** Open	**Z** No Device	**X** Diagnostic

1 **Cervical Vertebral Joint**
   Atlantoaxial joint
   Cervical facet joint
	3 Percutaneous
	4 Percutaneous Endoscopic
			Z No Qualifier

3 **Cervical Vertebral Disc**			
4 **Cervicothoracic Vertebral Joint** Cervicothoracic facet joint			
5 **Cervicothoracic Vertebral Disc**			

6 **Thoracic Vertebral Joint**
   Costotransverse joint
   Costovertebral joint
   Thoracic facet joint			

9 **Thoracic Vertebral Disc**			
A **Thoracolumbar Vertebral Joint** Thoracolumbar facet joint			
B **Thoracolumbar Vertebral Disc**			
C Temporomandibular Joint, Right			
D Temporomandibular Joint, Left			
E **Sternoclavicular Joint, Right**			
F **Sternoclavicular Joint, Left**			
G **Acromioclavicular Joint, Right**			
H **Acromioclavicular Joint, Left**			

J **Shoulder Joint, Right**
   Glenohumeral joint
   Glenoid ligament (labrum)			

K Shoulder Joint, Left *See J Shoulder Joint, Right*			

L **Elbow Joint, Right**
   Distal humerus, involving joint
   Humeroradial joint
   Humeroulnar joint
   Proximal radioulnar joint			

M Elbow Joint, Left *See L Elbow Joint, Right*			

N **Wrist Joint, Right**
   Distal radioulnar joint
   Radiocarpal joint			

P **Wrist Joint, Left** *See N Wrist Joint, Right*			

Q **Carpal Joint, Right**
   Intercarpal joint
   Midcarpal joint			

R **Carpal Joint, Left** *See Q Carpal Joint, Right*			
S **Carpometacarpal Joint, Right**			
T **Carpometacarpal Joint, Left**			
U **Metacarpophalangeal Joint, Right**			
V **Metacarpophalangeal Joint, Left**			
W **Finger Phalangeal Joint, Right** Interphalangeal (IP) joint			
X **Finger Phalangeal Joint, Left** *See W Finger Phalangeal Joint, Right*			

Non-OR   ØRB[Ø,1,3,4,5,6,9,A,B,E,F,G,H,J,K,L,M,N,P,Q,R,S,T,U,V,W,X][Ø,3,4]ZX

LC Limited Coverage   **NC** Noncovered   ⊞ Combination Member   HAC associated procedure   Combination Only   DRG Non-OR   Non-OR   New/Revised in GREEN

ICD-10-PCS 2021   581

ØRB–ØRB

Upper Joints

Ø   **Medical and Surgical**
R   **Upper Joints**
C   **Extirpation**   Definition: Taking or cutting out solid matter from a body part

Explanation: The solid matter may be an abnormal byproduct of a biological function or a foreign body; it may be imbedded in a body part or in the lumen of a tubular body part. The solid matter may or may not have been previously broken into pieces.

Body Part Character 4	Approach Character 5	Device Character 6	Qualifier Character 7
Ø Occipital-cervical Joint	**Ø Open**	**Z No Device**	**Z No Qualifier**
1 Cervical Vertebral Joint Atlantoaxial joint Cervical facet joint	**3 Percutaneous** **4 Percutaneous Endoscopic**		
3 Cervical Vertebral Disc			
4 Cervicothoracic Vertebral Joint Cervicothoracic facet joint			
5 Cervicothoracic Vertebral Disc			
6 Thoracic Vertebral Joint Costotransverse joint Costovertebral joint Thoracic facet joint			
9 Thoracic Vertebral Disc			
A Thoracolumbar Vertebral Joint Thoracolumbar facet joint			
B Thoracolumbar Vertebral Disc			
C Temporomandibular Joint, Right			
D Temporomandibular Joint, Left			
E Sternoclavicular Joint, Right			
F Sternoclavicular Joint, Left			
G Acromioclavicular Joint, Right			
H Acromioclavicular Joint, Left			
J Shoulder Joint, Right Glenohumeral joint Glenoid ligament (labrum)			
K Shoulder Joint, Left *See J Shoulder Joint, Right*			
L Elbow Joint, Right Distal humerus, involving joint Humeroradial joint Humeroulnar joint Proximal radioulnar joint			
M Elbow Joint, Left *See L Elbow Joint, Right*			
N Wrist Joint, Right Distal radioulnar joint Radiocarpal joint			
P Wrist Joint, Left *See N Wrist Joint, Right*			
Q Carpal Joint, Right Intercarpal joint Midcarpal joint			
R Carpal Joint, Left *See Q Carpal Joint, Right*			
S Carpometacarpal Joint, Right			
T Carpometacarpal Joint, Left			
U Metacarpophalangeal Joint, Right			
V Metacarpophalangeal Joint, Left			
W Finger Phalangeal Joint, Right Interphalangeal (IP) joint			
X Finger Phalangeal Joint, Left *See W Finger Phalangeal Joint, Right*			

LC Limited Coverage   NC Noncovered   ⊞ Combination Member   HAC associated procedure   Combination Only   DRG Non-OR   Non-OR   New/Revised in GREEN

582   ICD-10-PCS 2021

Upper Joints

Ø   Medical and Surgical
R   Upper Joints
G   Fusion   Definition: Joining together portions of an articular body part rendering the articular body part immobile
                     Explanation: The body part is joined together by fixation device, bone graft, or other means

Body Part Character 4	Approach Character 5	Device Character 6	Qualifier Character 7

Ø **Occipital-cervical Joint**
1 **Cervical Vertebral Joint**
    Atlantoaxial joint
    Cervical facet joint
2 **Cervical Vertebral Joints, 2 or more**
    Cervical facet joint
4 **Cervicothoracic Vertebral Joint**
    Cervicothoracic facet joint
6 **Thoracic Vertebral Joint**
    Costotransverse joint
    Costovertebral joint
    Thoracic facet joint
7 **Thoracic Vertebral Joints, 2 to 7** ⊞
8 **Thoracic Vertebral Joints, 8 or more**
A **Thoracolumbar Vertebral Joint**
    Thoracolumbar facet joint
	Ø Open
	3 Percutaneous
	4 Percutaneous Endoscopic
		7 Autologous Tissue Substitute
		J Synthetic Substitute
		K Nonautologous Tissue Substitute
			Ø Anterior Approach, Anterior Column
			1 Posterior Approach, Posterior Column
			J Posterior Approach, Anterior Column

Ø **Occipital-cervical Joint**
1 **Cervical Vertebral Joint**
    Atlantoaxial joint
    Cervical facet joint
2 **Cervical Vertebral Joints, 2 or more**
    Cervical facet joint
4 **Cervicothoracic Vertebral Joint**
    Cervicothoracic facet joint
6 **Thoracic Vertebral Joint**
    Costotransverse joint
    Costovertebral joint
    Thoracic facet joint
7 **Thoracic Vertebral Joints, 2 to 7** ⊞
8 **Thoracic Vertebral Joints, 8 or more**
A **Thoracolumbar Vertebral Joint**
    Thoracolumbar facet joint
	Ø Open
	3 Percutaneous
	4 Percutaneous Endoscopic
		A Interbody Fusion Device	**Ø** Anterior Approach, Anterior Column
			J Posterior Approach, Anterior Column

C **Temporomandibular Joint, Right**
D **Temporomandibular Joint, Left**
E **Sternoclavicular Joint, Right**
F **Sternoclavicular Joint, Left**
G **Acromioclavicular Joint, Right**
H **Acromioclavicular Joint, Left**
J **Shoulder Joint, Right**
    Glenohumeral joint
    Glenoid ligament (labrum)
K **Shoulder Joint, Left**
    See J Shoulder Joint, Right
	Ø Open
	3 Percutaneous
	4 Percutaneous Endoscopic
		4 Internal Fixation Device
		7 Autologous Tissue Substitute
		J Synthetic Substitute
		K Nonautologous Tissue Substitute
			Z No Qualifier

L **Elbow Joint, Right**
    Distal humerus, involving joint
    Humeroradial joint
    Humeroulnar joint
    Proximal radioulnar joint
M **Elbow Joint, Left**
    See L Elbow Joint, Right
N **Wrist Joint, Right**
    Distal radioulnar joint
    Radiocarpal joint
P **Wrist Joint, Left**
    See N Wrist Joint, Right
Q **Carpal Joint, Right**
    Intercarpal joint
    Midcarpal joint
 	
R **Carpal Joint, Left**
    See Q Carpal Joint, Right
S **Carpometacarpal Joint, Right**
T **Carpometacarpal Joint, Left**
U **Metacarpophalangeal Joint, Right**
V **Metacarpophalangeal Joint, Left**
W **Finger Phalangeal Joint, Right**
    Interphalangeal (IP) joint
X **Finger Phalangeal Joint, Left**
    See W Finger Phalangeal Joint, Right
	Ø Open
	3 Percutaneous
	4 Percutaneous Endoscopic
		3 Internal Fixation Device, Sustained Compression
		4 Internal Fixation Device
		5 External Fixation Device
		7 Autologous Tissue Substitute
		J Synthetic Substitute
		K Nonautologous Tissue Substitute
			Z No Qualifier

HAC   ØRG[Ø,1,2,4,6,7,8,A][Ø,3,4][7,J,K][Ø,1,J] when reported with SDx K68.11 or T81.4Ø–T81.49, T84.6Ø-T84.619, T84.63-T84.7 with 7th character A
HAC   ØRG[Ø,1,2,4,6,7,8,A][Ø,3,4]A[Ø,J] when reported with SDx K68.11 or T81.4Ø–T81.49, T84.6Ø-T84.619, T84.63-T84.7 with 7th character A
HAC   ØRG[E,F,G,H,J,K][Ø,3,4][4,7,J,K]Z when reported with SDx K68.11 or T81.4Ø–T81.49, T84.6Ø-T84.619, T84.63-T84.7 with 7th character A
HAC   ØRG[L,M][Ø,3,4][4,5,7,J,K]Z when reported with SDx K68.11 or T81.4Ø–T81.49, T84.6Ø-T84.619, T84.63-T84.7 with 7th character A

See Appendix L for Procedure Combinations
⊞   ØRG7[Ø,3,4][7,J,K][Ø,1,J]
⊞   ØRG7[Ø,3,4]A[Ø,J]

Ø **Medical and Surgical**
R **Upper Joints**
H **Insertion**   Definition: Putting in a nonbiological appliance that monitors, assists, performs, or prevents a physiological function but does not physically
                          take the place of a body part
                          Explanation: None

Body Part Character 4	Approach Character 5	Device Character 6	Qualifier Character 7

Ø Occipital-cervical Joint
1 Cervical Vertebral Joint
  Atlantoaxial joint
  Cervical facet joint
4 Cervicothoracic Vertebral Joint
  Cervicothoracic facet joint
6 Thoracic Vertebral Joint
  Costotransverse joint
  Costovertebral joint
  Thoracic facet joint
A Thoracolumbar Vertebral Joint
  Thoracolumbar facet joint
	Ø Open
	3 Percutaneous
	4 Percutaneous Endoscopic
		3 Infusion Device
		4 Internal Fixation Device
		8 Spacer
		B Spinal Stabilization Device,
		  Interspinous Process
		C Spinal Stabilization Device,
		  Pedicle-Based
		D Spinal Stabilization Device,
		  Facet Replacement
			Z No Qualifier

3 Cervical Vertebral Disc 5 Cervicothoracic Vertebral Disc 9 Thoracic Vertebral Disc B Thoracolumbar Vertebral Disc	Ø Open 3 Percutaneous 4 Percutaneous Endoscopic	3 Infusion Device	Z No Qualifier

C Temporomandibular Joint, Right
D Temporomandibular Joint, Left
E Sternoclavicular Joint, Right
F Sternoclavicular Joint, Left
G Acromioclavicular Joint, Right
H Acromioclavicular Joint, Left
J Shoulder Joint, Right
  Glenohumeral joint
  Glenoid ligament (labrum)
K Shoulder Joint, Left
  See J Shoulder Joint, Right
	Ø Open
	3 Percutaneous
	4 Percutaneous Endoscopic
		3 Infusion Device
		4 Internal Fixation Device
		8 Spacer
			Z No Qualifier

L Elbow Joint, Right
  Distal humerus, involving joint
  Humeroradial joint
  Humeroulnar joint
  Proximal radioulnar joint
M Elbow Joint, Left
  See L Elbow Joint, Right
N Wrist Joint, Right
  Distal radioulnar joint
  Radiocarpal joint
P Wrist Joint, Left
  See N Wrist Joint, Right
Q Carpal Joint, Right
  Intercarpal joint
  Midcarpal joint
R Carpal Joint, Left
  See Q Carpal Joint, Right
S Carpometacarpal Joint, Right
T Carpometacarpal Joint, Left
U Metacarpophalangeal Joint, Right
V Metacarpophalangeal Joint, Left
W Finger Phalangeal Joint, Right
  Interphalangeal (IP) joint
X Finger Phalangeal Joint, Left
  See W Finger Phalangeal Joint, Right
	Ø Open
	3 Percutaneous
	4 Percutaneous Endoscopic
		3 Infusion Device
		4 Internal Fixation Device
		5 External Fixation Device
		8 Spacer
			Z No Qualifier

Non-OR	ØRH[Ø,1,4,6,A][Ø,3,4][3,8]Z
Non-OR	ØRH[3,5,9,B][Ø,3,4]3Z
Non-OR	ØRH[C,D][Ø,4]8Z
Non-OR	ØRH[C,D]3[3,8]Z
Non-OR	ØRH[E,F,G,H,J,K][Ø,3,4][3,8]Z
Non-OR	ØRH[L,M,N,P,Q,R,S,T,U,V,W,X][Ø,3,4][3,8]Z

LC Limited Coverage   NC Noncovered   ⊞ Combination Member   HAC associated procedure   Combination Only   DRG Non-OR   Non-OR   New/Revised in GREEN
584   ICD-10-PCS 2021

ØRH–ØRH

Ø   Medical and Surgical
R   Upper Joints
J   Inspection   Definition: Visually and/or manually exploring a body part

Explanation: Visual exploration may be performed with or without optical instrumentation. Manual exploration may be performed directly or through intervening body layers.

Body Part Character 4	Approach Character 5	Device Character 6	Qualifier Character 7
Ø **Occipital-cervical Joint**	**Ø** Open	**Z** No Device	**Z** No Qualifier

1 **Cervical Vertebral Joint**
    Atlantoaxial joint
    Cervical facet joint
	3 Percutaneous
	4 Percutaneous Endoscopic
	X External		

3 **Cervical Vertebral Disc**			
4 **Cervicothoracic Vertebral Joint** Cervicothoracic facet joint			
5 **Cervicothoracic Vertebral Disc**			

6 **Thoracic Vertebral Joint**
    Costotransverse joint
    Costovertebral joint
    Thoracic facet joint			

9 **Thoracic Vertebral Disc**			
A **Thoracolumbar Vertebral Joint** Thoracolumbar facet joint			
B **Thoracolumbar Vertebral Disc**			
C **Temporomandibular Joint, Right**			
D **Temporomandibular Joint, Left**			
E **Sternoclavicular Joint, Right**			
F **Sternoclavicular Joint, Left**			
G **Acromioclavicular Joint, Right**			
H **Acromioclavicular Joint, Left**			

J **Shoulder Joint, Right**
    Glenohumeral joint
    Glenoid ligament (labrum)			

K **Shoulder Joint, Left** *See J Shoulder Joint, Right*			

L **Elbow Joint, Right**
    Distal humerus, involving joint
    Humeroradial joint
    Humeroulnar joint
    Proximal radioulnar joint			

M **Elbow Joint, Left** *See L Elbow Joint, Right*			

N **Wrist Joint, Right**
    Distal radioulnar joint
    Radiocarpal joint			

P **Wrist Joint, Left** *See N Wrist Joint, Right*			

Q **Carpal Joint, Right**
    Intercarpal joint
    Midcarpal joint			

R **Carpal Joint, Left** *See Q Carpal Joint, Right*			
S **Carpometacarpal Joint, Right**			
T **Carpometacarpal Joint, Left**			
U **Metacarpophalangeal Joint, Right**			
V **Metacarpophalangeal Joint, Left**			
W **Finger Phalangeal Joint, Right** Interphalangeal (IP) joint			
X **Finger Phalangeal Joint, Left** *See W Finger Phalangeal Joint, Right*			

Non-OR   ØRJ[Ø,1,3,4,5,6,9,A,B,C,D,E,F,G,H,J,K,L,M,N,P,Q,R,S,T,U,V,W,X][3,X]ZZ

LC Limited Coverage   NC Noncovered   ⊞ Combination Member   HAC associated procedure   Combination Only   DRG Non-OR   Non-OR   New/Revised in GREEN

ICD-10-PCS 2021   585

Upper Joints

Ø   **Medical and Surgical**
R   **Upper Joints**
N   **Release**   Definition: Freeing a body part from an abnormal physical constraint by cutting or by the use of force
                          Explanation: Some of the restraining tissue may be taken out but none of the body part is taken out

Body Part Character 4	Approach Character 5	Device Character 6	Qualifier Character 7
Ø **Occipital-cervical Joint**	**Ø** Open	**Z** No Device	**Z** No Qualifier
1 **Cervical Vertebral Joint**	**3** Percutaneous		
Atlantoaxial joint	**4** Percutaneous Endoscopic		
Cervical facet joint	**X** External		
3 **Cervical Vertebral Disc**			
4 **Cervicothoracic Vertebral Joint**			
Cervicothoracic facet joint			
5 **Cervicothoracic Vertebral Disc**			
6 **Thoracic Vertebral Joint**			
Costotransverse joint			
Costovertebral joint			
Thoracic facet joint			
9 **Thoracic Vertebral Disc**			
A **Thoracolumbar Vertebral Joint**			
Thoracolumbar facet joint			
B **Thoracolumbar Vertebral Disc**			
C **Temporomandibular Joint, Right**			
D **Temporomandibular Joint, Left**			
E **Sternoclavicular Joint, Right**			
F **Sternoclavicular Joint, Left**			
G **Acromioclavicular Joint, Right**			
H **Acromioclavicular Joint, Left**			
J **Shoulder Joint, Right**			
Glenohumeral joint			
Glenoid ligament (labrum)			
K **Shoulder Joint, Left**			
See J Shoulder Joint, Right			
L **Elbow Joint, Right**			
Distal humerus, involving joint			
Humeroradial joint			
Humeroulnar joint			
Proximal radioulnar joint			
M **Elbow Joint, Left**			
See L Elbow Joint, Right			
N **Wrist Joint, Right**			
Distal radioulnar joint			
Radiocarpal joint			
P **Wrist Joint, Left**			
See N Wrist Joint, Right			
Q **Carpal Joint, Right**			
Intercarpal joint			
Midcarpal joint			
R **Carpal Joint, Left**			
See Q Carpal Joint, Right			
S **Carpometacarpal Joint, Right**			
T **Carpometacarpal Joint, Left**			
U **Metacarpophalangeal Joint, Right**			
V **Metacarpophalangeal Joint, Left**			
W **Finger Phalangeal Joint, Right**			
Interphalangeal (IP) joint			
X **Finger Phalangeal Joint, Left**			
See W Finger Phalangeal Joint, Right			

Non-OR   ØRN[Ø,1,3,4,5,6,9,A,B,C,D,E,F,G,H,J,K,L,M,N,P,Q,R,S,T,U,V,W,X]XZZ

Ø   **Medical and Surgical**
R   **Upper Joints**
P   **Removal**   Definition: Taking out or off a device from a body part

Explanation: If a device is taken out and a similar device put in without cutting or puncturing the skin or mucous membrane, the procedure is coded to the root operation CHANGE. Otherwise, the procedure for taking out the device is coded to the root operation REMOVAL.

Body Part Character 4	Approach Character 5	Device Character 6	Qualifier Character 7

Ø Occipital-cervical Joint
1 Cervical Vertebral Joint
  Atlantoaxial joint
  Cervical facet joint
4 Cervicothoracic Vertebral Joint
  Cervicothoracic facet joint
6 Thoracic Vertebral Joint
  Costotransverse joint
  Costovertebral joint
  Thoracic facet joint
A Thoracolumbar Vertebral Joint
  Thoracolumbar facet joint
	Ø Open
	3 Percutaneous
	4 Percutaneous Endoscopic
		Ø Drainage Device
		3 Infusion Device
		4 Internal Fixation Device
		7 Autologous Tissue Substitute
		8 Spacer
		A Interbody Fusion Device
		J Synthetic Substitute
		K Nonautologous Tissue Substitute
			Z No Qualifier

Ø Occipital-cervical Joint
1 Cervical Vertebral Joint
  Atlantoaxial joint
  Cervical facet joint
4 Cervicothoracic Vertebral Joint
  Cervicothoracic facet joint
6 Thoracic Vertebral Joint
  Costotransverse joint
  Costovertebral joint
  Thoracic facet joint
A Thoracolumbar Vertebral Joint
  Thoracolumbar facet joint
	X External	Ø Drainage Device
		3 Infusion Device
		4 Internal Fixation Device
			Z No Qualifier

3 Cervical Vertebral Disc 5 Cervicothoracic Vertebral Disc 9 Thoracic Vertebral Disc B Thoracolumbar Vertebral Disc	Ø Open 3 Percutaneous 4 Percutaneous Endoscopic	Ø Drainage Device 3 Infusion Device 7 Autologous Tissue Substitute J Synthetic Substitute K Nonautologous Tissue Substitute	Z No Qualifier
3 Cervical Vertebral Disc 5 Cervicothoracic Vertebral Disc 9 Thoracic Vertebral Disc B Thoracolumbar Vertebral Disc	X External	Ø Drainage Device 3 Infusion Device	Z No Qualifier

C Temporomandibular Joint, Right
D Temporomandibular Joint, Left
E Sternoclavicular Joint, Right
F Sternoclavicular Joint, Left
G Acromioclavicular Joint, Right
H Acromioclavicular Joint, Left
J Shoulder Joint, Right
  Glenohumeral joint
  Glenoid ligament (labrum)
K Shoulder Joint, Left
  See J Shoulder Joint, Right
	Ø Open
	3 Percutaneous
	4 Percutaneous Endoscopic
		Ø Drainage Device
		3 Infusion Device
		4 Internal Fixation Device
		7 Autologous Tissue Substitute
		8 Spacer
		J Synthetic Substitute
		K Nonautologous Tissue Substitute
			Z No Qualifier

C Temporomandibular Joint, Right
D Temporomandibular Joint, Left
E Sternoclavicular Joint, Right
F Sternoclavicular Joint, Left
G Acromioclavicular Joint, Right
H Acromioclavicular Joint, Left
J Shoulder Joint, Right
  Glenohumeral joint
  Glenoid ligament (labrum)
K Shoulder Joint, Left
  See J Shoulder Joint, Right
	X External	Ø Drainage Device
		3 Infusion Device
		4 Internal Fixation Device
			Z No Qualifier

Non-OR	ØRP[Ø,1,4,6,A]3[Ø,3,8]Z
Non-OR	ØRP[Ø,1,4,6,A][Ø,4]8Z
Non-OR	ØRP[Ø,1,4,6,A]X[Ø,3,4]Z
Non-OR	ØRP[3,5,9,B]3[Ø,3]Z
Non-OR	ØRP[3,5,9,B]X[Ø,3]Z
Non-OR	ØRP[C,D,E,F,G,H,J,K]3[Ø,3,8]Z
Non-OR	ØRP[C,D,E,F,G,H,J,K][Ø,4]8Z
Non-OR	ØRP[C,D]X[Ø,3]Z
Non-OR	ØRP[E,F,G,H,J,K]X[Ø,3,4]Z

ØRP Continued on next page

LC Limited Coverage   NC Noncovered   ⊞ Combination Member   HAC associated procedure   Combination Only   DRG Non-OR   Non-OR   New/Revised in GREEN

Upper Joints

ØRP–ØRP

Ø   Medical and Surgical
R   Upper Joints
P   Removal

ØRP Continued

Definition: Taking out or off a device from a body part

Explanation: If a device is taken out and a similar device put in without cutting or puncturing the skin or mucous membrane, the procedure is coded to the root operation CHANGE. Otherwise, the procedure for taking out the device is coded to the root operation REMOVAL.

Body Part Character 4	Approach Character 5	Device Character 6	Qualifier Character 7
L Elbow Joint, Right Distal humerus, involving joint Humeroradial joint Humeroulnar joint Proximal radioulnar joint **M Elbow Joint, Left** *See L Elbow Joint, Right* **N Wrist Joint, Right** Distal radioulnar joint Radiocarpal joint **P Wrist Joint, Left** *See N Wrist Joint, Right* **Q Carpal Joint, Right** Intercarpal joint Midcarpal joint **R Carpal Joint, Left** *See Q Carpal Joint, Right* **S Carpometacarpal Joint, Right** **T Carpometacarpal Joint, Left** **U Metacarpophalangeal Joint, Right** **V Metacarpophalangeal Joint, Left** **W Finger Phalangeal Joint, Right** Interphalangeal (IP) joint **X Finger Phalangeal Joint, Left** *See W Finger Phalangeal Joint, Right*	**Ø Open** **3 Percutaneous** **4 Percutaneous Endoscopic**	**Ø Drainage Device** **3 Infusion Device** **4 Internal Fixation Device** **5 External Fixation Device** **7 Autologous Tissue Substitute** **8 Spacer** **J Synthetic Substitute** **K Nonautologous Tissue Substitute**	**Z No Qualifier**
L Elbow Joint, Right Distal humerus, involving joint Humeroradial joint Humeroulnar joint Proximal radioulnar joint **M Elbow Joint, Left** *See L Elbow Joint, Right* **N Wrist Joint, Right** Distal radioulnar joint Radiocarpal joint **P Wrist Joint, Left** *See N Wrist Joint, Right* **Q Carpal Joint, Right** Intercarpal joint Midcarpal joint **R Carpal Joint, Left** *See Q Carpal Joint, Right* **S Carpometacarpal Joint, Right** **T Carpometacarpal Joint, Left** **U Metacarpophalangeal Joint, Right** **V Metacarpophalangeal Joint, Left** **W Finger Phalangeal Joint, Right** Interphalangeal (IP) joint **X Finger Phalangeal Joint, Left** *See W Finger Phalangeal Joint, Right*	**X External**	**Ø Drainage Device** **3 Infusion Device** **4 Internal Fixation Device** **5 External Fixation Device**	**Z No Qualifier**

Non-OR   ØRP[L,M,N,P,Q,R,S,T,U,V,W,X]3[Ø,3,8]Z
Non-OR   ØRP[L,M,N,P,Q,R,S,T,U,V,W,X][Ø,4]8Z
Non-OR   ØRP[L,M,N,P,Q,R,S,T,U,V,W,X]X[Ø,3,4,5]Z

LC Limited Coverage   **NC** Noncovered   ⊞ Combination Member   HAC associated procedure   Combination Only   DRG Non-OR   Non-OR   New/Revised in GREEN

588   ICD-10-PCS 2021

Ø　**Medical and Surgical**
R　**Upper Joints**
Q　**Repair**　　Definition: Restoring, to the extent possible, a body part to its normal anatomic structure and function
　　　　　　　　Explanation: Used only when the method to accomplish the repair is not one of the other root operations

Body Part Character 4	Approach Character 5	Device Character 6	Qualifier Character 7
Ø　Occipital-cervical Joint	Ø　Open	Z　No Device	Z　No Qualifier
1　Cervical Vertebral Joint	3　Percutaneous		
Atlantoaxial joint	4　Percutaneous Endoscopic		
Cervical facet joint	X　External		
3　Cervical Vertebral Disc			
4　Cervicothoracic Vertebral Joint			
Cervicothoracic facet joint			
5　Cervicothoracic Vertebral Disc			
6　Thoracic Vertebral Joint			
Costotransverse joint			
Costovertebral joint			
Thoracic facet joint			
9　Thoracic Vertebral Disc			
A　Thoracolumbar Vertebral Joint			
Thoracolumbar facet joint			
B　Thoracolumbar Vertebral Disc			
C　Temporomandibular Joint, Right			
D　Temporomandibular Joint, Left			
E　Sternoclavicular Joint, Right			
F　Sternoclavicular Joint, Left			
G　Acromioclavicular Joint, Right			
H　Acromioclavicular Joint, Left			
J　Shoulder Joint, Right			
Glenohumeral joint			
Glenoid ligament (labrum)			
K　Shoulder Joint, Left			
See J Shoulder Joint, Right			
L　Elbow Joint, Right			
Distal humerus, involving joint			
Humeroradial joint			
Humeroulnar joint			
Proximal radioulnar joint			
M　Elbow Joint, Left			
See L Elbow Joint, Right			
N　Wrist Joint, Right			
Distal radioulnar joint			
Radiocarpal joint			
P　Wrist Joint, Left			
See N Wrist Joint, Right			
Q　Carpal Joint, Right			
Intercarpal joint			
Midcarpal joint			
R　Carpal Joint, Left			
See Q Carpal Joint, Right			
S　Carpometacarpal Joint, Right			
T　Carpometacarpal Joint, Left			
U　Metacarpophalangeal Joint, Right			
V　Metacarpophalangeal Joint, Left			
W　Finger Phalangeal Joint, Right			
Interphalangeal (IP) joint			
X　Finger Phalangeal Joint, Left			
See W Finger Phalangeal Joint, Right			

Non-OR　ØRQ[Ø,1,3,4,5,6,9,A,B,C,D,E,F,G,H,J,K,L,M,N,P,Q,R,S,T,U,V,W,X]XZZ
HAC　　ØRQ[E,F,G,H,J,K,L,M][Ø,3,4,X]ZZ when reported with SDx K68.11 or T81.4Ø–T81.49, T84.6Ø-T84.619, T84.63-T84.7 with 7th character A

Upper Joints

Ø Medical and Surgical
R Upper Joints
R Replacement Definition: Putting in or on biological or synthetic material that physically takes the place and/or function of all or a portion of a body part
Explanation: The body part may have been taken out or replaced, or may be taken out, physically eradicated, or rendered nonfunctional during the REPLACEMENT procedure. A REMOVAL procedure is coded for taking out the device used in a previous replacement procedure.

Body Part Character 4	Approach Character 5	Device Character 6	Qualifier Character 7
Ø Occipital-cervical Joint	**Ø Open**	**7 Autologous Tissue Substitute**	**Z No Qualifier**
1 Cervical Vertebral Joint Atlantoaxial joint Cervical facet joint		**J Synthetic Substitute**	
3 Cervical Vertebral Disc		**K Nonautologous Tissue Substitute**	
4 Cervicothoracic Vertebral Joint Cervicothoracic facet joint			
5 Cervicothoracic Vertebral Disc			
6 Thoracic Vertebral Joint Costotransverse joint Costovertebral joint Thoracic facet joint			
9 Thoracic Vertebral Disc			
A Thoracolumbar Vertebral Joint Thoracolumbar facet joint			
B Thoracolumbar Vertebral Disc			
C Temporomandibular Joint, Right			
D Temporomandibular Joint, Left			
E Sternoclavicular Joint, Right			
F Sternoclavicular Joint, Left			
G Acromioclavicular Joint, Right			
H Acromioclavicular Joint, Left			
L Elbow Joint, Right Distal humerus, involving joint Humeroradial joint Humeroulnar joint Proximal radioulnar joint			
M Elbow Joint, Left *See L Elbow Joint, Right*			
N Wrist Joint, Right Distal radioulnar joint Radiocarpal joint			
P Wrist Joint, Left *See N Wrist Joint, Right*			
Q Carpal Joint, Right Intercarpal joint Midcarpal joint			
R Carpal Joint, Left *See Q Carpal Joint, Right*			
S Carpometacarpal Joint, Right			
T Carpometacarpal Joint, Left			
U Metacarpophalangeal Joint, Right			
V Metacarpophalangeal Joint, Left			
W Finger Phalangeal Joint, Right Interphalangeal (IP) joint			
X Finger Phalangeal Joint, Left *See W Finger Phalangeal Joint, Right*			
J Shoulder Joint, Right Glenohumeral joint Glenoid ligament (labrum)	**Ø Open**	**Ø Synthetic Substitute, Reverse Ball and Socket**	**Z No Qualifier**
K Shoulder Joint, Left *See J Shoulder Joint, Right*		**7 Autologous Tissue Substitute**	
		K Nonautologous Tissue Substitute	
J Shoulder Joint, Right Glenohumeral joint Glenoid ligament (labrum)	**Ø Open**	**J Synthetic Substitute**	**6 Humeral Surface**
K Shoulder Joint, Left *See J Shoulder Joint, Right*			**7 Glenoid Surface**
			Z No Qualifier

Ø   **Medical and Surgical**
R   **Upper Joints**
S   **Reposition**   Definition: Moving to its normal location, or other suitable location, all or a portion of a body part

                         Explanation: The body part is moved to a new location from an abnormal location, or from a normal location where it is not functioning correctly. The body part may or may not be cut out or off to be moved to the new location.

Body Part Character 4	Approach Character 5	Device Character 6	Qualifier Character 7

Ø **Occipital-cervical Joint**
1 **Cervical Vertebral Joint**
    Atlantoaxial joint
    Cervical facet joint
4 **Cervicothoracic Vertebral Joint**
    Cervicothoracic facet joint
6 **Thoracic Vertebral Joint**
    Costotransverse joint
    Costovertebral joint
    Thoracic facet joint
A **Thoracolumbar Vertebral Joint**
    Thoracolumbar facet joint
C **Temporomandibular Joint, Right**
D **Temporomandibular Joint, Left**
E **Sternoclavicular Joint, Right**
F **Sternoclavicular Joint, Left**
G **Acromioclavicular Joint, Right**
H **Acromioclavicular Joint, Left**
J **Shoulder Joint, Right**
    Glenohumeral joint
    Glenoid ligament (labrum)
K **Shoulder Joint, Left**
    See J Shoulder Joint, Right
	Ø Open
	3 Percutaneous
	4 Percutaneous Endoscopic
	X External
		4 Internal Fixation Device
		Z No Device
			Z No Qualifier

L **Elbow Joint, Right**
    Distal humerus, involving joint
    Humeroradial joint
    Humeroulnar joint
    Proximal radioulnar joint
M **Elbow Joint, Left**
    See L Elbow Joint, Right
N **Wrist Joint, Right**
    Distal radioulnar joint
    Radiocarpal joint
P **Wrist Joint, Left**
    See N Wrist Joint, Right
Q **Carpal Joint, Right**
    Intercarpal joint
    Midcarpal joint
R **Carpal Joint, Left**
    See Q Carpal Joint, Right
S **Carpometacarpal Joint, Right**
T **Carpometacarpal Joint, Left**
U **Metacarpophalangeal Joint, Right**
V **Metacarpophalangeal Joint, Left**
W **Finger Phalangeal Joint, Right**
    Interphalangeal (IP) joint
X **Finger Phalangeal Joint, Left**
    See W Finger Phalangeal Joint, Right
	Ø Open
	3 Percutaneous
	4 Percutaneous Endoscopic
	X External
		4 Internal Fixation Device
		5 External Fixation Device
		Z No Device
			Z No Qualifier

Non-OR   ØRS[Ø,1,4,6,A,C,D,E,F,G,H,J,K][3,4,X][4,Z]Z
Non-OR   ØRS[L,M,N,P,Q,R,S,T,U,V,W,X][3,4,X][4,5,Z]Z

LC Limited Coverage   NC Noncovered   ⊞ Combination Member   HAC associated procedure   Combination Only   DRG Non-OR   Non-OR   New/Revised in GREEN

ICD-10-PCS 2021   591

ØRS–ØRS

Ø Medical and Surgical
R Upper Joints
T Resection   Definition: Cutting out or off, without replacement, all of a body part
               Explanation: None

Body Part Character 4	Approach Character 5	Device Character 6	Qualifier Character 7
3 Cervical Vertebral Disc	**Ø Open**	**Z No Device**	**Z No Qualifier**
4 Cervicothoracic Vertebral Joint Cervicothoracic facet joint			
5 Cervicothoracic Vertebral Disc			
9 Thoracic Vertebral Disc			
B Thoracolumbar Vertebral Disc			
C Temporomandibular Joint, Right			
D Temporomandibular Joint, Left			
E Sternoclavicular Joint, Right			
F Sternoclavicular Joint, Left			
G Acromioclavicular Joint, Right			
H Acromioclavicular Joint, Left			
J Shoulder Joint, Right Glenohumeral joint Glenoid ligament (labrum)			
K Shoulder Joint, Left *See J Shoulder Joint, Right*			
L Elbow Joint, Right Distal humerus, involving joint Humeroradial joint Humeroulnar joint Proximal radioulnar joint			
M Elbow Joint, Left *See L Elbow Joint, Right*			
N Wrist Joint, Right Distal radioulnar joint Radiocarpal joint			
P Wrist Joint, Left *See N Wrist Joint, Right*			
Q Carpal Joint, Right Intercarpal joint Midcarpal joint			
R Carpal Joint, Left *See Q Carpal Joint, Right*			
S Carpometacarpal Joint, Right			
T Carpometacarpal Joint, Left			
U Metacarpophalangeal Joint, Right			
V Metacarpophalangeal Joint, Left			
W Finger Phalangeal Joint, Right Interphalangeal (IP) joint			
X Finger Phalangeal Joint, Left *See W Finger Phalangeal Joint, Right*			

🄛 Limited Coverage   🄝 Noncovered   ⊞ Combination Member   HAC associated procedure   Combination Only   DRG Non-OR   Non-OR   New/Revised in GREEN

592   ICD-10-PCS 2021

Ø	**Medical and Surgical**
R	**Upper Joints**
U	**Supplement**

Definition: Putting in or on biological or synthetic material that physically reinforces and/or augments the function of a portion of a body part

Explanation: The biological material is non-living, or is living and from the same individual. The body part may have been previously replaced, and the SUPPLEMENT procedure is performed to physically reinforce and/or augment the function of the replaced body part.

Body Part Character 4	Approach Character 5	Device Character 6	Qualifier Character 7

Ø   **Occipital-cervical Joint**
 1   **Cervical Vertebral Joint**
     Atlantoaxial joint
     Cervical facet joint
 3   **Cervical Vertebral Disc**
 4   **Cervicothoracic Vertebral Joint**
     Cervicothoracic facet joint
 5   **Cervicothoracic Vertebral Disc**
 6   **Thoracic Vertebral Joint**
     Costotransverse joint
     Costovertebral joint
     Thoracic facet joint
 9   **Thoracic Vertebral Disc**
 A   **Thoracolumbar Vertebral Joint**
     Thoracolumbar facet joint
 B   **Thoracolumbar Vertebral Disc**
 C   **Temporomandibular Joint, Right**
 D   **Temporomandibular Joint, Left**
 E   **Sternoclavicular Joint, Right**
 F   **Sternoclavicular Joint, Left**
 G   **Acromioclavicular Joint, Right**
 H   **Acromioclavicular Joint, Left**
 J   **Shoulder Joint, Right**
     Glenohumeral joint
     Glenoid ligament (labrum)
 K   **Shoulder Joint, Left**
     See J Shoulder Joint, Right
 L   **Elbow Joint, Right**
     Distal humerus, involving joint
     Humeroradial joint
     Humeroulnar joint
     Proximal radioulnar joint
 M   **Elbow Joint, Left**
     See L Elbow Joint, Right
 N   **Wrist Joint, Right**
     Distal radioulnar joint
     Radiocarpal joint
 P   **Wrist Joint, Left**
     See N Wrist Joint, Right
 Q   **Carpal Joint, Right**
     Intercarpal joint
     Midcarpal joint
 R   **Carpal Joint, Left**
     See Q Carpal Joint, Right
 S   **Carpometacarpal Joint, Right**
 T   **Carpometacarpal Joint, Left**
 U   **Metacarpophalangeal Joint, Right**
 V   **Metacarpophalangeal Joint, Left**
 W   **Finger Phalangeal Joint, Right**
     Interphalangeal (IP) joint
 X   **Finger Phalangeal Joint, Left**
     See W Finger Phalangeal Joint, Right
	Ø **Open**
	 3 **Percutaneous**
	 4 **Percutaneous Endoscopic**
		7 **Autologous Tissue Substitute**
		 J **Synthetic Substitute**
		 K **Nonautologous Tissue Substitute**
			Z **No Qualifier**

HAC   ØRU[E,F,G,H,J,K,L,M][Ø,3,4][7,J,K]Z when reported with SDx K68.11 or T81.4Ø–T81.49, T84.6Ø-T84.619, T84.63-T84.7 with 7th character A

LC Limited Coverage   **NC** Noncovered   ⊞ Combination Member   HAC associated procedure   Combination Only   DRG Non-OR   Non-OR   New/Revised in GREEN

ICD-10-PCS 2021   593

ØRU–ØRU

Ø   Medical and Surgical
R   Upper Joints
W   Revision   Definition: Correcting, to the extent possible, a portion of a malfunctioning device or the position of a displaced device

Explanation: Revision can include correcting a malfunctioning or displaced device by taking out or putting in components of the device such as a screw or pin

Body Part Character 4	Approach Character 5	Device Character 6	Qualifier Character 7

Ø   **Occipital-cervical Joint**
1   **Cervical Vertebral Joint**
    Atlantoaxial joint
    Cervical facet joint
4   **Cervicothoracic Vertebral Joint**
    Cervicothoracic facet joint
6   **Thoracic Vertebral Joint**
    Costotransverse joint
    Costovertebral joint
    Thoracic facet joint
A   **Thoracolumbar Vertebral Joint**
    Thoracolumbar facet joint
	Ø Open
	3 Percutaneous
	4 Percutaneous Endoscopic
	X External
		Ø Drainage Device
		3 Infusion Device
		4 Internal Fixation Device
		7 Autologous Tissue
		    Substitute
		8 Spacer
		A Interbody Fusion Device
		J Synthetic Substitute
		K Nonautologous Tissue
		    Substitute
			Z No Qualifier

3   **Cervical Vertebral Disc**
5   **Cervicothoracic Vertebral Disc**
9   **Thoracic Vertebral Disc**
B   **Thoracolumbar Vertebral Disc**
	Ø Open
	3 Percutaneous
	4 Percutaneous Endoscopic
	X External
		Ø Drainage Device
		3 Infusion Device
		7 Autologous Tissue
		    Substitute
		J Synthetic Substitute
		K Nonautologous Tissue
		    Substitute
			Z No Qualifier

C   **Temporomandibular Joint, Right**
D   **Temporomandibular Joint, Left**
E   **Sternoclavicular Joint, Right**
F   **Sternoclavicular Joint, Left**
G   **Acromioclavicular Joint, Right**
H   **Acromioclavicular Joint, Left**
J   **Shoulder Joint, Right**
    Glenohumeral joint
    Glenoid ligament (labrum)
K   **Shoulder Joint, Left**
    See J Shoulder Joint, Right
	Ø Open
	3 Percutaneous
	4 Percutaneous Endoscopic
	X External
		Ø Drainage Device
		3 Infusion Device
		4 Internal Fixation Device
		7 Autologous Tissue
		    Substitute
		8 Spacer
		J Synthetic Substitute
		K Nonautologous Tissue
		    Substitute
			Z No Qualifier

L   **Elbow Joint, Right**
    Distal humerus, involving joint
    Humeroradial joint
    Humeroulnar joint
    Proximal radioulnar joint
M   **Elbow Joint, Left**
    See L Elbow Joint, Right
N   **Wrist Joint, Right**
    Distal radioulnar joint
    Radiocarpal joint
P   **Wrist Joint, Left**
    See N Wrist Joint, Right
Q   **Carpal Joint, Right**
    Intercarpal joint
    Midcarpal joint
R   **Carpal Joint, Left**
    See Q Carpal Joint, Right
S   **Carpometacarpal Joint, Right**
T   **Carpometacarpal Joint, Left**
U   **Metacarpophalangeal Joint, Right**
V   **Metacarpophalangeal Joint, Left**
W   **Finger Phalangeal Joint, Right**
    Interphalangeal (IP) joint
X   **Finger Phalangeal Joint, Left**
    See W Finger Phalangeal Joint, Right
	Ø Open
	3 Percutaneous
	4 Percutaneous Endoscopic
	X External
		Ø Drainage Device
		3 Infusion Device
		4 Internal Fixation Device
		5 External Fixation Device
		7 Autologous Tissue
		    Substitute
		8 Spacer
		J Synthetic Substitute
		K Nonautologous Tissue
		    Substitute
			Z No Qualifier

Non-OR	ØRW[Ø,1,4,6,A]X[Ø,3,4,7,8,A,J,K]Z
Non-OR	ØRW[3,5,9,B]X[Ø,3,7,J,K]Z
Non-OR	ØRW[C,D,E,F,G,H,J,K]X[Ø,3,4,7,8,J,K]Z
Non-OR	ØRW[L,M,N,P,Q,R,S,T,U,V,W,X]X[Ø,3,4,5,7,8,J,K]Z

LC Limited Coverage   **NC** Noncovered   ⊞ Combination Member   HAC associated procedure   Combination Only   DRG Non-OR   Non-OR   New/Revised in **GREEN**

594   ICD-10-PCS 2021

ØRW–ØRW

Lower Joints ØS2–ØSW

Character Meanings*

This Character Meaning table is provided as a guide to assist the user in the identification of character members that may be found in this section of code tables. It **SHOULD NOT** be used to build a PCS code.

Operation–Character 3	Body Part–Character 4	Approach–Character 5	Device–Character 6	Qualifier–Character 7
2 Change	Ø Lumbar Vertebral Joint	Ø Open	Ø Drainage Device OR Synthetic Substitute, Polyethylene	Ø Anterior Approach, Anterior Column
5 Destruction	1 Lumbar Vertebral Joint, 2 or more	3 Percutaneous	1 Synthetic Substitute, Metal	1 Posterior Approach, Posterior Column
9 Drainage	2 Lumbar Vertebral Disc	4 Percutaneous Endoscopic	2 Synthetic Substitute, Metal on Polyethylene	9 Cemented
B Excision	3 Lumbosacral Joint	X External	3 Infusion Device OR Internal Fixation Device, Sustained Compression OR Synthetic Substitute, Ceramic	A Uncemented
C Extirpation	4 Lumbosacral Disc		4 Internal Fixation Device OR Synthetic Substitute, Ceramic on Polyethylene	C Patellar Surface
G Fusion	5 Sacrococcygeal Joint		5 External Fixation Device	J Posterior Approach, Anterior Column
H Insertion	6 Coccygeal Joint		6 Synthetic Substitute, Oxidized Zirconium on Polyethylene	X Diagnostic
J Inspection	7 Sacroiliac Joint, Right		7 Autologous Tissue Substitute	Z No Qualifier
N Release	8 Sacroiliac Joint, Left		8 Spacer	
P Removal	9 Hip Joint, Right		9 Liner	
Q Repair	A Hip Joint, Acetabular Surface, Right		A Interbody Fusion Device	
R Replacement	B Hip Joint, Left		B Resurfacing Device OR Spinal Stabilization Device, Interspinous Process	
S Reposition	C Knee Joint, Right		C Spinal Stabilization Device, Pedicle-Based	
T Resection	D Knee Joint, Left		D Spinal Stabilization Device, Facet Replacement	
U Supplement	E Hip Joint, Acetabular Surface, Left		E Articulating Spacer	
W Revision	F Ankle Joint, Right		J Synthetic Substitute	
	G Ankle Joint, Left		K Nonautologous Tissue Substitute	
	H Tarsal Joint, Right		L Synthetic Substitute, Unicondylar Medial	
	J Tarsal Joint, Left		M Synthetic Substitute, Unicondylar Lateral	
	K Tarsometatarsal Joint, Right		N Synthetic Substitute, Patellofemoral	
	L Tarsometatarsal Joint, Left		Y Other Device	
	M Metatarsal-Phalangeal Joint, Right		Z No Device	
	N Metatarsal-Phalangeal Joint, Left			
	P Toe Phalangeal Joint, Right			
	Q Toe Phalangeal Joint, Left			
	R Hip Joint, Femoral Surface, Right			
	S Hip Joint, Femoral Surface, Left			
	T Knee Joint, Femoral Surface, Right			
	U Knee Joint, Femoral Surface, Left			
	V Knee Joint, Tibial Surface, Right			
	W Knee Joint, Tibial Surface, Left			
	Y Lower Joint			

* Includes synovial membrane.

AHA Coding Clinic for table 0S9
2018, 2Q, 17	Arthroscopic drainage of knee and nonexcisional debridement
2017, 1Q, 50	Dry aspiration of ankle joint

AHA Coding Clinic for table 0SB
2017, 4Q, 76	Radiolucent porous interbody fusion device
2016, 2Q, 16	Decompressive laminectomy/foraminotomy and lumbar discectomy
2016, 1Q, 20	Metatarsophalangeal joint resection arthroplasty
2015, 1Q, 34	Arthroscopic meniscectomy with debridement and abrasion chondroplasty
2014, 2Q, 6	Posterior lumbar fusion with discectomy

AHA Coding Clinic for table 0SG
2020, 2Q, 27	Spinal Fusion with NuVasive® VersaTie®
2020, 1Q, 33	Spinal fusion without use of bone graft
2019, 3Q, 35	Fusion procedures of the spine (guideline B3.10c)
2019, 1Q, 30	Spinal fusion performed at same level as decompressive laminectomy
2018, 4Q, 43	Joint fusion device value
2018, 1Q, 22	Spinal fusion procedures without bone graft
2017, 4Q, 76	Radiolucent porous interbody fusion device
2017, 2Q, 23	Decompression of spinal cord and placement of instrumentation
2014, 3Q, 30	Spinal fusion and fixation instrumentation
2014, 3Q, 36	Lumbar interbody fusion of two vertebral levels
2014, 2Q, 6	Posterior lumbar fusion with discectomy
2013, 3Q, 25	360-degree spinal fusion
2013, 2Q, 39	Ankle fusion, osteotomy, and removal of hardware
2013, 1Q, 21-23	Spinal fusion of thoracic and lumbar vertebrae

AHA Coding Clinic for table 0SH
2017, 2Q, 23	Decompression of spinal cord and placement of instrumentation

AHA Coding Clinic for table 0SJ
2017, 1Q, 50	Dry aspiration of ankle joint

AHA Coding Clinic for table 0SN
2020, 2Q, 26	Arthroscopic Manipulation and Nonexcisional Debridement of Knee Joint
2019, 1Q, 30	Spinal fusion performed at same level as decompressive laminectomy

AHA Coding Clinic for table 0SP
2018, 4Q, 43	Articulating spacer for hip and knee joint
2018, 2Q, 16	Exchange of tibial polyethylene component with stabilizing insert (tibial tray)
2017, 4Q, 107	Total ankle replacement versus revision
2016, 4Q, 110-112	Removal and revision of hip and knee devices
2015, 2Q, 18	Total knee revision
2015, 2Q, 19	Revision of femoral head and acetabular liner
2013, 2Q, 39	Ankle fusion, osteotomy, and removal of hardware

AHA Coding Clinic for table 0SQ
2014, 4Q, 25	Femoroacetabular impingement and labral tear with repair

AHA Coding Clinic for table 0SR
2018, 4Q, 43	Articulating spacer for hip and knee joint
2018, 2Q, 16	Exchange of tibial polyethylene component with stabilizing insert (tibial tray)
2017, 4Q, 38-39	Oxidized zirconium on polyethylene bearing surface
2017, 4Q, 107	Total ankle replacement versus revision
2017, 1Q, 22	Total knee replacement and patellar component
2016, 4Q, 110-111	Partial (unicondylar) knee replacement
2016, 4Q, 111-112	Removal and revision of hip and knee devices
2016, 3Q, 35	Use of cemented versus uncemented qualifier for joint replacement
2015, 3Q, 18	Total hip replacement with acetabular reconstruction
2015, 2Q, 18	Total knee revision
2015, 2Q, 19	Revision of femoral head and acetabular liner

AHA Coding Clinic for table 0SS
2016, 2Q, 31	Periacetabular ostectomy for repair of congenital hip dysplasia

AHA Coding Clinic for table 0ST
2016, 1Q, 20	Metatarsophalangeal joint resection arthroplasty
2014, 4Q, 29	Rotational osteosynthesis

AHA Coding Clinic for table 0SU
2018, 2Q, 16	Exchange of tibial polyethylene component with stabilizing insert (tibial tray)
2016, 4Q, 111	Removal and revision of hip and knee devices
2015, 2Q, 19	Revision of femoral head and acetabular liner

AHA Coding Clinic for table 0SW
2017, 4Q, 107	Total ankle replacement versus revision
2016, 4Q, 110-112	Removal and revision of hip and knee devices
2015, 2Q, 18	Total knee revision
2015, 2Q, 19	Revision of femoral head and acetabular liner

Lower Joints

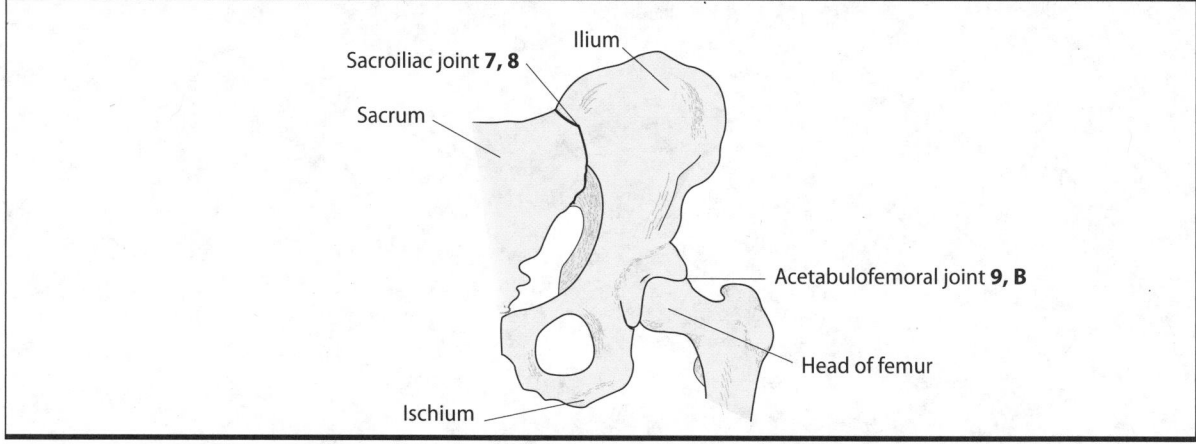

Sacroiliac **7, 8**

Lumbosacral **3**

Sacrococcygeal joint **5**

Hip **9, B**

Knee **C, D**

(Transverse) tarsal **H, J**

Metatarsal-phalangeal **M, N**

Ankle **F, G**

Hip Joint

Sacroiliac joint **7, 8**

Ilium

Sacrum

Acetabulofemoral joint **9, B**

Head of femur

Ischium

Knee Joint

Anterior view

Patella

Medial meniscus cartilage

Lateral meniscus cartilage

Lateral view

Femur

Synovial cavity

Patella

Tibia

Foot Joints

Phalanges

Tarsal joints **H, J**

Metatarso-phalangeal joints **M, N**

Tarsometatarsal joints **K, L**

Distal interphalangeal joint **P, Q**

Proximal interphalangeal joint **P, Q**

Tarsals

Metatarsals

Ø   Medical and Surgical
S   Lower Joints
2   Change   Definition: Taking out or off a device from a body part and putting back an identical or similar device in or on the same body part without cutting or puncturing the skin or a mucous membrane

Explanation: All CHANGE procedures are coded using the approach EXTERNAL

Body Part Character 4	Approach Character 5	Device Character 6	Qualifier Character 7
Y Lower Joint	X External	Ø Drainage Device Y Other Device	Z No Qualifier

Non-OR   All body part, approach, device, and qualifier values

Ø   Medical and Surgical
S   Lower Joints
5   Destruction   Definition: Physical eradication of all or a portion of a body part by the direct use of energy, force, or a destructive agent

Explanation: None of the body part is physically taken out

Body Part Character 4	Approach Character 5	Device Character 6	Qualifier Character 7
Ø **Lumbar Vertebral Joint** Lumbar facet joint 2 **Lumbar Vertebral Disc** 3 **Lumbosacral Joint** Lumbosacral facet joint 4 **Lumbosacral Disc** 5 **Sacrococcygeal Joint** Sacrococcygeal symphysis 6 **Coccygeal Joint** 7 **Sacroiliac Joint, Right** 8 **Sacroiliac Joint, Left** 9 **Hip Joint, Right** Acetabulofemoral joint B **Hip Joint, Left** *See 9 Hip Joint, Right* C **Knee Joint, Right** Femoropatellar joint Femorotibial joint Lateral meniscus Medial meniscus Patellofemoral joint Tibiofemoral joint D **Knee Joint, Left** *See C Knee Joint, Right* F **Ankle Joint, Right** Inferior tibiofibular joint Talocrural joint G **Ankle Joint, Left** *See F Ankle Joint, Right* H **Tarsal Joint, Right** Calcaneocuboid joint Cuboideonavicular joint Cuneonavicular joint Intercuneiform joint Subtalar (talocalcaneal) joint Talocalcaneal (subtalar) joint Talocalcaneonavicular joint J **Tarsal Joint, Left** *See H Tarsal Joint, Right* K **Tarsometatarsal Joint, Right** L **Tarsometatarsal Joint, Left** M **Metatarsal-Phalangeal Joint, Right** Metatarsophalangeal (MTP) joint N **Metatarsal-Phalangeal Joint, Left** *See M Metatarsal-Phalangeal Joint, Right* P **Toe Phalangeal Joint, Right** Interphalangeal (IP) joint Q **Toe Phalangeal Joint, Left** *See P Toe Phalangeal Joint, Right*	Ø Open 3 Percutaneous 4 Percutaneous Endoscopic	Z No Device	Z No Qualifier

LC Limited Coverage   **NC** Noncovered   ⊞ Combination Member   HAC associated procedure   Combination Only   DRG Non-OR   Non-OR   New/Revised in **GREEN**

ICD-10-PCS 2021   599

ØS2–ØS5

Ø Medical and Surgical
S Lower Joints
9 Drainage　　Definition: Taking or letting out fluids and/or gases from a body part
　　　　　　　　　　Explanation: The qualifier DIAGNOSTIC is used to identify drainage procedures that are biopsies

Body Part Character 4		Approach Character 5	Device Character 6	Qualifier Character 7
Ø Lumbar Vertebral Joint Lumbar facet joint **2 Lumbar Vertebral Disc** **3 Lumbosacral Joint** Lumbosacral facet joint **4 Lumbosacral Disc** **5 Sacrococcygeal Joint** Sacrococcygeal symphysis **6 Coccygeal Joint** **7 Sacroiliac Joint, Right** **8 Sacroiliac Joint, Left** **9 Hip Joint, Right** Acetabulofemoral joint **B Hip Joint, Left** *See 9 Hip Joint, Right* **C Knee Joint, Right** Femoropatellar joint Femorotibial joint Lateral meniscus Medial meniscus Patellofemoral joint Tibiofemoral joint **D Knee Joint, Left** *See C Knee Joint, Right* **F Ankle Joint, Right** Inferior tibiofibular joint Talocrural joint **G Ankle Joint, Left** *See F Ankle Joint, Right*	**H Tarsal Joint, Right** Calcaneocuboid joint Cuboideonavicular joint Cuneonavicular joint Intercuneiform joint Subtalar (talocalcaneal) joint Talocalcaneal (subtalar) 　joint Talocalcaneonavicular joint **J Tarsal Joint, Left** *See H Tarsal Joint, Right* **K Tarsometatarsal Joint, Right** **L Tarsometatarsal Joint, Left** **M Metatarsal-Phalangeal Joint, Right** Metatarsophalangeal (MTP) 　joint **N Metatarsal-Phalangeal Joint, Left** *See M Metatarsal-Phalangeal Joint, Right* **P Toe Phalangeal Joint, Right** Interphalangeal (IP) joint **Q Toe Phalangeal Joint, Left** *See P Toe Phalangeal Joint, Right*	**Ø Open** **3 Percutaneous** **4 Percutaneous Endoscopic**	**Ø Drainage Device**	**Z No Qualifier**
Ø Lumbar Vertebral Joint Lumbar facet joint **2 Lumbar Vertebral Disc** **3 Lumbosacral Joint** Lumbosacral facet joint **4 Lumbosacral Disc** **5 Sacrococcygeal Joint** Sacrococcygeal symphysis **6 Coccygeal Joint** **7 Sacroiliac Joint, Right** **8 Sacroiliac Joint, Left** **9 Hip Joint, Right** Acetabulofemoral joint **B Hip Joint, Left** *See 9 Hip Joint, Right* **C Knee Joint, Right** Femoropatellar joint Femorotibial joint Lateral meniscus Medial meniscus Patellofemoral joint Tibiofemoral joint **D Knee Joint, Left** *See C Knee Joint, Right* **F Ankle Joint, Right** Inferior tibiofibular joint Talocrural joint **G Ankle Joint, Left** *See F Ankle Joint, Right*	**H Tarsal Joint, Right** Calcaneocuboid joint Cuboideonavicular joint Cuneonavicular joint Intercuneiform joint Subtalar (talocalcaneal) joint Talocalcaneal (subtalar) 　joint Talocalcaneonavicular joint **J Tarsal Joint, Left** *See H Tarsal Joint, Right* **K Tarsometatarsal Joint, Right** **L Tarsometatarsal Joint, Left** **M Metatarsal-Phalangeal Joint, Right** Metatarsophalangeal (MTP) 　joint **N Metatarsal-Phalangeal Joint, Left** *See M Metatarsal-Phalangeal Joint, Right* **P Toe Phalangeal Joint, Right** Interphalangeal (IP) joint **Q Toe Phalangeal Joint, Left** *See P Toe Phalangeal Joint, Right*	**Ø Open** **3 Percutaneous** **4 Percutaneous Endoscopic**	**Z No Device**	**X Diagnostic** **Z No Qualifier**

Non-OR　ØS9[Ø,2,3,4,5,6,7,8,9,B,C,D,F,G,H,J,K,L,M,N,P,Q][3,4]ØZ
Non-OR　ØS9[Ø,2,3,4,5,6,7,8,9,B,C,D,F,G,H,J,K,L,M,N,P,Q][Ø,3,4]ZX
Non-OR　ØS9[Ø,2,3,4,5,6,7,8,9,B,C,D,F,G,H,J,K,L,M,N,P,Q][3,4]ZZ

Ø Medical and Surgical
S Lower Joints
B Excision　　Definition: Cutting out or off, without replacement, a portion of a body part
　　　　　　　　　　Explanation: The qualifier DIAGNOSTIC is used to identify excision procedures that are biopsies

Body Part Character 4		Approach Character 5	Device Character 6	Qualifier Character 7
Ø Lumbar Vertebral Joint Lumbar facet joint	**H Tarsal Joint, Right** Calcaneocuboid joint	**Ø Open** **3 Percutaneous** **4 Percutaneous Endoscopic**	**Z No Device**	**X Diagnostic** **Z No Qualifier**
2 Lumbar Vertebral Disc	Cuboideonavicular joint			
3 Lumbosacral Joint Lumbosacral facet joint	Cuneonavicular joint Intercuneiform joint			
4 Lumbosacral Disc	Subtalar (talocalcaneal) joint Talocalcaneal (subtalar)			
5 Sacrococcygeal Joint Sacrococcygeal symphysis	joint Talocalcaneonavicular joint			
6 Coccygeal Joint	**J Tarsal Joint, Left** *See H Tarsal Joint, Right*			
7 Sacroiliac Joint, Right	**K Tarsometatarsal Joint,**			
8 Sacroiliac Joint, Left	**Right**			
9 Hip Joint, Right Acetabulofemoral joint	**L Tarsometatarsal Joint, Left** **M Metatarsal-Phalangeal**			
B Hip Joint, Left *See 9 Hip Joint, Right*	**Joint, Right** Metatarsophalangeal (MTP)			
C Knee Joint, Right Femoropatellar joint	joint **N Metatarsal-Phalangeal**			
Femorotibial joint Lateral meniscus	**Joint, Left** *See M Metatarsal-Phalangeal*			
Medial meniscus Patellofemoral joint	*Joint, Right*			
Tibiofemoral joint	**P Toe Phalangeal Joint, Right**			
D Knee Joint, Left *See C Knee Joint, Right*	Interphalangeal (IP) joint **Q Toe Phalangeal Joint, Left**			
F Ankle Joint, Right Inferior tibiofibular joint	*See P Toe Phalangeal Joint,* *Right*			
Talocrural joint				
G Ankle Joint, Left *See F Ankle Joint, Right*				

Non-OR　ØSB[Ø,2,3,4,5,6,7,8,9,B,C,D,F,G,H,J,K,L,M,N,P,Q][Ø,3,4]ZX

Ø Medical and Surgical
S Lower Joints
C Extirpation　　Definition: Taking or cutting out solid matter from a body part
　　　　　　　　　　　Explanation: The solid matter may be an abnormal byproduct of a biological function or a foreign body; it may be imbedded in a body part or in the lumen of a tubular body part. The solid matter may or may not have been previously broken into pieces.

Body Part Character 4		Approach Character 5	Device Character 6	Qualifier Character 7
Ø Lumbar Vertebral Joint Lumbar facet joint	**H Tarsal Joint, Right** Calcaneocuboid joint	**Ø Open** **3 Percutaneous** **4 Percutaneous Endoscopic**	**Z No Device**	**Z No Qualifier**
2 Lumbar Vertebral Disc	Cuboideonavicular joint			
3 Lumbosacral Joint Lumbosacral facet joint	Cuneonavicular joint Intercuneiform joint			
4 Lumbosacral Disc	Subtalar (talocalcaneal) joint Talocalcaneal (subtalar)			
5 Sacrococcygeal Joint Sacrococcygeal symphysis	joint Talocalcaneonavicular joint			
6 Coccygeal Joint	**J Tarsal Joint, Left** *See H Tarsal Joint, Right*			
7 Sacroiliac Joint, Right	**K Tarsometatarsal Joint,**			
8 Sacroiliac Joint, Left	**Right**			
9 Hip Joint, Right Acetabulofemoral joint	**L Tarsometatarsal Joint, Left** **M Metatarsal-Phalangeal**			
B Hip Joint, Left *See 9 Hip Joint, Right*	**Joint, Right** Metatarsophalangeal (MTP)			
C Knee Joint, Right Femoropatellar joint	joint **N Metatarsal-Phalangeal**			
Femorotibial joint Lateral meniscus	**Joint, Left** *See M Metatarsal-Phalangeal*			
Medial meniscus Patellofemoral joint	*Joint, Right*			
Tibiofemoral joint	**P Toe Phalangeal Joint, Right**			
D Knee Joint, Left *See C Knee Joint, Right*	Interphalangeal (IP) joint **Q Toe Phalangeal Joint, Left**			
F Ankle Joint, Right Inferior tibiofibular joint	*See P Toe Phalangeal Joint,* *Right*			
Talocrural joint				
G Ankle Joint, Left *See F Ankle Joint, Right*				

Ø Medical and Surgical
S Lower Joints
G Fusion   Definition: Joining together portions of an articular body part rendering the articular body part immobile
                Explanation: The body part is joined together by fixation device, bone graft, or other means

Body Part Character 4	Approach Character 5	Device Character 6	Qualifier Character 7
Ø Lumbar Vertebral Joint Lumbar facet joint **1 Lumbar Vertebral Joints, 2 or more** ⊞ **3 Lumbosacral Joint** Lumbosacral facet joint	**Ø** Open **3** Percutaneous **4** Percutaneous Endoscopic	**7** Autologous Tissue Substitute **J** Synthetic Substitute **K** Nonautologous Tissue Substitute	**Ø** Anterior Approach, Anterior Column **1** Posterior Approach, Posterior Column **J** Posterior Approach, Anterior Column
Ø Lumbar Vertebral Joint Lumbar facet joint **1 Lumbar Vertebral Joints, 2 or more** ⊞ **3 Lumbosacral Joint** Lumbosacral facet joint	**Ø** Open **3** Percutaneous **4** Percutaneous Endoscopic	**A** Interbody Fusion Device	**Ø** Anterior Approach, Anterior Column **J** Posterior Approach, Anterior Column
5 Sacrococcygeal Joint Sacrococcygeal symphysis **6 Coccygeal Joint** **7 Sacroiliac Joint, Right** **8 Sacroiliac Joint, Left**	**Ø** Open **3** Percutaneous **4** Percutaneous Endoscopic	**4** Internal Fixation Device **7** Autologous Tissue Substitute **J** Synthetic Substitute **K** Nonautologous Tissue Substitute	**Z** No Qualifier
9 Hip Joint, Right Acetabulofemoral joint **B Hip Joint, Left** *See 9 Hip Joint, Right* **C Knee Joint, Right** Femoropatellar joint Femorotibial joint Lateral meniscus Medial meniscus Patellofemoral joint Tibiofemoral joint **D Knee Joint, Left** *See C Knee Joint, Right* **F Ankle Joint, Right** Inferior tibiofibular joint Talocrural joint **G Ankle Joint, Left** *See F Ankle Joint, Right* **H Tarsal Joint, Right** Calcaneocuboid joint Cuboideonavicular joint Cuneonavicular joint Intercuneiform joint Subtalar (talocalcaneal) joint Talocalcaneal (subtalar) joint Talocalcaneonavicular joint **J Tarsal Joint, Left** *See H Tarsal Joint, Right* **K Tarsometatarsal Joint, Right** **L Tarsometatarsal Joint, Left** **M Metatarsal-Phalangeal Joint, Right** Metatarsophalangeal (MTP) joint **N Metatarsal-Phalangeal Joint, Left** *See M Metatarsal-Phalangeal Joint, Right* **P Toe Phalangeal Joint, Right** Interphalangeal (IP) joint **Q Toe Phalangeal Joint, Left** *See P Toe Phalangeal Joint, Right*	**Ø** Open **3** Percutaneous **4** Percutaneous Endoscopic	**3** Internal Fixation Device, Sustained Compression **4** Internal Fixation Device **5** External Fixation Device **7** Autologous Tissue Substitute **J** Synthetic Substitute **K** Nonautologous Tissue Substitute	**Z** No Qualifier

HAC	ØSG[Ø,1,3][Ø,3,4][7,J,K][Ø,1,J] when reported with SDx K68.11 or T81.4Ø–T81.49, T84.6Ø-T84.619, T84.63-T84.7 with 7th character A
HAC	ØSG[Ø,1,3][Ø,3,4]A[Ø,J] when reported with SDx K68.11 or T81.4Ø–T81.49, T84.6Ø-T84.619, T84.63-T84.7 with 7th character A
HAC	ØSG[7,8][Ø,3,4][4,7,J,K]Z when reported with SDx K68.11 or T81.4Ø–T81.49, T84.6Ø-T84.619, T84.63-T84.7 with 7th character A

See Appendix L for Procedure Combinations
⊞   ØSG1[Ø,3,4][7,J,K][Ø,1,J]
⊞   ØSG1[Ø,3,4]A[Ø,J]

LC Limited Coverage   NC Noncovered   ⊞ Combination Member   HAC associated procedure   Combination Only   DRG Non-OR   Non-OR   New/Revised in **GREEN**

602   ICD-10-PCS 2021

Ø　Medical and Surgical
S　Lower Joints
H　Insertion　　Definition: Putting in a nonbiological appliance that monitors, assists, performs, or prevents a physiological function but does not physically take the place of a body part
　　　　　　　　　Explanation: None

Body Part Character 4	Approach Character 5	Device Character 6	Qualifier Character 7
Ø　Lumbar Vertebral Joint 　　Lumbar facet joint **3　Lumbosacral Joint** 　　Lumbosacral facet joint	**Ø　Open** **3　Percutaneous** **4　Percutaneous Endoscopic**	**3　Infusion Device** **4　Internal Fixation Device** **8　Spacer** **B　Spinal Stabilization Device, 　　Interspinous Process** **C　Spinal Stabilization Device, 　　Pedicle-Based** **D　Spinal Stabilization Device, Facet 　　Replacement**	**Z　No Qualifier**
2　Lumbar Vertebral Disc **4　Lumbosacral Disc**	**Ø　Open** **3　Percutaneous** **4　Percutaneous Endoscopic**	**3　Infusion Device** **8　Spacer**	**Z　No Qualifier**
5　Sacrococcygeal Joint 　　Sacrococcygeal symphysis **6　Coccygeal Joint** **7　Sacroiliac Joint, Right** **8　Sacroiliac Joint, Left**	**Ø　Open** **3　Percutaneous** **4　Percutaneous Endoscopic**	**3　Infusion Device** **4　Internal Fixation Device** **8　Spacer**	**Z　No Qualifier**
9　Hip Joint, Right 　　Acetabulofemoral joint **B　Hip Joint, Left** 　　*See 9 Hip Joint, Right* **C　Knee Joint, Right** 　　Femoropatellar joint 　　Femorotibial joint 　　Lateral meniscus 　　Medial meniscus 　　Patellofemoral joint 　　Tibiofemoral joint **D　Knee Joint, Left** 　　*See C Knee Joint, Right* **F　Ankle Joint, Right** 　　Inferior tibiofibular joint 　　Talocrural joint **G　Ankle Joint, Left** 　　*See F Ankle Joint, Right* **H　Tarsal Joint, Right** 　　Calcaneocuboid joint 　　Cuboideonavicular joint 　　Cuneonavicular joint 　　Intercuneiform joint 　　Subtalar (talocalcaneal) joint 　　Talocalcaneal (subtalar) joint 　　Talocalcaneonavicular joint **J　Tarsal Joint, Left** 　　*See H Tarsal Joint, Right* **K　Tarsometatarsal Joint, Right** **L　Tarsometatarsal Joint, Left** **M　Metatarsal-Phalangeal Joint, Right** 　　Metatarsophalangeal (MTP) joint **N　Metatarsal-Phalangeal Joint, Left** 　　*See M Metatarsal-Phalangeal Joint, Right* **P　Toe Phalangeal Joint, Right** 　　Interphalangeal (IP) joint **Q　Toe Phalangeal Joint, Left** 　　*See P Toe Phalangeal Joint, Right*	**Ø　Open** **3　Percutaneous** **4　Percutaneous Endoscopic**	**3　Infusion Device** **4　Internal Fixation Device** **5　External Fixation Device** **8　Spacer**	**Z　No Qualifier**

Non-OR	ØSH[Ø,3][Ø,3,4][3,8]Z
Non-OR	ØSH[2,4][Ø,3,4][3,8]Z
Non-OR	ØSH[5,6,7,8][Ø,3,4][3,8]Z
Non-OR	ØSH[9,B,C,D][Ø,3,4]3Z
Non-OR	ØSH[9,B,C,D][3,4]8Z
Non-OR	ØSH[F,G,H,J,K,L,M,N,P,Q][Ø,3,4][3,8]Z

LC Limited Coverage　　**NC** Noncovered　　⊞ Combination Member　　HAC associated procedure　　Combination Only　　DRG Non-OR　　Non-OR　　New/Revised in GREEN
ICD-10-PCS 2021　　　**603**

ØSH–ØSH

Lower Joints

Ø Medical and Surgical
S Lower Joints
J Inspection   Definition: Visually and/or manually exploring a body part

Explanation: Visual exploration may be performed with or without optical instrumentation. Manual exploration may be performed directly or through intervening body layers.

Body Part Character 4		Approach Character 5	Device Character 6	Qualifier Character 7
Ø **Lumbar Vertebral Joint** Lumbar facet joint	H **Tarsal Joint, Right** Calcaneocuboid joint Cuboideonavicular joint Cuneonavicular joint Intercuneiform joint Subtalar (talocalcaneal) joint Talocalcaneal (subtalar) joint Talocalcaneonavicular joint	Ø Open 3 Percutaneous 4 Percutaneous Endoscopic X External	Z No Device	Z No Qualifier
2 **Lumbar Vertebral Disc**				
3 **Lumbosacral Joint** Lumbosacral facet joint				
4 **Lumbosacral Disc**				
5 **Sacrococcygeal Joint** Sacrococcygeal symphysis				
6 **Coccygeal Joint**	J **Tarsal Joint, Left** *See H Tarsal Joint, Right*			
7 **Sacroiliac Joint, Right**	K **Tarsometatarsal Joint, Right**			
8 **Sacroiliac Joint, Left**	L **Tarsometatarsal Joint, Left**			
9 **Hip Joint, Right** Acetabulofemoral joint	M **Metatarsal-Phalangeal Joint, Right** Metatarsophalangeal (MTP) joint			
B **Hip Joint, Left** *See 9 Hip Joint, Right*				
C **Knee Joint, Right** Femoropatellar joint Femorotibial joint Lateral meniscus Medial meniscus Patellofemoral joint Tibiofemoral joint	N **Metatarsal-Phalangeal Joint, Left** *See M Metatarsal-Phalangeal Joint, Right*			
	P **Toe Phalangeal Joint, Right** Interphalangeal (IP) joint			
D **Knee Joint, Left** *See C Knee Joint, Right*	Q **Toe Phalangeal Joint, Left** *See P Toe Phalangeal Joint, Right*			
F **Ankle Joint, Right** Inferior tibiofibular joint Talocrural joint				
G **Ankle Joint, Left** *See F Ankle Joint, Right*				

Non-OR   ØSJ[Ø,2,3,4,5,6,7,8,9,B,C,D,F,G,H,J,K,L,M,N,P,Q][3,X]ZZ

Ø Medical and Surgical
S Lower Joints
N Release   Definition: Freeing a body part from an abnormal physical constraint by cutting or by the use of force

Explanation: Some of the restraining tissue may be taken out but none of the body part is taken out

Body Part Character 4		Approach Character 5	Device Character 6	Qualifier Character 7
Ø **Lumbar Vertebral Joint** Lumbar facet joint	H **Tarsal Joint, Right** Calcaneocuboid joint Cuboideonavicular joint Cuneonavicular joint Intercuneiform joint Subtalar (talocalcaneal) joint Talocalcaneal (subtalar) joint Talocalcaneonavicular joint	Ø Open 3 Percutaneous 4 Percutaneous Endoscopic X External	Z No Device	Z No Qualifier
2 **Lumbar Vertebral Disc**				
3 **Lumbosacral Joint** Lumbosacral facet joint				
4 **Lumbosacral Disc**				
5 **Sacrococcygeal Joint** Sacrococcygeal symphysis				
6 **Coccygeal Joint**	J **Tarsal Joint, Left** *See H Tarsal Joint, Right*			
7 **Sacroiliac Joint, Right**	K **Tarsometatarsal Joint, Right**			
8 **Sacroiliac Joint, Left**	L **Tarsometatarsal Joint, Left**			
9 **Hip Joint, Right** Acetabulofemoral joint	M **Metatarsal-Phalangeal Joint, Right** Metatarsophalangeal (MTP) joint			
B **Hip Joint, Left** *See 9 Hip Joint, Right*				
C **Knee Joint, Right** Femoropatellar joint Femorotibial joint Lateral meniscus Medial meniscus Patellofemoral joint Tibiofemoral joint	N **Metatarsal-Phalangeal Joint, Left** *See M Metatarsal-Phalangeal Joint, Right*			
	P **Toe Phalangeal Joint, Right** Interphalangeal (IP) joint			
D **Knee Joint, Left** *See C Knee Joint, Right*	Q **Toe Phalangeal Joint, Left** *See P Toe Phalangeal Joint, Right*			
F **Ankle Joint, Right** Inferior tibiofibular joint Talocrural joint				
G **Ankle Joint, Left** *See F Ankle Joint, Right*				

Non-OR   ØSN[Ø,2,3,4,5,6,7,8,9,B,C,D,F,G,H,J,K,L,M,N,P,Q]XZZ

LC Limited Coverage   NC Noncovered   ⊞ Combination Member   HAC associated procedure   Combination Only   DRG Non-OR   Non-OR   New/Revised in GREEN

604   ICD-10-PCS 2021

ØSJ–ØSN

Ø Medical and Surgical
S Lower Joints
P Removal   Definition: Taking out or off a device from a body part

Explanation: If a device is taken out and a similar device put in without cutting or puncturing the skin or mucous membrane, the procedure is coded to the root operation CHANGE. Otherwise, the procedure for taking out the device is coded to the root operation REMOVAL.

Body Part Character 4	Approach Character 5	Device Character 6	Qualifier Character 7
Ø Lumbar Vertebral Joint Lumbar facet joint **3 Lumbosacral Joint** Lumbosacral facet joint	**Ø** Open **3** Percutaneous **4** Percutaneous Endoscopic	**Ø** Drainage Device **3** Infusion Device **4** Internal Fixation Device **7** Autologous Tissue Substitute **8** Spacer **A** Interbody Fusion Device **J** Synthetic Substitute **K** Nonautologous Tissue Substitute	**Z** No Qualifier
Ø Lumbar Vertebral Joint Lumbar facet joint **3 Lumbosacral Joint** Lumbosacral facet joint	**X** External	**Ø** Drainage Device **3** Infusion Device **4** Internal Fixation Device	**Z** No Qualifier
2 Lumbar Vertebral Disc **4 Lumbosacral Disc**	**Ø** Open **3** Percutaneous **4** Percutaneous Endoscopic	**Ø** Drainage Device **3** Infusion Device **7** Autologous Tissue Substitute **J** Synthetic Substitute **K** Nonautologous Tissue Substitute	**Z** No Qualifier
2 Lumbar Vertebral Disc **4 Lumbosacral Disc**	**X** External	**Ø** Drainage Device **3** Infusion Device	**Z** No Qualifier
5 Sacrococcygeal Joint Sacrococcygeal symphysis **6 Coccygeal Joint** **7 Sacroiliac Joint, Right** **8 Sacroiliac Joint, Left**	**Ø** Open **3** Percutaneous **4** Percutaneous Endoscopic	**Ø** Drainage Device **3** Infusion Device **4** Internal Fixation Device **7** Autologous Tissue Substitute **8** Spacer **J** Synthetic Substitute **K** Nonautologous Tissue Substitute	**Z** No Qualifier
5 Sacrococcygeal Joint Sacrococcygeal symphysis **6 Coccygeal Joint** **7 Sacroiliac Joint, Right** **8 Sacroiliac Joint, Left**	**X** External	**Ø** Drainage Device **3** Infusion Device **4** Internal Fixation Device	**Z** No Qualifier
9 Hip Joint, Right ⊞ Acetabulofemoral joint **B Hip Joint, Left** ⊞ *See 9 Hip Joint, Right*	**Ø** Open	**Ø** Drainage Device **3** Infusion Device **4** Internal Fixation Device **5** External Fixation Device **7** Autologous Tissue Substitute **8** Spacer **9** Liner **B** Resurfacing Device **E** Articulating Spacer **J** Synthetic Substitute **K** Nonautologous Tissue Substitute	**Z** No Qualifier
9 Hip Joint, Right ⊞ Acetabulofemoral joint **B Hip Joint, Left** ⊞ *See 9 Hip Joint, Right*	**3** Percutaneous **4** Percutaneous Endoscopic	**Ø** Drainage Device **3** Infusion Device **4** Internal Fixation Device **5** External Fixation Device **7** Autologous Tissue Substitute **8** Spacer **J** Synthetic Substitute **K** Nonautologous Tissue Substitute	**Z** No Qualifier
9 Hip Joint, Right Acetabulofemoral joint **B Hip Joint, Left** *See 9 Hip Joint, Right*	**X** External	**Ø** Drainage Device **3** Infusion Device **4** Internal Fixation Device **5** External Fixation Device	**Z** No Qualifier

Non-OR	ØSP[Ø,3][Ø,3,4]8Z	**See Appendix L for Procedure Combinations**	
Non-OR	ØSP[Ø,3]3[Ø,3]Z	**Combo-only**	ØSP[9,B]48Z
Non-OR	ØSP[Ø,3]X[Ø,3,4]Z	⊞	ØSP[9,B][Ø,8,9,B,E,J]Z
Non-OR	ØSP[2,4]3[Ø,3]Z	⊞	ØSP[9,B]4JZ
Non-OR	ØSP[2,4]X[Ø,3]Z		
Non-OR	ØSP[5,6,7,8][Ø,3,4]8Z		
Non-OR	ØSP[5,6,7,8]3[Ø,3]Z		
Non-OR	ØSP[5,6,7,8]X[Ø,3,4]Z		
Non-OR	ØSP[9,B]3[Ø,3,8]Z		
Non-OR	ØSP[9,B]X[Ø,3,4,5]Z		

ØSP Continued on next page

⊡ Limited Coverage   ⊡ Noncovered   ⊞ Combination Member   HAC associated procedure   Combination Only   DRG Non-OR   Non-OR   New/Revised in GREEN

Ø Medical and Surgical
S Lower Joints
P Removal

Definition: Taking out or off a device from a body part
Explanation: If a device is taken out and a similar device put in without cutting or puncturing the skin or mucous membrane, the procedure is coded to the root operation CHANGE. Otherwise, the procedure for taking out the device is coded to the root operation REMOVAL.

Body Part Character 4	Approach Character 5	Device Character 6	Qualifier Character 7

A Hip Joint, Acetabular Surface, Right ⊞
E Hip Joint, Acetabular Surface, Left ⊞
R Hip Joint, Femoral Surface, Right ⊞
S Hip Joint, Femoral Surface, Left ⊞
T Knee Joint, Femoral Surface, Right ⊞
  Femoropatellar joint
  Patellofemoral joint
U Knee Joint, Femoral Surface, Left ⊞
  See T Knee Joint, Femoral Surface, Right
V Knee Joint, Tibial Surface, Right ⊞
  Femorotibial joint
  Tibiofemoral joint
W Knee Joint, Tibial Surface, Left ⊞
  See V Knee Joint, Tibial Surface, Right
	Ø Open
	3 Percutaneous
	4 Percutaneous Endoscopic
		J Synthetic Substitute	Z No Qualifier

C Knee Joint, Right ⊞
  Femoropatellar joint
  Femorotibial joint
  Lateral meniscus
  Medial meniscus
  Patellofemoral joint
  Tibiofemoral joint
D Knee Joint, Left ⊞
  See C Knee Joint, Right
	Ø Open	Ø Drainage Device
		3 Infusion Device
		4 Internal Fixation Device
		5 External Fixation Device
		7 Autologous Tissue Substitute
		8 Spacer
		9 Liner
		E Articulating Spacer
		K Nonautologous Tissue Substitute
		L Synthetic Substitute, Unicondylar Medial
		M Synthetic Substitute, Unicondylar Lateral
		N Synthetic Substitute, Patellofemoral
			Z No Qualifier

C Knee Joint, Right ⊞
  Femoropatellar joint
  Femorotibial joint
  Lateral meniscus
  Medial meniscus
  Patellofemoral joint
  Tibiofemoral joint
D Knee Joint, Left ⊞
  See C Knee Joint, Right
	Ø Open	J Synthetic Substitute	C Patellar Surface
			Z No Qualifier

C Knee Joint, Right ⊞
  Femoropatellar joint
  Femorotibial joint
  Lateral meniscus
  Medial meniscus
  Patellofemoral joint
  Tibiofemoral joint
D Knee Joint, Left ⊞
  See C Knee Joint, Right
	3 Percutaneous
	4 Percutaneous Endoscopic
		Ø Drainage Device
		3 Infusion Device
		4 Internal Fixation Device
		5 External Fixation Device
		7 Autologous Tissue Substitute
		8 Spacer
		K Nonautologous Tissue Substitute
		L Synthetic Substitute, Unicondylar Medial
		M Synthetic Substitute, Unicondylar Lateral
		N Synthetic Substitute, Patellofemoral
			Z No Qualifier

C Knee Joint, Right ⊞
  Femoropatellar joint
  Femorotibial joint
  Lateral meniscus
  Medial meniscus
  Patellofemoral joint
  Tibiofemoral joint
D Knee Joint, Left ⊞
  See C Knee Joint, Right
	3 Percutaneous
	4 Percutaneous Endoscopic
		J Synthetic Substitute	C Patellar Surface
			Z No Qualifier

Non-OR   ØSP[C,D]3[Ø,3]Z

See Appendix L for Procedure Combinations
Combo-only   ØSP[C,D][3,4]8Z   ⊞   ØSP[C,D]ØJ[C,Z]
⊞   ØSP[A,E,R,S,T,U,V,W][Ø,4]JZ   ⊞   ØSP[C,D]4[L,M,N]Z
⊞   ØSP[C,D]Ø[8,9,E,L,M,N]Z   ⊞   ØSP[C,D]4J[C,Z]

ØSP Continued on next page

Ø   Medical and Surgical
S   Lower Joints
P   Removal

ØSP Continued

Definition: Taking out or off a device from a body part

Explanation: If a device is taken out and a similar device put in without cutting or puncturing the skin or mucous membrane, the procedure is coded to the root operation CHANGE. Otherwise, the procedure for taking out the device is coded to the root operation REMOVAL.

Body Part Character 4	Approach Character 5	Device Character 6	Qualifier Character 7
C Knee Joint, Right Femoropatellar joint Femorotibial joint Lateral meniscus Medial meniscus Patellofemoral joint Tibiofemoral joint **D Knee Joint, Left** *See C Knee Joint, Right*	**X** External	**Ø** Drainage Device **3** Infusion Device **4** Internal Fixation Device **5** External Fixation Device	**Z** No Qualifier
F Ankle Joint, Right Inferior tibiofibular joint Talocrural joint **G Ankle Joint, Left** *See F Ankle Joint, Right* **H Tarsal Joint, Right** Calcaneocuboid joint Cuboideonavicular joint Cuneonavicular joint Intercuneiform joint Subtalar (talocalcaneal) joint Talocalcaneal (subtalar) joint Talocalcaneonavicular joint **J Tarsal Joint, Left** *See H Tarsal Joint, Right* **K Tarsometatarsal Joint, Right** **L Tarsometatarsal Joint, Left** **M Metatarsal-Phalangeal Joint, Right** Metatarsophalangeal (MTP) joint **N Metatarsal-Phalangeal Joint, Left** *See M Metatarsal-Phalangeal Joint, Right* **P Toe Phalangeal Joint, Right** Interphalangeal (IP) joint **Q Toe Phalangeal Joint, Left** *See P Toe Phalangeal Joint, Right*	**Ø** Open **3** Percutaneous **4** Percutaneous Endoscopic	**Ø** Drainage Device **3** Infusion Device **4** Internal Fixation Device **5** External Fixation Device **7** Autologous Tissue Substitute **8** Spacer **J** Synthetic Substitute **K** Nonautologous Tissue Substitute	**Z** No Qualifier
F Ankle Joint, Right Inferior tibiofibular joint Talocrural joint **G Ankle Joint, Left** *See F Ankle Joint, Right* **H Tarsal Joint, Right** Calcaneocuboid joint Cuboideonavicular joint Cuneonavicular joint Intercuneiform joint Subtalar (talocalcaneal) joint Talocalcaneal (subtalar) joint Talocalcaneonavicular joint **J Tarsal Joint, Left** *See H Tarsal Joint, Right* **K Tarsometatarsal Joint, Right** **L Tarsometatarsal Joint, Left** **M Metatarsal-Phalangeal Joint, Right** Metatarsophalangeal (MTP) joint **N Metatarsal-Phalangeal Joint, Left** *See M Metatarsal-Phalangeal Joint, Right* **P Toe Phalangeal Joint, Right** Interphalangeal (IP) joint **Q Toe Phalangeal Joint, Left** *See P Toe Phalangeal Joint, Right*	**X** External	**Ø** Drainage Device **3** Infusion Device **4** Internal Fixation Device **5** External Fixation Device	**Z** No Qualifier

Non-OR   ØSP[C,D]X[Ø,3,4,5]Z
Non-OR   ØSP[F,G,H,J,K,L,M,N,P,Q]3[Ø,3,8]Z
Non-OR   ØSP[F,G,H,J,K,L,M,N,P,Q][Ø,4]8Z
Non-OR   ØSP[F,G,H,J,K,L,M,N,P,Q]X[Ø,3,4,5]Z

LC Limited Coverage   NC Noncovered   ⊞ Combination Member   HAC associated procedure   Combination Only   DRG Non-OR   Non-OR   New/Revised in GREEN

ICD-10-PCS 2021   607

ØSP–ØSP

Ø   **Medical and Surgical**
S   **Lower Joints**
Q   **Repair**   Definition: Restoring, to the extent possible, a body part to its normal anatomic structure and function
                     Explanation: Used only when the method to accomplish the repair is not one of the other root operations

Body Part Character 4	Approach Character 5	Device Character 6	Qualifier Character 7
Ø Lumbar Vertebral Joint Lumbar facet joint **2 Lumbar Vertebral Disc** **3 Lumbosacral Joint** Lumbosacral facet joint **4 Lumbosacral Disc** **5 Sacrococcygeal Joint** Sacrococcygeal symphysis **6 Coccygeal Joint** **7 Sacroiliac Joint, Right** **8 Sacroiliac Joint, Left** **9 Hip Joint, Right** Acetabulofemoral joint **B Hip Joint, Left** *See* 9 Hip Joint, Right **C Knee Joint, Right** Femoropatellar joint Femorotibial joint Lateral meniscus Medial meniscus Patellofemoral joint Tibiofemoral joint **D Knee Joint, Left** *See* C Knee Joint, Right **F Ankle Joint, Right** Inferior tibiofibular joint Talocrural joint **G Ankle Joint, Left** *See* F Ankle Joint, Right **H Tarsal Joint, Right** Calcaneocuboid joint Cuboideonavicular joint Cuneonavicular joint Intercuneiform joint Subtalar (talocalcaneal) joint Talocalcaneal (subtalar) joint Talocalcaneonavicular joint **J Tarsal Joint, Left** *See* H Tarsal Joint, Right **K Tarsometatarsal Joint, Right** **L Tarsometatarsal Joint, Left** **M Metatarsal-Phalangeal Joint, Right** Metatarsophalangeal (MTP) joint **N Metatarsal-Phalangeal Joint, Left** *See* M Metatarsal-Phalangeal Joint, Right **P Toe Phalangeal Joint, Right** Interphalangeal (IP) joint **Q Toe Phalangeal Joint, Left** *See* P Toe Phalangeal Joint, Right	**Ø Open** **3 Percutaneous** **4 Percutaneous Endoscopic** **X External**	**Z No Device**	**Z No Qualifier**

Non-OR   ØSQ[Ø,2,3,4,5,6,7,8,9,B,C,D,F,G,H,J,K,L,M,N,P,Q]XZZ

LG Limited Coverage   NC Noncovered   ⊞ Combination Member   HAC associated procedure   Combination Only   DRG Non-OR   Non-OR   New/Revised in GREEN

608   ICD-10-PCS 2021

ØSQ–ØSQ

Ø Medical and Surgical
S Lower Joints
R Replacement

Definition: Putting in or on biological or synthetic material that physically takes the place and/or function of all or a portion of a body part

Explanation: The body part may have been taken out or replaced, or may be taken out, physically eradicated, or rendered nonfunctional during the REPLACEMENT procedure. A REMOVAL procedure is coded for taking out the device used in a previous replacement procedure.

Body Part Character 4	Approach Character 5	Device Character 6	Qualifier Character 7
Ø Lumbar Vertebral Joint Lumbar facet joint	**Ø Open**	**7 Autologous Tissue Substitute**	**Z No Qualifier**
2 Lumbar Vertebral Disc NC		**J Synthetic Substitute**	
3 Lumbosacral Joint Lumbosacral facet joint		**K Nonautologous Tissue Substitute**	
4 Lumbosacral Disc NC			
5 Sacrococcygeal Joint Sacrococcygeal symphysis			
6 Coccygeal Joint			
7 Sacroiliac Joint, Right			
8 Sacroiliac Joint, Left			
H Tarsal Joint, Right Calcaneocuboid joint Cuboideonavicular joint Cuneonavicular joint Intercuneiform joint Subtalar (talocalcaneal) joint Talocalcaneal (subtalar) joint Talocalcaneonavicular joint			
J Tarsal Joint, Left *See H Tarsal Joint, Right*			
K Tarsometatarsal Joint, Right			
L Tarsometatarsal Joint, Left			
M Metatarsal-Phalangeal Joint, Right Metatarsophalangeal (MTP) joint			
N Metatarsal-Phalangeal Joint, Left *See M Metatarsal-Phalangeal Joint, Right*			
P Toe Phalangeal Joint, Right Interphalangeal (IP) joint			
Q Toe Phalangeal Joint, Left *See P Toe Phalangeal Joint, Right*			
9 Hip Joint, Right ⊞ Acetabulofemoral joint **B Hip Joint, Left** ⊞ *See 9 Hip Joint, Right*	**Ø Open**	**1 Synthetic Substitute, Metal** **2 Synthetic Substitute, Metal on Polyethylene** **3 Synthetic Substitute, Ceramic** **4 Synthetic Substitute, Ceramic on Polyethylene** **6 Synthetic Substitute, Oxidized Zirconium on Polyethylene** **J Synthetic Substitute**	**9 Cemented** **A Uncemented** **Z No Qualifier**
9 Hip Joint, Right ⊞ Acetabulofemoral joint **B Hip Joint, Left** ⊞ *See 9 Hip Joint, Right*	**Ø Open**	**7 Autologous Tissue Substitute** **E Articulating Spacer** **K Nonautologous Tissue Substitute**	**Z No Qualifier**
A Hip Joint, Acetabular Surface, Right ⊞ **E Hip Joint, Acetabular Surface, Left** ⊞	**Ø Open**	**Ø Synthetic Substitute, Polyethylene** **1 Synthetic Substitute, Metal** **3 Synthetic Substitute, Ceramic** **J Synthetic Substitute**	**9 Cemented** **A Uncemented** **Z No Qualifier**
A Hip Joint, Acetabular Surface, Right **E Hip Joint, Acetabular Surface, Left**	**Ø Open**	**7 Autologous Tissue Substitute** **K Nonautologous Tissue Substitute**	**Z No Qualifier**

HAC   ØSR[9,B]Ø[1,2,3,4,6,J][9,A,Z] when reported with SDx of I26.02-I26.09, I26.92-I26.99, or I82.401-I82.4Z9

HAC   ØSR[9,B]Ø[7,E,K]Z when reported with SDx of I26.02-I26.09, I26.92-I26.99, or I82.401-I82.4Z9

HAC   ØSR[A,E]Ø[Ø,1,3,J][9,A,Z] when reported with SDx of I26.02-I26.09, I26.92-I26.99, or I82.401-I82.4Z9

HAC   ØSR[A,E]Ø[7,K]Z when reported with SDx of I26.02-I26.09, I26.92-I26.99, or I82.401-I82.4Z9

NC   ØSR[2,4]ØJZ when beneficiary age is over 60

See Appendix L for Procedure Combinations
⊞   ØSR[9,B]Ø[1,2,3,4,6,J][9,A,Z]
⊞   ØSR[9,B]ØEZ
⊞   ØSR[A,E]Ø[Ø,1,3,J][9,A,Z]

ØSR Continued on next page

ⓁⒸ Limited Coverage   NC Noncovered   ⊞ Combination Member   HAC associated procedure   Combination Only   DRG Non-OR   Non-OR   New/Revised in GREEN

ICD-10-PCS 2021   609

Ø   Medical and Surgical
S   Lower Joints
R   Replacement

ØSR Continued

Definition: Putting in or on biological or synthetic material that physically takes the place and/or function of all or a portion of a body part

Explanation: The body part may have been taken out or replaced, or may be taken out, physically eradicated, or rendered nonfunctional during the REPLACEMENT procedure. A REMOVAL procedure is coded for taking out the device used in a previous replacement procedure.

Body Part Character 4	Approach Character 5	Device Character 6	Qualifier Character 7
C Knee Joint, Right ⊞ Femoropatellar joint Femorotibial joint Lateral meniscus Medial meniscus Patellofemoral joint Tibiofemoral joint **D Knee Joint, Left** ⊞ *See C Knee Joint, Right*	**Ø Open**	**6** Synthetic Substitute, Oxidized Zirconium on Polyethylene **J** Synthetic Substitute **L** Synthetic Substitute, Unicondylar Medial **M** Synthetic Substitute, Unicondylar Lateral **N** Synthetic Substitute, Patellofemoral	**9** Cemented **A** Uncemented **Z** No Qualifier
C Knee Joint, Right ⊞ Femoropatellar joint Femorotibial joint Lateral meniscus Medial meniscus Patellofemoral joint Tibiofemoral joint **D Knee Joint, Left** ⊞ *See C Knee Joint, Right*	**Ø Open**	**7** Autologous Tissue Substitute **E** Articulating Spacer **K** Nonautologous Tissue Substitute	**Z** No Qualifier
F Ankle Joint, Right Inferior tibiofibular joint Talocrural joint **G Ankle Joint, Left** *See F Ankle Joint, Right* **T Knee Joint, Femoral Surface, Right** Femoropatellar joint Patellofemoral joint **U Knee Joint, Femoral Surface, Left** *See T Knee Joint, Femoral Surface, Right* **V Knee Joint, Tibial Surface, Right** Femorotibial joint Tibiofemoral joint **W Knee Joint, Tibial Surface, Left** *See V Knee Joint, Tibial Surface, Right*	**Ø Open**	**7** Autologous Tissue Substitute **K** Nonautologous Tissue Substitute	**Z** No Qualifier
F Ankle Joint, Right Inferior tibiofibular joint Talocrural joint **G Ankle Joint, Left** *See F Ankle Joint, Right* **T Knee Joint, Femoral Surface, Right** ⊞ Femoropatellar joint Patellofemoral joint **U Knee Joint, Femoral Surface, Left** ⊞ *See T Knee Joint, Femoral Surface, Right* **V Knee Joint, Tibial Surface, Right** ⊞ Femorotibial joint Tibiofemoral joint **W Knee Joint, Tibial Surface, Left** ⊞ *See V Knee Joint, Tibial Surface, Right*	**Ø Open**	**J** Synthetic Substitute	**9** Cemented **A** Uncemented **Z** No Qualifier
R Hip Joint, Femoral Surface, Right ⊞ **S Hip Joint, Femoral Surface, Left** ⊞	**Ø Open**	**1** Synthetic Substitute, Metal **3** Synthetic Substitute, Ceramic **J** Synthetic Substitute	**9** Cemented **A** Uncemented **Z** No Qualifier
R Hip Joint, Femoral Surface, Right **S Hip Joint, Femoral Surface, Left**	**Ø Open**	**7** Autologous Tissue Substitute **K** Nonautologous Tissue Substitute	**Z** No Qualifier

HAC   ØSR[C,D]Ø[6,J,L,M,N][9,A,Z] when reported with SDx of I26.Ø2-I26.Ø9, I26.92-I26.99 or I82.4Ø1-I82.4Z9

HAC   ØSR[C,D]Ø[7,E,K]Z when reported with SDx of I26.Ø2-I26.Ø9, I26.92-I26.99 or I82.4Ø1-I82.4Z9

HAC   ØSR[T,U,V,W]Ø[7,K]Z when reported with SDx of I26.Ø2-I26.Ø9, I26.92-I26.99 or I82.4Ø1-I82.4Z9

HAC   ØSR[T,U,V,W]ØJ[9,A,Z] when reported with SDx of I26.Ø2-I26.Ø9, I26.92-I26.99 or I82.4Ø1-I82.4Z9

HAC   ØSR[R,S]Ø[1,3,J][9,A,Z] when reported with SDx of I26.Ø2-I26.Ø9, I26.92-I26.99, or I82.4Ø1-I82.4Z9

HAC   ØSR[R,S]Ø[7,K]Z when reported with SDx of I26.Ø2-I26.Ø9, I26.92-I26.99, or I82.4Ø1-I82.4Z9

See Appendix L for Procedure Combinations
⊞   ØSR[C,D]Ø[6,J,L,M,N][9,A,Z]
⊞   ØSR[C,D]ØEZ
⊞   ØSR[T,U,V,W]ØJ[9,A,Z]
⊞   ØSR[R,S]Ø[1,3,J][9,A,Z]

LC Limited Coverage   **NC** Noncovered   ⊞ Combination Member   HAC associated procedure   Combination Only   DRG Non-OR   Non-OR   New/Revised in GREEN

610   ICD-10-PCS 2021

ØSR–ØSR

Ø Medical and Surgical
S Lower Joints
S Reposition

Definition: Moving to its normal location, or other suitable location, all or a portion of a body part

Explanation: The body part is moved to a new location from an abnormal location, or from a normal location where it is not functioning correctly. The body part may or may not be cut out or off to be moved to the new location.

Body Part Character 4		Approach Character 5	Device Character 6	Qualifier Character 7
Ø Lumbar Vertebral Joint Lumbar facet joint **3 Lumbosacral Joint** Lumbosacral facet joint **5 Sacrococcygeal Joint** Sacrococcygeal symphysis **6 Coccygeal Joint** **7 Sacroiliac Joint, Right** **8 Sacroiliac Joint, Left**		**Ø Open** **3 Percutaneous** **4 Percutaneous Endoscopic** **X External**	**4 Internal Fixation Device** **Z No Device**	**Z No Qualifier**
9 Hip Joint, Right Acetabulofemoral joint **B Hip Joint, Left** *See 9 Hip Joint, Right* **C Knee Joint, Right** Femoropatellar joint Femorotibial joint Lateral meniscus Medial meniscus Patellofemoral joint Tibiofemoral joint **D Knee Joint, Left** *See C Knee Joint, Right* **F Ankle Joint, Right** Inferior tibiofibular joint Talocrural joint **G Ankle Joint, Left** *See F Ankle Joint, Right* **H Tarsal Joint, Right** Calcaneocuboid joint Cuboideonavicular joint Cuneonavicular joint Intercuneiform joint Subtalar (talocalcaneal) joint Talocalcaneal (subtalar) joint Talocalcaneonavicular joint	**J Tarsal Joint, Left** *See H Tarsal Joint, Right* **K Tarsometatarsal Joint, Right** **L Tarsometatarsal Joint, Left** **M Metatarsal-Phalangeal Joint, Right** Metatarsophalangeal (MTP) joint **N Metatarsal-Phalangeal Joint, Left** *See M Metatarsal-Phalangeal Joint, Right* **P Toe Phalangeal Joint, Right** Interphalangeal (IP) joint **Q Toe Phalangeal Joint, Left** *See P Toe Phalangeal Joint, Right*	**Ø Open** **3 Percutaneous** **4 Percutaneous Endoscopic** **X External**	**4 Internal Fixation Device** **5 External Fixation Device** **Z No Device**	**Z No Qualifier**

Non-OR ØSS[Ø,3,5,6,7,8][3,4,X][4,Z]Z
Non-OR ØSS[9,B,C,D,F,G,H,J,K,L,M,N,P,Q][3,4,X][4,5,Z]Z

Ø Medical and Surgical
S Lower Joints
T Resection

Definition: Cutting out or off, without replacement, all of a body part

Explanation: None

Body Part Character 4		Approach Character 5	Device Character 6	Qualifier Character 7
2 Lumbar Vertebral Disc **4 Lumbosacral Disc** **5 Sacrococcygeal Joint** Sacrococcygeal symphysis **6 Coccygeal Joint** **7 Sacroiliac Joint, Right** **8 Sacroiliac Joint, Left** **9 Hip Joint, Right** Acetabulofemoral joint **B Hip Joint, Left** *See 9 Hip Joint, Right* **C Knee Joint, Right** Femoropatellar joint Femorotibial joint Lateral meniscus Medial meniscus Patellofemoral joint Tibiofemoral joint **D Knee Joint, Left** *See C Knee Joint, Right* **F Ankle Joint, Right** Inferior tibiofibular joint Talocrural joint **G Ankle Joint, Left** *See F Ankle Joint, Right*	**H Tarsal Joint, Right** Calcaneocuboid joint Cuboideonavicular joint Cuneonavicular joint Intercuneiform joint Subtalar (talocalcaneal) joint Talocalcaneal (subtalar) joint Talocalcaneonavicular joint **J Tarsal Joint, Left** *See H Tarsal Joint, Right* **K Tarsometatarsal Joint, Right** **L Tarsometatarsal Joint, Left** **M Metatarsal-Phalangeal Joint, Right** Metatarsophalangeal (MTP) joint **N Metatarsal-Phalangeal Joint, Left** *See M Metatarsal-Phalangeal Joint, Right* **P Toe Phalangeal Joint, Right** Interphalangeal (IP) joint **Q Toe Phalangeal Joint, Left** *See P Toe Phalangeal Joint, Right*	**Ø Open**	**Z No Device**	**Z No Qualifier**

LC Limited Coverage   **NC** Noncovered   ⊞ Combination Member   HAC associated procedure   Combination Only   DRG Non-OR   Non-OR   New/Revised in GREEN

ICD-10-PCS 2021

ØSS–ØST

611

Lower Joints

Ø   **Medical and Surgical**
S   **Lower Joints**
U   **Supplement**   Definition: Putting in or on biological or synthetic material that physically reinforces and/or augments the function of a portion of a body part

Explanation: The biological material is non-living, or is living and from the same individual. The body part may have been previously replaced, and the SUPPLEMENT procedure is performed to physically reinforce and/or augment the function of the replaced body part.

Body Part Character 4	Approach Character 5	Device Character 6	Qualifier Character 7
Ø Lumbar Vertebral Joint — Lumbar facet joint 2 Lumbar Vertebral Disc 3 Lumbosacral Joint — Lumbosacral facet joint 4 Lumbosacral Disc 5 Sacrococcygeal Joint — Sacrococcygeal symphysis 6 Coccygeal Joint 7 Sacroiliac Joint, Right 8 Sacroiliac Joint, Left F Ankle Joint, Right — Inferior tibiofibular joint — Talocrural joint G Ankle Joint, Left — *See F Ankle Joint, Right* H Tarsal Joint, Right — Calcaneocuboid joint — Cuboideonavicular joint — Cuneonavicular joint — Intercuneiform joint — Subtalar (talocalcaneal) joint — Talocalcaneal (subtalar) joint — Talocalcaneonavicular joint J Tarsal Joint, Left — *See H Tarsal Joint, Right* K Tarsometatarsal Joint, Right L Tarsometatarsal Joint, Left M Metatarsal-Phalangeal Joint, Right — Metatarsophalangeal (MTP) joint N Metatarsal-Phalangeal Joint, Left — *See M Metatarsal-Phalangeal Joint, Right* P Toe Phalangeal Joint, Right — Interphalangeal (IP) joint Q Toe Phalangeal Joint, Left — *See P Toe Phalangeal Joint, Right*	Ø Open 3 Percutaneous 4 Percutaneous Endoscopic	7 Autologous Tissue Substitute J Synthetic Substitute K Nonautologous Tissue Substitute	Z No Qualifier
9 Hip Joint, Right ⊞ — Acetabulofemoral joint B Hip Joint, Left ⊞ — *See 9 Hip Joint, Right*	Ø Open	7 Autologous Tissue Substitute 9 Liner B Resurfacing Device J Synthetic Substitute K Nonautologous Tissue Substitute	Z No Qualifier
9 Hip Joint, Right — Acetabulofemoral joint B Hip Joint, Left — *See 9 Hip Joint, Right*	3 Percutaneous 4 Percutaneous Endoscopic	7 Autologous Tissue Substitute J Synthetic Substitute K Nonautologous Tissue Substitute	Z No Qualifier
A Hip Joint, Acetabular Surface, Right ⊞ E Hip Joint, Acetabular Surface, Left ⊞ R Hip Joint, Femoral Surface, Right ⊞ S Hip Joint, Femoral Surface, Left ⊞	Ø Open	9 Liner B Resurfacing Device	Z No Qualifier
C Knee Joint, Right — Femoropatellar joint — Femorotibial joint — Lateral meniscus — Medial meniscus — Patellofemoral joint — Tibiofemoral joint D Knee Joint, Left — *See C Knee Joint, Right*	Ø Open	7 Autologous Tissue Substitute J Synthetic Substitute K Nonautologous Tissue Substitute	Z No Qualifier
C Knee Joint, Right — Femoropatellar joint — Femorotibial joint — Lateral meniscus — Medial meniscus — Patellofemoral joint — Tibiofemoral joint D Knee Joint, Left — *See C Knee Joint, Right*	Ø Open	9 Liner	C Patellar Surface Z No Qualifier

HAC   ØSU[9,B]ØBZ when reported with SDx of I26.Ø2-I26.Ø9, I26.92-I26.99, or I82.4Ø1-I82.4Z9
HAC   ØSU[A,E,R,S]ØBZ when reported with SDx of I26.Ø2-I26.Ø9, I26.92-I26.99, or I82.4Ø1-I82.4Z9

See Appendix L for Procedure Combinations
⊞   ØSU[9,B]Ø9Z
⊞   ØSU[A,E,R,S]Ø9Z

ØSU Continued on next page

LC Limited Coverage   NC Noncovered   ⊞ Combination Member   HAC associated procedure   Combination Only   DRG Non-OR   Non-OR   New/Revised in GREEN

Ø　Medical and Surgical
S　Lower Joints
U　Supplement

ØSU Continued

Definition: Putting in or on biological or synthetic material that physically reinforces and/or augments the function of a portion of a body part

Explanation: The biological material is non-living, or is living and from the same individual. The body part may have been previously replaced, and the SUPPLEMENT procedure is performed to physically reinforce and/or augment the function of the replaced body part.

Body Part Character 4	Approach Character 5	Device Character 6	Qualifier Character 7
C **Knee Joint, Right** 　Femoropatellar joint 　Femorotibial joint 　Lateral meniscus 　Medial meniscus 　Patellofemoral joint 　Tibiofemoral joint **D** **Knee Joint, Left** 　*See C Knee Joint, Right*	**3** Percutaneous **4** Percutaneous Endoscopic	**7** Autologous Tissue 　Substitute **J** Synthetic Substitute **K** Nonautologous Tissue 　Substitute	**Z** No Qualifier
T **Knee Joint, Femoral Surface, Right** 　Femoropatellar joint 　Patellofemoral joint **U** **Knee Joint, Femoral Surface, Left** 　*See T Knee Joint, Femoral Surface, Right* **V** **Knee Joint, Tibial Surface, Right** ⊞ 　Femorotibial joint 　Tibiofemoral joint **W** **Knee Joint, Tibial Surface, Left** ⊞ 　*See V Knee Joint, Tibial Surface, Right*	**Ø** Open	**9** Liner	**Z** No Qualifier

See Appendix L for Procedure Combinations
　⊞　　ØSU[V,W]Ø9Z

LC Limited Coverage　NC Noncovered　⊞ Combination Member　HAC associated procedure　Combination Only　DRG Non-OR　Non-OR　New/Revised in GREEN

ICD-10-PCS 2021　　　　　　　　　　　　　　　　　　　　　　　　　　　　　　　613

ØSU–ØSU

Lower Joints

Ø **Medical and Surgical**
S **Lower Joints**
W **Revision** Definition: Correcting, to the extent possible, a portion of a malfunctioning device or the position of a displaced device
Explanation: Revision can include correcting a malfunctioning or displaced device by taking out or putting in components of the device such as a screw or pin

Body Part Character 4	Approach Character 5	Device Character 6	Qualifier Character 7
Ø Lumbar Vertebral Joint Lumbar facet joint **3** Lumbosacral Joint Lumbosacral facet joint	**Ø** Open **3** Percutaneous **4** Percutaneous Endoscopic **X** External	**Ø** Drainage Device **3** Infusion Device **4** Internal Fixation Device **7** Autologous Tissue Substitute **8** Spacer **A** Interbody Fusion Device **J** Synthetic Substitute **K** Nonautologous Tissue Substitute	**Z** No Qualifier
2 Lumbar Vertebral Disc **4** Lumbosacral Disc	**Ø** Open **3** Percutaneous **4** Percutaneous Endoscopic **X** External	**Ø** Drainage Device **3** Infusion Device **7** Autologous Tissue Substitute **J** Synthetic Substitute **K** Nonautologous Tissue Substitute	**Z** No Qualifier
5 Sacrococcygeal Joint Sacrococcygeal symphysis **6** Coccygeal Joint **7** Sacroiliac Joint, Right **8** Sacroiliac Joint, Left	**Ø** Open **3** Percutaneous **4** Percutaneous Endoscopic **X** External	**Ø** Drainage Device **3** Infusion Device **4** Internal Fixation Device **7** Autologous Tissue Substitute **8** Spacer **J** Synthetic Substitute **K** Nonautologous Tissue Substitute	**Z** No Qualifier
9 Hip Joint, Right Acetabulofemoral joint **B** Hip Joint, Left *See 9 Hip Joint, Right*	**Ø** Open	**Ø** Drainage Device **3** Infusion Device **4** Internal Fixation Device **5** External Fixation Device **7** Autologous Tissue Substitute **8** Spacer **9** Liner **B** Resurfacing Device **J** Synthetic Substitute **K** Nonautologous Tissue Substitute	**Z** No Qualifier
9 Hip Joint, Right Acetabulofemoral joint **B** Hip Joint, Left *See 9 Hip Joint, Right*	**3** Percutaneous **4** Percutaneous Endoscopic **X** External	**Ø** Drainage Device **3** Infusion Device **4** Internal Fixation Device **5** External Fixation Device **7** Autologous Tissue Substitute **8** Spacer **J** Synthetic Substitute **K** Nonautologous Tissue Substitute	**Z** No Qualifier
A Hip Joint, Acetabular Surface, Right **E** Hip Joint, Acetabular Surface, Left **R** Hip Joint, Femoral Surface, Right **S** Hip Joint, Femoral Surface, Left **T** Knee Joint, Femoral Surface, Right Femoropatellar joint Patellofemoral joint **U** Knee Joint, Femoral Surface, Left *See T Knee Joint, Femoral Surface, Right* **V** Knee Joint, Tibial Surface, Right Femorotibial joint Tibiofemoral joint **W** Knee Joint, Tibial Surface, Left *See V Knee Joint, Tibial Surface, Right*	**Ø** Open **3** Percutaneous **4** Percutaneous Endoscopic **X** External	**J** Synthetic Substitute	**Z** No Qualifier
C Knee Joint, Right Femoropatellar joint Femorotibial joint Lateral meniscus Medial meniscus Patellofemoral joint Tibiofemoral joint **D** Knee Joint, Left *See C Knee Joint, Right*	**Ø** Open	**Ø** Drainage Device **3** Infusion Device **4** Internal Fixation Device **5** External Fixation Device **7** Autologous Tissue Substitute **8** Spacer **9** Liner **K** Nonautologous Tissue Substitute	**Z** No Qualifier

Non-OR ØSW[Ø,3]X[Ø,3,4,7,8,A,J,K]Z
Non-OR ØSW[2,4]X[Ø,3,7,J,K]Z
Non-OR ØSW[5,6,7,8]X[Ø,3,4,7,8,J,K]Z
Non-OR ØSW[9,B]X[Ø,3,4,5,7,8,J,K]Z
Non-OR ØSW[A,E,R,S,T,U,V,W]XJZ

ØSW Continued on next page

LC Limited Coverage   NC Noncovered   ⊞ Combination Member   HAC associated procedure   Combination Only   DRG Non-OR   Non-OR   New/Revised in GREEN

Ø   Medical and Surgical
S   Lower Joints
W   Revision

ØSW Continued

Definition: Correcting, to the extent possible, a portion of a malfunctioning device or the position of a displaced device

Explanation: Revision can include correcting a malfunctioning or displaced device by taking out or putting in components of the device such as a screw or pin

Body Part Character 4	Approach Character 5	Device Character 6	Qualifier Character 7
C Knee Joint, Right Femoropatellar joint Femorotibial joint Lateral meniscus Medial meniscus Patellofemoral joint Tibiofemoral joint **D Knee Joint, Left** *See C Knee Joint, Right*	**Ø** Open	**J** Synthetic Substitute	**C** Patellar Surface **Z** No Qualifier
C Knee Joint, Right Femoropatellar joint Femorotibial joint Lateral meniscus Medial meniscus Patellofemoral joint Tibiofemoral joint **D Knee Joint, Left** *See C Knee Joint, Right*	**3** Percutaneous **4** Percutaneous Endoscopic **X** External	**Ø** Drainage Device **3** Infusion Device **4** Internal Fixation Device **5** External Fixation Device **7** Autologous Tissue Substitute **8** Spacer **K** Nonautologous Tissue Substitute	**Z** No Qualifier
C Knee Joint, Right Femoropatellar joint Femorotibial joint Lateral meniscus Medial meniscus Patellofemoral joint Tibiofemoral joint **D Knee Joint, Left** *See C Knee Joint, Right*	**3** Percutaneous **4** Percutaneous Endoscopic **X** External	**J** Synthetic Substitute	**C** Patellar Surface **Z** No Qualifier
F Ankle Joint, Right Inferior tibiofibular joint Talocrural joint **G Ankle Joint, Left** *See F Ankle Joint, Right* **H Tarsal Joint, Right** Calcaneocuboid joint Cuboideonavicular joint Cuneonavicular joint Intercuneiform joint Subtalar (talocalcaneal) joint Talocalcaneal (subtalar) joint Talocalcaneonavicular joint **J Tarsal Joint, Left** *See H Tarsal Joint, Right* **K Tarsometatarsal Joint, Right** **L Tarsometatarsal Joint, Left** **M Metatarsal-Phalangeal Joint, Right** Metatarsophalangeal (MTP) joint **N Metatarsal-Phalangeal Joint, Left** *See M Metatarsal-Phalangeal Joint, Right* **P Toe Phalangeal Joint, Right** Interphalangeal (IP) joint **Q Toe Phalangeal Joint, Left** *See P Toe Phalangeal Joint, Right*	**Ø** Open **3** Percutaneous **4** Percutaneous Endoscopic **X** External	**Ø** Drainage Device **3** Infusion Device **4** Internal Fixation Device **5** External Fixation Device **7** Autologous Tissue Substitute **8** Spacer **J** Synthetic Substitute **K** Nonautologous Tissue Substitute	**Z** No Qualifier

Non-OR   ØSW[C,D]X[Ø,3,4,5,7,8,K]Z
Non-OR   ØSW[C,D]XJ[C,Z]
Non-OR   ØSW[F,G,H,J,K,L,M,N,P,Q]X[Ø,3,4,5,7,8,J,K]Z

LC Limited Coverage   NC Noncovered   ⊞ Combination Member   HAC associated procedure   Combination Only   DRG Non-OR   Non-OR   New/Revised in GREEN

ICD-10-PCS 2021   615

ØSW–ØSW

Urinary System ØT1–ØTY

Character Meanings

This Character Meaning table is provided as a guide to assist the user in the identification of character members that may be found in this section of code tables. It **SHOULD NOT** be used to build a PCS code.

Operation–Character 3		Body Part–Character 4		Approach–Character 5		Device–Character 6		Qualifier–Character 7	
1	Bypass	Ø	Kidney, Right	Ø	Open	Ø	Drainage Device	Ø	Allogeneic
2	Change	1	Kidney, Left	3	Percutaneous	1	Radioactive Element	1	Syngeneic
5	Destruction	2	Kidneys, Bilateral	4	Percutaneous Endoscopic	2	Monitoring Device	2	Zooplastic
7	Dilation	3	Kidney Pelvis, Right	7	Via Natural or Artificial Opening	3	Infusion Device	3	Kidney Pelvis, Right
8	Division	4	Kidney Pelvis, Left	8	Via Natural or Artificial Opening Endoscopic	7	Autologous Tissue Substitute	4	Kidney Pelvis, Left
9	Drainage	5	Kidney	X	External	C	Extraluminal Device	6	Ureter, Right
B	Excision	6	Ureter, Right			D	Intraluminal Device	7	Ureter, Left
C	Extirpation	7	Ureter, Left			J	Synthetic Substitute	8	Colon
D	Extraction	8	Ureters, Bilateral			K	Nonautologous Tissue Substitute	9	Colocutaneous
F	Fragmentation	9	Ureter			L	Artificial Sphincter	A	Ileum
H	Insertion	B	Bladder			M	Stimulator Lead	B	Bladder
J	Inspection	C	Bladder Neck			Y	Other Device	C	Ileocutaneous
L	Occlusion	D	Urethra			Z	No Device	D	Cutaneous
M	Reattachment							X	Diagnostic
N	Release							Z	No Qualifier
P	Removal								
Q	Repair								
R	Replacement								
S	Reposition								
T	Resection								
U	Supplement								
V	Restriction								
W	Revision								
Y	Transplantation								

AHA Coding Clinic for table ØT1
2017, 3Q, 20   Creation of Indiana pouch
2017, 3Q, 21   Augmentation cystoplasty with Indiana pouch and continent urinary diversion
2017, 1Q, 37   Perineal urethrostomy
2015, 3Q, 34   Redo urinary diversion surgery via left ureteral reimplantation

AHA Coding Clinic for table ØT7
2019, 2Q, 16   Reimplantation of ureters with insertion of tubes
2017, 4Q, 111   Exchange of ureteral stent
2016, 2Q, 27   Exchange of ureteral stents
2015, 2Q, 8   Urinary calculi fragmentation and evacuation
2013, 4Q, 123   Urolift® procedure

AHA Coding Clinic for table ØT9
2017, 3Q, 19   Ureteral stent placement for urinary leakage
2017, 3Q, 20   Creation of Indiana pouch
2017, 3Q, 21   Augmentation cystoplasty with Indiana pouch and continent urinary diversion

AHA Coding Clinic for table ØTB
2016, 1Q, 19   Biopsy of neobladder malignancy
2015, 3Q, 34   Excision of Mitrofanoff polyp
2014, 2Q, 8   Ileoscopy with excision of polyp of Ileal loop urinary diversion

AHA Coding Clinic for table ØTC
2019, 3Q, 4   Evacuation of clots from bladder dome
2016, 3Q, 23   Ureteral stone migrating into bladder
2015, 2Q, 7   Urinary calculi fragmentation and evacuation
2015, 2Q, 8   Urinary calculi fragmentation and evacuation
2013, 4Q, 122   Laser lithotripsy with removal of fragments

AHA Coding Clinic for table ØTF
2015, 2Q, 7   Urinary calculi fragmentation and evacuation
2013, 4Q, 122   Extracorporeal shock wave lithotripsy
2013, 4Q, 122   Laser lithotripsy with removal of fragments

AHA Coding Clinic for table ØTH
2019, 2Q, 16   Reimplantation of ureters with insertion of tubes

AHA Coding Clinic for table ØTP
2017, 4Q, 111   Exchange of ureteral stent
2016, 2Q, 27   Exchange of ureteral stents

AHA Coding Clinic for table ØTQ
2018, 2Q, 27   Dismembered pyeloplasty
2017, 1Q, 37   Perineal urethrostomy

AHA Coding Clinic for table ØTR
2017, 3Q, 20   Creation of Indiana pouch

AHA Coding Clinic for table ØTS
2019, 1Q, 29   Young-Dees-Leadbetter bladder neck reconstruction
2018, 2Q, 27   Dismembered pyeloplasty
2017, 1Q, 36   Dismembered pyeloplasty
2016, 1Q, 15   Pubovaginal sling placement

AHA Coding Clinic for table ØTT
2014, 3Q, 16   Hand-assisted laparoscopy nephroureterectomy

AHA Coding Clinic for table ØTU
2019, 1Q, 29   Young-Dees-Leadbetter bladder neck reconstruction
2017, 3Q, 21   Augmentation cystoplasty with Indiana pouch and continent urinary diversion

AHA Coding Clinic for table ØTV
2015, 2Q, 11   Cystourethroscopic Deflux® injection

Urinary System

Urinary System

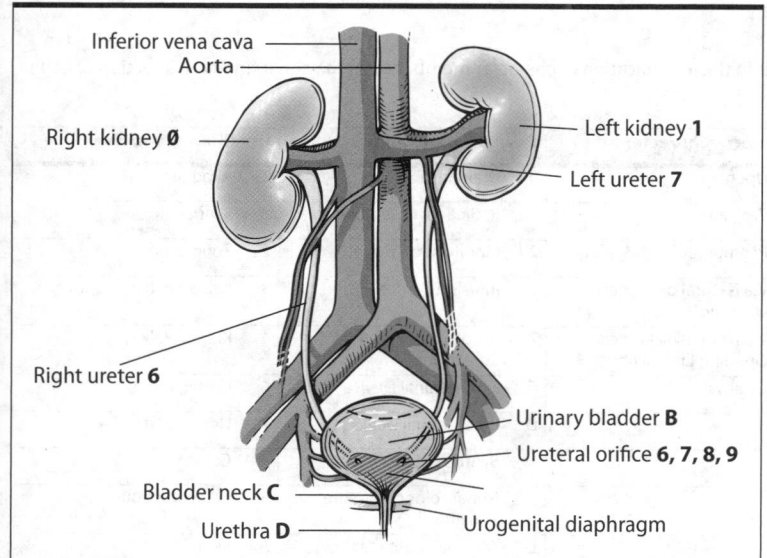

- Inferior vena cava
- Aorta
- Right kidney Ø
- Left kidney 1
- Left ureter 7
- Right ureter 6
- Urinary bladder B
- Ureteral orifice 6, 7, 8, 9
- Bladder neck C
- Urethra D
- Urogenital diaphragm

Kidney

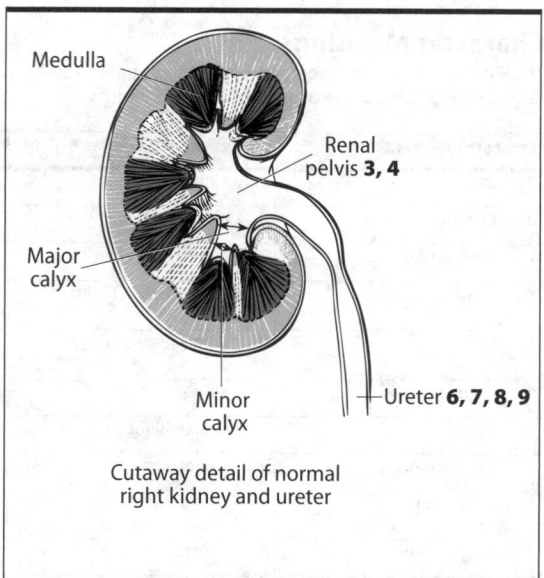

- Medulla
- Renal pelvis 3, 4
- Major calyx
- Minor calyx
- Ureter 6, 7, 8, 9

Cutaway detail of normal right kidney and ureter

Bladder

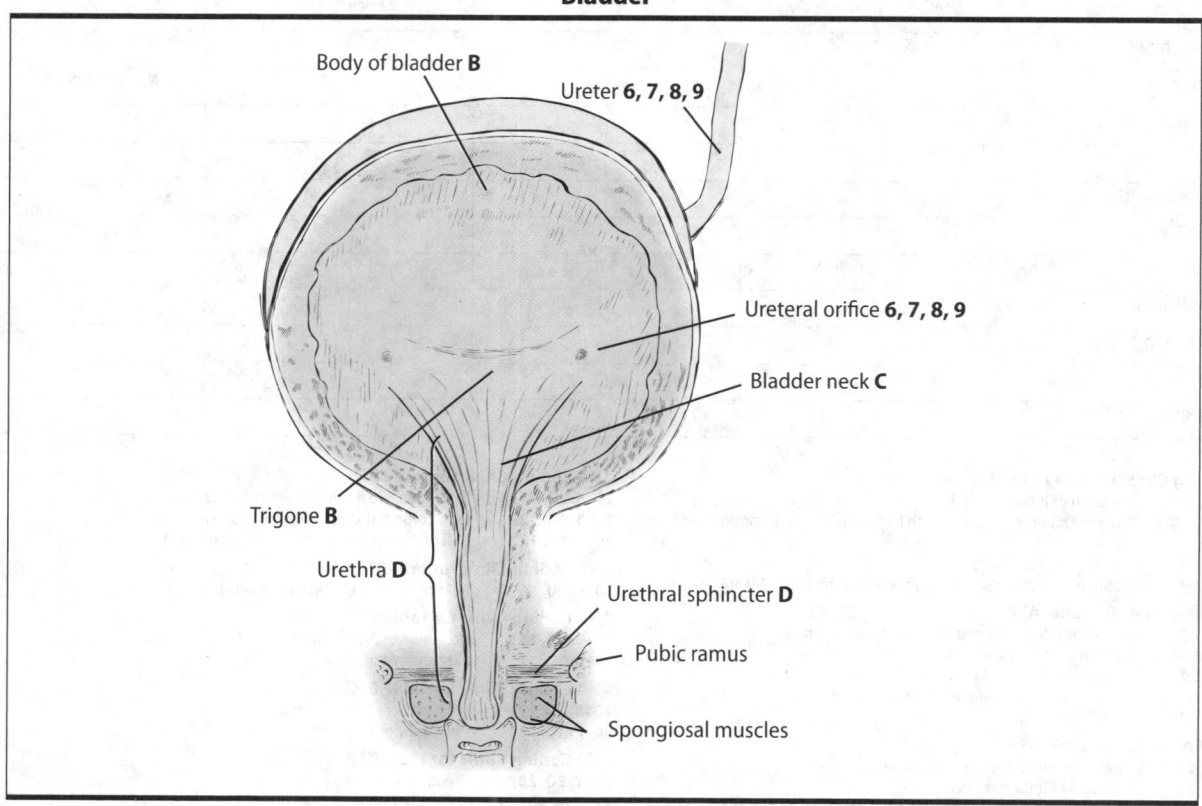

- Body of bladder B
- Ureter 6, 7, 8, 9
- Ureteral orifice 6, 7, 8, 9
- Bladder neck C
- Trigone B
- Urethra D
- Urethral sphincter D
- Pubic ramus
- Spongiosal muscles

Ø　**Medical and Surgical**
T　**Urinary System**
1　**Bypass**　　Definition: Altering the route of passage of the contents of a tubular body part

Explanation: Rerouting contents of a body part to a downstream area of the normal route, to a similar route and body part, or to an abnormal route and dissimilar body part. Includes one or more anastomoses, with or without the use of a device.

Body Part Character 4	Approach Character 5	Device Character 6	Qualifier Character 7
3　**Kidney Pelvis, Right** 　Ureteropelvic junction (UPJ) 4　**Kidney Pelvis, Left** 　*See 3 Kidney Pelvis, Right*	Ø　Open 4　Percutaneous Endoscopic	7　Autologous Tissue Substitute J　Synthetic Substitute K　Nonautologous Tissue Substitute Z　No Device	3　Kidney Pelvis, Right 4　Kidney Pelvis, Left 6　Ureter, Right 7　Ureter, Left 8　Colon 9　Colocutaneous A　Ileum B　Bladder C　Ileocutaneous D　Cutaneous
3　**Kidney Pelvis, Right** 　Ureteropelvic junction (UPJ) 4　**Kidney Pelvis, Left** 　*See 3 Kidney Pelvis, Right*	3　Percutaneous	J　Synthetic Substitute	D　Cutaneous
6　**Ureter, Right** 　Ureteral orifice 　Ureterovesical orifice 7　**Ureter, Left** 　*See 6 Ureter, Right* 8　**Ureters, Bilateral** 　*See 6 Ureter, Right*	Ø　Open 4　Percutaneous Endoscopic	7　Autologous Tissue Substitute J　Synthetic Substitute K　Nonautologous Tissue Substitute Z　No Device	6　Ureter, Right 7　Ureter, Left 8　Colon 9　Colocutaneous A　Ileum B　Bladder C　Ileocutaneous D　Cutaneous
6　**Ureter, Right** 　Ureteral orifice 　Ureterovesical orifice 7　**Ureter, Left** 　*See 6 Ureter, Right* 8　**Ureters, Bilateral** 　*See 6 Ureter, Right*	3　Percutaneous	J　Synthetic Substitute	D　Cutaneous
B　**Bladder** 　Trigone of bladder	Ø　Open 4　Percutaneous Endoscopic	7　Autologous Tissue Substitute J　Synthetic Substitute K　Nonautologous Tissue Substitute Z　No Device	9　Colocutaneous C　Ileocutaneous D　Cutaneous
B　**Bladder** 　Trigone of bladder	3　Percutaneous	J　Synthetic Substitute	D　Cutaneous

Ø　**Medical and Surgical**
T　**Urinary System**
2　**Change**　　Definition: Taking out or off a device from a body part and putting back an identical or similar device in or on the same body part without cutting or puncturing the skin or a mucous membrane

Explanation: All CHANGE procedures are coded using the approach EXTERNAL

Body Part Character 4	Approach Character 5	Device Character 6	Qualifier Character 7
5　**Kidney** 　Renal calyx 　Renal capsule 　Renal cortex 　Renal segment 9　**Ureter** 　Ureteral orifice 　Ureterovesical orifice B　**Bladder** 　Trigone of bladder D　**Urethra** 　Bulbourethral (Cowper's) gland 　Cowper's (bulbourethral) gland 　External urethral sphincter 　Internal urethral sphincter 　Membranous urethra 　Penile urethra 　Prostatic urethra	X　External	Ø　Drainage Device Y　Other Device	Z　No Qualifier

Non-OR　All body part, approach, device, and qualifier values

LC Limited Coverage　NC Noncovered　⊞ Combination Member　HAC associated procedure　Combination Only　DRG Non-OR　Non-OR　New/Revised in GREEN

ICD-10-PCS 2021　　　　　　　　　　　　　　　　　　　　　　　　　　　　　　　　619

ØT1–ØT2

Ø   Medical and Surgical
T   Urinary System
5   Destruction   Definition: Physical eradication of all or a portion of a body part by the direct use of energy, force, or a destructive agent

Explanation: None of the body part is physically taken out

Body Part Character 4	Approach Character 5	Device Character 6	Qualifier Character 7
Ø Kidney, Right Renal calyx Renal capsule Renal cortex Renal segment **1 Kidney, Left** *See Ø Kidney, Right* **3 Kidney Pelvis, Right** Ureteropelvic junction (UPJ) **4 Kidney Pelvis, Left** *See 3 Kidney Pelvis, Right* **6 Ureter, Right** Ureteral orifice Ureterovesical orifice **7 Ureter, Left** *See 6 Ureter, Right* **B Bladder** Trigone of bladder **C Bladder Neck**	**Ø Open** **3 Percutaneous** **4 Percutaneous Endoscopic** **7 Via Natural or Artificial Opening** **8 Via Natural or Artificial Opening Endoscopic**	**Z No Device**	**Z No Qualifier**
D Urethra Bulbourethral (Cowper's) gland Cowper's (bulbourethral) gland External urethral sphincter Internal urethral sphincter Membranous urethra Penile urethra Prostatic urethra	**Ø Open** **3 Percutaneous** **4 Percutaneous Endoscopic** **7 Via Natural or Artificial Opening** **8 Via Natural or Artificial Opening Endoscopic** **X External**	**Z No Device**	**Z No Qualifier**

Non-OR   ØT5D[Ø,3,4,7,8,X]ZZ

Ø   Medical and Surgical
T   Urinary System
7   Dilation   Definition: Expanding an orifice or the lumen of a tubular body part

Explanation: The orifice can be a natural orifice or an artificially created orifice. Accomplished by stretching a tubular body part using intraluminal pressure or by cutting part of the orifice or wall of the tubular body part.

Body Part Character 4	Approach Character 5	Device Character 6	Qualifier Character 7
3 Kidney Pelvis, Right Ureteropelvic junction (UPJ) **4 Kidney Pelvis, Left** *See 3 Kidney Pelvis, Right* **6 Ureter, Right** Ureteral orifice Ureterovesical orifice **7 Ureter, Left** *See 6 Ureter, Right* **8 Ureters, Bilateral** *See 6 Ureter, Right* **B Bladder** Trigone of bladder **C Bladder Neck** **D Urethra** Bulbourethral (Cowper's) gland Cowper's (bulbourethral) gland External urethral sphincter Internal urethral sphincter Membranous urethra Penile urethra Prostatic urethra	**Ø Open** **3 Percutaneous** **4 Percutaneous Endoscopic** **7 Via Natural or Artificial Opening** **8 Via Natural or Artificial Opening Endoscopic**	**D Intraluminal Device** **Z No Device**	**Z No Qualifier**

Non-OR   ØT7[6,7,8][Ø,3,4,7]DZ   Non-OR   ØT7B7[D,Z]Z   Non-OR   ØT7[C,D][7,8][D,Z]Z
Non-OR   ØT7[6,7,8]7ZZ   Non-OR   ØT7C[Ø,3,4]ZZ
Non-OR   ØT788ZZ   Non-OR   ØT7[C,D][Ø,3,4]DZ

Ø   Medical and Surgical
T   Urinary System
8   Division   Definition: Cutting into a body part, without draining fluids and/or gases from the body part, in order to separate or transect a body part

Explanation: All or a portion of the body part is separated into two or more portions

Body Part Character 4	Approach Character 5	Device Character 6	Qualifier Character 7
2 Kidneys, Bilateral Renal calyx Renal capsule Renal cortex Renal segment **C Bladder Neck**	**Ø Open** **3 Percutaneous** **4 Percutaneous Endoscopic**	**Z No Device**	**Z No Qualifier**

LC Limited Coverage   NC Noncovered   ⊞ Combination Member   HAC associated procedure   Combination Only   DRG Non-OR   Non-OR   New/Revised in GREEN

0   **Medical and Surgical**
T   **Urinary System**
9   **Drainage**   Definition: Taking or letting out fluids and/or gases from a body part
                                Explanation: The qualifier DIAGNOSTIC is used to identify drainage procedures that are biopsies

Body Part Character 4	Approach Character 5	Device Character 6	Qualifier Character 7

0 **Kidney, Right**
    Renal calyx
    Renal capsule
    Renal cortex
    Renal segment
1 **Kidney, Left**
    See 0 Kidney, Right
3 **Kidney Pelvis, Right**
    Ureteropelvic junction (UPJ)
4 **Kidney Pelvis, Left**
    See 3 Kidney Pelvis, Right
6 **Ureter, Right**
    Ureteral orifice
    Ureterovesical orifice
7 **Ureter, Left**
    See 6 Ureter, Right
8 **Ureters, Bilateral**
    See 6 Ureter, Right
B **Bladder**
    Trigone of bladder
C **Bladder Neck**
	0 Open
	3 Percutaneous
	4 Percutaneous Endoscopic
	7 Via Natural or Artificial Opening
	8 Via Natural or Artificial Opening
	    Endoscopic
		0 Drainage Device	**Z** No Qualifier

0 **Kidney, Right**
    Renal calyx
    Renal capsule
    Renal cortex
    Renal segment
1 **Kidney, Left**
    See 0 Kidney, Right
3 **Kidney Pelvis, Right**
    Ureteropelvic junction (UPJ)
4 **Kidney Pelvis, Left**
    See 3 Kidney Pelvis, Right
6 **Ureter, Right**
    Ureteral orifice
    Ureterovesical orifice
7 **Ureter, Left**
    See 6 Ureter, Right
8 **Ureters, Bilateral**
    See 6 Ureter, Right
B **Bladder**
    Trigone of bladder
C **Bladder Neck**
	0 Open
	3 Percutaneous
	4 Percutaneous Endoscopic
	7 Via Natural or Artificial Opening
	8 Via Natural or Artificial Opening
	    Endoscopic
		Z No Device	**X** Diagnostic
			Z No Qualifier

D **Urethra**
    Bulbourethral (Cowper's) gland
    Cowper's (bulbourethral) gland
    External urethral sphincter
    Internal urethral sphincter
    Membranous urethra
    Penile urethra
    Prostatic urethra
	0 Open
	3 Percutaneous
	4 Percutaneous Endoscopic
	7 Via Natural or Artificial Opening
	8 Via Natural or Artificial Opening
	    Endoscopic
	X External
		0 Drainage Device	**Z** No Qualifier

D **Urethra**
    Bulbourethral (Cowper's) gland
    Cowper's (bulbourethral) gland
    External urethral sphincter
    Internal urethral sphincter
    Membranous urethra
    Penile urethra
    Prostatic urethra
	0 Open
	3 Percutaneous
	4 Percutaneous Endoscopic
	7 Via Natural or Artificial Opening
	8 Via Natural or Artificial Opening
	    Endoscopic
	X External
		Z No Device	**X** Diagnostic
			Z No Qualifier

Non-OR	0T9[0,1,3,4]30Z
Non-OR	0T9[6,7,8][0,3,4,7,8]0Z
Non-OR	0T9[B,C][3,4,7,8]0Z
Non-OR	0T9[0,1,3,4,6,7,8][3,4,7,8]ZX
Non-OR	0T9[0,1,3,4][3,4]ZZ
Non-OR	0T9[6,7,8]3ZZ
Non-OR	0T9[B,C][3,4,7,8]ZZ
Non-OR	0T9D30Z
Non-OR	0T9D[0,3,4,7,8,X]ZX
Non-OR	0T9D3ZZ

LC Limited Coverage   **NC** Noncovered   ⊞ Combination Member   HAC associated procedure   Combination Only   DRG Non-OR   Non-OR   New/Revised in GREEN

ICD-10-PCS 2021   621

0T9–0T9

Ø   Medical and Surgical
T   Urinary System
B   Excision   Definition: Cutting out or off, without replacement, a portion of a body part
                      Explanation: The qualifier DIAGNOSTIC is used to identify excision procedures that are biopsies

Body Part Character 4	Approach Character 5	Device Character 6	Qualifier Character 7

Ø Kidney, Right
  Renal calyx
  Renal capsule
  Renal cortex
  Renal segment
1 Kidney, Left
  See Ø Kidney, Right
3 Kidney Pelvis, Right
  Ureteropelvic junction (UPJ)
4 Kidney Pelvis, Left
  See 3 Kidney Pelvis, Right
6 Ureter, Right
  Ureteral orifice
  Ureterovesical orifice
7 Ureter, Left
  See 6 Ureter, Right
B Bladder
  Trigone of bladder
C Bladder Neck
	Ø Open
	3 Percutaneous
	4 Percutaneous Endoscopic
	7 Via Natural or Artificial Opening
	8 Via Natural or Artificial Opening Endoscopic
		Z No Device	X Diagnostic
			Z No Qualifier

D Urethra
  Bulbourethral (Cowper's) gland
  Cowper's (bulbourethral) gland
  External urethral sphincter
  Internal urethral sphincter
  Membranous urethra
  Penile urethra
  Prostatic urethra
	Ø Open
	3 Percutaneous
	4 Percutaneous Endoscopic
	7 Via Natural or Artificial Opening
	8 Via Natural or Artificial Opening Endoscopic
	X External
		Z No Device	X Diagnostic
			Z No Qualifier

Non-OR ØTB[Ø,1,3,4,6,7][3,4,7,8]ZX
Non-OR ØTBD[Ø,3,4,7,8,X]ZX

Ø   Medical and Surgical
T   Urinary System
C   Extirpation   Definition: Taking or cutting out solid matter from a body part
                      Explanation: The solid matter may be an abnormal byproduct of a biological function or a foreign body; it may be imbedded in a body part or in the lumen of a tubular body part. The solid matter may or may not have been previously broken into pieces.

Body Part Character 4	Approach Character 5	Device Character 6	Qualifier Character 7

Ø Kidney, Right
  Renal calyx
  Renal capsule
  Renal cortex
  Renal segment
1 Kidney, Left
  See Ø Kidney, Right
3 Kidney Pelvis, Right
  Ureteropelvic junction (UPJ)
4 Kidney Pelvis, Left
  See 3 Kidney Pelvis, Right
6 Ureter, Right
  Ureteral orifice
  Ureterovesical orifice
7 Ureter, Left
  See 6 Ureter, Right
B Bladder
  Trigone of bladder
C Bladder Neck
	Ø Open
	3 Percutaneous
	4 Percutaneous Endoscopic
	7 Via Natural or Artificial Opening
	8 Via Natural or Artificial Opening Endoscopic
		Z No Device	Z No Qualifier

D Urethra
  Bulbourethral (Cowper's) gland
  Cowper's (bulbourethral) gland
  External urethral sphincter
  Internal urethral sphincter
  Membranous urethra
  Penile urethra
  Prostatic urethra
	Ø Open
	3 Percutaneous
	4 Percutaneous Endoscopic
	7 Via Natural or Artificial Opening
	8 Via Natural or Artificial Opening Endoscopic
	X External
		Z No Device	Z No Qualifier

Non-OR ØTC[B,C][7,8]ZZ
Non-OR ØTCD[7,8,X]ZZ

Ø   **Medical and Surgical**
T   **Urinary System**
D   **Extraction**   Definition: Pulling or stripping out or off all or a portion of a body part by the use of force
                      Explanation: The qualifier DIAGNOSTIC is used to identify extraction procedures that are biopsies

Body Part Character 4	Approach Character 5	Device Character 6	Qualifier Character 7

Ø **Kidney, Right**
   Renal calyx
   Renal capsule
   Renal cortex
   Renal segment
1 **Kidney, Left**
   See Ø Kidney, Right
	Ø Open
	3 Percutaneous
	4 Percutaneous Endoscopic
		Z No Device	Z No Qualifier

Ø   **Medical and Surgical**
T   **Urinary System**
F   **Fragmentation**   Definition: Breaking solid matter in a body part into pieces
                      Explanation: Physical force (e.g., manual, ultrasonic) applied directly or indirectly is used to break the solid matter into pieces. The solid matter may be an abnormal byproduct of a biological function or a foreign body. The pieces of solid matter are not taken out.

Body Part Character 4	Approach Character 5	Device Character 6	Qualifier Character 7

3 **Kidney Pelvis, Right**
   Ureteropelvic junction (UPJ)
4 **Kidney Pelvis, Left**
   See 3 Kidney Pelvis, Right
6 **Ureter, Right**
   Ureteral orifice
   Ureterovesical orifice
7 **Ureter, Left**
   See 6 Ureter, Right
B **Bladder**
   Trigone of bladder
C **Bladder Neck**
D **Urethra**   NC
   Bulbourethral (Cowper's) gland
   Cowper's (bulbourethral) gland
   External urethral sphincter
   Internal urethral sphincter
   Membranous urethra
   Penile urethra
   Prostatic urethra
	Ø Open
	3 Percutaneous
	4 Percutaneous Endoscopic
	7 Via Natural or Artificial Opening
	8 Via Natural or Artificial Opening
	   Endoscopic
	X External
		Z No Device	Z No Qualifier

Non-OR	ØTF[3,4][Ø,7,8]ZZ
Non-OR	ØTF[6,7,B,C,D][Ø,3,4,7,8]ZZ
Non-OR	ØTF[3,4,6,7,B,C,D]XZZ
NC	ØTFDXZZ

Urinary System

Ø   Medical and Surgical
T   Urinary System
H   Insertion

Definition: Putting in a nonbiological appliance that monitors, assists, performs, or prevents a physiological function but does not physically take the place of a body part

Explanation: None

Body Part Character 4	Approach Character 5	Device Character 6	Qualifier Character 7
5 Kidney Renal calyx Renal capsule Renal cortex Renal segment	**Ø** Open **3** Percutaneous **4** Percutaneous Endoscopic **7** Via Natural or Artificial Opening **8** Via Natural or Artificial Opening Endoscopic	**1** Radioactive Element **2** Monitoring Device **3** Infusion Device **Y** Other Device	**Z** No Qualifier
9 Ureter Ureteral orifice Ureterovesical orifice	**Ø** Open **3** Percutaneous **4** Percutaneous Endoscopic **7** Via Natural or Artificial Opening **8** Via Natural or Artificial Opening Endoscopic	**1** Radioactive Element **2** Monitoring Device **3** Infusion Device **M** Stimulator Lead **Y** Other Device	**Z** No Qualifier
B Bladder NC Trigone of bladder	**Ø** Open **3** Percutaneous **4** Percutaneous Endoscopic **7** Via Natural or Artificial Opening **8** Via Natural or Artificial Opening Endoscopic	**1** Radioactive Element **2** Monitoring Device **3** Infusion Device **L** Artificial Sphincter **M** Stimulator Lead **Y** Other Device	**Z** No Qualifier
C Bladder Neck	**Ø** Open **3** Percutaneous **4** Percutaneous Endoscopic **7** Via Natural or Artificial Opening **8** Via Natural or Artificial Opening Endoscopic	**L** Artificial Sphincter	**Z** No Qualifier
D Urethra Bulbourethral (Cowper's) gland Cowper's (bulbourethral) gland External urethral sphincter Internal urethral sphincter Membranous urethra Penile urethra Prostatic urethra	**Ø** Open **3** Percutaneous **4** Percutaneous Endoscopic **7** Via Natural or Artificial Opening **8** Via Natural or Artificial Opening Endoscopic	**1** Radioactive Element **2** Monitoring Device **3** Infusion Device **L** Artificial Sphincter **Y** Other Device	**Z** No Qualifier
D Urethra Bulbourethral (Cowper's) gland Cowper's (bulbourethral) gland External urethral sphincter Internal urethral sphincter Membranous urethra Penile urethra Prostatic urethra	**X** External	**2** Monitoring Device **3** Infusion Device **L** Artificial Sphincter	**Z** No Qualifier

Non-OR ØTH5Ø3Z		**Non-OR** ØTHB[3,4][3,Y]Z	
Non-OR ØTH5[3,4][3,Y]Z		**Non-OR** ØTHB7[2,3,Y]Z	
Non-OR ØTH57[2,3,Y]Z		**Non-OR** ØTHB8[2,3]Z	
Non-OR ØTH58[2,3]Z		**Non-OR** ØTHDØ3Z	
Non-OR ØTH9Ø3Z		**Non-OR** ØTHD[3,4][3,Y]Z	
Non-OR ØTH9[3,4][3,Y]Z		**Non-OR** ØTHD[7,8][2,3,Y]Z	
Non-OR ØTH97[2,3,Y]Z		**Non-OR** ØTHDX3Z	
Non-OR ØTH98[2,3]Z		**NC** ØTHB[Ø,3,4,7,8]MZ	
Non-OR ØTHBØ3Z			

Ø   Medical and Surgical
T   Urinary System
J   Inspection   Definition: Visually and/or manually exploring a body part

Explanation: Visual exploration may be performed with or without optical instrumentation. Manual exploration may be performed directly or through intervening body layers.

Body Part Character 4	Approach Character 5	Device Character 6	Qualifier Character 7
5 Kidney Renal calyx Renal capsule Renal cortex Renal segment **9 Ureter** Ureteral orifice Ureterovesical orifice **B Bladder** Trigone of bladder **D Urethra** Bulbourethral (Cowper's) gland Cowper's (bulbourethral) gland External urethral sphincter Internal urethral sphincter Membranous urethra Penile urethra Prostatic urethra	**Ø Open** **3 Percutaneous** **4 Percutaneous Endoscopic** **7 Via Natural or Artificial Opening** **8 Via Natural or Artificial Opening Endoscopic** **X External**	**Z No Device**	**Z No Qualifier**

Non-OR	ØTJ[5,9,D][3,4,7,8,X]ZZ
Non-OR	ØTJB[3,7,8,X]ZZ

Ø   Medical and Surgical
T   Urinary System
L   Occlusion   Definition: Completely closing an orifice or the lumen of a tubular body part

Explanation: The orifice can be a natural orifice or an artificially created orifice

Body Part Character 4	Approach Character 5	Device Character 6	Qualifier Character 7
3 Kidney Pelvis, Right Ureteropelvic junction (UPJ) **4 Kidney Pelvis, Left** *See 3 Kidney Pelvis, Right* **6 Ureter, Right** Ureteral orifice Ureterovesical orifice **7 Ureter, Left** *See 6 Ureter, Right* **B Bladder** Trigone of bladder **C Bladder Neck**	**Ø Open** **3 Percutaneous** **4 Percutaneous Endoscopic**	**C Extraluminal Device** **D Intraluminal Device** **Z No Device**	**Z No Qualifier**
3 Kidney Pelvis, Right Ureteropelvic junction (UPJ) **4 Kidney Pelvis, Left** *See 3 Kidney Pelvis, Right* **6 Ureter, Right** Ureteral orifice Ureterovesical orifice **7 Ureter, Left** *See 6 Ureter, Right* **B Bladder** Trigone of bladder **C Bladder Neck**	**7 Via Natural or Artificial Opening** **8 Via Natural or Artificial Opening Endoscopic**	**D Intraluminal Device** **Z No Device**	**Z No Qualifier**
D Urethra Bulbourethral (Cowper's) gland Cowper's (bulbourethral) gland External urethral sphincter Internal urethral sphincter Membranous urethra Penile urethra Prostatic urethra	**Ø Open** **3 Percutaneous** **4 Percutaneous Endoscopic** **X External**	**C Extraluminal Device** **D Intraluminal Device** **Z No Device**	**Z No Qualifier**
D Urethra Bulbourethral (Cowper's) gland Cowper's (bulbourethral) gland External urethral sphincter Internal urethral sphincter Membranous urethra Penile urethra Prostatic urethra	**7 Via Natural or Artificial Opening** **8 Via Natural or Artificial Opening Endoscopic**	**D Intraluminal Device** **Z No Device**	**Z No Qualifier**

Ø   Medical and Surgical
T   Urinary System
M   Reattachment   Definition: Putting back in or on all or a portion of a separated body part to its normal location or other suitable location

                        Explanation: Vascular circulation and nervous pathways may or may not be reestablished

Body Part Character 4	Approach Character 5	Device Character 6	Qualifier Character 7

Ø Kidney, Right
   Renal calyx
   Renal capsule
   Renal cortex
   Renal segment
1 Kidney, Left
   See Ø Kidney, Right
2 Kidneys, Bilateral
   See Ø Kidney, Right
3 Kidney Pelvis, Right
   Ureteropelvic junction (UPJ)
4 Kidney Pelvis, Left
   See 3 Kidney Pelvis, Right
6 Ureter, Right
   Ureteral orifice
   Ureterovesical orifice
7 Ureter, Left
   See 6 Ureter, Right
8 Ureters, Bilateral
   See 6 Ureter, Right
B Bladder
   Trigone of bladder
C Bladder Neck
D Urethra
   Bulbourethral (Cowper's) gland
   Cowper's (bulbourethral) gland
   External urethral sphincter
   Internal urethral sphincter
   Membranous urethra
   Penile urethra
   Prostatic urethra
	Ø Open
	4 Percutaneous Endoscopic
		Z No Device	**Z No Qualifier**

Ø   Medical and Surgical
T   Urinary System
N   Release   Definition: Freeing a body part from an abnormal physical constraint by cutting or by the use of force

                        Explanation: Some of the restraining tissue may be taken out but none of the body part is taken out

Body Part Character 4	Approach Character 5	Device Character 6	Qualifier Character 7

Ø Kidney, Right
   Renal calyx
   Renal capsule
   Renal cortex
   Renal segment
1 Kidney, Left
   See Ø Kidney, Right
3 Kidney Pelvis, Right
   Ureteropelvic junction (UPJ)
4 Kidney Pelvis, Left
   See 3 Kidney Pelvis, Right
6 Ureter, Right
   Ureteral orifice
   Ureterovesical orifice
7 Ureter, Left
   See 6 Ureter, Right
B Bladder
   Trigone of bladder
C Bladder Neck
	Ø Open
	3 Percutaneous
	4 Percutaneous Endoscopic
	7 Via Natural or Artificial Opening
	8 Via Natural or Artificial Opening
	   Endoscopic
		Z No Device	**Z No Qualifier**

D Urethra
   Bulbourethral (Cowper's) gland
   Cowper's (bulbourethral) gland
   External urethral sphincter
   Internal urethral sphincter
   Membranous urethra
   Penile urethra
   Prostatic urethra
	Ø Open
	3 Percutaneous
	4 Percutaneous Endoscopic
	7 Via Natural or Artificial Opening
	8 Via Natural or Artificial Opening
	   Endoscopic
	X External
		Z No Device	**Z No Qualifier**

🔵 Limited Coverage   🔵 Noncovered   ⊞ Combination Member   HAC associated procedure   Combination Only   DRG Non-OR   Non-OR   New/Revised in GREEN

626   ICD-10-PCS 2021

ØTM–ØTN

Ø   Medical and Surgical
T   Urinary System
P   Removal

Definition: Taking out or off a device from a body part

Explanation: If a device is taken out and a similar device put in without cutting or puncturing the skin or mucous membrane, the procedure is coded to the root operation CHANGE. Otherwise, the procedure for taking out the device is coded to the root operation REMOVAL.

Body Part Character 4	Approach Character 5	Device Character 6	Qualifier Character 7
5 Kidney Renal calyx Renal capsule Renal cortex Renal segment	**Ø** Open **3** Percutaneous **4** Percutaneous Endoscopic **7** Via Natural or Artificial Opening **8** Via Natural or Artificial Opening Endoscopic	**Ø** Drainage Device **2** Monitoring Device **3** Infusion Device **7** Autologous Tissue Substitute **C** Extraluminal Device **D** Intraluminal Device **J** Synthetic Substitute **K** Nonautologous Tissue Substitute **Y** Other Device	**Z** No Qualifier
5 Kidney Renal calyx Renal capsule Renal cortex Renal segment	**X** External	**Ø** Drainage Device **2** Monitoring Device **3** Infusion Device **D** Intraluminal Device	**Z** No Qualifier
9 Ureter Ureteral orifice Ureterovesical orifice	**Ø** Open **3** Percutaneous **4** Percutaneous Endoscopic **7** Via Natural or Artificial Opening **8** Via Natural or Artificial Opening Endoscopic	**Ø** Drainage Device **2** Monitoring Device **3** Infusion Device **7** Autologous Tissue Substitute **C** Extraluminal Device **D** Intraluminal Device **J** Synthetic Substitute **K** Nonautologous Tissue Substitute **M** Stimulator Lead **Y** Other Device	**Z** No Qualifier
9 Ureter Ureteral orifice Ureterovesical orifice	**X** External	**Ø** Drainage Device **2** Monitoring Device **3** Infusion Device **D** Intraluminal Device **M** Stimulator Lead	**Z** No Qualifier
B Bladder NC Trigone of bladder	**Ø** Open **3** Percutaneous **4** Percutaneous Endoscopic **7** Via Natural or Artificial Opening **8** Via Natural or Artificial Opening Endoscopic	**Ø** Drainage Device **2** Monitoring Device **3** Infusion Device **7** Autologous Tissue Substitute **C** Extraluminal Device **D** Intraluminal Device **J** Synthetic Substitute **K** Nonautologous Tissue Substitute **L** Artificial Sphincter **M** Stimulator Lead **Y** Other Device	**Z** No Qualifier
B Bladder Trigone of bladder	**X** External	**Ø** Drainage Device **2** Monitoring Device **3** Infusion Device **D** Intraluminal Device **L** Artificial Sphincter **M** Stimulator Lead	**Z** No Qualifier
D Urethra Bulbourethral (Cowper's) gland Cowper's (bulbourethral) gland External urethral sphincter Internal urethral sphincter Membranous urethra Penile urethra Prostatic urethra	**Ø** Open **3** Percutaneous **4** Percutaneous Endoscopic **7** Via Natural or Artificial Opening **8** Via Natural or Artificial Opening Endoscopic	**Ø** Drainage Device **2** Monitoring Device **3** Infusion Device **7** Autologous Tissue Substitute **C** Extraluminal Device **D** Intraluminal Device **J** Synthetic Substitute **K** Nonautologous Tissue Substitute **L** Artificial Sphincter **Y** Other Device	**Z** No Qualifier
D Urethra Bulbourethral (Cowper's) gland Cowper's (bulbourethral) gland External urethral sphincter Internal urethral sphincter Membranous urethra Penile urethra Prostatic urethra	**X** External	**Ø** Drainage Device **2** Monitoring Device **3** Infusion Device **D** Intraluminal Device **L** Artificial Sphincter	**Z** No Qualifier

Non-OR ØTP5[3,4,7]YZ	**Non-OR** ØTP9[7,8][Ø,2,3,D]Z	**Non-OR** ØTPB[7,8][Ø,2,3,D]Z	**Non-OR** ØTPD[7,8][Ø,2,3,D,Y]Z
Non-OR ØTP5[7,8][Ø,2,3,D]Z	**Non-OR** ØTP9X[Ø,2,3,D]Z	**Non-OR** ØTPBX[Ø,2,3,D,L]Z	**Non-OR** ØTPDX[Ø,2,3,D]Z
Non-OR ØTP5X[Ø,2,3,D]Z	**Non-OR** ØTPB[3,4,7]YZ	**Non-OR** ØTPD[3,4]YZ	**NC** ØTPB[Ø,3,4,7,8]MZ
Non-OR ØTP9[3,4,7]YZ			

LC Limited Coverage   **NC** Noncovered   ⊞ Combination Member   HAC associated procedure   Combination Only   DRG Non-OR   Non-OR   New/Revised in **GREEN**

ICD-10-PCS 2021   627

ØTP–ØTP

Ø   **Medical and Surgical**
T   **Urinary System**
Q   **Repair**   Definition: Restoring, to the extent possible, a body part to its normal anatomic structure and function
                       Explanation: Used only when the method to accomplish the repair is not one of the other root operations

Body Part Character 4	Approach Character 5	Device Character 6	Qualifier Character 7

Ø Kidney, Right
   Renal calyx
   Renal capsule
   Renal cortex
   Renal segment
1 Kidney, Left
   See Ø Kidney, Right
3 Kidney Pelvis, Right
   Ureteropelvic junction (UPJ)
4 Kidney Pelvis, Left
   See 3 Kidney Pelvis, Right
6 Ureter, Right
   Ureteral orifice
   Ureterovesical orifice
7 Ureter, Left
   See 6 Ureter, Right
B Bladder ⊞
   Trigone of bladder
C Bladder Neck
	Ø Open
	3 Percutaneous
	4 Percutaneous Endoscopic
	7 Via Natural or Artificial Opening
	**8 Via Natural or Artificial Opening
	   Endoscopic**
		Z No Device	**Z No Qualifier**

D Urethra
   Bulbourethral (Cowper's) gland
   Cowper's (bulbourethral) gland
   External urethral sphincter
   Internal urethral sphincter
   Membranous urethra
   Penile urethra
   Prostatic urethra
	Ø Open
	3 Percutaneous
	4 Percutaneous Endoscopic
	7 Via Natural or Artificial Opening
	**8 Via Natural or Artificial Opening
	   Endoscopic**
	X External
		Z No Device	**Z No Qualifier**

See Appendix L for Procedure Combinations
   ⊞   ØTQB[Ø,3,4]ZZ

Ø   **Medical and Surgical**
T   **Urinary System**
R   **Replacement**   Definition: Putting in or on biological or synthetic material that physically takes the place and/or function of all or a portion of a body part
                       Explanation: The body part may have been taken out or replaced, or may be taken out, physically eradicated, or rendered nonfunctional during the REPLACEMENT procedure. A REMOVAL procedure is coded for taking out the device used in a previous replacement procedure.

Body Part Character 4	Approach Character 5	Device Character 6	Qualifier Character 7

3 Kidney Pelvis, Right
   Ureteropelvic junction (UPJ)
4 Kidney Pelvis, Left
   See 3 Kidney Pelvis, Right
6 Ureter, Right
   Ureteral orifice
   Ureterovesical orifice
7 Ureter, Left
   See 6 Ureter, Right
B Bladder
   Trigone of bladder
C Bladder Neck
	Ø Open
	4 Percutaneous Endoscopic
	7 Via Natural or Artificial Opening
	**8 Via Natural or Artificial Opening
	   Endoscopic**
		7 Autologous Tissue Substitute
		J Synthetic Substitute
		K Nonautologous Tissue Substitute
			Z No Qualifier

D Urethra
   Bulbourethral (Cowper's) gland
   Cowper's (bulbourethral) gland
   External urethral sphincter
   Internal urethral sphincter
   Membranous urethra
   Penile urethra
   Prostatic urethra
	Ø Open
	4 Percutaneous Endoscopic
	7 Via Natural or Artificial Opening
	**8 Via Natural or Artificial Opening
	   Endoscopic**
	X External
		7 Autologous Tissue Substitute
		J Synthetic Substitute
		K Nonautologous Tissue Substitute
			Z No Qualifier

LC Limited Coverage   **NC** Noncovered   ⊞ Combination Member   HAC associated procedure   Combination Only   DRG Non-OR   Non-OR   New/Revised in **GREEN**

628   ICD-10-PCS 2021

Ø   **Medical and Surgical**
T   **Urinary System**
S   **Reposition**   Definition: Moving to its normal location, or other suitable location, all or a portion of a body part

Explanation: The body part is moved to a new location from an abnormal location, or from a normal location where it is not functioning correctly. The body part may or may not be cut out or off to be moved to the new location.

Body Part Character 4	Approach Character 5	Device Character 6	Qualifier Character 7
Ø Kidney, Right Renal calyx Renal capsule Renal cortex Renal segment **1 Kidney, Left** *See Ø Kidney, Right* **2 Kidneys, Bilateral** *See Ø Kidney, Right* **3 Kidney Pelvis, Right** Ureteropelvic junction (UPJ) **4 Kidney Pelvis, Left** *See 3 Kidney Pelvis, Right* **6 Ureter, Right** Ureteral orifice Ureterovesical orifice **7 Ureter, Left** *See 6 Ureter, Right* **8 Ureters, Bilateral** *See 6 Ureter, Right* **B Bladder** Trigone of bladder **C Bladder Neck** **D Urethra** Bulbourethral (Cowper's) gland Cowper's (bulbourethral) gland External urethral sphincter Internal urethral sphincter Membranous urethra Penile urethra Prostatic urethra	**Ø Open** **4 Percutaneous Endoscopic**	**Z No Device**	**Z No Qualifier**

Ø   **Medical and Surgical**
T   **Urinary System**
T   **Resection**   Definition: Cutting out or off, without replacement, all of a body part

Explanation: None

Body Part Character 4	Approach Character 5	Device Character 6	Qualifier Character 7
Ø Kidney, Right Renal calyx Renal capsule Renal cortex Renal segment **1 Kidney, Left** *See Ø Kidney, Right* **2 Kidneys, Bilateral** *See Ø Kidney, Right*	**Ø Open** **4 Percutaneous Endoscopic**	**Z No Device**	**Z No Qualifier**
3 Kidney Pelvis, Right Ureteropelvic junction (UPJ) **4 Kidney Pelvis, Left** *See 3 Kidney Pelvis, Right* **6 Ureter, Right** Ureteral orifice Ureterovesical orifice **7 Ureter, Left** *See 6 Ureter, Right* **B Bladder** ⊞ Trigone of bladder **C Bladder Neck** **D Urethra** Bulbourethral (Cowper's) gland Cowper's (bulbourethral) gland External urethral sphincter Internal urethral sphincter Membranous urethra Penile urethra Prostatic urethra	**Ø Open** **4 Percutaneous Endoscopic** **7 Via Natural or Artificial Opening** **8 Via Natural or Artificial Opening Endoscopic**	**Z No Device**	**Z No Qualifier**

Non-OR   ØTTD[4,7,8]ZZ

See Appendix L for Procedure Combinations
     Combo-only   ØTTDØZZ
     ⊞   ØTTBØZZ

LC Limited Coverage   NC Noncovered   ⊞ Combination Member   HAC associated procedure   Combination Only   DRG Non-OR   Non-OR   New/Revised in GREEN

ICD-10-PCS 2021   629

ØTS–ØTT

Ø   **Medical and Surgical**
T   **Urinary System**
U   **Supplement**   Definition: Putting in or on biological or synthetic material that physically reinforces and/or augments the function of a portion of a body part

                      Explanation: The biological material is non-living, or is living and from the same individual. The body part may have been previously replaced, and the SUPPLEMENT procedure is performed to physically reinforce and/or augment the function of the replaced body part.

Body Part Character 4	Approach Character 5	Device Character 6	Qualifier Character 7

3 **Kidney Pelvis, Right**
    Ureteropelvic junction (UPJ)
4 **Kidney Pelvis, Left**
    See 3 Kidney Pelvis, Right
6 **Ureter, Right**
    Ureteral orifice
    Ureterovesical orifice
7 **Ureter, Left**
    See 6 Ureter, Right
B **Bladder**
    Trigone of bladder
C **Bladder Neck**
	Ø Open
	4 Percutaneous Endoscopic
	7 Via Natural or Artificial Opening
	8 Via Natural or Artificial Opening
	    Endoscopic
		7 Autologous Tissue Substitute
		J Synthetic Substitute
		K Nonautologous Tissue Substitute
			Z No Qualifier

D **Urethra**
    Bulbourethral (Cowper's) gland
    Cowper's (bulbourethral) gland
    External urethral sphincter
    Internal urethral sphincter
    Membranous urethra
    Penile urethra
    Prostatic urethra
	Ø Open
	4 Percutaneous Endoscopic
	7 Via Natural or Artificial Opening
	8 Via Natural or Artificial Opening
	    Endoscopic
	X External
		7 Autologous Tissue Substitute
		J Synthetic Substitute
		K Nonautologous Tissue Substitute
			Z No Qualifier

Ø   **Medical and Surgical**
T   **Urinary System**
V   **Restriction**   Definition: Partially closing an orifice or the lumen of a tubular body part

                      Explanation: The orifice can be a natural orifice or an artificially created orifice

Body Part Character 4	Approach Character 5	Device Character 6	Qualifier Character 7

3 **Kidney Pelvis, Right**
    Ureteropelvic junction (UPJ)
4 **Kidney Pelvis, Left**
    See 3 Kidney Pelvis, Right
6 **Ureter, Right**
    Ureteral orifice
    Ureterovesical orifice
7 **Ureter, Left**
    See 6 Ureter, Right
B **Bladder**
    Trigone of bladder
C **Bladder Neck**
	Ø Open
	3 Percutaneous
	4 Percutaneous Endoscopic
		C Extraluminal Device
		D Intraluminal Device
		Z No Device
			Z No Qualifier

3 **Kidney Pelvis, Right**
    Ureteropelvic junction (UPJ)
4 **Kidney Pelvis, Left**
    See 3 Kidney Pelvis, Right
6 **Ureter, Right**
    Ureteral orifice
    Ureterovesical orifice
7 **Ureter, Left**
    See 6 Ureter, Right
B **Bladder**
    Trigone of bladder
C **Bladder Neck**
	7 Via Natural or Artificial Opening
	8 Via Natural or Artificial Opening
	    Endoscopic
		D Intraluminal Device
		Z No Device
			Z No Qualifier

D **Urethra**
    Bulbourethral (Cowper's) gland
    Cowper's (bulbourethral) gland
    External urethral sphincter
    Internal urethral sphincter
    Membranous urethra
    Penile urethra
    Prostatic urethra
	Ø Open
	3 Percutaneous
	4 Percutaneous Endoscopic
		C Extraluminal Device
		D Intraluminal Device
		Z No Device
			Z No Qualifier

D **Urethra**
    Bulbourethral (Cowper's) gland
    Cowper's (bulbourethral) gland
    External urethral sphincter
    Internal urethral sphincter
    Membranous urethra
    Penile urethra
    Prostatic urethra
	7 Via Natural or Artificial Opening
	8 Via Natural or Artificial Opening
	    Endoscopic
		D Intraluminal Device
		Z No Device
			Z No Qualifier

D **Urethra**
    Bulbourethral (Cowper's) gland
    Cowper's (bulbourethral) gland
    External urethral sphincter
    Internal urethral sphincter
    Membranous urethra
    Penile urethra
    Prostatic urethra
	X External	**Z** No Device	**Z** No Qualifier

Ø   **Medical and Surgical**
T   **Urinary System**
W   **Revision**   Definition: Correcting, to the extent possible, a portion of a malfunctioning device or the position of a displaced device

                Explanation: Revision can include correcting a malfunctioning or displaced device by taking out or putting in components of the device such as a screw or pin

Body Part Character 4	Approach Character 5	Device Character 6	Qualifier Character 7
5 Kidney Renal calyx Renal capsule Renal cortex Renal segment	**Ø** Open **3** Percutaneous **4** Percutaneous Endoscopic **7** Via Natural or Artificial Opening **8** Via Natural or Artificial Opening Endoscopic	**Ø** Drainage Device **2** Monitoring Device **3** Infusion Device **7** Autologous Tissue Substitute **C** Extraluminal Device **D** Intraluminal Device **J** Synthetic Substitute **K** Nonautologous Tissue Substitute **Y** Other Device	**Z** No Qualifier
5 Kidney Renal calyx Renal capsule Renal cortex Renal segment	**X** External	**Ø** Drainage Device **2** Monitoring Device **3** Infusion Device **7** Autologous Tissue Substitute **C** Extraluminal Device **D** Intraluminal Device **J** Synthetic Substitute **K** Nonautologous Tissue Substitute	**Z** No Qualifier
9 Ureter Ureteral orifice Ureterovesical orifice	**Ø** Open **3** Percutaneous **4** Percutaneous Endoscopic **7** Via Natural or Artificial Opening **8** Via Natural or Artificial Opening Endoscopic	**Ø** Drainage Device **2** Monitoring Device **3** Infusion Device **7** Autologous Tissue Substitute **C** Extraluminal Device **D** Intraluminal Device **J** Synthetic Substitute **K** Nonautologous Tissue Substitute **M** Stimulator Lead **Y** Other Device	**Z** No Qualifier
9 Ureter Ureteral orifice Ureterovesical orifice	**X** External	**Ø** Drainage Device **2** Monitoring Device **3** Infusion Device **7** Autologous Tissue Substitute **C** Extraluminal Device **D** Intraluminal Device **J** Synthetic Substitute **K** Nonautologous Tissue Substitute **M** Stimulator Lead	**Z** No Qualifier
B Bladder Trigone of bladder	**Ø** Open **3** Percutaneous **4** Percutaneous Endoscopic **7** Via Natural or Artificial Opening **8** Via Natural or Artificial Opening Endoscopic	**Ø** Drainage Device **2** Monitoring Device **3** Infusion Device **7** Autologous Tissue Substitute **C** Extraluminal Device **D** Intraluminal Device **J** Synthetic Substitute **K** Nonautologous Tissue Substitute **L** Artificial Sphincter **M** Stimulator Lead **Y** Other Device	**Z** No Qualifier
B Bladder Trigone of bladder	**X** External	**Ø** Drainage Device **2** Monitoring Device **3** Infusion Device **7** Autologous Tissue Substitute **C** Extraluminal Device **D** Intraluminal Device **J** Synthetic Substitute **K** Nonautologous Tissue Substitute **L** Artificial Sphincter **M** Stimulator Lead	**Z** No Qualifier

Non-OR   ØTW5[3,4,7]YZ
Non-OR   ØTW5X[Ø,2,3,7,C,D,J,K]Z
Non-OR   ØTW9[3,4,7]YZ

Non-OR   ØTW9X[Ø,2,3,7,C,D,J,K,M]Z
Non-OR   ØTWB[3,4,7]YZ
Non-OR   ØTWBX[Ø,2,3,7,C,D,J,K,L,M]Z

ØTW Continued on next page

LC Limited Coverage   NC Noncovered   ⊞ Combination Member   HAC associated procedure   Combination Only   DRG Non-OR   Non-OR   New/Revised in GREEN

Ø Medical and Surgical
T Urinary System
W Revision

Definition: Correcting, to the extent possible, a portion of a malfunctioning device or the position of a displaced device

Explanation: Revision can include correcting a malfunctioning or displaced device by taking out or putting in components of the device such as a screw or pin

Body Part Character 4	Approach Character 5	Device Character 6	Qualifier Character 7
D Urethra Bulbourethral (Cowper's) gland Cowper's (bulbourethral) gland External urethral sphincter Internal urethral sphincter Membranous urethra Penile urethra Prostatic urethra	**Ø** Open **3** Percutaneous **4** Percutaneous Endoscopic **7** Via Natural or Artificial Opening **8** Via Natural or Artificial Opening Endoscopic	**Ø** Drainage Device **2** Monitoring Device **3** Infusion Device **7** Autologous Tissue Substitute **C** Extraluminal Device **D** Intraluminal Device **J** Synthetic Substitute **K** Nonautologous Tissue Substitute **L** Artificial Sphincter **Y** Other Device	**Z** No Qualifier
D Urethra Bulbourethral (Cowper's) gland Cowper's (bulbourethral) gland External urethral sphincter Internal urethral sphincter Membranous urethra Penile urethra Prostatic urethra	**X** External	**Ø** Drainage Device **2** Monitoring Device **3** Infusion Device **7** Autologous Tissue Substitute **C** Extraluminal Device **D** Intraluminal Device **J** Synthetic Substitute **K** Nonautologous Tissue Substitute **L** Artificial Sphincter	**Z** No Qualifier

Non-OR ØTWD[3,4,7,8]YZ
Non-OR ØTWDX[Ø,2,3,7,C,D,J,K,L]Z

Ø Medical and Surgical
T Urinary System
Y Transplantation

Definition: Putting in or on all or a portion of a living body part taken from another individual or animal to physically take the place and/or function of all or a portion of a similar body part

Explanation: The native body part may or may not be taken out, and the transplanted body part may take over all or a portion of its function

Body Part Character 4	Approach Character 5	Device Character 6	Qualifier Character 7
Ø Kidney, Right LC ⊞ Renal calyx Renal capsule Renal cortex Renal segment **1 Kidney, Left** LC ⊞ *See Ø Kidney, Right*	**Ø** Open	**Z** No Device	**Ø** Allogeneic **1** Syngeneic **2** Zooplastic

LC ØTY[Ø,1]ØZ[Ø,1,2]

See Appendix L for Procedure Combinations
⊞ ØTY[Ø,1]ØZ[Ø,1,2]

Female Reproductive System ØU1–ØUY

Character Meanings

This Character Meaning table is provided as a guide to assist the user in the identification of character members that may be found in this section of code tables. It **SHOULD NOT** be used to build a PCS code.

Operation–Character 3	Body Part–Character 4	Approach–Character 5	Device–Character 6	Qualifier–Character 7
1　Bypass	Ø　Ovary, Right	Ø　Open	Ø　Drainage Device	Ø　Allogeneic
2　Change	1　Ovary, Left	3　Percutaneous	1　Radioactive Element	1　Syngeneic
5　Destruction	2　Ovaries, Bilateral	4　Percutaneous Endoscopic	3　Infusion Device	2　Zooplastic
7　Dilation	3　Ovary	7　Via Natural or Artificial Opening	7　Autologous Tissue Substitute	5　Fallopian Tube, Right
8　Division	4　Uterine Supporting Structure	8　Via Natural or Artificial Opening Endoscopic	C　Extraluminal Device	6　Fallopian Tube, Left
9　Drainage	5　Fallopian Tube, Right	F　Via Natural or Artificial Opening With Percutaneous Endoscopic Assistance	D　Intraluminal Device	9　Uterus
B　Excision	6　Fallopian Tube, Left	X　External	G　Intraluminal Device, Pessary	L　Supracervical
C　Extirpation	7　Fallopian Tubes, Bilateral		H　Contraceptive Device	X　Diagnostic
D　Extraction	8　Fallopian Tube		J　Synthetic Substitute	Z　No Qualifier
F　Fragmentation	9　Uterus		K　Nonautologous Tissue Substitute	
H　Insertion	B　Endometrium		Y　Other Device	
J　Inspection	C　Cervix		Z　No Device	
L　Occlusion	D　Uterus and Cervix			
M　Reattachment	F　Cul-de-sac			
N　Release	G　Vagina			
P　Removal	H　Vagina and Cul-de-sac			
Q　Repair	J　Clitoris			
S　Reposition	K　Hymen			
T　Resection	L　Vestibular Gland			
U　Supplement	M　Vulva			
V　Restriction	N　Ova			
W　Revision				
Y　Transplantation				

AHA Coding Clinic for table ØU5
2015, 3Q, 31　　　Tubal ligation for sterilization

AHA Coding Clinic for table ØU7
2020, 2Q, 30　　　Duhrssen Cervical Incision

AHA Coding Clinic for table ØU9
2016, 4Q, 58　　　Longitudinal vaginal septum

AHA Coding Clinic for table ØUB
2018, 1Q, 23　　　Tubal ligation procedure
2015, 3Q, 31　　　Laparoscopic partial salpingectomy for ectopic pregnancy
2015, 3Q, 31　　　Tubal ligation for sterilization
2014, 4Q, 16　　　Excision of multiple uterine fibroids
2014, 3Q, 12　　　Excision of skin tag from labia majora

AHA Coding Clinic for table ØUC
2015, 3Q, 30　　　Removal of cervical cerclage
2013, 2Q, 38　　　Evacuation of clot post-partum

AHA Coding Clinic for table ØUH
2018, 1Q, 25　　　Intrauterine brachytherapy & placement of tandems & ovoids
2013, 2Q, 34　　　Placement of intrauterine device via open approach

AHA Coding Clinic for table ØUJ
2015, 1Q, 33　　　Robotic-assisted laparoscopic hysterectomy converted to open procedure

AHA Coding Clinic for table ØUL
2018, 1Q, 23　　　Tubal ligation procedure
2015, 3Q, 31　　　Tubal ligation for sterilization

AHA Coding Clinic for table ØUQ
2014, 4Q, 18　　　Obstetrical periurethral laceration
2013, 4Q, 120　　Repair of clitoral obstetric laceration

AHA Coding Clinic for table ØUS
2016, 1Q, 9　　　Anteversion of retroverted pregnant uterus

AHA Coding Clinic for table ØUT
2017, 4Q, 68　　　New qualifier values - Supracervical hysterectomy
2015, 1Q, 33　　　Robotic-assisted laparoscopic hysterectomy converted to open procedure
2013, 3Q, 28　　　Total hysterectomy
2013, 1Q, 24　　　Excision versus Resection of remaining ovarian remnant following previous excision

AHA Coding Clinic for table ØUV
2015, 3Q, 30　　　Insertion of cervical cerclage

AHA Coding Clinic for table ØUY
2018, 4Q, 40　　　Uterus transplant

Female Reproductive System

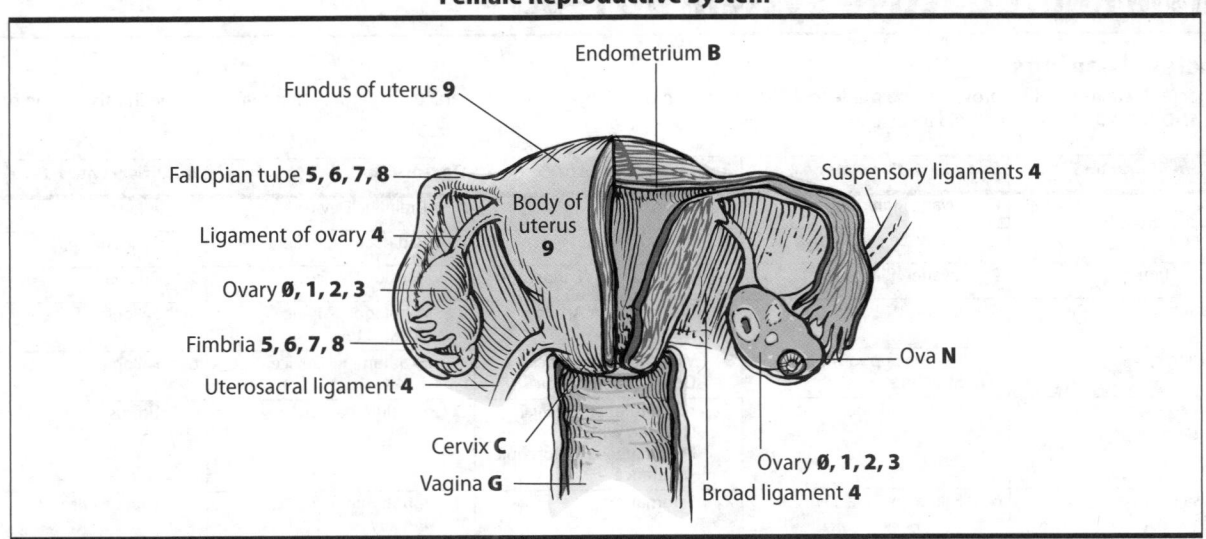

Endometrium **B**

Fundus of uterus **9**

Fallopian tube **5, 6, 7, 8**

Body of uterus **9**

Suspensory ligaments **4**

Ligament of ovary **4**

Ovary **Ø, 1, 2, 3**

Fimbria **5, 6, 7, 8**

Ova **N**

Uterosacral ligament **4**

Cervix **C**

Ovary **Ø, 1, 2, 3**

Vagina **G**

Broad ligament **4**

Female Internal/External Structures

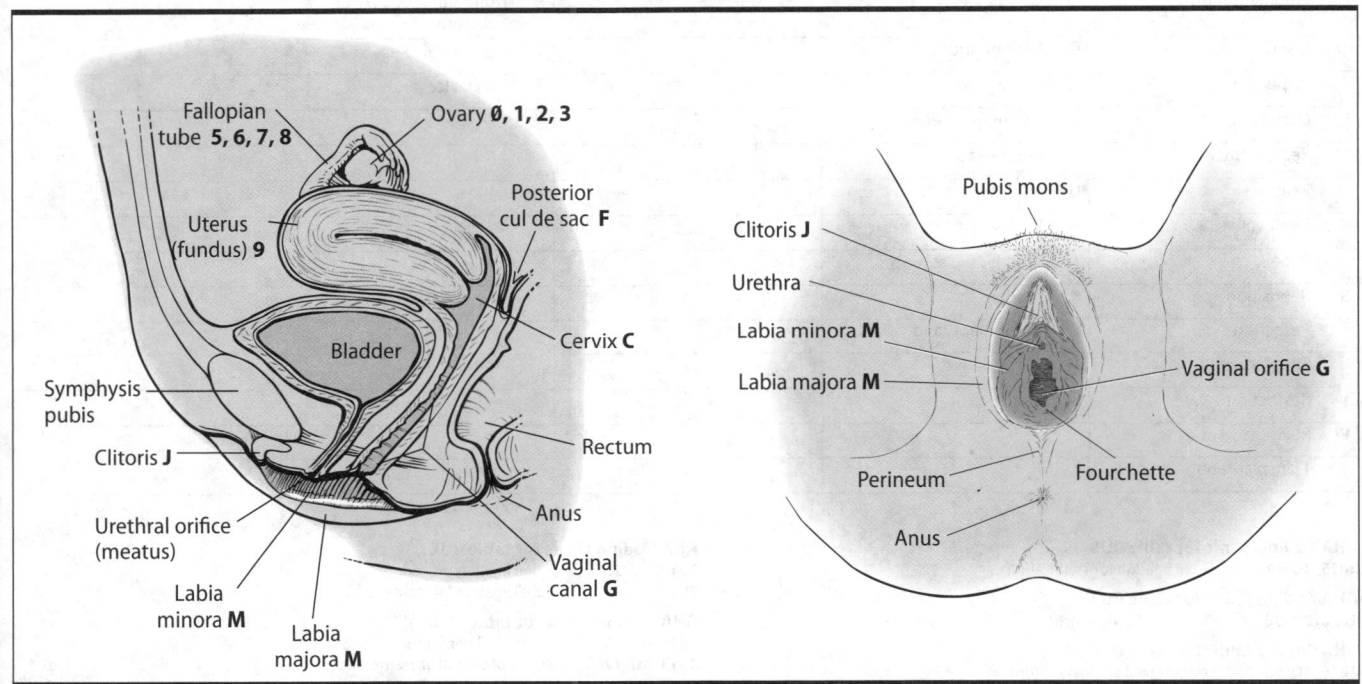

Fallopian tube **5, 6, 7, 8**

Ovary **Ø, 1, 2, 3**

Uterus (fundus) **9**

Posterior cul de sac **F**

Cervix **C**

Bladder

Symphysis pubis

Rectum

Clitoris **J**

Anus

Urethral orifice (meatus)

Vaginal canal **G**

Labia minora **M**

Labia majora **M**

Pubis mons

Clitoris **J**

Urethra

Labia minora **M**

Labia majora **M**

Vaginal orifice **G**

Perineum

Fourchette

Anus

Ø   Medical and Surgical
U   Female Reproductive System
1   Bypass   Definition: Altering the route of passage of the contents of a tubular body part

Explanation: Rerouting contents of a body part to a downstream area of the normal route, to a similar route and body part, or to an abnormal route and dissimilar body part. Includes one or more anastomoses, with or without the use of a device.

Body Part Character 4	Approach Character 5	Device Character 6	Qualifier Character 7

5 Fallopian Tube, Right   ♀
  Oviduct
  Salpinx
  Uterine tube
6 Fallopian Tube, Left   ♀
  See 5 Fallopian Tube, Right
	Ø Open
	4 Percutaneous Endoscopic
		7 Autologous Tissue Substitute
		J Synthetic Substitute
		K Nonautologous Tissue Substitute
		Z No Device
			5 Fallopian Tube, Right
			6 Fallopian Tube, Left
			9 Uterus

♀	All body part, approach, device, and qualifier values

Ø   Medical and Surgical
U   Female Reproductive System
2   Change   Definition: Taking out or off a device from a body part and putting back an identical or similar device in or on the same body part without cutting or puncturing the skin or a mucous membrane

Explanation: All CHANGE procedures are coded using the approach EXTERNAL

Body Part Character 4	Approach Character 5	Device Character 6	Qualifier Character 7

3 Ovary   ♀
8 Fallopian Tube   ♀
M Vulva   ♀
  Labia majora
  Labia minora
	X External	Ø Drainage Device
		Y Other Device
			Z No Qualifier

D Uterus and Cervix ♀	X External	Ø Drainage Device H Contraceptive Device Y Other Device	Z No Qualifier
H Vagina and Cul-de-sac ♀	X External	Ø Drainage Device G Intraluminal Device, Pessary Y Other Device	Z No Qualifier

Non-OR	All body part, approach, device, and qualifier values	♀	All body part, approach, device, and qualifier values

Female Reproductive System

Ø Medical and Surgical
U Female Reproductive System
5 Destruction   Definition: Physical eradication of all or a portion of a body part by the direct use of energy, force, or a destructive agent
                         Explanation: None of the body part is physically taken out

Body Part Character 4	Approach Character 5	Device Character 6	Qualifier Character 7

Ø Ovary, Right ♀
1 Ovary, Left ♀
2 Ovaries, Bilateral ♀
4 Uterine Supporting Structure ♀
  Broad ligament
  Infundibulopelvic ligament
  Ovarian ligament
  Round ligament of uterus
	Ø Open
	3 Percutaneous
	4 Percutaneous Endoscopic
	8 Via Natural or Artificial Opening
	  Endoscopic
		Z No Device	**Z** No Qualifier

5 Fallopian Tube, Right ♀
  Oviduct
  Salpinx
  Uterine tube
6 Fallopian Tube, Left ♀
  See 5 Fallopian Tube, Right
7 Fallopian Tubes, Bilateral [NC] ♀
9 Uterus ♀
  Fundus uteri
  Myometrium
  Perimetrium
  Uterine cornu
B Endometrium ♀
C Cervix ♀
F Cul-de-sac ♀
	Ø Open
	3 Percutaneous
	4 Percutaneous Endoscopic
	7 Via Natural or Artificial Opening
	8 Via Natural or Artificial Opening
	  Endoscopic
		Z No Device	**Z** No Qualifier

G Vagina ♀ **K** Hymen ♀	**Ø** Open **3** Percutaneous **4** Percutaneous Endoscopic **7** Via Natural or Artificial Opening **8** Via Natural or Artificial Opening Endoscopic **X** External	**Z** No Device	**Z** No Qualifier

J Clitoris ♀
L Vestibular Gland ♀
  Bartholin's (greater vestibular) gland
  Greater vestibular (Bartholin's) gland
  Paraurethral (Skene's) gland
  Skene's (paraurethral) gland
M Vulva ♀
  Labia majora
  Labia minora
	Ø Open
	X External
		Z No Device	**Z** No Qualifier

[NC]   ØU57[Ø,3,4,7,8]ZZ with principal or secondary diagnosis of Z30.2   ♀   All body part, approach, device, and qualifier values

[LC] Limited Coverage [NC] Noncovered [+] Combination Member HAC associated procedure Combination Only DRG Non-OR Non-OR New/Revised in GREEN

636   ICD-10-PCS 2021

Ø   Medical and Surgical
U   Female Reproductive System
7   Dilation   Definition: Expanding an orifice or the lumen of a tubular body part

Explanation: The orifice can be a natural orifice or an artificially created orifice. Accomplished by stretching a tubular body part using intraluminal pressure or by cutting part of the orifice or wall of the tubular body part.

Body Part Character 4		Approach Character 5	Device Character 6	Qualifier Character 7

5   **Fallopian Tube, Right**
    Oviduct
    Salpinx
    Uterine tube
6   **Fallopian Tube, Left**
    See 5 Fallopian Tube, Right
7   **Fallopian Tubes, Bilateral**
9   **Uterus**
    Fundus uteri
    Myometrium
    Perimetrium
    Uterine cornu
C   **Cervix**
G   **Vagina**
	♀
	
	♀
	
	♀
	♀
	
	♀
	♀
		Ø Open
		3 Percutaneous
		4 Percutaneous Endoscopic
		7 Via Natural or Artificial Opening
		8 Via Natural or Artificial Opening
		     Endoscopic
			D Intraluminal Device
			Z No Device
				Z No Qualifier

K **Hymen**	♀	**Ø** Open **3** Percutaneous **4** Percutaneous Endoscopic **7** Via Natural or Artificial Opening **8** Via Natural or Artificial Opening Endoscopic **X** External	**D** Intraluminal Device **Z** No Device	**Z** No Qualifier

Non-OR   ØU7C[Ø,3,4,7,8][D,Z]Z   ♀   All body part, approach, device, and qualifier values
Non-OR   ØU7G[7,8][D,Z]Z

Ø   Medical and Surgical
U   Female Reproductive System
8   Division   Definition: Cutting into a body part, without draining fluids and/or gases from the body part, in order to separate or transect a body part

Explanation: All or a portion of the body part is separated into two or more portions

Body Part Character 4		Approach Character 5	Device Character 6	Qualifier Character 7

Ø   **Ovary, Right**
1   **Ovary, Left**
2   **Ovaries, Bilateral**
4   **Uterine Supporting Structure**
    Broad ligament
    Infundibulopelvic ligament
    Ovarian ligament
    Round ligament of uterus
	♀
	♀
	♀
	♀
		Ø Open
		3 Percutaneous
		4 Percutaneous Endoscopic
			Z No Device	**Z** No Qualifier

K **Hymen**	♀	**7** Via Natural or Artificial Opening **8** Via Natural or Artificial Opening Endoscopic **X** External	**Z** No Device	**Z** No Qualifier

Non-OR   ØU8K[7,8,X]ZZ   ♀   All body part, approach, device, and qualifier values

LC Limited Coverage   **NC** Noncovered   ⊞ Combination Member   HAC associated procedure   Combination Only   DRG Non-OR   Non-OR   New/Revised in GREEN

ICD-10-PCS 2021   637

Ø   Medical and Surgical
U   Female Reproductive System
9   Drainage   Definition: Taking or letting out fluids and/or gases from a body part
                           Explanation: The qualifier DIAGNOSTIC is used to identify drainage procedures that are biopsies

Body Part Character 4	Approach Character 5	Device Character 6	Qualifier Character 7
Ø Ovary, Right ♀ 1 Ovary, Left ♀ 2 Ovaries, Bilateral ♀	Ø Open 3 Percutaneous 4 Percutaneous Endoscopic 8 Via Natural or Artificial Opening Endoscopic	Ø Drainage Device	Z No Qualifier
Ø Ovary, Right ♀ 1 Ovary, Left ♀ 2 Ovaries, Bilateral ♀	Ø Open 3 Percutaneous 4 Percutaneous Endoscopic 8 Via Natural or Artificial Opening Endoscopic	Z No Device	X Diagnostic Z No Qualifier
Ø Ovary, Right ♀ 1 Ovary, Left ♀ 2 Ovaries, Bilateral ♀	X External	Z No Device	Z No Qualifier

4 Uterine Supporting Structure ♀
   Broad ligament
   Infundibulopelvic ligament
   Ovarian ligament
   Round ligament of uterus
	Ø Open
	3 Percutaneous
	4 Percutaneous Endoscopic
	8 Via Natural or Artificial Opening
	    Endoscopic
		Ø Drainage Device	Z No Qualifier

4 Uterine Supporting Structure ♀
   Broad ligament
   Infundibulopelvic ligament
   Ovarian ligament
   Round ligament of uterus
	Ø Open
	3 Percutaneous
	4 Percutaneous Endoscopic
	8 Via Natural or Artificial Opening
	    Endoscopic
		Z No Device	X Diagnostic
			Z No Qualifier

5 Fallopian Tube, Right ♀
   Oviduct
   Salpinx
   Uterine tube
6 Fallopian Tube, Left ♀
   See 5 Fallopian Tube, Right
7 Fallopian Tubes, Bilateral ♀
9 Uterus ♀
   Fundus uteri
   Myometrium
   Perimetrium
   Uterine cornu
C Cervix ♀
F Cul-de-sac ♀
	Ø Open
	3 Percutaneous
	4 Percutaneous Endoscopic
	7 Via Natural or Artificial Opening
	8 Via Natural or Artificial Opening
	    Endoscopic
		Ø Drainage Device	Z No Qualifier

5 Fallopian Tube, Right ♀
   Oviduct
   Salpinx
   Uterine tube
6 Fallopian Tube, Left ♀
   See 5 Fallopian Tube, Right
7 Fallopian Tubes, Bilateral ♀
9 Uterus ♀
   Fundus uteri
   Myometrium
   Perimetrium
   Uterine cornu
C Cervix ♀
F Cul-de-sac ♀
	Ø Open
	3 Percutaneous
	4 Percutaneous Endoscopic
	7 Via Natural or Artificial Opening
	8 Via Natural or Artificial Opening
	    Endoscopic
		Z No Device	X Diagnostic
			Z No Qualifier

Non-OR ØU9[Ø,1,2][3,8]ØZ		**Non-OR** ØU9[5,6,7,9,C]3ØZ	
Non-OR ØU9[Ø,1,2][3,8]ZZ		**Non-OR** ØU9F[3,4]ØZ	
Non-OR ØU9[Ø,1,2]8ZX		**Non-OR** ØU9[5,6,7][3,4,7,8]ZZ	
Non-OR ØU94[3,8]ØZ		**Non-OR** ØU9[9,C]3ZZ	
Non-OR ØU94[3,8]ZZ		**Non-OR** ØU9F[3,4]ZZ	
Non-OR ØU948ZX		♀ All body part, approach, device, and qualifier values	

ØU9 Continued on next page

ØU9 Continued

Ø   **Medical and Surgical**
U   **Female Reproductive System**
9   **Drainage**   Definition: Taking or letting out fluids and/or gases from a body part
                        Explanation: The qualifier DIAGNOSTIC is used to identify drainage procedures that are biopsies

Body Part Character 4	Approach Character 5	Device Character 6	Qualifier Character 7
G Vagina ♀ K Hymen ♀	Ø Open 3 Percutaneous 4 Percutaneous Endoscopic 7 Via Natural or Artificial Opening 8 Via Natural or Artificial Opening Endoscopic X External	Ø Drainage Device	Z No Qualifier
G Vagina ♀ K Hymen ♀	Ø Open 3 Percutaneous 4 Percutaneous Endoscopic 7 Via Natural or Artificial Opening 8 Via Natural or Artificial Opening Endoscopic X External	Z No Device	X Diagnostic Z No Qualifier

J   Clitoris   ♀
L   Vestibular Gland   ♀
     Bartholin's (greater vestibular) gland
     Greater vestibular (Bartholin's) gland
     Paraurethral (Skene's) gland
     Skene's (paraurethral) gland
M   Vulva   ♀
     Labia majora
     Labia minora
	Ø Open
	X External
		Ø Drainage Device	Z No Qualifier

J   Clitoris   ♀
L   Vestibular Gland   ♀
     Bartholin's (greater vestibular) gland
     Greater vestibular (Bartholin's) gland
     Paraurethral (Skene's) gland
     Skene's (paraurethral) gland
M   Vulva   ♀
     Labia majora
     Labia minora
	Ø Open
	X External
		Z No Device	X Diagnostic
			Z No Qualifier

Non-OR ØU9G3ØZ	**Non-OR** ØU9L[Ø,X]ØZ
Non-OR ØU9K[Ø,3,4,7,8,X]ØZ	**Non-OR** ØU9L[Ø,X]ZZ
Non-OR ØU9G3ZZ	♀ All body part, approach, device, and qualifier values
Non-OR ØU9K[Ø,3,4,7,8,X]ZZ	

Female Reproductive System

Ø Medical and Surgical
U Female Reproductive System
B Excision Definition: Cutting out or off, without replacement, a portion of a body part
Explanation: The qualifier DIAGNOSTIC is used to identify excision procedures that are biopsies

Body Part Character 4	Approach Character 5	Device Character 6	Qualifier Character 7

Ø Ovary, Right ♀
1 Ovary, Left ♀
2 Ovaries, Bilateral ♀
4 Uterine Supporting Structure ♀
  Broad ligament
  Infundibulopelvic ligament
  Ovarian ligament
  Round ligament of uterus
5 Fallopian Tube, Right ♀
  Oviduct
  Salpinx
  Uterine tube
6 Fallopian Tube, Left ♀
  See 5 Fallopian Tube, Right
7 Fallopian Tubes, Bilateral ♀
9 Uterus ♀
  Fundus uteri
  Myometrium
  Perimetrium
  Uterine cornu
C Cervix ♀
F Cul-de-sac ♀
	Ø Open
	3 Percutaneous
	4 Percutaneous Endoscopic
	7 Via Natural or Artificial Opening
	8 Via Natural or Artificial Opening Endoscopic
		Z No Device	X Diagnostic
			Z No Qualifier

G Vagina ♀ K Hymen ♀	Ø Open 3 Percutaneous 4 Percutaneous Endoscopic 7 Via Natural or Artificial Opening 8 Via Natural or Artificial Opening Endoscopic X External	Z No Device	X Diagnostic Z No Qualifier

J Clitoris ♀
L Vestibular Gland ♀
  Bartholin's (greater vestibular) gland
  Greater vestibular (Bartholin's) gland
  Paraurethral (Skene's) gland
  Skene's (paraurethral) gland
M Vulva ♀
  Labia majora
  Labia minora
	Ø Open
	X External
		Z No Device	X Diagnostic
			Z No Qualifier

♀ All body part, approach, device, and qualifier values

Ø   Medical and Surgical
U   Female Reproductive System
C   Extirpation   Definition: Taking or cutting out solid matter from a body part

Explanation: The solid matter may be an abnormal byproduct of a biological function or a foreign body; it may be imbedded in a body part or in the lumen of a tubular body part. The solid matter may or may not have been previously broken into pieces.

Body Part Character 4	Approach Character 5	Device Character 6	Qualifier Character 7

Ø Ovary, Right   ♀
1 Ovary, Left   ♀
2 Ovaries, Bilateral   ♀
4 Uterine Supporting Structure   ♀
    Broad ligament
    Infundibulopelvic ligament
    Ovarian ligament
    Round ligament of uterus
	Ø Open
	3 Percutaneous
	4 Percutaneous Endoscopic
	8 Via Natural or Artificial Opening Endoscopic
		Z No Device	**Z** No Qualifier

5 Fallopian Tube, Right   ♀
    Oviduct
    Salpinx
    Uterine tube
6 Fallopian Tube, Left   ♀
    See 5 Fallopian Tube, Right
7 Fallopian Tubes, Bilateral   ♀
9 Uterus   ♀
    Fundus uteri
    Myometrium
    Perimetrium
    Uterine cornu
B Endometrium   ♀
C Cervix   ♀
F Cul-de-sac   ♀
	Ø Open
	3 Percutaneous
	4 Percutaneous Endoscopic
	7 Via Natural or Artificial Opening
	8 Via Natural or Artificial Opening Endoscopic
		Z No Device	**Z** No Qualifier

G Vagina ♀ **K** Hymen ♀	**Ø** Open **3** Percutaneous **4** Percutaneous Endoscopic **7** Via Natural or Artificial Opening **8** Via Natural or Artificial Opening Endoscopic **X** External	**Z** No Device	**Z** No Qualifier

J Clitoris   ♀
L Vestibular Gland   ♀
    Bartholin's (greater vestibular) gland
    Greater vestibular (Bartholin's) gland
    Paraurethral (Skene's) gland
    Skene's (paraurethral) gland
M Vulva   ♀
    Labia majora
    Labia minora
	Ø Open
	X External
		Z No Device	**Z** No Qualifier

Non-OR   ØUC9[7,8]ZZ
Non-OR   ØUCG[7,8,X]ZZ
Non-OR   ØUCK[Ø,3,4,7,8,X]ZZ

Non-OR   ØUCMXZZ
♀   All body part, approach, device, and qualifier values

Ø   Medical and Surgical
U   Female Reproductive System
D   Extraction   Definition: Pulling or stripping out or off all or a portion of a body part by the use of force

Explanation: The qualifier DIAGNOSTIC is used to identify extraction procedures that are biopsies

Body Part Character 4	Approach Character 5	Device Character 6	Qualifier Character 7
B Endometrium ♀	**7** Via Natural or Artificial Opening **8** Via Natural or Artificial Opening Endoscopic	**Z** No Device	**X** Diagnostic **Z** No Qualifier
N Ova ♀	**Ø** Open **3** Percutaneous **4** Percutaneous Endoscopic	**Z** No Device	**Z** No Qualifier

♀   All body part, approach, device, and qualifier values

Female Reproductive System

Ø   **Medical and Surgical**
U   **Female Reproductive System**
F   **Fragmentation**   Definition: Breaking solid matter in a body part into pieces

Explanation: Physical force (e.g., manual, ultrasonic) applied directly or indirectly is used to break the solid matter into pieces. The solid matter may be an abnormal byproduct of a biological function or a foreign body. The pieces of solid matter are not taken out.

Body Part Character 4	Approach Character 5	Device Character 6	Qualifier Character 7

5 Fallopian Tube, Right NC ♀
  Oviduct
  Salpinx
  Uterine tube
6 Fallopian Tube, Left NC ♀
  See 5 Fallopian Tube, Right
7 Fallopian Tubes, Bilateral NC ♀
9 Uterus NC ♀
  Fundus uteri
  Myometrium
  Perimetrium
  Uterine cornu
	Ø Open
	3 Percutaneous
	4 Percutaneous Endoscopic
	7 Via Natural or Artificial Opening
	8 Via Natural or Artificial Opening
	  Endoscopic
	X External
		Z No Device	Z No Qualifier

Non-OR   ØUF[5,6,7,9]XZZ   ♀   All body part, approach, device, and qualifier values
NC   ØUF[5,6,7,9]XZZ

Ø   **Medical and Surgical**
U   **Female Reproductive System**
H   **Insertion**   Definition: Putting in a nonbiological appliance that monitors, assists, performs, or prevents a physiological function but does not physically take the place of a body part

Explanation: None

Body Part Character 4	Approach Character 5	Device Character 6	Qualifier Character 7
3 Ovary ♀	Ø Open 3 Percutaneous 4 Percutaneous Endoscopic	1 Radioactive Element 3 Infusion Device Y Other Device	Z No Qualifier
3 Ovary ♀	7 Via Natural or Artificial Opening 8 Via Natural or Artificial Opening Endoscopic	1 Radioactive Element Y Other Device	Z No Qualifier
8 Fallopian Tube ♀ D Uterus and Cervix ♀ H Vagina and Cul-de-sac ♀	Ø Open 3 Percutaneous 4 Percutaneous Endoscopic 7 Via Natural or Artificial Opening 8 Via Natural or Artificial Opening Endoscopic	3 Infusion Device Y Other Device	Z No Qualifier

9 Uterus ♀
  Fundus uteri
  Myometrium
  Perimetrium
  Uterine cornu
	Ø Open
	7 Via Natural or Artificial Opening
	8 Via Natural or Artificial Opening
	  Endoscopic
		1 Radioactive Element
		H Contraceptive Device
			Z No Qualifier

C Cervix ♀	Ø Open 3 Percutaneous 4 Percutaneous Endoscopic	1 Radioactive Element	Z No Qualifier
C Cervix ♀	7 Via Natural or Artificial Opening 8 Via Natural or Artificial Opening Endoscopic	1 Radioactive Element H Contraceptive Device	Z No Qualifier
F Cul-de-sac ♀	7 Via Natural or Artificial Opening 8 Via Natural or Artificial Opening Endoscopic	G Intraluminal Device, Pessary	Z No Qualifier
G Vagina ♀	Ø Open 3 Percutaneous 4 Percutaneous Endoscopic X External	1 Radioactive Element	Z No Qualifier
G Vagina ♀	7 Via Natural or Artificial Opening 8 Via Natural or Artificial Opening Endoscopic	1 Radioactive Element G Intraluminal Device, Pessary	Z No Qualifier

Non-OR   ØUH3[Ø,3,4][3,Y]Z   **Non-OR**   ØUH9[Ø,7,8]HZ
Non-OR   ØUH3[7,8]YZ   **Non-OR**   ØUHC[7,8]HZ
Non-OR   ØUH[8,D][Ø,3,4,7,8][3,Y]Z   **Non-OR**   ØUHF[7,8]GZ
Non-OR   ØUHH[3,4]YZ   **Non-OR**   ØUHG[7,8]GZ
Non-OR   ØUHH[7,8][3,Y]Z   ♀   All body part, approach, device, and qualifier values

Ø **Medical and Surgical**
U **Female Reproductive System**
J **Inspection**   Definition: Visually and/or manually exploring a body part

Explanation: Visual exploration may be performed with or without optical instrumentation. Manual exploration may be performed directly or through intervening body layers.

Body Part Character 4	Approach Character 5	Device Character 6	Qualifier Character 7
3 Ovary ♀	Ø Open 3 Percutaneous 4 Percutaneous Endoscopic 8 Via Natural or Artificial Opening Endoscopic X External	Z No Device	Z No Qualifier
8 Fallopian Tube ♀ D Uterus and Cervix ♀ H Vagina and Cul-de-sac ♀	Ø Open 3 Percutaneous 4 Percutaneous Endoscopic 7 Via Natural or Artificial Opening 8 Via Natural or Artificial Opening Endoscopic X External	Z No Device	Z No Qualifier

M Vulva ♀
  Labia majora
  Labia minora
	Ø Open
	X External
		Z No Device	Z No Qualifier

Non-OR ØUJ3[3,8,X]ZZ
Non-OR ØUJ[8,D,H][3,7,8,X]ZZ

Non-OR ØUJMXZZ
♀ All body part, approach, device, and qualifier values

Ø **Medical and Surgical**
U **Female Reproductive System**
L **Occlusion**   Definition: Completely closing an orifice or the lumen of a tubular body part

Explanation: The orifice can be a natural orifice or an artificially created orifice

Body Part Character 4	Approach Character 5	Device Character 6	Qualifier Character 7

5 Fallopian Tube, Right ♀
  Oviduct
  Salpinx
  Uterine tube
6 Fallopian Tube, Left ♀
  See 5 Fallopian Tube, Right
7 Fallopian Tubes, Bilateral NC ♀
	Ø Open
	3 Percutaneous
	4 Percutaneous Endoscopic
		C Extraluminal Device
		D Intraluminal Device
		Z No Device
			Z No Qualifier

5 Fallopian Tube, Right ♀
  Oviduct
  Salpinx
  Uterine tube
6 Fallopian Tube, Left ♀
  See 5 Fallopian Tube, Right
7 Fallopian Tubes, Bilateral NC ♀
	7 Via Natural or Artificial Opening
	8 Via Natural or Artificial Opening Endoscopic
		D Intraluminal Device
		Z No Device
			Z No Qualifier

F Cul-de-sac ♀ G Vagina ♀	7 Via Natural or Artificial Opening 8 Via Natural or Artificial Opening Endoscopic	D Intraluminal Device Z No Device	Z No Qualifier

NC ØUL7[Ø,3,4][C,D,Z]Z with principal or secondary diagnosis of Z3Ø.2
NC ØUL7[7,8][D,Z]Z with principal or secondary diagnosis of Z3Ø.2

♀ All body part, approach, device, and qualifier values

LC Limited Coverage   NC Noncovered   ⊞ Combination Member   HAC associated procedure   Combination Only   DRG Non-OR   Non-OR   New/Revised in GREEN
ICD-10-PCS 2021   643

ØUJ–ØUL

Female Reproductive System

Ø   **Medical and Surgical**
U   **Female Reproductive System**
M   **Reattachment**   Definition: Putting back in or on all or a portion of a separated body part to its normal location or other suitable location
                      Explanation: Vascular circulation and nervous pathways may or may not be reestablished

Body Part Character 4	Approach Character 5	Device Character 6	Qualifier Character 7

Ø **Ovary, Right** ♀
1 **Ovary, Left** ♀
2 **Ovaries, Bilateral** ♀
4 **Uterine Supporting Structure** ♀
    Broad ligament
    Infundibulopelvic ligament
    Ovarian ligament
    Round ligament of uterus
5 **Fallopian Tube, Right** ♀
    Oviduct
    Salpinx
    Uterine tube
6 **Fallopian Tube, Left** ♀
    See 5 Fallopian Tube, Right
7 **Fallopian Tubes, Bilateral** ♀
9 **Uterus** ♀
    Fundus uteri
    Myometrium
    Perimetrium
    Uterine cornu
C **Cervix** ♀
F **Cul-de-sac** ♀
G **Vagina** ♀
	Ø Open
	4 Percutaneous Endoscopic
		Z No Device	**Z** No Qualifier

J **Clitoris** ♀
M **Vulva** ♀
    Labia majora
    Labia minora
	X External	**Z** No Device	**Z** No Qualifier

K **Hymen** ♀	**Ø** Open **4** Percutaneous Endoscopic **X** External	**Z** No Device	**Z** No Qualifier

♀   All body part, approach, device, and qualifier values

Ø   **Medical and Surgical**
U   **Female Reproductive System**
N   **Release**   Definition: Freeing a body part from an abnormal physical constraint by cutting or by the use of force
                          Explanation: Some of the restraining tissue may be taken out but none of the body part is taken out

Body Part Character 4	Approach Character 5	Device Character 6	Qualifier Character 7

Ø Ovary, Right ♀
1 Ovary, Left ♀
2 Ovaries, Bilateral ♀
4 Uterine Supporting Structure ♀
    Broad ligament
    Infundibulopelvic ligament
    Ovarian ligament
    Round ligament of uterus
	Ø Open
	3 Percutaneous
	4 Percutaneous Endoscopic
	8 Via Natural or Artificial Opening
	    Endoscopic
		Z No Device	**Z** No Qualifier

5 Fallopian Tube, Right ♀
    Oviduct
    Salpinx
    Uterine tube
6 Fallopian Tube, Left ♀
    See 5 Fallopian Tube, Right
7 Fallopian Tubes, Bilateral ♀
9 Uterus ♀
    Fundus uteri
    Myometrium
    Perimetrium
    Uterine cornu
C Cervix ♀
F Cul-de-sac ♀
	Ø Open
	3 Percutaneous
	4 Percutaneous Endoscopic
	7 Via Natural or Artificial Opening
	8 Via Natural or Artificial Opening
	    Endoscopic
		Z No Device	**Z** No Qualifier

G Vagina ♀ **K** Hymen ♀	**Ø** Open **3** Percutaneous **4** Percutaneous Endoscopic **7** Via Natural or Artificial Opening **8** Via Natural or Artificial Opening Endoscopic **X** External	**Z** No Device	**Z** No Qualifier

J Clitoris ♀
L Vestibular Gland ♀
    Bartholin's (greater vestibular) gland
    Greater vestibular (Bartholin's) gland
    Paraurethral (Skene's) gland
    Skene's (paraurethral) gland
M Vulva ♀
    Labia majora
    Labia minora
	Ø Open
	X External
		Z No Device	**Z** No Qualifier

    ♀   All body part, approach, device, and qualifier values

LC Limited Coverage   **NC** Noncovered   ⊞ Combination Member   HAC associated procedure   Combination Only   DRG Non-OR   Non-OR   New/Revised in **GREEN**

ICD-10-PCS 2021   **645**

Female Reproductive System

ØUP–ØUP

Ø   **Medical and Surgical**
U   **Female Reproductive System**
P   **Removal**   Definition: Taking out or off a device from a body part
                   Explanation: If a device is taken out and a similar device put in without cutting or puncturing the skin or mucous membrane, the procedure is coded to the root operation CHANGE. Otherwise, the procedure for taking out the device is coded to the root operation REMOVAL.

Body Part Character 4	Approach Character 5	Device Character 6	Qualifier Character 7
3 Ovary ♀	**Ø** Open **3** Percutaneous **4** Percutaneous Endoscopic	**Ø** Drainage Device **3** Infusion Device **Y** Other Device	**Z** No Qualifier
3 Ovary ♀	**7** Via Natural or Artificial Opening **8** Via Natural or Artificial Opening Endoscopic	**Y** Other Device	**Z** No Qualifier
3 Ovary ♀	**X** External	**Ø** Drainage Device **3** Infusion Device	**Z** No Qualifier
8 Fallopian Tube ♀	**Ø** Open **3** Percutaneous **4** Percutaneous Endoscopic **7** Via Natural or Artificial Opening **8** Via Natural or Artificial Opening Endoscopic	**Ø** Drainage Device **3** Infusion Device **7** Autologous Tissue Substitute **C** Extraluminal Device **D** Intraluminal Device **J** Synthetic Substitute **K** Nonautologous Tissue Substitute **Y** Other Device	**Z** No Qualifier
8 Fallopian Tube ♀	**X** External	**Ø** Drainage Device **3** Infusion Device **D** Intraluminal Device	**Z** No Qualifier
D Uterus and Cervix ♀	**Ø** Open **3** Percutaneous **4** Percutaneous Endoscopic **7** Via Natural or Artificial Opening **8** Via Natural or Artificial Opening Endoscopic	**Ø** Drainage Device **1** Radioactive Element **3** Infusion Device **7** Autologous Tissue Substitute **C** Extraluminal Device **D** Intraluminal Device **H** Contraceptive Device **J** Synthetic Substitute **K** Nonautologous Tissue Substitute **Y** Other Device	**Z** No Qualifier
D Uterus and Cervix ♀	**X** External	**Ø** Drainage Device **3** Infusion Device **D** Intraluminal Device **H** Contraceptive Device	**Z** No Qualifier
H Vagina and Cul-de-sac ♀	**Ø** Open **3** Percutaneous **4** Percutaneous Endoscopic **7** Via Natural or Artificial Opening **8** Via Natural or Artificial Opening Endoscopic	**Ø** Drainage Device **1** Radioactive Element **3** Infusion Device **7** Autologous Tissue Substitute **D** Intraluminal Device **J** Synthetic Substitute **K** Nonautologous Tissue Substitute **Y** Other Device	**Z** No Qualifier
H Vagina and Cul-de-sac ♀	**X** External	**Ø** Drainage Device **1** Radioactive Element **3** Infusion Device **D** Intraluminal Device	**Z** No Qualifier
M Vulva ♀ Labia majora Labia minora	**Ø** Open	**Ø** Drainage Device **7** Autologous Tissue Substitute **J** Synthetic Substitute **K** Nonautologous Tissue Substitute	**Z** No Qualifier
M Vulva ♀ Labia majora Labia minora	**X** External	**Ø** Drainage Device	**Z** No Qualifier

Non-OR ØUP3[3,4]YZ		**Non-OR** ØUPD[7,8][Ø,3,C,D,H,Y]Z	
Non-OR ØUP3[7,8]YZ		**Non-OR** ØUPDX[Ø,3,D,H]Z	
Non-OR ØUP3X[Ø,3]Z		**Non-OR** ØUPH[3,4]YZ	
Non-OR ØUP8[3,4]YZ		**Non-OR** ØUPH[7,8][Ø,3,D,Y]Z	
Non-OR ØUP8[7,8][Ø,3,D,Y]Z		**Non-OR** ØUPHX[Ø,1,3,D]Z	
Non-OR ØUP8X[Ø,3,D]Z		**Non-OR** ØUPMXØZ	
Non-OR ØUPD[3,4][C,Y]Z		♀ All body part, approach, device, and qualifier values	

LC Limited Coverage   **NC** Noncovered   ⊞ Combination Member   HAC associated procedure   Combination Only   DRG Non-OR   Non-OR   New/Revised in **GREEN**

646   ICD-10-PCS 2021

Female Reproductive System

Ø   Medical and Surgical
U   Female Reproductive System
Q   Repair   Definition: Restoring, to the extent possible, a body part to its normal anatomic structure and function

            Explanation: Used only when the method to accomplish the repair is not one of the other root operations

Body Part Character 4	Approach Character 5	Device Character 6	Qualifier Character 7

Ø   Ovary, Right ♀
1   Ovary, Left ♀
2   Ovaries, Bilateral ♀
4   Uterine Supporting Structure ♀
     Broad ligament
     Infundibulopelvic ligament
     Ovarian ligament
     Round ligament of uterus
	Ø Open
	3 Percutaneous
	4 Percutaneous Endoscopic
	8 Via Natural or Artificial Opening
	     Endoscopic
		Z No Device	Z No Qualifier

5   Fallopian Tube, Right ♀
     Oviduct
     Salpinx
     Uterine tube
6   Fallopian Tube, Left ♀
     See 5 Fallopian Tube, Right
7   Fallopian Tubes, Bilateral ♀
9   Uterus ♀
     Fundus uteri
     Myometrium
     Perimetrium
     Uterine cornu
C   Cervix ♀
F   Cul-de-sac ♀
	Ø Open
	3 Percutaneous
	4 Percutaneous Endoscopic
	7 Via Natural or Artificial Opening
	8 Via Natural or Artificial Opening
	     Endoscopic
		Z No Device	Z No Qualifier

G Vagina ♀ K Hymen ♀	Ø Open 3 Percutaneous 4 Percutaneous Endoscopic 7 Via Natural or Artificial Opening 8 Via Natural or Artificial Opening Endoscopic X External	Z No Device	Z No Qualifier

J   Clitoris ♀
L   Vestibular Gland ♀
     Bartholin's (greater vestibular) gland
     Greater vestibular (Bartholin's) gland
     Paraurethral (Skene's) gland
     Skene's (paraurethral) gland
M   Vulva ♀
     Labia majora
     Labia minora
	Ø Open
	X External
		Z No Device	Z No Qualifier

Non-OR	ØUQG[7,X]ZZ		Non-OR	ØUQMXZZ
Non-OR	ØUQKXZZ		♀	All body part, approach, device, and qualifier values

Ø   Medical and Surgical
U   Female Reproductive System
S   Reposition   Definition: Moving to its normal location, or other suitable location, all or a portion of a body part

            Explanation: The body part is moved to a new location from an abnormal location, or from a normal location where it is not functioning correctly. The body part may or may not be cut out or off to be moved to the new location.

Body Part Character 4	Approach Character 5	Device Character 6	Qualifier Character 7

Ø   Ovary, Right ♀
1   Ovary, Left ♀
2   Ovaries, Bilateral ♀
4   Uterine Supporting Structure ♀
     Broad ligament
     Infundibulopelvic ligament
     Ovarian ligament
     Round ligament of uterus
5   Fallopian Tube, Right ♀
     Oviduct
     Salpinx
     Uterine tube
6   Fallopian Tube, Left ♀
     See 5 Fallopian Tube, Right
7   Fallopian Tubes, Bilateral ♀
C   Cervix ♀
F   Cul-de-sac ♀
	Ø Open
	4 Percutaneous Endoscopic
	8 Via Natural or Artificial Opening
	     Endoscopic
		Z No Device	Z No Qualifier

9   Uterus ♀
     Fundus uteri
     Myometrium
     Perimetrium
     Uterine cornu
G   Vagina ♀
	Ø Open
	4 Percutaneous Endoscopic
	7 Via Natural or Artificial Opening
	8 Via Natural or Artificial Opening
	     Endoscopic
	X External
		Z No Device	Z No Qualifier

Non-OR	ØUS9XZZ		♀	All body part, approach, device, and qualifier values

LC Limited Coverage   NC Noncovered   ⊞ Combination Member   HAC associated procedure   Combination Only   DRG Non-OR   Non-OR   New/Revised in GREEN

Female Reproductive System

Ø   **Medical and Surgical**
U   **Female Reproductive System**
T   **Resection**   Definition: Cutting out or off, without replacement, all of a body part
                   Explanation: None

Body Part Character 4	Approach Character 5	Device Character 6	Qualifier Character 7

Ø Ovary, Right ♀
1 Ovary, Left ♀
2 Ovaries, Bilateral ⊞♀
5 Fallopian Tube, Right ♀
    Oviduct
    Salpinx
    Uterine tube
6 Fallopian Tube, Left ♀
    See 5 Fallopian Tube, Right
7 Fallopian Tubes, Bilateral ⊞♀
	Ø Open
	4 Percutaneous Endoscopic
	7 Via Natural or Artificial Opening
	8 Via Natural or Artificial Opening
	    Endoscopic
	F Via Natural or Artificial Opening
	    With Percutaneous Endoscopic
	    Assistance
		Z No Device	**Z** No Qualifier

4 Uterine Supporting Structure ⊞♀
    Broad ligament
    Infundibulopelvic ligament
    Ovarian ligament
    Round ligament of uterus
C Cervix ⊞♀
F Cul-de-sac ♀
G Vagina ⊞♀
	Ø Open
	4 Percutaneous Endoscopic
	7 Via Natural or Artificial Opening
	8 Via Natural or Artificial Opening
	    Endoscopic
		Z No Device	**Z** No Qualifier

9 Uterus ⊞♀
    Fundus uteri
    Myometrium
    Perimetrium
    Uterine cornu
	Ø Open
	4 Percutaneous Endoscopic
	7 Via Natural or Artificial Opening
	8 Via Natural or Artificial Opening
	    Endoscopic
	F Via Natural or Artificial Opening
	    With Percutaneous Endoscopic
	    Assistance
		Z No Device	**L** Supracervical
			Z No Qualifier

J Clitoris ♀
L Vestibular Gland ♀
    Bartholin's (greater vestibular)
       gland
    Greater vestibular (Bartholin's)
       gland
    Paraurethral (Skene's) gland
    Skene's (paraurethral) gland
M Vulva ⊞♀
    Labia majora
    Labia minora
	Ø Open
	X External
		Z No Device	**Z** No Qualifier

K Hymen ♀	**Ø** Open **4** Percutaneous Endoscopic **7** Via Natural or Artificial Opening **8** Via Natural or Artificial Opening Endoscopic **X** External	**Z** No Device	**Z** No Device

♀   All body part, approach, device, and qualifier values

See Appendix L for Procedure Combinations
⊞   ØUT[2,7]ØZZ
⊞   ØUT[4,C][Ø,4,7,8]ZZ
⊞   ØUTGØZZ
⊞   ØUT9[Ø,4,7,8,F]ZZ
⊞   ØUTM[Ø,X]ZZ

Ø   **Medical and Surgical**
U   **Female Reproductive System**
U   **Supplement**   Definition: Putting in or on biological or synthetic material that physically reinforces and/or augments the function of a portion of a body part

                       Explanation: The biological material is non-living, or is living and from the same individual. The body part may have been previously replaced, and the SUPPLEMENT procedure is performed to physically reinforce and/or augment the function of the replaced body part.

Body Part Character 4	Approach Character 5	Device Character 6	Qualifier Character 7

4   **Uterine Supporting Structure** ♀
    Broad ligament
    Infundibulopelvic ligament
    Ovarian ligament
    Round ligament of uterus
	Ø Open
	4 Percutaneous Endoscopic
		7 Autologous Tissue Substitute
		J Synthetic Substitute
		K Nonautologous Tissue Substitute
			Z No Qualifier

5   **Fallopian Tube, Right** ♀
    Oviduct
    Salpinx
    Uterine tube
6   **Fallopian Tube, Left** ♀
    See 5 Fallopian Tube, Right
7   **Fallopian Tubes, Bilateral** ♀
F   **Cul-de-sac** ♀
	Ø Open
	4 Percutaneous Endoscopic
	7 Via Natural or Artificial Opening
	8 Via Natural or Artificial Opening
	     Endoscopic
		7 Autologous Tissue Substitute
		J Synthetic Substitute
		K Nonautologous Tissue Substitute
			Z No Qualifier

G **Vagina** ♀ **K** **Hymen** ♀	**Ø** Open **4** Percutaneous Endoscopic **7** Via Natural or Artificial Opening **8** Via Natural or Artificial Opening Endoscopic **X** External	**7** Autologous Tissue Substitute **J** Synthetic Substitute **K** Nonautologous Tissue Substitute	**Z** No Qualifier

J   **Clitoris** ♀
M   **Vulva** ♀
    Labia majora
    Labia minora
	Ø Open
	X External
		7 Autologous Tissue Substitute
		J Synthetic Substitute
		K Nonautologous Tissue Substitute
			Z No Qualifier

     ♀   All body part, approach, device, and qualifier values

Ø   **Medical and Surgical**
U   **Female Reproductive System**
V   **Restriction**   Definition: Partially closing an orifice or the lumen of a tubular body part

                       Explanation: The orifice can be a natural orifice or an artificially created orifice

Body Part Character 4	Approach Character 5	Device Character 6	Qualifier Character 7
C Cervix ♀	**Ø** Open **3** Percutaneous **4** Percutaneous Endoscopic	**C** Extraluminal Device **D** Intraluminal Device **Z** No Device	**Z** No Qualifier
C Cervix ♀	**7** Via Natural or Artificial Opening **8** Via Natural or Artificial Opening Endoscopic	**D** Intraluminal Device **Z** No Device	**Z** No Qualifier

     ♀   All body part, approach, device, and qualifier values

Female Reproductive System

Ø   **Medical and Surgical**
U   **Female Reproductive System**
W   **Revision**   Definition: Correcting, to the extent possible, a portion of a malfunctioning device or the position of a displaced device
                        Explanation: Revision can include correcting a malfunctioning or displaced device by taking out or putting in components of the device such as a screw or pin

Body Part Character 4	Approach Character 5	Device Character 6	Qualifier Character 7
3 Ovary ♀	Ø Open 3 Percutaneous 4 Percutaneous Endoscopic	Ø Drainage Device 3 Infusion Device Y Other Device	Z No Qualifier
3 Ovary ♀	7 Via Natural or Artificial Opening 8 Via Natural or Artificial Opening Endoscopic	Y Other Device	Z No Qualifier
3 Ovary ♀	X External	Ø Drainage Device 3 Infusion Device	Z No Qualifier
8 Fallopian Tube ♀	Ø Open 3 Percutaneous 4 Percutaneous Endoscopic 7 Via Natural or Artificial Opening 8 Via Natural or Artificial Opening Endoscopic	Ø Drainage Device 3 Infusion Device 7 Autologous Tissue Substitute C Extraluminal Device D Intraluminal Device J Synthetic Substitute K Nonautologous Tissue Substitute Y Other Device	Z No Qualifier
8 Fallopian Tube ♀	X External	Ø Drainage Device 3 Infusion Device 7 Autologous Tissue Substitute C Extraluminal Device D Intraluminal Device J Synthetic Substitute K Nonautologous Tissue Substitute	Z No Qualifier
D Uterus and Cervix ♀	Ø Open 3 Percutaneous 4 Percutaneous Endoscopic 7 Via Natural or Artificial Opening 8 Via Natural or Artificial Opening Endoscopic	Ø Drainage Device 1 Radioactive Element 3 Infusion Device 7 Autologous Tissue Substitute C Extraluminal Device D Intraluminal Device H Contraceptive Device J Synthetic Substitute K Nonautologous Tissue Substitute Y Other Device	Z No Qualifier
D Uterus and Cervix ♀	X External	Ø Drainage Device 3 Infusion Device 7 Autologous Tissue Substitute C Extraluminal Device D Intraluminal Device H Contraceptive Device J Synthetic Substitute K Nonautologous Tissue Substitute	Z No Qualifier
H Vagina and Cul-de-sac ♀	Ø Open 3 Percutaneous 4 Percutaneous Endoscopic 7 Via Natural or Artificial Opening 8 Via Natural or Artificial Opening Endoscopic	Ø Drainage Device 1 Radioactive Element 3 Infusion Device 7 Autologous Tissue Substitute D Intraluminal Device J Synthetic Substitute K Nonautologous Tissue Substitute Y Other Device	Z No Qualifier
H Vagina and Cul-de-sac ♀	X External	Ø Drainage Device 3 Infusion Device 7 Autologous Tissue Substitute D Intraluminal Device J Synthetic Substitute K Nonautologous Tissue Substitute	Z No Qualifier
M Vulva ♀ Labia majora Labia minora	Ø Open X External	Ø Drainage Device 7 Autologous Tissue Substitute J Synthetic Substitute K Nonautologous Tissue Substitute	Z No Qualifier

Non-OR ØUW3[3,4]YZ	**Non-OR** ØUWDX[Ø,3,7,C,D,H,J,K]Z
Non-OR ØUW3[7,8]YZ	**Non-OR** ØUWH[3,4,7,8]YZ
Non-OR ØUW3X[Ø,3]Z	**Non-OR** ØUWHX[Ø,3,7,D,J,K]Z
Non-OR ØUW8[3,4,7,8]YZ	**Non-OR** ØUWMX[Ø,7,J,K]Z
Non-OR ØUW8X[Ø,3,7,C,D,J,K]Z	♀ All body part, approach, device, and qualifier values
Non-OR ØUWD[3,4,7,8]YZ	

Ø   **Medical and Surgical**
U   **Female Reproductive System**
Y   **Transplantation**   Definition: Putting in or on all or a portion of a living body part taken from another individual or animal to physically take the place and/or function of all or a portion of a similar body part

                        Explanation: The native body part may or may not be taken out, and the transplanted body part may take over all or a portion of its function

Body Part Character 4		Approach Character 5	Device Character 6	Qualifier Character 7
Ø Ovary, Right	♀	Ø Open	Z No Device	Ø Allogeneic
1 Ovary, Left	♀			1 Syngeneic
9 Uterus	♀			2 Zooplastic
♀ All body part, approach, device, and qualifier values				

Male Reproductive System ØV1–ØVX

Character Meanings

This Character Meaning table is provided as a guide to assist the user in the identification of character members that may be found in this section of code tables. It **SHOULD NOT** be used to build a PCS code.

Operation–Character 3	Body Part–Character 4	Approach–Character 5	Device–Character 6	Qualifier–Character 7
1　Bypass	Ø　Prostate	Ø　Open	Ø　Drainage Device	Ø　Allogeneic
2　Change	1　Seminal Vesicle, Right	3　Percutaneous	1　Radioactive Element	1　Syngeneic
5　Destruction	2　Seminal Vesicle, Left	4　Percutaneous Endoscopic	3　Infusion Device	2　Zooplastic
7　Dilation	3　Seminal Vesicles, Bilateral	7　Via Natural or Artificial Opening	7　Autologous Tissue Substitute	D　Urethra
9　Drainage	4　Prostate and Seminal Vesicles	8　Via Natural or Artificial Opening Endoscopic	C　Extraluminal Device	J　Epididymis, Right
B　Excision	5　Scrotum	X　External	D　Intraluminal Device	K　Epididymis, Left
C　Extirpation	6　Tunica Vaginalis, Right		J　Synthetic Substitute	N　Vas Deferens, Right
H　Insertion	7　Tunica Vaginalis, Left		K　Nonautologous Tissue Substitute	P　Vas Deferens, Left
J　Inspection	8　Scrotum and Tunica Vaginalis		Y　Other Device	S　Penis
L　Occlusion	9　Testis, Right		Z　No Device	X　Diagnostic
M　Reattachment	B　Testis, Left			Z　No Qualifier
N　Release	C　Testes, Bilateral			
P　Removal	D　Testis			
Q　Repair	F　Spermatic Cord, Right			
R　Replacement	G　Spermatic Cord, Left			
S　Reposition	H　Spermatic Cords, Bilateral			
T　Resection	J　Epididymis, Right			
U　Supplement	K　Epididymis, Left			
W　Revision	L　Epididymis, Bilateral			
X　Transfer	M　Epididymis and Spermatic Cord			
Y　Transplantation	N　Vas Deferens, Right			
	P　Vas Deferens, Left			
	Q　Vas Deferens, Bilateral			
	R　Vas Deferens			
	S　Penis			
	T　Prepuce			

AHA Coding Clinic for table ØV1
2018, 3Q, 12　　　Al-Ghorab distal penile shunt surgery

AHA Coding Clinic for table ØV9
2018, 3Q, 12　　　Al-Ghorab distal penile shunt surgery

AHA Coding Clinic for table ØVB
2020, 1Q, 31　　　Repair of buried penis
2019, 3Q, 18　　　Radical prostatectomy and lymph node dissection with biopsy of neurovascular bundle
2016, 1Q, 23　　　Transurethral resection of ejaculatory ducts
2014, 4Q, 33　　　Radical prostatectomy

AHA Coding Clinic for table ØVP
2016, 2Q, 28　　　Removal of multi-component inflatable penile prosthesis with placement of new malleable device

AHA Coding Clinic for table ØVQ
2018, 3Q, 12　　　Al-Ghorab distal penile shunt surgery

AHA Coding Clinic for table ØVT
2019, 3Q, 18　　　Radical prostatectomy and lymph node dissection with biopsy of neurovascular bundle
2014, 4Q, 33　　　Radical prostatectomy

AHA Coding Clinic for table ØVU
2020, 1Q, 31　　　Repair of buried penis
2016, 2Q, 28　　　Removal of multi-component inflatable penile prosthesis with placement of new malleable device
2015, 3Q, 25　　　Placement of inflatable penile prosthesis

AHA Coding Clinic for table ØVX
2018, 4Q, 40　　　Transfer of prepuce

Male Reproductive System

Penis

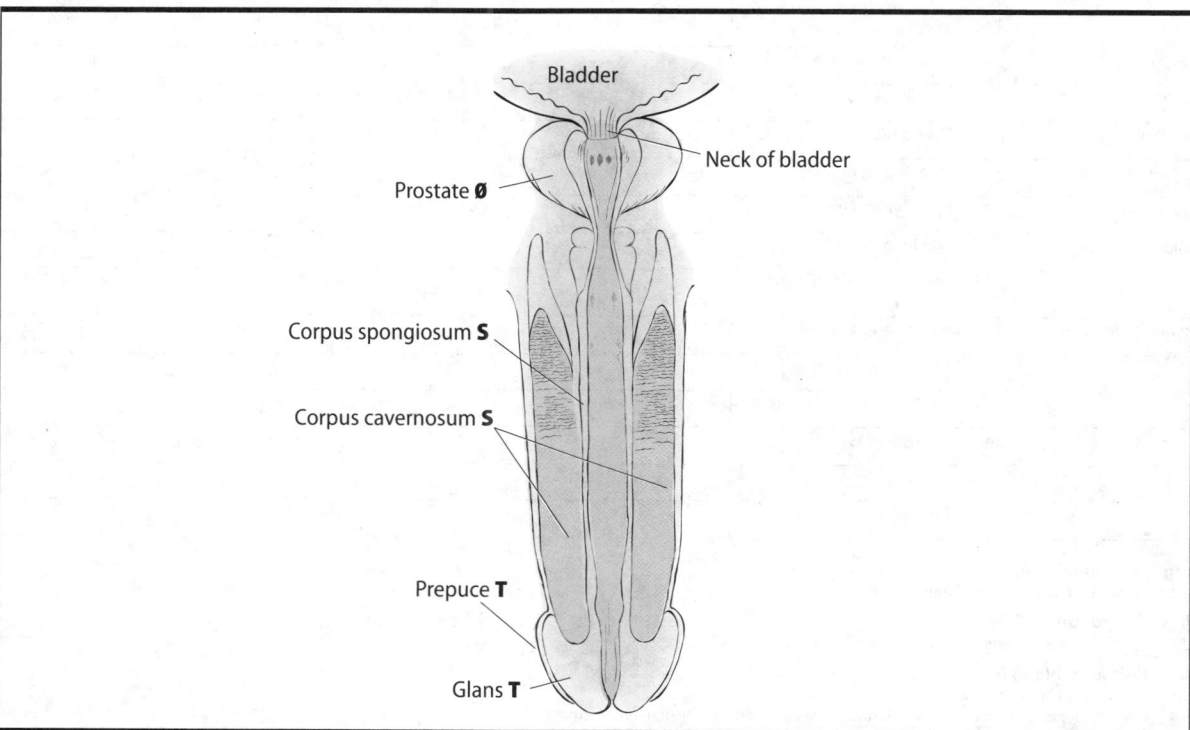

Ø   **Medical and Surgical**
V   **Male Reproductive System**
1   **Bypass**   Definition: Altering the route of passage of the contents of a tubular body part

                         Explanation: Rerouting contents of a body part to a downstream area of the normal route, to a similar route and body part, or to an abnormal route and dissimilar body part. Includes one or more anastomoses, with or without the use of a device.

Body Part Character 4	Approach Character 5	Device Character 6	Qualifier Character 7

N Vas Deferens, Right ♂
    Ductus deferens
    Ejaculatory duct
P Vas Deferens, Left ♂
    See N Vas Deferens, Right
Q Vas Deferens, Bilateral ♂
    See N Vas Deferens, Right
	Ø Open
	4 Percutaneous Endoscopic
		7 Autologous Tissue Substitute
		J Synthetic Substitute
		K Nonautologous Tissue Substitute
		Z No Device
			J Epididymis, Right
			K Epididymis, Left
			N Vas Deferens, Right
			P Vas Deferens, Left

    ♂   All body part, approach, device, and qualifier values

Ø   **Medical and Surgical**
V   **Male Reproductive System**
2   **Change**   Definition: Taking out or off a device from a body part and putting back an identical or similar device in or on the same body part without cutting or puncturing the skin or a mucous membrane

                         Explanation: All CHANGE procedures are coded using the approach EXTERNAL

Body Part Character 4	Approach Character 5	Device Character 6	Qualifier Character 7

4 Prostate and Seminal Vesicles ♂
8 Scrotum and Tunica Vaginalis ♂
D Testis ♂
M Epididymis and Spermatic Cord ♂
R Vas Deferens ♂
    Ductus deferens
    Ejaculatory duct
S Penis ♂
    Corpus cavernosum
    Corpus spongiosum
	X External	Ø Drainage Device
		Y Other Device
			Z No Qualifier

    Non-OR All body part, approach, device, and qualifier values   ♂   All body part, approach, device, and qualifier values

Ø   **Medical and Surgical**
V   **Male Reproductive System**
5   **Destruction**   Definition: Physical eradication of all or a portion of a body part by the direct use of energy, force, or a destructive agent

                         Explanation: None of the body part is physically taken out

Body Part Character 4	Approach Character 5	Device Character 6	Qualifier Character 7
Ø Prostate ♂	Ø Open 3 Percutaneous 4 Percutaneous Endoscopic 7 Via Natural or Artificial Opening 8 Via Natural or Artificial Opening Endoscopic	Z No Device	Z No Qualifier
1 Seminal Vesicle, Right ♂ 2 Seminal Vesicle, Left ♂ 3 Seminal Vesicles, Bilateral ♂ 6 Tunica Vaginalis, Right ♂ 7 Tunica Vaginalis, Left ♂ 9 Testis, Right ♂ B Testis, Left ♂ C Testes, Bilateral ♂	Ø Open 3 Percutaneous 4 Percutaneous Endoscopic	Z No Device	Z No Qualifier

5 Scrotum ♂
S Penis ♂
    Corpus cavernosum
    Corpus spongiosum
T Prepuce ♂
    Foreskin
    Glans penis
	Ø Open
	3 Percutaneous
	4 Percutaneous Endoscopic
	X External
		Z No Device	Z No Qualifier

F Spermatic Cord, Right ♂
G Spermatic Cord, Left ♂
H Spermatic Cords, Bilateral ♂
J Epididymis, Right ♂
K Epididymis, Left ♂
L Epididymis, Bilateral ♂
N Vas Deferens, Right NC ♂
    Ductus deferens
    Ejaculatory duct
P Vas Deferens, Left NC ♂
    See N Vas Deferens, Right
Q Vas Deferens, Bilateral NC ♂
    See N Vas Deferens, Right
	Ø Open
	3 Percutaneous
	4 Percutaneous Endoscopic
	8 Via Natural or Artificial Opening
	    Endoscopic
		Z No Device	Z No Qualifier

    Non-OR ØV55[Ø,3,4,X]ZZ
    Non-OR ØV5[N,P,Q][Ø,3,4,8]ZZ   NC ØV5[N,P,Q][Ø,3,4]ZZ with principal or secondary diagnosis of Z3Ø.2
                                          ♂   All body part, approach, device, and qualifier values

Male Reproductive System

Ø   Medical and Surgical
V   Male Reproductive System
7   Dilation   Definition: Expanding an orifice or the lumen of a tubular body part

Explanation: The orifice can be a natural orifice or an artificially created orifice. Accomplished by stretching a tubular body part using intraluminal pressure or by cutting part of the orifice or wall of the tubular body part.

Body Part Character 4		Approach Character 5	Device Character 6	Qualifier Character 7

N   Vas Deferens, Right
     Ductus deferens
     Ejaculatory duct
P   Vas Deferens, Left
     See N Vas Deferens, Right
Q   Vas Deferens, Bilateral
     See N Vas Deferens, Right
	♂
	
	♂
	
	♂
		Ø Open
		3 Percutaneous
		4 Percutaneous Endoscopic
			D Intraluminal Device
			Z No Device
				Z No Qualifier

♂   All body part, approach, device, and qualifier values

Ø   Medical and Surgical
V   Male Reproductive System
9   Drainage   Definition: Taking or letting out fluids and/or gases from a body part

Explanation: The qualifier DIAGNOSTIC is used to identify drainage procedures that are biopsies

Body Part Character 4		Approach Character 5	Device Character 6	Qualifier Character 7
Ø Prostate	♂	Ø Open 3 Percutaneous 4 Percutaneous Endoscopic 7 Via Natural or Artificial Opening 8 Via Natural or Artificial Opening Endoscopic	Ø Drainage Device	Z No Qualifier
Ø Prostate	♂	Ø Open 3 Percutaneous 4 Percutaneous Endoscopic 7 Via Natural or Artificial Opening 8 Via Natural or Artificial Opening Endoscopic	Z No Device	X Diagnostic Z No Qualifier

1   Seminal Vesicle, Right
2   Seminal Vesicle, Left
3   Seminal Vesicles, Bilateral
6   Tunica Vaginalis, Right
7   Tunica Vaginalis, Left
9   Testis, Right
B   Testis, Left
C   Testes, Bilateral
F   Spermatic Cord, Right
G   Spermatic Cord, Left
H   Spermatic Cords, Bilateral
J   Epididymis, Right
K   Epididymis, Left
L   Epididymis, Bilateral
N   Vas Deferens, Right
     Ductus deferens
     Ejaculatory duct
P   Vas Deferens, Left
     See N Vas Deferens, Right
Q   Vas Deferens, Bilateral
     See N Vas Deferens, Right
	♂
	♂
	♂
	♂
	♂
	♂
	♂
	♂
	♂
	♂
	♂
	♂
	♂
	♂
	♂
	
	♂
	
	♂
		Ø Open
		3 Percutaneous
		4 Percutaneous Endoscopic
			Ø Drainage Device	Z No Qualifier

Non-OR	ØV9Ø[3,4]ØZ	**Non-OR**	ØV9[6,7,F,G,H,N,P,Q][Ø,3,4]ØZ
Non-OR	ØV9Ø[3,4]Z[X,Z]	**Non-OR**	ØV9[J,K,L]3ØZ
Non-OR	ØV9Ø[7,8]ZX	♂	All body part, approach, device, and qualifier values
Non-OR	ØV9[1,2,3,9,B,C][3,4]ØZ		

ØV9 Continued on next page

Ø **Medical and Surgical**
V **Male Reproductive System**
9 **Drainage**   Definition: Taking or letting out fluids and/or gases from a body part
         Explanation: The qualifier DIAGNOSTIC is used to identify drainage procedures that are biopsies

Body Part Character 4	Approach Character 5	Device Character 6	Qualifier Character 7

1 Seminal Vesicle, Right ♂
2 Seminal Vesicle, Left ♂
3 Seminal Vesicles, Bilateral ♂
6 Tunica Vaginalis, Right ♂
7 Tunica Vaginalis, Left ♂
9 Testis, Right ♂
B Testis, Left ♂
C Testes, Bilateral ♂
F Spermatic Cord, Right ♂
G Spermatic Cord, Left ♂
H Spermatic Cords, Bilateral ♂
J Epididymis, Right ♂
K Epididymis, Left ♂
L Epididymis, Bilateral ♂
N Vas Deferens, Right ♂
  Ductus deferens
  Ejaculatory duct
P Vas Deferens, Left ♂
  See N Vas Deferens, Right
Q Vas Deferens, Bilateral ♂
  See N Vas Deferens, Right
	Ø Open
	3 Percutaneous
	4 Percutaneous Endoscopic
		Z No Device	X Diagnostic
			Z No Qualifier

5 Scrotum ♂
S Penis ♂
  Corpus cavernosum
  Corpus spongiosum
T Prepuce ♂
  Foreskin
  Glans penis
	Ø Open
	3 Percutaneous
	4 Percutaneous Endoscopic
	X External
		Ø Drainage Device	Z No Qualifier

5 Scrotum ♂
S Penis ♂
  Corpus cavernosum
  Corpus spongiosum
T Prepuce ♂
  Foreskin
  Glans penis
	Ø Open
	3 Percutaneous
	4 Percutaneous Endoscopic
	X External
		Z No Device	X Diagnostic
			Z No Qualifier

Non-OR   ØV9[1,2,3,9,B,C][3,4]Z[X,Z]
Non-OR   ØV9[6,7,F,G,H,J,K,L,N,P,Q][Ø,3,4]ZX
Non-OR   ØV9[6,7,F,G,H,N,P,Q][Ø,3,4]ZZ
Non-OR   ØV9[J,K,L]3ZZ
Non-OR   ØV95[Ø,3,4,X]ØZ

Non-OR   ØV9[S,T]3ØZ
Non-OR   ØV95ØZX
Non-OR   ØV95[3,4,X]Z[X,Z]
Non-OR   ØV9[S,T]3ZZ
♂   All body part, approach, device, and qualifier values

Male Reproductive System *(side tab)*

Ø Medical and Surgical
V Male Reproductive System
B Excision   Definition: Cutting out or off, without replacement, a portion of a body part
                     Explanation: The qualifier DIAGNOSTIC is used to identify excision procedures that are biopsies

Body Part Character 4	Approach Character 5	Device Character 6	Qualifier Character 7
Ø Prostate ♂	Ø Open 3 Percutaneous 4 Percutaneous Endoscopic 7 Via Natural or Artificial Opening 8 Via Natural or Artificial Opening Endoscopic	Z No Device	X Diagnostic Z No Qualifier
1 Seminal Vesicle, Right ♂ 2 Seminal Vesicle, Left ♂ 3 Seminal Vesicles, Bilateral ♂ 6 Tunica Vaginalis, Right ♂ 7 Tunica Vaginalis, Left ♂ 9 Testis, Right ♂ B Testis, Left ♂ C Testes, Bilateral ♂	Ø Open 3 Percutaneous 4 Percutaneous Endoscopic	Z No Device	X Diagnostic Z No Qualifier

5 Scrotum ♂
S Penis ♂
  Corpus cavernosum
  Corpus spongiosum
T Prepuce ♂
  Foreskin
  Glans penis
	Ø Open
	3 Percutaneous
	4 Percutaneous Endoscopic
	X External
		Z No Device	X Diagnostic
			Z No Qualifier

F Spermatic Cord, Right ♂
G Spermatic Cord, Left ♂
H Spermatic Cords, Bilateral ♂
J Epididymis, Right ♂
K Epididymis, Left ♂
L Epididymis, Bilateral ♂
N Vas Deferens, Right ＮＣ♂
  Ductus deferens
  Ejaculatory duct
P Vas Deferens, Left ＮＣ♂
  See N Vas Deferens, Right
Q Vas Deferens, Bilateral ＮＣ♂
  See N Vas Deferens, Right
	Ø Open
	3 Percutaneous
	4 Percutaneous Endoscopic
	8 Via Natural or Artificial Opening Endoscopic
		Z No Device	X Diagnostic
			Z No Qualifier

Non-OR ØVBØ[3,4,7,8]ZX	**Non-OR** ØVB[F,G,H,J,K,L][Ø,3,4,8]ZX
Non-OR ØVB[1,2,3,9,B,C][3,4]ZX	**Non-OR** ØVB[N,P,Q][Ø,3,4,8]Z[X,Z]
Non-OR ØVB[6,7][Ø,3,4]ZX	**ＮＣ** ØVB[N,P,Q][Ø,3,4]ZZ with principal or secondary diagnosis of Z3Ø.2
Non-OR ØVB5ØZX	♂ All body part, approach, device, and qualifier values
Non-OR ØVB5[3,4,X]Z[X,Z]	

Ø   **Medical and Surgical**
V   **Male Reproductive System**
C   **Extirpation**   Definition: Taking or cutting out solid matter from a body part
                      Explanation: The solid matter may be an abnormal byproduct of a biological function or a foreign body; it may be imbedded in a body part or in the lumen of a tubular body part. The solid matter may or may not have been previously broken into pieces.

Body Part Character 4	Approach Character 5	Device Character 6	Qualifier Character 7
Ø Prostate ♂	**Ø** Open **3** Percutaneous **4** Percutaneous Endoscopic **7** Via Natural or Artificial Opening **8** Via Natural or Artificial Opening Endoscopic	**Z** No Device	**Z** No Qualifier

1   Seminal Vesicle, Right ♂
2   Seminal Vesicle, Left ♂
3   Seminal Vesicles, Bilateral ♂
6   Tunica Vaginalis, Right ♂
7   Tunica Vaginalis, Left ♂
9   Testis, Right ♂
B   Testis, Left ♂
C   Testes, Bilateral ♂
F   Spermatic Cord, Right ♂
G   Spermatic Cord, Left ♂
H   Spermatic Cords, Bilateral ♂
J   Epididymis, Right ♂
K   Epididymis, Left ♂
L   Epididymis, Bilateral ♂
N   Vas Deferens, Right ♂
     Ductus deferens
     Ejaculatory duct
P   Vas Deferens, Left ♂
     See N Vas Deferens, Right
Q   Vas Deferens, Bilateral ♂
     See N Vas Deferens, Right
	Ø Open
	3 Percutaneous
	4 Percutaneous Endoscopic
		Z No Device	**Z** No Qualifier

5   Scrotum ♂
S   Penis ♂
     Corpus cavernosum
     Corpus spongiosum
T   Prepuce ♂
     Foreskin
     Glans penis
	Ø Open
	3 Percutaneous
	4 Percutaneous Endoscopic
	X External
		Z No Device	**Z** No Qualifier

Non-OR   ØVC[6,7,N,P,Q][Ø,3,4]ZZ
Non-OR   ØVC5[3,4,X]ZZ

Non-OR   ØVCSXZZ
♂   All body part, approach, device, and qualifier values

LC Limited Coverage   NC Noncovered   ⊞ Combination Member   HAC associated procedure   Combination Only   DRG Non-OR   Non-OR   New/Revised in GREEN

Ø **Medical and Surgical**
V **Male Reproductive System**
H **Insertion**   Definition: Putting in a nonbiological appliance that monitors, assists, performs, or prevents a physiological function but does not physically take the place of a body part
                         Explanation: None

Body Part Character 4	Approach Character 5	Device Character 6	Qualifier Character 7
Ø Prostate ♂	Ø Open 3 Percutaneous 4 Percutaneous Endoscopic 7 Via Natural or Artificial Opening 8 Via Natural or Artificial Opening Endoscopic	1 Radioactive Element	Z No Qualifier

4 Prostate and Seminal Vesicles ♂
8 Scrotum and Tunica Vaginalis ♂
M Epididymis and Spermatic Cord ♂
R Vas Deferens ♂
  Ductus deferens
  Ejaculatory duct
	Ø Open
	3 Percutaneous
	4 Percutaneous Endoscopic
	7 Via Natural or Artificial Opening
	8 Via Natural or Artificial Opening Endoscopic
		3 Infusion Device
		Y Other Device
			Z No Qualifier

D Testis ♂	Ø Open 3 Percutaneous 4 Percutaneous Endoscopic 7 Via Natural or Artificial Opening 8 Via Natural or Artificial Opening Endoscopic	1 Radioactive Element 3 Infusion Device Y Other Device	Z No Qualifier

S Penis ♂
  Corpus cavernosum
  Corpus spongiosum
	Ø Open
	3 Percutaneous
	4 Percutaneous Endoscopic
		3 Infusion Device
		Y Other Device
			Z No Qualifier

S Penis ♂
  Corpus cavernosum
  Corpus spongiosum
	7 Via Natural or Artificial Opening
	8 Via Natural or Artificial Opening Endoscopic
		Y Other Device	Z No Qualifier

S Penis ♂
  Corpus cavernosum
  Corpus spongiosum
	X External	3 Infusion Device	Z No Qualifier

Non-OR ØVH[4,8,M,R][Ø,3,4,7,8][3,Y]Z
Non-OR ØVHD[Ø,3,4,7,8][3,Y]Z
Non-OR ØVHS[Ø,3,4][3,Y]Z
Non-OR ØVHS[7,8]YZ
Non-OR ØVHSX3Z
♂ All body part, approach, device, and qualifier values

Ø **Medical and Surgical**
V **Male Reproductive System**
J **Inspection**   Definition: Visually and/or manually exploring a body part
                         Explanation: Visual exploration may be performed with or without optical instrumentation. Manual exploration may be performed directly or through intervening body layers.

Body Part Character 4	Approach Character 5	Device Character 6	Qualifier Character 7

4 Prostate and Seminal Vesicles ♂
8 Scrotum and Tunica Vaginalis ♂
D Testis ♂
M Epididymis and Spermatic Cord ♂
R Vas Deferens ♂
  Ductus deferens
  Ejaculatory duct
S Penis ♂
  Corpus cavernosum
  Corpus spongiosum
	Ø Open
	3 Percutaneous
	4 Percutaneous Endoscopic
	X External
		Z No Device	Z No Qualifier

Non-OR ØVJ[4,D,M,R][3,X]ZZ
Non-OR ØVJ8[Ø,3,4,X]ZZ
Non-OR ØVJS[3,4,X]ZZ
♂ All body part, approach, device, and qualifier values

Ø   **Medical and Surgical**
V   **Male Reproductive System**
L   **Occlusion**   Definition: Completely closing an orifice or the lumen of a tubular body part
                 Explanation: The orifice can be a natural orifice or an artificially created orifice

Body Part Character 4	Approach Character 5	Device Character 6	Qualifier Character 7

F   Spermatic Cord, Right   NC ♂
G   Spermatic Cord, Left   NC ♂
H   Spermatic Cords, Bilateral   NC ♂
N   Vas Deferens, Right   NC ♂
     Ductus deferens
     Ejaculatory duct
P   Vas Deferens, Left   NC ♂
     See N Vas Deferens, Right
Q   Vas Deferens, Bilateral   NC ♂
     See N Vas Deferens, Right
	Ø Open
	3 Percutaneous
	4 Percutaneous Endoscopic
	8 Via Natural or Artificial Opening
	     Endoscopic
		C Extraluminal Device
		D Intraluminal Device
		Z No Device
			Z No Qualifier

Non-OR ØVL[F,G,H][Ø,3,4,8][C,D,Z]Z **Non-OR** ØVL[N,P,Q][Ø,3,4,8][C,Z]Z		NC ØVL[F,G,H][Ø,3,4][C,D,Z]Z with principal or secondary diagnosis of Z3Ø.2 NC ØVL[N,P,Q][Ø,3,4][C,Z]Z with principal or secondary diagnosis of Z3Ø.2 ♂ All body part, approach, device, and qualifier values	

Ø   **Medical and Surgical**
V   **Male Reproductive System**
M   **Reattachment**   Definition: Putting back in or on all or a portion of a separated body part to its normal location or other suitable location
                     Explanation: Vascular circulation and nervous pathways may or may not be reestablished

Body Part Character 4	Approach Character 5	Device Character 6	Qualifier Character 7

5   Scrotum   ♂
S   Penis   ♂
     Corpus cavernosum
     Corpus spongiosum
	X External	Z No Device	Z No Qualifier

6 Tunica Vaginalis, Right ♂ 7 Tunica Vaginalis, Left ♂ 9 Testis, Right ♂ B Testis, Left ♂ C Testes, Bilateral ♂ F Spermatic Cord, Right ♂ G Spermatic Cord, Left ♂ H Spermatic Cords, Bilateral ♂	Ø Open 4 Percutaneous Endoscopic	Z No Device	Z No Qualifier

♂   All body part, approach, device, and qualifier values

LC Limited Coverage   NC Noncovered   ⊞ Combination Member   HAC associated procedure   Combination Only   DRG Non-OR   Non-OR   New/Revised in GREEN
ICD-10-PCS 2021   **661**

ØVL–ØVM

Male Reproductive System

Ø   **Medical and Surgical**
V   **Male Reproductive System**
N   **Release**   Definition: Freeing a body part from an abnormal physical constraint by cutting or by the use of force
                       Explanation: Some of the restraining tissue may be taken out but none of the body part is taken out

Body Part Character 4	Approach Character 5	Device Character 6	Qualifier Character 7
Ø Prostate ♂	Ø Open 3 Percutaneous 4 Percutaneous Endoscopic 7 Via Natural or Artificial Opening 8 Via Natural or Artificial Opening Endoscopic	Z No Device	Z No Qualifier
1 Seminal Vesicle, Right ♂ 2 Seminal Vesicle, Left ♂ 3 Seminal Vesicles, Bilateral ♂ 6 Tunica Vaginalis, Right ♂ 7 Tunica Vaginalis, Left ♂ 9 Testis, Right ♂ B Testis, Left ♂ C Testes, Bilateral ♂	Ø Open 3 Percutaneous 4 Percutaneous Endoscopic	Z No Device	Z No Qualifier

5 Scrotum ♂
S Penis ♂
   Corpus cavernosum
   Corpus spongiosum
T Prepuce ♂
   Foreskin
   Glans penis
	Ø Open
	3 Percutaneous
	4 Percutaneous Endoscopic
	X External
		Z No Device	Z No Qualifier

F Spermatic Cord, Right ♂
G Spermatic Cord, Left ♂
H Spermatic Cords, Bilateral ♂
J Epididymis, Right ♂
K Epididymis, Left ♂
L Epididymis, Bilateral ♂
N Vas Deferens, Right ♂
   Ductus deferens
   Ejaculatory duct
P Vas Deferens, Left ♂
   See N Vas Deferens, Right
Q Vas Deferens, Bilateral ♂
   See N Vas Deferens, Right
	Ø Open
	3 Percutaneous
	4 Percutaneous Endoscopic
	8 Via Natural or Artificial Opening Endoscopic
		Z No Device	Z No Qualifier

Non-OR   ØVN[9,B,C][Ø,3,4]ZZ   ♂   All body part, approach, device, and qualifier values
Non-OR   ØVNT[Ø,3,4,X]ZZ

LC Limited Coverage   **NC** Noncovered   ⊞ Combination Member   HAC associated procedure   Combination Only   DRG Non-OR   Non-OR   New/Revised in GREEN

662   ICD-10-PCS 2021

Ø   Medical and Surgical
V   Male Reproductive System
P   Removal   Definition: Taking out or off a device from a body part

Explanation: If a device is taken out and a similar device put in without cutting or puncturing the skin or mucous membrane, the procedure is coded to the root operation CHANGE. Otherwise, the procedure for taking out the device is coded to the root operation REMOVAL.

Body Part Character 4	Approach Character 5	Device Character 6	Qualifier Character 7
4 Prostate and Seminal Vesicles ♂	**Ø** Open **3** Percutaneous **4** Percutaneous Endoscopic **7** Via Natural or Artificial Opening **8** Via Natural or Artificial Opening Endoscopic	**Ø** Drainage Device **1** Radioactive Element **3** Infusion Device **7** Autologous Tissue Substitute **J** Synthetic Substitute **K** Nonautologous Tissue Substitute **Y** Other Device	**Z** No Qualifier
4 Prostate and Seminal Vesicles ♂	**X** External	**Ø** Drainage Device **1** Radioactive Element **3** Infusion Device	**Z** No Qualifier

8   Scrotum and Tunica Vaginalis ♂
D   Testis ♂
S   Penis ♂
     Corpus cavernosum
     Corpus spongiosum
	Ø Open
	3 Percutaneous
	4 Percutaneous Endoscopic
	7 Via Natural or Artificial Opening
	8 Via Natural or Artificial Opening Endoscopic
		Ø Drainage Device
		3 Infusion Device
		7 Autologous Tissue Substitute
		J Synthetic Substitute
		K Nonautologous Tissue Substitute
		Y Other Device
			Z No Qualifier

8   Scrotum and Tunica Vaginalis ♂
D   Testis ♂
S   Penis ♂
     Corpus cavernosum
     Corpus spongiosum
	X External	**Ø** Drainage Device
		3 Infusion Device
			Z No Qualifier

M Epididymis and Spermatic Cord ♂	**Ø** Open **3** Percutaneous **4** Percutaneous Endoscopic **7** Via Natural or Artificial Opening **8** Via Natural or Artificial Opening Endoscopic	**Ø** Drainage Device **3** Infusion Device **7** Autologous Tissue Substitute **C** Extraluminal Device **J** Synthetic Substitute **K** Nonautologous Tissue Substitute **Y** Other Device	**Z** No Qualifier
M Epididymis and Spermatic Cord ♂	**X** External	**Ø** Drainage Device **3** Infusion Device	**Z** No Qualifier

R   Vas Deferens ♂
     Ductus deferens
     Ejaculatory duct
	Ø Open
	3 Percutaneous
	4 Percutaneous Endoscopic
	7 Via Natural or Artificial Opening
	8 Via Natural or Artificial Opening Endoscopic
		Ø Drainage Device
		3 Infusion Device
		7 Autologous Tissue Substitute
		C Extraluminal Device
		D Intraluminal Device
		J Synthetic Substitute
		K Nonautologous Tissue Substitute
		Y Other Device
			Z No Qualifier

R   Vas Deferens ♂
     Ductus deferens
     Ejaculatory duct
	X External	**Ø** Drainage Device
		3 Infusion Device
		D Intraluminal Device
			Z No Qualifier

Non-OR ØVP4[3,4]YZ		**Non-OR** ØVPM[3,4]YZ	
Non-OR ØVP4[7,8][Ø,3,Y]Z		**Non-OR** ØVPM[7,8][Ø,3,Y]Z	
Non-OR ØVP4X[Ø,1,3]Z		**Non-OR** ØVPMX[Ø,3]Z	
Non-OR ØVP8[Ø,3,4,7,8][Ø,3,7,J,K,Y]Z		**Non-OR** ØVPR[Ø,3,4][Ø,3,7,C,J,K,Y]Z	
Non-OR ØVP[D,S][3,4]YZ		**Non-OR** ØVPR[7,8][Ø,3,7,C,D,J,K,Y]Z	
Non-OR ØVP[D,S][7,8][Ø,3,Y]Z		**Non-OR** ØVPRX[Ø,3,D]Z	
Non-OR ØVP[8,D,S]X[Ø,3]Z		♂ All body part, approach, device, and qualifier values	

LC Limited Coverage   NC Noncovered   ⊞ Combination Member   HAC associated procedure   Combination Only   DRG Non-OR   Non-OR   New/Revised in GREEN

ICD-10-PCS 2021   663

ØVP–ØVP

Male Reproductive System

Ø   **Medical and Surgical**
V   **Male Reproductive System**
Q   **Repair**   Definition: Restoring, to the extent possible, a body part to its normal anatomic structure and function
                    Explanation: Used only when the method to accomplish the repair is not one of the other root operations

Body Part Character 4	Approach Character 5	Device Character 6	Qualifier Character 7
Ø Prostate ♂	Ø Open 3 Percutaneous 4 Percutaneous Endoscopic 7 Via Natural or Artificial Opening 8 Via Natural or Artificial Opening Endoscopic	Z No Device	Z No Qualifier
1 Seminal Vesicle, Right ♂ 2 Seminal Vesicle, Left ♂ 3 Seminal Vesicles, Bilateral ♂ 6 Tunica Vaginalis, Right ♂ 7 Tunica Vaginalis, Left ♂ 9 Testis, Right ♂ B Testis, Left ♂ C Testes, Bilateral ♂	Ø Open 3 Percutaneous 4 Percutaneous Endoscopic	Z No Device	Z No Qualifier

5 Scrotum ♂
S Penis ♂
     Corpus cavernosum
     Corpus spongiosum
T Prepuce ♂
     Foreskin
     Glans penis
	Ø Open
	3 Percutaneous
	4 Percutaneous Endoscopic
	X External
		Z No Device	Z No Qualifier

F Spermatic Cord, Right ♂
G Spermatic Cord, Left ♂
H Spermatic Cords, Bilateral ♂
J Epididymis, Right ♂
K Epididymis, Left ♂
L Epididymis, Bilateral ♂
N Vas Deferens, Right ♂
     Ductus deferens
     Ejaculatory duct
P Vas Deferens, Left ♂
     See N Vas Deferens, Right
Q Vas Deferens, Bilateral ♂
     See N Vas Deferens, Right
	Ø Open
	3 Percutaneous
	4 Percutaneous Endoscopic
	8 Via Natural or Artificial Opening
	     Endoscopic
		Z No Device	Z No Qualifier

Non-OR   ØVQ[6,7][Ø,3,4]ZZ   ♂   All body part, approach, device, and qualifier values
Non-OR   ØVQ5[Ø,3,4,X]ZZ

Ø   **Medical and Surgical**
V   **Male Reproductive System**
R   **Replacement**   Definition: Putting in or on biological or synthetic material that physically takes the place and/or function of all or a portion of a body part
                    Explanation: The body part may have been taken out or replaced, or may be taken out, physically eradicated, or rendered nonfunctional during the REPLACEMENT procedure. A REMOVAL procedure is coded for taking out the device used in a previous replacement procedure.

Body Part Character 4	Approach Character 5	Device Character 6	Qualifier Character 7
9 Testis, Right ♂ B Testis, Left ♂ C Testes, Bilateral ♂	Ø Open	J Synthetic Substitute	Z No Qualifier

♂   All body part, approach, device, and qualifier values

Ø   **Medical and Surgical**
V   **Male Reproductive System**
S   **Reposition**   Definition: Moving to its normal location, or other suitable location, all or a portion of a body part
                    Explanation: The body part is moved to a new location from an abnormal location, or from a normal location where it is not functioning correctly. The body part may or may not be cut out or off to be moved to the new location.

Body Part Character 4	Approach Character 5	Device Character 6	Qualifier Character 7
9 Testis, Right ♂ B Testis, Left ♂ C Testes, Bilateral ♂ F Spermatic Cord, Right ♂ G Spermatic Cord, Left ♂ H Spermatic Cords, Bilateral ♂	Ø Open 3 Percutaneous 4 Percutaneous Endoscopic 8 Via Natural or Artificial Opening Endoscopic	Z No Device	Z No Qualifier

♂   All body part, approach, device, and qualifier values

Ø   Medical and Surgical
V   Male Reproductive System
T   Resection   Definition: Cutting out or off, without replacement, all of a body part
                   Explanation: None

Body Part Character 4	Approach Character 5	Device Character 6	Qualifier Character 7
Ø Prostate ⊞♂	Ø Open 4 Percutaneous Endoscopic 7 Via Natural or Artificial Opening 8 Via Natural or Artificial Opening Endoscopic	Z No Device	Z No Qualifier

1   Seminal Vesicle, Right   ♂
2   Seminal Vesicle, Left   ♂
3   Seminal Vesicles, Bilateral   ⊞♂
6   Tunica Vaginalis, Right   ♂
7   Tunica Vaginalis, Left   ♂
9   Testis, Right   ♂
B   Testis, Left   ♂
C   Testes, Bilateral   ♂
F   Spermatic Cord, Right   ♂
G   Spermatic Cord, Left   ♂
H   Spermatic Cords, Bilateral   ♂
J   Epididymis, Right   ♂
K   Epididymis, Left   ♂
L   Epididymis, Bilateral   ♂
N   Vas Deferens, Right   NC♂
      Ductus deferens
      Ejaculatory duct
P   Vas Deferens, Left   NC♂
      See N Vas Deferens, Right
Q   Vas Deferens, Bilateral   NC♂
      See N Vas Deferens, Right
	Ø Open
	4 Percutaneous Endoscopic
		Z No Device	Z No Qualifier

5   Scrotum   ♂
S   Penis   ♂
      Corpus cavernosum
      Corpus spongiosum
T   Prepuce   ♂
      Foreskin
      Glans penis
	Ø Open
	4 Percutaneous Endoscopic
	X External
		Z No Device	Z No Qualifier

Non-OR	ØVT[N,P,Q][Ø,4]ZZ	**See Appendix L for Procedure Combinations**
Non-OR	ØVT[5,T][Ø,4,X]ZZ	⊞ ØVTØ[Ø,4,7,8]ZZ
NC	ØVT[N,P,Q][Ø,4]ZZ with principal or secondary diagnosis of Z3Ø.2	⊞ ØVT3[Ø,4]ZZ
♂	All body part, approach, device, and qualifier values	

LC Limited Coverage   NC Noncovered   ⊞ Combination Member   HAC associated procedure   Combination Only   DRG Non-OR   Non-OR   New/Revised in GREEN

ICD-10-PCS 2021   665

Ø　Medical and Surgical
V　Male Reproductive System
U　Supplement　Definition: Putting in or on biological or synthetic material that physically reinforces and/or augments the function of a portion of a body part
　　　　　　　　Explanation: The biological material is non-living, or is living and from the same individual. The body part may have been previously replaced, and the SUPPLEMENT procedure is performed to physically reinforce and/or augment the function of the replaced body part.

Body Part Character 4		Approach Character 5	Device Character 6	Qualifier Character 7
1　Seminal Vesicle, Right 2　Seminal Vesicle, Left 3　Seminal Vesicles, Bilateral 6　Tunica Vaginalis, Right 7　Tunica Vaginalis, Left F　Spermatic Cord, Right G　Spermatic Cord, Left H　Spermatic Cords, Bilateral J　Epididymis, Right K　Epididymis, Left L　Epididymis, Bilateral N　Vas Deferens, Right 　　Ductus deferens 　　Ejaculatory duct P　Vas Deferens, Left 　　*See N Vas Deferens, Right* Q　Vas Deferens, Bilateral 　　*See N Vas Deferens, Right*	♂ ♂ ♂ ♂ ♂ ♂ ♂ ♂ ♂ ♂ ♂ ♂ ♂ ♂	Ø　Open 4　Percutaneous Endoscopic 8　Via Natural or Artificial Opening 　　Endoscopic	7　Autologous Tissue Substitute J　Synthetic Substitute K　Nonautologous Tissue Substitute	Z　No Qualifier
5　Scrotum S　Penis 　　Corpus cavernosum 　　Corpus spongiosum T　Prepuce 　　Foreskin 　　Glans penis	♂ ♂ ♂	Ø　Open 4　Percutaneous Endoscopic X　External	7　Autologous Tissue Substitute J　Synthetic Substitute K　Nonautologous Tissue Substitute	Z　No Qualifier
9　Testis, Right B　Testis, Left C　Testes, Bilateral	♂ ♂ ♂	Ø　Open	7　Autologous Tissue Substitute J　Synthetic Substitute K　Nonautologous Tissue Substitute	Z　No Qualifier

Non-OR　ØVUSX[7,J,K]Z　　　　　　　　　　　　　　♂　　All body part, approach, device, and qualifier values

Ø Medical and Surgical
V Male Reproductive System
W Revision　　Definition: Correcting, to the extent possible, a portion of a malfunctioning device or the position of a displaced device
　　　　　　Explanation: Revision can include correcting a malfunctioning or displaced device by taking out or putting in components of the device such as a screw or pin

Body Part Character 4		Approach Character 5	Device Character 6	Qualifier Character 7
4 Prostate and Seminal Vesicles ♂ 8 Scrotum and Tunica Vaginalis ♂ D Testis ♂ S Penis 　Corpus cavernosum 　Corpus spongiosum		Ø Open 3 Percutaneous 4 Percutaneous Endoscopic 7 Via Natural or Artificial Opening 8 Via Natural or Artificial Opening 　Endoscopic	Ø Drainage Device 3 Infusion Device 7 Autologous Tissue Substitute J Synthetic Substitute K Nonautologous Tissue Substitute Y Other Device	Z No Qualifier
4 Prostate and Seminal Vesicles ♂ 8 Scrotum and Tunica Vaginalis ♂ D Testis ♂ S Penis ♂ 　Corpus cavernosum 　Corpus spongiosum		X External	Ø Drainage Device 3 Infusion Device 7 Autologous Tissue Substitute J Synthetic Substitute K Nonautologous Tissue Substitute	Z No Qualifier
M Epididymis and Spermatic Cord ♂		Ø Open 3 Percutaneous 4 Percutaneous Endoscopic 7 Via Natural or Artificial Opening 8 Via Natural or Artificial Opening 　Endoscopic	Ø Drainage Device 3 Infusion Device 7 Autologous Tissue Substitute C Extraluminal Device J Synthetic Substitute K Nonautologous Tissue Substitute Y Other Device	Z No Qualifier
M Epididymis and Spermatic Cord ♂		X External	Ø Drainage Device 3 Infusion Device 7 Autologous Tissue Substitute C Extraluminal Device J Synthetic Substitute K Nonautologous Tissue Substitute	Z No Qualifier
R Vas Deferens ♂ 　Ductus deferens 　Ejaculatory duct		Ø Open 3 Percutaneous 4 Percutaneous Endoscopic 7 Via Natural or Artificial Opening 8 Via Natural or Artificial Opening 　Endoscopic	Ø Drainage Device 3 Infusion Device 7 Autologous Tissue Substitute C Extraluminal Device D Intraluminal Device J Synthetic Substitute K Nonautologous Tissue Substitute Y Other Device	Z No Qualifier
R Vas Deferens ♂ 　Ductus deferens 　Ejaculatory duct		X External	Ø Drainage Device 3 Infusion Device 7 Autologous Tissue Substitute C Extraluminal Device D Intraluminal Device J Synthetic Substitute K Nonautologous Tissue Substitute	Z No Qualifier

Non-OR ØVW[4,D,S][3,4,7,8]YZ
Non-OR ØVW8[Ø,3,4,7,8][Ø,3,7,J,K,Y]Z
Non-OR ØVW[4,8,D,S]X[Ø,3,7,J,K]Z
Non-OR ØVWM[3,4,7,8]YZ

Non-OR ØVWMX[Ø,3,7,C,J,K]Z
Non-OR ØVWR[Ø,3,4,7,8][Ø,3,7,C,D,J,K,Y]Z
Non-OR ØVWRX[Ø,3,7,C,D,J,K]Z
♂ All body part, approach, device, and qualifier values

Ø Medical and Surgical
V Male Reproductive System
X Transfer　　Definition: Moving, without taking out, all or a portion of a body part to another location to take over the function of all or a portion of a body part
　　　　　　Explanation: The body part transferred remains connected to its vascular and nervous supply

Body Part Character 4	Approach Character 5	Device Character 6	Qualifier Character 7
T Prepuce 　Foreskin 　Glans penis	Ø Open X External	Z No Device	D Urethra S Penis

LC Limited Coverage　NC Noncovered　⊞ Combination Member　HAC associated procedure　Combination Only　DRG Non-OR　Non-OR　New/Revised in GREEN

Ø   Medical and Surgical
V   Male Reproductive System
Y   Transplantation   Definition: Putting in or on all or a portion of a living body part taken from another individual or animal to physically take the place and/or
function of all or a portion of a similar body part
                 Explanation: The native body part may or may not be taken out, and the transplanted body part may take over all or a portion of its function

Body Part Character 4	Approach Character 5	Device Character 6	Qualifier Character 7

5   Scrotum   ♂
S   Penis   ♂
     Corpus cavernosum
     Corpus spongiosum
	Ø Open	Z No Device	Ø Allogeneic
			1 Syngeneic
			2 Zooplastic

     ♂   All body part, approach, device, and qualifier values

LC Limited Coverage   **NC** Noncovered   ⊞ Combination Member   HAC associated procedure   Combination Only   DRG Non-OR   Non-OR   New/Revised in GREEN

668   ICD-10-PCS 2021

Anatomical Regions, General ØWØ–ØWY

Character Meanings

This Character Meaning table is provided as a guide to assist the user in the identification of character members that may be found in this section of code tables. It **SHOULD NOT** be used to build a PCS code.

Operation–Character 3	Body Region–Character 4	Approach–Character 5	Device–Character 6	Qualifier–Character 7
Ø Alteration	Ø Head	Ø Open	Ø Drainage Device	Ø Vagina OR Allogeneic
1 Bypass	1 Cranial Cavity	3 Percutaneous	1 Radioactive Element	1 Penis OR Syngeneic
2 Change	2 Face	4 Percutaneous Endoscopic	3 Infusion Device	2 Stoma
3 Control	3 Oral Cavity and Throat	7 Via Natural or Artificial Opening	7 Autologous Tissue Substitute	4 Cutaneous
4 Creation	4 Upper Jaw	8 Via Natural or Artificial Opening Endoscopic	J Synthetic Substitute	6 Bladder
8 Division	5 Lower Jaw	X External	K Nonautologous Tissue Substitute	9 Pleural Cavity, Right
9 Drainage	6 Neck		Y Other Device	B Pleural Cavity, Left
B Excision	8 Chest Wall		Z No Device	G Peritoneal Cavity
C Extirpation	9 Pleural Cavity, Right			J Pelvic Cavity
F Fragmentation	B Pleural Cavity, Left			W Upper Vein
H Insertion	C Mediastinum			X Diagnostic
J Inspection	D Pericardial Cavity			Y Lower Vein
M Reattachment	F Abdominal Wall			Z No Qualifier
P Removal	G Peritoneal Cavity			
Q Repair	H Retroperitoneum			
U Supplement	J Pelvic Cavity			
W Revision	K Upper Back			
Y Transplantation	L Lower Back			
	M Perineum, Male			
	N Perineum, Female			
	P Gastrointestinal Tract			
	Q Respiratory Tract			
	R Genitourinary Tract			

AHA Coding Clinic for table ØWØ
2015, 1Q, 31   Bilateral browpexy

AHA Coding Clinic for table ØW1
2018, 4Q, 41-42   Anatomical regions bypass qualifiers
2015, 2Q, 36   Insertion of infusion device into peritoneal cavity
2013, 4Q, 126-127 Creation of percutaneous cutaneoperitoneal fistula

AHA Coding Clinic for table ØW3
2019, 3Q, 4   Evacuation of subdural hematoma and control of bleeding artery
2018, 4Q, 38   Control of epistaxis
2018, 1Q, 19   Argon plasma coagulation of duodenal arteriovenous malformation
2018, 1Q, 19   Control of epistaxis via silver nitrate cauterization
2017, 4Q, 57-58   Added approach values - Transorifice esophageal vein banding
2017, 4Q, 105   Control of gastrointestinal bleeding
2017, 4Q, 106   Control of bleeding of external naris using suture
2017, 4Q, 106   Nasal packing for epistaxis
2016, 4Q, 99-100   Root operation Control
2014, 4Q, 44   Bakri balloon for control of postpartum hemorrhage
2013, 3Q, 23   Control of intraoperative bleeding

AHA Coding Clinic for table ØW4
2019, 4Q, 30   Transfer large intestine to vagina
2016, 4Q, 101   Root operation Creation

AHA Coding Clinic for table ØW9
2017, 3Q, 12   Therapeutic and diagnostic paracentesis
2017, 2Q, 16   Incision and drainage of floor of mouth

AHA Coding Clinic for table ØWB
2019, 1Q, 27   Excision of pelvic sidewall mass
2017, 2Q, 16   Excision of floor of mouth
2016, 1Q, 21   Excision of urachal mass
2013, 4Q, 119   Excision of inclusion cyst of perineum

AHA Coding Clinic for table ØWC
2019, 4Q, 35   Extirpation of jaw
2017, 2Q, 16   Excision of floor of mouth

AHA Coding Clinic for table ØWH
2019, 4Q, 43   Unidirectional source brachytherapy
2018, 1Q, 25   Intrauterine brachytherapy & placement of tandems & ovoids
2017, 4Q, 104   Intrauterine brachytherapy & placement of tandems & ovoids
2016, 2Q, 14   Insertion of peritoneal totally implantable venous access device
2015, 2Q, 36   Insertion of infusion device into peritoneal cavity

AHA Coding Clinic for table ØWJ
2019, 1Q, 3-8   Whipple procedure
2019, 1Q, 25   Laparoscopic appendectomy converted to open procedure
2018, 3Q, 29   Decommissioning of left ventricular assist device with exploration of mediastinum
2016, 4Q, 58   Longitudinal vaginal septum
2013, 2Q, 36   Insertion of ventriculoperitoneal shunt with laparoscopic assistance

AHA Coding Clinic for table ØWQ
2017, 4Q, 106   Control of bleeding of external naris using suture
2017, 3Q, 8   Removal of silo and closure of gastroschisis
2016, 3Q, 3-7   Stoma creation & takedown procedures
2014, 4Q, 38   Abdominoplasty and abdominal wall plication for hernia repair
2014, 3Q, 28   Ileostomy takedown and parastomal hernia repair

AHA Coding Clinic for table ØWU
2017, 3Q, 8   First stage of gastroschisis repair with silo placement
2016, 3Q, 40   Omentoplasty
2015, 2Q, 29   Placement of Ioban™ antimicrobial drape over surgical wound
2014, 4Q, 39   Abdominal component release with placement of mesh for hernia repair
2012, 4Q, 101   Rib resection with reconstruction of anterior chest wall

AHA Coding Clinic for table ØWW
2015, 2Q, 9   Revision of ventriculoperitoneal (VP) shunt

AHA Coding Clinic for table ØWY
2016, 4Q, 112-113 Transplantation

Anatomical Regions, General

Ø   **Medical and Surgical**
W   **Anatomical Regions, General**
Ø   **Alteration**   Definition: Modifying the anatomic structure of a body part without affecting the function of the body part
                        Explanation: Principal purpose is to improve appearance

Body Part Character 4	Approach Character 5	Device Character 6	Qualifier Character 7
Ø Head 2 Face 4 Upper Jaw 5 Lower Jaw 6 Neck 8 Chest Wall F Abdominal Wall K Upper Back L Lower Back M Perineum, Male ♂ N Perineum, Female ♀	Ø Open 3 Percutaneous 4 Percutaneous Endoscopic	7 Autologous Tissue Substitute J Synthetic Substitute K Nonautologous Tissue Substitute Z No Device	Z No Qualifier

    ♂   ØWØM[Ø,3,4][7,J,K,Z]Z
    ♀   ØWØN[Ø,3,4][7,J,K,Z]Z

Ø   **Medical and Surgical**
W   **Anatomical Regions, General**
1   **Bypass**   Definition: Altering the route of passage of the contents of a tubular body part
                        Explanation: Rerouting contents of a body part to a downstream area of the normal route, to a similar route and body part, or to an abnormal route and dissimilar body part. Includes one or more anastomoses, with or without the use of a device.

Body Part Character 4	Approach Character 5	Device Character 6	Qualifier Character 7
1 Cranial Cavity	Ø Open	J Synthetic Substitute	9 Pleural Cavity, Right B Pleural Cavity, Left G Peritoneal Cavity J Pelvic Cavity
9 Pleural Cavity, Right B Pleural Cavity, Left J Pelvic Cavity Retropubic space	Ø Open 3 Percutaneous 4 Percutaneous Endoscopic	J Synthetic Substitute	4 Cutaneous 9 Pleural Cavity, Right B Pleural Cavity, Left G Peritoneal Cavity J Pelvic Cavity W Upper Vein Y Lower Vein
G Peritoneal Cavity	Ø Open 3 Percutaneous 4 Percutaneous Endoscopic	J Synthetic Substitute	4 Cutaneous 6 Bladder 9 Pleural Cavity, Right B Pleural Cavity, Left G Peritoneal Cavity J Pelvic Cavity W Upper Vein Y Lower Vein

   Non-OR   ØW1[9,B][Ø,3,4]J[4,G,W,Y]
   Non-OR   ØW1J[Ø,3,4]J[4,W,Y]
   Non-OR   ØW1G[Ø,3,4]J[9,B,G,J]

LC Limited Coverage   **NC** Noncovered   ⊞ Combination Member   HAC associated procedure   Combination Only   DRG Non-OR   Non-OR   New/Revised in GREEN

670   ICD-10-PCS 2021

Ø   Medical and Surgical
W   Anatomical Regions, General
2   Change   Definition: Taking out or off a device from a body part and putting back an identical or similar device in or on the same body part without cutting or puncturing the skin or a mucous membrane

                        Explanation: All CHANGE procedures are coded using the approach EXTERNAL

Body Part Character 4	Approach Character 5	Device Character 6	Qualifier Character 7

Ø Head
1 Cranial Cavity
2 Face
4 Upper Jaw
5 Lower Jaw
6 Neck
8 Chest Wall
9 Pleural Cavity, Right
B Pleural Cavity, Left
C Mediastinum
     Mediastinal cavity
     Mediastinal space
D Pericardial Cavity
F Abdominal Wall
G Peritoneal Cavity
H Retroperitoneum
     Retroperitoneal cavity
     Retroperitoneal space
J Pelvic Cavity
     Retropubic space
K Upper Back
L Lower Back
M Perineum, Male   ♂
N Perineum, Female   ♀
	X External	Ø Drainage Device
		Y Other Device
			Z No Qualifier

Non-OR	All body part, approach, device, and qualifier values	♂ ♀	ØW2MX[Ø,Y]Z ØW2NX[Ø,Y]Z

🔲 Limited Coverage   🔲 Noncovered   ⊞ Combination Member   HAC associated procedure   Combination Only   DRG Non-OR   Non-OR   New/Revised in GREEN

ICD-10-PCS 2021   671

Ø   Medical and Surgical
W   Anatomical Regions, General
3   Control   Definition: Stopping, or attempting to stop, postprocedural or other acute bleeding
                Explanation: None

Body Part Character 4	Approach Character 5	Device Character 6	Qualifier Character 7

Ø   Head
1   Cranial Cavity
2   Face
4   Upper Jaw
5   Lower Jaw
6   Neck
8   Chest Wall
9   Pleural Cavity, Right
B   Pleural Cavity, Left
C   Mediastinum
     Mediastinal cavity
     Mediastinal space
D   Pericardial Cavity
F   Abdominal Wall
G   Peritoneal Cavity
H   Retroperitoneum
     Retroperitoneal cavity
     Retroperitoneal space
J   Pelvic Cavity
     Retropubic space
K   Upper Back
L   Lower Back
M   Perineum, Male   ♂
N   Perineum, Female   ♀
	Ø Open
	3 Percutaneous
	4 Percutaneous Endoscopic
		Z No Device	Z No Qualifier

3 Oral Cavity and Throat	Ø Open 3 Percutaneous 4 Percutaneous Endoscopic 7 Via Natural or Artificial Opening 8 Via Natural or Artificial Opening Endoscopic X External	Z No Device	Z No Qualifier
P Gastrointestinal Tract Q Respiratory Tract R Genitourinary Tract	Ø Open 3 Percutaneous 4 Percutaneous Endoscopic 7 Via Natural or Artificial Opening 8 Via Natural or Artificial Opening Endoscopic	Z No Device	Z No Qualifier

Non-OR   ØW3P8ZZ   ♂   ØW3M[Ø,3,4]ZZ
                                                ♀   ØW3N[Ø,3,4]ZZ

Ø   Medical and Surgical
W   Anatomical Regions, General
4   Creation   Definition: Putting in or on biological or synthetic material to form a new body part that to the extent possible replicates the anatomic
                structure or function of an absent body part
                Explanation: Used for gender reassignment surgery and corrective procedures in individuals with congenital anomalies

Body Part Character 4	Approach Character 5	Device Character 6	Qualifier Character 7
M Perineum, Male ♂	Ø Open	7 Autologous Tissue Substitute J Synthetic Substitute K Nonautologous Tissue Substitute	Ø Vagina
N Perineum, Female ♀	Ø Open	7 Autologous Tissue Substitute J Synthetic Substitute K Nonautologous Tissue Substitute	1 Penis

    ♂   ØW4MØ[7,J,K]Ø
    ♀   ØW4NØ[7,J,K]1

Ø   Medical and Surgical
W   Anatomical Regions, General
8   Division   Definition: Cutting into a body part, without draining fluids and/or gases from the body part, in order to separate or transect a body part
                Explanation: All or a portion of the body part is separated into two or more portions

Body Part Character 4	Approach Character 5	Device Character 6	Qualifier Character 7
N Perineum, Female ♀	X External	Z No Device	Z No Qualifier

Non-OR   ØW8NXZZ   ♀   ØW8NXZZ

LC Limited Coverage   NC Noncovered   ⊞ Combination Member   HAC associated procedure   Combination Only   DRG Non-OR   Non-OR   New/Revised in GREEN

672   ICD-10-PCS 2021

Ø   **Medical and Surgical**
W   **Anatomical Regions, General**
9   **Drainage**   Definition: Taking or letting out fluids and/or gases from a body part
                        Explanation: The qualifier DIAGNOSTIC is used to identify drainage procedures that are biopsies

Body Part Character 4	Approach Character 5	Device Character 6	Qualifier Character 7

Ø Head
1 Cranial Cavity
2 Face
3 Oral Cavity and Throat
4 Upper Jaw
5 Lower Jaw
6 Neck
8 Chest Wall
9 Pleural Cavity, Right
B Pleural Cavity, Left
C Mediastinum
     Mediastinal cavity
     Mediastinal space
D Pericardial Cavity
F Abdominal Wall
G Peritoneal Cavity
H Retroperitoneum
     Retroperitoneal cavity
     Retroperitoneal space
K Upper Back
L Lower Back
M Perineum, Male ♂
N Perineum, Female ♀
	Ø Open
	3 Percutaneous
	4 Percutaneous Endoscopic
		Ø Drainage Device	**Z** No Qualifier

Ø Head
1 Cranial Cavity
2 Face
3 Oral Cavity and Throat
4 Upper Jaw
5 Lower Jaw
6 Neck
8 Chest Wall
9 Pleural Cavity, Right
B Pleural Cavity, Left
C Mediastinum
     Mediastinal cavity
     Mediastinal space
D Pericardial Cavity
F Abdominal Wall
G Peritoneal Cavity
H Retroperitoneum
     Retroperitoneal cavity
     Retroperitoneal space
K Upper Back
L Lower Back
M Perineum, Male ♂
N Perineum, Female ♀
	Ø Open
	3 Percutaneous
	4 Percutaneous Endoscopic
		Z No Device	**X** Diagnostic
			Z No Qualifier

J Pelvic Cavity
     Retropubic space
	Ø Open
	3 Percutaneous
	4 Percutaneous Endoscopic
	7 Via Natural or Artificial Opening
	8 Via Natural or Artificial Opening
	     Endoscopic
		Ø Drainage Device	**Z** No Qualifier

J Pelvic Cavity
     Retropubic space
	Ø Open
	3 Percutaneous
	4 Percutaneous Endoscopic
	7 Via Natural or Artificial Opening
	8 Via Natural or Artificial Opening
	     Endoscopic
		Z No Device	**X** Diagnostic
			Z No Qualifier

Non-OR	ØW9[Ø,8,9,B,K,L,M]ØØZ	♂	ØW9M[Ø,3,4]ØZ
Non-OR	ØW9[Ø,1,2,3,4,5,6,8,9,B,C,D,F,G,H,K,L,M,N]3ØZ	♂	ØW9M[Ø,3,4]Z[X,Z]
Non-OR	ØW9[Ø,1,8,F,K,L,M]4ØZ	♀	ØW9N[Ø,3,4]ØZ
Non-OR	ØW9[Ø,2,3,4,5,6,8,9,B,K,L,M,N]ØZX	♀	ØW9N[Ø,3]Z[X,Z]
Non-OR	ØW9[Ø,1,2,3,4,5,6,8,9,B,C,D,G,K,L,M,N]3ZX	♀	ØW9N4ZZ
Non-OR	ØW9[Ø,1,2,3,4,5,6,8,C,K,L,M,N]4ZX		
Non-OR	ØW9[Ø,8,9,B,K,L,M]ØZZ		
Non-OR	ØW9[Ø,1,2,3,4,5,6,8,9,B,C,D,F,G,H,K,L,M,N]3ZZ		
Non-OR	ØW9[Ø,1,8,F,K,L,M]4ZZ		
Non-OR	ØW9J[3,7,8]ØZ		
Non-OR	ØW9J[3,7,8]Z[X,Z]		

LC Limited Coverage   NC Noncovered   ⊞ Combination Member   HAC associated procedure   Combination Only   DRG Non-OR   Non-OR   New/Revised in GREEN

ICD-10-PCS 2021   673

Ø Medical and Surgical
W Anatomical Regions, General
B Excision   Definition: Cutting out or off, without replacement, a portion of a body part

         Explanation: The qualifier DIAGNOSTIC is used to identify excision procedures that are biopsies

Body Part Character 4	Approach Character 5	Device Character 6	Qualifier Character 7
Ø Head 2 Face 3 Oral Cavity and Throat 4 Upper Jaw 5 Lower Jaw 8 Chest Wall K Upper Back L Lower Back M Perineum, Male ♂ N Perineum, Female ♀	Ø Open 3 Percutaneous 4 Percutaneous Endoscopic X External	Z No Device	X Diagnostic Z No Qualifier
6 Neck F Abdominal Wall	Ø Open 3 Percutaneous 4 Percutaneous Endoscopic	Z No Device	X Diagnostic Z No Qualifier
6 Neck F Abdominal Wall	X External	Z No Device	2 Stoma X Diagnostic Z No Qualifier

C Mediastinum
  Mediastinal cavity
  Mediastinal space
H Retroperitoneum
  Retroperitoneal cavity
  Retroperitoneal space
	Ø Open
	3 Percutaneous
	4 Percutaneous Endoscopic
		Z No Device	X Diagnostic
			Z No Qualifier

Non-OR	ØWB[Ø,2,4,5,8,K,L,M][Ø,3,4,X]ZX	♂	ØWBM[Ø,3,4,X]Z[X,Z]
Non-OR	ØWB6[Ø,3,4]ZX	♀	ØWBN[Ø,3,4,X]Z[X,Z]
Non-OR	ØWB6XZX		
Non-OR	ØWBH[3,4]ZX		

Ø Medical and Surgical
W Anatomical Regions, General
C Extirpation   Definition: Taking or cutting out solid matter from a body part

         Explanation: The solid matter may be an abnormal byproduct of a biological function or a foreign body; it may be imbedded in a body part or in the lumen of a tubular body part. The solid matter may or may not have been previously broken into pieces.

Body Part Character 4	Approach Character 5	Device Character 6	Qualifier Character 7

1 Cranial Cavity
3 Oral Cavity and Throat
9 Pleural Cavity, Right
B Pleural Cavity, Left
C Mediastinum
  Mediastinal cavity
  Mediastinal space
D Pericardial Cavity
G Peritoneal Cavity
H Retroperitoneum
  Retroperitoneal cavity
  Retroperitoneal space
J Pelvic Cavity
  Retropubic space
	Ø Open
	3 Percutaneous
	4 Percutaneous Endoscopic
	X External
		Z No Device	Z No Qualifier

4 Upper Jaw 5 Lower Jaw	Ø Open 3 Percutaneous 4 Percutaneous Endoscopic	Z No Device	Z No Qualifier
P Gastrointestinal Tract Q Respiratory Tract R Genitourinary Tract	Ø Open 3 Percutaneous 4 Percutaneous Endoscopic 7 Via Natural or Artificial Opening 8 Via Natural or Artificial Opening Endoscopic X External	Z No Device	Z No Qualifier

Non-OR	ØWC[1,3]XZZ
Non-OR	ØWC[9,B][Ø,3,4,X]ZZ
Non-OR	ØWC[C,D,G,H,J]XZZ
Non-OR	ØWC[4,5][Ø,3,4]ZZ
Non-OR	ØWC[P,R][7,8,X]ZZ
Non-OR	ØWCQ[Ø,3,4,X]ZZ

LC Limited Coverage   NC Noncovered   ⊞ Combination Member   HAC associated procedure   Combination Only   DRG Non-OR   Non-OR   New/Revised in GREEN

674   ICD-10-PCS 2021

Ø   **Medical and Surgical**
W   **Anatomical Regions, General**
F   **Fragmentation**   Definition: Breaking solid matter in a body part into pieces

Explanation: Physical force (e.g., manual, ultrasonic) applied directly or indirectly is used to break the solid matter into pieces. The solid matter may be an abnormal byproduct of a biological function or a foreign body. The pieces of solid matter are not taken out.

Body Part Character 4	Approach Character 5	Device Character 6	Qualifier Character 7

1 Cranial Cavity   `NC`
3 Oral Cavity and Throat   `NC`
9 Pleural Cavity, Right   `NC`
B Pleural Cavity, Left   `NC`
C Mediastinum   `NC`
   Mediastinal cavity
   Mediastinal space
D Pericardial Cavity
G Peritoneal Cavity   `NC`
J Pelvic Cavity   `NC`
   Retropubic space
	Ø Open
	3 Percutaneous
	4 Percutaneous Endoscopic
	X External
		Z No Device	Z No Qualifier

P Gastrointestinal Tract `NC` Q Respiratory Tract `NC` R Genitourinary Tract	Ø Open 3 Percutaneous 4 Percutaneous Endoscopic 7 Via Natural or Artificial Opening 8 Via Natural or Artificial Opening Endoscopic X External	Z No Device	Z No Qualifier

Non-OR	ØWF[1,3,9,B,C,G]XZZ	`NC`	ØWF[1,3,9,B,C,G,J]XZZ
Non-OR	ØWFJ[Ø,3,4,X]ZZ	`NC`	ØWF[P,Q]XZZ
Non-OR	ØWFP[Ø,3,4,7,8,X]ZZ		
Non-OR	ØWFQXZZ		
Non-OR	ØWFR[Ø,3,4,7,8,X]ZZ		

Ø   **Medical and Surgical**
W   **Anatomical Regions, General**
H   **Insertion**   Definition: Putting in a nonbiological appliance that monitors, assists, performs, or prevents a physiological function but does not physically take the place of a body part

Explanation: None

Body Part Character 4	Approach Character 5	Device Character 6	Qualifier Character 7

Ø Head
1 Cranial Cavity
2 Face
3 Oral Cavity and Throat
4 Upper Jaw
5 Lower Jaw
6 Neck
8 Chest Wall
9 Pleural Cavity, Right
B Pleural Cavity, Left
C Mediastinum
   Mediastinal cavity
   Mediastinal space
D Pericardial Cavity
F Abdominal Wall
G Peritoneal Cavity
H Retroperitoneum
   Retroperitoneal cavity
   Retroperitoneal space
J Pelvic Cavity
   Retropubic space
K Upper Back
L Lower Back
M Perineum, Male
N Perineum, Female   ♀
	Ø Open
	3 Percutaneous
	4 Percutaneous Endoscopic
		1 Radioactive Element
		3 Infusion Device
		Y Other Device
			Z No Qualifier

P Gastrointestinal Tract Q Respiratory Tract R Genitourinary Tract	Ø Open 3 Percutaneous 4 Percutaneous Endoscopic 7 Via Natural or Artificial Opening 8 Via Natural or Artificial Opening Endoscopic	1 Radioactive Element 3 Infusion Device Y Other Device	Z No Qualifier

DRG Non-OR	ØWH[Ø,2,4,5,6,K,L,M][Ø,3,4][3,Y]Z	Non-OR	ØWHP[3,4,7,8][3,Y]Z
Non-OR	ØWH1[Ø,3,4]3Z	Non-OR	ØWHQ[Ø,7,8][3,Y]Z
Non-OR	ØWH[8,9,B][Ø,3,4][3,Y]Z	Non-OR	ØWHR[Ø,3,4,7,8][3,Y]Z
Non-OR	ØWHPØYZ	♀	ØWHN[Ø,3,4][3,Y]Z

`LC` Limited Coverage `NC` Noncovered ⊞ Combination Member HAC associated procedure Combination Only DRG Non-OR Non-OR New/Revised in GREEN

ICD-10-PCS 2021   675

Ø   Medical and Surgical
W   Anatomical Regions, General
J   Inspection   Definition: Visually and/or manually exploring a body part

Explanation: Visual exploration may be performed with or without optical instrumentation. Manual exploration may be performed directly or through intervening body layers.

Body Part Character 4	Approach Character 5	Device Character 6	Qualifier Character 7
Ø Head 2 Face 3 Oral Cavity and Throat 4 Upper Jaw 5 Lower Jaw 6 Neck 8 Chest Wall F Abdominal Wall K Upper Back L Lower Back M Perineum, Male ♂ N Perineum, Female ♀	Ø Open 3 Percutaneous 4 Percutaneous Endoscopic X External	Z No Device	Z No Qualifier

1   Cranial Cavity
9   Pleural Cavity, Right
B   Pleural Cavity, Left
C   Mediastinum
     Mediastinal cavity
     Mediastinal space
D   Pericardial Cavity
G   Peritoneal Cavity
H   Retroperitoneum
     Retroperitoneal cavity
     Retroperitoneal space
J   Pelvic Cavity
     Retropubic space
	Ø Open
	3 Percutaneous
	4 Percutaneous Endoscopic
		Z No Device	Z No Qualifier

P Gastrointestinal Tract Q Respiratory Tract R Genitourinary Tract	Ø Open 3 Percutaneous 4 Percutaneous Endoscopic 7 Via Natural or Artificial Opening 8 Via Natural or Artificial Opening Endoscopic	Z No Device	Z No Qualifier

DRG Non-OR	ØWJ[Ø,2,4,5,K,L]ØZZ	♂	ØWJM[Ø,3,4,X]ZZ
DRG Non-OR	ØWJM[Ø,4]ZZ	♀	ØWJN[Ø,3,4,X]ZZ
Non-OR	ØWJ3ØZZ		
Non-OR	ØWJ[Ø,2,3,4,5,6,8,F,K,L,M,N][3,X]ZZ		
Non-OR	ØWJ[Ø,2,3,4,5,K,L]4ZZ		
Non-OR	ØWJDØZZ		
Non-OR	ØWJ[1,9,B,C,D,G,H,J]3ZZ		
Non-OR	ØWJ[P,Q,R][3,7,8]ZZ		

Ø   Medical and Surgical
W   Anatomical Regions, General
M   Reattachment   Definition: Putting back in or on all or a portion of a separated body part to its normal location or other suitable location

Explanation: Vascular circulation and nervous pathways may or may not be reestablished

Body Part Character 4	Approach Character 5	Device Character 6	Qualifier Character 7
2 Face 4 Upper Jaw 5 Lower Jaw 6 Neck 8 Chest Wall F Abdominal Wall K Upper Back L Lower Back M Perineum, Male ♂ N Perineum, Female ♀	Ø Open	Z No Device	Z No Qualifier

♂	ØWMMØZZ
♀	ØWMNØZZ

LC Limited Coverage   **NC** Noncovered   ⊞ Combination Member   HAC associated procedure   Combination Only   DRG Non-OR   Non-OR   New/Revised in GREEN

676   ICD-10-PCS 2021

Ø   **Medical and Surgical**
W   **Anatomical Regions, General**
P   **Removal**   Definition: Taking out or off a device from a body part

                     Explanation: If a device is taken out and a similar device put in without cutting or puncturing the skin or mucous membrane, the procedure is coded to the root operation CHANGE. Otherwise, the procedure for taking out the device is coded to the root operation REMOVAL.

Body Part Character 4	Approach Character 5	Device Character 6	Qualifier Character 7

Ø Head
2 Face
4 Upper Jaw
5 Lower Jaw
6 Neck
8 Chest Wall
C Mediastinum
   Mediastinal cavity
   Mediastinal space
F Abdominal Wall
K Upper Back
L Lower Back
M Perineum, Male   ♂
N Perineum, Female   ♀
	Ø Open
	3 Percutaneous
	4 Percutaneous Endoscopic
	X External
		Ø Drainage Device
		1 Radioactive Element
		3 Infusion Device
		7 Autologous Tissue Substitute
		J Synthetic Substitute
		K Nonautologous Tissue Substitute
		Y Other Device
			Z No Qualifier

1 Cranial Cavity 9 Pleural Cavity, Right B Pleural Cavity, Left G Peritoneal Cavity J Pelvic Cavity Retropubic space	Ø Open 3 Percutaneous 4 Percutaneous Endoscopic	Ø Drainage Device 1 Radioactive Element 3 Infusion Device J Synthetic Substitute Y Other Device	Z No Qualifier
1 Cranial Cavity 9 Pleural Cavity, Right B Pleural Cavity, Left G Peritoneal Cavity J Pelvic Cavity Retropubic space	X External	Ø Drainage Device 1 Radioactive Element 3 Infusion Device	Z No Qualifier

D Pericardial Cavity
H Retroperitoneum
   Retroperitoneal cavity
   Retroperitoneal space
	Ø Open
	3 Percutaneous
	4 Percutaneous Endoscopic
		Ø Drainage Device
		1 Radioactive Element
		3 Infusion Device
		Y Other Device
			Z No Qualifier

D Pericardial Cavity
H Retroperitoneum
   Retroperitoneal cavity
   Retroperitoneal space
	X External	Ø Drainage Device
		1 Radioactive Element
		3 Infusion Device
			Z No Qualifier

P Gastrointestinal Tract Q Respiratory Tract R Genitourinary Tract	Ø Open 3 Percutaneous 4 Percutaneous Endoscopic 7 Via Natural or Artificial Opening 8 Via Natural or Artificial Opening Endoscopic X External	1 Radioactive Element 3 Infusion Device Y Other Device	Z No Qualifier

Non-OR	ØWP[Ø,2,4,5,6,8][Ø,3,4,X][Ø,1,3,7,J,K,Y]Z	♂	ØWPM[Ø,3,4,X][Ø,1,3,7,J,K,Y]Z
Non-OR	ØWP[C,F]X[Ø,1,3,7,J,K,Y]Z	♀	ØWPN[Ø,3,4,X][Ø,1,3,7,J,K,Y]Z
Non-OR	ØWP[K,L][Ø,3,4,X][Ø,1,3,7,J,K,Y]Z		
Non-OR	ØWPM[Ø,3,4][Ø,1,3,J,Y]Z		
Non-OR	ØWPMX[Ø,1,3,Y]Z		
Non-OR	ØWPNX[Ø,1,3,7,J,K,Y]Z		
Non-OR	ØWP1[Ø,3,4]3Z		
Non-OR	ØWP[9,B,J][Ø,3,4][Ø,1,3,J,Y]Z		
Non-OR	ØWP[1,9,B,G,J]X[Ø,1,3]Z		
Non-OR	ØWP[D,H]X[Ø,1,3]Z		
Non-OR	ØWPP[3,4,7,8,X][1,3,Y]Z		
Non-OR	ØWPQ73Z		
Non-OR	ØWPQ8[3,Y]Z		
Non-OR	ØWPQ[Ø,X][1,3,Y]Z		
Non-OR	ØWPR[Ø,3,4,7,8,X][1,3,Y]Z		

Ø   Medical and Surgical
W   Anatomical Regions, General
Q   Repair   Definition: Restoring, to the extent possible, a body part to its normal anatomic structure and function
                 Explanation: Used only when the method to accomplish the repair is not one of the other root operations

Body Part Character 4	Approach Character 5	Device Character 6	Qualifier Character 7
Ø Head 2 Face 3 Oral Cavity and Throat 4 Upper Jaw 5 Lower Jaw 8 Chest Wall K Upper Back L Lower Back M Perineum, Male ♂ N Perineum, Female ♀	Ø Open 3 Percutaneous 4 Percutaneous Endoscopic X External	Z No Device	Z No Qualifier
6 Neck F Abdominal Wall	Ø Open 3 Percutaneous 4 Percutaneous Endoscopic	Z No Device	Z No Qualifier
6 Neck F Abdominal Wall ⊞	X External	Z No Device	2 Stoma Z No Qualifier

C Mediastinum
    Mediastinal cavity
    Mediastinal space
	Ø Open
	3 Percutaneous
	4 Percutaneous Endoscopic
		Z No Device	Z No Qualifier

Non-OR	ØWQNXZZ
♂	ØWQM[Ø,3,4,X]ZZ
♀	ØWQN[Ø,3,4,X]ZZ

See Appendix L for Procedure Combinations
⊞   ØWQFXZ[2,Z]

Ø   Medical and Surgical
W   Anatomical Regions, General
U   Supplement   Definition: Putting in or on biological or synthetic material that physically reinforces and/or augments the function of a portion of a body part
                 Explanation: The biological material is non-living, or is living and from the same individual. The body part may have been previously replaced, and the SUPPLEMENT procedure is performed to physically reinforce and/or augment the function of the replaced body part.

Body Part Character 4	Approach Character 5	Device Character 6	Qualifier Character 7

Ø Head
2 Face
4 Upper Jaw
5 Lower Jaw
6 Neck
8 Chest Wall
C Mediastinum
    Mediastinal cavity
    Mediastinal space
F Abdominal Wall
K Upper Back
L Lower Back
M Perineum, Male   ♂
N Perineum, Female   ♀
	Ø Open
	4 Percutaneous Endoscopic
		7 Autologous Tissue Substitute
		J Synthetic Substitute
		K Nonautologous Tissue Substitute
			Z No Qualifier

♂	ØWUM[Ø,4][7,J,K]Z
♀	ØWUN[Ø,4][7,J,K]Z

LC Limited Coverage   **NC** Noncovered   ⊞ Combination Member   HAC associated procedure   Combination Only   DRG Non-OR   Non-OR   New/Revised in GREEN

678   ICD-10-PCS 2021

Ø   Medical and Surgical
W   Anatomical Regions, General
W   Revision   Definition: Correcting, to the extent possible, a portion of a malfunctioning device or the position of a displaced device

                     Explanation: Revision can include correcting a malfunctioning or displaced device by taking out or putting in components of the device such as a screw or pin

Body Part Character 4	Approach Character 5	Device Character 6	Qualifier Character 7

Ø Head
2 Face
4 Upper Jaw
5 Lower Jaw
6 Neck
8 Chest Wall
C Mediastinum
     Mediastinal cavity
     Mediastinal space
F Abdominal Wall
K Upper Back
L Lower Back
M Perineum, Male   ♂
N Perineum, Female   ♀
	Ø Open
	3 Percutaneous
	4 Percutaneous Endoscopic
	X External
		Ø Drainage Device
		1 Radioactive Element
		3 Infusion Device
		7 Autologous Tissue Substitute
		J Synthetic Substitute
		K Nonautologous Tissue Substitute
		Y Other Device
			Z No Qualifier

1 Cranial Cavity 9 Pleural Cavity, Right B Pleural Cavity, Left G Peritoneal Cavity J Pelvic Cavity Retropubic space	Ø Open 3 Percutaneous 4 Percutaneous Endoscopic X External	Ø Drainage Device 1 Radioactive Element 3 Infusion Device J Synthetic Substitute Y Other Device	Z No Qualifier

D Pericardial Cavity
H Retroperitoneum
     Retroperitoneal cavity
     Retroperitoneal space
	Ø Open
	3 Percutaneous
	4 Percutaneous Endoscopic
	X External
		Ø Drainage Device
		1 Radioactive Element
		3 Infusion Device
		Y Other Device
			Z No Qualifier

P Gastrointestinal Tract Q Respiratory Tract R Genitourinary Tract	Ø Open 3 Percutaneous 4 Percutaneous Endoscopic 7 Via Natural or Artificial Opening 8 Via Natural or Artificial Opening Endoscopic X External	1 Radioactive Element 3 Infusion Device Y Other Device	Z No Qualifier

DRG Non-OR	ØWW[Ø,2,4,5,6,K,L][Ø,3,4][Ø,1,3,7,J,K,Y]Z	♂	ØWWM[Ø,3,4,X][Ø,1,3,7,K,Y]Z
DRG Non-OR	ØWWM[Ø,3,4][Ø,1,3,J,Y]Z	♀	ØWWN[Ø,3,4,X][Ø,1,3,7,K,Y]Z
Non-OR	ØWW[Ø,2,4,5,6,C,F,K,L,M,N]X[Ø,1,3,7,J,K,Y]Z		
Non-OR	ØWW8[Ø,3,4,X][Ø,1,3,7,J,K,Y]Z		
Non-OR	ØWW[1,G,J]X[Ø,1,3,J,Y]Z		
Non-OR	ØWW[9,B][Ø,3,4,X][Ø,1,3,J,Y]Z		
Non-OR	ØWW[D,H]X[Ø,1,3,Y]Z		
Non-OR	ØWWP[3,4,7,8,X][1,3,Y]Z		
Non-OR	ØWWQ[Ø,X][1,3,Y]Z		
Non-OR	ØWWR[Ø,3,4,7,8,X][1,3,Y]Z		

Ø   Medical and Surgical
W   Anatomical Regions, General
Y   Transplantation   Definition: Putting in or on all or a portion of a living body part taken from another individual or animal to physically take the place and/or function of all or a portion of a similar body part

                     Explanation: The native body part may or may not be taken out, and the transplanted body part may take over all or a portion of its function

Body Part Character 4	Approach Character 5	Device Character 6	Qualifier Character 7
2 Face	Ø Open	Z No Device	Ø Allogeneic 1 Syngeneic

LC Limited Coverage   **NC** Noncovered   ⊞ Combination Member   HAC associated procedure   Combination Only   DRG Non-OR   Non-OR   New/Revised in **GREEN**

ICD-10-PCS 2021   **679**

Anatomical Regions, Upper Extremities ØXØ–ØXY

Character Meanings

This Character Meaning table is provided as a guide to assist the user in the identification of character members that may be found in this section of code tables. It **SHOULD NOT** be used to build a PCS code.

Operation–Character 3	Body Part–Character 4	Approach–Character 5	Device–Character 6	Qualifier–Character 7
Ø Alteration	Ø Forequarter, Right	Ø Open	Ø Drainage Device	Ø Allogeneic OR Complete
2 Change	1 Forequarter, Left	3 Percutaneous	1 Radioactive Element	1 High OR Syngeneic
3 Control	2 Shoulder Region, Right	4 Percutaneous Endoscopic	3 Infusion Device	2 Mid
6 Detachment	3 Shoulder Region, Left	X External	7 Autologous Tissue Substitute	3 Low
9 Drainage	4 Axilla, Right		J Synthetic Substitute	4 Complete 1st Ray
B Excision	5 Axilla, Left		K Nonautologous Tissue Substitute	5 Complete 2nd Ray
H Insertion	6 Upper Extremity, Right		Y Other Device	6 Complete 3rd Ray
J Inspection	7 Upper Extremity, Left		Z No Device	7 Complete 4th Ray
M Reattachment	8 Upper Arm, Right			8 Complete 5th Ray
P Removal	9 Upper Arm, Left			9 Partial 1st Ray
Q Repair	B Elbow Region, Right			B Partial 2nd Ray
R Replacement	C Elbow Region, Left			C Partial 3rd Ray
U Supplement	D Lower Arm, Right			D Partial 4th Ray
W Revision	F Lower Arm, Left			F Partial 5th Ray
X Transfer	G Wrist Region, Right			L Thumb, Right
Y Transplantation	H Wrist Region, Left			M Thumb, Left
	J Hand, Right			N Toe, Right
	K Hand, Left			P Toe, Left
	L Thumb, Right			X Diagnostic
	M Thumb, Left			Z No Qualifier
	N Index Finger, Right			
	P Index Finger, Left			
	Q Middle Finger, Right			
	R Middle Finger, Left			
	S Ring Finger, Right			
	T Ring Finger, Left			
	V Little Finger, Right			
	W Little Finger, Left			

AHA Coding Clinic for table ØX3

2016, 4Q, 99	Root operation Control
2015, 1Q, 35	Evacuation of hematoma for control of postprocedural bleeding
2013, 3Q, 23	Control of intraoperative bleeding

AHA Coding Clinic for table ØX6

2017, 2Q, 3-4	Qualifiers for the root operation detachment
2017, 2Q, 18	Removal of polydactyl digits
2017, 1Q, 52	Further distal phalangeal amputation
2016, 3Q, 33	Traumatic amputation of fingers with further revision amputation

AHA Coding Clinic for table ØXH

2017, 2Q, 20	Exchange of intramedullary antibiotic impregnated spacer

AHA Coding Clinic for table ØXP

2017, 2Q, 20	Exchange of intramedullary antibiotic impregnated spacer

AHA Coding Clinic for table ØXY

2016, 4Q, 112-113	Transplantation

Detachment Qualifier Descriptions

Qualifier Definition	Upper Arm	Lower Arm
1 **High:** Amputation at the proximal portion of the shaft of the:	Humerus	Radius/Ulna
2 **Mid:** Amputation at the middle portion of the shaft of the:	Humerus	Radius/Ulna
3 **Low:** Amputation at the distal portion of the shaft of the:	Humerus	Radius/Ulna

Qualifier Definition	Hand
Ø Complete 1st through 5th Rays Ray: digit of hand or foot with corresponding metacarpus or metatarsus	Through carpo-metacarpal joint, **Wrist**
4 Complete 1st Ray	Through carpo-metacarpal joint, **Thumb**
5 Complete 2nd Ray	Through carpo-metacarpal joint, **Index Finger**
6 Complete 3rd Ray	Through carpo-metacarpal joint, **Middle Finger**
7 Complete 4th Ray	Through carpo-metacarpal joint, **Ring Finger**
8 Complete 5th Ray	Through carpo-metacarpal joint, **Little Finger**
9 Partial 1st Ray	Anywhere along shaft or head of metacarpal bone, **Thumb**
B Partial 2nd Ray	Anywhere along shaft or head of metacarpal bone, **Index Finger**
C Partial 3rd Ray	Anywhere along shaft or head of metacarpal bone, **Middle Finger**
D Partial 4th Ray	Anywhere along shaft or head of metacarpal bone, **Ring Finger**
F Partial 5th Ray	Anywhere along shaft or head of metacarpal bone, **Little Finger**

Qualifier Definition	Thumb/Finger
Ø Complete	At the metacarpophalangeal joint
1 High	Anywhere along the proximal phalanx
2 Mid	Through the proximal interphalangeal joint or anywhere along the middle phalanx
3 Low	Through the distal interphalangeal joint or anywhere along the distal phalanx

Ø   **Medical and Surgical**
X   **Anatomical Regions, Upper Extremities**
Ø   **Alteration**   Definition: Modifying the anatomic structure of a body part without affecting the function of the body part
           Explanation: Principal purpose is to improve appearance

Body Part Character 4	Approach Character 5	Device Character 6	Qualifier Character 7
2 Shoulder Region, Right 3 Shoulder Region, Left 4 Axilla, Right 5 Axilla, Left 6 Upper Extremity, Right 7 Upper Extremity, Left 8 Upper Arm, Right 9 Upper Arm, Left B Elbow Region, Right C Elbow Region, Left D Lower Arm, Right F Lower Arm, Left G Wrist Region, Right H Wrist Region, Left	Ø Open 3 Percutaneous 4 Percutaneous Endoscopic	7 Autologous Tissue Substitute J Synthetic Substitute K Nonautologous Tissue Substitute Z No Device	Z No Qualifier

Ø   **Medical and Surgical**
X   **Anatomical Regions, Upper Extremities**
2   **Change**   Definition: Taking out or off a device from a body part and putting back an identical or similar device in or on the same body part without cutting or puncturing the skin or a mucous membrane
           Explanation: All CHANGE procedures are coded using the approach EXTERNAL

Body Part Character 4	Approach Character 5	Device Character 6	Qualifier Character 7
6 Upper Extremity, Right 7 Upper Extremity, Left	X External	Ø Drainage Device Y Other Device	Z No Qualifier

Non-OR   All body part, approach, device, and qualifier values

Ø   **Medical and Surgical**
X   **Anatomical Regions, Upper Extremities**
3   **Control**   Definition: Stopping, or attempting to stop, postprocedural or other acute bleeding
           Explanation: None

Body Part Character 4	Approach Character 5	Device Character 6	Qualifier Character 7
2 Shoulder Region, Right 3 Shoulder Region, Left 4 Axilla, Right 5 Axilla, Left 6 Upper Extremity, Right 7 Upper Extremity, Left 8 Upper Arm, Right 9 Upper Arm, Left B Elbow Region, Right C Elbow Region, Left D Lower Arm, Right F Lower Arm, Left G Wrist Region, Right H Wrist Region, Left J Hand, Right K Hand, Left	Ø Open 3 Percutaneous 4 Percutaneous Endoscopic	Z No Device	Z No Qualifier

Anatomical Regions, Upper Extremities

ØX6–ØX6

Ø   **Medical and Surgical**
X   **Anatomical Regions, Upper Extremities**
6   **Detachment**   Definition: Cutting off all or a portion of the upper or lower extremities

                                Explanation: The body part value is the site of the detachment, with a qualifier if applicable to further specify the level where the extremity was detached

Body Part Character 4	Approach Character 5	Device Character 6	Qualifier Character 7
Ø Forequarter, Right **1** Forequarter, Left **2** Shoulder Region, Right **3** Shoulder Region, Left **B** Elbow Region, Right **C** Elbow Region, Left	**Ø** Open	**Z** No Device	**Z** No Qualifier
8 Upper Arm, Right **9** Upper Arm, Left **D** Lower Arm, Right **F** Lower Arm, Left	**Ø** Open	**Z** No Device	**1** High **2** Mid **3** Low
J Hand, Right **K** Hand, Left	**Ø** Open	**Z** No Device	**Ø** Complete **4** Complete 1st Ray **5** Complete 2nd Ray **6** Complete 3rd Ray **7** Complete 4th Ray **8** Complete 5th Ray **9** Partial 1st Ray **B** Partial 2nd Ray **C** Partial 3rd Ray **D** Partial 4th Ray **F** Partial 5th Ray
L Thumb, Right **M** Thumb, Left **N** Index Finger, Right **P** Index Finger, Left **Q** Middle Finger, Right **R** Middle Finger, Left **S** Ring Finger, Right **T** Ring Finger, Left **V** Little Finger, Right **W** Little Finger, Left	**Ø** Open	**Z** No Device	**Ø** Complete **1** High **2** Mid **3** Low

LC Limited Coverage   NC Noncovered   ⊞ Combination Member   HAC associated procedure   Combination Only   DRG Non-OR   Non-OR   New/Revised in GREEN

684   ICD-10-PCS 2021

Ø   **Medical and Surgical**
X   **Anatomical Regions, Upper Extremities**
9   **Drainage**   Definition: Taking or letting out fluids and/or gases from a body part
                       Explanation: The qualifier DIAGNOSTIC is used to identify drainage procedures that are biopsies

Body Part Character 4	Approach Character 5	Device Character 6	Qualifier Character 7
2 Shoulder Region, Right 3 Shoulder Region, Left 4 Axilla, Right 5 Axilla, Left 6 Upper Extremity, Right 7 Upper Extremity, Left 8 Upper Arm, Right 9 Upper Arm, Left B Elbow Region, Right C Elbow Region, Left D Lower Arm, Right F Lower Arm, Left G Wrist Region, Right H Wrist Region, Left J Hand, Right K Hand, Left	Ø Open 3 Percutaneous 4 Percutaneous Endoscopic	Ø Drainage Device	Z No Qualifier
2 Shoulder Region, Right 3 Shoulder Region, Left 4 Axilla, Right 5 Axilla, Left 6 Upper Extremity, Right 7 Upper Extremity, Left 8 Upper Arm, Right 9 Upper Arm, Left B Elbow Region, Right C Elbow Region, Left D Lower Arm, Right F Lower Arm, Left G Wrist Region, Right H Wrist Region, Left J Hand, Right K Hand, Left	Ø Open 3 Percutaneous 4 Percutaneous Endoscopic	Z No Device	X Diagnostic Z No Qualifier

Non-OR   All body part, approach, device, and qualifier values

Ø   **Medical and Surgical**
X   **Anatomical Regions, Upper Extremities**
B   **Excision**   Definition: Cutting out or off, without replacement, a portion of a body part
                       Explanation: The qualifier DIAGNOSTIC is used to identify excision procedures that are biopsies

Body Part Character 4	Approach Character 5	Device Character 6	Qualifier Character 7
2 Shoulder Region, Right 3 Shoulder Region, Left 4 Axilla, Right 5 Axilla, Left 6 Upper Extremity, Right 7 Upper Extremity, Left 8 Upper Arm, Right 9 Upper Arm, Left B Elbow Region, Right C Elbow Region, Left D Lower Arm, Right F Lower Arm, Left G Wrist Region, Right H Wrist Region, Left J Hand, Right K Hand, Left	Ø Open 3 Percutaneous 4 Percutaneous Endoscopic	Z No Device	X Diagnostic Z No Qualifier

Non-OR   ØXB[2,3,4,5,6,7,8,9,B,C,D,F,G,H,J,K][Ø,3,4]ZX

Anatomical Regions, Upper Extremities *(left margin)*

Ø   **Medical and Surgical**
X   **Anatomical Regions, Upper Extremities**
H   **Insertion**   Definition: Putting in a nonbiological appliance that monitors, assists, performs, or prevents a physiological function but does not physically take the place of a body part

                 Explanation: None

Body Part Character 4	Approach Character 5	Device Character 6	Qualifier Character 7
2 Shoulder Region, Right 3 Shoulder Region, Left 4 Axilla, Right 5 Axilla, Left 6 Upper Extremity, Right 7 Upper Extremity, Left 8 Upper Arm, Right 9 Upper Arm, Left B Elbow Region, Right C Elbow Region, Left D Lower Arm, Right F Lower Arm, Left G Wrist Region, Right H Wrist Region, Left J Hand, Right K Hand, Left	Ø Open 3 Percutaneous 4 Percutaneous Endoscopic	1 Radioactive Element 3 Infusion Device Y Other Device	Z No Qualifier

DRG Non-OR   ØXH[2,3,4,5,6,7,8,9,B,C,D,F,G,H,J,K][Ø,3,4][3,Y]Z

Ø   **Medical and Surgical**
X   **Anatomical Regions, Upper Extremities**
J   **Inspection**   Definition: Visually and/or manually exploring a body part

                 Explanation: Visual exploration may be performed with or without optical instrumentation. Manual exploration may be performed directly or through intervening body layers.

Body Part Character 4	Approach Character 5	Device Character 6	Qualifier Character 7
2 Shoulder Region, Right 3 Shoulder Region, Left 4 Axilla, Right 5 Axilla, Left 6 Upper Extremity, Right 7 Upper Extremity, Left 8 Upper Arm, Right 9 Upper Arm, Left B Elbow Region, Right C Elbow Region, Left D Lower Arm, Right F Lower Arm, Left G Wrist Region, Right H Wrist Region, Left J Hand, Right K Hand, Left	Ø Open 3 Percutaneous 4 Percutaneous Endoscopic X External	Z No Device	Z No Qualifier

DRG Non-OR   ØXJ[2,3,4,5,6,7,8,9,B,C,D,F,G,H,J,K]ØZZ
Non-OR   ØXJ[2,3,4,5,6,7,8,9,B,C,D,F,G,H][3,4,X]ZZ
Non-OR   ØXJ[J,K][3,X]ZZ

LC Limited Coverage   NC Noncovered   ⊞ Combination Member   HAC associated procedure   Combination Only   DRG Non-OR   Non-OR   New/Revised in GREEN

686   ICD-10-PCS 2021

Ø   **Medical and Surgical**
X   **Anatomical Regions, Upper Extremities**
M   **Reattachment**   Definition: Putting back in or on all or a portion of a separated body part to its normal location or other suitable location

           Explanation: Vascular circulation and nervous pathways may or may not be reestablished

Body Part Character 4	Approach Character 5	Device Character 6	Qualifier Character 7
Ø Forequarter, Right 1 Forequarter, Left 2 Shoulder Region, Right 3 Shoulder Region, Left 4 Axilla, Right 5 Axilla, Left 6 Upper Extremity, Right 7 Upper Extremity, Left 8 Upper Arm, Right 9 Upper Arm, Left B Elbow Region, Right C Elbow Region, Left D Lower Arm, Right F Lower Arm, Left G Wrist Region, Right H Wrist Region, Left J Hand, Right K Hand, Left L Thumb, Right M Thumb, Left N Index Finger, Right P Index Finger, Left Q Middle Finger, Right R Middle Finger, Left S Ring Finger, Right T Ring Finger, Left V Little Finger, Right W Little Finger, Left	Ø Open	Z No Device	Z No Qualifier

Ø   **Medical and Surgical**
X   **Anatomical Regions, Upper Extremities**
P   **Removal**   Definition: Taking out or off a device from a body part

           Explanation: If a device is taken out and a similar device put in without cutting or puncturing the skin or mucous membrane, the procedure is coded to the root operation CHANGE. Otherwise, the procedure for taking out the device is coded to the root operation REMOVAL.

Body Part Character 4	Approach Character 5	Device Character 6	Qualifier Character 7
6 Upper Extremity, Right 7 Upper Extremity, Left	Ø Open 3 Percutaneous 4 Percutaneous Endoscopic X External	Ø Drainage Device 1 Radioactive Element 3 Infusion Device 7 Autologous Tissue Substitute J Synthetic Substitute K Nonautologous Tissue Substitute Y Other Device	Z No Qualifier

Non-OR   All body part, approach, device, and qualifier values

LC Limited Coverage   **NC** Noncovered   ⊞ Combination Member   HAC associated procedure   Combination Only   DRG Non-OR   Non-OR   New/Revised in GREEN

ICD-10-PCS 2021   **687**

Ø Medical and Surgical
X Anatomical Regions, Upper Extremities
Q Repair   Definition: Restoring, to the extent possible, a body part to its normal anatomic structure and function

Explanation: Used only when the method to accomplish the repair is not one of the other root operations

Body Part Character 4	Approach Character 5	Device Character 6	Qualifier Character 7
2 Shoulder Region, Right	Ø Open	Z No Device	Z No Qualifier
3 Shoulder Region, Left	3 Percutaneous		
4 Axilla, Right	4 Percutaneous Endoscopic		
5 Axilla, Left	X External		
6 Upper Extremity, Right			
7 Upper Extremity, Left			
8 Upper Arm, Right			
9 Upper Arm, Left			
B Elbow Region, Right			
C Elbow Region, Left			
D Lower Arm, Right			
F Lower Arm, Left			
G Wrist Region, Right			
H Wrist Region, Left			
J Hand, Right			
K Hand, Left			
L Thumb, Right			
M Thumb, Left			
N Index Finger, Right			
P Index Finger, Left			
Q Middle Finger, Right			
R Middle Finger, Left			
S Ring Finger, Right			
T Ring Finger, Left			
V Little Finger, Right			
W Little Finger, Left			

Ø Medical and Surgical
X Anatomical Regions, Upper Extremities
R Replacement   Definition: Putting in or on biological or synthetic material that physically takes the place and/or function of all or a portion of a body part

Explanation: The body part may have been taken out or replaced, or may be taken out, physically eradicated, or rendered nonfunctional during the REPLACEMENT procedure. A REMOVAL procedure is coded for taking out the device used in a previous replacement procedure.

Body Part Character 4	Approach Character 5	Device Character 6	Qualifier Character 7
L Thumb, Right	Ø Open	7 Autologous Tissue Substitute	N Toe, Right
M Thumb, Left	4 Percutaneous Endoscopic		P Toe, Left

LC Limited Coverage   NC Noncovered   ⊞ Combination Member   HAC associated procedure   Combination Only   DRG Non-OR   Non-OR   New/Revised in GREEN

688   ICD-10-PCS 2021

Ø   **Medical and Surgical**
X   **Anatomical Regions, Upper Extremities**
U   **Supplement**   Definition: Putting in or on biological or synthetic material that physically reinforces and/or augments the function of a portion of a body part

Explanation: The biological material is non-living, or is living and from the same individual. The body part may have been previously replaced, and the SUPPLEMENT procedure is performed to physically reinforce and/or augment the function of the replaced body part.

Body Part Character 4	Approach Character 5	Device Character 6	Qualifier Character 7
2 Shoulder Region, Right 3 Shoulder Region, Left 4 Axilla, Right 5 Axilla, Left 6 Upper Extremity, Right 7 Upper Extremity, Left 8 Upper Arm, Right 9 Upper Arm, Left B Elbow Region, Right C Elbow Region, Left D Lower Arm, Right F Lower Arm, Left G Wrist Region, Right H Wrist Region, Left J Hand, Right K Hand, Left L Thumb, Right M Thumb, Left N Index Finger, Right P Index Finger, Left Q Middle Finger, Right R Middle Finger, Left S Ring Finger, Right T Ring Finger, Left V Little Finger, Right W Little Finger, Left	Ø Open 4 Percutaneous Endoscopic	7 Autologous Tissue Substitute J Synthetic Substitute K Nonautologous Tissue Substitute	Z No Qualifier

Ø   **Medical and Surgical**
X   **Anatomical Regions, Upper Extremities**
W   **Revision**   Definition: Correcting, to the extent possible, a portion of a malfunctioning device or the position of a displaced device

Explanation: Revision can include correcting a malfunctioning or displaced device by taking out or putting in components of the device such as a screw or pin

Body Part Character 4	Approach Character 5	Device Character 6	Qualifier Character 7
6 Upper Extremity, Right 7 Upper Extremity, Left	Ø Open 3 Percutaneous 4 Percutaneous Endoscopic X External	Ø Drainage Device 3 Infusion Device 7 Autologous Tissue Substitute J Synthetic Substitute K Nonautologous Tissue Substitute Y Other Device	Z No Qualifier

DRG Non-OR	ØXW[6,7][Ø,3,4][Ø,3,7,J,K,Y]Z
Non-OR	ØXW[6,7]X[Ø,3,7,J,K,Y]Z

Ø   **Medical and Surgical**
X   **Anatomical Regions, Upper Extremities**
X   **Transfer**   Definition: Moving, without taking out, all or a portion of a body part to another location to take over the function of all or a portion of a body part

Explanation: The body part transferred remains connected to its vascular and nervous supply

Body Part Character 4	Approach Character 5	Device Character 6	Qualifier Character 7
N Index Finger, Right	Ø Open	Z No Device	L Thumb, Right
P Index Finger, Left	Ø Open	Z No Device	M Thumb, Left

Ø   **Medical and Surgical**
X   **Anatomical Regions, Upper Extremities**
Y   **Transplantation**   Definition: Putting in or on all or a portion of a living body part taken from another individual or animal to physically take the place and/or function of all or a portion of a similar body part

Explanation: The native body part may or may not be taken out, and the transplanted body part may take over all or a portion of its function

Body Part Character 4	Approach Character 5	Device Character 6	Qualifier Character 7
J Hand, Right K Hand, Left	Ø Open	Z No Device	Ø Allogeneic 1 Syngeneic

Anatomical Regions, Lower Extremities ØYØ–ØYW

Character Meanings

This Character Meaning table is provided as a guide to assist the user in the identification of character members that may be found in this section of code tables. It **SHOULD NOT** be used to build a PCS code.

Operation–Character 3	Body Part–Character 4	Approach–Character 5	Device–Character 6	Qualifier–Character 7
Ø Alteration	Ø Buttock, Right	Ø Open	Ø Drainage Device	Ø Complete
2 Change	1 Buttock, Left	3 Percutaneous	1 Radioactive Element	1 High
3 Control	2 Hindquarter, Right	4 Percutaneous Endoscopic	3 Infusion Device	2 Mid
6 Detachment	3 Hindquarter, Left	X External	7 Autologous Tissue Substitute	3 Low
9 Drainage	4 Hindquarter, Bilateral		J Synthetic Substitute	4 Complete 1st Ray
B Excision	5 Inguinal Region, Right		K Nonautologous Tissue Substitute	5 Complete 2nd Ray
H Insertion	6 Inguinal Region, Left		Y Other Device	6 Complete 3rd Ray
J Inspection	7 Femoral Region, Right		Z No Device	7 Complete 4th Ray
M Reattachment	8 Femoral Region, Left			8 Complete 5th Ray
P Removal	9 Lower Extremity, Right			9 Partial 1st Ray
Q Repair	A Inguinal Region, Bilateral			B Partial 2nd Ray
U Supplement	B Lower Extremity, Left			C Partial 3rd Ray
W Revision	C Upper Leg, Right			D Partial 4th Ray
	D Upper Leg, Left			F Partial 5th Ray
	E Femoral Region, Bilateral			X Diagnostic
	F Knee Region, Right			Z No Qualifier
	G Knee Region, Left			
	H Lower Leg, Right			
	J Lower Leg, Left			
	K Ankle Region, Right			
	L Ankle Region, Left			
	M Foot, Right			
	N Foot, Left			
	P 1st Toe, Right			
	Q 1st Toe, Left			
	R 2nd Toe, Right			
	S 2nd Toe, Left			
	T 3rd Toe, Right			
	U 3rd Toe, Left			
	V 4th Toe, Right			
	W 4th Toe, Left			
	X 5th Toe, Right			
	Y 5th Toe, Left			

AHA Coding Clinic for table ØY3
2016, 4Q, 99   Root operation Control
2013, 3Q, 23   Control of intraoperative bleeding

AHA Coding Clinic for table ØY6
2019, 2Q, 17   Cryoamputation of lower leg
2017, 2Q, 3-4   Qualifiers for the root operation detachment
2017, 1Q, 22   Chopart amputation of foot
2015, 2Q, 28   Partial amputation of hallux at interphalangeal Joint
2015, 1Q, 28   Mid-foot amputation

AHA Coding Clinic for table ØY9
2015, 1Q, 22   Incision and drainage of abscess of femoropopliteal bypass site
2015, 1Q, 22   Incision and drainage of groin abscess

Detachment Qualifier Descriptions

Qualifier Definition	Upper Leg	Lower Leg
1 **High:** Amputation at the proximal portion of the shaft of the:	Femur	Tibia/Fibula
2 **Mid:** Amputation at the middle portion of the shaft of the:	Femur	Tibia/Fibula
3 **Low:** Amputation at the distal portion of the shaft of the:	Femur	Tibia/Fibula

Qualifier Definition	Foot
Ø Complete 1st through 5th Rays Ray: digit of hand or foot with corresponding metacarpus or metatarsus	Through tarso-metatarsal Joint, **Ankle**
4 Complete 1st Ray	Through tarso-metatarsal joint, **Great Toe**
5 Complete 2nd Ray	Through tarso-metatarsal joint, **2nd Toe**
6 Complete 3rd Ray	Through tarso-metatarsal joint, **3rd Toe**
7 Complete 4th Ray	Through tarso-metatarsal joint, **4th Toe**
8 Complete 5th Ray	Through tarso-metatarsal joint, **Little Toe**
9 Partial 1st Ray	Anywhere along shaft or head of metatarsal bone, **Great Toe**
B Partial 2nd Ray	Anywhere along shaft or head of metatarsal bone, **2nd Toe**
C Partial 3rd Ray	Anywhere along shaft or head of metatarsal bone, **3rd Toe**
D Partial 4th Ray	Anywhere along shaft or head of metatarsal bone, **4th Toe**
F Partial 5th Ray	Anywhere along shaft or head of metatarsal bone, **Little Toe**

Qualifier Definition	Toe
Ø Complete	At the metatarsal-phalangeal joint
1 High	Anywhere along the proximal phalanx
2 Mid	Through the proximal interphalangeal joint or anywhere along the middle phalanx
3 Low	Through the distal interphalangeal joint or anywhere along the distal phalanx

Ø   **Medical and Surgical**
Y   **Anatomical Regions, Lower Extremities**
Ø   **Alteration**   Definition: Modifying the anatomic structure of a body part without affecting the function of the body part
                        Explanation: Principal purpose is to improve appearance

Body Part Character 4	Approach Character 5	Device Character 6	Qualifier Character 7
Ø Buttock, Right 1 Buttock, Left 9 Lower Extremity, Right B Lower Extremity, Left C Upper Leg, Right D Upper Leg, Left F Knee Region, Right G Knee Region, Left H Lower Leg, Right J Lower Leg, Left K Ankle Region, Right L Ankle Region, Left	Ø Open 3 Percutaneous 4 Percutaneous Endoscopic	7 Autologous Tissue Substitute J Synthetic Substitute K Nonautologous Tissue Substitute Z No Device	Z No Qualifier

Ø   **Medical and Surgical**
Y   **Anatomical Regions, Lower Extremities**
2   **Change**   Definition: Taking out or off a device from a body part and putting back an identical or similar device in or on the same body part without
                        cutting or puncturing the skin or a mucous membrane
                        Explanation: All CHANGE procedures are coded using the approach EXTERNAL

Body Part Character 4	Approach Character 5	Device Character 6	Qualifier Character 7
9 Lower Extremity, Right B Lower Extremity, Left	X External	Ø Drainage Device Y Other Device	Z No Qualifier

Non-OR   All body part, approach, device, and qualifier values

Ø   **Medical and Surgical**
Y   **Anatomical Regions, Lower Extremities**
3   **Control**   Definition: Stopping, or attempting to stop, postprocedural or other acute bleeding
                        Explanation: None

Body Part Character 4	Approach Character 5	Device Character 6	Qualifier Character 7

Ø Buttock, Right
1 Buttock, Left
5 Inguinal Region, Right
    Inguinal canal
    Inguinal triangle
6 Inguinal Region, Left
    See 5 Inguinal Region, Right
7 Femoral Region, Right
8 Femoral Region, Left
9 Lower Extremity, Right
B Lower Extremity, Left
C Upper Leg, Right
D Upper Leg, Left
F Knee Region, Right
G Knee Region, Left
H Lower Leg, Right
J Lower Leg, Left
K Ankle Region, Right
L Ankle Region, Left
M Foot, Right
N Foot, Left
	Ø Open
	3 Percutaneous
	4 Percutaneous Endoscopic
		Z No Device	Z No Qualifier

Anatomical Regions, Lower Extremities

Ø   **Medical and Surgical**
Y   **Anatomical Regions, Lower Extremities**
6   **Detachment**   Definition: Cutting off all or a portion of the upper or lower extremities

                 Explanation: The body part value is the site of the detachment, with a qualifier if applicable to further specify the level where the extremity was detached

Body Part Character 4	Approach Character 5	Device Character 6	Qualifier Character 7
2 Hindquarter, Right 3 Hindquarter, Left 4 Hindquarter, Bilateral 7 Femoral Region, Right 8 Femoral Region, Left F Knee Region, Right G Knee Region, Left	Ø Open	Z No Device	Z No Qualifier
C Upper Leg, Right D Upper Leg, Left H Lower Leg, Right J Lower Leg, Left	Ø Open	Z No Device	1 High 2 Mid 3 Low
M Foot, Right N Foot, Left	Ø Open	Z No Device	Ø Complete 4 Complete 1st Ray 5 Complete 2nd Ray 6 Complete 3rd Ray 7 Complete 4th Ray 8 Complete 5th Ray 9 Partial 1st Ray B Partial 2nd Ray C Partial 3rd Ray D Partial 4th Ray F Partial 5th Ray

P 1st Toe, Right
   Hallux
Q 1st Toe, Left
   See 1st Toe, Right
R 2nd Toe, Right
S 2nd Toe, Left
T 3rd Toe, Right
U 3rd Toe, Left
V 4th Toe, Right
W 4th Toe, Left
X 5th Toe, Right
Y 5th Toe, Left
	Ø Open	Z No Device	Ø Complete
			1 High
			2 Mid
			3 Low

LC Limited Coverage   NC Noncovered   ⊞ Combination Member   HAC associated procedure   Combination Only   DRG Non-OR   Non-OR   New/Revised in GREEN

694   ICD-10-PCS 2021

Ø **Medical and Surgical**
Y **Anatomical Regions, Lower Extremities**
9 **Drainage**   Definition: Taking or letting out fluids and/or gases from a body part
                         Explanation: The qualifier DIAGNOSTIC is used to identify drainage procedures that are biopsies

Body Part Character 4	Approach Character 5	Device Character 6	Qualifier Character 7

Ø Buttock, Right
1 Buttock, Left
5 Inguinal Region, Right
   Inguinal canal
   Inguinal triangle
6 Inguinal Region, Left
   See 5 Inguinal Region, Right
7 Femoral Region, Right
8 Femoral Region, Left
9 Lower Extremity, Right
B Lower Extremity, Left
C Upper Leg, Right
D Upper Leg, Left
F Knee Region, Right
G Knee Region, Left
H Lower Leg, Right
J Lower Leg, Left
K Ankle Region, Right
L Ankle Region, Left
M Foot, Right
N Foot, Left
	Ø Open
	3 Percutaneous
	4 Percutaneous Endoscopic
		Ø Drainage Device	Z No Qualifier

Ø Buttock, Right
1 Buttock, Left
5 Inguinal Region, Right
   Inguinal canal
   Inguinal triangle
6 Inguinal Region, Left
   See 5 Inguinal Region, Right
7 Femoral Region, Right
8 Femoral Region, Left
9 Lower Extremity, Right
B Lower Extremity, Left
C Upper Leg, Right
D Upper Leg, Left
F Knee Region, Right
G Knee Region, Left
H Lower Leg, Right
J Lower Leg, Left
K Ankle Region, Right
L Ankle Region, Left
M Foot, Right
N Foot, Left
	Ø Open
	3 Percutaneous
	4 Percutaneous Endoscopic
		Z No Device	X Diagnostic
			Z No Qualifier

Non-OR ØY9[Ø,1,7,8,9,B,C,D,F,G,H,J,K,L,M,N][Ø,3,4]ØZ
Non-OR ØY9[5,6]3ØZ
Non-OR ØY9[Ø,1,7,8,9,B,C,D,F,G,H,J,K,L,M,N][Ø,3,4]Z[X,Z]
Non-OR ØY9[5,6]3ZZ

Ø   **Medical and Surgical**
Y   **Anatomical Regions, Lower Extremities**
B   **Excision**   Definition: Cutting out or off, without replacement, a portion of a body part
                            Explanation: The qualifier DIAGNOSTIC is used to identify excision procedures that are biopsies

Body Part Character 4	Approach Character 5	Device Character 6	Qualifier Character 7

Ø Buttock, Right
1 Buttock, Left
5 Inguinal Region, Right
   Inguinal canal
   Inguinal triangle
6 Inguinal Region, Left
   See 5 Inguinal Region, Right
7 Femoral Region, Right
8 Femoral Region, Left
9 Lower Extremity, Right
B Lower Extremity, Left
C Upper Leg, Right
D Upper Leg, Left
F Knee Region, Right
G Knee Region, Left
H Lower Leg, Right
J Lower Leg, Left
K Ankle Region, Right
L Ankle Region, Left
M Foot, Right
N Foot, Left
	Ø Open
	3 Percutaneous
	4 Percutaneous Endoscopic
		Z No Device	X Diagnostic
			Z No Qualifier

Non-OR   ØYB[Ø,1,9,B,C,D,F,G,H,J,K,L,M,N][Ø,3,4]ZX

Ø   **Medical and Surgical**
Y   **Anatomical Regions, Lower Extremities**
H   **Insertion**   Definition: Putting in a nonbiological appliance that monitors, assists, performs, or prevents a physiological function but does not physically
                            take the place of a body part
                            Explanation: None

Body Part Character 4	Approach Character 5	Device Character 6	Qualifier Character 7

Ø Buttock, Right
1 Buttock, Left
5 Inguinal Region, Right
   Inguinal canal
   Inguinal triangle
6 Inguinal Region, Left
   See 5 Inguinal Region, Right
7 Femoral Region, Right
8 Femoral Region, Left
9 Lower Extremity, Right
B Lower Extremity, Left
C Upper Leg, Right
D Upper Leg, Left
F Knee Region, Right
G Knee Region, Left
H Lower Leg, Right
J Lower Leg, Left
K Ankle Region, Right
L Ankle Region, Left
M Foot, Right
N Foot, Left
	Ø Open
	3 Percutaneous
	4 Percutaneous Endoscopic
		1 Radioactive Element
		3 Infusion Device
		Y Other Device
			Z No Qualifier

DRG Non-OR   ØYH[Ø,1,5,6,7,8,9,B,C,D,F,G,H,J,K,L,M,N][Ø,3,4][3,Y]Z

Ø   **Medical and Surgical**
Y   **Anatomical Regions, Lower Extremities**
J   **Inspection**   Definition: Visually and/or manually exploring a body part

                     Explanation: Visual exploration may be performed with or without optical instrumentation. Manual exploration may be performed directly or through intervening body layers.

Body Part Character 4	Approach Character 5	Device Character 6	Qualifier Character 7

Ø   Buttock, Right
1   Buttock, Left
5   Inguinal Region, Right
     Inguinal canal
     Inguinal triangle
6   Inguinal Region, Left
     See 5 Inguinal Region, Right
7   Femoral Region, Right
8   Femoral Region, Left
9   Lower Extremity, Right
A   Inguinal Region, Bilateral
     See 5 Inguinal Region, Right
B   Lower Extremity, Left
C   Upper Leg, Right
D   Upper Leg, Left
E   Femoral Region, Bilateral
F   Knee Region, Right
G   Knee Region, Left
H   Lower Leg, Right
J   Lower Leg, Left
K   Ankle Region, Right
L   Ankle Region, Left
M   Foot, Right
N   Foot, Left
	Ø Open
	3 Percutaneous
	4 Percutaneous Endoscopic
	X External
		Z No Device	Z No Qualifier

DRG Non-OR	ØYJ[Ø,1,8,9,B,C,D,E,F,G,H,J,K,L,M,N]ØZZ
Non-OR	ØYJ[Ø,1,9,B,C,D,F,G,H,J,K,L,M,N][3,4,X]ZZ
Non-OR	ØYJ[5,6,7,8,A,E][3,X]ZZ

LC Limited Coverage   NC Noncovered   ⊞ Combination Member   HAC associated procedure   Combination Only   DRG Non-OR   Non-OR   New/Revised in GREEN

ICD-10-PCS 2021   **697**

Ø Medical and Surgical
Y Anatomical Regions, Lower Extremities
M Reattachment   Definition: Putting back in or on all or a portion of a separated body part to its normal location or other suitable location

Explanation: Vascular circulation and nervous pathways may or may not be reestablished

Body Part Character 4	Approach Character 5	Device Character 6	Qualifier Character 7
Ø Buttock, Right	Ø Open	Z No Device	Z No Qualifier
1 Buttock, Left			
2 Hindquarter, Right			
3 Hindquarter, Left			
4 Hindquarter, Bilateral			
5 Inguinal Region, Right Inguinal canal Inguinal triangle			
6 Inguinal Region, Left See 5 Inguinal Region, Right			
7 Femoral Region, Right			
8 Femoral Region, Left			
9 Lower Extremity, Right			
B Lower Extremity, Left			
C Upper Leg, Right			
D Upper Leg, Left			
F Knee Region, Right			
G Knee Region, Left			
H Lower Leg, Right			
J Lower Leg, Left			
K Ankle Region, Right			
L Ankle Region, Left			
M Foot, Right			
N Foot, Left			
P 1st Toe, Right Hallux			
Q 1st Toe, Left See 1st Toe, Right			
R 2nd Toe, Right			
S 2nd Toe, Left			
T 3rd Toe, Right			
U 3rd Toe, Left			
V 4th Toe, Right			
W 4th Toe, Left			
X 5th Toe, Right			
Y 5th Toe, Left			

Ø Medical and Surgical
Y Anatomical Regions, Lower Extremities
P Removal   Definition: Taking out or off a device from a body part

Explanation: If a device is taken out and a similar device put in without cutting or puncturing the skin or mucous membrane, the procedure is coded to the root operation CHANGE. Otherwise, the procedure for taking out the device is coded to the root operation REMOVAL.

Body Part Character 4	Approach Character 5	Device Character 6	Qualifier Character 7
9 Lower Extremity, Right	Ø Open	Ø Drainage Device	Z No Qualifier
B Lower Extremity, Left	3 Percutaneous	1 Radioactive Element	
	4 Percutaneous Endoscopic	3 Infusion Device	
	X External	7 Autologous Tissue Substitute	
		J Synthetic Substitute	
		K Nonautologous Tissue Substitute	
		Y Other Device	

Non-OR   All body part, approach, device, and qualifier values

Ø Medical and Surgical
Y Anatomical Regions, Lower Extremities
Q Repair   Definition: Restoring, to the extent possible, a body part to its normal anatomic structure and function
                            Explanation: Used only when the method to accomplish the repair is not one of the other root operations

Body Part Character 4	Approach Character 5	Device Character 6	Qualifier Character 7
Ø Buttock, Right	Ø Open	Z No Device	Z No Qualifier
1 Buttock, Left	3 Percutaneous		
5 Inguinal Region, Right	4 Percutaneous Endoscopic		
Inguinal canal	X External		
Inguinal triangle			
6 Inguinal Region, Left			
See 5 Inguinal Region, Right			
7 Femoral Region, Right			
8 Femoral Region, Left			
9 Lower Extremity, Right			
A Inguinal Region, Bilateral			
See 5 Inguinal Region, Right			
B Lower Extremity, Left			
C Upper Leg, Right			
D Upper Leg, Left			
E Femoral Region, Bilateral			
F Knee Region, Right			
G Knee Region, Left			
H Lower Leg, Right			
J Lower Leg, Left			
K Ankle Region, Right			
L Ankle Region, Left			
M Foot, Right			
N Foot, Left			
P 1st Toe, Right			
Hallux			
Q 1st Toe, Left			
See 1st Toe, Right			
R 2nd Toe, Right			
S 2nd Toe, Left			
T 3rd Toe, Right			
U 3rd Toe, Left			
V 4th Toe, Right			
W 4th Toe, Left			
X 5th Toe, Right			
Y 5th Toe, Left			

Non-OR   ØYQ[5,6,7,8,A,E]XZZ

Anatomical Regions, Lower Extremities *(left margin)*

Ø   **Medical and Surgical**
Y   **Anatomical Regions, Lower Extremities**
U   **Supplement**   Definition: Putting in or on biological or synthetic material that physically reinforces and/or augments the function of a portion of a body part

Explanation: The biological material is non-living, or is living and from the same individual. The body part may have been previously replaced, and the SUPPLEMENT procedure is performed to physically reinforce and/or augment the function of the replaced body part.

Body Part Character 4	Approach Character 5	Device Character 6	Qualifier Character 7

Ø Buttock, Right
1 Buttock, Left
5 Inguinal Region, Right
   Inguinal canal
   Inguinal triangle
6 Inguinal Region, Left
   See 5 Inguinal Region, Right
7 Femoral Region, Right
8 Femoral Region, Left
9 Lower Extremity, Right
A Inguinal Region, Bilateral
   See 5 Inguinal Region, Right
B Lower Extremity, Left
C Upper Leg, Right
D Upper Leg, Left
E Femoral Region, Bilateral
F Knee Region, Right
G Knee Region, Left
H Lower Leg, Right
J Lower Leg, Left
K Ankle Region, Right
L Ankle Region, Left
M Foot, Right
N Foot, Left
P 1st Toe, Right
   Hallux
Q 1st Toe, Left
   See 1st Toe, Right
R 2nd Toe, Right
S 2nd Toe, Left
T 3rd Toe, Right
U 3rd Toe, Left
V 4th Toe, Right
W 4th Toe, Left
X 5th Toe, Right
Y 5th Toe, Left
	Ø Open
	4 Percutaneous Endoscopic
		7 Autologous Tissue Substitute
		J Synthetic Substitute
		K Nonautologous Tissue Substitute
			Z No Qualifier

Ø   **Medical and Surgical**
Y   **Anatomical Regions, Lower Extremities**
W   **Revision**   Definition: Correcting, to the extent possible, a portion of a malfunctioning device or the position of a displaced device

Explanation: Revision can include correcting a malfunctioning or displaced device by taking out or putting in components of the device such as a screw or pin

Body Part Character 4	Approach Character 5	Device Character 6	Qualifier Character 7
9 Lower Extremity, Right B Lower Extremity, Left	Ø Open 3 Percutaneous 4 Percutaneous Endoscopic X External	Ø Drainage Device 3 Infusion Device 7 Autologous Tissue Substitute J Synthetic Substitute K Nonautologous Tissue Substitute Y Other Device	Z No Qualifier

DRG Non-OR   ØYW[9,B][Ø,3,4][Ø,3,7,J,K,Y]Z
Non-OR   ØYW[9,B]X[Ø,3,7,J,K,Y]Z

Obstetrics 1Ø2–1ØY

Character Meanings

This Character Meaning table is provided as a guide to assist the user in the identification of character members that may be found in this section of code tables. It **SHOULD NOT** be used to build a PCS code.

Ø: Pregnancy

Operation–Character 3		Body Part–Character 4		Approach–Character 5		Device–Character 6		Qualifier–Character 7	
2	Change	Ø	Products of Conception	Ø	Open	3	Monitoring Electrode	Ø	High
9	Drainage	1	Products of Conception, Retained	3	Percutaneous	Y	Other Device	1	Low
A	Abortion	2	Products of Conception, Ectopic	4	Percutaneous Endoscopic	Z	No Device	2	Extraperitoneal
D	Extraction			7	Via Natural or Artificial Opening			3	Low Forceps
E	Delivery			8	Via Natural or Artificial Opening Endoscopic			4	Mid Forceps
H	Insertion			X	External			5	High Forceps
J	Inspection							6	Vacuum
P	Removal							7	Internal Version
Q	Repair							8	Other
S	Reposition							9	Fetal Blood OR Manual
T	Resection							A	Fetal Cerebrospinal Fluid
Y	Transplantation							B	Fetal Fluid, Other
								C	Amniotic Fluid, Therapeutic
								D	Fluid, Other
								E	Nervous System
								F	Cardiovascular System
								G	Lymphatics & Hemic
								H	Eye
								J	Ear, Nose & Sinus
								K	Respiratory System
								L	Mouth & Throat
								M	Gastrointestinal System
								N	Hepatobiliary & Pancreas
								P	Endocrine System
								Q	Skin
								R	Musculoskeletal System
								S	Urinary System
								T	Female Reproductive System
								U	Amniotic Fluid, Diagnostic
								V	Male Reproductive System
								W	Laminaria
								X	Abortifacient
								Y	Other Body System
								Z	No Qualifier

AHA Coding Clinic for table 1Ø9

| 2014, 3Q, 12 | Fetoscopic laser photocoagulation and laser microseptostomy for twin-twin transfusion syndrome |
| 2014, 2Q, 9 | Pitocin administration to augment labor |

AHA Coding Clinic for table 1ØD

2018, 4Q, 49-51	Revised qualifier values for root operation "extraction" (cesarean delivery)
2018, 2Q, 17	High transverse cesarean section
2016, 1Q, 9	Vaginal delivery assisted by vacuum and low forceps extraction
2014, 4Q, 43	Cesarean delivery assisted by vacuum extraction
2014, 4Q, 43	Vacuum dilation and curettage for blighted ovum

AHA Coding Clinic for table 1ØE

2017, 3Q, 5	Delivery of placenta
2016, 2Q, 34	Assisted vaginal delivery
2014, 4Q, 17	RH (D) alloimmunization (sensitization)
2014, 2Q, 9	Pitocin administration to augment labor

AHA Coding Clinic for table 1ØH

| 2013, 2Q, 36 | Intrauterine pressure monitor |

AHA Coding Clinic for table 1ØQ

| 2014, 3Q, 12 | Fetoscopic laser photocoagulation and laser microseptostomy for twin-twin transfusion syndrome |

AHA Coding Clinic for table 1ØT

| 2015, 3Q, 31 | Laparoscopic partial salpingectomy for ectopic pregnancy |

1 Obstetrics
Ø Pregnancy
2 Change

Definition: Taking out or off a device from a body part and putting back an identical or similar device in or on the same body part without cutting or puncturing the skin or a mucous membrane

Explanation: None

Body Part Character 4	Approach Character 5	Device Character 6	Qualifier Character 7
Ø Products of Conception ♀	7 Via Natural or Artificial Opening	3 Monitoring Electrode Y Other Device	Z No Qualifier

Non-OR	All body part, approach, device, and qualifier values	♀ All body part, approach, device, and qualifier values

1 Obstetrics
Ø Pregnancy
9 Drainage

Definition: Taking or letting out fluids and/or gases from a body part

Explanation: None

Body Part Character 4	Approach Character 5	Device Character 6	Qualifier Character 7
Ø Products of Conception ♀	Ø Open 3 Percutaneous 4 Percutaneous Endoscopic 7 Via Natural or Artificial Opening 8 Via Natural or Artificial Opening Endoscopic	Z No Device	9 Fetal Blood A Fetal Cerebrospinal Fluid B Fetal Fluid, Other C Amniotic Fluid, Therapeutic D Fluid, Other U Amniotic Fluid, Diagnostic

Non-OR	All body part, approach, device, and qualifier values	♀ All body part, approach, device, and qualifier values

1 Obstetrics
Ø Pregnancy
A Abortion

Definition: Artificially terminating a pregnancy

Explanation: None

Body Part Character 4	Approach Character 5	Device Character 6	Qualifier Character 7
Ø Products of Conception ♀	Ø Open 3 Percutaneous 4 Percutaneous Endoscopic 8 Via Natural or Artificial Opening Endoscopic	Z No Device	Z No Qualifier
Ø Products of Conception ♀	7 Via Natural or Artificial Opening	Z No Device	6 Vacuum W Laminaria X Abortifacient Z No Qualifier

Non-OR	1ØAØ7Z[6,W,X]	♀ All body part, approach, device, and qualifier values

1 Obstetrics
Ø Pregnancy
D Extraction

Definition: Pulling or stripping out or off all or a portion of a body part by the use of force

Explanation: None

Body Part Character 4	Approach Character 5	Device Character 6	Qualifier Character 7
Ø Products of Conception 🅀ᴬ ♀	Ø Open	Z No Device	Ø High 1 Low 2 Extraperitoneal
Ø Products of Conception 🅀ᴬ ♀	7 Via Natural or Artificial Opening	Z No Device	3 Low Forceps 4 Mid Forceps 5 High Forceps 6 Vacuum 7 Internal Version 8 Other
1 Products of Conception, Retained ♀	7 Via Natural or Artificial Opening 8 Via Natural or Artificial Opening Endoscopic	Z No Device	9 Manual Z No Qualifier
2 Products of Conception, Ectopic ♀	Ø Open 4 Percutaneous Endoscopic 7 Via Natural or Artificial Opening 8 Via Natural or Artificial Opening Endoscopic	Z No Device	Z No Qualifier

DRG Non-OR	1ØDØ7Z[3,4,5,6,7,8]	♀ All body part, approach, device, and qualifier values
🅀ᴬ	1ØDØØZ[Ø,1,2] except when a corresponding SDX of Z37.Ø-Z37.9 is also reported	
🅀ᴬ	1ØDØ7Z[3,4,5,7] except when a corresponding SDX of Z37.Ø-Z37.9 is also reported	

🄻🄲 Limited Coverage   🄽🄲 Noncovered   🅀ᴬ Questionable Admit   ⊞ Combination Member   HAC   Combination Only   DRG Non-OR   Non-OR   New/Revised in GREEN

702   ICD-10-PCS 2021

1Ø2–1ØD

1   Obstetrics
Ø   Pregnancy
E   Delivery   Definition: Assisting the passage of the products of conception from the genital canal

                     Explanation: None

Body Part Character 4	Approach Character 5	Device Character 6	Qualifier Character 7
Ø Products of Conception 0A ♀	X External	Z No Device	Z No Qualifier

DRG Non-OR 10EØXZZ		♀ All body part, approach, device, and qualifier values	
0A 10EØXZZ except when a corresponding SDX of Z37.Ø-Z37.9 is also reported			

1   Obstetrics
Ø   Pregnancy
H   Insertion   Definition: Putting in a nonbiological appliance that monitors, assists, performs, or prevents a physiological function but does not physically take the place of a body part

                     Explanation: None

Body Part Character 4	Approach Character 5	Device Character 6	Qualifier Character 7
Ø Products of Conception ♀	Ø Open 7 Via Natural or Artificial Opening	3 Monitoring Electrode Y Other Device	Z No Qualifier

Non-OR All body part, approach, device, and qualifier values		♀ All body part, approach, device, and qualifier values	

1   Obstetrics
Ø   Pregnancy
J   Inspection   Definition: Visually and/or manually exploring a body part

                     Explanation: Visual exploration may be performed with or without optical instrumentation. Manual exploration may be performed directly or through intervening body layers.

Body Part Character 4	Approach Character 5	Device Character 6	Qualifier Character 7
Ø Products of Conception ♀ 1 Products of Conception, Retained ♀ 2 Products of Conception, Ectopic ♀	Ø Open 3 Percutaneous 4 Percutaneous Endoscopic 7 Via Natural or Artificial Opening 8 Via Natural or Artificial Opening Endoscopic X External	Z No Device	Z No Qualifier

Non-OR All body part, approach, device, and qualifier values		♀ All body part, approach, device, and qualifier values	

1   Obstetrics
Ø   Pregnancy
P   Removal   Definition: Taking out or off a device from a body part, region or orifice

                     Explanation: If a device is taken out and a similar device put in without cutting or puncturing the skin or mucous membrane, the procedure is coded to the root operation CHANGE. Otherwise, the procedure for taking out a device is coded to the root operation REMOVAL.

Body Part Character 4	Approach Character 5	Device Character 6	Qualifier Character 7
Ø Products of Conception ♀	Ø Open 7 Via Natural or Artificial Opening	3 Monitoring Electrode Y Other Device	Z No Qualifier

Non-OR All body part, approach, device, and qualifier values		♀ All body part, approach, device, and qualifier values	

1   Obstetrics
Ø   Pregnancy
Q   Repair   Definition: Restoring, to the extent possible, a body part to its normal anatomic structure and function

                     Explanation: Used only when the method to accomplish the repair is not one of the other root operations

Body Part Character 4	Approach Character 5	Device Character 6	Qualifier Character 7
Ø Products of Conception ♀	Ø Open 3 Percutaneous 4 Percutaneous Endoscopic 7 Via Natural or Artificial Opening 8 Via Natural or Artificial Opening Endoscopic	Y Other Device Z No Device	E Nervous System F Cardiovascular System G Lymphatics and Hemic H Eye J Ear, Nose and Sinus K Respiratory System L Mouth and Throat M Gastrointestinal System N Hepatobiliary and Pancreas P Endocrine System Q Skin R Musculoskeletal System S Urinary System T Female Reproductive System V Male Reproductive System Y Other Body System

Non-OR All body part, approach, device, and qualifier values		♀ All body part, approach, device, and qualifier values	

1 **Obstetrics**
Ø **Pregnancy**
S **Reposition** Definition: Moving to its normal location, or other suitable location, all or a portion of a body part

Explanation: The body part is moved to a new location from an abnormal location, or from a normal location where it is not functioning correctly. The body part may or may not be cut out or off to be moved to the new location.

Body Part Character 4	Approach Character 5	Device Character 6	Qualifier Character 7
Ø Products of Conception ♀	7 Via Natural or Artificial Opening X External	Z No Device	Z No Qualifier
2 Products of Conception, Ectopic ♀	Ø Open 3 Percutaneous 4 Percutaneous Endoscopic 7 Via Natural or Artificial Opening 8 Via Natural or Artificial Opening Endoscopic	Z No Device	Z No Qualifier

Non-OR 10SØ[7,X]ZZ   ♀ All body part, approach, device, and qualifier values

1 **Obstetrics**
Ø **Pregnancy**
T **Resection** Definition: Cutting out or off, without replacement, all of a body part

Explanation: None

Body Part Character 4	Approach Character 5	Device Character 6	Qualifier Character 7
2 Products of Conception, Ectopic ♀	Ø Open 3 Percutaneous 4 Percutaneous Endoscopic 7 Via Natural or Artificial Opening 8 Via Natural or Artificial Opening Endoscopic	Z No Device	Z No Qualifier

♀ All body part, approach, device, and qualifier values

1 **Obstetrics**
Ø **Pregnancy**
Y **Transplantation** Definition: Putting in or on all or a portion of a living body part taken from another individual or animal to physically take the place and/or function of all or a portion of a similar body part

Explanation: The native body part may or may not be taken out, and the transplanted body part may take over all or a portion of its function

Body Part Character 4	Approach Character 5	Device Character 6	Qualifier Character 7
Ø Products of Conception ♀	3 Percutaneous 4 Percutaneous Endoscopic 7 Via Natural or Artificial Opening	Z No Device	E Nervous System F Cardiovascular System G Lymphatics and Hemic H Eye J Ear, Nose and Sinus K Respiratory System L Mouth and Throat M Gastrointestinal System N Hepatobiliary and Pancreas P Endocrine System Q Skin R Musculoskeletal System S Urinary System T Female Reproductive System V Male Reproductive System Y Other Body System

Non-OR All body part, approach, device, and qualifier values   ♀ All body part, approach, device, and qualifier values

Placement 2W0–2Y5

AHA Coding Clinic for table 2W6

2015, 2Q, 35	Application of tongs to reduce and stabilize cervical fracture
2013, 2Q, 39	Application of cervical tongs for reduction of cervical fracture

AHA Coding Clinic for table 2Y4

2018, 4Q, 38	Control of epistaxis
2017, 4Q, 106	Nasal packing for epistaxis

2   **Placement**
W   **Anatomical Regions**
Ø   **Change**   Definition: Taking out or off a device from a body part and putting back an identical or similar device in or on the same body part without cutting or puncturing the skin or a mucous membrane

Body Region Character 4	Approach Character 5	Device Character 6	Qualifier Character 7
Ø Head 2 Neck 3 Abdominal Wall 4 Chest Wall 5 Back 6 Inguinal Region, Right 7 Inguinal Region, Left 8 Upper Extremity, Right 9 Upper Extremity, Left A Upper Arm, Right B Upper Arm, Left C Lower Arm, Right D Lower Arm, Left E Hand, Right F Hand, Left G Thumb, Right H Thumb, Left J Finger, Right K Finger, Left L Lower Extremity, Right M Lower Extremity, Left N Upper Leg, Right P Upper Leg, Left Q Lower Leg, Right R Lower Leg, Left S Foot, Right T Foot, Left U Toe, Right V Toe, Left	X External	Ø Traction Apparatus 1 Splint 2 Cast 3 Brace 4 Bandage 5 Packing Material 6 Pressure Dressing 7 Intermittent Pressure Device Y Other Device	Z No Qualifier
1 Face	X External	Ø Traction Apparatus 1 Splint 2 Cast 3 Brace 4 Bandage 5 Packing Material 6 Pressure Dressing 7 Intermittent Pressure Device 9 Wire Y Other Device	Z No Qualifier

Placement *(side tab)*

2 Placement
W Anatomical Regions
1 Compression   Definition: Putting pressure on a body region

Body Region Character 4	Approach Character 5	Device Character 6	Qualifier Character 7
Ø Head	X External	6 Pressure Dressing	Z No Qualifier
1 Face		7 Intermittent Pressure Device	
2 Neck			
3 Abdominal Wall			
4 Chest Wall			
5 Back			
6 Inguinal Region, Right			
7 Inguinal Region, Left			
8 Upper Extremity, Right			
9 Upper Extremity, Left			
A Upper Arm, Right			
B Upper Arm, Left			
C Lower Arm, Right			
D Lower Arm, Left			
E Hand, Right			
F Hand, Left			
G Thumb, Right			
H Thumb, Left			
J Finger, Right			
K Finger, Left			
L Lower Extremity, Right			
M Lower Extremity, Left			
N Upper Leg, Right			
P Upper Leg, Left			
Q Lower Leg, Right			
R Lower Leg, Left			
S Foot, Right			
T Foot, Left			
U Toe, Right			
V Toe, Left			

2 Placement
W Anatomical Regions
2 Dressing   Definition: Putting material on a body region for protection

Body Region Character 4	Approach Character 5	Device Character 6	Qualifier Character 7
Ø Head	X External	4 Bandage	Z No Qualifier
1 Face			
2 Neck			
3 Abdominal Wall			
4 Chest Wall			
5 Back			
6 Inguinal Region, Right			
7 Inguinal Region, Left			
8 Upper Extremity, Right			
9 Upper Extremity, Left			
A Upper Arm, Right			
B Upper Arm, Left			
C Lower Arm, Right			
D Lower Arm, Left			
E Hand, Right			
F Hand, Left			
G Thumb, Right			
H Thumb, Left			
J Finger, Right			
K Finger, Left			
L Lower Extremity, Right			
M Lower Extremity, Left			
N Upper Leg, Right			
P Upper Leg, Left			
Q Lower Leg, Right			
R Lower Leg, Left			
S Foot, Right			
T Foot, Left			
U Toe, Right			
V Toe, Left			

2   Placement
W   Anatomical Regions
3   Immobilization   Definition: Limiting or preventing motion of a body region

Body Region Character 4	Approach Character 5	Device Character 6	Qualifier Character 7
Ø Head 2 Neck 3 Abdominal Wall 4 Chest Wall 5 Back 6 Inguinal Region, Right 7 Inguinal Region, Left 8 Upper Extremity, Right 9 Upper Extremity, Left A Upper Arm, Right B Upper Arm, Left C Lower Arm, Right D Lower Arm, Left E Hand, Right F Hand, Left G Thumb, Right H Thumb, Left J Finger, Right K Finger, Left L Lower Extremity, Right M Lower Extremity, Left N Upper Leg, Right P Upper Leg, Left Q Lower Leg, Right R Lower Leg, Left S Foot, Right T Foot, Left U Toe, Right V Toe, Left	X External	1 Splint 2 Cast 3 Brace Y Other Device	Z No Qualifier
1 Face	X External	1 Splint 2 Cast 3 Brace 9 Wire Y Other Device	Z No Qualifier

2   Placement
W   Anatomical Regions
4   Packing   Definition: Putting material in a body region or orifice

Body Region Character 4	Approach Character 5	Device Character 6	Qualifier Character 7
Ø Head 1 Face 2 Neck 3 Abdominal Wall 4 Chest Wall 5 Back 6 Inguinal Region, Right 7 Inguinal Region, Left 8 Upper Extremity, Right 9 Upper Extremity, Left A Upper Arm, Right B Upper Arm, Left C Lower Arm, Right D Lower Arm, Left E Hand, Right F Hand, Left G Thumb, Right H Thumb, Left J Finger, Right K Finger, Left L Lower Extremity, Right M Lower Extremity, Left N Upper Leg, Right P Upper Leg, Left Q Lower Leg, Right R Lower Leg, Left S Foot, Right T Foot, Left U Toe, Right V Toe, Left	X External	5 Packing Material	Z No Qualifier

2 Placement
W Anatomical Regions
5 Removal   Definition: Taking out or off a device from a body part

Body Region Character 4	Approach Character 5	Device Character 6	Qualifier Character 7
Ø Head	X External	Ø Traction Apparatus	Z No Qualifier
2 Neck		1 Splint	
3 Abdominal Wall		2 Cast	
4 Chest Wall		3 Brace	
5 Back		4 Bandage	
6 Inguinal Region, Right		5 Packing Material	
7 Inguinal Region, Left		6 Pressure Dressing	
8 Upper Extremity, Right		7 Intermittent Pressure Device	
9 Upper Extremity, Left		Y Other Device	
A Upper Arm, Right			
B Upper Arm, Left			
C Lower Arm, Right			
D Lower Arm, Left			
E Hand, Right			
F Hand, Left			
G Thumb, Right			
H Thumb, Left			
J Finger, Right			
K Finger, Left			
L Lower Extremity, Right			
M Lower Extremity, Left			
N Upper Leg, Right			
P Upper Leg, Left			
Q Lower Leg, Right			
R Lower Leg, Left			
S Foot, Right			
T Foot, Left			
U Toe, Right			
V Toe, Left			
1 Face	X External	Ø Traction Apparatus	Z No Qualifier
		1 Splint	
		2 Cast	
		3 Brace	
		4 Bandage	
		5 Packing Material	
		6 Pressure Dressing	
		7 Intermittent Pressure Device	
		9 Wire	
		Y Other Device	

2   Placement
W   Anatomical Regions
6   Traction   Definition: Exerting a pulling force on a body region in a distal direction

Body Region Character 4	Approach Character 5	Device Character 6	Qualifier Character 7
Ø Head 1 Face 2 Neck 3 Abdominal Wall 4 Chest Wall 5 Back 6 Inguinal Region, Right 7 Inguinal Region, Left 8 Upper Extremity, Right 9 Upper Extremity, Left A Upper Arm, Right B Upper Arm, Left C Lower Arm, Right D Lower Arm, Left E Hand, Right F Hand, Left G Thumb, Right H Thumb, Left J Finger, Right K Finger, Left L Lower Extremity, Right M Lower Extremity, Left N Upper Leg, Right P Upper Leg, Left Q Lower Leg, Right R Lower Leg, Left S Foot, Right T Foot, Left U Toe, Right V Toe, Left	X External	Ø Traction Apparatus Z No Device	Z No Qualifier

2   Placement
Y   Anatomical Orifices
Ø   Change   Definition: Taking out or off a device from a body part and putting back an identical or similar device in or on the same body part without cutting or puncturing the skin or a mucous membrane

Body Region Character 4	Approach Character 5	Device Character 6	Qualifier Character 7
Ø Mouth and Pharynx 1 Nasal 2 Ear 3 Anorectal 4 Female Genital Tract ♀ 5 Urethra	X External	5 Packing Material	Z No Qualifier

♀   2YØ4X5Z

2   Placement
Y   Anatomical Orifices
4   Packing   Definition: Putting material in a body region or orifice

Body Region Character 4	Approach Character 5	Device Character 6	Qualifier Character 7
Ø Mouth and Pharynx 1 Nasal 2 Ear 3 Anorectal 4 Female Genital Tract ♀ 5 Urethra	X External	5 Packing Material	Z No Qualifier

♀   2Y44X5Z

2   Placement
Y   Anatomical Orifices
5   Removal   Definition: Taking out or off a device from a body part

Body Region Character 4	Approach Character 5	Device Character 6	Qualifier Character 7
Ø Mouth and Pharynx 1 Nasal 2 Ear 3 Anorectal 4 Female Genital Tract ♀ 5 Urethra	X External	5 Packing Material	Z No Qualifier

♀   2Y54X5Z

Administration 3Ø2–3E1

AHA Coding Clinic for table 3Ø2

2019, 4Q, 35	Transfusion of blood products
2019, 4Q, 36	T-cell depleted hematopoietic stem cells for transplantation
2016, 4Q, 113	Bone marrow and stem cell transfusion (Transplantation)

AHA Coding Clinic for table 3EØ

2019, 4Q, 36-37	Hyperthermic antineoplastic chemotherapy
2018, 3Q, 7	Coronary brachytherapy with angioplasty
2018, 1Q, 8	Placement of bone morphogenetic protein & spinal fusion surgery
2017, 2Q, 14	Infusion of tPA into pleural cavity
2017, 1Q, 37	Injection of glue into enteric fistula tract
2016, 4Q, 113-114	Substances applied to cranial cavity and brain
2016, 3Q, 29	Closure of bilateral alveolar clefts
2016, 1Q, 20	Metatarsophalangeal joint resection arthroplasty
2015, 3Q, 24	Esophagogastroduodenoscopy with epinephrine injection for control of bleeding
2015, 3Q, 29	Placement of adhesion barrier
2015, 2Q, 29	Insertion of nasogastric tube for drainage and feeding
2015, 2Q, 31	Thoracoscopic talc pleurodesis

AHA Coding Clinic for table 3EØ (Continued)

2015, 1Q, 31	Intrathecal chemotherapy
2015, 1Q, 38	Chemoembolization of the hepatic artery
2014, 4Q, 16	Administration of RH (D) immunoglobulin
2014, 4Q, 17	RH (D) alloimmunization (sensitization)
2014, 4Q, 19	Ultrasound accelerated thrombolysis
2014, 4Q, 34	Resection of brain malignancy with implantation of chemotherapeutic wafer
2014, 4Q, 38	Placement of saline and seprafilm solution into abdominal cavity
2014, 3Q, 26	Coil embolization of gastroduodenal artery with chemoembolization of hepatic artery
2014, 2Q, 8	Medical induction of labor with Cervidil tampon insertion
2014, 2Q, 10	Prophylactic Neulasta injection for infection prevention
2013, 4Q, 124	Administration of tPA for stroke treatment prior to transfer
2013, 1Q, 27	Injection of sclerosing agent into an esophageal varix

AHA Coding Clinic for table 3E1

2019, 4Q, 38	Irrigation of joint using irrigating substance
2017, 3Q, 14	Bronchoscopy with suctioning and washings for removal of mucus plug

3   Administration
Ø   Circulatory
2   Transfusion   Definition: Putting in blood or blood products

Body System/Region Character 4	Approach Character 5	Substance Character 6	Qualifier Character 7
3 Peripheral Vein NC 4 Central Vein NC	Ø Open 3 Percutaneous	A Stem Cells, Embryonic	Z No Qualifier
3 Peripheral Vein 4 Central Vein	Ø Open 3 Percutaneous	C Hematopoietic Stem/Progenitor Cells, Genetically Modified	Ø Autologous
3 Peripheral Vein NC 4 Central Vein NC	Ø Open 3 Percutaneous	G Bone Marrow X Stem Cells, Cord Blood Y Stem Cells, Hematopoietic	Ø Autologous 2 Allogeneic, Related 3 Allogeneic, Unrelated 4 Allogeneic, Unspecified
3 Peripheral Vein 4 Central Vein	Ø Open 3 Percutaneous	H Whole Blood J Serum Albumin K Frozen Plasma L Fresh Plasma M Plasma Cryoprecipitate N Red Blood Cells P Frozen Red Cells Q White Cells R Platelets S Globulin T Fibrinogen V Antihemophilic Factors W Factor IX	Ø Autologous 1 Nonautologous
3 Peripheral Vein 4 Central Vein	Ø Open 3 Percutaneous	U Stem Cells, T-cell Depleted Hematopoietic	2 Allogeneic, Related 3 Allogeneic, Unrelated 4 Allogeneic, Unspecified
7 Products of Conception, Circulatory ♀	3 Percutaneous 7 Via Natural or Artificial Opening	H Whole Blood J Serum Albumin K Frozen Plasma L Fresh Plasma M Plasma Cryoprecipitate N Red Blood Cells P Frozen Red Cells Q White Cells R Platelets S Globulin T Fibrinogen V Antihemophilic Factors W Factor IX	1 Nonautologous
8 Vein	Ø Open 3 Percutaneous	B 4-Factor Prothrombin Complex Concentrate	1 Nonautologous

DRG-Non-OR   3Ø2[3,4][Ø,3]AZ
DRG-Non-OR   3Ø2[3,4][Ø,3][G,X,Y][Ø,2,3,4]
DRG-Non-OR   3Ø2[3,4][Ø,3]U[2,3,4]

NC   3Ø2[3,4][Ø,3]AZ Only when reported with PDx or SDx of C91.ØØ, C92.ØØ, C92.1Ø, C92.11, C92.4Ø, C92.5Ø, C92.6Ø, C92.AØ, C93.ØØ, C94.ØØ, C95.ØØ
NC   3Ø2[3,4][Ø,3][G,Y]Ø Only when reported with PDx or SDx of C91.ØØ, C92.ØØ, C92.1Ø, C92.11, C92.4Ø, C92.5Ø, C92.6Ø, C92.AØ, C93.ØØ, C94.ØØ, C95.ØØ
NC   3Ø2[3,4][Ø,3][G,Y][2,3,4]
♀   3Ø27[3,7][H,J,K,L,M,N,P,Q,R,S,T,V,W]1

3   Administration
C   Indwelling Device
1   Irrigation   Definition: Putting in or on a cleansing substance

Body System/Region Character 4	Approach Character 5	Substance Character 6	Qualifier Character 7
Z None	X External	8 Irrigating Substance	Z No Qualifier

LC Limited Coverage   NC Noncovered   ⊞ Combination Member   HAC   Valid OR   Combination Only   DRG Non-OR   New/Revised in GREEN

Administration

3 Administration
E Physiological Systems and Anatomical Regions
Ø Introduction   Definition: Putting in or on a therapeutic, diagnostic, nutritional, physiological, or prophylactic substance except blood or blood products

Body System/Region Character 4	Approach Character 5	Substance Character 6	Qualifier Character 7
Ø Skin and Mucous Membranes	X External	Ø Antineoplastic	5 Other Antineoplastic M Monoclonal Antibody
Ø Skin and Mucous Membranes	X External	2 Anti-infective	8 Oxazolidinones 9 Other Anti-infective
Ø Skin and Mucous Membranes	X External	3 Anti-inflammatory 4 Serum, Toxoid and Vaccine B Anesthetic Agent K Other Diagnostic Substance M Pigment N Analgesics, Hypnotics, Sedatives T Destructive Agent	Z No Qualifier
Ø Skin and Mucous Membranes	X External	G Other Therapeutic Substance	C Other Substance
1 Subcutaneous Tissue	Ø Open	2 Anti-infective	A Anti-Infective Envelope
1 Subcutaneous Tissue	3 Percutaneous	Ø Antineoplastic	5 Other Antineoplastic M Monoclonal Antibody
1 Subcutaneous Tissue	3 Percutaneous	2 Anti-infective	8 Oxazolidinones 9 Other Anti-infective A Anti-Infective Envelope
1 Subcutaneous Tissue	3 Percutaneous	3 Anti-inflammatory 6 Nutritional Substance 7 Electrolytic and Water Balance Substance B Anesthetic Agent H Radioactive Substance K Other Diagnostic Substance N Analgesics, Hypnotics, Sedatives T Destructive Agent	Z No Qualifier
1 Subcutaneous Tissue	3 Percutaneous	4 Serum, Toxoid and Vaccine	Ø Influenza Vaccine Z No Qualifier
1 Subcutaneous Tissue	3 Percutaneous	G Other Therapeutic Substance	C Other Substance
1 Subcutaneous Tissue	3 Percutaneous	V Hormone	G Insulin J Other Hormone
2 Muscle	3 Percutaneous	Ø Antineoplastic	5 Other Antineoplastic M Monoclonal Antibody
2 Muscle	3 Percutaneous	2 Anti-infective	8 Oxazolidinones 9 Other Anti-infective
2 Muscle	3 Percutaneous	3 Anti-inflammatory 6 Nutritional Substance 7 Electrolytic and Water Balance Substance B Anesthetic Agent H Radioactive Substance K Other Diagnostic Substance N Analgesics, Hypnotics, Sedatives T Destructive Agent	Z No Qualifier
2 Muscle	3 Percutaneous	4 Serum, Toxoid and Vaccine	Ø Influenza Vaccine Z No Qualifier
2 Muscle	3 Percutaneous	G Other Therapeutic Substance	C Other Substance
3 Peripheral Vein	Ø Open	Ø Antineoplastic	2 High-dose Interleukin-2 3 Low-dose Interleukin-2 5 Other Antineoplastic M Monoclonal Antibody P Clofarabine
3 Peripheral Vein	Ø Open	1 Thrombolytic	6 Recombinant Human-activated Protein C 7 Other Thrombolytic
3 Peripheral Vein	Ø Open	2 Anti-infective	8 Oxazolidinones 9 Other Anti-infective

DRG Non-OR   3E03002
DRG Non-OR   3E03017

3EØ Continued on next page

3E0 Continued

3   **Administration**
E   **Physiological Systems and Anatomical Regions**
0   **Introduction**   Definition: Putting in or on a therapeutic, diagnostic, nutritional, physiological, or prophylactic substance except blood or blood products

Body System/Region Character 4	Approach Character 5	Substance Character 6	Qualifier Character 7
3 Peripheral Vein	0 Open	3 Anti-inflammatory 4 Serum, Toxoid and Vaccine 6 Nutritional Substance 7 Electrolytic and Water Balance Substance F Intracirculatory Anesthetic H Radioactive Substance K Other Diagnostic Substance N Analgesics, Hypnotics, Sedatives P Platelet Inhibitor R Antiarrhythmic T Destructive Agent X Vasopressor	Z No Qualifier
3 Peripheral Vein	0 Open	G Other Therapeutic Substance	C Other Substance N Blood Brain Barrier Disruption
3 Peripheral Vein	0 Open	U Pancreatic Islet Cells	0 Autologous 1 Nonautologous
3 Peripheral Vein	0 Open	V Hormone	G Insulin H Human B-type Natriuretic Peptide J Other Hormone
3 Peripheral Vein	0 Open	W Immunotherapeutic	K Immunostimulator L Immunosuppressive
3 Peripheral Vein	3 Percutaneous	0 Antineoplastic	2 High-dose Interleukin-2 3 Low-dose Interleukin-2 5 Other Antineoplastic M Monoclonal Antibody P Clofarabine
3 Peripheral Vein	3 Percutaneous	1 Thrombolytic	6 Recombinant Human- activated Protein C 7 Other Thrombolytic
3 Peripheral Vein	3 Percutaneous	2 Anti-infective	8 Oxazolidinones 9 Other Anti-infective
3 Peripheral Vein	3 Percutaneous	3 Anti-inflammatory 4 Serum, Toxoid and Vaccine 6 Nutritional Substance 7 Electrolytic and Water Balance Substance F Intracirculatory Anesthetic H Radioactive Substance K Other Diagnostic Substance N Analgesics, Hypnotics, Sedatives P Platelet Inhibitor R Antiarrhythmic T Destructive Agent X Vasopressor	Z No Qualifier
3 Peripheral Vein	3 Percutaneous	G Other Therapeutic Substance	C Other Substance N Blood Brain Barrier Disruption Q Glucarpidase
3 Peripheral Vein	3 Percutaneous	U Pancreatic Islet Cells	0 Autologous 1 Nonautologous
3 Peripheral Vein	3 Percutaneous	V Hormone	G Insulin H Human B-type Natriuretic Peptide J Other Hormone
3 Peripheral Vein	3 Percutaneous	W Immunotherapeutic	K Immunostimulator L Immunosuppressive
4 Central Vein	0 Open	0 Antineoplastic	2 High-dose Interleukin-2 3 Low-dose Interleukin-2 5 Other Antineoplastic M Monoclonal Antibody P Clofarabine
4 Central Vein	0 Open	1 Thrombolytic	6 Recombinant Human- activated Protein C 7 Other Thrombolytic

Valid OR 3E030TZ		**DRG Non-OR** 3E033U[0,1]	
DRG Non-OR 3E030U[0,1]		**DRG Non-OR** 3E04002	
DRG Non-OR 3E03302		**DRG Non-OR** 3E04017	
DRG Non-OR 3E03317			

3E0 Continued on next page

LC Limited Coverage   NC Noncovered   ⊞ Combination Member   HAC   Valid OR   Combination Only   DRG Non-OR   New/Revised in GREEN

3 **Administration**
E **Physiological Systems and Anatomical Regions**
Ø **Introduction**   Definition: Putting in or on a therapeutic, diagnostic, nutritional, physiological, or prophylactic substance except blood or blood products

3EØ Continued

Body System/Region Character 4	Approach Character 5	Substance Character 6	Qualifier Character 7
4 Central Vein	**Ø** Open	**2** Anti-infective	**8** Oxazolidinones **9** Other Anti-infective
4 Central Vein	**Ø** Open	**3** Anti-inflammatory **4** Serum, Toxoid and Vaccine **6** Nutritional Substance **7** Electrolytic and Water Balance Substance **F** Intracirculatory Anesthetic **H** Radioactive Substance **K** Other Diagnostic Substance **N** Analgesics, Hypnotics, Sedatives **P** Platelet Inhibitor **R** Antiarrhythmic **T** Destructive Agent **X** Vasopressor	**Z** No Qualifier
4 Central Vein	**Ø** Open	**G** Other Therapeutic Substance	**C** Other Substance **N** Blood Brain Barrier Disruption
4 Central Vein	**Ø** Open	**V** Hormone	**G** Insulin **H** Human B-type Natriuretic Peptide **J** Other Hormone
4 Central Vein	**Ø** Open	**W** Immunotherapeutic	**K** Immunostimulator **L** Immunosuppressive
4 Central Vein	**3** Percutaneous	**Ø** Antineoplastic	**2** High-dose Interleukin-2 **3** Low-dose Interleukin-2 **5** Other Antineoplastic **M** Monoclonal Antibody **P** Clofarabine
4 Central Vein	**3** Percutaneous	**1** Thrombolytic	**6** Recombinant Human- activated Protein C **7** Other Thrombolytic
4 Central Vein	**3** Percutaneous	**2** Anti-infective	**8** Oxazolidinones **9** Other Anti-infective
4 Central Vein	**3** Percutaneous	**3** Anti-inflammatory **4** Serum, Toxoid and Vaccine **6** Nutritional Substance **7** Electrolytic and Water Balance Substance **F** Intracirculatory Anesthetic **H** Radioactive Substance **K** Other Diagnostic Substance **N** Analgesics, Hypnotics, Sedatives **P** Platelet Inhibitor **R** Antiarrhythmic **T** Destructive Agent **X** Vasopressor	**Z** No Qualifier
4 Central Vein	**3** Percutaneous	**G** Other Therapeutic Substance	**C** Other Substance **N** Blood Brain Barrier Disruption **Q** Glucarpidase
4 Central Vein	**3** Percutaneous	**V** Hormone	**G** Insulin **H** Human B-type Natriuretic Peptide **J** Other Hormone
4 Central Vein	**3** Percutaneous	**W** Immunotherapeutic	**K** Immunostimulator **L** Immunosuppressive
5 Peripheral Artery **6** Central Artery	**Ø** Open **3** Percutaneous	**Ø** Antineoplastic	**2** High-dose Interleukin-2 **3** Low-dose Interleukin-2 **5** Other Antineoplastic **M** Monoclonal Antibody **P** Clofarabine
5 Peripheral Artery **6** Central Artery	**Ø** Open **3** Percutaneous	**1** Thrombolytic	**6** Recombinant Human- activated Protein C **7** Other Thrombolytic
5 Peripheral Artery **6** Central Artery	**Ø** Open **3** Percutaneous	**2** Anti-infective	**8** Oxazolidinones **9** Other Anti-infective

Valid OR 3EØ4ØTZ		**DRG Non-OR** 3EØ[5,6][Ø,3]Ø2	
DRG Non-OR 3EØ43Ø2		**DRG Non-OR** 3EØ[5,6][Ø,3]17	
DRG Non-OR 3EØ4317			

3EØ Continued on next page

LC Limited Coverage   **NC** Noncovered   ⊞ Combination Member   HAC   Valid OR   Combination Only   DRG Non-OR   New/Revised in GREEN

714   ICD-10-PCS 2021

3EØ Continued

3   **Administration**
E   **Physiological Systems and Anatomical Regions**
Ø   **Introduction**   Definition: Putting in or on a therapeutic, diagnostic, nutritional, physiological, or prophylactic substance except blood or blood products

Body System/Region Character 4	Approach Character 5	Substance Character 6	Qualifier Character 7
5 Peripheral Artery 6 Central Artery	Ø Open 3 Percutaneous	3 Anti-inflammatory 4 Serum, Toxoid and Vaccine 6 Nutritional Substance 7 Electrolytic and Water Balance Substance F Intracirculatory Anesthetic H Radioactive Substance K Other Diagnostic Substance N Analgesics, Hypnotics, Sedatives P Platelet Inhibitor R Antiarrhythmic T Destructive Agent X Vasopressor	Z No Qualifier
5 Peripheral Artery 6 Central Artery	Ø Open 3 Percutaneous	G Other Therapeutic Substance	C Other Substance N Blood Brain Barrier Disruption
5 Peripheral Artery 6 Central Artery	Ø Open 3 Percutaneous	V Hormone	G Insulin H Human B-type Natriuretic Peptide J Other Hormone
5 Peripheral Artery 6 Central Artery	Ø Open 3 Percutaneous	W Immunotherapeutic	K Immunostimulator L Immunosuppressive
7 Coronary Artery 8 Heart	Ø Open 3 Percutaneous	1 Thrombolytic	6 Recombinant Human- activated Protein C 7 Other Thrombolytic
7 Coronary Artery 8 Heart	Ø Open 3 Percutaneous	G Other Therapeutic Substance	C Other Substance
7 Coronary Artery 8 Heart	Ø Open 3 Percutaneous	K Other Diagnostic Substance P Platelet Inhibitor	Z No Qualifier
7 Coronary Artery 8 Heart	4 Percutaneous Endoscopic	G Other Therapeutic Substance	C Other Substance
9 Nose	3 Percutaneous 7 Via Natural or Artificial Opening X External	Ø Antineoplastic	5 Other Antineoplastic M Monoclonal Antibody
9 Nose	3 Percutaneous 7 Via Natural or Artificial Opening X External	2 Anti-infective	8 Oxazolidinones 9 Other Anti-infective
9 Nose	3 Percutaneous 7 Via Natural or Artificial Opening X External	3 Anti-inflammatory 4 Serum, Toxoid and Vaccine B Anesthetic Agent H Radioactive Substance K Other Diagnostic Substance N Analgesics, Hypnotics, Sedatives T Destructive Agent	Z No Qualifier
9 Nose	3 Percutaneous 7 Via Natural or Artificial Opening X External	G Other Therapeutic Substance	C Other Substance
A Bone Marrow	3 Percutaneous	Ø Antineoplastic	5 Other Antineoplastic M Monoclonal Antibody
A Bone Marrow	3 Percutaneous	G Other Therapeutic Substance	C Other Substance
B Ear	3 Percutaneous 7 Via Natural or Artificial Opening X External	Ø Antineoplastic	4 Liquid Brachytherapy Radioisotope 5 Other Antineoplastic M Monoclonal Antibody
B Ear	3 Percutaneous 7 Via Natural or Artificial Opening X External	2 Anti-infective	8 Oxazolidinones 9 Other Anti-infective
B Ear	3 Percutaneous 7 Via Natural or Artificial Opening X External	3 Anti-inflammatory B Anesthetic Agent H Radioactive Substance K Other Diagnostic Substance N Analgesics, Hypnotics, Sedatives T Destructive Agent	Z No Qualifier
B Ear	3 Percutaneous 7 Via Natural or Artificial Opening X External	G Other Therapeutic Substance	C Other Substance

DRG Non-OR   3EØ8[Ø,3]17

3EØ Continued on next page

Administration

3E0 Continued

3   **Administration**
E   **Physiological Systems and Anatomical Regions**
0   **Introduction**   Definition: Putting in or on a therapeutic, diagnostic, nutritional, physiological, or prophylactic substance except blood or blood products

Body System/Region Character 4	Approach Character 5	Substance Character 6	Qualifier Character 7
C Eye	**3** Percutaneous **7** Via Natural or Artificial Opening **X** External	**0** Antineoplastic	**4** Liquid Brachytherapy Radioisotope **5** Other Antineoplastic **M** Monoclonal Antibody
C Eye	**3** Percutaneous **7** Via Natural or Artificial Opening **X** External	**2** Anti-infective	**8** Oxazolidinones **9** Other Anti-infective
C Eye	**3** Percutaneous **7** Via Natural or Artificial Opening **X** External	**3** Anti-inflammatory **B** Anesthetic Agent **H** Radioactive Substance **K** Other Diagnostic Substance **M** Pigment **N** Analgesics, Hypnotics, Sedatives **T** Destructive Agent	**Z** No Qualifier
C Eye	**3** Percutaneous **7** Via Natural or Artificial Opening **X** External	**G** Other Therapeutic Substance	**C** Other Substance
C Eye	**3** Percutaneous **7** Via Natural or Artificial Opening **X** External	**S** Gas	**F** Other Gas
D Mouth and Pharynx	**3** Percutaneous **7** Via Natural or Artificial Opening **X** External	**0** Antineoplastic	**4** Liquid Brachytherapy Radioisotope **5** Other Antineoplastic **M** Monoclonal Antibody
D Mouth and Pharynx	**3** Percutaneous **7** Via Natural or Artificial Opening **X** External	**2** Anti-infective	**8** Oxazolidinones **9** Other Anti-infective
D Mouth and Pharynx	**3** Percutaneous **7** Via Natural or Artificial Opening **X** External	**3** Anti-inflammatory **4** Serum, Toxoid and Vaccine **6** Nutritional Substance **7** Electrolytic and Water Balance Substance **B** Anesthetic Agent **H** Radioactive Substance **K** Other Diagnostic Substance **N** Analgesics, Hypnotics, Sedatives **R** Antiarrhythmic **T** Destructive Agent	**Z** No Qualifier
D Mouth and Pharynx	**3** Percutaneous **7** Via Natural or Artificial Opening **X** External	**G** Other Therapeutic Substance	**C** Other Substance
E Products of Conception ♀ **G** Upper GI **H** Lower GI **K** Genitourinary Tract **N** Male Reproductive ♂	**3** Percutaneous **7** Via Natural or Artificial Opening **8** Via Natural or Artificial Opening Endoscopic	**0** Antineoplastic	**4** Liquid Brachytherapy Radioisotope **5** Other Antineoplastic **M** Monoclonal Antibody
E Products of Conception ♀ **G** Upper GI **H** Lower GI **K** Genitourinary Tract **N** Male Reproductive ♂	**3** Percutaneous **7** Via Natural or Artificial Opening **8** Via Natural or Artificial Opening Endoscopic	**2** Anti-infective	**8** Oxazolidinones **9** Other Anti-infective

E Products of Conception ♀
G Upper GI
H Lower GI
K Genitourinary Tract
N Male Reproductive ♂
	3 Percutaneous
	7 Via Natural or Artificial Opening
	8 Via Natural or Artificial Opening
	    Endoscopic
		3 Anti-inflammatory
		6 Nutritional Substance
		7 Electrolytic and Water Balance
		    Substance
		B Anesthetic Agent
		H Radioactive Substance
		K Other Diagnostic Substance
		N Analgesics, Hypnotics, Sedatives
		T Destructive Agent
			Z No Qualifier

E Products of Conception ♀ **G** Upper GI **H** Lower GI **K** Genitourinary Tract **N** Male Reproductive ♂	**3** Percutaneous **7** Via Natural or Artificial Opening **8** Via Natural or Artificial Opening Endoscopic	**G** Other Therapeutic Substance	**C** Other Substance

♂   All approach, substance, and qualifier values for body system/region (character 4) with this icon
♀   All approach, substance, and qualifier values for body system/region (character 4) with this icon

3E0 Continued on next page

LC Limited Coverage   **NC** Noncovered   ⊞ Combination Member   HAC   Valid OR   Combination Only   DRG Non-OR   New/Revised in GREEN

716   ICD-10-PCS 2021

3E0 Continued

3   **Administration**
E   **Physiological Systems and Anatomical Regions**
0   **Introduction**   Definition: Putting in or on a therapeutic, diagnostic, nutritional, physiological, or prophylactic substance except blood or blood products

Body System/Region Character 4	Approach Character 5	Substance Character 6	Qualifier Character 7
E Products of Conception ♀ G Upper GI H Lower GI K Genitourinary Tract N Male Reproductive ♂	3 Percutaneous 7 Via Natural or Artificial Opening 8 Via Natural or Artificial Opening Endoscopic	S Gas	F Other Gas
E Products of Conception ♀ G Upper GI H Lower GI K Genitourinary Tract N Male Reproductive ♂	4 Percutaneous Endoscopic	G Other Therapeutic Substance	C Other Substance
F Respiratory Tract	3 Percutaneous 7 Via Natural or Artificial Opening 8 Via Natural or Artificial Opening Endoscopic	0 Antineoplastic	4 Liquid Brachytherapy Radioisotope 5 Other Antineoplastic M Monoclonal Antibody
F Respiratory Tract	3 Percutaneous 7 Via Natural or Artificial Opening 8 Via Natural or Artificial Opening Endoscopic	2 Anti-infective	8 Oxazolidinones 9 Other Anti-infective
F Respiratory Tract	3 Percutaneous 7 Via Natural or Artificial Opening 8 Via Natural or Artificial Opening Endoscopic	3 Anti-inflammatory 6 Nutritional Substance 7 Electrolytic and Water Balance Substance B Anesthetic Agent H Radioactive Substance K Other Diagnostic Substance N Analgesics, Hypnotics, Sedatives T Destructive Agent	Z No Qualifier
F Respiratory Tract	3 Percutaneous 7 Via Natural or Artificial Opening 8 Via Natural or Artificial Opening Endoscopic	G Other Therapeutic Substance	C Other Substance
F Respiratory Tract	3 Percutaneous 7 Via Natural or Artificial Opening 8 Via Natural or Artificial Opening Endoscopic	S Gas	D Nitric Oxide F Other Gas
F Respiratory Tract	4 Percutaneous Endoscopic	G Other Therapeutic Substance	C Other Substance
J Biliary and Pancreatic Tract	3 Percutaneous 7 Via Natural or Artificial Opening 8 Via Natural or Artificial Opening Endoscopic	0 Antineoplastic	4 Liquid Brachytherapy Radioisotope 5 Other Antineoplastic M Monoclonal Antibody
J Biliary and Pancreatic Tract	3 Percutaneous 7 Via Natural or Artificial Opening 8 Via Natural or Artificial Opening Endoscopic	2 Anti-infective	8 Oxazolidinones 9 Other Anti-infective
J Biliary and Pancreatic Tract	3 Percutaneous 7 Via Natural or Artificial Opening 8 Via Natural or Artificial Opening Endoscopic	3 Anti-inflammatory 6 Nutritional Substance 7 Electrolytic and Water Balance Substance B Anesthetic Agent H Radioactive Substance K Other Diagnostic Substance N Analgesics, Hypnotics, Sedatives T Destructive Agent	Z No Qualifier
J Biliary and Pancreatic Tract	3 Percutaneous 7 Via Natural or Artificial Opening 8 Via Natural or Artificial Opening Endoscopic	G Other Therapeutic Substance	C Other Substance
J Biliary and Pancreatic Tract	3 Percutaneous 7 Via Natural or Artificial Opening 8 Via Natural or Artificial Opening Endoscopic	S Gas	F Other Gas

♂   All approach, substance, and qualifier values for body system/region (character 4) with this icon
♀   All approach, substance, and qualifier values for body system/region (character 4) with this icon

3E0 Continued on next page

LC Limited Coverage   **NC** Noncovered   ⊞ Combination Member   **HAC**   **Valid OR**   **Combination Only**   **DRG Non-OR**   New/Revised in GREEN

ICD-10-PCS 2021   717

Administration

3E0 Continued

3   **Administration**
E   **Physiological Systems and Anatomical Regions**
0   **Introduction**   Definition: Putting in or on a therapeutic, diagnostic, nutritional, physiological, or prophylactic substance except blood or blood products

Body System/Region Character 4	Approach Character 5	Substance Character 6	Qualifier Character 7
J Biliary and Pancreatic Tract	3 Percutaneous 7 Via Natural or Artificial Opening 8 Via Natural or Artificial Opening Endoscopic	U Pancreatic Islet Cells	0 Autologous 1 Nonautologous
J Biliary and Pancreatic Tract	4 Percutaneous Endoscopic	G Other Therapeutic Substance	C Other Substance
L Pleural Cavity	0 Open	5 Adhesion Barrier	Z No Qualifier
L Pleural Cavity	3 Percutaneous	0 Antineoplastic	4 Liquid Brachytherapy Radioisotope 5 Other Antineoplastic M Monoclonal Antibody
L Pleural Cavity	3 Percutaneous	2 Anti-infective	8 Oxazolidinones 9 Other Anti-infective
L Pleural Cavity	3 Percutaneous	3 Anti-inflammatory 5 Adhesion Barrier 6 Nutritional Substance 7 Electrolytic and Water Balance Substance B Anesthetic Agent H Radioactive Substance K Other Diagnostic Substance N Analgesics, Hypnotics, Sedatives T Destructive Agent	Z No Qualifier
L Pleural Cavity	3 Percutaneous	G Other Therapeutic Substance	C Other Substance
L Pleural Cavity	3 Percutaneous	S Gas	F Other Gas
L Pleural Cavity	4 Percutaneous Endoscopic	5 Adhesion Barrier	Z No Qualifier
L Pleural Cavity	4 Percutaneous Endoscopic	G Other Therapeutic Substance	C Other Substance
L Pleural Cavity	7 Via Natural or Artificial Opening	0 Antineoplastic	4 Liquid Brachytherapy Radioisotope 5 Other Antineoplastic M Monoclonal Antibody
L Pleural Cavity	7 Via Natural or Artificial Opening	S Gas	F Other Gas
M Peritoneal Cavity	0 Open	5 Adhesion Barrier	Z No Qualifier
M Peritoneal Cavity	3 Percutaneous	0 Antineoplastic	4 Liquid Brachytherapy Radioisotope 5 Other Antineoplastic M Monoclonal Antibody Y Hyperthermic
M Peritoneal Cavity	3 Percutaneous	2 Anti-infective	8 Oxazolidinones 9 Other Anti-infective
M Peritoneal Cavity	3 Percutaneous	3 Anti-inflammatory 5 Adhesion Barrier 6 Nutritional Substance 7 Electrolytic and Water Balance Substance B Anesthetic Agent H Radioactive Substance K Other Diagnostic Substance N Analgesics, Hypnotics, Sedatives T Destructive Agent	Z No Qualifier
M Peritoneal Cavity	3 Percutaneous	G Other Therapeutic Substance	C Other Substance
M Peritoneal Cavity	3 Percutaneous	S Gas	F Other Gas
M Peritoneal Cavity	4 Percutaneous Endoscopic	5 Adhesion Barrier	Z No Qualifier
M Peritoneal Cavity	4 Percutaneous Endoscopic	G Other Therapeutic Substance	C Other Substance
M Peritoneal Cavity	7 Via Natural or Artificial Opening	0 Antineoplastic	4 Liquid Brachytherapy Radioisotope 5 Other Antineoplastic M Monoclonal Antibody
M Peritoneal Cavity	7 Via Natural or Artificial Opening	S Gas	F Other Gas
P Female Reproductive ♀	0 Open	5 Adhesion Barrier	Z No Qualifier
P Female Reproductive ♀	3 Percutaneous	0 Antineoplastic	4 Liquid Brachytherapy Radioisotope 5 Other Antineoplastic M Monoclonal Antibody
P Female Reproductive ♀	3 Percutaneous	2 Anti-infective	8 Oxazolidinones 9 Other Anti-infective

Valid OR   3E0L4GC
DRG Non-OR   3E0J[3,7,8]U[0,1]
♀   All approach, substance, and qualifier values for body system/region (character 4) with this icon

3E0 Continued on next page

3EØ Continued

3   **Administration**
E   **Physiological Systems and Anatomical Regions**
Ø   **Introduction**   Definition: Putting in or on a therapeutic, diagnostic, nutritional, physiological, or prophylactic substance except blood or blood products

Body System/Region Character 4		Approach Character 5	Substance Character 6	Qualifier Character 7
P Female Reproductive	♀	3 Percutaneous	3 Anti-inflammatory 5 Adhesion Barrier 6 Nutritional Substance 7 Electrolytic and Water Balance Substance B Anesthetic Agent H Radioactive Substance K Other Diagnostic Substance L Sperm N Analgesics, Hypnotics, Sedatives T Destructive Agent V Hormone	Z No Qualifier
P Female Reproductive	♀	3 Percutaneous	G Other Therapeutic Substance	C Other Substance
P Female Reproductive	♀	3 Percutaneous	Q Fertilized Ovum	Ø Autologous 1 Nonautologous
P Female Reproductive	♀	3 Percutaneous	S Gas	F Other Gas
P Female Reproductive	♀	4 Percutaneous Endoscopic	5 Adhesion Barrier	Z No Qualifier
P Female Reproductive	♀	4 Percutaneous Endoscopic	G Other Therapeutic Substance	C Other Substance
P Female Reproductive	♀	7 Via Natural or Artificial Opening	Ø Antineoplastic	4 Liquid Brachytherapy Radioisotope 5 Other Antineoplastic M Monoclonal Antibody
P Female Reproductive	♀	7 Via Natural or Artificial Opening	2 Anti-infective	8 Oxazolidinones 9 Other Anti-infective
P Female Reproductive	♀	7 Via Natural or Artificial Opening	3 Anti-inflammatory 6 Nutritional Substance 7 Electrolytic and Water Balance Substance B Anesthetic Agent H Radioactive Substance K Other Diagnostic Substance L Sperm N Analgesics, Hypnotics, Sedatives T Destructive Agent V Hormone	Z No Qualifier
P Female Reproductive	♀	7 Via Natural or Artificial Opening	G Other Therapeutic Substance	C Other Substance
P Female Reproductive	♀	7 Via Natural or Artificial Opening	Q Fertilized Ovum	Ø Autologous 1 Nonautologous
P Female Reproductive	♀	7 Via Natural or Artificial Opening	S Gas	F Other Gas
P Female Reproductive	♀	8 Via Natural or Artificial Opening Endoscopic	Ø Antineoplastic	4 Liquid Brachytherapy Radioisotope 5 Other Antineoplastic M Monoclonal Antibody
P Female Reproductive	♀	8 Via Natural or Artificial Opening Endoscopic	2 Anti-infective	8 Oxazolidinones 9 Other Anit-infection
P Female Reproductive	♀	8 Via Natural or Artificial Opening Endoscopic	3 Anti-inflammatory 6 Nutritional Substance 7 Electrolytic and Water Balance Substance B Anesthetic Agent H Radioactive Substance K Other Diagnostic Substance N Analgesics, Hypnotics, Sedative T Destructive Agent	Z No Qualifier
P Female Reproductive	♀	8 Via Natural or Artificial Opening Endoscopic	G Other Therapeutic Substance	C Other Substance
P Female Reproductive	♀	8 Via Natural or Artificial Opening Endoscopic	S Gas	F Other Gas
Q Cranial Cavity and Brain		Ø Open 3 Percutaneous	Ø Antineoplastic	4 Liquid Brachytherapy Radioisotope 5 Other Antineoplastic M Monoclonal Antibody
Q Cranial Cavity and Brain		Ø Open 3 Percutaneous	2 Anti-infective	8 Oxazolidinones 9 Other Anti-infective

Valid OR	3EØP3Q[Ø,1]
Valid OR	3EØP7Q[Ø,1]
DRG Non-OR	3EØQ[Ø,3]Ø5
♀	All approach, substance, and qualifier values for body system/region (character 4) with this icon

3EØ Continued on next page

3   **Administration**
E   **Physiological Systems and Anatomical Regions**
Ø   **Introduction**   Definition: Putting in or on a therapeutic, diagnostic, nutritional, physiological, or prophylactic substance except blood or blood products

3EØ Continued

Body System/Region Character 4	Approach Character 5	Substance Character 6	Qualifier Character 7
Q Cranial Cavity and Brain	Ø Open 3 Percutaneous	3 Anti-inflammatory 6 Nutritional Substance 7 Electrolytic and Water Balance Substance A Stem Cells, Embryonic B Anesthetic Agent H Radioactive Substance K Other Diagnostic Substance N Analgesics, Hypnotics, Sedatives T Destructive Agent	Z No Qualifier
Q Cranial Cavity and Brain	Ø Open 3 Percutaneous	E Stem Cells, Somatic	Ø Autologous 1 Nonautologous
Q Cranial Cavity and Brain	Ø Open 3 Percutaneous	G Other Therapeutic Substance	C Other Substance
Q Cranial Cavity and Brain	Ø Open 3 Percutaneous	S Gas	F Other Gas
Q Cranial Cavity and Brain	7 Via Natural or Artificial Opening	Ø Antineoplastic	4 Liquid Brachytherapy Radioisotope 5 Other Antineoplastic M Monoclonal Antibody
Q Cranial Cavity and Brain	7 Via Natural or Artificial Opening	S Gas	F Other Gas
R Spinal Canal	Ø Open	A Stem Cells, Embryonic	Z No Qualifier
R Spinal Canal	Ø Open	E Stem Cells, Somatic	Ø Autologous 1 Nonautologous
R Spinal Canal	3 Percutaneous	Ø Antineoplastic	2 High-dose Interleukin-2 3 Low-dose Interleukin-2 4 Liquid Brachytherapy Radioisotope 5 Other Antineoplastic M Monoclonal Antibody
R Spinal Canal	3 Percutaneous	2 Anti-infective	8 Oxazolidinones 9 Other Anti-infective
R Spinal Canal	3 Percutaneous	3 Anti-inflammatory 6 Nutritional Substance 7 Electrolytic and Water Balance Substance A Stem Cells, Embryonic B Anesthetic Agent H Radioactive Substance K Other Diagnostic Substance N Analgesics, Hypnotics, Sedatives T Destructive Agent	Z No Qualifier
R Spinal Canal	3 Percutaneous	E Stem Cells, Somatic	Ø Autologous 1 Nonautologous
R Spinal Canal	3 Percutaneous	G Other Therapeutic Substance	C Other Substance
R Spinal Canal	3 Percutaneous	S Gas	F Other Gas
R Spinal Canal	7 Via Natural or Artificial Opening	S Gas	F Other Gas
S Epidural Space	3 Percutaneous	Ø Antineoplastic	2 High-dose Interleukin-2 3 Low-dose Interleukin-2 4 Liquid Brachytherapy Radioisotope 5 Other Antineoplastic M Monoclonal Antibody
S Epidural Space	3 Percutaneous	2 Anti-infective	8 Oxazolidinones 9 Other Anti-infective
S Epidural Space	3 Percutaneous	3 Anti-inflammatory 6 Nutritional Substance 7 Electrolytic and Water Balance Substance B Anesthetic Agent H Radioactive Substance K Other Diagnostic Substance N Analgesics, Hypnotics, Sedatives T Destructive Agent	Z No Qualifier

DRG Non-OR   3EØQ7Ø5
DRG Non-OR   3EØR3Ø2
DRG Non-OR   3EØS3Ø2

3EØ Continued on next page

LC Limited Coverage   NC Noncovered   ⊞ Combination Member   HAC   Valid OR   Combination Only   DRG Non-OR   New/Revised in GREEN

3E0 Continued

3   **Administration**
E   **Physiological Systems and Anatomical Regions**
0   **Introduction**   Definition: Putting in or on a therapeutic, diagnostic, nutritional, physiological, or prophylactic substance except blood or blood products

Body System/Region Character 4	Approach Character 5	Substance Character 6	Qualifier Character 7
S Epidural Space	**3** Percutaneous	**G** Other Therapeutic Substance	**C** Other Substance
S Epidural Space	**3** Percutaneous	**S** Gas	**F** Other Gas
S Epidural Space	**7** Via Natural or Artificial Opening	**S** Gas	**F** Other Gas
T Peripheral Nerves and Plexi **X** Cranial Nerves	**3** Percutaneous	**3** Anti-inflammatory **B** Anesthetic Agent **T** Destructive Agent	**Z** No Qualifier
T Peripheral Nerves and Plexi **X** Cranial Nerves	**3** Percutaneous	**G** Other Therapeutic Substance	**C** Other Substance
U Joints	**0** Open	**2** Anti-infective	**8** Oxazolidinones **9** Other Anti-infective
U Joints	**0** Open	**G** Other Therapeutic Substance	**B** Recombinant Bone Morphogenetic Protein
U Joints	**3** Percutaneous	**0** Antineoplastic	**4** Liquid Brachytherapy Radioisotope **5** Other Antineoplastic **M** Monoclonal Antibody
U Joints	**3** Percutaneous	**2** Anti-infective	**8** Oxazolidinones **9** Other Anti-infective
U Joints	**3** Percutaneous	**3** Anti-inflammatory **6** Nutritional Substance **7** Electrolytic and Water Balance Substance **B** Anesthetic Agent **H** Radioactive Substance **K** Other Diagnostic Substance **N** Analgesics, Hypnotics, Sedatives **T** Destructive Agent	**Z** No Qualifier
U Joints	**3** Percutaneous	**G** Other Therapeutic Substance	**B** Recombinant Bone Morphogenetic Protein **C** Other Substance
U Joints	**3** Percutaneous	**S** Gas	**F** Other Gas
U Joints	**4** Percutaneous Endoscopic	**G** Other Therapeutic Substance	**C** Other Substance
V Bones	**0** Open	**G** Other Therapeutic Substance	**B** Recombinant Bone Morphogenetic Protein
V Bones	**3** Percutaneous	**0** Antineoplastic	**5** Other Antineoplastic **M** Monoclonal Antibody
V Bones	**3** Percutaneous	**2** Anti-infective	**8** Oxazolidinones **9** Other Anti-infective
V Bones	**3** Percutaneous	**3** Anti-inflammatory **6** Nutritional Substance **7** Electrolytic and Water Balance Substance **B** Anesthetic Agent **H** Radioactive Substance **K** Other Diagnostic Substance **N** Analgesics, Hypnotics, Sedatives **T** Destructive Agent	**Z** No Qualifier
V Bones	**3** Percutaneous	**G** Other Therapeutic Substance	**B** Recombinant Bone Morphogenetic Protein **C** Other Substance
W Lymphatics	**3** Percutaneous	**0** Antineoplastic	**5** Other Antineoplastic **M** Monoclonal Antibody
W Lymphatics	**3** Percutaneous	**2** Anti-infective	**8** Oxazolidinones **9** Other Anti-infective
W Lymphatics	**3** Percutaneous	**3** Anti-inflammatory **6** Nutritional Substance **7** Electrolytic and Water Balance Substance **B** Anesthetic Agent **H** Radioactive Substance **K** Other Diagnostic Substance **N** Analgesics, Hypnotics, Sedatives **T** Destructive Agent	**Z** No Qualifier
W Lymphatics	**3** Percutaneous	**G** Other Therapeutic Substance	**C** Other Substance

3E0 Continued on next page

Administration

3   **Administration**
E   **Physiological Systems and Anatomical Regions**
0   **Introduction**   Definition: Putting in or on a therapeutic, diagnostic, nutritional, physiological, or prophylactic substance except blood or blood products

Body System/Region Character 4	Approach Character 5	Substance Character 6	Qualifier Character 7
Y Pericardial Cavity	3 Percutaneous	0 Antineoplastic	4 Liquid Brachytherapy Radioisotope 5 Other Antineoplastic M Monoclonal Antibody
Y Pericardial Cavity	3 Percutaneous	2 Anti-infective	8 Oxazolidinones 9 Other Anti-infective
Y Pericardial Cavity	3 Percutaneous	3 Anti-inflammatory 6 Nutritional Substance 7 Electrolytic and Water Balance Substance B Anesthetic Agent H Radioactive Substance K Other Diagnostic Substance N Analgesics, Hypnotics, Sedatives T Destructive Agent	Z No Qualifier
Y Pericardial Cavity	3 Percutaneous	G Other Therapeutic Substance	C Other Substance
Y Pericardial Cavity	3 Percutaneous	S Gas	F Other Gas
Y Pericardial Cavity	4 Percutaneous Endoscopic	G Other Therapeutic Substance	C Other Substance
Y Pericardial Cavity	7 Via Natural or Artificial Opening	0 Antineoplastic	4 Liquid Brachytherapy Radioisotope 5 Other Antineoplastic M Monoclonal Antibody
Y Pericardial Cavity	7 Via Natural or Artificial Opening	S Gas	F Other Gas

3   **Administration**
E   **Physiological Systems and Anatomical Regions**
1   **Irrigation**   Definition: Putting in or on a cleansing substance

Body System/Region Character 4	Approach Character 5	Substance Character 6	Qualifier Character 7
0 Skin and Mucous Membranes C Eye	3 Percutaneous X External	8 Irrigating Substance	X Diagnostic Z No Qualifier
9 Nose B Ear F Respiratory Tract G Upper GI H Lower GI J Biliary and Pancreatic Tract K Genitourinary Tract N Male Reproductive ♂ P Female Reproductive ♀	3 Percutaneous 7 Via Natural or Artificial Opening 8 Via Natural or Artificial Opening Endoscopic	8 Irrigating Substance	X Diagnostic Z No Qualifier
L Pleural Cavity Q Cranial Cavity and Brain R Spinal Canal S Epidural Space Y Pericardial Cavity	3 Percutaneous	8 Irrigating Substance	X Diagnostic Z No Qualifier
M Peritoneal Cavity	3 Percutaneous	8 Irrigating Substance	X Diagnostic Z No Qualifier
M Peritoneal Cavity	3 Percutaneous	9 Dialysate	Z No Qualifier
U Joints	3 Percutaneous 4 Percutaneous Endoscopic	8 Irrigating Substance	X Diagnostic Z No Qualifier

♂   3E1N[3,7,8]8[X,Z]
♀   3E1P[3,7,8]8[X,Z]

Measurement and Monitoring 4A0–4B0

AHA Coding Clinic for table 4A0

2019, 3Q, 32	Endomyocardial biopsy and right heart catheterization
2018, 1Q, 12	Percutaneous balloon valvuloplasty & cardiac catheterization with ventriculogram
2016, 3Q, 37	Fractional flow reserve
2015, 3Q, 29	Approach value for esophageal electrophysiology study

AHA Coding Clinic for table 4A1

2019, 4Q, 38-39	Intraoperative fluorescence lymphatic mapping using Indocyanine green dye
2016, 4Q, 114	Fluorescence vascular angiography
2016, 2Q, 29	Decompressive craniectomy with cryopreservation and storage of bone flap
2016, 2Q, 33	Monitoring of arterial pressure & pulse
2015, 3Q, 35	Swan Ganz catheterization
2015, 2Q, 14	Intraoperative EMG monitoring via endotracheal tube
2015, 1Q, 26	Intraoperative monitoring using Sentio MMG®
2014, 4Q, 28	Removal and replacement of displaced growing rods

4   **Measurement and Monitoring**
A   **Physiological Systems**
0   **Measurement**   Definition: Determining the level of a physiological or physical function at a point in time

Body System Character 4	Approach Character 5	Function/Device Character 6	Qualifier Character 7
0 Central Nervous	**0** Open	**2** Conductivity **4** Electrical Activity **B** Pressure	**Z** No Qualifier
0 Central Nervous	**3** Percutaneous **7** Via Natural or Artificial Opening **8** Via Natural or Artificial Opening Endoscopic	**4** Electrical Activity	**Z** No Qualifier
0 Central Nervous	**3** Percutaneous **7** Via Natural or Artificial Opening **8** Via Natural or Artificial Opening Endoscopic	**B** Pressure **K** Temperature **R** Saturation	**D** Intracranial
0 Central Nervous	**X** External	**2** Conductivity **4** Electrical Activity	**Z** No Qualifier
1 Peripheral Nervous	**0** Open **3** Percutaneous **7** Via Natural or Artificial Opening **8** Via Natural or Artificial Opening Endoscopic **X** External	**2** Conductivity	**9** Sensory **B** Motor
1 Peripheral Nervous	**0** Open **3** Percutaneous **7** Via Natural or Artificial Opening **8** Via Natural or Artificial Opening Endoscopic **X** External	**4** Electrical Activity	**Z** No Qualifier
2 Cardiac	**0** Open **3** Percutaneous **7** Via Natural or Artificial Opening **8** Via Natural or Artificial Opening Endoscopic	**4** Electrical Activity **9** Output **C** Rate **F** Rhythm **H** Sound **P** Action Currents	**Z** No Qualifier
2 Cardiac	**0** Open **3** Percutaneous **7** Via Natural or Artificial Opening **8** Via Natural or Artificial Opening Endoscopic	**N** Sampling and Pressure	**6** Right Heart **7** Left Heart **8** Bilateral
2 Cardiac	**X** External	**4** Electrical Activity	**A** Guidance **Z** No Qualifier
2 Cardiac	**X** External	**9** Output **C** Rate **F** Rhythm **H** Sound **P** Action Currents	**Z** No Qualifier
2 Cardiac	**X** External	**M** Total Activity	**4** Stress
3 Arterial	**0** Open **3** Percutaneous	**5** Flow **J** Pulse	**1** Peripheral **3** Pulmonary **C** Coronary
3 Arterial	**0** Open **3** Percutaneous	**B** Pressure	**1** Peripheral **3** Pulmonary **C** Coronary **F** Other Thoracic

DRG Non-OR   4A02[3,7,8]FZ
DRG Non-OR   4A02[0,3,7,8]N[6,7,8]

4A0 Continued on next page

Measurement and Monitoring

4 Measurement and Monitoring
A Physiological Systems
Ø Measurement   Definition: Determining the level of a physiological or physical function at a point in time

4AØ Continued

Body System Character 4	Approach Character 5	Function/Device Character 6	Qualifier Character 7
3 Arterial	Ø Open 3 Percutaneous	H Sound R Saturation	1 Peripheral
3 Arterial	X External	5 Flow	1 Peripheral D Intracranial
3 Arterial	X External	B Pressure H Sound J Pulse R Saturation	1 Peripheral
4 Venous	Ø Open 3 Percutaneous	5 Flow B Pressure J Pulse	Ø Central 1 Peripheral 2 Portal 3 Pulmonary
4 Venous	Ø Open 3 Percutaneous	R Saturation	1 Peripheral
4 Venous	4 Percutaneous Endoscopic	B Pressure	2 Portal
4 Venous	X External	5 Flow B Pressure J Pulse R Saturation	1 Peripheral
5 Circulatory	X External	L Volume	Z No Qualifier
6 Lymphatic	Ø Open 3 Percutaneous 7 Via Natural or Artificial Opening 8 Via Natural or Artificial Opening Endoscopic	5 Flow B Pressure	Z No Qualifier
7 Visual	X External	Ø Acuity 7 Mobility B Pressure	Z No Qualifier
8 Olfactory	X External	Ø Acuity	Z No Qualifier
9 Respiratory	7 Via Natural or Artificial Opening 8 Via Natural or Artificial Opening Endoscopic X External	1 Capacity 5 Flow C Rate D Resistance L Volume M Total Activity	Z No Qualifier
B Gastrointestinal	7 Via Natural or Artificial Opening 8 Via Natural or Artificial Opening Endoscopic	8 Motility B Pressure G Secretion	Z No Qualifier
C Biliary	3 Percutaneous 4 Percutaneous Endoscopic 7 Via Natural or Artificial Opening 8 Via Natural or Artificial Opening Endoscopic	5 Flow B Pressure	Z No Qualifier
D Urinary	7 Via Natural or Artificial Opening 8 Via Natural or Artificial Opening Endoscopic	3 Contractility 5 Flow B Pressure D Resistance L Volume	Z No Qualifier
F Musculoskeletal	3 Percutaneous	3 Contractility	Z No Qualifier
F Musculoskeletal	3 Percutaneous	B Pressure	E Compartment
F Musculoskeletal	X External	3 Contractility	Z No Qualifier
H Products of Conception, Cardiac ♀	7 Via Natural or Artificial Opening 8 Via Natural or Artificial Opening Endoscopic X External	4 Electrical Activity C Rate F Rhythm H Sound	Z No Qualifier
J Products of Conception, Nervous ♀	7 Via Natural or Artificial Opening 8 Via Natural or Artificial Opening Endoscopic X External	2 Conductivity 4 Electrical Activity B Pressure	Z No Qualifier
Z None	7 Via Natural or Artificial Opening	6 Metabolism K Temperature	Z No Qualifier
Z None	X External	6 Metabolism K Temperature Q Sleep	Z No Qualifier

Valid OR	4AØ6Ø[5,B]Z	♀	4AØH[7,8,X][4,C,F,H]Z
Valid OR	4AØC4[5,B]Z	♀	4AØJ[7,8,X][2,4,B]Z

4 Measurement and Monitoring
A Physiological Systems
1 Monitoring   Definition: Determining the level of a physiological or physical function repetitively over a period of time

Body System Character 4		Approach Character 5		Function/Device Character 6		Qualifier Character 7	
Ø	Central Nervous	Ø	Open	2 B	Conductivity Pressure	Z	No Qualifier
Ø	Central Nervous	Ø	Open	4	Electrical Activity	G Z	Intraoperative No Qualifier
Ø	Central Nervous	3 7 8	Percutaneous Via Natural or Artificial Opening Via Natural or Artificial Opening Endoscopic	4	Electrical Activity	G Z	Intraoperative No Qualifier
Ø	Central Nervous	3 7 8	Percutaneous Via Natural or Artificial Opening Via Natural or Artificial Opening Endoscopic	B K R	Pressure Temperature Saturation	D	Intracranial
Ø	Central Nervous	X	External	2	Conductivity	Z	No Qualifier
Ø	Central Nervous	X	External	4	Electrical Activity	G Z	Intraoperative No Qualifier
1	Peripheral Nervous	Ø 3 7 8 X	Open Percutaneous Via Natural or Artificial Opening Via Natural or Artificial Opening Endoscopic External	2	Conductivity	9 B	Sensory Motor
1	Peripheral Nervous	Ø 3 7 8 X	Open Percutaneous Via Natural or Artificial Opening Via Natural or Artificial Opening Endoscopic External	4	Electrical Activity	G Z	Intraoperative No Qualifier
2	Cardiac	Ø 3 7 8	Open Percutaneous Via Natural or Artificial Opening Via Natural or Artificial Opening Endoscopic	4 9 C F H	Electrical Activity Output Rate Rhythm Sound	Z	No Qualifier
2	Cardiac	X	External	4	Electrical Activity	5 Z	Ambulatory No Qualifier
2	Cardiac	X	External	9 C F H	Output Rate Rhythm Sound	Z	No Qualifier
2	Cardiac	X	External	M	Total Activity	4	Stress
2	Cardiac	X	External	S	Vascular Perfusion	H	Indocyanine Green Dye
3	Arterial	Ø 3	Open Percutaneous	5 B J	Flow Pressure Pulse	1 3 C	Peripheral Pulmonary Coronary
3	Arterial	Ø 3	Open Percutaneous	H R	Sound Saturation	1	Peripheral
3	Arterial	X	External	5 B H J R	Flow Pressure Sound Pulse Saturation	1	Peripheral
4	Venous	Ø 3	Open Percutaneous	5 B J	Flow Pressure Pulse	Ø 1 2 3	Central Peripheral Portal Pulmonary
4	Venous	Ø 3	Open Percutaneous	R	Saturation	Ø 2 3	Central Portal Pulmonary
4	Venous	X	External	5 B J	Flow Pressure Pulse	1	Peripheral
6	Lymphatic	Ø 3 7 8	Open Percutaneous Via Natural or Artificial Opening Via Natural or Artificial Opening Endoscopic	5	Flow	H Z	Indocyanine Green Dye No Qualifier

Valid OR   4A16Ø5Z

4A1 Continued on next page

LC Limited Coverage   **NC** Noncovered   ⊞ Combination Member   HAC   Valid OR   Combination Only   DRG Non-OR   New/Revised in GREEN

ICD-10-PCS 2021   725

4   **Measurement and Monitoring**
A   **Physiological Systems**
1   **Monitoring**   Definition: Determining the level of a physiological or physical function repetitively over a period of time

4A1 Continued

Body System Character 4	Approach Character 5	Function/Device Character 6	Qualifier Character 7
6 Lymphatic	Ø Open 3 Percutaneous 7 Via Natural or Artificial Opening 8 Via Natural or Artificial Opening Endoscopic	B Pressure	Z No Qualifier
9 Respiratory	7 Via Natural or Artificial Opening X External	1 Capacity 5 Flow C Rate D Resistance L Volume	Z No Qualifier
B Gastrointestinal	7 Via Natural or Artificial Opening 8 Via Natural or Artificial Opening Endoscopic	8 Motility B Pressure G Secretion	Z No Qualifier
B Gastrointestinal	X External	S Vascular Perfusion	H Indocyanine Green Dye
D Urinary	7 Via Natural or Artificial Opening 8 Via Natural or Artificial Opening Endoscopic	3 Contractility 5 Flow B Pressure D Resistance L Volume	Z No Qualifier
G Skin and Breast	X External	S Vascular Perfusion	H Indocyanine Green Dye

H   Products of Conception, ♀
     Cardiac
	7 Via Natural or Artificial Opening
	8 Via Natural or Artificial Opening
	     Endoscopic
	X External
		4 Electrical Activity
		C Rate
		F Rhythm
		H Sound
			Z No Qualifier

J   Products of Conception, ♀
     Nervous
	7 Via Natural or Artificial Opening
	8 Via Natural or Artificial Opening
	     Endoscopic
	X External
		2 Conductivity
		4 Electrical Activity
		B Pressure
			Z No Qualifier

Z None	7 Via Natural or Artificial Opening	K Temperature	Z No Qualifier
Z None	X External	K Temperature Q Sleep	Z No Qualifier

Valid OR   4A16ØBZ
♀   4A1H[7,8,X][4,C,F,H]Z
♀   4A1J[7,8,X][2,4,B]Z

4   **Measurement and Monitoring**
B   **Physiological Devices**
Ø   **Measurement**   Definition: Determining the level of a physiological or physical function at a point in time

Body System Character 4	Approach Character 5	Function/Device Character 6	Qualifier Character 7
Ø Central Nervous 1 Peripheral Nervous F Musculoskeletal	X External	V Stimulator	Z No Qualifier
2 Cardiac	X External	S Pacemaker T Defibrillator	Z No Qualifier
9 Respiratory	X External	S Pacemaker	Z No Qualifier

LC Limited Coverage   **NC** Noncovered   ⊞ Combination Member   HAC   Valid OR   Combination Only   DRG Non-OR   New/Revised in GREEN

726   ICD-10-PCS 2021

Extracorporeal or Systemic Assistance and Performance 5A0–5A2

AHA Coding Clinic for table 5A0

2020, 1Q, 10	Intermittent use of continuous positive airway pressure
2018, 2Q, 3-5	Intra-aortic balloon pump
2017, 4Q, 43-44	Insertion of external heart assist devices
2017, 3Q, 18	Intra-aortic balloon pump removal
2017, 1Q, 10-11	External heart assist device
2017, 1Q, 29	Newborn resuscitation using positive pressure ventilation
2017, 1Q, 29	Newborn noninvasive ventilation
2016, 4Q, 137-139	Heart assist device systems
2014, 4Q, 9	Mechanical ventilation
2014, 3Q, 19	Ablation of ventricular tachycardia with Impella® support
2013, 3Q, 18	Heart transplant surgery

AHA Coding Clinic for table 5A1

2019, 4Q, 39-41	Intraoperative extracorporeal membrane oxygenation
2019, 3Q, 19	Insertion of left ventricular catheter
2019, 3Q, 20	Removal and revision of ECMO component
2019, 3Q, 21	Exchange of extracorporeal membrane oxygenation component (oxygenator)
2019, 2Q, 36	Veno-arterial extracorporeal membrane oxygenation via sternotomy

AHA Coding Clinic for table 5A1 (Continued)

2019, 3Q, 22	Extracorporeal membrane oxygenation and Centrimag™ pump
2019, 3Q, 22	Extracorporeal membrane oxygenation transfers
2018, 4Q, 52-54	Percutaneous extracorporeal membrane oxygenation
2018, 1Q, 13	Mechanical ventilation using patient's equipment
2017, 4Q, 71-73	Hemodialysis and renal replacement therapy
2017, 3Q, 7	Senning procedure (arterial switch)
2017, 1Q, 19	Norwood Sano procedure
2016, 1Q, 27	Aortocoronary bypass graft utilizing Y-graft
2016, 1Q, 28	Extracorporeal liver assist device
2016, 1Q, 29	Duration of hemodialysis
2015, 4Q, 22-24	Congenital heart corrective procedures
2014, 4Q, 3-10	Mechanical ventilation
2014, 1Q, 11-15	Sequencing of mechanical ventilation with other procedures
2014, 3Q, 16	Repair of Tetralogy of Fallot
2014, 3Q, 20	MAZE procedure performed with coronary artery bypass graft
2014, 1Q, 10	Repair of thoracic aortic aneurysm & coronary artery bypass graft
2013, 3Q, 18	Heart transplant surgery

5   Extracorporeal or Systemic Assistance and Performance
A   Physiological Systems
Ø   Assistance   Definition: Taking over a portion of a physiological function by extracorporeal means

Body System Character 4	Duration Character 5	Function Character 6	Qualifier Character 7
2 Cardiac	1 Intermittent 2 Continuous	1 Output	Ø Balloon Pump 5 Pulsatile Compression 6 Other Pump D Impeller Pump
5 Circulatory	1 Intermittent 2 Continuous	2 Oxygenation	1 Hyperbaric C Supersaturated
9 Respiratory	2 Continuous	Ø Filtration	Z No Qualifier
9 Respiratory	3 Less than 24 Consecutive Hours 4 24-96 Consecutive Hours 5 Greater than 96 Consecutive Hours	5 Ventilation	7 Continuous Positive Airway Pressure 8 Intermittent Positive Airway Pressure 9 Continuous Negative Airway Pressure A High Nasal Flow/Velocity B Intermittent Negative Airway Pressure Z No Qualifier

Valid OR   5A02[1,2]1[Ø,6,D]

5   Extracorporeal or Systemic Assistance and Performance
A   Physiological Systems
1   Performance   Definition: Completely taking over a physiological function by extracorporeal means

Body System Character 4	Duration Character 5	Function Character 6	Qualifier Character 7
2 Cardiac	Ø Single	1 Output	2 Manual
2 Cardiac	1 Intermittent	3 Pacing	Z No Qualifier
2 Cardiac	2 Continuous	1 Output 3 Pacing	Z No Qualifier
5 Circulatory	2 Continuous A Intraoperative	2 Oxygenation	F Membrane, Central G Membrane, Peripheral Veno-arterial H Membrane, Peripheral Veno-venous
9 Respiratory	Ø Single	5 Ventilation	4 Nonmechanical
9 Respiratory	3 Less than 24 Consecutive Hours 4 24-96 Consecutive Hours 5 Greater than 96 Consecutive Hours	5 Ventilation	Z No Qualifier
C Biliary	Ø Single 6 Multiple	Ø Filtration	Z No Qualifier
D Urinary	7 Intermittent, Less than 6 Hours per day 8 Prolonged Intermittent, 6-18 Hours per day 9 Continuous, Greater than 18 Hours per day	Ø Filtration	Z No Qualifier

Valid OR   5A1522F
DRG Non-OR   5A1522[G,H]
DRG Non-OR   5A19[3,4]5Z
DRG Non-OR   5A1955Z Length of stay must be > 4 consecutive days.
DRG Non-OR   5A1D[7,8,9]ØZ

LC Limited Coverage   **NC** Noncovered   ⊞ Combination Member   HAC   Valid OR   Combination Only   DRG Non-OR   New/Revised in GREEN

ICD-10-PCS 2021   727

Extracorporeal or Systemic Assistance and Performance

5A0–5A1

5   Extracorporeal or Systemic Assistance and Performance
A   Physiological Systems
2   Restoration   Definition: Returning, or attempting to return, a physiological function to its original state by extracorporeal means.

Body System Character 4	Duration Character 5	Function Character 6	Qualifier Character 7
2 Cardiac	Ø Single	4 Rhythm	Z No Qualifier

Extracorporeal or Systemic Therapies 6A0–6AB

AHA Coding Clinic for table 6A4
2019, 2Q, 17   Cryoamputation of lower leg

AHA Coding Clinic for table 6A7
2014, 4Q, 19   Ultrasound accelerated thrombolysis

AHA Coding Clinic for table 6AB
2016, 4Q, 115   Donor organ perfusion

6   Extracorporeal or Systemic Therapies
A   Physiological Systems
0   Atmospheric Control   Definition: Extracorporeal control of atmospheric pressure and composition

Body System Character 4	Duration Character 5	Qualifier Character 6	Qualifier Character 7
Z None	0 Single 1 Multiple	Z No Qualifier	Z No Qualifier

6   Extracorporeal or Systemic Therapies
A   Physiological Systems
1   Decompression   Definition: Extracorporeal elimination of undissolved gas from body fluids

Body System Character 4	Duration Character 5	Qualifier Character 6	Qualifier Character 7
5 Circulatory	0 Single 1 Multiple	Z No Qualifier	Z No Qualifier

6   Extracorporeal or Systemic Therapies
A   Physiological Systems
2   Electromagnetic Therapy   Definition: Extracorporeal treatment by electromagnetic rays

Body System Character 4	Duration Character 5	Qualifier Character 6	Qualifier Character 7
1 Urinary 2 Central Nervous	0 Single 1 Multiple	Z No Qualifier	Z No Qualifier

6   Extracorporeal or Systemic Therapies
A   Physiological Systems
3   Hyperthermia   Definition: Extracorporeal raising of body temperature

Body System Character 4	Duration Character 5	Qualifier Character 6	Qualifier Character 7
Z None	0 Single 1 Multiple	Z No Qualifier	Z No Qualifier

6   Extracorporeal or Systemic Therapies
A   Physiological Systems
4   Hypothermia   Definition: Extracorporeal lowering of body temperature

Body System Character 4	Duration Character 5	Qualifier Character 6	Qualifier Character 7
Z None	0 Single 1 Multiple	Z No Qualifier	Z No Qualifier

6   Extracorporeal or Systemic Therapies
A   Physiological Systems
5   Pheresis   Definition: Extracorporeal separation of blood products

Body System Character 4	Duration Character 5	Qualifier Character 6	Qualifier Character 7
5 Circulatory	0 Single 1 Multiple	Z No Qualifier	0 Erythrocytes 1 Leukocytes 2 Platelets 3 Plasma T Stem Cells, Cord Blood V Stem Cells, Hematopoietic

6   Extracorporeal or Systemic Therapies
A   Physiological Systems
6   Phototherapy   Definition: Extracorporeal treatment by light rays

Body System Character 4	Duration Character 5	Qualifier Character 6	Qualifier Character 7
0 Skin 5 Circulatory	0 Single 1 Multiple	Z No Qualifier	Z No Qualifier

6　Extracorporeal or Systemic Therapies
A　Physiological Systems
7　Ultrasound Therapy　　　Definition: Extracorporeal treatment by ultrasound

Body System Character 4	Duration Character 5	Qualifier Character 6	Qualifier Character 7
5　Circulatory	Ø　Single 1　Multiple	Z　No Qualifier	4　Head and Neck Vessels 5　Heart 6　Peripheral Vessels 7　Other Vessels Z　No Qualifier

6　Extracorporeal or Systemic Therapies
A　Physiological Systems
8　Ultraviolet Light Therapy　　　Definition: Extracorporeal treatment by ultraviolet light

Body System Character 4	Duration Character 5	Qualifier Character 6	Qualifier Character 7
Ø　Skin	Ø　Single 1　Multiple	Z　No Qualifier	Z　No Qualifier

6　Extracorporeal or Systemic Therapies
A　Physiological Systems
9　Shock Wave Therapy　　　Definition: Extracorporeal treatment by shock waves

Body System Character 4	Duration Character 5	Qualifier Character 6	Qualifier Character 7
3　Musculoskeletal	Ø　Single 1　Multiple	Z　No Qualifier	Z　No Qualifier

6　Extracorporeal or Systemic Therapies
A　Physiological Systems
B　Perfusion　　　Definition: Extracorporeal treatment by diffusion of therapeutic fluid

Body System Character 4	Duration Character 5	Qualifier Character 6	Qualifier Character 7
5　Circulatory B　Respiratory System F　Hepatobiliary System and Pancreas T　Urinary System	Ø　Single	B　Donor Organ	Z　No Qualifier

Osteopathic 7WØ

7   **Osteopathic**
W   **Anatomical Regions**
Ø   **Treatment**   Definition: Manual treatment to eliminate or alleviate somatic dysfunction and related disorders

Body Region Character 4	Approach Character 5	Method Character 6	Qualifier Character 7
Ø Head	X External	Ø Articulatory-Raising	Z None
1 Cervical		1 Fascial Release	
2 Thoracic		2 General Mobilization	
3 Lumbar		3 High Velocity-Low Amplitude	
4 Sacrum		4 Indirect	
5 Pelvis		5 Low Velocity-High Amplitude	
6 Lower Extremities		6 Lymphatic Pump	
7 Upper Extremities		7 Muscle Energy-Isometric	
8 Rib Cage		8 Muscle Energy-Isotonic	
9 Abdomen		9 Other Method	

Other Procedures 8C0–8E0

AHA Coding Clinic for table 8E0

2019, 4Q, 41-42	Intraoperative fluorescence guidance
2019, 1Q, 30	Laparoscopic-assisted rectopexy with manual reduction of prolapse
2015, 1Q, 33	Robotic-assisted laparoscopic hysterectomy converted to open procedure
2014, 4Q, 33	Radical prostatectomy

8   Other Procedures
C   Indwelling Device
0   Other Procedures   Definition: Methodologies which attempt to remediate or cure a disorder or disease

Body Region Character 4	Approach Character 5	Method Character 6	Qualifier Character 7
1 Nervous System	X External	6 Collection	J Cerebrospinal Fluid L Other Fluid
2 Circulatory System	X External	6 Collection	K Blood L Other Fluid

8   Other Procedures
E   Physiological Systems and Anatomical Regions
0   Other Procedures   Definition: Methodologies which attempt to remediate or cure a disorder or disease

Body Region Character 4	Approach Character 5	Method Character 6	Qualifier Character 7
1 Nervous System U Female Reproductive System ♀	X External	Y Other Method	7 Examination
2 Circulatory System	3 Percutaneous X External	D Near Infrared Spectroscopy	Z No Qualifier
9 Head and Neck Region	0 Open	C Robotic Assisted Procedure	Z No Qualifier
9 Head and Neck Region	0 Open	E Fluorescence Guided Procedure	M Aminolevulinic Acid Z No Qualifier
9 Head and Neck Region	3 Percutaneous 4 Percutaneous Endoscopic 7 Via Natural or Artificial Opening 8 Via Natural or Artificial Opening Endoscopic	C Robotic Assisted Procedure E Fluorescence Guided Procedure	Z No Qualifier
9 Head and Neck Region	X External	B Computer Assisted Procedure	F With Fluoroscopy G With Computerized Tomography H With Magnetic Resonance Imaging Z No Qualifier
9 Head and Neck Region	X External	C Robotic Assisted Procedure	Z No Qualifier
9 Head and Neck Region	X External	Y Other Method	8 Suture Removal
H Integumentary System and Breast	3 Percutaneous	0 Acupuncture	0 Anesthesia Z No Qualifier
H Integumentary System and Breast ♀	X External	6 Collection	2 Breast Milk
H Integumentary System and Breast	X External	Y Other Method	9 Piercing
K Musculoskeletal System	X External	1 Therapeutic Massage	Z No Qualifier
K Musculoskeletal System	X External	Y Other Method	7 Examination
V Male Reproductive System ♂	X External	1 Therapeutic Massage	C Prostate D Rectum
V Male Reproductive System ♂	X External	6 Collection	3 Sperm
W Trunk Region	0 Open 3 Percutaneous 4 Percutaneous Endoscopic 7 Via Natural or Artificial Opening 8 Via Natural or Artificial Opening Endoscopic	C Robotic Assisted Procedure E Fluorescence Guided Procedure	Z No Qualifier
W Trunk Region	X External	B Computer Assisted Procedure	F With Fluoroscopy G With Computerized Tomography H With Magnetic Resonance Imaging Z No Qualifier
W Trunk Region	X External	C Robotic Assisted Procedure	Z No Qualifier
W Trunk Region	X External	Y Other Method	8 Suture Removal
X Upper Extremity Y Lower Extremity	0 Open 3 Percutaneous 4 Percutaneous Endoscopic	C Robotic Assisted Procedure E Fluorescence Guided Procedure	Z No Qualifier

♂   8E0VX1C
♂   8E0VX63
♀   8E0UXY7
♀   8E0HX62

8E0 Continued on next page

LC Limited Coverage   **NC** Noncovered   ⊞ Combination Member   HAC   Valid OR   Combination Only   DRG Non-OR   New/Revised in **GREEN**

ICD-10-PCS 2021   **733**

8C0–8E0

8   **Other Procedures**
E   **Physiological Systems and Anatomical Regions**
Ø   **Other Procedures**   Definition: Methodologies which attempt to remediate or cure a disorder or disease

Body Region Character 4	Approach Character 5	Method Character 6	Qualifier Character 7
X Upper Extremity **Y** Lower Extremity	**X** External	**B** Computer Assisted Procedure	**F** With Fluoroscopy **G** With Computerized Tomography **H** With Magnetic Resonance Imaging **Z** No Qualifier
X Upper Extremity **Y** Lower Extremity	**X** External	**C** Robotic Assisted Procedure	**Z** No Qualifier
X Upper Extremity **Y** Lower Extremity	**X** External	**Y** Other Method	**8** Suture Removal
Z None	**X** External	**Y** Other Method	**1** In Vitro Fertilization **4** Yoga Therapy **5** Meditation **6** Isolation

Chiropractic 9WB

9   Chiropractic
W   Anatomical Regions
B   Manipulation   Definition: Manual procedure that involves a directed thrust to move a joint past the physiological range of motion, without exceeding the anatomical limit

Body Region Character 4	Approach Character 5	Method Character 6	Qualifier Character 7
Ø Head 1 Cervical 2 Thoracic 3 Lumbar 4 Sacrum 5 Pelvis 6 Lower Extremities 7 Upper Extremities 8 Rib Cage 9 Abdomen	X External	B Non-Manual C Indirect Visceral D Extra-Articular F Direct Visceral G Long Lever Specific Contact H Short Lever Specific Contact J Long and Short Lever Specific Contact K Mechanically Assisted L Other Method	Z None

LC Limited Coverage   **NC** Noncovered   ⊞ Combination Member   HAC   Valid OR   Combination Only   DRG Non-OR   New/Revised in GREEN

ICD-10-PCS 2021   735

Imaging BØØ–BY4

AHA Coding Clinic for table B21
2018, 1Q, 12   Percutaneous balloon valvuloplasty & cardiac catheterization with ventriculogram
2016, 3Q, 36   Type of contrast medium for angiography (high osmolar, low osmolar, and other)

AHA Coding Clinic for table B41
2015, 3Q, 9   Aborted endovascular stenting of superficial femoral artery

AHA Coding Clinic for table B51
2015, 4Q, 30   Vascular access devices

AHA Coding Clinic for table BF4
2014, 3Q, 15   Drainage of pancreatic pseudocyst

B   Imaging
Ø   Central Nervous System
Ø   Plain Radiography   Definition: Planar display of an image developed from the capture of external ionizing radiation on photographic or photoconductive plate

Body Part Character 4	Contrast Character 5	Qualifier Character 6	Qualifier Character 7
B Spinal Cord	Ø High Osmolar 1 Low Osmolar Y Other Contrast Z None	Z None	Z None

B   Imaging
Ø   Central Nervous System
1   Fluoroscopy   Definition: Single plane or bi-plane real time display of an image developed from the capture of external ionizing radioation on a fluorescent screen. The image may also be stored by either digital or analog means.

Body Part Character 4	Contrast Character 5	Qualifier Character 6	Qualifier Character 7
B Spinal Cord	Ø High Osmolar 1 Low Osmolar Y Other Contrast Z None	Z None	Z None

B   Imaging
Ø   Central Nervous System
2   Computerized Tomography (CT Scan)   Definition: Computer reformatted digital display of multiplanar images developed from the capture of multiple exposures of external ionizing radiation

Body Part Character 4	Contrast Character 5	Qualifier Character 6	Qualifier Character 7
Ø Brain 7 Cisterna 8 Cerebral Ventricle(s) 9 Sella Turcica/Pituitary Gland B Spinal Cord	Ø High Osmolar 1 Low Osmolar Y Other Contrast	Ø Unenhanced and Enhanced Z None	Z None
Ø Brain 7 Cisterna 8 Cerebral Ventricle(s) 9 Sella Turcica/Pituitary Gland B Spinal Cord	Z None	Z None	Z None

B   Imaging
Ø   Central Nervous System
3   Magnetic Resonance Imaging (MRI)   Definition: Computer reformatted digital display of multiplanar images developed from the capture of radio-frequency signals emitted by nuclei in a body site excited within a magnetic field

Body Part Character 4	Contrast Character 5	Qualifier Character 6	Qualifier Character 7
Ø Brain 9 Sella Turcica/Pituitary Gland B Spinal Cord C Acoustic Nerves	Y Other Contrast	Ø Unenhanced and Enhanced Z None	Z None
Ø Brain 9 Sella Turcica/Pituitary Gland B Spinal Cord C Acoustic Nerves	Z None	Z None	Z None

LC Limited Coverage   **NC** Noncovered   ⊞ Combination Member   HAC   Valid OR   Combination Only   DRG Non-OR   New/Revised in GREEN
ICD-10-PCS 2021   737

BØØ–BØ3

B   **Imaging**
Ø   **Central Nervous System**
4   **Ultrasonography**   Definition: Real time display of images of anatomy or flow information developed from the capture of relected and attenuated high frequency sound waves

Body Part Character 4	Contrast Character 5	Qualifier Character 6	Qualifier Character 7
Ø Brain B Spinal Cord	Z None	Z None	Z None

B   **Imaging**
2   **Heart**
Ø   **Plain Radiography**   Definition: Planar display of an image developed from the capture of external ionizing radiation on photographic or photoconductive plate

Body Part Character 4	Contrast Character 5	Qualifier Character 6	Qualifier Character 7
Ø Coronary Artery, Single 1 Coronary Arteries, Multiple 2 Coronary Artery Bypass Graft, Single 3 Coronary Artery Bypass Grafts, Multiple 4 Heart, Right 5 Heart, Left 6 Heart, Right and Left 7 Internal Mammary Bypass Graft, Right 8 Internal Mammary Bypass Graft, Left F Bypass Graft, Other	Ø High Osmolar 1 Low Osmolar Y Other Contrast	Z None	Z None

DRG Non-OR   All body part, contrast, and qualifier values

B   **Imaging**
2   **Heart**
1   **Fluoroscopy**   Definition: Single plane or bi-plane real time display of an image developed from the capture of external ionizing radioation on a fluorescent screen. The image may also be stored by either digital or analog means.

Body Part Character 4	Contrast Character 5	Qualifier Character 6	Qualifier Character 7
Ø Coronary Artery, Single 1 Coronary Arteries, Multiple 2 Coronary Artery Bypass Graft, Single 3 Coronary Artery Bypass Grafts, Multiple	Ø High Osmolar 1 Low Osmolar Y Other Contrast	1 Laser	Ø Intraoperative
Ø Coronary Artery, Single 1 Coronary Arteries, Multiple 2 Coronary Artery Bypass Graft, Single 3 Coronary Artery Bypass Grafts, Multiple	Ø High Osmolar 1 Low Osmolar Y Other Contrast	Z None	Z None
4 Heart, Right 5 Heart, Left 6 Heart, Right and Left 7 Internal Mammary Bypass Graft, Right 8 Internal Mammary Bypass Graft, Left F Bypass Graft, Other	Ø High Osmolar 1 Low Osmolar Y Other Contrast	Z None	Z None

DRG Non-OR   All body part, contrast, and qualifier values

B   **Imaging**
2   **Heart**
2   **Computerized Tomography (CT Scan)**   Definition: Computer reformatted digital display of multiplanar images developed from the capture of multiple exposures of external ionizing radiation

Body Part Character 4	Contrast Character 5	Qualifier Character 6	Qualifier Character 7
1 Coronary Arteries, Multiple 3 Coronary Artery Bypass Grafts, Multiple 6 Heart, Right and Left	Ø High Osmolar 1 Low Osmolar Y Other Contrast	Ø Unenhanced and Enhanced Z None	Z None
1 Coronary Arteries, Multiple 3 Coronary Artery Bypass Grafts, Multiple 6 Heart, Right and Left	Z None	2 Intravascular Optical Coherence Z None	Z None

LC Limited Coverage   **NC** Noncovered   ⊞ Combination Member   HAC   Valid OR   Combination Only   DRG Non-OR   New/Revised in GREEN

738   ICD-10-PCS 2021

B   **Imaging**
2   **Heart**
3   **Magnetic Resonance Imaging (MRI)**   Definition: Computer reformatted digital display of multiplanar images developed from the capture of radio-frequency signals emitted by nuclei in a body site excited within a magnetic field

Body Part Character 4	Contrast Character 5	Qualifier Character 6	Qualifier Character 7
1 Coronary Arteries, Multiple 3 Coronary Artery Bypass Grafts, Multiple 6 Heart, Right and Left	Y Other Contrast	Ø Unenhanced and Enhanced Z None	Z None
1 Coronary Arteries, Multiple 3 Coronary Artery Bypass Grafts, Multiple 6 Heart, Right and Left	Z None	Z None	Z None

B   **Imaging**
2   **Heart**
4   **Ultrasonography**   Definition: Real time display of images of anatomy or flow information developed from the capture of relected and attenuated high frequency sound waves

Body Part Character 4	Contrast Character 5	Qualifier Character 6	Qualifier Character 7
Ø Coronary Artery, Single 1 Coronary Arteries, Multiple 4 Heart, Right 5 Heart, Left 6 Heart, Right and Left B Heart with Aorta C Pericardium D Pediatric Heart	Y Other Contrast	Z None	Z None
Ø Coronary Artery, Single 1 Coronary Arteries, Multiple 4 Heart, Right 5 Heart, Left 6 Heart, Right and Left B Heart with Aorta C Pericardium D Pediatric Heart	Z None	Z None	3 Intravascular 4 Transesophageal Z None

B   **Imaging**
3   **Upper Arteries**
Ø   **Plain Radiography**   Definition: Planar display of an image developed from the capture of external ionizing radiation on photographic or photoconductive plate

Body Part Character 4	Contrast Character 5	Qualifier Character 6	Qualifier Character 7
Ø Thoracic Aorta 1 Brachiocephalic-Subclavian Artery, Right 2 Subclavian Artery, Left 3 Common Carotid Artery, Right 4 Common Carotid Artery, Left 5 Common Carotid Arteries, Bilateral 6 Internal Carotid Artery, Right 7 Internal Carotid Artery, Left 8 Internal Carotid Arteries, Bilateral 9 External Carotid Artery, Right B External Carotid Artery, Left C External Carotid Arteries, Bilateral D Vertebral Artery, Right F Vertebral Artery, Left G Vertebral Arteries, Bilateral H Upper Extremity Arteries, Right J Upper Extremity Arteries, Left K Upper Extremity Arteries, Bilateral L Intercostal and Bronchial Arteries M Spinal Arteries N Upper Arteries, Other P Thoraco-Abdominal Aorta Q Cervico-Cerebral Arch R Intracranial Arteries S Pulmonary Artery, Right T Pulmonary Artery, Left	Ø High Osmolar 1 Low Osmolar Y Other Contrast Z None	Z None	Z None

B Imaging
3 Upper Arteries
1 Fluoroscopy   Definition: Single plane or bi-plane real time display of an image developed from the capture of external ionizing radiation on a fluorescent screen. The image may also be stored by either digital or analog means.

Body Part Character 4	Contrast Character 5	Qualifier Character 6	Qualifier Character 7
Ø Thoracic Aorta 1 Brachiocephalic-Subclavian Artery, Right 2 Subclavian Artery, Left 3 Common Carotid Artery, Right 4 Common Carotid Artery, Left 5 Common Carotid Arteries, Bilateral 6 Internal Carotid Artery, Right 7 Internal Carotid Artery, Left 8 Internal Carotid Arteries, Bilateral 9 External Carotid Artery, Right B External Carotid Artery, Left C External Carotid Arteries, Bilateral D Vertebral Artery, Right F Vertebral Artery, Left G Vertebral Arteries, Bilateral H Upper Extremity Arteries, Right J Upper Extremity Arteries, Left K Upper Extremity Arteries, Bilateral L Intercostal and Bronchial Arteries M Spinal Arteries N Upper Arteries, Other P Thoraco-Abdominal Aorta Q Cervico-Cerebral Arch R Intracranial Arteries S Pulmonary Artery, Right T Pulmonary Artery, Left U Pulmonary Trunk	Ø High Osmolar 1 Low Osmolar Y Other Contrast	1 Laser	Ø Intraoperative
Ø Thoracic Aorta 1 Brachiocephalic-Subclavian Artery, Right 2 Subclavian Artery, Left 3 Common Carotid Artery, Right 4 Common Carotid Artery, Left 5 Common Carotid Arteries, Bilateral 6 Internal Carotid Artery, Right 7 Internal Carotid Artery, Left 8 Internal Carotid Arteries, Bilateral 9 External Carotid Artery, Right B External Carotid Artery, Left C External Carotid Arteries, Bilateral D Vertebral Artery, Right F Vertebral Artery, Left G Vertebral Arteries, Bilateral H Upper Extremity Arteries, Right J Upper Extremity Arteries, Left K Upper Extremity Arteries, Bilateral L Intercostal and Bronchial Arteries M Spinal Arteries N Upper Arteries, Other P Thoraco-Abdominal Aorta Q Cervico-Cerebral Arch R Intracranial Arteries S Pulmonary Artery, Right T Pulmonary Artery, Left U Pulmonary Trunk	Ø High Osmolar 1 Low Osmolar Y Other Contrast	Z None	Z None

B31 Continued on next page

B31 Continued

B   **Imaging**
3   **Upper Arteries**
1   **Fluoroscopy**   Definition: Single plane or bi-plane real time display of an image developed from the capture of external ionizing radiation on a fluorescent screen. The image may also be stored by either digital or analog means.

Body Part Character 4	Contrast Character 5	Qualifier Character 6	Qualifier Character 7
Ø Thoracic Aorta	Z None	Z None	Z None
1 Brachiocephalic-Subclavian Artery, Right			
2 Subclavian Artery, Left			
3 Common Carotid Artery, Right			
4 Common Carotid Artery, Left			
5 Common Carotid Arteries, Bilateral			
6 Internal Carotid Artery, Right			
7 Internal Carotid Artery, Left			
8 Internal Carotid Arteries, Bilateral			
9 External Carotid Artery, Right			
B External Carotid Artery, Left			
C External Carotid Arteries, Bilateral			
D Vertebral Artery, Right			
F Vertebral Artery, Left			
G Vertebral Arteries, Bilateral			
H Upper Extremity Arteries, Right			
J Upper Extremity Arteries, Left			
K Upper Extremity Arteries, Bilateral			
L Intercostal and Bronchial Arteries			
M Spinal Arteries			
N Upper Arteries, Other			
P Thoraco-Abdominal Aorta			
Q Cervico-Cerebral Arch			
R Intracranial Arteries			
S Pulmonary Artery, Right			
T Pulmonary Artery, Left			
U Pulmonary Trunk			

B   **Imaging**
3   **Upper Arteries**
2   **Computerized Tomography (CT Scan)**   Definition: Computer reformatted digital display of multiplanar images developed from the capture of multiple exposures of external ionizing radiation

Body Part Character 4	Contrast Character 5	Qualifier Character 6	Qualifier Character 7
Ø Thoracic Aorta	Ø High Osmolar	Z None	Z None
5 Common Carotid Arteries, Bilateral	1 Low Osmolar		
8 Internal Carotid Arteries, Bilateral	Y Other Contrast		
G Vertebral Arteries, Bilateral			
R Intracranial Arteries			
S Pulmonary Artery, Right			
T Pulmonary Artery, Left			
Ø Thoracic Aorta	Z None	2 Intravascular Optical Coherence	Z None
5 Common Carotid Arteries, Bilateral		Z None	
8 Internal Carotid Arteries, Bilateral			
G Vertebral Arteries, Bilateral			
R Intracranial Arteries			
S Pulmonary Artery, Right			
T Pulmonary Artery, Left			

B Imaging
3 Upper Arteries
3 Magnetic Resonance Imaging (MRI) Definition: Computer reformatted digital display of multiplanar images developed from the capture of radio-frequency signals emitted by nuclei in a body site excited within a magnetic field

Body Part Character 4	Contrast Character 5	Qualifier Character 6	Qualifier Character 7
Ø Thoracic Aorta 5 Common Carotid Arteries, Bilateral 8 Internal Carotid Arteries, Bilateral G Vertebral Arteries, Bilateral H Upper Extremity Arteries, Right J Upper Extremity Arteries, Left K Upper Extremity Arteries, Bilateral M Spinal Arteries Q Cervico-Cerebral Arch R Intracranial Arteries	Y Other Contrast	Ø Unenhanced and Enhanced Z None	Z None
Ø Thoracic Aorta 5 Common Carotid Arteries, Bilateral 8 Internal Carotid Arteries, Bilateral G Vertebral Arteries, Bilateral H Upper Extremity Arteries, Right J Upper Extremity Arteries, Left K Upper Extremity Arteries, Bilateral M Spinal Arteries Q Cervico-Cerebral Arch R Intracranial Arteries	Z None	Z None	Z None

B Imaging
3 Upper Arteries
4 Ultrasonography Definition: Real time display of images of anatomy or flow information developed from the capture of relected and attenuated high frequency sound waves

Body Part Character 4	Contrast Character 5	Qualifier Character 6	Qualifier Character 7
Ø Thoracic Aorta 1 Brachiocephalic-Subclavian Artery, Right 2 Subclavian Artery, Left 3 Common Carotid Artery, Right 4 Common Carotid Artery, Left 5 Common Carotid Arteries, Bilateral 6 Internal Carotid Artery, Right 7 Internal Carotid Artery, Left 8 Internal Carotid Arteries, Bilateral H Upper Extremity Arteries, Right J Upper Extremity Arteries, Left K Upper Extremity Arteries, Bilateral R Intracranial Arteries S Pulmonary Artery, Right T Pulmonary Artery, Left V Ophthalmic Arteries	Z None	Z None	3 Intravascular Z None

B Imaging
4 Lower Arteries
Ø Plain Radiography Definition: Planar display of an image developed from the capture of external ionizing radiation on photographic or photoconductive plate

Body Part Character 4	Contrast Character 5	Qualifier Character 6	Qualifier Character 7
Ø Abdominal Aorta 2 Hepatic Artery 3 Splenic Arteries 4 Superior Mesenteric Artery 5 Inferior Mesenteric Artery 6 Renal Artery, Right 7 Renal Artery, Left 8 Renal Arteries, Bilateral 9 Lumbar Arteries B Intra-Abdominal Arteries, Other C Pelvic Arteries D Aorta and Bilateral Lower Extremity Arteries F Lower Extremity Arteries, Right G Lower Extremity Arteries, Left J Lower Arteries, Other M Renal Artery Transplant	Ø High Osmolar 1 Low Osmolar Y Other Contrast	Z None	Z None

B   Imaging
4   Lower Arteries
1   Fluoroscopy   Definition: Single plane or bi-plane real time display of an image developed from the capture of external ionizing radiation on a fluorescent screen. The image may also be stored by either digital or analog means.

Body Part Character 4	Contrast Character 5	Qualifier Character 6	Qualifier Character 7
Ø Abdominal Aorta 2 Hepatic Artery 3 Splenic Arteries 4 Superior Mesenteric Artery 5 Inferior Mesenteric Artery 6 Renal Artery, Right 7 Renal Artery, Left 8 Renal Arteries, Bilateral 9 Lumbar Arteries B Intra-Abdominal Arteries, Other C Pelvic Arteries D Aorta and Bilateral Lower Extremity Arteries F Lower Extremity Arteries, Right G Lower Extremity Arteries, Left J Lower Arteries, Other	Ø High Osmolar 1 Low Osmolar Y Other Contrast	1 Laser	Ø Intraoperative
Ø Abdominal Aorta 2 Hepatic Artery 3 Splenic Arteries 4 Superior Mesenteric Artery 5 Inferior Mesenteric Artery 6 Renal Artery, Right 7 Renal Artery, Left 8 Renal Arteries, Bilateral 9 Lumbar Arteries B Intra-Abdominal Arteries, Other C Pelvic Arteries D Aorta and Bilateral Lower Extremity Arteries F Lower Extremity Arteries, Right G Lower Extremity Arteries, Left J Lower Arteries, Other	Ø High Osmolar 1 Low Osmolar Y Other Contrast	Z None	Z None
Ø Abdominal Aorta 2 Hepatic Artery 3 Splenic Arteries 4 Superior Mesenteric Artery 5 Inferior Mesenteric Artery 6 Renal Artery, Right 7 Renal Artery, Left 8 Renal Arteries, Bilateral 9 Lumbar Arteries B Intra-Abdominal Arteries, Other C Pelvic Arteries D Aorta and Bilateral Lower Extremity Arteries F Lower Extremity Arteries, Right G Lower Extremity Arteries, Left J Lower Arteries, Other	Z None	Z None	Z None

B **Imaging**
4 **Lower Arteries**
2 **Computerized Tomography (CT Scan)** Definition: Computer reformatted digital display of multiplanar images developed from the capture of multiple exposures of external ionizing radiation

Body Part Character 4	Contrast Character 5	Qualifier Character 6	Qualifier Character 7
Ø Abdominal Aorta 1 Celiac Artery 4 Superior Mesenteric Artery 8 Renal Arteries, Bilateral C Pelvic Arteries F Lower Extremity Arteries, Right G Lower Extremity Arteries, Left H Lower Extremity Arteries, Bilateral M Renal Artery Transplant	Ø High Osmolar 1 Low Osmolar Y Other Contrast	Z None	Z None
Ø Abdominal Aorta 1 Celiac Artery 4 Superior Mesenteric Artery 8 Renal Arteries, Bilateral C Pelvic Arteries F Lower Extremity Arteries, Right G Lower Extremity Arteries, Left H Lower Extremity Arteries, Bilateral M Renal Artery Transplant	Z None	2 Intravascular Optical Coherence Z None	Z None

B **Imaging**
4 **Lower Arteries**
3 **Magnetic Resonance Imaging (MRI)** Definition: Computer reformatted digital display of multiplanar images developed from the capture of radio-frequency signals emitted by nuclei in a body site excited within a magnetic field

Body Part Character 4	Contrast Character 5	Qualifier Character 6	Qualifier Character 7
Ø Abdominal Aorta 1 Celiac Artery 4 Superior Mesenteric Artery 8 Renal Arteries, Bilateral C Pelvic Arteries F Lower Extremity Arteries, Right G Lower Extremity Arteries, Left H Lower Extremity Arteries, Bilateral	Y Other Contrast	Ø Unenhanced and Enhanced Z None	Z None
Ø Abdominal Aorta 1 Celiac Artery 4 Superior Mesenteric Artery 8 Renal Arteries, Bilateral C Pelvic Arteries F Lower Extremity Arteries, Right G Lower Extremity Arteries, Left H Lower Extremity Arteries, Bilateral	Z None	Z None	Z None

B **Imaging**
4 **Lower Arteries**
4 **Ultrasonography** Definition: Real time display of images of anatomy or flow information developed from the capture of relected and attenuated high frequency sound waves

Body Part Character 4	Contrast Character 5	Qualifier Character 6	Qualifier Character 7
Ø Abdominal Aorta 4 Superior Mesenteric Artery 5 Inferior Mesenteric Artery 6 Renal Artery, Right 7 Renal Artery, Left 8 Renal Arteries, Bilateral B Intra-Abdominal Arteries, Other F Lower Extremity Arteries, Right G Lower Extremity Arteries, Left H Lower Extremity Arteries, Bilateral K Celiac and Mesenteric Arteries L Femoral Artery N Penile Arteries	Z None	Z None	3 Intravascular Z None

LC Limited Coverage **NC** Noncovered ⊞ Combination Member HAC Valid OR Combination Only DRG Non-OR New/Revised in GREEN

744

ICD-10-PCS 2021

B42–B44

B   **Imaging**
5   **Veins**
Ø   **Plain Radiography**   Definition: Planar display of an image developed from the capture of external ionizing radiation on photographic or photoconductive plate

Body Part Character 4	Contrast Character 5	Qualifier Character 6	Qualifier Character 7
Ø Epidural Veins	Ø High Osmolar	Z None	Z None
1 Cerebral and Cerebellar Veins	1 Low Osmolar		
2 Intracranial Sinuses	Y Other Contrast		
3 Jugular Veins, Right			
4 Jugular Veins, Left			
5 Jugular Veins, Bilateral			
6 Subclavian Vein, Right			
7 Subclavian Vein, Left			
8 Superior Vena Cava			
9 Inferior Vena Cava			
B Lower Extremity Veins, Right			
C Lower Extremity Veins, Left			
D Lower Extremity Veins, Bilateral			
F Pelvic (Iliac) Veins, Right			
G Pelvic (Iliac) Veins, Left			
H Pelvic (Iliac) Veins, Bilateral			
J Renal Vein, Right			
K Renal Vein, Left			
L Renal Veins, Bilateral			
M Upper Extremity Veins, Right			
N Upper Extremity Veins, Left			
P Upper Extremity Veins, Bilateral			
Q Pulmonary Vein, Right			
R Pulmonary Vein, Left			
S Pulmonary Veins, Bilateral			
T Portal and Splanchnic Veins			
V Veins, Other			
W Dialysis Shunt/Fistula			

B   **Imaging**
5   **Veins**
1   **Fluoroscopy**   Definition: Single plane or bi-plane real time display of an image developed from the capture of external ionizing radioation on a fluorescent screen. The image may also be stored by either digital or analog means.

Body Part Character 4	Contrast Character 5	Qualifier Character 6	Qualifier Character 7
Ø Epidural Veins	Ø High Osmolar	Z None	A Guidance
1 Cerebral and Cerebellar Veins	1 Low Osmolar		Z None
2 Intracranial Sinuses	Y Other Contrast		
3 Jugular Veins, Right	Z None		
4 Jugular Veins, Left			
5 Jugular Veins, Bilateral			
6 Subclavian Vein, Right			
7 Subclavian Vein, Left			
8 Superior Vena Cava			
9 Inferior Vena Cava			
B Lower Extremity Veins, Right			
C Lower Extremity Veins, Left			
D Lower Extremity Veins, Bilateral			
F Pelvic (Iliac) Veins, Right			
G Pelvic (Iliac) Veins, Left			
H Pelvic (Iliac) Veins, Bilateral			
J Renal Vein, Right			
K Renal Vein, Left			
L Renal Veins, Bilateral			
M Upper Extremity Veins, Right			
N Upper Extremity Veins, Left			
P Upper Extremity Veins, Bilateral			
Q Pulmonary Vein, Right			
R Pulmonary Vein, Left			
S Pulmonary Veins, Bilateral			
T Portal and Splanchnic Veins			
V Veins, Other			
W Dialysis Shunt/Fistula			

LC Limited Coverage   **NC** Noncovered   ⊞ Combination Member   **HAC**   Valid OR   Combination Only   DRG Non-OR   New/Revised in GREEN

ICD-10-PCS 2021   745

B5Ø–B51

B   **Imaging**
5   **Veins**
2   **Computerized Tomography (CT Scan)** Definition: Computer reformatted digital display of multiplanar images developed from the capture of multiple exposures of external ionizing radiation

Body Part Character 4	Contrast Character 5	Qualifier Character 6	Qualifier Character 7
2 Intracranial Sinuses 8 Superior Vena Cava 9 Inferior Vena Cava F Pelvic (Iliac) Veins, Right G Pelvic (Iliac) Veins, Left H Pelvic (Iliac) Veins, Bilateral J Renal Vein, Right K Renal Vein, Left L Renal Veins, Bilateral Q Pulmonary Vein, Right R Pulmonary Vein, Left S Pulmonary Veins, Bilateral T Portal and Splanchnic Veins	Ø High Osmolar 1 Low Osmolar Y Other Contrast	Ø Unenhanced and Enhanced Z None	Z None
2 Intracranial Sinuses 8 Superior Vena Cava 9 Inferior Vena Cava F Pelvic (Iliac) Veins, Right G Pelvic (Iliac) Veins, Left H Pelvic (Iliac) Veins, Bilateral J Renal Vein, Right K Renal Vein, Left L Renal Veins, Bilateral Q Pulmonary Vein, Right R Pulmonary Vein, Left S Pulmonary Veins, Bilateral T Portal and Splanchnic Veins	Z None	2 Intravascular Optical Coherence Z None	Z None

B   **Imaging**
5   **Veins**
3   **Magnetic Resonance Imaging (MRI)** Definition: Computer reformatted digital display of multiplanar images developed from the capture of radio-frequency signals emitted by nuclei in a body site excited within a magnetic field

Body Part Character 4	Contrast Character 5	Qualifier Character 6	Qualifier Character 7
1 Cerebral and Cerebellar Veins 2 Intracranial Sinuses 5 Jugular Veins, Bilateral 8 Superior Vena Cava 9 Inferior Vena Cava B Lower Extremity Veins, Right C Lower Extremity Veins, Left D Lower Extremity Veins, Bilateral H Pelvic (Iliac) Veins, Bilateral L Renal Veins, Bilateral M Upper Extremity Veins, Right N Upper Extremity Veins, Left P Upper Extremity Veins, Bilateral S Pulmonary Veins, Bilateral T Portal and Splanchnic Veins V Veins, Other	Y Other Contrast	Ø Unenhanced and Enhanced Z None	Z None
1 Cerebral and Cerebellar Veins 2 Intracranial Sinuses 5 Jugular Veins, Bilateral 8 Superior Vena Cava 9 Inferior Vena Cava B Lower Extremity Veins, Right C Lower Extremity Veins, Left D Lower Extremity Veins, Bilateral H Pelvic (Iliac) Veins, Bilateral L Renal Veins, Bilateral M Upper Extremity Veins, Right N Upper Extremity Veins, Left P Upper Extremity Veins, Bilateral S Pulmonary Veins, Bilateral T Portal and Splanchnic Veins V Veins, Other	Z None	Z None	Z None

B　Imaging
5　Veins
4　Ultrasonography　Definition: Real time display of images of anatomy or flow information developed from the capture of relected and attenuated high frequency sound waves

Body Part Character 4	Contrast Character 5	Qualifier Character 6	Qualifier Character 7
3　Jugular Veins, Right 4　Jugular Veins, Left 6　Subclavian Vein, Right 7　Subclavian Vein, Left 8　Superior Vena Cava 9　Inferior Vena Cava B　Lower Extremity Veins, Right C　Lower Extremity Veins, Left D　Lower Extremity Veins, Bilateral J　Renal Vein, Right K　Renal Vein, Left L　Renal Veins, Bilateral M　Upper Extremity Veins, Right N　Upper Extremity Veins, Left P　Upper Extremity Veins, Bilateral T　Portal and Splanchnic Veins	Z　None	Z　None	3　Intravascular A　Guidance Z　None

B　Imaging
7　Lymphatic System
Ø　Plain Radiography　Definition: Planar display of an image developed from the capture of external ionizing radiation on photographic or photoconductive plate

Body Part Character 4	Contrast Character 5	Qualifier Character 6	Qualifier Character 7
Ø　Abdominal/Retroperitoneal 　　Lymphatics, Unilateral 1　Abdominal/Retroperitoneal 　　Lymphatics, Bilateral 4　Lymphatics, Head and Neck 5　Upper Extremity Lymphatics, Right 6　Upper Extremity Lymphatics, Left 7　Upper Extremity Lymphatics, 　　Bilateral 8　Lower Extremity Lymphatics, Right 9　Lower Extremity Lymphatics, Left B　Lower Extremity Lymphatics, 　　Bilateral C　Lymphatics, Pelvic	Ø　High Osmolar 1　Low Osmolar Y　Other Contrast	Z　None	Z　None

B　Imaging
8　Eye
Ø　Plain Radiography　Definition: Planar display of an image developed from the capture of external ionizing radiation on photographic or photoconductive plate

Body Part Character 4	Contrast Character 5	Qualifier Character 6	Qualifier Character 7
Ø　Lacrimal Duct, Right 1　Lacrimal Duct, Left 2　Lacrimal Ducts, Bilateral	Ø　High Osmolar 1　Low Osmolar Y　Other Contrast	Z　None	Z　None
3　Optic Foramina, Right 4　Optic Foramina, Left 5　Eye, Right 6　Eye, Left 7　Eyes, Bilateral	Z　None	Z　None	Z　None

B　Imaging
8　Eye
2　Computerized Tomography (CT Scan)　Definition: Computer reformatted digital display of multiplanar images developed from the capture of multiple exposures of external ionizing radiation

Body Part Character 4	Contrast Character 5	Qualifier Character 6	Qualifier Character 7
5　Eye, Right 6　Eye, Left 7　Eyes, Bilateral	Ø　High Osmolar 1　Low Osmolar Y　Other Contrast	Ø　Unenhanced and Enhanced Z　None	Z　None
5　Eye, Right 6　Eye, Left 7　Eyes, Bilateral	Z　None	Z　None	Z　None

B **Imaging**
8 **Eye**
3 **Magnetic Resonance Imaging (MRI)**   Definition: Computer reformatted digital display of multiplanar images developed from the capture of radio-frequency signals emitted by nuclei in a body site excited within a magnetic field

Body Part Character 4	Contrast Character 5	Qualifier Character 6	Qualifier Character 7
5 Eye, Right 6 Eye, Left 7 Eyes, Bilateral	Y Other Contrast	Ø Unenhanced and Enhanced Z None	Z None
5 Eye, Right 6 Eye, Left 7 Eyes, Bilateral	Z None	Z None	Z None

B **Imaging**
8 **Eye**
4 **Ultrasonography**   Definition: Real time display of images of anatomy or flow information developed from the capture of relected and attenuated high frequency sound waves

Body Part Character 4	Contrast Character 5	Qualifier Character 6	Qualifier Character 7
5 Eye, Right 6 Eye, Left 7 Eyes, Bilateral	Z None	Z None	Z None

B **Imaging**
9 **Ear, Nose, Mouth and Throat**
Ø **Plain Radiography**   Definition: Planar display of an image developed from the capture of external ionizing radiation on photographic or photoconductive plate

Body Part Character 4	Contrast Character 5	Qualifier Character 6	Qualifier Character 7
2 Paranasal Sinuses F Nasopharynx/Oropharynx H Mastoids	Z None	Z None	Z None
4 Parotid Gland, Right 5 Parotid Gland, Left 6 Parotid Glands, Bilateral 7 Submandibular Gland, Right 8 Submandibular Gland, Left 9 Submandibular Glands, Bilateral B Salivary Gland, Right C Salivary Gland, Left D Salivary Glands, Bilateral	Ø High Osmolar 1 Low Osmolar Y Other Contrast	Z None	Z None

B **Imaging**
9 **Ear, Nose, Mouth and Throat**
1 **Fluoroscopy**   Definition: Single plane or bi-plane real time display of an image developed from the capture of external ionizing radioation on a fluorescent screen. The image may also be stored by either digital or analog means.

Body Part Character 4	Contrast Character 5	Qualifier Character 6	Qualifier Character 7
G Pharynx and Epiglottis J Larynx	Y Other Contrast Z None	Z None	Z None

B **Imaging**
9 **Ear, Nose, Mouth and Throat**
2 **Computerized Tomography (CT Scan)**   Definition: Computer reformatted digital display of multiplanar images developed from the capture of multiple exposures of external ionizing radiation

Body Part Character 4	Contrast Character 5	Qualifier Character 6	Qualifier Character 7
Ø Ear 2 Paranasal Sinuses 6 Parotid Glands, Bilateral 9 Submandibular Glands, Bilateral D Salivary Glands, Bilateral F Nasopharynx/Oropharynx J Larynx	Ø High Osmolar 1 Low Osmolar Y Other Contrast	Ø Unenhanced and Enhanced Z None	Z None
Ø Ear 2 Paranasal Sinuses 6 Parotid Glands, Bilateral 9 Submandibular Glands, Bilateral D Salivary Glands, Bilateral F Nasopharynx/Oropharynx J Larynx	Z None	Z None	Z None

LC Limited Coverage   NC Noncovered   ⊞ Combination Member   HAC   Valid OR   Combination Only   DRG Non-OR   New/Revised in GREEN
748   ICD-10-PCS 2021

B83–B92

B   Imaging
9   Ear, Nose, Mouth and Throat
3   Magnetic Resonance Imaging (MRI)   Definition: Computer reformatted digital display of multiplanar images developed from the capture of radio-frequency signals emitted by nuclei in a body site excited within a magnetic field

Body Part Character 4	Contrast Character 5	Qualifier Character 6	Qualifier Character 7
Ø Ear 2 Paranasal Sinuses 6 Parotid Glands, Bilateral 9 Submandibular Glands, Bilateral D Salivary Glands, Bilateral F Nasopharynx/Oropharynx J Larynx	Y Other Contrast	Ø Unenhanced and Enhanced Z None	Z None
Ø Ear 2 Paranasal Sinuses 6 Parotid Glands, Bilateral 9 Submandibular Glands, Bilateral D Salivary Glands, Bilateral F Nasopharynx/Oropharynx J Larynx	Z None	Z None	Z None

B   Imaging
B   Respiratory System
Ø   Plain Radiography   Definition: Planar display of an image developed from the capture of external ionizing radiation on photographic or photoconductive plate

Body Part Character 4	Contrast Character 5	Qualifier Character 6	Qualifier Character 7
7 Tracheobronchial Tree, Right 8 Tracheobronchial Tree, Left 9 Tracheobronchial Trees, Bilateral	Y Other Contrast	Z None	Z None
D Upper Airways	Z None	Z None	Z None

B   Imaging
B   Respiratory System
1   Fluoroscopy   Definition: Single plane or bi-plane real time display of an image developed from the capture of external ionizing radioation on a fluorescent screen. The image may also be stored by either digital or analog means.

Body Part Character 4	Contrast Character 5	Qualifier Character 6	Qualifier Character 7
2 Lung, Right 3 Lung, Left 4 Lungs, Bilateral 6 Diaphragm C Mediastinum D Upper Airways	Z None	Z None	Z None
7 Tracheobronchial Tree, Right 8 Tracheobronchial Tree, Left 9 Tracheobronchial Trees, Bilateral	Y Other Contrast	Z None	Z None

B   Imaging
B   Respiratory System
2   Computerized Tomography (CT Scan)   Definition: Computer reformatted digital display of multiplanar images developed from the capture of multiple exposures of external ionizing radiation

Body Part Character 4	Contrast Character 5	Qualifier Character 6	Qualifier Character 7
4 Lungs, Bilateral 7 Tracheobronchial Tree, Right 8 Tracheobronchial Tree, Left 9 Tracheobronchial Trees, Bilateral F Trachea/Airways	Ø High Osmolar 1 Low Osmolar Y Other Contrast	Ø Unenhanced and Enhanced Z None	Z None
4 Lungs, Bilateral 7 Tracheobronchial Tree, Right 8 Tracheobronchial Tree, Left 9 Tracheobronchial Trees, Bilateral F Trachea/Airways	Z None	Z None	Z None

B   Imaging
B   Respiratory System
3   Magnetic Resonance Imaging (MRI)   Definition: Computer reformatted digital display of multiplanar images developed from the capture of radio-frequency signals emitted by nuclei in a body site excited within a magnetic field

Body Part Character 4	Contrast Character 5	Qualifier Character 6	Qualifier Character 7
G Lung Apices	Y Other Contrast	0 Unenhanced and Enhanced Z None	Z None
G Lung Apices	Z None	Z None	Z None

B   Imaging
B   Respiratory System
4   Ultrasonography   Definition: Real time display of images of anatomy or flow information developed from the capture of relected and attenuated high frequency sound waves

Body Part Character 4	Contrast Character 5	Qualifier Character 6	Qualifier Character 7
B Pleura C Mediastinum	Z None	Z None	Z None

B   Imaging
D   Gastrointestinal System
1   Fluoroscopy   Definition: Single plane or bi-plane real time display of an image developed from the capture of external ionizing radioation on a fluorescent screen. The image may also be stored by either digital or analog means.

Body Part Character 4	Contrast Character 5	Qualifier Character 6	Qualifier Character 7
1 Esophagus 2 Stomach 3 Small Bowel 4 Colon 5 Upper GI 6 Upper GI and Small Bowel 9 Duodenum B Mouth/Oropharynx	Y Other Contrast Z None	Z None	Z None

B   Imaging
D   Gastrointestinal System
2   Computerized Tomography (CT Scan)   Definition: Computer reformatted digital display of multiplanar images developed from the capture of multiple exposures of external ionizing radiation

Body Part Character 4	Contrast Character 5	Qualifier Character 6	Qualifier Character 7
4 Colon	0 High Osmolar 1 Low Osmolar Y Other Contrast	0 Unenhanced and Enhanced Z None	Z None
4 Colon	Z None	Z None	Z None

B   Imaging
D   Gastrointestinal System
4   Ultrasonography   Definition: Real time display of images of anatomy or flow information developed from the capture of relected and attenuated high frequency sound waves

Body Part Character 4	Contrast Character 5	Qualifier Character 6	Qualifier Character 7
1 Esophagus 2 Stomach 7 Gastrointestinal Tract 8 Appendix 9 Duodenum C Rectum	Z None	Z None	Z None

B   Imaging
F   Hepatobiliary System and Pancreas
0   Plain Radiography   Definition: Planar display of an image developed from the capture of external ionizing radiation on photographic or photoconductive plate

Body Part Character 4	Contrast Character 5	Qualifier Character 6	Qualifier Character 7
0 Bile Ducts 3 Gallbladder and Bile Ducts C Hepatobiliary System, All	0 High Osmolar 1 Low Osmolar Y Other Contrast	Z None	Z None

B Imaging
F Hepatobiliary System and Pancreas
1 Fluoroscopy Definition: Single plane or bi-plane real time display of an image developed from the capture of external ionizing radioation on a fluorescent screen. The image may also be stored by either digital or analog means.

Body Part Character 4	Contrast Character 5	Qualifier Character 6	Qualifier Character 7
Ø Bile Ducts 1 Biliary and Pancreatic Ducts 2 Gallbladder 3 Gallbladder and Bile Ducts 4 Gallbladder, Bile Ducts and Pancreatic Ducts 8 Pancreatic Ducts	Ø High Osmolar 1 Low Osmolar Y Other Contrast	Z None	Z None

B Imaging
F Hepatobiliary System and Pancreas
2 Computerized Tomography (CT Scan) Definition: Computer reformatted digital display of multiplanar images developed from the capture of multiple exposures of external ionizing radiation

Body Part Character 4	Contrast Character 5	Qualifier Character 6	Qualifier Character 7
5 Liver 6 Liver and Spleen 7 Pancreas C Hepatobiliary System, All	Ø High Osmolar 1 Low Osmolar Y Other Contrast	Ø Unenhanced and Enhanced Z None	Z None
5 Liver 6 Liver and Spleen 7 Pancreas C Hepatobiliary System, All	Z None	Z None	Z None

B Imaging
F Hepatobiliary System and Pancreas
3 Magnetic Resonance Imaging (MRI) Definition: Computer reformatted digital display of multiplanar images developed from the capture of radio-frequency signals emitted by nuclei in a body site excited within a magnetic field

Body Part Character 4	Contrast Character 5	Qualifier Character 6	Qualifier Character 7
5 Liver 6 Liver and Spleen 7 Pancreas	Y Other Contrast	Ø Unenhanced and Enhanced Z None	Z None
5 Liver 6 Liver and Spleen 7 Pancreas	Z None	Z None	Z None

B Imaging
F Hepatobiliary System and Pancreas
4 Ultrasonography Definition: Real time display of images of anatomy or flow information developed from the capture of relected and attenuated high frequency sound waves

Body Part Character 4	Contrast Character 5	Qualifier Character 6	Qualifier Character 7
Ø Bile Ducts 2 Gallbladder 3 Gallbladder and Bile Ducts 5 Liver 6 Liver and Spleen 7 Pancreas C Hepatobiliary System, All	Z None	Z None	Z None

B Imaging
F Hepatobiliary System and Pancreas
5 Other Imaging Definition: Other specified modality for visualizing a body part

Body Part Character 4	Contrast Character 5	Qualifier Character 6	Qualifier Character 7
Ø Bile Ducts 2 Gallbladder 3 Gallbladder and Bile Ducts 5 Liver 6 Liver and Spleen 7 Pancreas C Hepatobiliary System, All	2 Fluorescing Agent	Ø Indocyanine Green Dye Z None	Ø Intraoperative Z None

LC Limited Coverage   **NC** Noncovered   ⊞ Combination Member   HAC   Valid OR   Combination Only   DRG Non-OR   New/Revised in GREEN

ICD-10-PCS 2021

751

BF1–BF5

B   Imaging
G   Endocrine System
2   Computerized Tomography (CT Scan) Definition: Computer reformatted digital display of multiplanar images developed from the capture of multiple exposures of external ionizing radiation

Body Part Character 4	Contrast Character 5	Qualifier Character 6	Qualifier Character 7
2 Adrenal Glands, Bilateral 3 Parathyroid Glands 4 Thyroid Gland	Ø High Osmolar 1 Low Osmolar Y Other Contrast	Ø Unenhanced and Enhanced Z None	Z None
2 Adrenal Glands, Bilateral 3 Parathyroid Glands 4 Thyroid Gland	Z None	Z None	Z None

B   Imaging
G   Endocrine System
3   Magnetic Resonance Imaging (MRI)   Definition: Computer reformatted digital display of multiplanar images developed from the capture of radio-frequency signals emitted by nuclei in a body site excited within a magnetic field

Body Part Character 4	Contrast Character 5	Qualifier Character 6	Qualifier Character 7
2 Adrenal Glands, Bilateral 3 Parathyroid Glands 4 Thyroid Gland	Y Other Contrast	Ø Unenhanced and Enhanced Z None	Z None
2 Adrenal Glands, Bilateral 3 Parathyroid Glands 4 Thyroid Gland	Z None	Z None	Z None

B   Imaging
G   Endocrine System
4   Ultrasonography   Definition: Real time display of images of anatomy or flow information developed from the capture of relected and attenuated high frequency sound waves

Body Part Character 4	Contrast Character 5	Qualifier Character 6	Qualifier Character 7
Ø Adrenal Gland, Right 1 Adrenal Gland, Left 2 Adrenal Glands, Bilateral 3 Parathyroid Glands 4 Thyroid Gland	Z None	Z None	Z None

B   Imaging
H   Skin, Subcutaneous Tissue and Breast
Ø   Plain Radiography   Definition: Planar display of an image developed from the capture of external ionizing radiation on photographic or photoconductive plate

Body Part Character 4	Contrast Character 5	Qualifier Character 6	Qualifier Character 7
Ø Breast, Right 1 Breast, Left 2 Breasts, Bilateral	Z None	Z None	Z None
3 Single Mammary Duct, Right 4 Single Mammary Duct, Left 5 Multiple Mammary Ducts, Right 6 Multiple Mammary Ducts, Left	Ø High Osmolar 1 Low Osmolar Y Other Contrast Z None	Z None	Z None

B   Imaging
H   Skin, Subcutaneous Tissue and Breast
3   Magnetic Resonance Imaging (MRI)   Definition: Computer reformatted digital display of multiplanar images developed from the capture of radio-frequency signals emitted by nuclei in a body site excited within a magnetic field

Body Part Character 4	Contrast Character 5	Qualifier Character 6	Qualifier Character 7
Ø Breast, Right 1 Breast, Left 2 Breasts, Bilateral D Subcutaneous Tissue, Head/Neck F Subcutaneous Tissue, Upper Extremity G Subcutaneous Tissue, Thorax H Subcutaneous Tissue, Abdomen and Pelvis J Subcutaneous Tissue, Lower Extremity	Y Other Contrast	Ø Unenhanced and Enhanced Z None	Z None
Ø Breast, Right 1 Breast, Left 2 Breasts, Bilateral D Subcutaneous Tissue, Head/Neck F Subcutaneous Tissue, Upper Extremity G Subcutaneous Tissue, Thorax H Subcutaneous Tissue, Abdomen and Pelvis J Subcutaneous Tissue, Lower Extremity	Z None	Z None	Z None

B   Imaging
H   Skin, Subcutaneous Tissue and Breast
4   Ultrasonography   Definition: Real time display of images of anatomy or flow information developed from the capture of relected and attenuated high frequency sound waves

Body Part Character 4	Contrast Character 5	Qualifier Character 6	Qualifier Character 7
Ø Breast, Right 1 Breast, Left 2 Breasts, Bilateral 7 Extremity, Upper 8 Extremity, Lower 9 Abdominal Wall B Chest Wall C Head and Neck	Z None	Z None	Z None

B   Imaging
L   Connective Tissue
3   Magnetic Resonance Imaging (MRI)   Definition: Computer reformatted digital display of multiplanar images developed from the capture of radio-frequency signals emitted by nuclei in a body site excited within a magnetic field

Body Part Character 4	Contrast Character 5	Qualifier Character 6	Qualifier Character 7
Ø Connective Tissue, Upper Extremity 1 Connective Tissue, Lower Extremity 2 Tendons, Upper Extremity 3 Tendons, Lower Extremity	Y Other Contrast	Ø Unenhanced and Enhanced Z None	Z None
Ø Connective Tissue, Upper Extremity 1 Connective Tissue, Lower Extremity 2 Tendons, Upper Extremity 3 Tendons, Lower Extremity	Z None	Z None	Z None

B   Imaging
L   Connective Tissue
4   Ultrasonography   Definition: Real time display of images of anatomy or flow information developed from the capture of relected and attenuated high frequency sound waves

Body Part Character 4	Contrast Character 5	Qualifier Character 6	Qualifier Character 7
Ø Connective Tissue, Upper Extremity 1 Connective Tissue, Lower Extremity 2 Tendons, Upper Extremity 3 Tendons, Lower Extremity	Z None	Z None	Z None

LC Limited Coverage   NC Noncovered   ⊞ Combination Member   HAC   Valid OR   Combination Only   DRG Non-OR   New/Revised in GREEN

B   **Imaging**
N   **Skull and Facial Bones**
0   **Plain Radiography**   Definition: Planar display of an image developed from the capture of external ionizing radiation on photographic or photoconductive plate

Body Part Character 4	Contrast Character 5	Qualifier Character 6	Qualifier Character 7
0 Skull **1** Orbit, Right **2** Orbit, Left **3** Orbits, Bilateral **4** Nasal Bones **5** Facial Bones **6** Mandible **B** Zygomatic Arch, Right **C** Zygomatic Arch, Left **D** Zygomatic Arches, Bilateral **G** Tooth, Single **H** Teeth, Multiple **J** Teeth, All	**Z** None	**Z** None	**Z** None
7 Temporomandibular Joint, Right **8** Temporomandibular Joint, Left **9** Temporomandibular Joints, Bilateral	**0** High Osmolar **1** Low Osmolar **Y** Other Contrast **Z** None	**Z** None	**Z** None

B   **Imaging**
N   **Skull and Facial Bones**
1   **Fluoroscopy**   Definition: Single plane or bi-plane real time display of an image developed from the capture of external ionizing radioation on a fluorescent screen. The image may also be stored by either digital or analog means.

Body Part Character 4	Contrast Character 5	Qualifier Character 6	Qualifier Character 7
7 Temporomandibular Joint, Right **8** Temporomandibular Joint, Left **9** Temporomandibular Joints, Bilateral	**0** High Osmolar **1** Low Osmolar **Y** Other Contrast **Z** None	**Z** None	**Z** None

B   **Imaging**
N   **Skull and Facial Bones**
2   **Computerized Tomography (CT Scan)**   Definition: Computer reformatted digital display of multiplanar images developed from the capture of multiple exposures of external ionizing radiation

Body Part Character 4	Contrast Character 5	Qualifier Character 6	Qualifier Character 7
0 Skull **3** Orbits, Bilateral **5** Facial Bones **6** Mandible **9** Temporomandibular Joints, Bilateral **F** Temporal Bones	**0** High Osmolar **1** Low Osmolar **Y** Other Contrast **Z** None	**Z** None	**Z** None

B   **Imaging**
N   **Skull and Facial Bones**
3   **Magnetic Resonance Imaging (MRI)**   Definition: Computer reformatted digital display of multiplanar images developed from the capture of radio-frequency signals emitted by nuclei in a body site excited within a magnetic field

Body Part Character 4	Contrast Character 5	Qualifier Character 6	Qualifier Character 7
9 Temporomandibular Joints, Bilateral	**Y** Other Contrast **Z** None	**Z** None	**Z** None

LC Limited Coverage   **NC** Noncovered   ⊞ Combination Member   HAC   Valid OR   Combination Only   DRG Non-OR   New/Revised in GREEN

754   ICD-10-PCS 2021

BN0–BN3

B   Imaging
P   Non-Axial Upper Bones
Ø   Plain Radiography   Definition: Planar display of an image developed from the capture of external ionizing radiation on photographic or photoconductive plate

Body Part Character 4	Contrast Character 5	Qualifier Character 6	Qualifier Character 7
Ø Sternoclavicular Joint, Right 1 Sternoclavicular Joint, Left 2 Sternoclavicular Joints, Bilateral 3 Acromioclavicular Joints, Bilateral 4 Clavicle, Right 5 Clavicle, Left 6 Scapula, Right 7 Scapula, Left A Humerus, Right B Humerus, Left E Upper Arm, Right F Upper Arm, Left J Forearm, Right K Forearm, Left N Hand, Right P Hand, Left R Finger(s), Right S Finger(s), Left X Ribs, Right Y Ribs, Left	Z None	Z None	Z None
8 Shoulder, Right 9 Shoulder, Left C Hand/Finger Joint, Right D Hand/Finger Joint, Left G Elbow, Right H Elbow, Left L Wrist, Right M Wrist, Left	Ø High Osmolar 1 Low Osmolar Y Other Contrast Z None	Z None	Z None

B   Imaging
P   Non-Axial Upper Bones
1   Fluoroscopy   Definition: Single plane or bi-plane real time display of an image developed from the capture of external ionizing radioation on a fluorescent screen. The image may also be stored by either digital or analog means.

Body Part Character 4	Contrast Character 5	Qualifier Character 6	Qualifier Character 7
Ø Sternoclavicular Joint, Right 1 Sternoclavicular Joint, Left 2 Sternoclavicular Joints, Bilateral 3 Acromioclavicular Joints, Bilateral 4 Clavicle, Right 5 Clavicle, Left 6 Scapula, Right 7 Scapula, Left A Humerus, Right B Humerus, Left E Upper Arm, Right F Upper Arm, Left J Forearm, Right K Forearm, Left N Hand, Right P Hand, Left R Finger(s), Right S Finger(s), Left X Ribs, Right Y Ribs, Left	Z None	Z None	Z None
8 Shoulder, Right 9 Shoulder, Left L Wrist, Right M Wrist, Left	Ø High Osmolar 1 Low Osmolar Y Other Contrast Z None	Z None	Z None
C Hand/Finger Joint, Right D Hand/Finger Joint, Left G Elbow, Right H Elbow, Left	Ø High Osmolar 1 Low Osmolar Y Other Contrast	Z None	Z None

Imaging

B   Imaging
P   Non-Axial Upper Bones
2   Computerized Tomography (CT Scan) Definition: Computer reformatted digital display of multiplanar images developed from the capture of multiple exposures of external ionizing radiation

Body Part Character 4	Contrast Character 5	Qualifier Character 6	Qualifier Character 7
Ø Sternoclavicular Joint, Right 1 Sternoclavicular Joint, Left W Thorax	Ø High Osmolar 1 Low Osmolar Y Other Contrast	Z None	Z None
2 Sternoclavicular Joints, Bilateral 3 Acromioclavicular Joints, Bilateral 4 Clavicle, Right 5 Clavicle, Left 6 Scapula, Right 7 Scapula, Left 8 Shoulder, Right 9 Shoulder, Left A Humerus, Right B Humerus, Left E Upper Arm, Right F Upper Arm, Left G Elbow, Right H Elbow, Left J Forearm, Right K Forearm, Left L Wrist, Right M Wrist, Left N Hand, Right P Hand, Left Q Hands and Wrists, Bilateral R Finger(s), Right S Finger(s), Left T Upper Extremity, Right U Upper Extremity, Left V Upper Extremities, Bilateral X Ribs, Right Y Ribs, Left	Ø High Osmolar 1 Low Osmolar Y Other Contrast Z None	Z None	Z None
C Hand/Finger Joint, Right D Hand/Finger Joint, Left	Z None	Z None	Z None

B   Imaging
P   Non-Axial Upper Bones
3   Magnetic Resonance Imaging (MRI) Definition: Computer reformatted digital display of multiplanar images developed from the capture of radio-frequency signals emitted by nuclei in a body site excited within a magnetic field

Body Part Character 4	Contrast Character 5	Qualifier Character 6	Qualifier Character 7
8 Shoulder, Right 9 Shoulder, Left C Hand/Finger Joint, Right D Hand/Finger Joint, Left E Upper Arm, Right F Upper Arm, Left G Elbow, Right H Elbow, Left J Forearm, Right K Forearm, Left L Wrist, Right M Wrist, Left	Y Other Contrast	Ø Unenhanced and Enhanced Z None	Z None
8 Shoulder, Right 9 Shoulder, Left C Hand/Finger Joint, Right D Hand/Finger Joint, Left E Upper Arm, Right F Upper Arm, Left G Elbow, Right H Elbow, Left J Forearm, Right K Forearm, Left L Wrist, Right M Wrist, Left	Z None	Z None	Z None

B   **Imaging**
P   **Non-Axial Upper Bones**
4   **Ultrasonography**   Definition: Real time display of images of anatomy or flow information developed from the capture of relected and attenuated high frequency sound waves

Body Part Character 4	Contrast Character 5	Qualifier Character 6	Qualifier Character 7
8 Shoulder, Right 9 Shoulder, Left G Elbow, Right H Elbow, Left L Wrist, Right M Wrist, Left N Hand, Right P Hand, Left	Z None	Z None .	1 Densitometry Z None

B   **Imaging**
Q   **Non-Axial Lower Bones**
Ø   **Plain Radiography**   Definition: Planar display of an image developed from the capture of external ionizing radiation on photographic or photoconductive plate

Body Part Character 4	Contrast Character 5	Qualifier Character 6	Qualifier Character 7
Ø Hip, Right 1 Hip, Left	Ø High Osmolar 1 Low Osmolar Y Other Contrast	Z None	Z None
Ø Hip, Right 1 Hip, Left	Z None	Z None	1 Densitometry Z None
3 Femur, Right 4 Femur, Left	Z None	Z None	1 Densitometry Z None
7 Knee, Right 8 Knee, Left G Ankle, Right H Ankle, Left	Ø High Osmolar 1 Low Osmolar Y Other Contrast Z None	Z None	Z None
D Lower Leg, Right F Lower Leg, Left J Calcaneus, Right K Calcaneus, Left L Foot, Right M Foot, Left P Toe(s), Right Q Toe(s), Left V Patella, Right W Patella, Left	Z None	Z None	Z None
X Foot/Toe Joint, Right Y Foot/Toe Joint, Left	Ø High Osmolar 1 Low Osmolar Y Other Contrast	Z None	Z None

B   **Imaging**
Q   **Non-Axial Lower Bones**
1   **Fluoroscopy**   Definition: Single plane or bi-plane real time display of an image developed from the capture of external ionizing radioation on a fluorescent screen. The image may also be stored by either digital or analog means.

Body Part Character 4	Contrast Character 5	Qualifier Character 6	Qualifier Character 7
Ø Hip, Right 1 Hip, Left 7 Knee, Right 8 Knee, Left G Ankle, Right H Ankle, Left X Foot/Toe Joint, Right Y Foot/Toe Joint, Left	Ø High Osmolar 1 Low Osmolar Y Other Contrast Z None	Z None	Z None
3 Femur, Right 4 Femur, Left D Lower Leg, Right F Lower Leg, Left J Calcaneus, Right K Calcaneus, Left L Foot, Right M Foot, Left P Toe(s), Right Q Toe(s), Left V Patella, Right W Patella, Left	Z None	Z None	Z None

B   **Imaging**
Q   **Non-Axial Lower Bones**
2   **Computerized Tomography (CT Scan)**   Definition: Computer reformatted digital display of multiplanar images developed from the capture of multiple exposures of external ionizing radiation

Body Part Character 4	Contrast Character 5	Qualifier Character 6	Qualifier Character 7
Ø Hip, Right 1 Hip, Left 3 Femur, Right 4 Femur, Left 7 Knee, Right 8 Knee, Left D Lower Leg, Right F Lower Leg, Left G Ankle, Right H Ankle, Left J Calcaneus, Right K Calcaneus, Left L Foot, Right M Foot, Left P Toe(s), Right Q Toe(s), Left R Lower Extremity, Right S Lower Extremity, Left V Patella, Right W Patella, Left X Foot/Toe Joint, Right Y Foot/Toe Joint, Left	Ø High Osmolar 1 Low Osmolar Y Other Contrast Z None	Z None	Z None
B Tibia/Fibula, Right C Tibia/Fibula, Left	Ø High Osmolar 1 Low Osmolar Y Other Contrast	Z None	Z None

B   **Imaging**
Q   **Non-Axial Lower Bones**
3   **Magnetic Resonance Imaging (MRI)**   Definition: Computer reformatted digital display of multiplanar images developed from the capture of radio-frequency signals emitted by nuclei in a body site excited within a magnetic field

Body Part Character 4	Contrast Character 5	Qualifier Character 6	Qualifier Character 7
Ø Hip, Right 1 Hip, Left 3 Femur, Right 4 Femur, Left 7 Knee, Right 8 Knee, Left D Lower Leg, Right F Lower Leg, Left G Ankle, Right H Ankle, Left J Calcaneus, Right K Calcaneus, Left L Foot, Right M Foot, Left P Toe(s), Right Q Toe(s), Left V Patella, Right W Patella, Left	Y Other Contrast	Ø Unenhanced and Enhanced Z None	Z None
Ø Hip, Right 1 Hip, Left 3 Femur, Right 4 Femur, Left 7 Knee, Right 8 Knee, Left D Lower Leg, Right F Lower Leg, Left G Ankle, Right H Ankle, Left J Calcaneus, Right K Calcaneus, Left L Foot, Right M Foot, Left P Toe(s), Right Q Toe(s), Left V Patella, Right W Patella, Left	Z None	Z None	Z None

B   **Imaging**
Q   **Non-Axial Lower Bones**
4   **Ultrasonography**   Definition: Real time display of images of anatomy or flow information developed from the capture of relected and attenuated high frequency sound waves

Body Part Character 4	Contrast Character 5	Qualifier Character 6	Qualifier Character 7
Ø Hip, Right 1 Hip, Left 2 Hips, Bilateral 7 Knee, Right 8 Knee, Left 9 Knees, Bilateral	Z None	Z None	Z None

B   **Imaging**
R   **Axial Skeleton, Except Skull and Facial Bones**
Ø   **Plain Radiography**   Definition: Planar display of an image developed from the capture of external ionizing radiation on photographic or photoconductive plate

Body Part Character 4	Contrast Character 5	Qualifier Character 6	Qualifier Character 7
Ø Cervical Spine 7 Thoracic Spine 9 Lumbar Spine G Whole Spine	Z None	Z None	1 Densitometry Z None
1 Cervical Disc(s) 2 Thoracic Disc(s) 3 Lumbar Disc(s) 4 Cervical Facet Joint(s) 5 Thoracic Facet Joint(s) 6 Lumbar Facet Joint(s) D Sacroiliac Joints	Ø High Osmolar 1 Low Osmolar Y Other Contrast Z None	Z None	Z None
8 Thoracolumbar Joint B Lumbosacral Joint C Pelvis F Sacrum and Coccyx H Sternum	Z None	Z None	Z None

B   **Imaging**
R   **Axial Skeleton, Except Skull and Facial Bones**
1   **Fluoroscopy**   Definition: Single plane or bi-plane real time display of an image developed from the capture of external ionizing radioation on a fluorescent screen. The image may also be stored by either digital or analog means.

Body Part Character 4	Contrast Character 5	Qualifier Character 6	Qualifier Character 7
Ø Cervical Spine 1 Cervical Disc(s) 2 Thoracic Disc(s) 3 Lumbar Disc(s) 4 Cervical Facet Joint(s) 5 Thoracic Facet Joint(s) 6 Lumbar Facet Joint(s) 7 Thoracic Spine 8 Thoracolumbar Joint 9 Lumbar Spine B Lumbosacral Joint C Pelvis D Sacroiliac Joints F Sacrum and Coccyx G Whole Spine H Sternum	Ø High Osmolar 1 Low Osmolar Y Other Contrast Z None	Z None	Z None

B   **Imaging**
R   **Axial Skeleton, Except Skull and Facial Bones**
2   **Computerized Tomography (CT Scan)**   Definition: Computer reformatted digital display of multiplanar images developed from the capture of multiple exposures of external ionizing radiation

Body Part Character 4	Contrast Character 5	Qualifier Character 6	Qualifier Character 7
Ø Cervical Spine 7 Thoracic Spine 9 Lumbar Spine C Pelvis D Sacroiliac Joints F Sacrum and Coccyx	Ø High Osmolar 1 Low Osmolar Y Other Contrast Z None	Z None	Z None

LC Limited Coverage   **NC** Noncovered   ⊞ Combination Member   HAC   Valid OR   Combination Only   DRG Non-OR   New/Revised in GREEN

ICD-10-PCS 2021   759

BQ4–BR2

B **Imaging**
R **Axial Skeleton, Except Skull and Facial Bones**
3 **Magnetic Resonance Imaging (MRI)**　Definition: Computer reformatted digital display of multiplanar images developed from the capture of radio-frequency signals emitted by nuclei in a body site excited within a magnetic field

Body Part Character 4	Contrast Character 5	Qualifier Character 6	Qualifier Character 7
Ø Cervical Spine 1 Cervical Disc(s) 2 Thoracic Disc(s) 3 Lumbar Disc(s) 7 Thoracic Spine 9 Lumbar Spine C Pelvis F Sacrum and Coccyx	Y Other Contrast	Ø Unenhanced and Enhanced Z None	Z None
Ø Cervical Spine 1 Cervical Disc(s) 2 Thoracic Disc(s) 3 Lumbar Disc(s) 7 Thoracic Spine 9 Lumbar Spine C Pelvis F Sacrum and Coccyx	Z None	Z None	Z None

B **Imaging**
R **Axial Skeleton, Except Skull and Facial Bones**
4 **Ultrasonography**　Definition: Real time display of images of anatomy or flow information developed from the capture of relected and attenuated high frequency sound waves

Body Part Character 4	Contrast Character 5	Qualifier Character 6	Qualifier Character 7
Ø Cervical Spine 7 Thoracic Spine 9 Lumbar Spine F Sacrum and Coccyx	Z None	Z None	Z None

B **Imaging**
T **Urinary System**
Ø **Plain Radiography**　Definition: Planar display of an image developed from the capture of external ionizing radiation on photographic or photoconductive plate

Body Part Character 4	Contrast Character 5	Qualifier Character 6	Qualifier Character 7
Ø Bladder 1 Kidney, Right 2 Kidney, Left 3 Kidneys, Bilateral 4 Kidneys, Ureters and Bladder 5 Urethra 6 Ureter, Right 7 Ureter, Left 8 Ureters, Bilateral B Bladder and Urethra C Ileal Diversion Loop	Ø High Osmolar 1 Low Osmolar Y Other Contrast Z None	Z None	Z None

B **Imaging**
T **Urinary System**
1 **Fluoroscopy**　Definition: Single plane or bi-plane real time display of an image developed from the capture of external ionizing radioation on a fluorescent screen. The image may also be stored by either digital or analog means.

Body Part Character 4	Contrast Character 5	Qualifier Character 6	Qualifier Character 7
Ø Bladder 1 Kidney, Right 2 Kidney, Left 3 Kidneys, Bilateral 4 Kidneys, Ureters and Bladder 5 Urethra 6 Ureter, Right 7 Ureter, Left B Bladder and Urethra C Ileal Diversion Loop D Kidney, Ureter and Bladder, Right F Kidney, Ureter and Bladder, Left G Ileal Loop, Ureters and Kidneys	Ø High Osmolar 1 Low Osmolar Y Other Contrast Z None	Z None	Z None

B   Imaging
T   Urinary System
2   Computerized Tomography (CT Scan) Definition: Computer reformatted digital display of multiplanar images developed from the capture of multiple exposures of external ionizing radiation

Body Part Character 4	Contrast Character 5	Qualifier Character 6	Qualifier Character 7
0 Bladder 1 Kidney, Right 2 Kidney, Left 3 Kidneys, Bilateral 9 Kidney Transplant	0 High Osmolar 1 Low Osmolar Y Other Contrast	0 Unenhanced and Enhanced Z None	Z None
0 Bladder 1 Kidney, Right 2 Kidney, Left 3 Kidneys, Bilateral 9 Kidney Transplant	Z None	Z None	Z None

B   Imaging
T   Urinary System
3   Magnetic Resonance Imaging (MRI) Definition: Computer reformatted digital display of multiplanar images developed from the capture of radio-frequency signals emitted by nuclei in a body site excited within a magnetic field

Body Part Character 4	Contrast Character 5	Qualifier Character 6	Qualifier Character 7
0 Bladder 1 Kidney, Right 2 Kidney, Left 3 Kidneys, Bilateral 9 Kidney Transplant	Y Other Contrast	0 Unenhanced and Enhanced Z None	Z None
0 Bladder 1 Kidney, Right 2 Kidney, Left 3 Kidneys, Bilateral 9 Kidney Transplant	Z None	Z None	Z None

B   Imaging
T   Urinary System
4   Ultrasonography Definition: Real time display of images of anatomy or flow information developed from the capture of relected and attenuated high frequency sound waves

Body Part Character 4	Contrast Character 5	Qualifier Character 6	Qualifier Character 7
0 Bladder 1 Kidney, Right 2 Kidney, Left 3 Kidneys, Bilateral 5 Urethra 6 Ureter, Right 7 Ureter, Left 8 Ureters, Bilateral 9 Kidney Transplant J Kidneys and Bladder	Z None	Z None	Z None

B   Imaging
U   Female Reproductive System
0   Plain Radiography Definition: Planar display of an image developed from the capture of external ionizing radiation on photographic or photoconductive plate

Body Part Character 4	Contrast Character 5	Qualifier Character 6	Qualifier Character 7
0 Fallopian Tube, Right ♀ 1 Fallopian Tube, Left ♀ 2 Fallopian Tubes, Bilateral ♀ 6 Uterus ♀ 8 Uterus and Fallopian Tubes ♀ 9 Vagina ♀	0 High Osmolar 1 Low Osmolar Y Other Contrast	Z None	Z None

♀   All body part, contrast, and qualifier values

B   **Imaging**
U   **Female Reproductive System**
1   **Fluoroscopy**   Definition: Single plane or bi-plane real time display of an image developed from the capture of external ionizing radioation on a fluorescent screen. The image may also be stored by either digital or analog means.

Body Part Character 4	Contrast Character 5	Qualifier Character 6	Qualifier Character 7
0 Fallopian Tube, Right ♀ 1 Fallopian Tube, Left ♀ 2 Fallopian Tubes, Bilateral ♀ 6 Uterus ♀ 8 Uterus and Fallopian Tubes ♀ 9 Vagina ♀	0 High Osmolar 1 Low Osmolar Y Other Contrast Z None	Z None	Z None

♀   All body part, contrast, and qualifier values

B   **Imaging**
U   **Female Reproductive System**
3   **Magnetic Resonance Imaging (MRI)**   Definition: Computer reformatted digital display of multiplanar images developed from the capture of radio-frequency signals emitted by nuclei in a body site excited within a magnetic field

Body Part Character 4	Contrast Character 5	Qualifier Character 6	Qualifier Character 7
3 Ovary, Right ♀ 4 Ovary, Left ♀ 5 Ovaries, Bilateral ♀ 6 Uterus ♀ 9 Vagina ♀ B Pregnant Uterus ♀ C Uterus and Ovaries ♀	Y Other Contrast	0 Unenhanced and Enhanced Z None	Z None
3 Ovary, Right ♀ 4 Ovary, Left ♀ 5 Ovaries, Bilateral ♀ 6 Uterus ♀ 9 Vagina ♀ B Pregnant Uterus ♀ C Uterus and Ovaries ♀	Z None	Z None	Z None

♀   All body part, contrast, and qualifier values

B   **Imaging**
U   **Female Reproductive System**
4   **Ultrasonography**   Definition: Real time display of images of anatomy or flow information developed from the capture of relected and attenuated high frequency sound waves

Body Part Character 4	Contrast Character 5	Qualifier Character 6	Qualifier Character 7
0 Fallopian Tube, Right ♀ 1 Fallopian Tube, Left ♀ 2 Fallopian Tubes, Bilateral ♀ 3 Ovary, Right ♀ 4 Ovary, Left ♀ 5 Ovaries, Bilateral ♀ 6 Uterus ♀ C Uterus and Ovaries ♀	Y Other Contrast Z None	Z None	Z None

♀   All body part, contrast, and qualifier values

B   **Imaging**
V   **Male Reproductive System**
0   **Plain Radiography**   Definition: Planar display of an image developed from the capture of external ionizing radiation on photographic or photoconductive plate

Body Part Character 4	Contrast Character 5	Qualifier Character 6	Qualifier Character 7
0 Corpora Cavernosa ♂ 1 Epididymis, Right ♂ 2 Epididymis, Left ♂ 3 Prostate ♂ 5 Testicle, Right ♂ 6 Testicle, Left ♂ 8 Vasa Vasorum ♂	0 High Osmolar 1 Low Osmolar Y Other Contrast	Z None	Z None

♂   All body part, contrast, and qualifier values

LC Limited Coverage   **NC** Noncovered   ⊞ Combination Member   HAC   Valid OR   Combination Only   DRG Non-OR   New/Revised in GREEN

762   ICD-10-PCS 2021

BU1–BV0

B   Imaging
V   Male Reproductive System
1   Fluoroscopy   Definition: Single plane or bi-plane real time display of an image developed from the capture of external ionizing radioation on a fluorescent screen. The image may also be stored by either digital or analog means.

Body Part Character 4		Contrast Character 5	Qualifier Character 6	Qualifier Character 7
Ø Corpora Cavernosa 8 Vasa Vasorum	♂ ♂	Ø High Osmolar 1 Low Osmolar Y Other Contrast Z None	Z None	Z None

    ♂   All body part, contrast, and qualifier values

B   Imaging
V   Male Reproductive System
2   Computerized Tomography (CT Scan)   Definition: Computer reformatted digital display of multiplanar images developed from the capture of multiple exposures of external ionizing radiation

Body Part Character 4		Contrast Character 5	Qualifier Character 6	Qualifier Character 7
3 Prostate	♂	Ø High Osmolar 1 Low Osmolar Y Other Contrast	Ø Unenhanced and Enhanced Z None	Z None
3 Prostate	♂	Z None	Z None	Z None

    ♂   BV23[Ø,Y][Ø,Z]Z   ♂   BV23ZZZ
    ♂   BV231ØZ

B   Imaging
V   Male Reproductive System
3   Magnetic Resonance Imaging (MRI)   Definition: Computer reformatted digital display of multiplanar images developed from the capture of radio-frequency signals emitted by nuclei in a body site excited within a magnetic field

Body Part Character 4		Contrast Character 5	Qualifier Character 6	Qualifier Character 7
Ø Corpora Cavernosa 3 Prostate 4 Scrotum 5 Testicle, Right 6 Testicle, Left 7 Testicles, Bilateral	♂ ♂ ♂ ♂ ♂ ♂	Y Other Contrast	Ø Unenhanced and Enhanced Z None	Z None
Ø Corpora Cavernosa 3 Prostate 4 Scrotum 5 Testicle, Right 6 Testicle, Left 7 Testicles, Bilateral	♂ ♂ ♂ ♂ ♂ ♂	Z None	Z None	Z None

    ♂   All body part, contrast, and qualifier values

B   Imaging
V   Male Reproductive System
4   Ultrasonography   Definition: Real time display of images of anatomy or flow information developed from the capture of relected and attenuated high frequency sound waves

Body Part Character 4		Contrast Character 5	Qualifier Character 6	Qualifier Character 7
4 Scrotum 9 Prostate and Seminal Vesicles B Penis	♂ ♂ ♂	Z None	Z None	Z None

    ♂   All body part, contrast, and qualifier values

B   Imaging
W   Anatomical Regions
Ø   Plain Radiography   Definition: Planar display of an image developed from the capture of external ionizing radiation on photographic or photoconductive plate

Body Part Character 4	Contrast Character 5	Qualifier Character 6	Qualifier Character 7
Ø Abdomen 1 Abdomen and Pelvis 3 Chest B Long Bones, All C Lower Extremity J Upper Extremity K Whole Body L Whole Skeleton M Whole Body, Infant	Z None	Z None	Z None

LC Limited Coverage   **NC** Noncovered   ⊞ Combination Member   HAC   Valid OR   Combination Only   DRG Non-OR   New/Revised in GREEN

ICD-10-PCS 2021   763

BV1–BWØ

B   **Imaging**
W   **Anatomical Regions**
1   **Fluoroscopy**   Definition: Single plane or bi-plane real time display of an image developed from the capture of external ionizing radioation on a fluorescent screen. The image may also be stored by either digital or analog means.

Body Part Character 4	Contrast Character 5	Qualifier Character 6	Qualifier Character 7
1 Abdomen and Pelvis 9 Head and Neck C Lower Extremity J Upper Extremity	Ø High Osmolar 1 Low Osmolar Y Other Contrast Z None	Z None	Z None

B   **Imaging**
W   **Anatomical Regions**
2   **Computerized Tomography (CT Scan)**   Definition: Computer reformatted digital display of multiplanar images developed from the capture of multiple exposures of external ionizing radiation

Body Part Character 4	Contrast Character 5	Qualifier Character 6	Qualifier Character 7
Ø Abdomen 1 Abdomen and Pelvis 4 Chest and Abdomen 5 Chest, Abdomen and Pelvis 8 Head 9 Head and Neck F Neck G Pelvic Region	Ø High Osmolar 1 Low Osmolar Y Other Contrast	Ø Unenhanced and Enhanced Z None	Z None
Ø Abdomen 1 Abdomen and Pelvis 4 Chest and Abdomen 5 Chest, Abdomen and Pelvis 8 Head 9 Head and Neck F Neck G Pelvic Region	Z None	Z None	Z None

B   **Imaging**
W   **Anatomical Regions**
3   **Magnetic Resonance Imaging (MRI)**   Definition: Computer reformatted digital display of multiplanar images developed from the capture of radio-frequency signals emitted by nuclei in a body site excited within a magnetic field

Body Part Character 4	Contrast Character 5	Qualifier Character 6	Qualifier Character 7
Ø Abdomen 8 Head F Neck G Pelvic Region H Retroperitoneum P Brachial Plexus	Y Other Contrast	Ø Unenhanced and Enhanced Z None	Z None
Ø Abdomen 8 Head F Neck G Pelvic Region H Retroperitoneum P Brachial Plexus	Z None	Z None	Z None
3 Chest	Y Other Contrast	Ø Unenhanced and Enhanced Z None	Z None

B   **Imaging**
W   **Anatomical Regions**
4   **Ultrasonography**   Definition: Real time display of images of anatomy or flow information developed from the capture of relected and attenuated high frequency sound waves

Body Part Character 4	Contrast Character 5	Qualifier Character 6	Qualifier Character 7
Ø Abdomen 1 Abdomen and Pelvis F Neck G Pelvic Region	Z None	Z None	Z None

B   **Imaging**
W   **Anatomical Regions**
5   **Other Imaging**   Definition: Other specified modality for visualizing a body part

Body Part Character 4	Contrast Character 5	Qualifier Character 6	Qualifier Character 7
2 Trunk 9 Head and Neck C Lower Extremity J Upper Extremity	Z None	1 Bacterial Autofluorescence	Z None

B   **Imaging**
Y   **Fetus and Obstetrical**
3   **Magnetic Resonance Imaging (MRI)**   Definition: Computer reformatted digital display of multiplanar images developed from the capture of radio-frequency signals emitted by nuclei in a body site excited within a magnetic field

Body Part Character 4	Contrast Character 5	Qualifier Character 6	Qualifier Character 7
0 Fetal Head ♀ 1 Fetal Heart ♀ 2 Fetal Thorax ♀ 3 Fetal Abdomen ♀ 4 Fetal Spine ♀ 5 Fetal Extremities ♀ 6 Whole Fetus ♀	Y Other Contrast	0 Unenhanced and Enhanced Z None	Z None
0 Fetal Head ♀ 1 Fetal Heart ♀ 2 Fetal Thorax ♀ 3 Fetal Abdomen ♀ 4 Fetal Spine ♀ 5 Fetal Extremities ♀ 6 Whole Fetus ♀	Z None	Z None	Z None

♀   BY3[0,1,2,3,5,6]Y[0,Z]Z
♀   BY34YZZ
♀   BY3[0,1,2,3,4,5,6]ZZZ

B   **Imaging**
Y   **Fetus and Obstetrical**
4   **Ultrasonography**   Definition: Real time display of images of anatomy or flow information developed from the capture of relected and attenuated high frequency sound waves

Body Part Character 4	Contrast Character 5	Qualifier Character 6	Qualifier Character 7
7 Fetal Umbilical Cord ♀ 8 Placenta ♀ 9 First Trimester, Single Fetus ♀ B First Trimester, Multiple Gestation ♀ C Second Trimester, Single Fetus ♀ D Second Trimester, Multiple Gestation ♀ F Third Trimester, Single Fetus ♀ G Third Trimester, Multiple Gestation ♀	Z None	Z None	Z None

♀   All body part, contrast, and qualifier values

LC Limited Coverage   **NC** Noncovered   ⊞ Combination Member   HAC   Valid OR   Combination Only   DRG Non-OR   New/Revised in GREEN

ICD-10-PCS 2021   **765**

BW5–BY4

Nuclear Medicine C01–CW7

C   **Nuclear Medicine**
0   **Central Nervous System**
1   **Planar Nuclear Medicine Imaging**   Definition: Introduction of radioactive materials into the body for single plane display of images developed from the capture of radioactive emissions

Body Part Character 4	Radionuclide Character 5	Qualifier Character 6	Qualifier Character 7
0 Brain	1 Technetium 99m (Tc-99m) Y Other Radionuclide	Z None	Z None
5 Cerebrospinal Fluid	D Indium 111 (In-111) Y Other Radionuclide	Z None	Z None
Y Central Nervous System	Y Other Radionuclide	Z None	Z None

C   **Nuclear Medicine**
0   **Central Nervous System**
2   **Tomographic (Tomo) Nuclear Medicine Imaging**   Definition: Introduction of radioactive materials into the body for three dimensional display of images developed from the capture of radioactive emissions

Body Part Character 4	Radionuclide Character 5	Qualifier Character 6	Qualifier Character 7
0 Brain	1 Technetium 99m (Tc-99m) F Iodine 123 (I-123) S Thallium 201 (Tl-201) Y Other Radionuclide	Z None	Z None
5 Cerebrospinal Fluid	D Indium 111 (In-111) Y Other Radionuclide	Z None	Z None
Y Central Nervous System	Y Other Radionuclide	Z None	Z None

C   **Nuclear Medicine**
0   **Central Nervous System**
3   **Positron Emission Tomographic (PET) Imaging**   Definition: Introduction of radioactive materials into the body for three dimensional display of images developed from the simultaneous capture, 180 degrees apart, of radioactive emissions

Body Part Character 4	Radionuclide Character 5	Qualifier Character 6	Qualifier Character 7
0 Brain	B Carbon 11 (C-11) K Fluorine 18 (F-18) M Oxygen 15 (O-15) Y Other Radionuclide	Z None	Z None
Y Central Nervous System	Y Other Radionuclide	Z None	Z None

C   **Nuclear Medicine**
0   **Central Nervous System**
5   **Nonimaging Nuclear Medicine Probe**   Definition: Introduction of radioactive materials into the body for the study of distribution and fate of certain substances by the detection of radioactive emissions; or, alternatively, measurement of absorption of radioactive emissions from an external source

Body Part Character 4	Radionuclide Character 5	Qualifier Character 6	Qualifier Character 7
0 Brain	V Xenon 133 (Xe-133) Y Other Radionuclide	Z None	Z None
Y Central Nervous System	Y Other Radionuclide	Z None	Z None

C   **Nuclear Medicine**
2   **Heart**
1   **Planar Nuclear Medicine Imaging**   Definition: Introduction of radioactive materials into the body for single plane display of images developed from the capture of radioactive emissions

Body Part Character 4	Radionuclide Character 5	Qualifier Character 6	Qualifier Character 7
6 Heart, Right and Left	1 Technetium 99m (Tc-99m) Y Other Radionuclide	Z None	Z None
G Myocardium	1 Technetium 99m (Tc-99m) D Indium 111 (In-111) S Thallium 201 (Tl-201) Y Other Radionuclide Z None	Z None	Z None
Y Heart	Y Other Radionuclide	Z None	Z None

ⒾⒸ Limited Coverage   ⓃⒸ Noncovered   ⊞ Combination Member   HAC   Valid OR   Combination Only   DRG Non-OR   New/Revised in GREEN
ICD-10-PCS 2021   767

C01–C21

Nuclear Medicine

C Nuclear Medicine
2 Heart
2 Tomographic (Tomo) Nuclear Medicine Imaging   Definition: Introduction of radioactive materials into the body for three dimensional display of images developed from the capture of radioactive emissions

Body Part Character 4	Radionuclide Character 5	Qualifier Character 6	Qualifier Character 7
6 Heart, Right and Left	1 Technetium 99m (Tc-99m) Y Other Radionuclide	Z None	Z None
G Myocardium	1 Technetium 99m (Tc-99m) D Indium 111 (In-111) K Fluorine 18 (F-18) S Thallium 201 (Tl-201) Y Other Radionuclide Z None	Z None	Z None
Y Heart	Y Other Radionuclide	Z None	Z None

C Nuclear Medicine
2 Heart
3 Positron Emission Tomographic (PET) Imaging   Definition: Introduction of radioactive materials into the body for three dimensional display of images developed from the simultaneous capture, 180 degrees apart, of radioactive emissions

Body Part Character 4	Radionuclide Character 5	Qualifier Character 6	Qualifier Character 7
G Myocardium	K Fluorine 18 (F-18) M Oxygen 15 (O-15) Q Rubidium 82 (Rb-82) R Nitrogen 13 (N-13) Y Other Radionuclide	Z None	Z None
Y Heart	Y Other Radionuclide	Z None	Z None

C Nuclear Medicine
2 Heart
5 Nonimaging Nuclear Medicine Probe   Definition: Introduction of radioactive materials into the body for the study of distribution and fate of certain substances by the detection of radioactive emissions; or, alternatively, measurement of absorption of radioactive emissions from an external source

Body Part Character 4	Radionuclide Character 5	Qualifier Character 6	Qualifier Character 7
6 Heart, Right and Left	1 Technetium 99m (Tc-99m) Y Other Radionuclide	Z None	Z None
Y Heart	Y Other Radionuclide	Z None	Z None

C Nuclear Medicine
5 Veins
1 Planar Nuclear Medicine Imaging   Definition: Introduction of radioactive materials into the body for single plane display of images developed from the capture of radioactive emissions

Body Part Character 4	Radionuclide Character 5	Qualifier Character 6	Qualifier Character 7
B Lower Extremity Veins, Right C Lower Extremity Veins, Left D Lower Extremity Veins, Bilateral N Upper Extremity Veins, Right P Upper Extremity Veins, Left Q Upper Extremity Veins, Bilateral R Central Veins	1 Technetium 99m (Tc-99m) Y Other Radionuclide	Z None	Z None
Y Veins	Y Other Radionuclide	Z None	Z None

C   **Nuclear Medicine**
7   **Lymphatic and Hematologic System**
1   **Planar Nuclear Medicine Imaging**   Definition: Introduction of radioactive materials into the body for single plane display of images developed from the capture of radioactive emissions

Body Part Character 4	Radionuclide Character 5	Qualifier Character 6	Qualifier Character 7
0 Bone Marrow	1 Technetium 99m (Tc-99m) D Indium 111 (In-111) Y Other Radionuclide	Z None	Z None
2 Spleen 5 Lymphatics, Head and Neck D Lymphatics, Pelvic J Lymphatics, Head K Lymphatics, Neck L Lymphatics, Upper Chest M Lymphatics, Trunk N Lymphatics, Upper Extremity P Lymphatics, Lower Extremity	1 Technetium 99m (Tc-99m) Y Other Radionuclide	Z None	Z None
3 Blood	D Indium 111 (In-111) Y Other Radionuclide	Z None	Z None
Y Lymphatic and Hematologic System	Y Other Radionuclide	Z None	Z None

C   **Nuclear Medicine**
7   **Lymphatic and Hematologic System**
2   **Tomographic (Tomo) Nuclear Medicine Imaging**   Definition: Introduction of radioactive materials into the body for three dimensional display of images developed from the capture of radioactive emissions

Body Part Character 4	Radionuclide Character 5	Qualifier Character 6	Qualifier Character 7
2 Spleen	1 Technetium 99m (Tc-99m) Y Other Radionuclide	Z None	Z None
Y Lymphatic and Hematologic System	Y Other Radionuclide	Z None	Z None

C   **Nuclear Medicine**
7   **Lymphatic and Hematologic System**
5   **Nonimaging Nuclear Medicine Probe**   Definition: Introduction of radioactive materials into the body for the study of distribution and fate of certain substances by the detection of radioactive emissions; or, alternatively, measurement of absorption of radioactive emissions from an external source

Body Part Character 4	Radionuclide Character 5	Qualifier Character 6	Qualifier Character 7
5 Lymphatics, Head and Neck D Lymphatics, Pelvic J Lymphatics, Head K Lymphatics, Neck L Lymphatics, Upper Chest M Lymphatics, Trunk N Lymphatics, Upper Extremity P Lymphatics, Lower Extremity	1 Technetium 99m (Tc-99m) Y Other Radionuclide	Z None	Z None
Y Lymphatic and Hematologic System	Y Other Radionuclide	Z None	Z None

C   **Nuclear Medicine**
7   **Lymphatic and Hematologic System**
6   **Nonimaging Nuclear Medicine Assay**   Definition: Introduction of radioactive materials into the body for the study of body fluids and blood elements, by the detection of radioactive emissions

Body Part Character 4	Radionuclide Character 5	Qualifier Character 6	Qualifier Character 7
3 Blood	1 Technetium 99m (Tc-99m) 7 Cobalt 58 (Co-58) C Cobalt 57 (Co-57) D Indium 111 (In-111) H Iodine 125 (I-125) W Chromium (Cr-51) Y Other Radionuclide	Z None	Z None
Y Lymphatic and Hematologic System	Y Other Radionuclide	Z None	Z None

LC Limited Coverage   **NC** Noncovered   ⊞ Combination Member   **HAC**   Valid OR   Combination Only   DRG Non-OR   New/Revised in GREEN

ICD-10-PCS 2021   769

C71–C76

C Nuclear Medicine
8 Eye
1 Planar Nuclear Medicine Imaging   Definition: Introduction of radioactive materials into the body for single plane display of images developed from the capture of radioactive emissions

Body Part Character 4	Radionuclide Character 5	Qualifier Character 6	Qualifier Character 7
9 Lacrimal Ducts, Bilateral	1 Technetium 99m (Tc-99m) Y Other Radionuclide	Z None	Z None
Y Eye	Y Other Radionuclide	Z None	Z None

C Nuclear Medicine
9 Ear, Nose, Mouth and Throat
1 Planar Nuclear Medicine Imaging   Definition: Introduction of radioactive materials into the body for single plane display of images developed from the capture of radioactive emissions

Body Part Character 4	Radionuclide Character 5	Qualifier Character 6	Qualifier Character 7
B Salivary Glands, Bilateral	1 Technetium 99m (Tc-99m) Y Other Radionuclide	Z None	Z None
Y Ear, Nose, Mouth and Throat	Y Other Radionuclide	Z None	Z None

C Nuclear Medicine
B Respiratory System
1 Planar Nuclear Medicine Imaging   Definition: Introduction of radioactive materials into the body for single plane display of images developed from the capture of radioactive emissions

Body Part Character 4	Radionuclide Character 5	Qualifier Character 6	Qualifier Character 7
2 Lungs and Bronchi	1 Technetium 99m (Tc-99m) 9 Krypton (Kr-81m) T Xenon 127 (Xe-127) V Xenon 133 (Xe-133) Y Other Radionuclide	Z None	Z None
Y Respiratory System	Y Other Radionuclide	Z None	Z None

C Nuclear Medicine
B Respiratory System
2 Tomographic (Tomo) Nuclear Medicine Imaging Definition: Introduction of radioactive materials into the body for three dimensional display of images developed from the capture of radioactive emissions

Body Part Character 4	Radionuclide Character 5	Qualifier Character 6	Qualifier Character 7
2 Lungs and Bronchi	1 Technetium 99m (Tc-99m) 9 Krypton (Kr-81m) Y Other Radionuclide	Z None	Z None
Y Respiratory System	Y Other Radionuclide	Z None	Z None

C Nuclear Medicine
B Respiratory System
3 Positron Emission Tomographic (PET) Imaging   Definition: Introduction of radioactive materials into the body for three dimensional display of images developed from the simultaneous capture, 180 degrees apart, of radioactive emissions

Body Part Character 4	Radionuclide Character 5	Qualifier Character 6	Qualifier Character 7
2 Lungs and Bronchi	K Fluorine 18 (F-18) Y Other Radionuclide	Z None	Z None
Y Respiratory System	Y Other Radionuclide	Z None	Z None

C Nuclear Medicine
D Gastrointestinal System
1 Planar Nuclear Medicine Imaging   Definition: Introduction of radioactive materials into the body for single plane display of images developed from the capture of radioactive emissions

Body Part Character 4	Radionuclide Character 5	Qualifier Character 6	Qualifier Character 7
5 Upper Gastrointestinal Tract 7 Gastrointestinal Tract	1 Technetium 99m (Tc-99m) D Indium 111 (In-111) Y Other Radionuclide	Z None	Z None
Y Digestive System	Y Other Radionuclide	Z None	Z None

C   **Nuclear Medicine**
D   **Gastrointestinal System**
2   **Tomographic (Tomo) Nuclear Medicine Imaging**   Definition: Introduction of radioactive materials into the body for three dimensional display of images developed from the capture of radioactive emissions

Body Part Character 4	Radionuclide Character 5	Qualifier Character 6	Qualifier Character 7
7 Gastrointestinal Tract	1 Technetium 99m (Tc-99m) D Indium 111 (In-111) Y Other Radionuclide	Z None	Z None
Y Digestive System	Y Other Radionuclide	Z None	Z None

C   **Nuclear Medicine**
F   **Hepatobiliary System and Pancreas**
1   **Planar Nuclear Medicine Imaging**   Definition: Introduction of radioactive materials into the body for single plane display of images developed from the capture of radioactive emissions

Body Part Character 4	Radionuclide Character 5	Qualifier Character 6	Qualifier Character 7
4 Gallbladder 5 Liver 6 Liver and Spleen C Hepatobiliary System, All	1 Technetium 99m (Tc-99m) Y Other Radionuclide	Z None	Z None
Y Hepatobiliary System and Pancreas	Y Other Radionuclide	Z None	Z None

C   **Nuclear Medicine**
F   **Hepatobiliary System and Pancreas**
2   **Tomographic (Tomo) Nuclear Medicine Imaging**   Definition: Introduction of radioactive materials into the body for three dimensional display of images developed from the capture of radioactive emissions

Body Part Character 4	Radionuclide Character 5	Qualifier Character 6	Qualifier Character 7
4 Gallbladder 5 Liver 6 Liver and Spleen	1 Technetium 99m (Tc-99m) Y Other Radionuclide	Z None	Z None
Y Hepatobiliary System and Pancreas	Y Other Radionuclide	Z None	Z None

C   **Nuclear Medicine**
G   **Endocrine System**
1   **Planar Nuclear Medicine Imaging**   Definition: Introduction of radioactive materials into the body for single plane display of images developed from the capture of radioactive emissions

Body Part Character 4	Radionuclide Character 5	Qualifier Character 6	Qualifier Character 7
1 Parathyroid Glands	1 Technetium 99m (Tc-99m) S Thallium 201 (Tl-201) Y Other Radionuclide	Z None	Z None
2 Thyroid Gland	1 Technetium 99m (Tc-99m) F Iodine 123 (I-123) G Iodine 131 (I-131) Y Other Radionuclide	Z None	Z None
4 Adrenal Glands, Bilateral	G Iodine 131 (I-131) Y Other Radionuclide	Z None	Z None
Y Endocrine System	Y Other Radionuclide	Z None	Z None

C   **Nuclear Medicine**
G   **Endocrine System**
2   **Tomographic (Tomo) Nuclear Medicine Imaging**   Definition: Introduction of radioactive materials into the body for three dimensional display of images developed from the capture of radioactive emissions

Body Part Character 4	Radionuclide Character 5	Qualifier Character 6	Qualifier Character 7
1 Parathyroid Glands	1 Technetium 99m (Tc-99m) S Thallium 201 (Tl-201) Y Other Radionuclide	Z None	Z None
Y Endocrine System	Y Other Radionuclide	Z None	Z None

Nuclear Medicine

C　Nuclear Medicine
G　Endocrine System
4　Nonimaging Nuclear Medicine Uptake　　Definition: Introduction of radioactive materials into the body for measurements of organ function, from the detection of radioactive emmissions

Body Part Character 4	Radionuclide Character 5	Qualifier Character 6	Qualifier Character 7
2　Thyroid Gland	1　Technetium 99m (Tc-99m) F　Iodine 123 (I-123) G　Iodine 131 (I-131) Y　Other Radionuclide	Z　None	Z　None
Y　Endocrine System	Y　Other Radionuclide	Z　None	Z　None

C　Nuclear Medicine
H　Skin, Subcutaneous Tissue and Breast
1　Planar Nuclear Medicine Imaging　　Definition: Introduction of radioactive materials into the body for single plane display of images developed from the capture of radioactive emissions

Body Part Character 4	Radionuclide Character 5	Qualifier Character 6	Qualifier Character 7
Ø　Breast, Right 1　Breast, Left 2　Breasts, Bilateral	1　Technetium 99m (Tc-99m) S　Thallium 201 (Tl-201) Y　Other Radionuclide	Z　None	Z　None
Y　Skin, Subcutaneous Tissue and Breast	Y　Other Radionuclide	Z　None	Z　None

C　Nuclear Medicine
H　Skin, Subcutaneous Tissue and Breast
2　Tomographic (Tomo) Nuclear Medicine Imaging　Definition: Introduction of radioactive materials into the body for three dimensional display of images developed from the capture of radioactive emissions

Body Part Character 4	Radionuclide Character 5	Qualifier Character 6	Qualifier Character 7
Ø　Breast, Right 1　Breast, Left 2　Breasts, Bilateral	1　Technetium 99m (Tc-99m) S　Thallium 201 (Tl-201) Y　Other Radionuclide	Z　None	Z　None
Y　Skin, Subcutaneous Tissue and Breast	Y　Other Radionuclide	Z　None	Z　None

C　Nuclear Medicine
P　Musculoskeletal System
1　Planar Nuclear Medicine Imaging　　Definition: Introduction of radioactive materials into the body for single plane display of images developed from the capture of radioactive emissions

Body Part Character 4	Radionuclide Character 5	Qualifier Character 6	Qualifier Character 7
1　Skull 4　Thorax 5　Spine 6　Pelvis 7　Spine and Pelvis 8　Upper Extremity, Right 9　Upper Extremity, Left B　Upper Extremities, Bilateral C　Lower Extremity, Right D　Lower Extremity, Left F　Lower Extremities, Bilateral Z　Musculoskeletal System, All	1　Technetium 99m (Tc-99m) Y　Other Radionuclide	Z　None	Z　None
Y　Musculoskeletal System, Other	Y　Other Radionuclide	Z　None	Z　None

C Nuclear Medicine
P Musculoskeletal System
2 Tomographic (Tomo) Nuclear Medicine Imaging Definition: Introduction of radioactive materials into the body for three dimensional display of images developed from the capture of radioactive emissions

Body Part Character 4	Radionuclide Character 5	Qualifier Character 6	Qualifier Character 7
1 Skull 2 Cervical Spine 3 Skull and Cervical Spine 4 Thorax 6 Pelvis 7 Spine and Pelvis 8 Upper Extremity, Right 9 Upper Extremity, Left B Upper Extremities, Bilateral C Lower Extremity, Right D Lower Extremity, Left F Lower Extremities, Bilateral G Thoracic Spine H Lumbar Spine J Thoracolumbar Spine	1 Technetium 99m (Tc-99m) Y Other Radionuclide	Z None	Z None
Y Musculoskeletal System, Other	Y Other Radionuclide	Z None	Z None

C Nuclear Medicine
P Musculoskeletal System
5 Nonimaging Nuclear Medicine Probe Definition: Introduction of radioactive materials into the body for the study of distribution and fate of certain substances by the detection of radioactive emissions; or, alternatively, measurement of absorption of radioactive emissions from an external source

Body Part Character 4	Radionuclide Character 5	Qualifier Character 6	Qualifier Character 7
5 Spine N Upper Extremities P Lower Extremities	Z None	Z None	Z None
Y Musculoskeletal System, Other	Y Other Radionuclide	Z None	Z None

C Nuclear Medicine
T Urinary System
1 Planar Nuclear Medicine Imaging Definition: Introduction of radioactive materials into the body for single plane display of images developed from the capture of radioactive emissions

Body Part Character 4	Radionuclide Character 5	Qualifier Character 6	Qualifier Character 7
3 Kidneys, Ureters and Bladder	1 Technetium 99m (Tc-99m) F Iodine 123 (I-123) G Iodine 131 (I-131) Y Other Radionuclide	Z None	Z None
H Bladder and Ureters	1 Technetium 99m (Tc-99m) Y Other Radionuclide	Z None	Z None
Y Urinary System	Y Other Radionuclide	Z None	Z None

C Nuclear Medicine
T Urinary System
2 Tomographic (Tomo) Nuclear Medicine Imaging Definition: Introduction of radioactive materials into the body for three dimensional display of images developed from the capture of radioactive emissions

Body Part Character 4	Radionuclide Character 5	Qualifier Character 6	Qualifier Character 7
3 Kidneys, Ureters and Bladder	1 Technetium 99m (Tc-99m) Y Other Radionuclide	Z None	Z None
Y Urinary System	Y Other Radionuclide	Z None	Z None

C Nuclear Medicine
T Urinary System
6 Nonimaging Nuclear Medicine Assay Definition: Introduction of radioactive materials into the body for the study of body fluids and blood elements, by the detection of radioactive emissions

Body Part Character 4	Radionuclide Character 5	Qualifier Character 6	Qualifier Character 7
3 Kidneys, Ureters and Bladder	1 Technetium 99m (Tc-99m) F Iodine 123 (I-123) G Iodine 131 (I-131) H Iodine 125 (I-125) Y Other Radionuclide	Z None	Z None
Y Urinary System	Y Other Radionuclide	Z None	Z None

C   **Nuclear Medicine**
V   **Male Reproductive System**
1   **Planar Nuclear Medicine Imaging**   Definition: Introduction of radioactive materials into the body for single plane display of images developed from the capture of radioactive emissions

Body Part Character 4	Radionuclide Character 5	Qualifier Character 6	Qualifier Character 7
9 Testicles, Bilateral ♂	1 Technetium 99m (Tc-99m) Y Other Radionuclide	Z None	Z None
Y Male Reproductive System ♂	Y Other Radionuclide	Z None	Z None

♂   All body part, radionuclide, and qualifier values

C   **Nuclear Medicine**
W   **Anatomical Regions**
1   **Planar Nuclear Medicine Imaging**   Definition: Introduction of radioactive materials into the body for single plane display of images developed from the capture of radioactive emissions

Body Part Character 4	Radionuclide Character 5	Qualifier Character 6	Qualifier Character 7
Ø Abdomen 1 Abdomen and Pelvis 4 Chest and Abdomen 6 Chest and Neck B Head and Neck D Lower Extremity J Pelvic Region M Upper Extremity N Whole Body	1 Technetium 99m (Tc-99m) D Indium 111 (In-111) F Iodine 123 (I-123) G Iodine 131 (I-131) L Gallium 67 (Ga-67) S Thallium 201 (Tl-201) Y Other Radionuclide	Z None	Z None
3 Chest	1 Technetium 99m (Tc-99m) D Indium 111 (In-111) F Iodine 123 (I-123) G Iodine 131 (I-131) K Fluorine 18 (F-18) L Gallium 67 (Ga-67) S Thallium 201 (Tl-201) Y Other Radionuclide	Z None	Z None
Y Anatomical Regions, Multiple	Y Other Radionuclide	Z None	Z None
Z Anatomical Region, Other	Z None	Z None	Z None

C   **Nuclear Medicine**
W   **Anatomical Regions**
2   **Tomographic (Tomo) Nuclear Medicine Imaging**   Definition: Introduction of radioactive materials into the body for three dimensional display of images developed from the capture of radioactive emissions

Body Part Character 4	Radionuclide Character 5	Qualifier Character 6	Qualifier Character 7
Ø Abdomen 1 Abdomen and Pelvis 3 Chest 4 Chest and Abdomen 6 Chest and Neck B Head and Neck D Lower Extremity J Pelvic Region M Upper Extremity	1 Technetium 99m (Tc-99m) D Indium 111 (In-111) F Iodine 123 (I-123) G Iodine 131 (I-131) K Fluorine 18 (F-18) L Gallium 67 (Ga-67) S Thallium 201 (Tl-201) Y Other Radionuclide	Z None	Z None
Y Anatomical Regions, Multiple	Y Other Radionuclide	Z None	Z None

C   **Nuclear Medicine**
W   **Anatomical Regions**
3   **Positron Emission Tomographic (PET) Imaging**   Definition: Introduction of radioactive materials into the body for three dimensional display of images developed from the simultaneous capture, 180 degrees apart, of radioactive emissions

Body Part Character 4	Radionuclide Character 5	Qualifier Character 6	Qualifier Character 7
N Whole Body	Y Other Radionuclide	Z None	Z None

C   **Nuclear Medicine**
W   **Anatomical Regions**
5   **Nonimaging Nuclear Medicine Probe**   Definition: Introduction of radioactive materials into the body for the study of distribution and fate of certain substances by the detection of radioactive emissions; or, alternatively, measurement of absorption of radioactive emissions from an external source

Body Part Character 4	Radionuclide Character 5	Qualifier Character 6	Qualifier Character 7
Ø Abdomen 1 Abdomen and Pelvis 3 Chest 4 Chest and Abdomen 6 Chest and Neck B Head and Neck D Lower Extremity J Pelvic Region M Upper Extremity	1 Technetium 99m (Tc-99m) D Indium 111 (In-111) Y Other Radionuclide	Z None	Z None

C   **Nuclear Medicine**
W   **Anatomical Regions**
7   **Systemic Nuclear Medicine Therapy**   Definition: Introduction of unsealed radioactive materials into the body for treatment

Body Part Character 4	Radionuclide Character 5	Qualifier Character 6	Qualifier Character 7
Ø Abdomen 3 Chest	N Phosphorus 32 (P-32) Y Other Radionuclide	Z None	Z None
G Thyroid	G Iodine 131 (I-131) Y Other Radionuclide	Z None	Z None
N Whole Body	8 Samarium 153 (Sm-153) G Iodine 131 (I-131) N Phosphorus 32 (P-32) P Strontium 89 (Sr-89) Y Other Radionuclide	Z None	Z None
Y Anatomical Regions, Multiple	Y Other Radionuclide	Z None	Z None

Radiation Therapy D00–DWY

AHA Coding Clinic for table D01
2019, 4Q, 42-44   Unidirectional source brachytherapy

AHA Coding Clinic for table D71
2019, 4Q, 42-44   Unidirectional source brachytherapy

AHA Coding Clinic for table D81
2019, 4Q, 42-44   Unidirectional source brachytherapy

AHA Coding Clinic for table D91
2019, 4Q, 42-44   Unidirectional source brachytherapy

AHA Coding Clinic for table DB1
2019, 4Q, 42-44   Unidirectional source brachytherapy

AHA Coding Clinic for table DD1
2019, 4Q, 42-44   Unidirectional source brachytherapy

AHA Coding Clinic for table DF1
2019, 4Q, 42-44   Unidirectional source brachytherapy

AHA Coding Clinic for table DG1
2019, 4Q, 42-44   Unidirectional source brachytherapy

AHA Coding Clinic for table DM1
2019, 4Q, 42-44   Unidirectional source brachytherapy

AHA Coding Clinic for table DT1
2019, 4Q, 42-44   Unidirectional source brachytherapy

AHA Coding Clinic for table DU1
2019, 4Q, 42-44   Unidirectional source brachytherapy
2017, 4Q, 104   Intrauterine brachytherapy & placement of tandems & ovoids

AHA Coding Clinic for table DV1
2019, 4Q, 42-44   Unidirectional source brachytherapy

AHA Coding Clinic for table DW1
2019, 4Q, 42-44   Unidirectional source brachytherapy

AHA Coding Clinic for table DWY
2019, 4Q, 37   Hyperthermic antineoplastic chemotherapy

D   **Radiation Therapy**
0   **Central and Peripheral Nervous System**
0   **Beam Radiation**

Treatment Site Character 4	Modality Qualifier Character 5	Isotope Character 6	Qualifier Character 7
0 Brain 1 Brain Stem 6 Spinal Cord 7 Peripheral Nerve	0 Photons <1 MeV 1 Photons 1- 10 MeV 2 Photons >10 MeV 4 Heavy Particles (Protons, Ions) 5 Neutrons 6 Neutron Capture	Z None	Z None
0 Brain 1 Brain Stem 6 Spinal Cord 7 Peripheral Nerve	3 Electrons	Z None	0 Intraoperative Z None

D   **Radiation Therapy**
0   **Central and Peripheral Nervous System**
1   **Brachytherapy**

Treatment Site Character 4	Modality Qualifier Character 5	Isotope Character 6	Qualifier Character 7
0 Brain 1 Brain Stem 6 Spinal Cord 7 Peripheral Nerve	9 High Dose Rate (HDR)	7 Cesium 137 (Cs-137) 8 Iridium 192 (Ir-192) 9 Iodine 125 (I-125) B Palladium 103 (Pd-103) C Californium 252 (Cf-252) Y Other Isotope	Z None
0 Brain 1 Brain Stem 6 Spinal Cord 7 Peripheral Nerve	B Low Dose Rate (LDR)	6 Cesium 131 (Cs-131) 7 Cesium 137 (Cs-137) 8 Iridium 192 (Ir-192) 9 Iodine 125 (I-125) C Californium 252 (Cf-252) Y Other Isotope	Z None
0 Brain 1 Brain Stem 6 Spinal Cord 7 Peripheral Nerve	B Low Dose Rate (LDR)	B Palladium 103 (Pd-103)	1 Unidirectional Source Z None

D   **Radiation Therapy**
0   **Central and Peripheral Nervous System**
2   **Stereotactic Radiosurgery**

Treatment Site Character 4	Modality Qualifier Character 5	Isotope Character 6	Qualifier Character 7
0 Brain 1 Brain Stem 6 Spinal Cord 7 Peripheral Nerve	D Stereotactic Other Photon Radiosurgery H Stereotactic Particulate Radiosurgery J Stereotactic Gamma Beam Radiosurgery	Z None	Z None

DRG Non-OR All treatment site, modality, isotope, and qualifier values

D   **Radiation Therapy**
Ø   **Central and Peripheral Nervous System**
Y   **Other Radiation**

Treatment Site Character 4	Modality Qualifier Character 5	Isotope Character 6	Qualifier Character 7
Ø Brain 1 Brain Stem 6 Spinal Cord 7 Peripheral Nerve	7 Contact Radiation 8 Hyperthermia C Intraoperative Radiation Therapy (IORT) F Plaque Radiation K Laser Interstitial Thermal Therapy	Z None	Z None

Valid OR   DØY[Ø,1,6,7]KZZ

D   **Radiation Therapy**
7   **Lymphatic and Hematologic System**
Ø   **Beam Radiation**

Treatment Site Character 4	Modality Qualifier Character 5	Isotope Character 6	Qualifier Character 7
Ø Bone Marrow 1 Thymus 2 Spleen 3 Lymphatics, Neck 4 Lymphatics, Axillary 5 Lymphatics, Thorax 6 Lymphatics, Abdomen 7 Lymphatics, Pelvis 8 Lymphatics, Inguinal	Ø Photons <1 MeV 1 Photons 1- 10 MeV 2 Photons >10 MeV 4 Heavy Particles (Protons, Ions) 5 Neutrons 6 Neutron Capture	Z None	Z None
Ø Bone Marrow 1 Thymus 2 Spleen 3 Lymphatics, Neck 4 Lymphatics, Axillary 5 Lymphatics, Thorax 6 Lymphatics, Abdomen 7 Lymphatics, Pelvis 8 Lymphatics, Inguinal	3 Electrons	Z None	Ø Intraoperative Z None

D   **Radiation Therapy**
7   **Lymphatic and Hematologic System**
1   **Brachytherapy**

Treatment Site Character 4	Modality Qualifier Character 5	Isotope Character 6	Qualifier Character 7
Ø Bone Marrow 1 Thymus 2 Spleen 3 Lymphatics, Neck 4 Lymphatics, Axillary 5 Lymphatics, Thorax 6 Lymphatics, Abdomen 7 Lymphatics, Pelvis 8 Lymphatics, Inguinal	9 High Dose Rate (HDR)	7 Cesium 137 (Cs-137) 8 Iridium 192 (Ir-192) 9 Iodine 125 (I-125) B Palladium 103 (Pd-103) C Californium 252 (Cf-252) Y Other Isotope	Z None
Ø Bone Marrow 1 Thymus 2 Spleen 3 Lymphatics, Neck 4 Lymphatics, Axillary 5 Lymphatics, Thorax 6 Lymphatics, Abdomen 7 Lymphatics, Pelvis 8 Lymphatics, Inguinal	B Low Dose Rate (LDR)	6 Cesium 131 (Cs-131) 7 Cesium 137 (Cs-137) 8 Iridium 192 (Ir-192) 9 Iodine 125 (I-125) C Californium 252 (Cf-252) Y Other Isotope	Z None
Ø Bone Marrow 1 Thymus 2 Spleen 3 Lymphatics, Neck 4 Lymphatics, Axillary 5 Lymphatics, Thorax 6 Lymphatics, Abdomen 7 Lymphatics, Pelvis 8 Lymphatics, Inguinal	B Low Dose Rate (LDR)	B Palladium 103 (Pd-103)	1 Unidirectional Source Z None

D   **Radiation Therapy**
7   **Lymphatic and Hematologic System**
2   **Stereotactic Radiosurgery**

Treatment Site Character 4	Modality Qualifier Character 5	Isotope Character 6	Qualifier Character 7

Ø Bone Marrow
1 Thymus
2 Spleen
3 Lymphatics, Neck
4 Lymphatics, Axillary
5 Lymphatics, Thorax
6 Lymphatics, Abdomen
7 Lymphatics, Pelvis
8 Lymphatics, Inguinal
	D Stereotactic Other Photon
	    Radiosurgery
	H Stereotactic Particulate
	    Radiosurgery
	J Stereotactic Gamma Beam
	    Radiosurgery
		Z None	**Z** None

DRG Non-OR   All treatment site, modality, isotope, and qualifier values

D   **Radiation Therapy**
7   **Lymphatic and Hematologic System**
Y   **Other Radiation**

Treatment Site Character 4	Modality Qualifier Character 5	Isotope Character 6	Qualifier Character 7
Ø Bone Marrow **1** Thymus **2** Spleen **3** Lymphatics, Neck **4** Lymphatics, Axillary **5** Lymphatics, Thorax **6** Lymphatics, Abdomen **7** Lymphatics, Pelvis **8** Lymphatics, Inguinal	**8** Hyperthermia **F** Plaque Radiation	**Z** None	**Z** None

D   **Radiation Therapy**
8   **Eye**
Ø   **Beam Radiation**

Treatment Site Character 4	Modality Qualifier Character 5	Isotope Character 6	Qualifier Character 7
Ø Eye	**Ø** Photons <1 MeV **1** Photons 1- 10 MeV **2** Photons >10 MeV **4** Heavy Particles (Protons, Ions) **5** Neutrons **6** Neutron Capture	**Z** None	**Z** None
Ø Eye	**3** Electrons	**Z** None	**Ø** Intraoperative **Z** None

D   **Radiation Therapy**
8   **Eye**
1   **Brachytherapy**

Treatment Site Character 4	Modality Qualifier Character 5	Isotope Character 6	Qualifier Character 7
Ø Eye	**9** High Dose Rate (HDR)	**7** Cesium 137 (Cs-137) **8** Iridium 192 (Ir-192) **9** Iodine 125 (I-125) **B** Palladium 103 (Pd-103) **C** Californium 252 (Cf-252) **Y** Other Isotope	**Z** None
Ø Eye	**B** Low Dose Rate (LDR)	**6** Cesium 131 (Cs-131) **7** Cesium 137 (Cs-137) **8** Iridium 192 (Ir-192) **9** Iodine 125 (I-125) **C** Californium 252 (Cf-252) **Y** Other Isotope	**Z** None
Ø Eye	**B** Low Dose Rate (LDR)	**B** Palladium 103 (Pd-103)	**1** Unidirectional Source **Z** None

LC Limited Coverage   **NC** Noncovered   ⊞ Combination Member   **HAC**   Valid OR   Combination Only   DRG Non-OR   New/Revised in **GREEN**

ICD-10-PCS 2021   779

D72–D81

Radiation Therapy

D   **Radiation Therapy**
8   **Eye**
2   **Stereotactic Radiosurgery**

Treatment Site Character 4	Modality Qualifier Character 5	Isotope Character 6	Qualifier Character 7
Ø Eye	D Stereotactic Other Photon Radiosurgery H Stereotactic Particulate Radiosurgery J Stereotactic Gamma Beam Radiosurgery	Z None	Z None

DRG Non-OR   All treatment site, modality, isotope, and qualifier values

D   **Radiation Therapy**
8   **Eye**
Y   **Other Radiation**

Treatment Site Character 4	Modality Qualifier Character 5	Isotope Character 6	Qualifier Character 7
Ø Eye	7 Contact Radiation 8 Hyperthermia F Plaque Radiation	Z None	Z None

D   **Radiation Therapy**
9   **Ear, Nose, Mouth and Throat**
Ø   **Beam Radiation**

Treatment Site Character 4	Modality Qualifier Character 5	Isotope Character 6	Qualifier Character 7
Ø Ear 1 Nose 3 Hypopharynx 4 Mouth 5 Tongue 6 Salivary Glands 7 Sinuses 8 Hard Palate 9 Soft Palate B Larynx D Nasopharynx F Oropharynx	Ø Photons <1 MeV 1 Photons 1- 10 MeV 2 Photons >10 MeV 4 Heavy Particles (Protons, Ions) 5 Neutrons 6 Neutron Capture	Z None	Z None
Ø Ear 1 Nose 3 Hypopharynx 4 Mouth 5 Tongue 6 Salivary Glands 7 Sinuses 8 Hard Palate 9 Soft Palate B Larynx D Nasopharynx F Oropharynx	3 Electrons	Z None	Ø Intraoperative Z None

D   **Radiation Therapy**
9   **Ear, Nose, Mouth and Throat**
1   **Brachytherapy**

Treatment Site Character 4	Modality Qualifier Character 5	Isotope Character 6	Qualifier Character 7
Ø Ear 1 Nose 3 Hypopharynx 4 Mouth 5 Tongue 6 Salivary Glands 7 Sinuses 8 Hard Palate 9 Soft Palate B Larynx D Nasopharynx F Oropharynx	9 High Dose Rate (HDR)	7 Cesium 137 (Cs-137) 8 Iridium 192 (Ir-192) 9 Iodine 125 (I-125) B Palladium 103 (Pd-103) C Californium 252 (Cf-252) Y Other Isotope	Z None
Ø Ear 1 Nose 3 Hypopharynx 4 Mouth 5 Tongue 6 Salivary Glands 7 Sinuses 8 Hard Palate 9 Soft Palate B Larynx D Nasopharynx F Oropharynx	B Low Dose Rate (LDR)	6 Cesium 131 (Cs-131) 7 Cesium 137 (Cs-137) 8 Iridium 192 (Ir-192) 9 Iodine 125 (I-125) C Californium 252 (Cf-252) Y Other Isotope	Z None
Ø Ear 1 Nose 3 Hypopharynx 4 Mouth 5 Tongue 6 Salivary Glands 7 Sinuses 8 Hard Palate 9 Soft Palate B Larynx D Nasopharynx F Oropharynx	B Low Dose Rate (LDR)	B Palladium 103 (Pd-103)	1 Unidirectional Source Z None

D   **Radiation Therapy**
9   **Ear, Nose, Mouth and Throat**
2   **Stereotactic Radiosurgery**

Treatment Site Character 4	Modality Qualifier Character 5	Isotope Character 6	Qualifier Character 7
Ø Ear 1 Nose 4 Mouth 5 Tongue 6 Salivary Glands 7 Sinuses 8 Hard Palate 9 Soft Palate B Larynx C Pharynx D Nasopharynx	D Stereotactic Other Photon Radiosurgery H Stereotactic Particulate Radiosurgery J Stereotactic Gamma Beam Radiosurgery	Z None	Z None

DRG Non-OR   All treatment site, modality, isotope, and qualifier values

Radiation Therapy

D   Radiation Therapy
9   Ear, Nose, Mouth and Throat
Y   Other Radiation

Treatment Site Character 4	Modality Qualifier Character 5	Isotope Character 6	Qualifier Character 7
Ø Ear 1 Nose 5 Tongue 6 Salivary Glands 7 Sinuses 8 Hard Palate 9 Soft Palate	7 Contact Radiation 8 Hyperthermia F Plaque Radiation	Z None	Z None
3 Hypopharynx F Oropharynx	7 Contact Radiation 8 Hyperthermia	Z None	Z None
4 Mouth B Larynx D Nasopharynx	7 Contact Radiation 8 Hyperthermia C Intraoperative Radiation Therapy (IORT) F Plaque Radiation	Z None	Z None
C Pharynx	C Intraoperative Radiation Therapy (IORT) F Plaque Radiation	Z None	Z None

D   Radiation Therapy
B   Respiratory System
Ø   Beam Radiation

Treatment Site Character 4	Modality Qualifier Character 5	Isotope Character 6	Qualifier Character 7
Ø Trachea 1 Bronchus 2 Lung 5 Pleura 6 Mediastinum 7 Chest Wall 8 Diaphragm	Ø Photons <1 MeV 1 Photons 1- 10 MeV 2 Photons >10 MeV 4 Heavy Particles (Protons, Ions) 5 Neutrons 6 Neutron Capture	Z None	Z None
Ø Trachea 1 Bronchus 2 Lung 5 Pleura 6 Mediastinum 7 Chest Wall 8 Diaphragm	3 Electrons	Z None	Ø Intraoperative Z None

D   Radiation Therapy
B   Respiratory System
1   Brachytherapy

Treatment Site Character 4	Modality Qualifier Character 5	Isotope Character 6	Qualifier Character 7
Ø Trachea 1 Bronchus 2 Lung 5 Pleura 6 Mediastinum 7 Chest Wall 8 Diaphragm	9 High Dose Rate (HDR)	7 Cesium 137 (Cs-137) 8 Iridium 192 (Ir-192) 9 Iodine 125 (I-125) B Palladium 103 (Pd-103) C Californium 252 (Cf-252) Y Other Isotope	Z None
Ø Trachea 1 Bronchus 2 Lung 5 Pleura 6 Mediastinum 7 Chest Wall 8 Diaphragm	B Low Dose Rate (LDR)	6 Cesium 131 (Cs-131) 7 Cesium 137 (Cs-137) 8 Iridium 192 (Ir-192) 9 Iodine 125 (I-125) C Californium 252 (Cf-252) Y Other Isotope	Z None
Ø Trachea 1 Bronchus 2 Lung 5 Pleura 6 Mediastinum 7 Chest Wall 8 Diaphragm	B Low Dose Rate (LDR)	B Palladium 103 (Pd-103)	1 Unidirectional Source Z None

D   **Radiation Therapy**
B   **Respiratory System**
2   **Stereotactic Radiosurgery**

Treatment Site Character 4	Modality Qualifier Character 5	Isotope Character 6	Qualifier Character 7

0   Trachea
1   Bronchus
2   Lung
5   Pleura
6   Mediastinum
7   Chest Wall
8   Diaphragm
	D Stereotactic Other Photon
	     Radiosurgery
	H Stereotactic Particulate
	     Radiosurgery
	J Stereotactic Gamma Beam
	     Radiosurgery
		Z None	Z None

DRG Non-OR   All treatment site, modality, isotope, and qualifier values

D   **Radiation Therapy**
B   **Respiratory System**
Y   **Other Radiation**

Treatment Site Character 4	Modality Qualifier Character 5	Isotope Character 6	Qualifier Character 7
0 Trachea 1 Bronchus 2 Lung 5 Pleura 6 Mediastinum 7 Chest Wall 8 Diaphragm	7 Contact Radiation 8 Hyperthermia F Plaque Radiation K Laser Interstitial Thermal Therapy	Z None	Z None

Valid OR   DBY[0,1,2,5,6,7,8]KZZ

D   **Radiation Therapy**
D   **Gastrointestinal System**
0   **Beam Radiation**

Treatment Site Character 4	Modality Qualifier Character 5	Isotope Character 6	Qualifier Character 7
0 Esophagus 1 Stomach 2 Duodenum 3 Jejunum 4 Ileum 5 Colon 7 Rectum	0 Photons <1 MeV 1 Photons 1- 10 MeV 2 Photons >10 MeV 4 Heavy Particles (Protons, Ions) 5 Neutrons 6 Neutron Capture	Z None	Z None
0 Esophagus 1 Stomach 2 Duodenum 3 Jejunum 4 Ileum 5 Colon 7 Rectum	3 Electrons	Z None	0 Intraoperative Z None

Radiation Therapy

D   **Radiation Therapy**
D   **Gastrointestinal System**
1   **Brachytherapy**

Treatment Site Character 4	Modality Qualifier Character 5	Isotope Character 6	Qualifier Character 7
Ø Esophagus 1 Stomach 2 Duodenum 3 Jejunum 4 Ileum 5 Colon 7 Rectum	9 High Dose Rate (HDR)	7 Cesium 137 (Cs-137) 8 Iridium 192 (Ir-192) 9 Iodine 125 (I-125) B Palladium 103 (Pd-103) C Californium 252 (Cf-252) Y Other Isotope	Z None
Ø Esophagus 1 Stomach 2 Duodenum 3 Jejunum 4 Ileum 5 Colon 7 Rectum	B Low Dose Rate (LDR)	6 Cesium 131 (Cs-131) 7 Cesium 137 (Cs-137) 8 Iridium 192 (Ir-192) 9 Iodine 125 (I-125) C Californium 252 (Cf-252) Y Other Isotope	Z None
Ø Esophagus 1 Stomach 2 Duodenum 3 Jejunum 4 Ileum 5 Colon 7 Rectum	B Low Dose Rate (LDR)	B Palladium 103 (Pd-103)	1 Unidirectional Source Z None

D   **Radiation Therapy**
D   **Gastrointestinal System**
2   **Stereotactic Radiosurgery**

Treatment Site Character 4	Modality Qualifier Character 5	Isotope Character 6	Qualifier Character 7

Ø Esophagus
1 Stomach
2 Duodenum
3 Jejunum
4 Ileum
5 Colon
7 Rectum
	D Stereotactic Other Photon
	   Radiosurgery
	H Stereotactic Particulate
	   Radiosurgery
	J Stereotactic Gamma Beam
	   Radiosurgery
		Z None	Z None

DRG Non-OR   All treatment site, modality, isotope, and qualifier values

D   **Radiation therapy**
D   **Gastrointestinal System**
Y   **Other Radiation**

Treatment Site Character 4	Modality Qualifier Character 5	Isotope Character 6	Qualifier Character 7
Ø Esophagus	7 Contact Radiation 8 Hyperthermia F Plaque Radiation K Laser Interstitial Thermal Therapy	Z None	Z None
1 Stomach 2 Duodenum 3 Jejunum 4 Ileum 5 Colon 7 Rectum	7 Contact Radiation 8 Hyperthermia C Intraoperative Radiation Therapy (IORT) F Plaque Radiation K Laser Interstitial Thermal Therapy	Z None	Z None
8 Anus	C Intraoperative Radiation Therapy (IORT) F Plaque Radiation K Laser Interstitial Thermal Therapy	Z None	Z None

Valid OR   DDYØKZZ
Valid OR   DDY[1,2,3,4,5,7]KZZ
Valid OR   DDY8KZZ

D   Radiation Therapy
F   Hepatobiliary System and Pancreas
0   Beam Radiation

Treatment Site Character 4	Modality Qualifier Character 5	Isotope Character 6	Qualifier Character 7
0 Liver 1 Gallbladder 2 Bile Ducts 3 Pancreas	0 Photons <1 MeV 1 Photons 1- 10 MeV 2 Photons >10 MeV 4 Heavy Particles (Protons, Ions) 5 Neutrons 6 Neutron Capture	Z None	Z None
0 Liver 1 Gallbladder 2 Bile Ducts 3 Pancreas	3 Electrons	Z None	0 Intraoperative Z None

D   Radiation Therapy
F   Hepatobiliary System and Pancreas
1   Brachytherapy

Treatment Site Character 4	Modality Qualifier Character 5	Isotope Character 6	Qualifier Character 7
0 Liver 1 Gallbladder 2 Bile Ducts 3 Pancreas	9 High Dose Rate (HDR)	7 Cesium 137 (Cs-137) 8 Iridium 192 (Ir-192) 9 Iodine 125 (I-125) B Palladium 103 (Pd-103) C Californium 252 (Cf-252) Y Other Isotope	Z None
0 Liver 1 Gallbladder 2 Bile Ducts 3 Pancreas	B Low Dose Rate (LDR)	6 Cesium 131 (Cs-131) 7 Cesium 137 (Cs-137) 8 Iridium 192 (Ir-192) 9 Iodine 125 (I-125) C Californium 252 (Cf-252) Y Other Isotope	Z None
0 Liver 1 Gallbladder 2 Bile Ducts 3 Pancreas	B Low Dose Rate (LDR)	B Palladium 103 (Pd-103)	1 Unidirectional Source Z None

D   Radiation Therapy
F   Hepatobiliary System and Pancreas
2   Stereotactic Radiosurgery

Treatment Site Character 4	Modality Qualifier Character 5	Isotope Character 6	Qualifier Character 7

0 Liver
1 Gallbladder
2 Bile Ducts
3 Pancreas
	D Stereotactic Other Photon
	   Radiosurgery
	H Stereotactic Particulate
	   Radiosurgery
	J Stereotactic Gamma Beam
	   Radiosurgery
		Z None	Z None

DRG Non-OR   All treatment site, modality, isotope, and qualifier values

D   Radiation Therapy
F   Hepatobiliary System and Pancreas
Y   Other Radiation

Treatment Site Character 4	Modality Qualifier Character 5	Isotope Character 6	Qualifier Character 7
0 Liver 1 Gallbladder 2 Bile Ducts 3 Pancreas	7 Contact Radiation 8 Hyperthermia C Intraoperative Radiation Therapy (IORT) F Plaque Radiation K Laser Interstitial Thermal Therapy	Z None	Z None

Valid OR   DFY[0,1,2,3]KZZ

D Radiation Therapy
G Endocrine System
Ø Beam Radiation

Treatment Site Character 4	Modality Qualifier Character 5	Isotope Character 6	Qualifier Character 7
Ø Pituitary Gland 1 Pineal Body 2 Adrenal Glands 4 Parathyroid Glands 5 Thyroid	Ø Photons <1 MeV 1 Photons 1- 10 MeV 2 Photons >10 MeV 5 Neutrons 6 Neutron Capture	Z None	Z None
Ø Pituitary Gland 1 Pineal Body 2 Adrenal Glands 4 Parathyroid Glands 5 Thyroid	3 Electrons	Z None	Ø Intraoperative Z None

D Radiation Therapy
G Endocrine System
1 Brachytherapy

Treatment Site Character 4	Modality Qualifier Character 5	Isotope Character 6	Qualifier Character 7
Ø Pituitary Gland 1 Pineal Body 2 Adrenal Glands 4 Parathyroid Glands 5 Thyroid	9 High Dose Rate (HDR)	7 Cesium 137 (Cs-137) 8 Iridium 192 (Ir-192) 9 Iodine 125 (I-125) B Palladium 103 (Pd-103) C Californium 252 (Cf-252) Y Other Isotope	Z None
Ø Pituitary Gland 1 Pineal Body 2 Adrenal Glands 4 Parathyroid Glands 5 Thyroid	B Low Dose Rate (LDR)	6 Cesium 131 (Cs-131) 7 Cesium 137 (Cs-137) 8 Iridium 192 (Ir-192) 9 Iodine 125 (I-125) C Californium 252 (Cf-252) Y Other Isotope	Z None
Ø Pituitary Gland 1 Pineal Body 2 Adrenal Glands 4 Parathyroid Glands 5 Thyroid	B Low Dose Rate (LDR)	B Palladium 103 (Pd-103)	1 Unidirectional Source Z None

D Radiation Therapy
G Endocrine System
2 Stereotactic Radiosurgery

Treatment Site Character 4	Modality Qualifier Character 5	Isotope Character 6	Qualifier Character 7
Ø Pituitary Gland 1 Pineal Body 2 Adrenal Glands 4 Parathyroid Glands 5 Thyroid	D Stereotactic Other Photon Radiosurgery H Stereotactic Particulate Radiosurgery J Stereotactic Gamma Beam Radiosurgery	Z None	Z None

DRG Non-OR All treatment site, modality, isotope, and qualifier values

D Radiation therapy
G Endocrine System
Y Other Radiation

Treatment Site Character 4	Modality Qualifier Character 5	Isotope Character 6	Qualifier Character 7
Ø Pituitary Gland 1 Pineal Body 2 Adrenal Glands 4 Parathyroid Glands 5 Thyroid	7 Contact Radiation 8 Hyperthermia F Plaque Radiation K Laser Interstitial Thermal Therapy	Z None	Z None

Valid OR DGY[Ø,1,2,4,5]KZZ

Radiation Therapy

D Radiation Therapy
H Skin
Ø Beam Radiation

Treatment Site Character 4	Modality Qualifier Character 5	Isotope Character 6	Qualifier Character 7
2 Skin, Face 3 Skin, Neck 4 Skin, Arm 6 Skin, Chest 7 Skin, Back 8 Skin, Abdomen 9 Skin, Buttock B Skin, Leg	Ø Photons <1 MeV 1 Photons 1- 10 MeV 2 Photons >10 MeV 4 Heavy Particles (Protons, Ions) 5 Neutrons 6 Neutron Capture	Z None	Z None
2 Skin, Face 3 Skin, Neck 4 Skin, Arm 6 Skin, Chest 7 Skin, Back 8 Skin, Abdomen 9 Skin, Buttock B Skin, Leg	3 Electrons	Z None	Ø Intraoperative Z None

D Radiation Therapy
H Skin
Y Other Radiation

Treatment Site Character 4	Modality Qualifier Character 5	Isotope Character 6	Qualifier Character 7
2 Skin, Face 3 Skin, Neck 4 Skin, Arm 6 Skin, Chest 7 Skin, Back 8 Skin, Abdomen 9 Skin, Buttock B Skin, Leg	7 Contact Radiation 8 Hyperthermia F Plaque Radiation	Z None	Z None
5 Skin, Hand C Skin, Foot	F Plaque Radiation	Z None	Z None

D Radiation Therapy
M Breast
Ø Beam Radiation

Treatment Site Character 4	Modality Qualifier Character 5	Isotope Character 6	Qualifier Character 7
Ø Breast, Left 1 Breast, Right	Ø Photons <1 MeV 1 Photons 1- 10 MeV 2 Photons >10 MeV 4 Heavy Particles (Protons, Ions) 5 Neutrons 6 Neutron Capture	Z None	Z None
Ø Breast, Left 1 Breast, Right	3 Electrons	Z None	Ø Intraoperative Z None

D Radiation Therapy
M Breast
1 Brachytherapy

Treatment Site Character 4	Modality Qualifier Character 5	Isotope Character 6	Qualifier Character 7
Ø Breast, Left 1 Breast, Right	9 High Dose Rate (HDR)	7 Cesium 137 (Cs-137) 8 Iridium 192 (Ir-192) 9 Iodine 125 (I-125) B Palladium 103 (Pd-103) C Californium 252 (Cf-252) Y Other Isotope	Z None
Ø Breast, Left 1 Breast, Right	B Low Dose Rate (LDR)	6 Cesium 131 (Cs-131) 7 Cesium 137 (Cs-137) 8 Iridium 192 (Ir-192) 9 Iodine 125 (I-125) C Californium 252 (Cf-252) Y Other Isotope	Z None
Ø Breast, Left 1 Breast, Right	B Low Dose Rate (LDR)	B Palladium 103 (Pd-103)	1 Unidirectional Source Z None

Radiation Therapy (side tab)

D   **Radiation Therapy**
M   **Breast**
2   **Stereotactic Radiosurgery**

Treatment Site Character 4	Modality Qualifier Character 5	Isotope Character 6	Qualifier Character 7

Ø   Breast, Left
1   Breast, Right
	D Stereotactic Other Photon
	     Radiosurgery
	H Stereotactic Particulate
	     Radiosurgery
	J Stereotactic Gamma Beam
	     Radiosurgery
		Z None	Z None

DRG Non-OR   All treatment site, modality, isotope, and qualifier values

D   **Radiation Therapy**
M   **Breast**
Y   **Other Radiation**

Treatment Site Character 4	Modality Qualifier Character 5	Isotope Character 6	Qualifier Character 7
Ø Breast, Left 1 Breast, Right	7 Contact Radiation 8 Hyperthermia F Plaque Radiation K Laser Interstitial Thermal Therapy	Z None	Z None

Valid OR   DMY[Ø,1]KZZ

D   **Radiation Therapy**
P   **Musculoskeletal System**
Ø   **Beam Radiation**

Treatment Site Character 4	Modality Qualifier Character 5	Isotope Character 6	Qualifier Character 7
Ø Skull 2 Maxilla 3 Mandible 4 Sternum 5 Rib(s) 6 Humerus 7 Radius/Ulna 8 Pelvic Bones 9 Femur B Tibia/Fibula C Other Bone	Ø Photons <1 MeV 1 Photons 1- 10 MeV 2 Photons >10 MeV 4 Heavy Particles (Protons, Ions) 5 Neutrons 6 Neutron Capture	Z None	Z None
Ø Skull 2 Maxilla 3 Mandible 4 Sternum 5 Rib(s) 6 Humerus 7 Radius/Ulna 8 Pelvic Bones 9 Femur B Tibia/Fibula C Other Bone	3 Electrons	Z None	Ø Intraoperative Z None

D   **Radiation Therapy**
P   **Musculoskeletal System**
Y   **Other Radiation**

Treatment Site Character 4	Modality Qualifier Character 5	Isotope Character 6	Qualifier Character 7
Ø Skull 2 Maxilla 3 Mandible 4 Sternum 5 Rib(s) 6 Humerus 7 Radius/Ulna 8 Pelvic Bones 9 Femur B Tibia/Fibula C Other Bone	7 Contact Radiation 8 Hyperthermia F Plaque Radiation	Z None	Z None

D   Radiation Therapy
T   Urinary System
Ø   Beam Radiation

Treatment Site Character 4	Modality Qualifier Character 5	Isotope Character 6	Qualifier Character 7
Ø Kidney 1 Ureter 2 Bladder 3 Urethra	Ø Photons <1 MeV 1 Photons 1- 10 MeV 2 Photons >10 MeV 4 Heavy Particles (Protons, Ions) 5 Neutrons 6 Neutron Capture	Z None	Z None
Ø Kidney 1 Ureter 2 Bladder 3 Urethra	3 Electrons	Z None	Ø Intraoperative Z None

D   Radiation Therapy
T   Urinary System
1   Brachytherapy

Treatment Site Character 4	Modality Qualifier Character 5	Isotope Character 6	Qualifier Character 7
Ø Kidney 1 Ureter 2 Bladder 3 Urethra	9 High Dose Rate (HDR)	7 Cesium 137 (Cs-137) 8 Iridium 192 (Ir-192) 9 Iodine 125 (I-125) B Palladium 103 (Pd-103) C Californium 252 (Cf-252) Y Other Isotope	Z None
Ø Kidney 1 Ureter 2 Bladder 3 Urethra	B Low Dose Rate (LDR)	6 Cesium 131 (Cs-131) 7 Cesium 137 (Cs-137) 8 Iridium 192 (Ir-192) 9 Iodine 125 (I-125) C Californium 252 (Cf-252) Y Other Isotope	Z None
Ø Kidney 1 Ureter 2 Bladder 3 Urethra	B Low Dose Rate (LDR)	B Palladium 103 (Pd-103)	1 Unidirectional Source Z None

D   Radiation Therapy
T   Urinary System
2   Stereotactic Radiosurgery

Treatment Site Character 4	Modality Qualifier Character 5	Isotope Character 6	Qualifier Character 7
Ø Kidney 1 Ureter 2 Bladder 3 Urethra	D Stereotactic Other Photon Radiosurgery H Stereotactic Particulate Radiosurgery J Stereotactic Gamma Beam Radiosurgery	Z None	Z None

DRG Non-OR All treatment site, modality, isotope, and qualifier values

D   Radiation Therapy
T   Urinary System
Y   Other Radiation

Treatment Site Character 4	Modality Qualifier Character 5	Isotope Character 6	Qualifier Character 7
Ø Kidney 1 Ureter 2 Bladder 3 Urethra	7 Contact Radiation 8 Hyperthermia C Intraoperative Radiation Therapy (IORT) F Plaque Radiation	Z None	Z None

LC Limited Coverage   NC Noncovered   ⊞ Combination Member   HAC   Valid OR   Combination Only   DRG Non-OR   New/Revised in GREEN
ICD-10-PCS 2021   789

DTØ–DTY

Radiation Therapy (side tab)

D Radiation Therapy
U Female Reproductive System
Ø Beam Radiation

Treatment Site Character 4	Modality Qualifier Character 5	Isotope Character 6	Qualifier Character 7
Ø Ovary ♀ 1 Cervix ♀ 2 Uterus ♀	Ø Photons <1 MeV 1 Photons 1- 10 MeV 2 Photons >10 MeV 4 Heavy Particles (Protons, Ions) 5 Neutrons 6 Neutron Capture	Z None	Z None
Ø Ovary ♀ 1 Cervix ♀ 2 Uterus ♀	3 Electrons	Z None	Ø Intraoperative Z None

♀ All treatment site, modality, isotope, and qualifier values

D Radiation Therapy
U Female Reproductive System
1 Brachytherapy

Treatment Site Character 4	Modality Qualifier Character 5	Isotope Character 6	Qualifier Character 7
Ø Ovary ♀ 1 Cervix ♀ 2 Uterus ♀	9 High Dose Rate (HDR)	7 Cesium 137 (Cs-137) 8 Iridium 192 (Ir-192) 9 Iodine 125 (I-125) B Palladium 103 (Pd-103) C Californium 252 (Cf-252) Y Other Isotope	Z None
Ø Ovary ♀ 1 Cervix ♀ 2 Uterus ♀	B Low Dose Rate (LDR)	6 Cesium 131 (Cs-131) 7 Cesium 137 (Cs-137) 8 Iridium 192 (Ir-192) 9 Iodine 125 (I-125) C Californium 252 (Cf-252) Y Other Isotope	Z None
Ø Ovary ♀ 1 Cervix ♀ 2 Uterus ♀	B Low Dose Rate (LDR)	B Palladium 103 (Pd-103)	1 Unidirectional Source Z None

♀ All treatment site, modality, isotope, and qualifier values

D Radiation Therapy
U Female Reproductive System
2 Stereotactic Radiosurgery

Treatment Site Character 4	Modality Qualifier Character 5	Isotope Character 6	Qualifier Character 7
Ø Ovary ♀ 1 Cervix ♀ 2 Uterus ♀	D Stereotactic Other Photon Radiosurgery H Stereotactic Particulate Radiosurgery J Stereotactic Gamma Beam Radiosurgery	Z None	Z None

DRG Non-OR All treatment site, modality, isotope, and qualifier values
♀ All treatment site, modality, isotope, and qualifier values

D Radiation Therapy
U Female Reproductive System
Y Other Radiation

Treatment Site Character 4	Modality Qualifier Character 5	Isotope Character 6	Qualifier Character 7
Ø Ovary ♀ 1 Cervix ♀ 2 Uterus ♀	7 Contact Radiation 8 Hyperthermia C Intraoperative Radiation Therapy (IORT) F Plaque Radiation	Z None	Z None

♀ All treatment site, modality, isotope, and qualifier values

D Radiation Therapy
V Male Reproductive System
Ø Beam Radiation

Treatment Site Character 4		Modality Qualifier Character 5	Isotope Character 6	Qualifier Character 7
Ø Prostate	♂	Ø Photons <1 MeV	Z None	Z None
1 Testis	♂	1 Photons 1- 10 MeV		
		2 Photons >10 MeV		
		4 Heavy Particles (Protons, Ions)		
		5 Neutrons		
		6 Neutron Capture		
Ø Prostate	♂	3 Electrons	Z None	Ø Intraoperative
1 Testis	♂			Z None

♂   All treatment site, modality, isotope, and qualifier values

D Radiation Therapy
V Male Reproductive System
1 Brachytherapy

Treatment Site Character 4		Modality Qualifier Character 5	Isotope Character 6	Qualifier Character 7
Ø Prostate	♂	9 High Dose Rate (HDR)	7 Cesium 137 (Cs-137)	Z None
1 Testis	♂		8 Iridium 192 (Ir-192)	
			9 Iodine 125 (I-125)	
			B Palladium 103 (Pd-103)	
			C Californium 252 (Cf-252)	
			Y Other Isotope	
Ø Prostate	♂	B Low Dose Rate (LDR)	6 Cesium 131 (Cs-131)	Z None
1 Testis	♂		7 Cesium 137 (Cs-137)	
			8 Iridium 192 (Ir-192)	
			9 Iodine 125 (I-125)	
			C Californium 252 (Cf-252)	
			Y Other Isotope	
Ø Prostate	♂	B Low Dose Rate (LDR)	B Palladium 103 (Pd-103)	1 Unidirectional Source
1 Testis	♂			Z None

♂   All treatment site, modality, isotope, and qualifier values

D Radiation Therapy
V Male Reproductive System
2 Stereotactic Radiosurgery

Treatment Site Character 4		Modality Qualifier Character 5	Isotope Character 6	Qualifier Character 7
Ø Prostate	♂	D Stereotactic Other Photon Radiosurgery	Z None	Z None
1 Testis	♂	H Stereotactic Particulate Radiosurgery		
		J Stereotactic Gamma Beam Radiosurgery		

DRG Non-OR   All treatment site, modality, isotope, and qualifier values
♂   All treatment site, modality, isotope, and qualifier values

D Radiation Therapy
V Male Reproductive System
Y Other Radiation

Treatment Site Character 4		Modality Qualifier Character 5	Isotope Character 6	Qualifier Character 7
Ø Prostate	♂	7 Contact Radiation	Z None	Z None
		8 Hyperthermia		
		C Intraoperative Radiation Therapy (IORT)		
		F Plaque Radiation		
		K Laser Interstitial Thermal Therapy		
1 Testis	♂	7 Contact Radiation	Z None	Z None
		8 Hyperthermia		
		F Plaque Radiation		

Valid OR   DVYØKZZ
♂   All treatment site, modality, isotope, and qualifier values

D Radiation Therapy
W Anatomical Regions
0 Beam Radiation

Treatment Site Character 4	Modality Qualifier Character 5	Isotope Character 6	Qualifier Character 7
1 Head and Neck 2 Chest 3 Abdomen 4 Hemibody 5 Whole Body 6 Pelvic Region	0 Photons <1 MeV 1 Photons 1- 10 MeV 2 Photons >10 MeV 4 Heavy Particles (Protons, Ions) 5 Neutrons 6 Neutron Capture	Z None	Z None
1 Head and Neck 2 Chest 3 Abdomen 4 Hemibody 5 Whole Body 6 Pelvic Region	3 Electrons	Z None	0 Intraoperative Z None

D Radiation Therapy
W Anatomical Regions
1 Brachytherapy

Treatment Site Character 4	Modality Qualifier Character 5	Isotope Character 6	Qualifier Character 7
0 Cranial Cavity K Upper Back L Lower Back P Gastrointestinal Tract Q Respiratory Tract R Genitourinary Tract X Upper Extremity Y Lower Extremity	B Low Dose Rate (LDR)	B Palladium 103 (Pd-103)	1 Unidirectional Source Z None
1 Head and Neck 2 Chest 3 Abdomen 6 Pelvic Region	9 High Dose Rate (HDR)	7 Cesium 137 (Cs-137) 8 Iridium 192 (Ir-192) 9 Iodine 125 (I-125) B Palladium 103 (Pd-103) C Californium 252 (Cf-252) Y Other Isotope	Z None
1 Head and Neck 2 Chest 3 Abdomen 6 Pelvic Region	B Low Dose Rate (LDR)	6 Cesium 131 (Cs-131) 7 Cesium 137 (Cs-137) 8 Iridium 192 (Ir-192) 9 Iodine 125 (I-125) C Californium 252 (Cf-252) Y Other Isotope	Z None
1 Head and Neck 2 Chest 3 Abdomen 6 Pelvic Region	B Low Dose Rate (LDR)	B Palladium 103 (Pd-103)	1 Unidirectional Source Z None

D Radiation Therapy
W Anatomical Regions
2 Stereotactic Radiosurgery

Treatment Site Character 4	Modality Qualifier Character 5	Isotope Character 6	Qualifier Character 7
1 Head and Neck 2 Chest 3 Abdomen 6 Pelvic Region	D Stereotactic Other Photon Radiosurgery H Stereotactic Particulate Radiosurgery J Stereotactic Gamma Beam Radiosurgery	Z None	Z None

DRG Non-OR All treatment site, modality, isotope, and qualifier values

D   Radiation Therapy
W   Anatomical Regions
Y   Other Radiation

Treatment Site Character 4	Modality Qualifier Character 5	Isotope Character 6	Qualifier Character 7
1 Head and Neck **2** Chest **3** Abdomen **4** Hemibody **6** Pelvic Region	**7** Contact Radiation **8** Hyperthermia **F** Plaque Radiation	**Z** None	**Z** None
5 Whole Body	**7** Contact Radiation **8** Hyperthermia **F** Plaque Radiation	**Z** None	**Z** None
5 Whole Body	**G** Isotope Administration	**D** Iodine 131 (I-131) **F** Phosphorus 32 (P-32) **G** Strontium 89 (Sr-89) **H** Strontium 90 (Sr-90) **Y** Other Isotope	**Z** None

Physical Rehabilitation and Diagnostic Audiology F00–F15

F   **Physical Rehabilitation and Diagnostic Audiology**
0   **Rehabilitation**
0   **Speech Assessment**   Definition: Measurement of speech and related functions

Body System/Region Character 4	Type Qualifier Character 5	Equipment Character 6	Qualifier Character 7
3 Neurological System - Whole Body	G Communicative/Cognitive Integration Skills	K Audiovisual M Augmentative / Alternative Communication P Computer Y Other Equipment Z None	Z None
Z None	0 Filtered Speech 3 Staggered Spondaic Word Q Performance Intensity Phonetically Balanced Speech Discrimination R Brief Tone Stimuli S Distorted Speech T Dichotic Stimuli V Temporal Ordering of Stimuli W Masking Patterns	1 Audiometer 2 Sound Field / Booth K Audiovisual Z None	Z None
Z None	1 Speech Threshold 2 Speech/Word Recognition	1 Audiometer 2 Sound Field / Booth 9 Cochlear Implant K Audiovisual Z None	Z None
Z None	4 Sensorineural Acuity Level	1 Audiometer 2 Sound Field / Booth Z None	Z None
Z None	5 Synthetic Sentence Identification	1 Audiometer 2 Sound Field / Booth 9 Cochlear Implant K Audiovisual	Z None
Z None	6 Speech and/or Language Screening 7 Nonspoken Language 8 Receptive/Expressive Language C Aphasia G Communicative/Cognitive Integration Skills L Augmentative/Alternative Communication System	K Audiovisual M Augmentative / Alternative Communication P Computer Y Other Equipment Z None	Z None
Z None	9 Articulation/Phonology	K Audiovisual P Computer Q Speech Analysis Y Other Equipment Z None	Z None
Z None	B Motor Speech	K Audiovisual N Biosensory Feedback P Computer Q Speech Analysis T Aerodynamic Function Y Other Equipment Z None	Z None
Z None	D Fluency	K Audiovisual N Biosensory Feedback P Computer Q Speech Analysis S Voice Analysis T Aerodynamic Function Y Other Equipment Z None	Z None
Z None	F Voice	K Audiovisual N Biosensory Feedback P Computer S Voice Analysis T Aerodynamic Function Y Other Equipment Z None	Z None

DRG Non-OR   All body system/region, type qualifier, equipment, and qualifier values

F00 Continued on next page

F   **Physical Rehabilitation and Diagnostic Audiology**
0   **Rehabilitation**
0   **Speech Assessment**   Definition: Measurement of speech and related functions

Body System/Region Character 4	Type Qualifier Character 5	Equipment Character 6	Qualifier Character 7
Z None	H Bedside Swallowing and Oral Function P Oral Peripheral Mechanism	Y Other Equipment Z None	Z None
Z None	J Instrumental Swallowing and Oral Function	T Aerodynamic Function W Swallowing Y Other Equipment	Z None
Z None	K Orofacial Myofunctional	K Audiovisual P Computer Y Other Equipment Z None	Z None
Z None	M Voice Prosthetic	K Audiovisual P Computer S Voice Analysis V Speech Prosthesis Y Other Equipment Z None	Z None
Z None	N Non-invasive Instrumental Status	N Biosensory Feedback P Computer Q Speech Analysis S Voice Analysis T Aerodynamic Function Y Other Equipment	Z None
Z None	X Other Specified Central Auditory Processing	Z None	Z None

DRG Non-OR   All body system/region, type qualifier, equipment, and qualifier values

F   **Physical Rehabilitation and Diagnostic Audiology**
0   **Rehabilitation**
1   **Motor and/or Nerve Function Assessment**   Definition: Measurement of motor, nerve, and related functions

Body System/Region Character 4	Type Qualifier Character 5	Equipment Character 6	Qualifier Character 7
0 Neurological System - Head and Neck 1 Neurological System - Upper Back/ Upper Extremity 2 Neurological System - Lower Back/ Lower Extremity 3 Neurological System - Whole Body	0 Muscle Performance	E Orthosis F Assistive, Adaptive, Supportive or Protective U Prosthesis Y Other Equipment Z None	Z None
0 Neurological System - Head and Neck 1 Neurological System - Upper Back/ Upper Extremity 2 Neurological System - Lower Back/ Lower Extremity 3 Neurological System - Whole Body	1 Integumentary Integrity 3 Coordination/Dexterity 4 Motor Function G Reflex Integrity	Z None	Z None
0 Neurological System - Head and Neck 1 Neurological System - Upper Back/ Upper Extremity 2 Neurological System - Lower Back/ Lower Extremity 3 Neurological System - Whole Body	5 Range of Motion and Joint Integrity 6 Sensory Awareness/Processing/ Integrity	Y Other Equipment Z None	Z None
D Integumentary System - Head and Neck F Integumentary System - Upper Back/ Upper Extremity G Integumentary System - Lower Back/ Lower Extremity H Integumentary System - Whole Body J Musculoskeletal System - Head and Neck K Musculoskeletal System - Upper Back/ Upper Extremity L Musculoskeletal System - Lower Back/ Lower Extremity M Musculoskeletal System - Whole Body	0 Muscle Performance	E Orthosis F Assistive, Adaptive, Supportive or Protective U Prosthesis Y Other Equipment Z None	Z None

DRG Non-OR   All body system/region, type qualifier, equipment, and qualifier values

F01 Continued on next page

F   Physical Rehabilitation and Diagnostic Audiology
Ø   Rehabilitation
1   Motor and/or Nerve Function Assessment   Definition: Measurement of motor, nerve, and related functions

FØ1 Continued

Body System/Region Character 4	Type Qualifier Character 5	Equipment Character 6	Qualifier Character 7
D Integumentary System - Head and Neck **F** Integumentary System - Upper Back/ Upper Extremity **G** Integumentary System - Lower Back/ Lower Extremity **H** Integumentary System - Whole Body **J** Musculoskeletal System - Head and Neck **K** Musculoskeletal System - Upper Back/ Upper Extremity **L** Musculoskeletal System - Lower Back/ Lower Extremity **M** Musculoskeletal System - Whole Body	**1** Integumentary Integrity	**Z** None	**Z** None
D Integumentary System - Head and Neck **F** Integumentary System - Upper Back/ Upper Extremity **G** Integumentary System - Lower Back/ Lower Extremity **H** Integumentary System - Whole Body **J** Musculoskeletal System - Head and Neck **K** Musculoskeletal System - Upper Back/ Upper Extremity **L** Musculoskeletal System - Lower Back/ Lower Extremity **M** Musculoskeletal System - Whole Body	**5** Range of Motion and Joint Integrity **6** Sensory Awareness/Processing/ Integrity	**Y** Other Equipment **Z** None	**Z** None
N Genitourinary System	**Ø** Muscle Performance	**E** Orthosis **F** Assistive, Adaptive, Supportive or Protective **U** Prosthesis **Y** Other Equipment **Z** None	**Z** None
Z None	**2** Visual Motor Integration	**K** Audiovisual **M** Augmentative / Alternative Communication **N** Biosensory Feedback **P** Computer **Q** Speech Analysis **S** Voice Analysis **Y** Other Equipment **Z** None	**Z** None
Z None	**7** Facial Nerve Function	**7** Electrophysiologic	**Z** None
Z None	**9** Somatosensory Evoked Potentials	**J** Somatosensory	**Z** None
Z None	**B** Bed Mobility **C** Transfer **F** Wheelchair Mobility	**E** Orthosis **F** Assistive, Adaptive, Supportive or Protective **U** Prosthesis **Z** None	**Z** None
Z None	**D** Gait and/or Balance	**E** Orthosis **F** Assistive, Adaptive, Supportive or Protective **U** Prosthesis **Y** Other Equipment **Z** None	**Z** None

DRG Non-OR   All body system/region, type qualifier, equipment, and qualifier values

LC Limited Coverage   NC Noncovered   ⊞ Combination Member   HAC   Valid OR   Combination Only   DRG Non-OR   New/Revised in GREEN

F   Physical Rehabilitation and Diagnostic Audiology
0   Rehabilitation
2   Activities of Daily Living Assessment   Definition: Measurement of functional level for activities of daily living

Body System/Region Character 4	Type Qualifier Character 5	Equipment Character 6	Qualifier Character 7
0 Neurological System - Head and Neck	**9** Cranial Nerve Integrity **D** Neuromotor Development	**Y** Other Equipment **Z** None	**Z** None
1 Neurological System - Upper Back/ Upper Extremity **2** Neurological System - Lower Back/ Lower Extremity **3** Neurological System - Whole Body	**D** Neuromotor Development	**Y** Other Equipment **Z** None	**Z** None
4 Circulatory System - Head and Neck **5** Circulatory System - Upper Back/ Upper Extremity **6** Circulatory System - Lower Back/ Lower Extremity **8** Respiratory System - Head and Neck **9** Respiratory System - Upper Back/ Upper Extremity **B** Respiratory System - Lower Back/ Lower Extremity	**G** Ventilation, Respiration and Circulation	**C** Mechanical **G** Aerobic Endurance and Conditioning **Y** Other Equipment **Z** None	**Z** None
7 Circulatory System - Whole Body **C** Respiratory System - Whole Body	**7** Aerobic Capacity and Endurance	**E** Orthosis **G** Aerobic Endurance and Conditioning **U** Prosthesis **Y** Other Equipment **Z** None	**Z** None
7 Circulatory System - Whole Body **C** Respiratory System - Whole Body	**G** Ventilation, Respiration and Circulation	**C** Mechanical **G** Aerobic Endurance and Conditioning **Y** Other Equipment **Z** None	**Z** None
Z None	**0** Bathing/Showering **1** Dressing **3** Grooming/Personal Hygiene **4** Home Management	**E** Orthosis **F** Assistive, Adaptive, Supportive or Protective **U** Prosthesis **Z** None	**Z** None
Z None	**2** Feeding/Eating **8** Anthropometric Characteristics **F** Pain	**Y** Other Equipment **Z** None	**Z** None
Z None	**5** Perceptual Processing	**K** Audiovisual **M** Augmentative / Alternative Communication **N** Biosensory Feedback **P** Computer **Q** Speech Analysis **S** Voice Analysis **Y** Other Equipment **Z** None	**Z** None
Z None	**6** Psychosocial Skills	**Z** None	**Z** None
Z None	**B** Environmental, Home and Work Barriers **C** Ergonomics and Body Mechanics	**E** Orthosis **F** Assistive, Adaptive, Supportive or Protective **U** Prosthesis **Y** Other Equipment **Z** None	**Z** None
Z None	**H** Vocational Activities and Functional Community or Work Reintegration Skills	**E** Orthosis **F** Assistive, Adaptive, Supportive or Protective **G** Aerobic Endurance and Conditioning **U** Prosthesis **Y** Other Equipment **Z** None	**Z** None

DRG Non-OR   All body system/region, type qualifier, equipment, and qualifier values

F   **Physical Rehabilitation and Diagnostic Audiology**
Ø   **Rehabilitation**
6   **Speech Treatment**   Definition: Application of techniques to improve, augment, or compensate for speech and related functional impairment

Body System/Region Character 4	Type Qualifier Character 5	Equipment Character 6	Qualifier Character 7
3 Neurological System - Whole Body	6 Communicative/Cognitive Integration Skills	K Audiovisual M Augmentative / Alternative Communication P Computer Y Other Equipment Z None	Z None
Z None	Ø Nonspoken Language 3 Aphasia 6 Communicative/Cognitive Integration Skills	K Audiovisual M Augmentative / Alternative Communication P Computer Y Other Equipment Z None	Z None
Z None	1 Speech-Language Pathology and Related Disorders Counseling 2 Speech-Language Pathology and Related Disorders Prevention	K Audiovisual Z None	Z None
Z None	4 Articulation/Phonology	K Audiovisual P Computer Q Speech Analysis T Aerodynamic Function Y Other Equipment Z None	Z None
Z None	5 Aural Rehabilitation	K Audiovisual L Assistive Listening M Augmentative / Alternative Communication N Biosensory Feedback P Computer Q Speech Analysis S Voice Analysis Y Other Equipment Z None	Z None
Z None	7 Fluency	4 Electroacoustic Immitance / Acoustic Reflex K Audiovisual N Biosensory Feedback Q Speech Analysis S Voice Analysis T Aerodynamic Function Y Other Equipment Z None	Z None
Z None	8 Motor Speech	K Audiovisual N Biosensory Feedback P Computer Q Speech Analysis S Voice Analysis T Aerodynamic Function Y Other Equipment Z None	Z None
Z None	9 Orofacial Myofunctional	K Audiovisual P Computer Y Other Equipment Z None	Z None
Z None	B Receptive/Expressive Language	K Audiovisual L Assistive Listening M Augmentative / Alternative Communication P Computer Y Other Equipment Z None	Z None

DRG Non-OR   All body system/region, type qualifier, equipment, and qualifier values

FØ6 Continued on next page

LC Limited Coverage   NC Noncovered   ⊞ Combination Member   HAC   Valid OR   Combination Only   DRG Non-OR   New/Revised in GREEN

F   Physical Rehabilitation and Diagnostic Audiology
Ø   Rehabilitation
6   Speech Treatment   Definition: Application of techniques to improve, augment, or compensate for speech and related functional impairment

F06 Continued

Body System/Region Character 4	Type Qualifier Character 5	Equipment Character 6	Qualifier Character 7
Z None	C Voice	K Audiovisual N Biosensory Feedback P Computer S Voice Analysis T Aerodynamic Function V Speech Prosthesis Y Other Equipment Z None	Z None
Z None	D Swallowing Dysfunction	M Augmentative / Alternative Communication T Aerodynamic Function V Speech Prosthesis Y Other Equipment Z None	Z None

DRG Non-OR   All body system/region, type qualifier, equipment, and qualifier values

F   Physical Rehabilitation and Diagnostic Audiology
Ø   Rehabilitation
7   Motor Treatment   Definition: Exercise or activities to increase or facilitate motor function

Body System/Region Character 4	Type Qualifier Character 5	Equipment Character 6	Qualifier Character 7
Ø Neurological System - Head and Neck 1 Neurological System - Upper Back/Upper Extremity 2 Neurological System - Lower Back/Lower Extremity 3 Neurological System - Whole Body D Integumentary System - Head and Neck F Integumentary System - Upper Back/Upper Extremity G Integumentary System - Lower Back/Lower Extremity H Integumentary System - Whole Body J Musculoskeletal System - Head and Neck K Musculoskeletal System - Upper Back/Upper Extremity L Musculoskeletal System - Lower Back/Lower Extremity M Musculoskeletal System - Whole Body	Ø Range of Motion and Joint Mobility 1 Muscle Performance 2 Coordination/Dexterity 3 Motor Function	E Orthosis F Assistive, Adaptive, Supportive or Protective U Prosthesis Y Other Equipment Z None	Z None
Ø Neurological System - Head and Neck 1 Neurological System - Upper Back/Upper Extremity 2 Neurological System - Lower Back/Lower Extremity 3 Neurological System - Whole Body D Integumentary System - Head and Neck F Integumentary System - Upper Back/Upper Extremity G Integumentary System - Lower Back/Lower Extremity H Integumentary System - Whole Body J Musculoskeletal System - Head and Neck K Musculoskeletal System - Upper Back/Upper Extremity L Musculoskeletal System - Lower Back/Lower Extremity M Musculoskeletal System - Whole Body	6 Therapeutic Exercise	B Physical Agents C Mechanical D Electrotherapeutic E Orthosis F Assistive, Adaptive, Supportive or Protective G Aerobic Endurance and Conditioning H Mechanical or Electromechanical U Prosthesis Y Other Equipment Z None	Z None

DRG Non-OR   All body system/region, type qualifier, equipment, and qualifier values

F07 Continued on next page

LC Limited Coverage   **NC** Noncovered   ⊞ Combination Member   **HAC**   Valid OR   Combination Only   DRG Non-OR   New/Revised in **GREEN**

F07 Continued

F   **Physical Rehabilitation and Diagnostic Audiology**
0   **Rehabilitation**
7   **Motor Treatment**   Definition: Exercise or activities to increase or facilitate motor function

Body System/Region Character 4	Type Qualifier Character 5	Equipment Character 6	Qualifier Character 7
0 Neurological System - Head and Neck 1 Neurological System - Upper Back/Upper Extremity 2 Neurological System - Lower Back/Lower Extremity 3 Neurological System - Whole Body D Integumentary System - Head and Neck F Integumentary System - Upper Back/Upper Extremity G Integumentary System - Lower Back/Lower Extremity H Integumentary System - Whole Body J Musculoskeletal System - Head and Neck K Musculoskeletal System - Upper Back/Upper Extremity L Musculoskeletal System - Lower Back/Lower Extremity M Musculoskeletal System - Whole Body	7 Manual Therapy Techniques	Z None	Z None
4 Circulatory System - Head and Neck 5 Circulatory System - Upper Back / Upper Extremity 6 Circulatory System - Lower Back / Lower Extremity 7 Circulatory System - Whole Body 8 Respiratory System - Head and Neck 9 Respiratory System - Upper Back / Upper Extremity B Respiratory System - Lower Back / Lower Extremity C Respiratory System - Whole Body	6 Therapeutic Exercise	B Physical Agents C Mechanical D Electrotherapeutic E Orthosis F Assistive, Adaptive, Supportive or Protective G Aerobic Endurance and Conditioning H Mechanical or Electromechanical U Prosthesis Y Other Equipment Z None	Z None
N Genitourinary System	1 Muscle Performance	E Orthosis F Assistive, Adaptive, Supportive or Protective U Prosthesis Y Other Equipment Z None	Z None
N Genitourinary System	6 Therapeutic Exercise	B Physical Agents C Mechanical D Electrotherapeutic E Orthosis F Assistive, Adaptive, Supportive or Protective G Aerobic Endurance and Conditioning H Mechanical or Electromechanical U Prosthesis Y Other Equipment Z None	Z None
Z None	4 Wheelchair Mobility	D Electrotherapeutic E Orthosis F Assistive, Adaptive, Supportive or Protective U Prosthesis Y Other Equipment Z None	Z None
Z None	5 Bed Mobility	C Mechanical E Orthosis F Assistive, Adaptive, Supportive or Protective U Prosthesis Y Other Equipment Z None	Z None

DRG Non-OR All body system/region, type qualifier, equipment, and qualifier values

F   Physical Rehabilitation and Diagnostic Audiology
Ø   Rehabilitation
8   Activities of Daily Living Treatment   Definition: Exercise or activities to facilitate functional competence for activities of daily living

Body System/Region Character 4	Type Qualifier Character 5	Equipment Character 6	Qualifier Character 7
Z None	8 Transfer Training	C Mechanical D Electrotherapeutic E Orthosis F Assistive, Adaptive, Supportive or Protective U Prosthesis Y Other Equipment Z None	Z None
Z None	9 Gait Training/Functional Ambulation	C Mechanical D Electrotherapeutic E Orthosis F Assistive, Adaptive, Supportive or Protective G Aerobic Endurance and Conditioning U Prosthesis Y Other Equipment Z None	Z None
D Integumentary System - Head and Neck F Integumentary System - Upper Back/Upper Extremity G Integumentary System - Lower Back/Lower Extremity H Integumentary System - Whole Body J Musculoskeletal System - Head and Neck K Musculoskeletal System - Upper Back/Upper Extremity L Musculoskeletal System - Lower Back/Lower Extremity M Musculoskeletal System - Whole Body	5 Wound Management	B Physical Agents C Mechanical D Electrotherapeutic E Orthosis F Assistive, Adaptive, Supportive or Protective U Prosthesis Y Other Equipment Z None	Z None
Z None	Ø Bathing/Showering Techniques 1 Dressing Techniques 2 Grooming/Personal Hygiene	E Orthosis F Assistive, Adaptive, Supportive or Protective U Prosthesis Y Other Equipment Z None	Z None
Z None	3 Feeding/Eating	C Mechanical D Electrotherapeutic E Orthosis F Assistive, Adaptive, Supportive or Protective U Prosthesis Y Other Equipment Z None	Z None
Z None	4 Home Management	D Electrotherapeutic E Orthosis F Assistive, Adaptive, Supportive or Protective U Prosthesis Y Other Equipment Z None	Z None
Z None	6 Psychosocial Skills	Z None	Z None
Z None	7 Vocational Activities and Functional Community or Work Reintegration Skills	B Physical Agents C Mechanical D Electrotherapeutic E Orthosis F Assistive, Adaptive, Supportive or Protective G Aerobic Endurance and Conditioning U Prosthesis Y Other Equipment Z None	Z None

DRG Non-OR All body system/region, type qualifier, equipment, and qualifier values

F   **Physical Rehabilitation and Diagnostic Audiology**
Ø   **Rehabilitation**
9   **Hearing Treatment**   Definition: Application of techniques to improve, augment, or compensate for hearing and related functional impairment

Body System/Region Character 4	Type Qualifier Character 5	Equipment Character 6	Qualifier Character 7
Z None	**Ø** Hearing and Related Disorders Counseling **1** Hearing and Related Disorders Prevention	**K** Audiovisual **Z** None	**Z** None
Z None	**2** Auditory Processing	**K** Audiovisual **L** Assistive Listening **P** Computer **Y** Other Equipment **Z** None	**Z** None
Z None	**3** Cerumen Management	**X** Cerumen Management **Z** None	**Z** None

DRG Non-OR   All body system/region, type qualifier, equipment, and qualifier values

---

F   **Physical Rehabilitation and Diagnostic Audiology**
Ø   **Rehabilitation**
B   **Cochlear Implant Treatment**   Definition: Application of techniques to improve the communication abilities of individuals with cochlear implant

Body System/Region Character 4	Type Qualifier Character 5	Equipment Character 6	Qualifier Character 7
Z None	**Ø** Cochlear Implant Rehabilitation	**1** Audiometer **2** Sound Field / Booth **9** Cochlear Implant **K** Audiovisual **P** Computer **Y** Other Equipment	**Z** None

DRG Non-OR   All body system/region, type qualifier, equipment, and qualifier values

---

F   **Physical Rehabilitation and Diagnostic Audiology**
Ø   **Rehabilitation**
C   **Vestibular Treatment**   Definition: Application of techniques to improve, augment, or compensate for vestibular and related functional impairment

Body System/Region Character 4	Type Qualifier Character 5	Equipment Character 6	Qualifier Character 7
3 Neurological System - Whole Body **H** Integumentary System - Whole Body **M** Musculoskeletal System - Whole Body	**3** Postural Control	**E** Orthosis **F** Assistive, Adaptive, Supportive or Protective **U** Prosthesis **Y** Other Equipment **Z** None	**Z** None
Z None	**Ø** Vestibular	**8** Vestibular / Balance **Z** None	**Z** None
Z None	**1** Perceptual Processing **2** Visual Motor Integration	**K** Audiovisual **L** Assistive Listening **N** Biosensory Feedback **P** Computer **Q** Speech Analysis **S** Voice Analysis **T** Aerodynamic Function **Y** Other Equipment **Z** None	**Z** None

DRG Non-OR   All body system/region, type qualifier, equipment, and qualifier values

---

LC Limited Coverage   **NC** Noncovered   ⊞ Combination Member   HAC   Valid OR   Combination Only   DRG Non-OR   New/Revised in GREEN

ICD-10-PCS 2021   803

Physical Rehabilitation and Diagnostic Audiology

F   **Physical Rehabilitation and Diagnostic Audiology**
0   **Rehabilitation**
D   **Device Fitting**   Definition: Fitting of a device designed to facilitate or support achievement of a higher level of function

Body System/Region Character 4	Type Qualifier Character 5	Equipment Character 6	Qualifier Character 7
Z None	0 Tinnitus Masker	5 Hearing Aid Selection / Fitting / Test Z None	Z None
Z None	1 Monaural Hearing Aid 2 Binaural Hearing Aid 5 Assistive Listening Device	1 Audiometer 2 Sound Field / Booth 5 Hearing Aid Selection / Fitting / Test K Audiovisual L Assistive Listening Z None	Z None
Z None	3 Augmentative/Alternative Communication System	M Augmentative / Alternative Communication	Z None
Z None	4 Voice Prosthetic	S Voice Analysis V Speech Prosthesis	Z None
Z None	6 Dynamic Orthosis 7 Static Orthosis 8 Prosthesis 9 Assistive, Adaptive, Supportive or Protective Devices	E Orthosis F Assistive, Adaptive, Supportive or Protective U Prosthesis Z None	Z None

DRG Non-OR	F0DZ0[5,Z]Z
DRG Non-OR	F0DZ[1, 2,5][1,2,5, K,L,Z]Z
DRG Non-OR	F0DZ3MZ
DRG Non-OR	F0DZ4[S,V]Z
DRG Non-OR	F0DZ[6,7][E,F,U,Z]Z
DRG Non-OR	F0DZ8[E,F,U]Z

F   **Physical Rehabilitation and Diagnostic Audiology**
0   **Rehabilitation**
F   **Caregiver Training**   Definition: Training in activities to support patient's optimal level of function

Body System/Region Character 4	Type Qualifier Character 5	Equipment Character 6	Qualifier Character 7
Z None	0 Bathing/Showering Technique 1 Dressing 2 Feeding and Eating 3 Grooming/Personal Hygiene 4 Bed Mobility 5 Transfer 6 Wheelchair Mobility 7 Therapeutic Exercise 8 Airway Clearance Techniques 9 Wound Management B Vocational Activities and Functional Community or Work Reintegration Skills C Gait Training/Functional Ambulation D Application, Proper Use and Care of Devices F Application, Proper Use and Care of Orthoses G Application, Proper Use and Care of Prosthesis H Home Management	E Orthosis F Assistive, Adaptive, Supportive or Protective U Prosthesis Z None	Z None
Z None	J Communication Skills	K Audiovisual L Assistive Listening M Augmentative / Alternative Communication P Computer Z None	Z None

DRG Non-OR	All body system/region, type qualifier, equipment, and qualifier values

F   Physical Rehabilitation and Diagnostic Audiology
1   Diagnostic Audiology
3   Hearing Assessment   Definition: Measurement of hearing and related functions

Body System/Region Character 4	Type Qualifier Character 5	Equipment Character 6	Qualifier Character 7
Z None	Ø Hearing Screening	Ø Occupational Hearing 1 Audiometer 2 Sound Field / Booth 3 Tympanometer 8 Vestibular / Balance 9 Cochlear Implant Z None	Z None
Z None	1 Pure Tone Audiometry, Air 2 Pure Tone Audiometry, Air and Bone	Ø Occupational Hearing 1 Audiometer 2 Sound Field / Booth Z None	Z None
Z None	3 Bekesy Audiometry 6 Visual Reinforcement Audiometry 9 Short Increment Sensitivity Index B Stenger C Pure Tone Stenger	1 Audiometer 2 Sound Field / Booth Z None	Z None
Z None	4 Conditioned Play Audiometry 5 Select Picture Audiometry	1 Audiometer 2 Sound Field / Booth K Audiovisual Z None	Z None
Z None	7 Alternate Binaural or Monaural Loudness Balance	1 Audiometer K Audiovisual Z None	Z None
Z None	8 Tone Decay D Tympanometry F Eustachian Tube Function G Acoustic Reflex Patterns H Acoustic Reflex Threshold J Acoustic Reflex Decay	3 Tympanometer 4 Electroacoustic Immitance / Acoustic Reflex Z None	Z None
Z None	K Electrocochleography L Auditory Evoked Potentials	7 Electrophysiologic Z None	Z None

Z None	M Evoked Otoacoustic Emissions,
	    Screening
	N Evoked Otoacoustic Emissions,
	    Diagnostic
		6 Otoacoustic Emission (OAE)
		Z None
			Z None

Z None	P Aural Rehabilitation Status	1 Audiometer 2 Sound Field / Booth 4 Electroacoustic Immitance / Acoustic Reflex 9 Cochlear Implant K Audiovisual L Assistive Listening P Computer Z None	Z None
Z None	Q Auditory Processing	K Audiovisual P Computer Y Other Equipment Z None	Z None

LC Limited Coverage   **NC** Noncovered   ⊞ Combination Member   HAC   Valid OR   Combination Only   DRG Non-OR   New/Revised in GREEN

ICD-10-PCS 2021   805

F13–F13

F Physical Rehabilitation and Diagnostic Audiology
1 Diagnostic Audiology
4 Hearing Aid Assessment   Definition: Measurement of the appropriateness and/or effectiveness of a hearing device

Body System/Region Character 4	Type Qualifier Character 5	Equipment Character 6	Qualifier Character 7
Z None	Ø Cochlear Implant	1 Audiometer 2 Sound Field / Booth 3 Tympanometer 4 Electroacoustic Immitance / Acoustic Reflex 5 Hearing Aid Selection / Fitting / Test 7 Electrophysiologic 9 Cochlear Implant K Audiovisual L Assistive Listening P Computer Y Other Equipment Z None	Z None

Z None	1 Ear Canal Probe Microphone
	6 Binaural Electroacoustic Hearing
	   Aid Check
	8 Monaural Electroacoustic Hearing
	   Aid Check
		5 Hearing Aid Selection / Fitting / Test
		Z None
			Z None

Z None	2 Monaural Hearing Aid 3 Binaural Hearing Aid	1 Audiometer 2 Sound Field / Booth 3 Tympanometer 4 Electroacoustic Immitance / Acoustic Reflex 5 Hearing Aid Selection / Fitting / Test K Audiovisual L Assistive Listening P Computer Z None	Z None

Z None	4 Assistive Listening System/Device
	   Selection
		1 Audiometer
		2 Sound Field / Booth
		3 Tympanometer
		4 Electroacoustic Immitance /
		   Acoustic Reflex
		K Audiovisual
		L Assistive Listening
		Z None
			Z None

Z None	5 Sensory Aids	1 Audiometer 2 Sound Field / Booth 3 Tympanometer 4 Electroacoustic Immitance / Acoustic Reflex 5 Hearing Aid Selection / Fitting / Test K Audiovisual L Assistive Listening Z None	Z None
Z None	7 Ear Protector Attentuation	Ø Occupational Hearing Z None	Z None

F Physical Rehabilitation and Diagnostic Audiology
1 Diagnostic Audiology
5 Vestibular Assessment   Definition: Measurement of the vestibular system and related functions

Body System/Region Character 4	Type Qualifier Character 5	Equipment Character 6	Qualifier Character 7

Z None	Ø Bithermal, Binaural Caloric
	   Irrigation
	1 Bithermal, Monaural Caloric
	   Irrigation
	2 Unithermal Binaural Screen
	3 Oscillating Tracking
	4 Sinusoidal Vertical Axis Rotational
	5 Dix-Hallpike Dynamic
	6 Computerized Dynamic
	   Posturography
		8 Vestibular / Balance
		Z None
			Z None

Z None	7 Tinnitus Masker	5 Hearing Aid Selection / Fitting / Test Z None	Z None

Mental Health GZ1–GZJ

G   **Mental Health**
Z   **None**
1   **Psychological Tests**   Definition: The administration and interpretation of standardized psychological tests and measurement instruments for the assessment of psychological function

Qualifier Character 4	Qualifier Character 5	Qualifier Character 6	Qualifier Character 7
Ø Developmental 1 Personality and Behavioral 2 Intellectual and Psychoeducational 3 Neuropsychological 4 Neurobehavioral and Cognitive Status	Z None	Z None	Z None

G   **Mental Health**
Z   **None**
2   **Crisis Intervention**   Definition: Treatment of a traumatized, acutely disturbed or distressed individual for the purpose of short-term stabilization

Qualifier Character 4	Qualifier Character 5	Qualifier Character 6	Qualifier Character 7
Z None	Z None	Z None	Z None

G   **Mental Health**
Z   **None**
3   **Medication Management**   Definition: Monitoring and adjusting the use of medications for the treatment of a mental health disorder

Qualifier Character 4	Qualifier Character 5	Qualifier Character 6	Qualifier Character 7
Z None	Z None	Z None	Z None

G   **Mental Health**
Z   **None**
5   **Individual Psychotherapy**   Definition: Treatment of an individual with a mental health disorder by behavioral, cognitive, psychoanalytic, psychodynamic or psychophysiological means to improve functioning or well-being

Qualifier Character 4	Qualifier Character 5	Qualifier Character 6	Qualifier Character 7
Ø Interactive 1 Behavioral 2 Cognitive 3 Interpersonal 4 Psychoanalysis 5 Psychodynamic 6 Supportive 8 Cognitive-Behavioral 9 Psychophysiological	Z None	Z None	Z None

G   **Mental Health**
Z   **None**
6   **Counseling**   Definition: The application of psychological methods to treat an individual with normal developmental issues and psychological problems in order to increase function, improve well-being, alleviate distress, maladjustment or resolve crises

Qualifier Character 4	Qualifier Character 5	Qualifier Character 6	Qualifier Character 7
Ø Educational 1 Vocational 3 Other Counseling	Z None	Z None	Z None

G   **Mental Health**
Z   **None**
7   **Family Psychotherapy**   Definition: Treatment that includes one or more family members of an individual with a mental health disorder by behavioral, cognitive, psychoanalytic, psychodynamic or psychophysiological means to improve functioning or well-being

     Explanation: Remediation of emotional or behavioral problems presented by one or more family members in cases where psychotherapy with more than one family member is indicated

Qualifier Character 4	Qualifier Character 5	Qualifier Character 6	Qualifier Character 7
2 Other Family Psychotherapy	Z None	Z None	Z None

Mental Health

G   **Mental Health**
Z   **None**
B   **Electroconvulsive Therapy**   Definition: The application of controlled electrical voltages to treat a mental health disorder

Qualifier Character 4	Qualifier Character 5	Qualifier Character 6	Qualifier Character 7
0 Unilateral-Single Seizure 1 Unilateral-Multiple Seizure 2 Bilateral-Single Seizure 3 Bilateral-Multiple Seizure 4 Other Electroconvulsive Therapy	Z None	Z None	Z None

G   **Mental Health**
Z   **None**
C   **Biofeedback**   Definition: Provision of information from the monitoring and regulating of physiological processes in conjunction with cognitive-behavioral techniques to improve patient functioning or well-being

Qualifier Character 4	Qualifier Character 5	Qualifier Character 6	Qualifier Character 7
9 Other Biofeedback	Z None	Z None	Z None

G   **Mental Health**
Z   **None**
F   **Hypnosis**   Definition: Induction of a state of heightened suggestibility by auditory, visual and tactile techniques to elicit an emotional or behavioral response

Qualifier Character 4	Qualifier Character 5	Qualifier Character 6	Qualifier Character 7
Z None	Z None	Z None	Z None

G   **Mental Health**
Z   **None**
G   **Narcosynthesis**   Definition: Administration of intravenous barbiturates in order to release suppressed or repressed thoughts

Qualifier Character 4	Qualifier Character 5	Qualifier Character 6	Qualifier Character 7
Z None	Z None	Z None	Z None

G   **Mental Health**
Z   **None**
H   **Group Psychotherapy**   Definition: Treatment of two or more individuals with a mental health disorder by behavioral, cognitive, psychoanalytic, psychodynamic or psychophysiological means to improve functioning or well-being

Qualifier Character 4	Qualifier Character 5	Qualifier Character 6	Qualifier Character 7
Z None	Z None	Z None	Z None

G   **Mental Health**
Z   **None**
J   **Light Therapy**   Definition: Application of specialized light treatments to improve functioning or well-being

Qualifier Character 4	Qualifier Character 5	Qualifier Character 6	Qualifier Character 7
Z None	Z None	Z None	Z None

Substance Abuse Treatment HZ2–HZ9

AHA Coding Clinic for table HZ2
2020, 1Q, 21   Inpatient detoxification services

AHA Coding Clinic for table HZ9
2020, 1Q, 21   Inpatient detoxification services

H   **Substance Abuse Treatment**
Z   **None**
2   **Detoxification Services**   Definition: Detoxification from alcohol and/or drugs

Explanation: Not a treatment modality, but helps the patient stabilize physically and psychologically until the body becomes free of drugs and the effects of alcohol

Qualifier Character 4	Qualifier Character 5	Qualifier Character 6	Qualifier Character 7
Z None	Z None	Z None	Z None

H   **Substance Abuse Treatment**
Z   **None**
3   **Individual Counseling**   Definition: The application of psychological methods to treat an individual with addictive behavior

Explanation: Comprised of several different techniques, which apply various strategies to address drug addiction

Qualifier Character 4	Qualifier Character 5	Qualifier Character 6	Qualifier Character 7
Ø Cognitive 1 Behavioral 2 Cognitive-Behavioral 3 12-Step 4 Interpersonal 5 Vocational 6 Psychoeducation 7 Motivational Enhancement 8 Confrontational 9 Continuing Care B Spiritual C Pre/Post-Test Infectious Disease	Z None	Z None	Z None

DRG Non-OR   HZ3[Ø,1,2,3,4,5,6,7,8,9,B]ZZZ

H   **Substance Abuse Treatment**
Z   **None**
4   **Group Counseling**   Definition: The application of psychological methods to treat two or more individuals with addictive behavior

Explanation: Provides structured group counseling sessions and healing power through the connection with others

Qualifier Character 4	Qualifier Character 5	Qualifier Character 6	Qualifier Character 7
Ø Cognitive 1 Behavioral 2 Cognitive-Behavioral 3 12-Step 4 Interpersonal 5 Vocational 6 Psychoeducation 7 Motivational Enhancement 8 Confrontational 9 Continuing Care B Spiritual C Pre/Post-Test Infectious Disease	Z None	Z None	Z None

DRG Non-OR   HZ4[Ø,1,2,3,4,5,6,7,8,9,B]ZZZ

Substance Abuse Treatment

H   Substance Abuse Treatment
Z   None
5   Individual Psychotherapy   Definition: Treatment of an individual with addictive behavior by behavioral, cognitive, psychoanalytic, psychodynamic or psychophysiological means

Qualifier Character 4	Qualifier Character 5	Qualifier Character 6	Qualifier Character 7
Ø Cognitive 1 Behavioral 2 Cognitive-Behavioral 3 12-Step 4 Interpersonal 5 Interactive 6 Psychoeducation 7 Motivational Enhancement 8 Confrontational 9 Supportive B Psychoanalysis C Psychodynamic D Psychophysiological	Z None	Z None	Z None

DRG Non-OR   For all qualifier values

H   Substance Abuse Treatment
Z   None
6   Family Counseling   Definition: The application of psychological methods that includes one or more family members to treat an individual with addictive behavior

     Explanation: Provides support and education for family members of addicted individuals. Family member participation is seen as a critical area of substance abuse treatment

Qualifier Character 4	Qualifier Character 5	Qualifier Character 6	Qualifier Character 7
3 Other Family Counseling	Z None	Z None	Z None

H   Substance Abuse Treatment
Z   None
8   Medication Management   Definition: Monitoring or adjusting the use of replacement medications for the treatment of addiction

Qualifier Character 4	Qualifier Character 5	Qualifier Character 6	Qualifier Character 7
Ø Nicotine Replacement 1 Methadone Maintenance 2 Levo-alpha-acetyl-methadol (LAAM) 3 Antabuse 4 Naltrexone 5 Naloxone 6 Clonidine 7 Bupropion 8 Psychiatric Medication 9 Other Replacement Medication	Z None	Z None	Z None

H   Substance Abuse Treatment
Z   None
9   Pharmacotherapy   Definition: The use of replacement medications for the treatment of addiction

Qualifier Character 4	Qualifier Character 5	Qualifier Character 6	Qualifier Character 7
Ø Nicotine Replacement 1 Methadone Maintenance 2 Levo-alpha-acetyl-methadol (LAAM) 3 Antabuse 4 Naltrexone 5 Naloxone 6 Clonidine 7 Bupropion 8 Psychiatric Medication 9 Other Replacement Medication	Z None	Z None	Z None

New Technology X27–XY0

AHA Coding Clinic for all tables in the New Technology Section
2015, 4Q, 8-11   New Section X codes - New Technology procedures

AHA Coding Clinic for table X27
2019, 4Q, 45-46   Sustained released drug-eluting stent

AHA Coding Clinic for table X2A
2019, 4Q, 46   Cerebral embolic filtration
2016, 4Q, 115-116 Cerebral embolic filtration

AHA Coding Clinic for table X2C
2016, 4Q, 82-83   Coronary artery, number of arteries
2015, 4Q, 8-14   New Section X codes—New Technology procedures

AHA Coding Clinic for table X2R
2016, 4Q, 116   Aortic valve rapid deployment
2015, 4Q, 8-12   New Section X codes—New Technology procedures

AHA Coding Clinic for table XHR
2016, 4Q, 116   Application of wound matrix

AHA Coding Clinic for table XK0
2017, 4Q, 74   Intramuscular autologous bone marrow cell therapy

AHA Coding Clinic for table XNS
2017, 4Q, 74-75   Magnetic growth rods
2016, 4Q, 117   Placement of magnetic growth rods

AHA Coding Clinic for table XRG
2017, 4Q, 76   Radiolucent porous interbody fusion device

AHA Coding Clinic for table XT2
2019, 4Q, 46-47   Renal function monitoring

AHA Coding Clinic for table XV5
2018, 4Q, 55   Robotic waterjet ablation

AHA Coding Clinic for table XW0
2019, 4Q, 47-50   New therapeutic substances
2018, 4Q, 56   New therapeutic substances
2015, 4Q, 8-15   New Section X codes—New Technology procedures

AHA Coding Clinic for table XXE
2019, 4Q, 50-51   Whole blood nucleic acid-base microbial detection

AHA Coding Clinic for table XY0
2017, 4Q, 78   Intraoperative treatment of vascular grafts

X   **New Technology**
2   **Cardiovascular System**
7   **Dilation**   Definition: Expanding an orifice or the lumen of a tubular body part

Explanation: The orifice can be a natural orifice or an artificially created orifice. Accomplished by stretching a tubular body part using intraluminal pressure or by cutting part of the orifice or wall of the tubular body part.

Body Part Character 4	Approach Character 5	Device/Substance/Technology Character 6	Qualifier Character 7
H Femoral Artery, Right J Femoral Artery, Left K Popliteal Artery, Proximal Right L Popliteal Artery, Proximal Left M Popliteal Artery, Distal Right N Popliteal Artery, Distal Left P Anterior Tibial Artery, Right Q Anterior Tibial Artery, Left R Posterior Tibial Artery, Right S Posterior Tibial Artery, Left T Peroneal Artery, Right U Peroneal Artery, Left	3 Percutaneous	8 Intraluminal Device, Sustained Release Drug-eluting 9 Intraluminal Device, Sustained Release Drug-eluting, Two B Intraluminal Device, Sustained Release Drug-eluting, Three C Intraluminal Device, Sustained Release Drug-eluting, Four or More	5 New Technology Group 5

Valid OR   All body part, approach, device/substance/technology, and qualifier values

X   **New Technology**
2   **Cardiovascular System**
A   **Assistance**   Definition: Taking over a portion of a physiological function by extracorporeal means

Explanation: None

Body Part Character 4	Approach Character 5	Device/Substance/Technology Character 6	Qualifier Character 7
5 Innominate Artery and Left Common Carotid Artery	3 Percutaneous	1 Cerebral Embolic Filtration, Dual Filter	2 New Technology Group 2
6 Aortic Arch	3 Percutaneous	2 Cerebral Embolic Filtration, Single Deflection Filter	5 New Technology Group 5
H Common Carotid Artery, Right J Common Carotid Artery, Left	3 Percutaneous	3 Cerebral Embolic Filtration, Extracorporeal Flow Reversal Circuit	6 New Technology Group 6

X   **New Technology**
2   **Cardiovascular System**
C   **Extirpation**   Definition: Taking or cutting out solid matter from a body part

Explanation: The solid matter may be an abnormal byproduct of a biological function or a foreign body; it may be imbedded in a body part or in the lumen of a tubular body part. The solid matter may or may not have been previously broken into pieces.

Body Part Character 4	Approach Character 5	Device/Substance/Technology Character 6	Qualifier Character 7
0 Coronary Artery, One Artery 1 Coronary Artery, Two Arteries 2 Coronary Artery, Three Arteries 3 Coronary Artery, Four or More Arteries	3 Percutaneous	6 Orbital Atherectomy Technology	1 New Technology Group 1

Valid OR   All body part, approach, device/substance/technology, and qualifier values

X   **New Technology**
2   **Cardiovascular System**
R   **Replacement**   Definition: Putting in or on biological or synthetic material that physically takes the place and/or function of all or a portion of a body part

Explanation: The body part may have been taken out or replaced, or may be taken out, physically eradicated, or rendered nonfunctional during the REPLACEMENT procedure. A REMOVAL procedure is coded for taking out the device used in a previous replacement procedure

Body Part Character 4	Approach Character 5	Device/Substance/Technology Character 6	Qualifier Character 7
F Aortic Valve	Ø Open 3 Percutaneous 4 Percutaneous Endoscopic	3 Zooplastic Tissue, Rapid Deployment Technique	2 New Technology Group 2

Valid OR   All body part, approach, device/substance/technology, and qualifier values

X   **New Technology**
H   **Skin, Subcutaneous Tissue, Fascia and Breast**
R   **Replacement**   Definition: Putting in or on biological or synthetic material that physically takes the place and/or function of all or a portion of a body part

Explanation: The body part may have been taken out or replaced, or may be taken out, physically eradicated, or rendered nonfunctional during the REPLACEMENT procedure. A REMOVAL procedure is coded for taking out the device used in a previous replacement procedure

Body Part Character 4	Approach Character 5	Device/Substance/Technology Character 6	Qualifier Character 7
P Skin	X External	L Skin Substitute, Porcine Liver Derived	2 New Technology Group 2

Valid OR   All body part, approach, device/substance/technology, and qualifier values

X   **New Technology**
K   **Muscles, Tendons, Bursae and Ligaments**
Ø   **Introduction**   Definition: Putting in or on a therapeutic, diagnostic, nutritional, physiological, or prophylactic substance except blood or blood products

Explanation: None

Body Part Character 4	Approach Character 5	Device/Substance/Technology Character 6	Qualifier Character 7
2 Muscle	3 Percutaneous	Ø Concentrated Bone Marrow Aspirate	3 New Technology Group 3

X   **New Technology**
N   **Bones**
S   **Reposition**   Definition: Moving to its normal location, or other suitable location, all or a portion of a body part

Explanation: The body part is moved to a new location from an abnormal location, or from a normal location where it is not functioning correctly. The body part may or may not be cut out or off to be moved to the new location.

Body Part Character 4	Approach Character 5	Device/Substance/Technology Character 6	Qualifier Character 7
Ø Lumbar Vertebra 3 Cervical Vertebra 4 Thoracic Vertebra	Ø Open 3 Percutaneous	3 Magnetically Controlled Growth Rod(s)	2 New Technology Group 2

Valid OR   All body part, approach, device/substance/technology, and qualifier values

X   **New Technology**
N   **Bones**
U   **Supplement**   Definition: Putting in or on biological or synthetic material that physically reinforces and/or augments the function of a portion of a body part

Explanation: None

Body Part Character 4	Approach Character 5	Device/Substance/Technology Character 6	Qualifier Character 7
Ø Lumbar Vertebra 4 Thoracic Vertebra	3 Percutaneous	5 Synthetic Substitute, Mechanically Expandable (Paired)	6 New Technology Group 6

X   **New Technology**
R   **Joints**
2   **Monitoring**   Definition: Determining the level of a physiological or physical function repetitively over a period of time

Explanation: None

Body Part Character 4	Approach Character 5	Device/Substance/Technology Character 6	Qualifier Character 7
G Knee Joint, Right H Knee Joint, Left	Ø Open	2 Intraoperative Knee Replacement Sensor	1 New Technology Group 1

Valid OR   All body part, approach, device/substance/technology, and qualifier values

X   **New Technology**
R   **Joints**
G   **Fusion**   Definition: Joining together portions of an articular body part rendering the articular body part immobile
                 Explanation: The body part is joined together by fixation device, bone graft, or other means

Body Part Character 4	Approach Character 5	Device/Substance/Technology Character 6	Qualifier Character 7
Ø Occipital-cervical Joint	Ø Open	9 Interbody Fusion Device, Nanotextured Surface	2 New Technology Group 2
Ø Occipital-cervical Joint	Ø Open	F Interbody Fusion Device, Radiolucent Porous	3 New Technology Group 3
1 Cervical Vertebral Joint	Ø Open	9 Interbody Fusion Device, Nanotextured Surface	2 New Technology Group 2
1 Cervical Vertebral Joint	Ø Open	F Interbody Fusion Device, Radiolucent Porous	3 New Technology Group 3
2 Cervical Vertebral Joints, 2 or more	Ø Open	9 Interbody Fusion Device, Nanotextured Surface	2 New Technology Group 2
2 Cervical Vertebral Joints, 2 or more	Ø Open	F Interbody Fusion Device, Radiolucent Porous	3 New Technology Group 3
4 Cervicothoracic Vertebral Joint	Ø Open	9 Interbody Fusion Device, Nanotextured Surface	2 New Technology Group 2
4 Cervicothoracic Vertebral Joint	Ø Open	F Interbody Fusion Device, Radiolucent Porous	3 New Technology Group 3
6 Thoracic Vertebral Joint	Ø Open	9 Interbody Fusion Device, Nanotextured Surface	2 New Technology Group 2
6 Thoracic Vertebral Joint	Ø Open	F Interbody Fusion Device, Radiolucent Porous	3 New Technology Group 3
7 Thoracic Vertebral Joints, 2 to 7 ⊞	Ø Open	9 Interbody Fusion Device, Nanotextured Surface	2 New Technology Group 2
7 Thoracic Vertebral Joints, 2 to 7 ⊞	Ø Open	F Interbody Fusion Device, Radiolucent Porous	3 New Technology Group 3
8 Thoracic Vertebral Joints, 8 or more	Ø Open	9 Interbody Fusion Device, Nanotextured Surface	2 New Technology Group 2
8 Thoracic Vertebral Joints, 8 or more	Ø Open	F Interbody Fusion Device, Radiolucent Porous	3 New Technology Group 3
A Thoracolumbar Vertebral Joint	Ø Open	9 Interbody Fusion Device, Nanotextured Surface	2 New Technology Group 2
A Thoracolumbar Vertebral Joint	Ø Open	F Interbody Fusion Device, Radiolucent Porous	3 New Technology Group 3
B Lumbar Vertebral Joint	Ø Open	9 Interbody Fusion Device, Nanotextured Surface	2 New Technology Group 2
B Lumbar Vertebral Joint	Ø Open	F Interbody Fusion Device, Radiolucent Porous	3 New Technology Group 3
C Lumbar Vertebral Joints, 2 or more ⊞	Ø Open	9 Interbody Fusion Device, Nanotextured Surface	2 New Technology Group 2
C Lumbar Vertebral Joints, 2 or more ⊞	Ø Open	F Interbody Fusion Device, Radiolucent Porous	3 New Technology Group 3
D Lumbosacral Joint	Ø Open	9 Interbody Fusion Device, Nanotextured Surface	2 New Technology Group 2
D Lumbosacral Joint	Ø Open	F Interbody Fusion Device, Radiolucent Porous	3 New Technology Group 3

Valid OR   All body part, approach, device/substance/technology, and qualifier values
HAC   XRG[Ø,1,2,4,6,7,8,A,B,C,D]Ø92 when reported with SDx K68.11 or
        T81.4Ø–T81.49, T84.6Ø-T84.619, T84.63-T84.7 with 7th character A
HAC   XRG[Ø,1,2,4,6,7,8,A,B,C,D]ØF3 when reported with SDx K68.11 or
        T81.4Ø–T81.49, T84.6Ø-T84.619, T84.63-T84.7 with 7th character A

See Appendix L for Procedure Combinations
⊞   XRG7Ø92
⊞   XRG7ØF3
⊞   XRGCØ92
⊞   XRGCØF3

X   **New Technology**
T   **Urinary System**
2   **Monitoring**   Definition: Determining the level of a physiological or physical function repetitively over a period of time
                 Explanation: None

Body Part Character 4	Approach Character 5	Device/Substance/Technology Character 6	Qualifier Character 7
5 Kidney	X External	E Fluorescent Pyrazine	5 New Technology Group 5

X   **New Technology**
V   **Male Reproductive System**
5   **Destruction**   Definition: Physical eradication of all or a portion of a body part by the direct use of energy, force, or a destructive agent
                 Explanation: None of the body part is physically taken out

Body Part Character 4	Approach Character 5	Device/Substance/Technology Character 6	Qualifier Character 7
Ø Prostate	8 Via Natural or Artificial Opening Endoscopic	A Robotic Waterjet Ablation	4 New Technology Group 4

Valid OR   All body part, approach, device/substance/technology, and qualifier values

---

New Technology

X New Technology
W Anatomical Regions
Ø Introduction   Definition: Putting in or on a therapeutic, diagnostic, nutritional, physiological, or prophylactic substance except blood or blood products
Explanation: None

Body Part Character 4	Approach Character 5	Device/Substance/Technology Character 6	Qualifier Character 7
1 Subcutaneous Tissue	3 Percutaneous	W Caplacizumab	5 New Technology Group 5
3 Peripheral Vein	3 Percutaneous	Ø Brexanolone	6 New Technology Group 6
3 Peripheral Vein	3 Percutaneous	2 Ceftazidime-Avibactam Anti-infective	1 New Technology Group 1
3 Peripheral Vein	3 Percutaneous	2 Nerinitide	6 New Technology Group 6
3 Peripheral Vein	3 Percutaneous	3 Idarucizumab, Dabigatran Reversal Agent	1 New Technology Group 1
3 Peripheral Vein	3 Percutaneous	3 Durvalumab Antineoplastic	6 New Technology Group 6
3 Peripheral Vein	3 Percutaneous	4 Isavuconazole Anti-infective 5 Blinatumomab Antineoplastic Immunotherapy	1 New Technology Group 1
3 Peripheral Vein	3 Percutaneous	6 Lefamulin Anti-infective	6 New Technology Group 6
3 Peripheral Vein	3 Percutaneous	7 Coagulation Factor Xa, Inactivated 9 Defibrotide Sodium Anticoagulant	2 New Technology Group 2
3 Peripheral Vein	3 Percutaneous	9 Ceftolozane/Tazobacatam Anti-infective	6 New Technology Group 6
3 Peripheral Vein	3 Percutaneous	A Bezlotoxumab Monoclonal Antibody	3 New Technology Group 3
3 Peripheral Vein	3 Percutaneous	A Cefiderocol Anti-infective	6 New Technology Group 6
3 Peripheral Vein	3 Percutaneous	B Cytarabine and Daunorubicin Liposome Antineoplastic	3 New Technology Group 3
3 Peripheral Vein	3 Percutaneous	B Omadacycline Anti-infective	6 New Technology Group 6
3 Peripheral Vein	3 Percutaneous	C Engineered Autologous Chimeric Antigen Receptor T-cell Immunotherapy	3 New Technology Group 3
3 Peripheral Vein	3 Percutaneous	C Eculizumab D Atezolizumab Antineoplastic	6 New Technology Group 6
3 Peripheral Vein	3 Percutaneous	F Other New Technology Therapeutic Substance	3 New Technology Group 3
3 Peripheral Vein	3 Percutaneous	G Plazomicin Anti-infective H Synthetic Human Angiotensin II	4 New Technology Group 4
3 Peripheral Vein	3 Percutaneous	K Fosfomycin Anti-infective N Meropenem-vaborbactam Anti-infective Q Tagraxofusp-erzs Antineoplastic S Iobenguane I-131 Antineoplastic U Imipenem-cilastatin-relebactam Anti-infective W Caplacizumab	5 New Technology Group 5
4 Central Vein	3 Percutaneous	Ø Brexanolone	6 New Technology Group 6
4 Central Vein	3 Percutaneous	2 Ceftazidime-Avibactam Anti-infective	1 New Technology Group 1
4 Central Vein	3 Percutaneous	2 Nerinitide	6 New Technology Group 6
4 Central Vein	3 Percutaneous	3 Idarucizumab, Dabigatran Reversal Agent	1 New Technology Group 1
4 Central Vein	3 Percutaneous	3 Durvalumab Antineoplastic	6 New Technology Group 6
4 Central Vein	3 Percutaneous	4 Isavuconazole Anti-infective 5 Blinatumomab Antineoplastic Immunotherapy	1 New Technology Group 1
4 Central Vein	3 Percutaneous	6 Lefamulin Anti-infective	6 New Technology Group 6
4 Central Vein	3 Percutaneous	7 Coagulation Factor Xa, Inactivated 9 Defibrotide Sodium Anticoagulant	2 New Technology Group 2
4 Central Vein	3 Percutaneous	9 Ceftolozane/Tazobacatam Anti-infective	6 New Technology Group 6
4 Central Vein	3 Percutaneous	A Bezlotoxumab Monoclonal Antibody	3 New Technology Group 3
4 Central Vein	3 Percutaneous	A Cefiderocol Anti-infective	6 New Technology Group 6
4 Central Vein	3 Percutaneous	B Cytarabine and Daunorubicin Liposome Antineoplastic	3 New Technology Group 3
4 Central Vein	3 Percutaneous	B Omadacycline Anti-infective	6 New Technology Group 6

DRG Non-OR XWØ33C3

XWØ Continued on next page

XWØ Continued

X New Technology
W Anatomical Regions
Ø Introduction   Definition: Putting in or on a therapeutic, diagnostic, nutritional, physiological, or prophylactic substance except blood or blood products
Explanation: None

Body Part Character 4	Approach Character 5	Device/Substance/Technology Character 6	Qualifier Character 7
4 Central Vein	3 Percutaneous	C Engineered Autologous Chimeric Antigen Receptor T-cell Immunotherapy	3 New Technology Group 3
4 Central Vein	3 Percutaneous	C Eculizumab D Atezolizumab Antineoplastic	6 New Technology Group 6
4 Central Vein	3 Percutaneous	F Other New Technology Therapeutic Substance	3 New Technology Group 3
4 Central Vein	3 Percutaneous	G Plazomicin Anti-infective H Synthetic Human Angiotensin II	4 New Technology Group 4
4 Central Vein	3 Percutaneous	K Fosfomycin Anti-infective N Meropenem-vaborbactam Anti-infective Q Tagraxofusp-erzs Antineoplastic S Iobenguane I-131 Antineoplastic U Imipenem-cilastatin-relebactam Anti-infective W Caplacizumab	5 New Technology Group 5
9 Nose	7 Via Natural or Artificial Opening	M Esketamine Hydrochloride	5 New Technology Group 5
D Mouth and Pharynx	X External	6 Lefamulin Anti-infective	6 New Technology Group 6
D Mouth and Pharynx	X External	8 Uridine Triacetate	2 New Technology Group 2
D Mouth and Pharynx	X External	J Apalutamide Antineoplastic L Erdafitinib Antineoplastic R Venetoclax Antineoplastic T Ruxolitinib V Gilteritinib Antineoplastic	5 New Technology Group 5
G Upper GI H Lower GI	8 Via Natural or Artificial Opening Endoscopic	8 Mineral-based Topical Hemostatic Agent	6 New Technology Group 6
Q Cranial Cavity and Brain	3 Percutaneous	1 Eladocagene exuparvovec	6 New Technology Group 6

DRG Non-OR XWØ43C3

X New Technology
W Anatomical Regions
2 Transfusion   Definition: Putting in blood or blood products
Explanation: None

Body Part Character 4	Approach Character 5	Device/Substance/Technology Character 6	Qualifier Character 7
3 Peripheral Vein 4 Central Vein	3 Percutaneous	4 Brexucabtagene Autoleucel Immunotherapy 7 Lisocabtagene Maraleucel Immunotherapy	6 New Technology Group 6

X New Technology
X Physiological Systems
E Measurement   Definition: Determining the level of a physiological or physical function at a point in time
Explanation: None

Body Part Character 4	Approach Character 5	Device/Substance/Technology Character 6	Qualifier Character 7
5 Circulatory	X External	M Infection, Whole Blood Nucleic Acid-base Microbial Detection	5 New Technology Group 5
5 Circulatory	X External	N Infection, Positive Blood Culture Fluorescence Hybridization for Organism Identification, Concentration and Susceptibility	6 New Technology Group 6
B Respiratory	X External	Q Infection, Lower Respiratory Fluid Nucleic Acid-base Microbial Detection	6 New Technology Group 6

X New Technology
Y Extracorporeal
Ø Introduction   Definition: Putting in or on a therapeutic, diagnostic, nutritional, physiological, or prophylactic substance except blood or blood products
Explanation: None

Body Part Character 4	Approach Character 5	Device/Substance/Technology Character 6	Qualifier Character 7
V Vein Graft	X External	8 Endothelial Damage Inhibitor	3 New Technology Group 3

ICD Limited Coverage   NC Noncovered   ⊞ Combination Member   HAC   Valid OR   Combination Only   DRG Non-OR   New/Revised in GREEN
ICD-10-PCS 2021   815

XWØ–XYØ

Appendixes

Appendix A: Components of the Medical and Surgical Approach Definitions

ICD-10-PCS Value	Definition	Access Location	Method	Type of Instrumentation	Example
Open (Ø)	Cutting through the skin or mucous membrane and any other body layers necessary to expose the site of the procedure	Skin or mucous membrane, any other body layers	Cutting	None	Abdominal hysterectomy
Percutaneous (3)	Entry, by puncture or minor incision, of instrumentation through the skin or mucous membrane and any other body layers necessary to reach the site of the procedure	Skin or mucous membrane, any other body layers	Puncture or minor incision	Without visualization	Needle biopsy of liver, Liposuction
Percutaneous endoscopic (4)	Entry, by puncture or minor incision, of instrumentation through the skin or mucous membrane and any other body layers necessary to reach and visualize the site of the procedure	Skin or mucous membrane, any other body layers	Puncture or minor incision	With visualization	Arthroscopy, Laparoscopic cholecystectomy
Via natural or artificial opening (7)	Entry of instrumentation through a natural or artificial external opening to reach the site of the procedure	Natural or artificial external opening	Direct entry	Without visualization	Endotracheal tube insertion, Foley catheter placement
Via natural or artificial opening endoscopic (8)	Entry of instrumentation through a natural or artificial external opening to reach and visualize the site of the procedure	Natural or artificial external opening	Direct entry	With visualization	Sigmoidoscopy, EGD, ERCP
Via natural or artificial opening with percutaneous endoscopic assistance (F)	Entry of instrumentation through a natural or artificial external opening and entry, by puncture or minor incision, of instrumentation through the skin or mucous membrane and any other body layers necessary to aid in the performance of the procedure	Skin or mucous membrane, any other body layers	Direct entry with puncture or minor incision for instrumentation only	With visualization	Laparoscopic-assisted vaginal hysterectomy
External (X)	Procedures performed directly on the skin or mucous membrane and procedures performed indirectly by the application of external force through the skin or mucous membrane	Skin or mucous membrane	Direct or indirect application	None	Closed fracture reduction, Resection of tonsils

Appendix A: Components of the Medical and Surgical Approach Definitions

Open (Ø)

Abdominal wall

Retractors

Percutaneous (3)

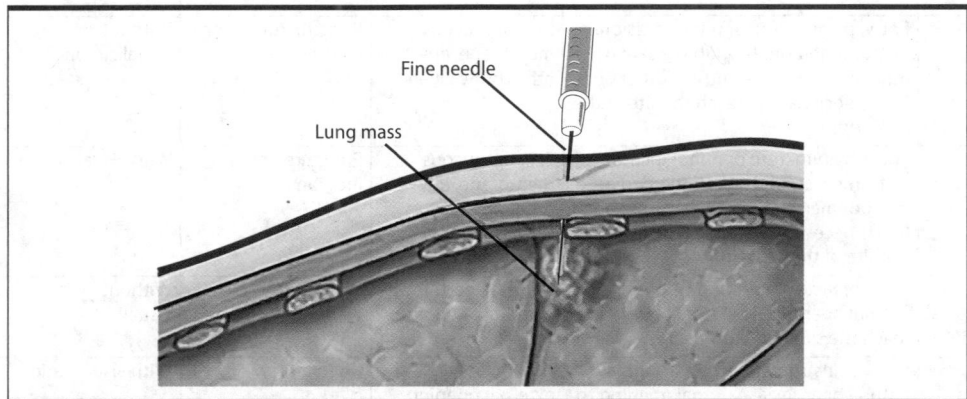

Fine needle

Lung mass

Percutaneous Endoscopic (4)

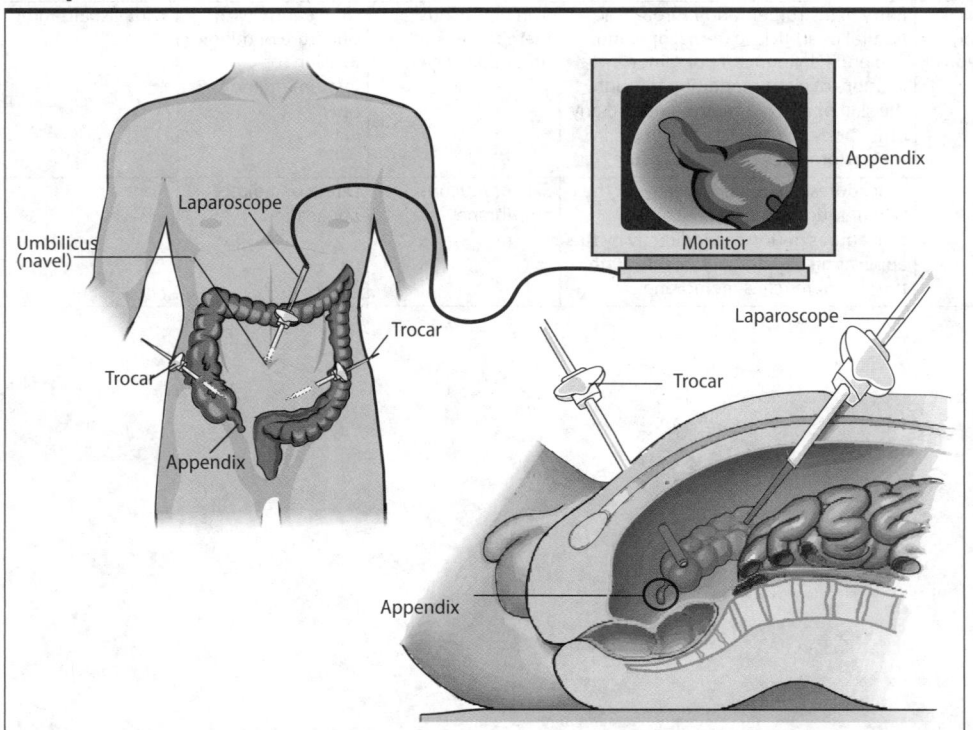

Laparoscope

Umbilicus (navel)

Trocar

Appendix

Trocar

Appendix

Monitor

Laparoscope

Trocar

Appendix

Via Natural or Artificial Opening (7)

Via Natural or Artificial Opening, Endoscopic (8)

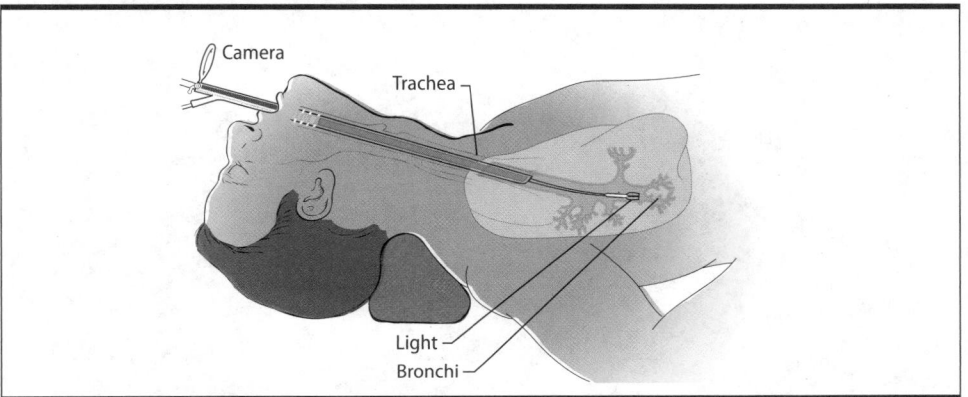

Via Natural or Artificial Opening with Percutaneous Endoscopic Assistance (F)

External (X)

The character 3 value in the Medical and Surgical section (Ø) and the Medical and Surgical-related sections (1-9) represents the root operation. This resource provides each root operation (character 3) value, found in sections Ø-9, as well as their associated definition, explanation, and examples, where applicable. The Ancillary sections (B-H) do not include root operations; instead the character 3 value represents the type of procedure performed with additional detail provided by the character 4 or 5 value, when applicable. For the character 3, character 4, and character 5 values used in the Ancillary sections of B-H, along with their definitions, see appendix J.

Ø	Medical and Surgical		
ICD-10-PCS Value			**Definition**
Ø	Alteration	Definition:	Modifying the anatomic structure of a body part without affecting the function of the body part
		Explanation:	Principal purpose is to improve appearance
		Examples:	Face lift, breast augmentation
1	Bypass	Definition:	Altering the route of passage of the contents of a tubular body part
		Explanation:	Rerouting contents of a body part to a downstream area of the normal route, to a similar route and body part, or to an abnormal route and dissimilar body part. Includes one or more anastomoses, with or without the use of a device.
		Examples:	Coronary artery bypass, colostomy formation
2	Change	Definition:	Taking out or off a device from a body part and putting back an identical or similar device in or on the same body part without cutting or puncturing the skin or a mucous membrane
		Explanation:	All CHANGE procedures are coded using the approach EXTERNAL
		Example:	Urinary catheter change, gastrostomy tube change
3	Control	Definition:	Stopping, or attempting to stop, postprocedural or other acute bleeding
		Explanation:	None
		Examples:	Control of post-prostatectomy hemorrhage, control of intracranial subdural hemorrhage, control of bleeding duodenal ulcer, control of retroperitoneal hemorrhage
4	Creation	Definition:	Putting in or on biological or synthetic material to form a new body part that to the extent possible replicates the anatomic structure or function of an absent body part
		Explanation:	Used for gender reassignment surgery and corrective procedures in individuals with congenital anomalies
		Examples:	Creation of vagina in a male, creation of right and left atrioventricular valve from common atrioventricular valve
5	Destruction	Definition:	Physical eradication of all or a portion of a body part by the direct use of energy, force, or a destructive agent
		Explanation:	None of the body part is physically taken out
		Examples:	Fulguration of rectal polyp, cautery of skin lesion
6	Detachment	Definition:	Cutting off all or a portion of the upper or lower extremities
		Explanation:	The body part value is the site of the detachment, with a qualifier if applicable to further specify the level where the extremity was detached
		Examples:	Below knee amputation, disarticulation of shoulder
7	Dilation	Definition:	Expanding an orifice or the lumen of a tubular body part
		Explanation:	The orifice can be a natural orifice or an artificially created orifice. Accomplished by stretching a tubular body part using intraluminal pressure or by cutting part of the orifice or wall of the tubular body part.
		Examples:	Percutaneous transluminal angioplasty, internal urethrotomy
8	Division	Definition:	Cutting into a body part, without draining fluids and/or gases from the body part, in order to separate or transect a body part
		Explanation:	All or a portion of the body part is separated into two or more portions
		Examples:	Spinal cordotomy, osteotomy
9	Drainage	Definition:	Taking or letting out fluids and/or gases from a body part
		Explanation:	The qualifier DIAGNOSTIC is used to identify drainage procedures that are biopsies
		Examples:	Thoracentesis, incision and drainage
B	Excision	Definition:	Cutting out or off, without replacement, a portion of a body part
		Explanation:	The qualifier DIAGNOSTIC is used to identify excision procedures that are biopsies
		Examples:	Partial nephrectomy, liver biopsy

Continued on next page

Ø	**Medical and Surgical**			*Continued from previous page*

ICD-10-PCS Value			Definition
C	Extirpation	Definition:	Taking or cutting out solid matter from a body part
		Explanation:	The solid matter may be an abnormal byproduct of a biological function or a foreign body; it may be imbedded in a body part or in the lumen of a tubular body part. The solid matter may or may not have been previously broken into pieces.
		Examples:	Thrombectomy, choledocholithotomy
D	Extraction	Definition:	Pulling or stripping out or off all or a portion of a body part by the use of force
		Explanation:	The qualifier DIAGNOSTIC is used to identify extractions that are biopsies
		Examples:	Dilation and curettage, vein stripping
F	Fragmentation	Definition:	Breaking solid matter in a body part into pieces
		Explanation:	Physical force (e.g., manual, ultrasonic) applied directly or indirectly is used to break the solid matter into pieces. The solid matter may be an abnormal byproduct of a biological function or a foreign body. The pieces of solid matter are not taken out.
		Examples:	Extracorporeal shockwave lithotripsy, transurethral lithotripsy
G	Fusion	Definition:	Joining together portions of an articular body part rendering the articular body part immobile
		Explanation:	The body part is joined together by fixation device, bone graft, or other means
		Examples:	Spinal fusion, ankle arthrodesis
H	Insertion	Definition:	Putting in a nonbiological appliance that monitors, assists, performs, or prevents a physiological function but does not physically take the place of a body part
		Explanation:	None
		Examples:	Insertion of radioactive implant, insertion of central venous catheter
J	Inspection	Definition:	Visually and/or manually exploring a body part
		Explanation:	Visual exploration may be performed with or without optical instrumentation. Manual exploration may be performed directly or through intervening body layers.
		Examples:	Diagnostic arthroscopy, exploratory laparotomy
K	Map	Definition:	Locating the route of passage of electrical impulses and/or locating functional areas in a body part
		Explanation:	Applicable only to the cardiac conduction mechanism and the central nervous system
		Examples:	Cardiac mapping, cortical mapping
L	Occlusion	Definition:	Completely closing an orifice or lumen of a tubular body part
		Explanation:	The orifice can be a natural orifice or an artificially created orifice
		Examples:	Fallopian tube ligation, ligation of inferior vena cava
M	Reattachment	Definition:	Putting back in or on all or a portion of a separated body part to its normal location or other suitable location
		Explanation:	Vascular circulation and nervous pathways may or may not be reestablished
		Examples:	Reattachment of hand, reattachment of avulsed kidney
N	Release	Definition:	Freeing a body part from an abnormal physical constraint by cutting or by use of force
		Explanation:	Some of the restraining tissue may be taken out but none of the body part is taken out
		Examples:	Adhesiolysis, carpal tunnel release
P	Removal	Definition:	Taking out or off a device from a body part
		Explanation:	If a device is taken out and a similar device put in without cutting or puncturing the skin or mucous membrane, the procedure is coded to the root operation CHANGE. Otherwise, the procedure for taking out a device is coded to the root operation REMOVAL.
		Examples:	Drainage tube removal, cardiac pacemaker removal
Q	Repair	Definition:	Restoring, to the extent possible, a body part to its normal anatomic structure and function
		Explanation:	Used only when the method to accomplish the repair is not one of the other root operations
		Examples:	Colostomy takedown, suture of laceration
R	Replacement	Definition:	Putting in or on biological or synthetic material that physically takes the place and/or function of all or a portion of a body part
		Explanation:	The body part may have been taken out or replaced, or may be taken out, physically eradicated, or rendered nonfunctional during the REPLACEMENT procedure. A REMOVAL procedure is coded for taking out the device used in a previous replacement procedure.
		Examples:	Total hip replacement, bone graft, free skin graft

Continued on next page

Ø   Medical and Surgical

Continued from previous page

ICD-10-PCS Value		Definition
S	Reposition	**Definition:** Moving to its normal location, or other suitable location, all or a portion of a body part
		Explanation: The body part is moved to a new location from an abnormal location, or from a normal location where it is not functioning correctly. The body part may or may not be cut out or off to be moved to the new location.
		Examples: Reposition of undescended testicle, fracture reduction
T	Resection	**Definition:** Cutting out or off, without replacement, all of a body part
		Explanation: None
		Examples: Total nephrectomy, total lobectomy of lung
V	Restriction	**Definition:** Partially closing an orifice or the lumen of a tubular body part
		Explanation: The orifice can be a natural orifice or an artificially created orifice
		Examples: Esophagogastric fundoplication, cervical cerclage
W	Revision	**Definition:** Correcting, to the extent possible, a portion of a malfunctioning device or the position of a displaced device
		Explanation: Revision can include correcting a malfunctioning or displaced device by taking out or putting in components of the device such as a screw or pin
		Examples: Adjustment of position of pacemaker lead, recementing of hip prosthesis
U	Supplement	**Definition:** Putting in or on biological or synthetic material that physically reinforces and/or augments the function of a portion of a body part
		Explanation: The biological material is non-living, or is living and from the same individual. The body part may have been previously replaced, and the SUPPLEMENT procedure is performed to physically reinforce and/or augment the function of the replaced body part.
		Examples: Herniorrhaphy using mesh, mitral valve ring annuloplasty, put a new acetabular liner in a previous hip replacement
X	Transfer	**Definition:** Moving, without taking out, all or a portion of a body part to another location to take over the function of all or a portion of a body part
		Explanation: The body part transferred remains connected to its vascular and nervous supply
		Examples: Tendon transfer, skin pedicle flap transfer
Y	Transplantation	**Definition:** Putting in or on all or a portion of a living body part taken from another individual or animal to physically take the place and/or function of all or a portion of a similar body part
		Explanation: The native body part may or may not be taken out, and the transplanted body part may take over all or a portion of its function
		Examples: Kidney transplant, heart transplant

Root Operation Definitions for Other Sections

1   Obstetrics

ICD-10-PCS Value		Definition
2	Change	**Definition:** Taking out or off a device from a body part and putting back an identical or similar device in or on the same body part without cutting or puncturing the skin or a mucous membrane
		Explanation: None
		Examples: Replacement of fetal scalp electrode
9	Drainage	**Definition:** Taking or letting out fluids and/or gases from a body part
		Explanation: None
		Examples: Biopsy of amniotic fluid
A	Abortion	**Definition:** Artificially terminating a pregnancy
		Explanation: None
		Examples: Transvaginal abortion using vacuum aspiration technique
D	Extraction	**Definition:** Pulling or stripping out or off all or a portion of a body part by the use of force
		Explanation: None
		Examples: Low-transverse C-section
E	Delivery	**Definition:** Assisting the passage of the products of conception from the genital canal
		Explanation: None
		Examples: Manually-assisted delivery

Continued on next page

1   Obstetrics

Continued from previous page

ICD-10-PCS Value			Definition
H	Insertion	Definition:	Putting in a nonbiological appliance that monitors, assists, performs, or prevents a physiological function but does not physically take the place of a body part
		Explanation:	None
		Examples:	Placement of fetal scalp electrode
J	Inspection	Definition:	Visually and/or manually exploring a body part
		Explanation:	Visual exploration may be performed with or without optical instrumentation. Manual exploration may be performed directly or through intervening body layers.
		Examples:	Bimanual pregnancy exam
P	Removal	Definition:	Taking out or off a device from a body part, region or orifice
		Explanation:	If a device is taken out and a similar device put in without cutting or puncturing the skin or mucous membrane, the procedure is coded to the root operation CHANGE. Otherwise, the procedure for taking out a device is coded to the root operation REMOVAL.
		Examples:	Removal of fetal monitoring electrode
Q	Repair	Definition:	Restoring, to the extent possible, a body part to its normal anatomic structure and function
		Explanation:	Used only when the method to accomplish the repair is not one of the other root operations
		Examples:	In utero repair of congenital diaphragmatic hernia
S	Reposition	Definition:	Moving to its normal location, or other suitable location, all or a portion of a body part
		Explanation:	The body part is moved to a new location from an abnormal location, or from a normal location where it is not functioning correctly. The body part may or may not be cut out or off to be moved to the new location.
		Examples:	External version of fetus
T	Resection	Definition:	Cutting out or off, without replacement, all of a body part
		Explanation:	None
		Examples:	Total excision of tubal pregnancy
Y	Transplantation	Definition:	Putting in or on all or a portion of a living body part taken from another individual or animal to physically take the place and/or function of all or a portion of a similar body part
		Explanation:	The native body part may or may not be taken out, and the transplanted body part may take over all or a portion of its function
		Examples:	In utero fetal kidney transplant

2   Placement

ICD-10-PCS Value			Definition
Ø	Change	Definition:	Taking out or off a device from a body part and putting back an identical or similar device in or on the same body part without cutting or puncturing the skin or a mucous membrane
		Examples:	Change of vaginal packing
1	Compression	Definition:	Putting pressure on a body region
		Examples:	Placement of pressure dressing on abdominal wall
2	Dressing	Definition:	Putting material on a body region for protection
		Examples:	Application of sterile dressing to head wound
3	Immobilization	Definition:	Limiting or preventing motion of a body region
		Examples:	Placement of splint on left finger
4	Packing	Definition:	Putting material in a body region or orifice
		Examples:	Placement of nasal packing
5	Removal	Definition:	Taking out or off a device from a body part
		Examples:	Removal of stereotactic head frame
6	Traction	Definition:	Exerting a pulling force on a body region in a distal direction
		Examples:	Lumbar traction using motorized split-traction table

3   Administration

ICD-10-PCS Value		Definition	
Ø	Introduction	Definition:	Putting in or on a therapeutic, diagnostic, nutritional, physiological, or prophylactic substance except blood or blood products
		Examples:	Nerve block injection to median nerve
1	Irrigation	Definition:	Putting in or on a cleansing substance
		Examples:	Flushing of eye
2	Transfusion	Definition:	Putting in blood or blood products
		Examples:	Transfusion of cell saver red cells into central venous line

4   Measurement and Monitoring

ICD-10-PCS Value		Definition	
Ø	Measurement	Definition:	Determining the level of a physiological or physical function at a point in time
		Examples:	External electrocardiogram(EKG), single reading
1	Monitoring	Definition:	Determining the level of a physiological or physical function repetitively over a period of time
		Examples:	Urinary pressure monitoring

5   Extracorporeal or Systemic Assistance and Performance

ICD-10-PCS Value		Definition	
Ø	Assistance	Definition:	Taking over a portion of a physiological function by extracorporeal means
		Examples:	Hyperbaric oxygenation of wound
1	Performance	Definition:	Completely taking over a physiological function by extracorporeal means
		Examples:	Cardiopulmonary bypass in conjunction with CABG
2	Restoration	Definition:	Returning, or attempting to return, a physiological function to its original state by extracorporeal means
		Examples:	Attempted cardiac defibrillation, unsuccessful

6   Extracorporeal or Systemic Therapies

ICD-10-PCS Value		Definition	
Ø	Atmospheric Control	Definition:	Extracorporeal control of atmospheric pressure and composition
		Examples:	Antigen-free air conditioning, series treatment
1	Decompression	Definition:	Extracorporeal elimination of undissolved gas from body fluids
		Examples:	Hyperbaric decompression treatment, single
2	Electromagnetic Therapy	Definition:	Extracorporeal treatment by electromagnetic rays
		Examples:	TMS (transcranial magnetic stimulation), series treatment
3	Hyperthermia	Definition:	Extracorporeal raising of body temperature
		Examples:	None
4	Hypothermia	Definition:	Extracorporeal lowering of body temperature
		Examples:	Whole body hypothermia treatment for temperature imbalances, series
5	Pheresis	Definition:	Extracorporeal separation of blood products
		Examples:	Therapeutic leukopheresis, single treatment
6	Phototherapy	Definition:	Extracorporeal treatment by light rays
		Examples:	Phototherapy of circulatory system, series treatment
7	Ultrasound Therapy	Definition:	Extracorporeal treatment by ultrasound
		Examples:	Therapeutic ultrasound of peripheral vessels, single treatment
8	Ultraviolet Light Therapy	Definition:	Extracorporeal treatment by ultraviolet light
		Examples:	Ultraviolet light phototherapy, series treatment
9	Shock Wave Therapy	Definition:	Extracorporeal treatment by shock waves
		Examples:	Shockwave therapy of plantar fascia, single treatment
B	Perfusion	Definition:	Extracorporeal treatment by diffusion of therapeutic fluid
		Examples:	Perfusion of donor liver while preparing transplant patient

7 Osteopathic

ICD-10-PCS Value			Definition
Ø	Treatment	Definition:	Manual treatment to eliminate or alleviate somatic dysfunction and related disorders
		Examples:	Fascial release of abdomen, osteopathic treatment

8 Other Procedures

ICD-10-PCS Value			Definition
Ø	Other Procedures	Definition:	Methodologies which attempt to remediate or cure a disorder or disease
		Examples:	Acupuncture, yoga therapy

9 Chiropractic

ICD-10-PCS Value			Definition
B	Manipulation	Definition:	Manual procedure that involves a directed thrust to move a joint past the physiological range of motion, without exceeding the anatomical limit
		Examples:	Chiropractic treatment of cervical spine, short lever specific contact

Appendix C: Comparison of Medical and Surgical Root Operations

Note: the character associated with each operation appears in parentheses after its title.

Procedures That Take Out Some or All of a Body Part

Root Operation	Objective of Procedure	Site of Procedure	Example
Destruction (5)	Eradicating without taking out or replacement	Some/all of a body part	Fulguration of endometrium
Detachment (6)	Cutting out/off without replacement	Extremity only, any level	Amputation above elbow
Excision (B)	Cutting out/off without replacement	Some of a body part	Breast lumpectomy
Extraction (D)	Pulling out or off without replacement	Some/all of a body part	Suction D&C
Resection (T)	Cutting out/off without replacement	All of a body part	Total mastectomy

Procedures That Put in/Put Back or Move Some/All of a Body Part

Root Operation	Objective of Procedure	Site of Procedure	Example
Reattachment (M)	Putting back a detached body part	Some/all of a body part	Reattach finger
Reposition (S)	Moving a body part to normal or other suitable location	Some/all of a body part	Move undescended testicle
Transfer (X)	Moving a body part to function for a similar body part	Some/all of a body part	Skin pedicle transfer flap
Transplantation (Y)	Putting in a living body part from a person/animal	Some/all of a body part	Kidney transplant

Procedures That Take Out or Eliminate Solid Matter, Fluids, or Gases From a Body Part

Root Operation	Objective of Procedure	Site of Procedure	Example
Drainage (9)	Taking or letting out	Fluids and/or gases from a body part	Incision and drainage
Extirpation (C)	Taking or cutting out	Solid matter in a body part	Thrombectomy
Fragmentation (F)	Breaking into pieces	Solid matter within a body part	Lithotripsy

Procedures That Involve Only Examination of Body Parts and Regions

Root Operation	Objective of Procedure	Site of Procedure	Example
Inspection (J)	Visual/manual exploration	Some/all of a body part	Diagnostic cystoscopy Exploratory laparoscopy
Map (K)	Locating electrical impulse route/functional areas	Brain/cardiac conduction mechanism	Cardiac mapping

Procedures That Alter the Diameter/Route of a Tubular Body Part

Root Operation	Objective of Procedure	Site of Procedure	Example
Bypass (1)	Altering route of passage of contents	Tubular body part	Coronary artery bypass graft (CABG)
Dilation (7)	Expanding natural or artificially created orifice/lumen	Tubular body part	Percutaneous transluminal coronary angioplasty (PTCA)
Occlusion (L)	Completely closing natural or artificially created orifice/lumen	Tubular body part	Fallopian tube ligation
Restriction (V)	Partially closing natural or artificially created orifice/lumen	Tubular body part	Gastroesophageal fundoplication

Procedures That Always Involve Devices

Root Operation		Objective of Procedure	Site of Procedure	Example
Change (2)	DVC	Exchanging device w/out cutting/puncturing	In/on a body part	Gastrostomy tube change
Insertion (H)	DVC	Putting in nonbiological device	In/on a body part	Central line insertion
Removal (P)	DVC	Taking out device	In/on a body part	Central line removal
Replacement (R)	DVC	Putting in device that replaces a body part	Some/all of a body part	Total hip replacement
Revision (W)	DVC	Correcting a malfunctioning/displaced device	In/on a body part	Revision of pacemaker
Supplement (U)	DVC	Putting in device that reinforces or augments a body part	In/on a body part	Abdominal wall herniorrhaphy using mesh

DVC = Device involved in root operation

Procedures Involving Cutting or Separation Only

Root Operation	Objective of Procedure	Site of Procedure	Example
Division (8)	Cutting into/separating	A body part	Neurotomy
Release (N)	Freeing a body part from constraint	Around a body part	Adhesiolysis

Procedures That Define Other Repairs

Root Operation	Objective of Procedure	Site of Procedure	Example
Control (3)	Stopping/attempting to stop postprocedural or other acute bleeding	Anatomical region or nasal mucosa/soft tissue	Post-prostatectomy bleeding control, control subdural hemorrhage, bleeding ulcer, retroperitoneal hemorrhage
Repair (Q)	Restoring body part to its normal structure/function	Some/all of a body part	Suture laceration

Procedures That Define Other Objectives

Root Operation	Objective of Procedure	Site of Procedure	Example
Alteration (Ø)	Modifying body part for cosmetic purposes without affecting function	Some/all of a body part	Face lift
Creation (4)	Using biological or synthetic material to form a new body part that replicates the anatomic structure or function of a missing body part	Perineum, valve	Sex change/artificial vagina/penis, atrioventricular valve creation
Fusion (G)	Unification or immobilization	Joint or articular body part	Spinal fusion

Appendix D: Body Part Key

Term	ICD-10-PCS Value
Abdominal aortic plexus	Abdominal Sympathetic Nerve
Abdominal esophagus	Esophagus, Lower
Abductor hallucis muscle	Foot Muscle, Right
	Foot Muscle, Left
Accessory cephalic vein	Cephalic Vein, Right
	Cephalic Vein, Left
Accessory obturator nerve	Lumbar Plexus
Accessory phrenic nerve	Phrenic nerve
Accessory spleen	Spleen
Acetabulofemoral joint	Hip Joint, Right
	Hip Joint, Left
Achilles tendon	Lower Leg Tendon, Right
	Lower Leg Tendon, Left
Acromioclavicular ligament	Shoulder Bursa and Ligament, Right
	Shoulder Bursa and Ligament, Left
Acromion (process)	Scapula, Right
	Scapula, Left
Adductor brevis muscle	Upper Leg Muscle, Right
	Upper Leg Muscle, Left
Adductor hallucis muscle	Foot Muscle, Right
	Foot Muscle, Left
Adductor longus muscle	Upper Leg Muscle, Right
	Upper Leg Muscle, Left
Adductor magnus muscle	Upper Leg Muscle, Right
	Upper Leg Muscle, Left
Adenohypophysis	Pituitary Gland
Alar ligament of axis	Head and Neck Bursa and Ligament
Alveolar process of mandible	Mandible, Right
	Mandible, Left
Alveolar process of maxilla	Maxilla
Anal orifice	Anus
Anatomical snuffbox	Lower Arm and Wrist Muscle, Right
	Lower Arm and Wrist Muscle, Left
Angular artery	Face Artery
Angular vein	Face Vein, Right
	Face Vein, Left
Annular ligament	Elbow Bursa and Ligament, Right
	Elbow Bursa and Ligament, Left
Anorectal junction	Rectum
Ansa cervicalis	Cervical Plexus
Antebrachial fascia	Subcutaneous Tissue and Fascia, Right Lower Arm
	Subcutaneous Tissue and Fascia, Left Lower Arm
Anterior (pectoral) lymph node	Lymphatic, Right Axillary
	Lymphatic, Left Axillary
Anterior cerebral artery	Intracranial Artery
Anterior cerebral vein	Intracranial Vein
Anterior choroidal artery	Intracranial Artery
Anterior circumflex humeral artery	Axillary Artery, Right
	Axillary Artery, Left
Anterior communicating artery	Intracranial Artery

Term	ICD-10-PCS Value
Anterior cruciate ligament (ACL)	Knee Bursa and Ligament, Right
	Knee Bursa and Ligament, Left
Anterior crural nerve	Femoral Nerve
Anterior facial vein	Face Vein, Right
	Face Vein, Left
Anterior intercostal artery	Internal Mammary Artery, Right
	Internal Mammary Artery, Left
Anterior interosseous nerve	Median Nerve
Anterior lateral malleolar artery	Anterior Tibial Artery, Right
	Anterior Tibial Artery, Left
Anterior lingual gland	Minor Salivary Gland
Anterior medial malleolar artery	Anterior Tibial Artery, Right
	Anterior Tibial Artery, Left
Anterior spinal artery	Vertebral Artery, Right
	Vertebral Artery, Left
Anterior tibial recurrent artery	Anterior Tibial Artery, Right
	Anterior Tibial Artery, Left
Anterior ulnar recurrent artery	Ulnar Artery, Right
	Ulnar Artery, Left
Anterior vagal trunk	Vagus Nerve
Anterior vertebral muscle	Neck Muscle, Right
	Neck Muscle, Left
Antihelix	External Ear, Right
	External Ear, Left
	External Ear, Bilateral
Antitragus	External Ear, Right
	External Ear, Left
	External Ear, Bilateral
Antrum of Highmore	Maxillary Sinus, Right
	Maxillary Sinus, Left
Aortic annulus	Aortic Valve
Aortic arch	Thoracic Aorta, Ascending/Arch
Aortic intercostal artery	Upper Artery
Apical (subclavicular) lymph node	Lymphatic, Right Axillary
	Lymphatic, Left Axillary
Apneustic center	Pons
Aqueduct of Sylvius	Cerebral Ventricle
Aqueous humour	Anterior Chamber, Right
	Anterior Chamber, Left
Arachnoid mater, intracranial	Cerebral Meninges
Arachnoid mater, spinal	Spinal Meninges
Arcuate artery	Foot Artery, Right
	Foot Artery, Left
Areola	Nipple, Right
	Nipple, Left
Arterial canal (duct)	Pulmonary Artery, Left
Aryepiglottic fold	Larynx
Arytenoid cartilage	Larynx
Arytenoid muscle	Neck Muscle, Right
	Neck Muscle, Left
Ascending aorta	Thoracic Aorta, Ascending/Arch
Ascending palatine artery	Face Artery

Appendix D: Body Part Key

Term	ICD-10-PCS Value
Ascending pharyngeal artery	External Carotid Artery, Right
	External Carotid Artery, Left
Atlantoaxial joint	Cervical Vertebral Joint
Atrioventricular node	Conduction Mechanism
Atrium dextrum cordis	Atrium, Right
Atrium pulmonale	Atrium, Left
Auditory tube	Eustachian Tube, Right
	Eustachian Tube, Left
Auerbach's (myenteric)plexus	Abdominal Sympathetic Nerve
Auricle	External Ear, Right
	External Ear, Left
	External Ear, Bilateral
Auricularis muscle	Head Muscle
Axillary fascia	Subcutaneous Tissue and Fascia, Right Upper Arm
	Subcutaneous Tissue and Fascia, Left Upper Arm
Axillary nerve	Brachial Plexus
Bartholin's (greater vestibular) gland	Vestibular Gland
Basal (internal) cerebral vein	Intracranial Vein
Basal nuclei	Basal Ganglia
Base of tongue	Pharynx
Basilar artery	Intracranial Artery
Basis pontis	Pons
Biceps brachii muscle	Upper Arm Muscle, Right
	Upper Arm Muscle, Left
Biceps femoris muscle	Upper Leg Muscle, Right
	Upper Leg Muscle, Left
Bicipital aponeurosis	Subcutaneous Tissue and Fascia, Right Lower Arm
	Subcutaneous Tissue and Fascia, Left Lower Arm
Bicuspid valve	Mitral Valve
Body of femur	Femoral Shaft, Right
	Femoral Shaft, Left
Body of fibula	Fibula, Right
	Fibula, Left
Bony labyrinth	Inner Ear, Right
	Inner Ear, Left
Bony orbit	Orbit, Right
	Orbit, Left
Bony vestibule	Inner Ear, Right
	Inner Ear, Left
Botallo's duct	Pulmonary Artery, Left
Brachial (lateral) lymph node	Lymphatic, Right Axillary
	Lymphatic, Left Axillary
Brachialis muscle	Upper Arm Muscle, Right
	Upper Arm Muscle, Left
Brachiocephalic artery	Innominate Artery
Brachiocephalic trunk	Innominate Artery
Brachiocephalic vein	Innominate Vein, Right
	Innominate Vein, Left
Brachioradialis muscle	Lower Arm and Wrist Muscle, Right
	Lower Arm and Wrist Muscle, Left

Term	ICD-10-PCS Value
Breast procedures, skin only	Skin, Chest
Broad ligament	Uterine Supporting Structure
Bronchial artery	Upper Artery
Bronchus intermedius	Main Bronchus, Right
Buccal gland	Buccal Mucosa
Buccinator lymph node	Lymphatic, Head
Buccinator muscle	Facial Muscle
Bulbospongiosus muscle	Perineum Muscle
Bulbourethral (Cowper's) gland	Urethra
Bundle of His	Conduction Mechanism
Bundle of Kent	Conduction Mechanism
Calcaneocuboid joint	Tarsal Joint, Right
	Tarsal Joint, Left
Calcaneocuboid ligament	Foot Bursa and Ligament, Right
	Foot Bursa and Ligament, Left
Calcaneofibular ligament	Ankle Bursa and Ligament, Right
	Ankle Bursa and Ligament, Left
Calcaneus	Tarsal, Right
	Tarsal, Left
Capitate bone	Carpal, Right
	Carpal, Left
Cardia	Esophagogastric Junction
Cardiac plexus	Thoracic Sympathetic Nerve
Cardioesophageal junction	Esophagogastric Junction
Caroticotympanic artery	Internal Carotid Artery, Right
	Internal Carotid Artery, Left
Carotid glomus	Carotid Body, Right
	Carotid Body, Left
	Carotid Bodies, Bilateral
Carotid sinus	Internal Carotid Artery, Right
	Internal Carotid Artery, Left
Carotid sinus nerve	Glossopharyngeal Nerve
Carpometacarpal ligament	Hand Bursa and Ligament, Right
	Hand Bursa and Ligament, Left
Cauda equina	Lumbar Spinal Cord
Cavernous plexus	Head and Neck Sympathetic Nerve
Celiac ganglion	Abdominal Sympathetic Nerve
Celiac (solar) plexus	Abdominal Sympathetic Nerve
Celiac lymph node	Lymphatic, Aortic
Celiac trunk	Celiac Artery
Central axillary lymph node	Lymphatic, Right Axillary
	Lymphatic, Left Axillary
Cerebral aqueduct (Sylvius)	Cerebral Ventricle
Cerebrum	Brain
Cervical esophagus	Esophagus, Upper
Cervical facet joint	Cervical Vertebral Joint
	Cervical Vertebral Joints, 2 or more
Cervical ganglion	Head and Neck Sympathetic Nerve
Cervical interspinous ligament	Head and Neck Bursa and Ligament
Cervical intertransverse ligament	Head and Neck Bursa and Ligament
Cervical ligamentum flavum	Head and Neck Bursa and Ligament

Term	ICD-10-PCS Value
Cervical lymph node	Lymphatic, Right Neck
	Lymphatic, Left Neck
Cervicothoracic facet joint	Cervicothoracic Vertebral Joint
Choana	Nasopharynx
Chondroglossus muscle	Tongue, Palate, Pharynx Muscle
Chorda tympani	Facial Nerve
Choroid plexus	Cerebral Ventricle
Ciliary body	Eye, Right
	Eye, Left
Ciliary ganglion	Head and Neck Sympathetic Nerve
Circle of Willis	Intracranial Artery
Circumflex iliac artery	Femoral Artery, Right
	Femoral Artery, Left
Claustrum	Basal Ganglia
Coccygeal body	Coccygeal Glomus
Coccygeus muscle	Trunk Muscle, Right
	Trunk Muscle, Left
Cochlea	Inner Ear, Right
	Inner Ear, Left
Cochlear nerve	Acoustic Nerve
Columella	Nasal Mucosa and Soft Tissue
Common digital vein	Foot Vein, Right
	Foot Vein, Left
Common facial vein	Face Vein, Right
	Face Vein, Left
Common fibular nerve	Peroneal Nerve
Common hepatic artery	Hepatic Artery
Common iliac (subaortic) lymph node	Lymphatic, Pelvis
Common interosseous artery	Ulnar Artery, Right
	Ulnar Artery, Left
Common peroneal nerve	Peroneal Nerve
Condyloid process	Mandible, Right
	Mandible, Left
Conus arteriosus	Ventricle, Right
Conus medullaris	Lumbar Spinal Cord
Coracoacromial ligament	Shoulder Bursa and Ligament, Right
	Shoulder Bursa and Ligament, Left
Coracobrachialis muscle	Upper Arm Muscle, Right
	Upper Arm Muscle, Left
Coracoclavicular ligament	Shoulder Bursa and Ligament, Right
	Shoulder Bursa and Ligament, Left
Coracohumeral ligament	Shoulder Bursa and Ligament, Right
	Shoulder Bursa and Ligament, Left
Coracoid process	Scapula, Right
	Scapula, Left
Corniculate cartilage	Larynx
Corpus callosum	Brain
Corpus cavernosum	Penis
Corpus spongiosum	Penis
Corpus striatum	Basal Ganglia
Corrugator supercilii muscle	Facial Muscle
Costocervical trunk	Subclavian Artery, Right
	Subclavian Artery, Left

Term	ICD-10-PCS Value
Costoclavicular ligament	Shoulder Bursa and Ligament, Right
	Shoulder Bursa and Ligament, Left
Costotransverse joint	Thoracic Vertebral Joint
Costotransverse ligament	Rib(s) Bursa and Ligament
Costovertebral joint	Thoracic Vertebral Joint
Costoxiphoid ligament	Sternum Bursa and Ligament
Cowper's (bulbourethral) gland	Urethra
Cremaster muscle	Perineum Muscle
Cribriform plate	Ethmoid Bone, Right
	Ethmoid Bone, Left
Cricoid cartilage	Trachea
Cricothyroid artery	Thyroid Artery, Right
	Thyroid Artery, Left
Cricothyroid muscle	Neck Muscle, Right
	Neck Muscle, Left
Crural fascia	Subcutaneous Tissue and Fascia, Right Upper Leg
	Subcutaneous Tissue and Fascia, Left Upper Leg
Cubital lymph node	Lymphatic, Right Upper Extremity
	Lymphatic, Left Upper Extremity
Cubital nerve	Ulnar Nerve
Cuboid bone	Tarsal, Right
	Tarsal, Left
Cuboideonavicular joint	Tarsal Joint, Right
	Tarsal Joint, Left
Culmen	Cerebellum
Cuneiform cartilage	Larynx
Cuneonavicular joint	Tarsal Joint, Right
	Tarsal Joint, Left
Cuneonavicular ligament	Foot Bursa and Ligament, Right
	Foot Bursa and Ligament, Left
Cutaneous (transverse) cervical nerve	Cervical Plexus
Deep cervical fascia	Subcutaneous Tissue and Fascia, Right Neck
	Subcutaneous Tissue and Fascia, Left Neck
Deep cervical vein	Vertebral Vein, Right
	Vertebral Vein, Left
Deep circumflex iliac artery	External Iliac Artery, Right
	External Iliac Artery, Left
Deep facial vein	Face Vein, Right
	Face Vein, Left
Deep femoral artery	Femoral Artery, Right
	Femoral Artery, Left
Deep femoral (profunda femoris) vein	Femoral Vein, Right
	Femoral Vein, Left
Deep palmar arch	Hand Artery, Right
	Hand Artery, Left
Deep transverse perineal muscle	Perineum Muscle
Deferential artery	Internal Iliac Artery, Right
	Internal Iliac Artery, Left

Term	ICD-10-PCS Value
Deltoid fascia	Subcutaneous Tissue and Fascia, Right Upper Arm
	Subcutaneous Tissue and Fascia, Left Upper Arm
Deltoid ligament	Ankle Bursa and Ligament, Right
	Ankle Bursa and Ligament, Left
Deltoid muscle	Shoulder Muscle, Right
	Shoulder Muscle, Left
Deltopectoral (infraclavicular) lymph node	Lymphatic, Right Upper Extremity
	Lymphatic, Left Upper Extremity
Dens	Cervical Vertebra
Denticulate (dentate) ligament	Spinal Meninges
Depressor anguli oris muscle	Facial Muscle
Depressor labii inferioris muscle	Facial Muscle
Depressor septi nasi muscle	Facial Muscle
Depressor supercilii muscle	Facial Muscle
Dermis	Skin
Descending genicular artery	Femoral Artery, Right
	Femoral Artery, Left
Diaphragma sellae	Dura Mater
Distal humerus	Humeral Shaft, Right
	Humeral Shaft, Left
Distal humerus, involving joint	Elbow Joint, Right
	Elbow Joint, Left
Distal radioulnar joint	Wrist Joint, Right
	Wrist Joint, Left
Dorsal digital nerve	Radial Nerve
Dorsal metacarpal vein	Hand Vein, Right
	Hand Vein, Left
Dorsal metatarsal artery	Foot Artery, Right
	Foot Artery, Left
Dorsal metatarsal vein	Foot Vein, Right
	Foot Vein, Left
Dorsal scapular artery	Subclavian Artery, Right
	Subclavian Artery, Left
Dorsal scapular nerve	Brachial Plexus
Dorsal venous arch	Foot Vein, Right
	Foot Vein, Left
Dorsalis pedis artery	Anterior Tibial Artery, Right
	Anterior Tibial Artery, Left
Duct of Santorini	Pancreatic Duct, Accessory
Duct of Wirsung	Pancreatic Duct
Ductus deferens	Vas Deferens, Right
	Vas Deferens, Left
	Vas Deferens, Bilateral
	Vas Deferens
Duodenal ampulla	Ampulla of Vater
Duodenojejunal flexure	Jejunum
Dura mater, intracranial	Dura Mater
Dura mater, spinal	Spinal Meninges
Dural venous sinus	Intracranial Vein

Term	ICD-10-PCS Value
Earlobe	External Ear, Right
	External Ear, Left
	External Ear, Bilateral
Eighth cranial nerve	Acoustic Nerve
Ejaculatory duct	Vas Deferens, Right
	Vas Deferens, Left
	Vas Deferens, Bilateral
	Vas Deferens
Eleventh cranial nerve	Accessory Nerve
Encephalon	Brain
Ependyma	Cerebral Ventricle
Epidermis	Skin
Epidural space, spinal	Spinal Canal
Epiploic foramen	Peritoneum
Epithalamus	Thalamus
Epitroclear lymph node	Lymphatic, Right Upper Extremity
	Lymphatic, Left Upper Extremity
Erector spinae muscle	Trunk Muscle, Right
	Trunk Muscle, Left
Esophageal artery	Upper Artery
Esophageal plexus	Thoracic Sympathetic Nerve
Ethmoidal air cell	Ethmoid Sinus, Right
	Ethmoid Sinus, Left
Extensor carpi radialis muscle	Lower Arm and Wrist Muscle, Right
	Lower Arm and Wrist Muscle, Left
Extensor carpi ulnaris muscle	Lower Arm and Wrist Muscle, Right
	Lower Arm and Wrist Muscle, Left
Extensor digitorum brevis muscle	Foot Muscle, Right
	Foot Muscle, Left
Extensor digitorum longus muscle	Lower Leg Muscle, Right
	Lower Leg Muscle, Left
Extensor hallucis brevis muscle	Foot Muscle, Right
	Foot Muscle, Left
Extensor hallucis longus muscle	Lower Leg Muscle, Right
	Lower Leg Muscle, Left
External anal sphincter	Anal Sphincter
External auditory meatus	External Auditory Canal, Right
	External Auditory Canal, Left
External maxillary artery	Face Artery
External naris	Nasal Mucosa and Soft Tissue
External oblique aponeurosis	Subcutaneous Tissue and Fascia, Trunk
External oblique muscle	Abdomen Muscle, Right
	Abdomen Muscle, Left
External popliteal nerve	Peroneal Nerve
External pudendal artery	Femoral Artery, Right
	Femoral Artery, Left
External pudenal vein	Saphenous Vein, Right
	Saphenous Vein, Left
External urethral sphincter	Urethra
Extradural space, intracranial	Epidural Space, Intracranial
Extradural space, spinal	Spinal Canal
Facial artery	Face Artery
False vocal cord	Larynx
Falx cerebri	Dura Mater

Term	ICD-10-PCS Value
Fascia lata	Subcutaneous Tissue and Fascia, Right Upper Leg
	Subcutaneous Tissue and Fascia, Left Upper Leg
Femoral head	Upper Femur, Right
	Upper Femur, Left
Femoral lymph node	Lymphatic, Right Lower Extremity
	Lymphatic, Left Lower Extremity
Femoropatellar joint	Knee Joint, Right
	Knee Joint, Left
	Knee Joint, Femoral Surface, Right
	Knee Joint, Femoral Surface, Left
Femorotibial joint	Knee Joint, Right
	Knee Joint, Left
	Knee Joint, Tibial Surface, Right
	Knee Joint, Tibial Surface, Left
Fibular artery	Peroneal Artery, Right
	Peroneal Artery, Left
Fibularis brevis muscle	Lower Leg Muscle, Right
	Lower Leg Muscle, Left
Fibularis longus muscle	Lower Leg Muscle, Right
	Lower Leg Muscle, Left
Fifth cranial nerve	Trigeminal Nerve
Filum terminale	Spinal Meninges
First cranial nerve	Olfactory Nerve
First intercostal nerve	Brachial Plexus
Flexor carpi radialis muscle	Lower Arm and Wrist Muscle, Right
	Lower Arm and Wrist Muscle, Left
Flexor carpi ulnaris muscle	Lower Arm and Wrist Muscle, Right
	Lower Arm and Wrist Muscle, Left
Flexor digitorum brevis muscle	Foot Muscle, Right
	Foot Muscle, Left
Flexor digitorum longus muscle	Lower Leg Muscle, Right
	Lower Leg Muscle, Left
Flexor hallucis brevis muscle	Foot Muscle, Right
	Foot Muscle, Left
Flexor hallucis longus muscle	Lower Leg Muscle, Right
	Lower Leg Muscle, Left
Flexor pollicis longus muscle	Lower Arm and Wrist Muscle, Right
	Lower Arm and Wrist Muscle, Left
Foramen magnum	Occipital Bone
Foramen of Monro (intraventricular)	Cerebral Ventricle
Foreskin	Prepuce
Fossa of Rosenmuller	Nasopharynx
Fourth cranial nerve	Trochlear Nerve
Fourth ventricle	Cerebral Ventricle
Fovea	Retina, Right
	Retina, Left
Frenulum labii inferioris	Lower Lip
Frenulum labii superioris	Upper Lip
Frenulum linguae	Tongue
Frontal lobe	Cerebral Hemisphere
Frontal vein	Face Vein, Right
	Face Vein, Left
Fundus uteri	Uterus

Term	ICD-10-PCS Value
Galea aponeurotica	Subcutaneous Tissue and Fascia, Scalp
Ganglion impar (ganglion of Walther)	Sacral Sympathetic Nerve
Gasserian ganglion	Trigeminal Nerve
Gastric lymph node	Lymphatic, Aortic
Gastric plexus	Abdominal Sympathetic Nerve
Gastrocnemius muscle	Lower Leg Muscle, Right
	Lower Leg Muscle, Left
Gastrocolic ligament	Omentum
Gastrocolic omentum	Omentum
Gastroduodenal artery	Hepatic Artery
Gastroesophageal (GE) junction	Esophagogastric Junction
Gastrohepatic omentum	Omentum
Gastrophrenic ligament	Omentum
Gastrosplenic ligament	Omentum
Gemellus muscle	Hip Muscle, Right
	Hip Muscle, Left
Geniculate ganglion	Facial Nerve
Geniculate nucleus	Thalamus
Genioglossus muscle	Tongue, Palate, Pharynx Muscle
Genitofemoral nerve	Lumbar Plexus
Glans penis	Prepuce
Glenohumeral joint	Shoulder Joint, Right
	Shoulder Joint, Left
Glenohumeral ligament	Shoulder Bursa and Ligament, Right
	Shoulder Bursa and Ligament, Left
Glenoid fossa (of scapula)	Glenoid Cavity, Right
	Glenoid Cavity, Left
Glenoid ligament (labrum)	Shoulder Joint, Right
	Shoulder Joint, Left
Globus pallidus	Basal Ganglia
Glossoepiglottic fold	Epiglottis
Glottis	Larynx
Gluteal lymph node	Lymphatic, Pelvis
Gluteal vein	Hypogastric Vein, Right
	Hypogastric Vein, Left
Gluteus maximus muscle	Hip Muscle, Right
	Hip Muscle, Left
Gluteus medius muscle	Hip Muscle, Right
	Hip Muscle, Left
Gluteus minimus muscle	Hip Muscle, Right
	Hip Muscle, Left
Gracilis muscle	Upper Leg Muscle, Right
	Upper Leg Muscle, Left
Great auricular nerve	Cervical Plexus
Great cerebral vein	Intracranial Vein
Great(er) saphenous vein	Saphenous Vein, Right
	Saphenous Vein, Left
Greater alar cartilage	Nasal Mucosa and Soft Tissue
Greater occipital nerve	Cervical Nerve
Greater omentum	Omentum
Greater splanchnic nerve	Thoracic Sympathetic Nerve
Greater superficial petrosal nerve	Facial Nerve

Term	ICD-10-PCS Value
Greater trochanter	Upper Femur, Right
	Upper Femur, Left
Greater tuberosity	Humeral Head, Right
	Humeral Head, Left
Greater vestibular (Bartholin's) gland	Vestibular Gland
Greater wing	Sphenoid Bone
Hallux	1st Toe, Right
	1st Toe, Left
Hamate bone	Carpal, Right
	Carpal, Left
Head of fibula	Fibula, Right
	Fibula, Left
Helix	External Ear, Right
	External Ear, Left
	External Ear, Bilateral
Hepatic artery proper	Hepatic Artery
Hepatic flexure	Transverse Colon
Hepatic lymph node	Lymphatic, Aortic
Hepatic plexus	Abdominal Sympathetic Nerve
Hepatic portal vein	Portal Vein
Hepatogastric ligament	Omentum
Hepatopancreatic ampulla	Ampulla of Vater
Humeroradial joint	Elbow Joint, Right
	Elbow Joint, Left
Humeroulnar joint	Elbow Joint, Right
	Elbow Joint, Left
Humerus, distal	Humeral Shaft, Right
	Humeral Shaft, Left
Hyoglossus muscle	Tongue, Palate, Pharynx Muscle
Hyoid artery	Thyroid Artery, Right
	Thyroid Artery, Left
Hypogastric artery	Internal Iliac Artery, Right
	Internal Iliac Artery, Left
Hypopharynx	Pharynx
Hypophysis	Pituitary Gland
Hypothenar muscle	Hand Muscle, Right
	Hand Muscle, Left
Ileal artery	Superior Mesenteric Artery
Ileocolic artery	Superior Mesenteric Artery
Ileocolic vein	Colic Vein
Iliac crest	Pelvic Bone, Right
	Pelvic Bone, Left
Iliac fascia	Subcutaneous Tissue and Fascia, Right Upper Leg
	Subcutaneous Tissue and Fascia, Left Upper Leg
Iliac lymph node	Lymphatic, Pelvis
Iliacus muscle	Hip Muscle, Right
	Hip Muscle, Left
Iliofemoral ligament	Hip Bursa and Ligament, Right
	Hip Bursa and Ligament, Left
Iliohypogastric nerve	Lumbar Plexus
Ilioinguinal nerve	Lumbar Plexus
Iliolumbar artery	Internal Iliac Artery, Right
	Internal Iliac Artery, Left

Term	ICD-10-PCS Value
Iliolumbar ligament	Lower Spine Bursa and Ligament
Iliotibial tract (band)	Subcutaneous Tissue and Fascia, Right Upper Leg
	Subcutaneous Tissue and Fascia, Left Upper Leg
Ilium	Pelvic Bone, Right
	Pelvic Bone, Left
Incus	Auditory Ossicle, Right
	Auditory Ossicle, Left
Inferior cardiac nerve	Thoracic Sympathetic Nerve
Inferior cerebellar vein	Intracranial Vein
Inferior cerebral vein	Intracranial Vein
Inferior epigastric artery	External Iliac Artery, Right
	External Iliac Artery, Left
Inferior epigastric lymph node	Lymphatic, Pelvis
Inferior genicular artery	Popliteal Artery, Right
	Popliteal Artery, Left
Inferior gluteal artery	Internal Iliac Artery, Right
	Internal Iliac Artery, Left
Inferior gluteal nerve	Sacral Plexus
Inferior hypogastric plexus	Abdominal Sympathetic Nerve
Inferior labial artery	Face Artery
Inferior longitudinal muscle	Tongue, Palate, Pharynx Muscle
Inferior mesenteric ganglion	Abdominal Sympathetic Nerve
Inferior mesenteric lymph node	Lymphatic, Mesenteric
Inferior mesenteric plexus	Abdominal Sympathetic Nerve
Inferior oblique muscle	Extraocular Muscle, Right
	Extraocular Muscle, Left
Inferior pancreaticoduo-denal artery	Superior Mesenteric Artery
Inferior phrenic artery	Abdominal Aorta
Inferior rectus muscle	Extraocular Muscle, Right
	Extraocular Muscle, Left
Inferior suprarenal artery	Renal Artery, Right
	Renal Artery, Left
Inferior tarsal plate	Lower Eyelid, Right
	Lower Eyelid, Left
Inferior thyroid vein	Innominate Vein, Right
	Innominate Vein, Left
Inferior tibiofibular joint	Ankle Joint, Right
	Ankle Joint, Left
Inferior turbinate	Nasal Turbinate
Inferior ulnar collateral artery	Brachial Artery, Right
	Brachial Artery, Left
Inferior vesical artery	Internal Iliac Artery, Right
	Internal Iliac Artery, Left
Infraauricular lymph node	Lymphatic, Head
Infraclavicular (deltopectoral) lymph node	Lymphatic, Right Upper Extremity
	Lymphatic, Left Upper Extremity
Infrahyoid muscle	Neck Muscle, Right
	Neck Muscle, Left
Infraparotid lymph node	Lymphatic, Head

Term	ICD-10-PCS Value
Infraspinatus fascia	Subcutaneous Tissue and Fascia, Right Upper Arm
	Subcutaneous Tissue and Fascia, Left Upper Arm
Infraspinatus muscle	Shoulder Muscle, Right
	Shoulder Muscle, Left
Infundibulopelvic ligament	Uterine Supporting Structure
Inguinal canal	Inguinal Region, Right
	Inguinal Region, Left
	Inguinal Region, Bilateral
Inguinal triangle	Inguinal Region, Right
	Inguinal Region, Left
	Inguinal Region, Bilateral
Interatrial septum	Atrial Septum
Intercarpal joint	Carpal Joint, Right
	Carpal Joint, Left
Intercarpal ligament	Hand Bursa and Ligament, Right
	Hand Bursa and Ligament, Left
Interclavicular ligament	Shoulder Bursa and Ligament, Right
	Shoulder Bursa and Ligament, Left
Intercostal lymph node	Lymphatic, Thorax
Intercostal muscle	Thorax Muscle, Right
	Thorax Muscle, Left
Intercostal nerve	Thoracic Nerve
Intercostobrachial nerve	Thoracic Nerve
Intercuneiform joint	Tarsal Joint, Right
	Tarsal Joint, Left
Intercuneiform ligament	Foot Bursa and Ligament, Right
	Foot Bursa and Ligament, Left
Intermediate bronchus	Main Bronchus, Right
Intermediate cuneiform bone	Tarsal, Right
	Tarsal, Left
Internal anal sphincter	Anal Sphincter
Internal (basal) cerebral vein	Intracranial Vein
Internal carotid artery, intracranial portion	Intracranial Artery
Internal carotid plexus	Head and Neck Sympathetic Nerve
Internal iliac vein	Hypogastric Vein, Right
	Hypogastric Vein, Left
Internal maxillary artery	External Carotid Artery, Right
	External Carotid Artery, Left
Internal naris	Nasal Mucosa and Soft Tissue
Internal oblique muscle	Abdomen Muscle, Right
	Abdomen Muscle, Left
Internal pudendal artery	Internal Iliac Artery, Right
	Internal Iliac Artery, Left
Internal pudendal vein	Hypogastric Vein, Right
	Hypogastric Vein, Left
Internal thoracic artery	Internal Mammary Artery, Right
	Internal Mammary Artery, Left
	Subclavian Artery, Right
	Subclavian Artery, Left
Internal urethral sphincter	Urethra

Term	ICD-10-PCS Value
Interphalangeal (IP) joint	Finger Phalangeal Joint, Right
	Finger Phalangeal Joint, Left
	Toe Phalangeal Joint, Right
	Toe Phalangeal Joint, Left
Interphalangeal ligament	Foot Bursa and Ligament, Right
	Foot Bursa and Ligament, Left
	Hand Bursa and Ligament, Right
	Hand Bursa and Ligament, Left
Interspinalis muscle	Trunk Muscle, Right
	Trunk Muscle, Left
Interspinous ligament, cervical	Head and Neck Bursa and Ligament
Interspinous ligament, lumbar	Lower Spine Bursa and Ligament
Interspinous ligament, thoracic	Upper Spine Bursa and Ligament
Intertransversarius muscle	Trunk Muscle, Right
	Trunk Muscle, Left
Intertransverse ligament, cervical	Head and Neck Bursa and Ligament
Intertransverse ligament, lumbar	Lower Spine Bursa and Ligament
Intertransverse ligament, thoracic	Upper Spine Bursa and Ligament
Interventricular foramen (Monro)	Cerebral Ventricle
Interventricular septum	Ventricular Septum
Intestinal lymphatic trunk	Cisterna Chyli
Ischiatic nerve	Sciatic Nerve
Ischiocavernosus muscle	Perineum Muscle
Ischiofemoral ligament	Hip Bursa and Ligament, Right
	Hip Bursa and Ligament, Left
Ischium	Pelvic Bone, Right
	Pelvic Bone, Left
Jejunal artery	Superior Mesenteric Artery
Jugular body	Glomus Jugulare
Jugular lymph node	Lymphatic, Right Neck
	Lymphatic, Left Neck
Labia majora	Vulva
Labia minora	Vulva
Labial gland	Upper Lip
	Lower Lip
Lacrimal canaliculus	Lacrimal Duct, Right
	Lacrimal Duct, Left
Lacrimal punctum	Lacrimal Duct, Right
	Lacrimal Duct, Left
Lacrimal sac	Lacrimal Duct, Right
	Lacrimal Duct, Left
Laryngopharynx	Pharynx
Lateral (brachial) lymph node	Lymphatic, Right Axillary
	Lymphatic, Left Axillary
Lateral canthus	Upper Eyelid, Right
	Upper Eyelid, Left
Lateral collateral ligament (LCL)	Knee Bursa and Ligament, Right
	Knee Bursa and Ligament, Left
Lateral condyle of femur	Lower Femur, Right
	Lower Femur, Left

Term	ICD-10-PCS Value
Lateral condyle of tibia	Tibia, Right
	Tibia, Left
Lateral cuneiform bone	Tarsal, Right
	Tarsal, Left
Lateral epicondyle of femur	Lower Femur, Right
	Lower Femur, Left
Lateral epicondyle of humerus	Humeral Shaft, Right
	Humeral Shaft, Left
Lateral femoral cutaneous nerve	Lumbar Plexus
Lateral malleolus	Fibula, Right
	Fibula, Left
Lateral meniscus	Knee Joint, Right
	Knee Joint, Left
Lateral nasal cartilage	Nasal Mucosa and Soft Tissue
Lateral plantar artery	Foot Artery, Right
	Foot Artery, Left
Lateral plantar nerve	Tibial Nerve
Lateral rectus muscle	Extraocular Muscle, Right
	Extraocular Muscle, Left
Lateral sacral artery	Internal Iliac Artery, Right
	Internal Iliac Artery, Left
Lateral sacral vein	Hypogastric Vein, Right
	Hypogastric Vein, Left
Lateral sural cutaneous nerve	Peroneal Nerve
Lateral tarsal artery	Foot Artery, Right
	Foot Artery, Left
Lateral temporo-mandibular ligament	Head and Neck Bursa and Ligament
Lateral thoracic artery	Axillary Artery, Right
	Axillary Artery, Left
Latissimus dorsi muscle	Trunk Muscle, Right
	Trunk Muscle, Left
Least splanchnic nerve	Thoracic Sympathetic Nerve
Left ascending lumbar vein	Hemiazygos Vein
Left atrioventricular valve	Mitral Valve
Left auricular appendix	Atrium, Left
Left colic vein	Colic Vein
Left coronary sulcus	Heart, Left
Left gastric artery	Gastric Artery
Left gastroepiploic artery	Splenic Artery
Left gastroepiploic vein	Splenic Vein
Left inferior phrenic vein	Renal Vein, Left
Left inferior pulmonary vein	Pulmonary Vein, Left
Left jugular trunk	Thoracic Duct
Left lateral ventricle	Cerebral Ventricle
Left ovarian vein	Renal Vein, Left
Left second lumbar vein	Renal Vein, Left
Left subclavian trunk	Thoracic Duct
Left subcostal vein	Hemiazygos Vein
Left superior pulmonary vein	Pulmonary Vein, Left
Left suprarenal vein	Renal Vein, Left
Left testicular vein	Renal Vein, Left

Term	ICD-10-PCS Value
Leptomeninges, intracranial	Cerebral Meninges
Leptomeninges, spinal	Spinal Meninges
Lesser alar cartilage	Nasal Mucosa and Soft Tissue
Lesser occipital nerve	Cervical Plexus
Lesser omentum	Omentum
Lesser saphenous vein	Saphenous Vein, Right
	Saphenous Vein, Left
Lesser splanchnic nerve	Thoracic Sympathetic Nerve
Lesser trochanter	Upper Femur, Right
	Upper Femur, Left
Lesser tuberosity	Humeral Head, Right
	Humeral Head, Left
Lesser wing	Sphenoid Bone
Levator anguli oris muscle	Facial Muscle
Levator ani muscle	Perineum Muscle
Levator labii superioris alaeque nasi muscle	Facial Muscle
Levator labii superioris muscle	Facial Muscle
Levator palpebrae superioris muscle	Upper Eyelid, Right
	Upper Eyelid, Left
Levator scapulae muscle	Neck Muscle, Right
	Neck Muscle, Left
Levator veli palatini muscle	Tongue, Palate, Pharynx Muscle
Levatores costarum muscle	Thorax Muscle, Right
	Thorax Muscle, Left
Ligament of head of fibula	Knee Bursa and Ligament, Right
	Knee Bursa and Ligament, Left
Ligament of the lateral malleolus	Ankle Bursa and Ligament, Right
	Ankle Bursa and Ligament, Left
Ligamentum flavum, cervical	Head and Neck Bursa and Ligament
Ligamentum flavum, lumbar	Lower Spine Bursa and Ligament
Ligamentum flavum, thoracic	Upper Spine Bursa and Ligament
Lingual artery	External Carotid Artery, Right
	External Carotid Artery, Left
Lingual tonsil	Pharynx
Locus ceruleus	Pons
Long thoracic nerve	Brachial Plexus
Lumbar artery	Abdominal Aorta
Lumbar facet joint	Lumbar Vertebral Joint
Lumbar ganglion	Lumbar Sympathetic Nerve
Lumbar lymph node	Lymphatic, Aortic
Lumbar lymphatic trunk	Cisterna Chyli
Lumbar splanchnic nerve	Lumbar Sympathetic Nerve
Lumbosacral facet joint	Lumbosacral Joint
Lumbosacral trunk	Lumbar Nerve
Lunate bone	Carpal, Right
	Carpal, Left
Lunotriquetral ligament	Hand Bursa and Ligament, Right
	Hand Bursa and Ligament, Left
Macula	Retina, Right
	Retina, Left

Term	ICD-10-PCS Value
Malleus	Auditory Ossicle, Right
	Auditory Ossicle, Left
Mammary duct	Breast, Right
	Breast, Left
	Breast, Bilateral
Mammary gland	Breast, Right
	Breast, Left
	Breast, Bilateral
Mammillary body	Hypothalamus
Mandibular nerve	Trigeminal Nerve
Mandibular notch	Mandible, Right
	Mandible, Left
Manubrium	Sternum
Masseter muscle	Head Muscle
Masseteric fascia	Subcutaneous Tissue and Fascia, Face
Mastoid (postauricular) lymph node	Lymphatic, Right Neck
	Lymphatic, Left Neck
Mastoid air cells	Mastoid Sinus, Right
	Mastoid Sinus, Left
Mastoid process	Temporal Bone, Right
	Temporal Bone, Left
Maxillary artery	External Carotid Artery, Right
	External Carotid Artery, Left
Maxillary nerve	Trigeminal Nerve
Medial canthus	Lower Eyelid, Right
	Lower Eyelid, Left
Medial collateral ligament (MCL)	Knee Bursa and Ligament, Right
	Knee Bursa and Ligament, Left
Medial condyle of femur	Lower Femur, Right
	Lower Femur, Left
Medial condyle of tibia	Tibia, Right
	Tibia, Left
Medial cuneiform bone	Tarsal, Right
	Tarsal, Left
Medial epicondyle of femur	Lower Femur, Right
	Lower Femur, Left
Medial epicondyle of humerus	Humeral Shaft, Right
	Humeral Shaft, Left
Medial malleolus	Tibia, Right
	Tibia, Left
Medial meniscus	Knee Joint, Right
	Knee Joint, Left
Medial plantar artery	Foot Artery, Right
	Foot Artery, Left
Medial plantar nerve	Tibial Nerve
Medial popliteal nerve	Tibial Nerve
Medial rectus muscle	Extraocular Muscle, Right
	Extraocular Muscle, Left
Medial sural cutaneous nerve	Tibial Nerve
Median antebrachial vein	Basilic Vein, Right
	Basilic Vein, Left
Median cubital vein	Basilic Vein, Right
	Basilic Vein, Left
Median sacral artery	Abdominal Aorta

Term	ICD-10-PCS Value
Mediastinal cavity	Mediastinum
Mediastinal lymph node	Lymphatic, Thorax
Mediastinal space	Mediastinum
Meissner's (submucous) plexus	Abdominal Sympathetic Nerve
Membranous urethra	Urethra
Mental foramen	Mandible, Right
	Mandible, Left
Mentalis muscle	Facial Muscle
Mesoappendix	Mesentery
Mesocolon	Mesentery
Metacarpal ligament	Hand Bursa and Ligament, Right
	Hand Bursa and Ligament, Left
Metacarpophalangeal ligament	Hand Bursa and Ligament, Right
	Hand Bursa and Ligament, Left
Metatarsal ligament	Foot Bursa and Ligament, Right
	Foot Bursa and Ligament, Left
Metatarsophalangeal ligament	Foot Bursa and Ligament, Right
	Foot Bursa and Ligament, Left
Metatarsophalangeal (MTP) joint	Metatarsal-Phalangeal Joint, Right
	Metatarsal-Phalangeal Joint, Left
Metathalamus	Thalamus
Midcarpal joint	Carpal Joint, Right
	Carpal Joint, Left
Middle cardiac nerve	Thoracic Sympathetic Nerve
Middle cerebral artery	Intracranial Artery
Middle cerebral vein	Intracranial Vein
Middle colic vein	Colic Vein
Middle genicular artery	Popliteal Artery, Right
	Popliteal Artery, Left
Middle hemorrhoidal vein	Hypogastric Vein, Right
	Hypogastric Vein, Left
Middle rectal artery	Internal Iliac Artery, Right
	Internal Iliac Artery, Left
Middle suprarenal artery	Abdominal Aorta
Middle temporal artery	Temporal Artery, Right
	Temporal Artery, Left
Middle turbinate	Nasal Turbinate
Mitral annulus	Mitral Valve
Molar gland	Buccal Mucosa
Musculocutaneous nerve	Brachial Plexus
Musculophrenic artery	Internal Mammary Artery, Right
	Internal Mammary Artery, Left
Musculospiral nerve	Radial Nerve
Myelencephalon	Medulla Oblongata
Myenteric (Auerbach's) plexus	Abdominal Sympathetic Nerve
Myometrium	Uterus
Nail bed	Finger Nail
	Toe Nail
Nail plate	Finger Nail
	Toe Nail
Nasal cavity	Nasal Mucosa and Soft Tissue
Nasal concha	Nasal Turbinate
Nasalis muscle	Facial Muscle

Term	ICD-10-PCS Value
Nasolacrimal duct	Lacrimal Duct, Right
	Lacrimal Duct, Left
Navicular bone	Tarsal, Right
	Tarsal, Left
Neck of femur	Upper Femur, Right
	Upper Femur, Left
Neck of humerus (anatomical) (surgical)	Humeral Head, Right
	Humeral Head, Left
Nerve to the stapedius	Facial Nerve
Neurohypophysis	Pituitary Gland
Ninth cranial nerve	Glossopharyngeal Nerve
Nostril	Nasal Mucosa and Soft Tissue
Obturator artery	Internal Iliac Artery, Right
	Internal Iliac Artery, Left
Obturator lymph node	Lymphatic, Pelvis
Obturator muscle	Hip Muscle, Right
	Hip Muscle, Left
Obturator nerve	Lumbar Plexus
Obturator vein	Hypogastric Vein, Right
	Hypogastric Vein, Left
Obtuse margin	Heart, Left
Occipital artery	External Carotid Artery, Right
	External Carotid Artery, Left
Occipital lobe	Cerebral Hemisphere
Occipital lymph node	Lymphatic, Right Neck
	Lymphatic, Left Neck
Occipitofrontalis muscle	Facial Muscle
Odontoid process	Cervical Vertebra
Olecranon bursa	Elbow Bursa and Ligament, Right
	Elbow Bursa and Ligament, Left
Olecranon process	Ulna, Right
	Ulna, Left
Olfactory bulb	Olfactory Nerve
Ophthalmic artery	Intracranial Artery
Ophthalmic nerve	Trigeminal Nerve
Ophthalmic vein	Intracranial Vein
Optic chiasma	Optic Nerve
Optic disc	Retina, Right
	Retina, Left
Optic foramen	Sphenoid Bone
Orbicularis oculi muscle	Upper Eyelid, Right
	Upper Eyelid, Left
Orbicularis oris muscle	Facial Muscle
Orbital fascia	Subcutaneous Tissue and Fascia, Face
Orbital portion of ethmoid bone	Orbit, Right
	Orbit, Left
Orbital portion of frontal bone	Orbit, Right
	Orbit, Left
Orbital portion of lacrimal bone	Orbit, Right
	Orbit, Left
Orbital portion of maxilla	Orbit, Right
	Orbit, Left
Orbital portion of palatine bone	Orbit, Right
	Orbit, Left

Term	ICD-10-PCS Value
Orbital portion of sphenoid bone	Orbit, Right
	Orbit, Left
Orbital portion of zygomatic bone	Orbit, Right
	Orbit, Left
Oropharynx	Pharynx
Otic ganglion	Head and Neck Sympathetic Nerve
Oval window	Middle Ear, Right
	Middle Ear, Left
Ovarian artery	Abdominal Aorta
Ovarian ligament	Uterine Supporting Structure
Oviduct	Fallopian Tube, Right
	Fallopian Tube, Left
Palatine gland	Buccal Mucosa
Palatine tonsil	Tonsils
Palatine uvula	Uvula
Palatoglossal muscle	Tongue, Palate, Pharynx Muscle
Palatopharyngeal muscle	Tongue, Palate, Pharynx Muscle
Palmar (volar) digital vein	Hand Vein, Right
	Hand Vein, Left
Palmar (volar) metacarpal vein	Hand Vein, Right
	Hand Vein, Left
Palmar cutaneous nerve	Median Nerve
	Radial Nerve
Palmar fascia (aponeurosis)	Subcutaneous Tissue and Fascia, Right Hand
	Subcutaneous Tissue and Fascia, Left Hand
Palmar interosseous muscle	Hand Muscle, Right
	Hand Muscle, Left
Palmar ulnocarpal ligament	Wrist Bursa and Ligament, Right
	Wrist Bursa and Ligament, Left
Palmaris longus muscle	Lower Arm and Wrist Muscle, Right
	Lower Arm and Wrist Muscle, Left
Pancreatic artery	Splenic Artery
Pancreatic plexus	Abdominal Sympathetic Nerve
Pancreatic vein	Splenic Vein
Pancreaticosplenic lymph node	Lymphatic, Aortic
Paraaortic lymph node	Lymphatic, Aortic
Pararectal lymph node	Lymphatic, Mesenteric
Parasternal lymph node	Lymphatic, Thorax
Paratracheal lymph node	Lymphatic, Thorax
Paraurethral (Skene's) gland	Vestibular Gland
Parietal lobe	Cerebral Hemisphere
Parotid lymph node	Lymphatic, Head
Parotid plexus	Facial Nerve
Pars flaccida	Tympanic Membrane, Right
	Tympanic Membrane, Left
Patellar ligament	Knee Bursa and Ligament, Right
	Knee Bursa and Ligament, Left
Patellar tendon	Knee Tendon, Right
	Knee Tendon, Left
Patellofemoral joint	Knee Joint, Right
	Knee Joint, Left
	Knee Joint, Femoral Surface, Right
	Knee Joint, Femoral Surface, Left

Term	ICD-10-PCS Value
Pectineus muscle	Upper Leg Muscle, Right
	Upper Leg Muscle, Left
Pectoral (anterior) lymph node	Lymphatic, Right Axillary
	Lymphatic, Left Axillary
Pectoral fascia	Subcutaneous Tissue and Fascia, Chest
Pectoralis major muscle	Thorax Muscle, Right
	Thorax Muscle, Left
Pectoralis minor muscle	Thorax Muscle, Right
	Thorax Muscle, Left
Pelvic splanchnic nerve	Abdominal Sympathetic Nerve
	Sacral Sympathetic Nerve
Penile urethra	Urethra
Pericardiophrenic artery	Internal Mammary Artery, Right
	Internal Mammary Artery, Left
Perimetrium	Uterus
Peroneus brevis muscle	Lower Leg Muscle, Right
	Lower Leg Muscle, Left
Peroneus longus muscle	Lower Leg Muscle, Right
	Lower Leg Muscle, Left
Petrous part of temporal bone	Temporal Bone, Right
	Temporal Bone, Left
Pharyngeal constrictor muscle	Tongue, Palate, Pharynx Muscle
Pharyngeal plexus	Vagus Nerve
Pharyngeal recess	Nasopharynx
Pharyngeal tonsil	Adenoids
Pharyngotympanic tube	Eustachian Tube, Right
	Eustachian Tube, Left
Pia mater, intracranial	Cerebral Meninges
Pia mater, spinal	Spinal Meninges
Pinna	External Ear, Right
	External Ear, Left
	External Ear, Bilateral
Piriform recess (sinus)	Pharynx
Piriformis muscle	Hip Muscle, Right
	Hip Muscle, Left
Pisiform bone	Carpal, Right
	Carpal, Left
Pisohamate ligament	Hand Bursa and Ligament, Right
	Hand Bursa and Ligament, Left
Pisometacarpal ligament	Hand Bursa and Ligament, Right
	Hand Bursa and Ligament, Left
Plantar digital vein	Foot Vein, Right
	Foot Vein, Left
Plantar fascia (aponeurosis)	Subcutaneous Tissue and Fascia, Right Foot
	Subcutaneous Tissue and Fascia, Left Foot
Plantar metatarsal vein	Foot Vein, Right
	Foot Vein, Left
Plantar venous arch	Foot Vein, Right
	Foot Vein, Left
Platysma muscle	Neck Muscle, Right
	Neck Muscle, Left
Plica semilunaris	Conjunctiva, Right
	Conjunctiva, Left
Pneumogastric nerve	Vagus Nerve

Term	ICD-10-PCS Value
Pneumotaxic center	Pons
Pontine tegmentum	Pons
Popliteal ligament	Knee Bursa and Ligament, Right
	Knee Bursa and Ligament, Left
Popliteallymph node	Lymphatic, Left Lower Extremity
	Lymphatic, Right Lower Extremity
Popliteal vein	Femoral Vein, Right
	Femoral Vein, Left
Popliteus muscle	Lower Leg Muscle, Right
	Lower Leg Muscle, Left
Postauricular (mastoid) lymph node	Lymphatic, Right Neck
	Lymphatic, Left Neck
Postcava	Inferior Vena Cava
Posterior (subscapular) lymph node	Lymphatic, Right Axillary
	Lymphatic, Left Axillary
Posterior auricular artery	External Carotid Artery, Right
	External Carotid Artery, Left
Posterior auricular nerve	Facial Nerve
Posterior auricular vein	External Jugular Vein, Right
	External Jugular Vein, Left
Posterior cerebral artery	Intracranial Artery
Posterior chamber	Eye, Right
	Eye, Left
Posterior circumflex humeral artery	Axillary Artery, Right
	Axillary Artery, Left
Posterior communicating artery	Intracranial Artery
Posterior cruciate ligament (PCL)	Knee Bursa and Ligament, Right
	Knee Bursa and Ligament, Left
Posterior facial (retromandibular) vein	Face Vein, Right
	Face Vein, Left
Posterior femoral cutaneous nerve	Sacral Plexus
Posterior inferior cerebellar artery (PICA)	Intracranial Artery
Posterior interosseous nerve	Radial Nerve
Posterior labial nerve	Pudendal Nerve
Posterior scrotal nerve	Pudendal Nerve
Posterior spinal artery	Vertebral Artery, Right
	Vertebral Artery, Left
Posterior tibial recurrent artery	Anterior Tibial Artery, Right
	Anterior Tibial Artery, Left
Posterior ulnar recurrent artery	Ulnar Artery, Right
	Ulnar Artery, Left
Posterior vagal trunk	Vagus Nerve
Preauricular lymph node	Lymphatic, Head
Precava	Superior Vena Cava
Prepatellar bursa	Knee Bursa and Ligament, Right
	Knee Bursa and Ligament, Left
Pretracheal fascia	Subcutaneous Tissue and Fascia, Right Neck
	Subcutaneous Tissue and Fascia, Left Neck
Prevertebral fascia	Subcutaneous Tissue and Fascia, Right Neck
	Subcutaneous Tissue and Fascia, Left Neck

Term	ICD-10-PCS Value
Princeps pollicis artery	Hand Artery, Right
	Hand Artery, Left
Procerus muscle	Facial Muscle
Profunda brachii	Brachial Artery, Right
	Brachial Artery, Left
Profunda femoris (deep femoral) vein	Femoral Vein, Right
	Femoral Vein, Left
Pronator quadratus muscle	Lower Arm and Wrist Muscle, Right
	Lower Arm and Wrist Muscle, Left
Pronator teres muscle	Lower Arm and Wrist Muscle, Right
	Lower Arm and Wrist Muscle, Left
Prostatic urethra	Urethra
Proximal radioulnar joint	Elbow Joint, Right
	Elbow Joint, Left
Psoas muscle	Hip Muscle, Right
	Hip Muscle, Left
Pterygoid muscle	Head Muscle
Pterygoid process	Sphenoid Bone
Pterygopalatine (sphenopalatine) ganglion	Head and Neck Sympathetic Nerve
Pubis	Pelvic Bone, Right
	Pelvic Bone, Left
Pubofemoral ligament	Hip Bursa and Ligament, Right
	Hip Bursa and Ligament, Left
Pudendal nerve	Sacral Plexus
Pulmoaortic canal	Pulmonary Artery, Left
Pulmonary annulus	Pulmonary Valve
Pulmonary plexus	Thoracic Sympathetic Nerve
	Vagus Nerve
Pulmonic valve	Pulmonary Valve
Pulvinar	Thalamus
Pyloric antrum	Stomach, Pylorus
Pyloric canal	Stomach, Pylorus
Pyloric sphincter	Stomach, Pylorus
Pyramidalis muscle	Abdomen Muscle, Right
	Abdomen Muscle, Left
Quadrangular cartilage	Nasal Septum
Quadrate lobe	Liver
Quadratus femoris muscle	Hip Muscle, Right
	Hip Muscle, Left
Quadratus lumborum muscle	Trunk Muscle, Right
	Trunk Muscle, Left
Quadratus plantae muscle	Foot Muscle, Right
	Foot Muscle, Left
Quadriceps (femoris)	Upper Leg Muscle, Right
	Upper Leg Muscle, Left
Radial collateral carpal ligament	Wrist Bursa and Ligament, Right
	Wrist Bursa and Ligament, Left
Radial collateral ligament	Elbow Bursa and Ligament, Right
	Elbow Bursa and Ligament, Left
Radial notch	Ulna, Right
	Ulna, Left
Radial recurrent artery	Radial Artery, Right
	Radial Artery, Left

Term	ICD-10-PCS Value
Radial vein	Brachial Vein, Right
	Brachial Vein, Left
Radialis indicis	Hand Artery, Right
	Hand Artery, Left
Radiocarpal joint	Wrist Joint, Right
	Wrist Joint, Left
Radiocarpal ligament	Wrist Bursa and Ligament, Right
	Wrist Bursa and Ligament, Left
Radioulnar ligament	Wrist Bursa and Ligament, Right
	Wrist Bursa and Ligament, Left
Rectosigmoid junction	Sigmoid Colon
Rectus abdominis muscle	Abdomen Muscle, Right
	Abdomen Muscle, Left
Rectus femoris muscle	Upper Leg Muscle, Right
	Upper Leg Muscle, Left
Recurrent laryngeal nerve	Vagus Nerve
Renal calyx	Kidney, Right
	Kidney, Left
	Kidneys, Bilateral
	Kidney
Renal capsule	Kidney, Right
	Kidney, Left
	Kidneys, Bilateral
	Kidney
Renal cortex	Kidney, Right
	Kidney, Left
	Kidneys, Bilateral
	Kidney
Renal nerve	Abdominal sympathetic Nerve
Renal plexus	Abdominal Sympathetic Nerve
Renal segment	Kidney, Right
	Kidney, Left
	Kidneys, Bilateral
	Kidney
Renal segmental artery	Renal Artery, Right
	Renal Artery, Left
Retroperitoneal cavity	Retroperitoneum
Retroperitoneal lymph node	Lymphatic, Aortic
Retroperitoneal space	Retroperitoneum
Retropharyngeal lymph node	Lymphatic, Right Neck
	Lymphatic, Left Neck
Retropubic space	Pelvic Cavity
Rhinopharynx	Nasopharynx
Rhomboid major muscle	Trunk Muscle, Right
	Trunk Muscle, Left
Rhomboid minor muscle	Trunk Muscle, Right
	Trunk Muscle, Left
Right ascending lumbar vein	Azygos Vein
Right atrioventricular valve	Tricuspid Valve
Right auricular appendix	Atrium, Right
Right colic vein	Colic Vein
Right coronary sulcus	Heart, Right
Right gastric artery	Gastric Artery

Term	ICD-10-PCS Value
Right gastroepiploic vein	Superior Mesenteric Vein
Right inferior phrenic vein	Inferior Vena Cava
Right inferior pulmonary vein	Pulmonary Vein, Right
Right jugular trunk	Lymphatic, Right Neck
Right lateral ventricle	Cerebral Ventricle
Right lymphatic duct	Lymphatic, Right Neck
Right ovarian vein	Inferior Vena Cava
Right second lumbar vein	Inferior Vena Cava
Right subclavian trunk	Lymphatic, Right Neck
Right subcostal vein	Azygos Vein
Right superior pulmonary vein	Pulmonary Vein, Right
Right suprarenal vein	Inferior Vena Cava
Right testicular vein	Inferior Vena Cava
Rima glottidis	Larynx
Risorius muscle	Facial Muscle
Round ligament of uterus	Uterine Supporting Structure
Round window	Inner Ear, Right
	Inner Ear, Left
Sacral ganglion	Sacral Sympathetic Nerve
Sacral lymph node	Lymphatic, Pelvis
Sacral splanchnic nerve	Sacral Sympathetic Nerve
Sacrococcygeal ligament	Lower Spine Bursa and Ligament
Sacrococcygeal symphysis	Sacrococcygeal Joint
Sacroiliac ligament	Lower Spine Bursa and Ligament
Sacrospinous ligament	Lower Spine Bursa and Ligament
Sacrotuberous ligament	Lower Spine Bursa and Ligament
Salpingopharyngeus muscle	Tongue, Palate, Pharynx Muscle
Salpinx	Fallopian Tube, Right
	Fallopian Tube, Left
Saphenous nerve	Femoral Nerve
Sartorius muscle	Upper Leg Muscle, Right
	Upper Leg Muscle, Left
Scalene muscle	Neck Muscle, Right
	Neck Muscle, Left
Scaphoid bone	Carpal, Right
	Carpal, Left
Scapholunate ligament	Wrist Bursa and Ligament, Right
	Wrist Bursa and Ligament, Left
Scaphotrapezium ligament	Hand Bursa and Ligament, Right
	Hand Bursa and Ligament, Left
Scarpa's (vestibular) ganglion	Acoustic Nerve
Sebaceous gland	Skin
Second cranial nerve	Optic Nerve
Sella turcica	Sphenoid Bone
Semicircular canal	Inner Ear, Right
	Inner Ear, Left
Semimembranosus muscle	Upper Leg Muscle, Right
	Upper Leg Muscle, Left
Semitendinosus muscle	Upper Leg Muscle, Right
	Upper Leg Muscle, Left
Septal cartilage	Nasal Septum

Term	ICD-10-PCS Value
Serratus anterior muscle	Thorax Muscle, Right
	Thorax Muscle, Left
Serratus posterior muscle	Trunk Muscle, Right
	Trunk Muscle, Left
Seventh cranial nerve	Facial Nerve
Short gastric artery	Splenic Artery
Sigmoid artery	Inferior Mesenteric Artery
Sigmoid flexure	Sigmoid Colon
Sigmoid vein	Inferior Mesenteric Vein
Sinoatrial node	Conduction Mechanism
Sinus venosus	Atrium, Right
Sixth cranial nerve	Abducens Nerve
Skene's (paraurethral) gland	Vestibular Gland
Small saphenous vein	Saphenous Vein, Right
	Saphenous Vein, Left
Solar (celiac) plexus	Abdominal Sympathetic Nerve
Soleus muscle	Lower Leg Muscle, Right
	Lower Leg Muscle, Left
Sphenomandibular ligament	Head and Neck Bursa and Ligament
Sphenopalatine (pterygopalatine) ganglion	Head and Neck Sympathetic Nerve
Spinal nerve, cervical	Cervical Nerve
Spinal nerve, lumbar	Lumbar Nerve
Spinal nerve, sacral	Sacral Nerve
Spinal nerve, thoracic	Thoracic Nerve
Spinous process	Cervical Vertebra
	Lumbar Vertebra
	Thoracic Vertebra
Spiral ganglion	Acoustic Nerve
Splenic flexure	Transverse Colon
Splenic plexus	Abdominal Sympathetic Nerve
Splenius capitis muscle	Head Muscle
Splenius cervicis muscle	Neck Muscle, Right
	Neck Muscle, Left
Stapes	Auditory Ossicle, Right
	Auditory Ossicle, Left
Stellate ganglion	Head and Neck Sympathetic Nerve
Stensen's duct	Parotid Duct, Right
	Parotid Duct, Left
Sternoclavicular ligament	Shoulder Bursa and Ligament, Right
	Shoulder Bursa and Ligament, Left
Sternocleidomastoid artery	Thyroid Artery, Right
	Thyroid Artery, Left
Sternocleidomastoid muscle	Neck Muscle, Right
	Neck Muscle, Left
Sternocostal ligament	Sternum Bursa and Ligament
Styloglossus muscle	Tongue, Palate, Pharynx Muscle
Stylomandibular ligament	Head and Neck Bursa and Ligament
Stylopharyngeus muscle	Tongue, Palate, Pharynx Muscle
Subacromial bursa	Shoulder Bursa and Ligament, Right
	Shoulder Bursa and Ligament, Left
Subaortic (common iliac) lymph node	Lymphatic, Pelvis
Subarachnoid space, spinal	Spinal Canal

Term	ICD-10-PCS Value
Subclavicular (apical) lymph node	Lymphatic, Right Axillary
	Lymphatic, Left Axillary
Subclavius muscle	Thorax Muscle, Right
	Thorax Muscle, Left
Subclavius nerve	Brachial Plexus
Subcostal artery	Upper Artery
Subcostal muscle	Thorax Muscle, Right
	Thorax Muscle, Left
Subcostal nerve	Thoracic Nerve
Subdural space, spinal	Spinal Canal
Submandibular ganglion	Facial Nerve
	Head and Neck Sympathetic Nerve
Submandibular gland	Submaxillary Gland, Right
	Submaxillary Gland, Left
Submandibular lymph node	Lymphatic, Head
Submandibular space	Subcutaneous Tissue and Fascia, Face
Submaxillary ganglion	Head and Neck Sympathetic Nerve
Submaxillary lymph node	Lymphatic, Head
Submental artery	Face Artery
Submental lymph node	Lymphatic, Head
Submucous (Meissner's) plexus	Abdominal Sympathetic Nerve
Suboccipital nerve	Cervical Nerve
Suboccipital venous plexus	Vertebral Vein, Right
	Vertebral Vein, Left
Subparotid lymph node	Lymphatic, Head
Subscapular aponeurosis	Subcutaneous Tissue and Fascia, Right Upper Arm
	Subcutaneous Tissue and Fascia, Left Upper Arm
Subscapular artery	Axillary Artery, Right
	Axillary Artery, Left
Subscapular (posterior) lymph node	Lymphatic, Right Axillary
	Lymphatic, Left Axillary
Subscapularis muscle	Shoulder Muscle, Right
	Shoulder Muscle, Left
Substantia nigra	Basal Ganglia
Subtalar (talocalcaneal) joint	Tarsal Joint, Right
	Tarsal Joint, Left
Subtalar ligament	Foot Bursa and Ligament, Right
	Foot Bursa and Ligament, Left
Subthalamic nucleus	Basal Ganglia
Superficial circumflex iliac vein	Saphenous Vein, Right
	Saphenous Vein, Left
Superficial epigastric artery	Femoral Artery, Right
	Femoral Artery, Left
Superficial epigastric vein	Saphenous Vein, Right
	Saphenous Vein, Left
Superficial palmar arch	Hand Artery, Right
	Hand Artery, Left
Superficial palmar venous arch	Hand Vein, Right
	Hand Vein, Left
Superficial temporal artery	Temporal Artery, Right
	Temporal Artery, Left

Term	ICD-10-PCS Value
Superficial transverse perineal muscle	Perineum Muscle
Superior cardiac nerve	Thoracic Sympathetic Nerve
Superior cerebellar vein	Intracranial Vein
Superior cerebral vein	Intracranial Vein
Superior clunic (cluneal) nerve	Lumbar Nerve
Superior epigastric artery	Internal Mammary Artery, Right
	Internal Mammary Artery, Left
Superior genicular artery	Popliteal Artery, Right
	Popliteal Artery, Left
Superior gluteal artery	Internal Iliac Artery, Right
	Internal Iliac Artery, Left
Superior gluteal nerve	Lumbar Plexus
Superior hypogastric plexus	Abdominal Sympathetic Nerve
Superior labial artery	Face Artery
Superior laryngeal artery	Thyroid Artery, Right
	Thyroid Artery, Left
Superior laryngeal nerve	Vagus Nerve
Superior longitudinal muscle	Tongue, Palate, Pharynx Muscle
Superior mesenteric ganglion	Abdominal Sympathetic Nerve
Superior mesenteric lymph node	Lymphatic, Mesenteric
Superior mesenteric plexus	Abdominal Sympathetic Nerve
Superior oblique muscle	Extraocular Muscle, Right
	Extraocular Muscle, Left
Superior olivary nucleus	Pons
Superior rectal artery	Inferior Mesenteric Artery
Superior rectal vein	Inferior Mesenteric Vein
Superior rectus muscle	Extraocular Muscle, Right
	Extraocular Muscle, Left
Superior tarsal plate	Upper Eyelid, Right
	Upper Eyelid, Left
Superior thoracic artery	Axillary Artery, Right
	Axillary Artery, Left
Superior thyroid artery	External Carotid Artery, Right
	External Carotid Artery, Left
	Thyroid Artery, Right
	Thyroid Artery, Left
Superior turbinate	Nasal Turbinate
Superior ulnar collateral artery	Brachial Artery, Right
	Brachial Artery, Left
Supraclavicular nerve	Cervical Plexus
Supraclavicular (Virchow's) lymph node	Lymphatic, Right Neck
	Lymphatic, Left Neck
Suprahyoid lymph node	Lymphatic, Head
Suprahyoid muscle	Neck Muscle, Right
	Neck Muscle, Left
Suprainguinal lymph node	Lymphatic, Pelvis
Supraorbital vein	Face Vein, Right
	Face Vein, Left

Term	ICD-10-PCS Value
Suprarenal gland	Adrenal Gland, Right
	Adrenal Gland, Left
	Adrenal Glands, Bilateral
	Adrenal Gland
Suprarenal plexus	Abdominal Sympathetic Nerve
Suprascapular nerve	Brachial Plexus
Supraspinatus fascia	Subcutaneous Tissue and Fascia, Right Upper Arm
	Subcutaneous Tissue and Fascia, Left Upper Arm
Supraspinatus muscle	Shoulder Muscle, Right
	Shoulder Muscle, Left
Supraspinous ligament	Upper Spine Bursa and Ligament
	Lower Spine Bursa and Ligament
Suprasternal notch	Sternum
Supratrochlear lymph node	Lymphatic, Right Upper Extremity
	Lymphatic, Left Upper Extremity
Sural artery	Popliteal Artery, Right
	Popliteal Artery, Left
Sweat gland	Skin
Talocalcaneal ligament	Foot Bursa and Ligament, Right
	Foot Bursa and Ligament, Left
Talocalcaneal (subtalar) joint	Tarsal Joint, Right
	Tarsal Joint, Left
Talocalcaneonavicular joint	Tarsal Joint, Right
	Tarsal Joint, Left
Talocalcaneonavicular ligament	Foot Bursa and Ligament, Right
	Foot Bursa and Ligament, Left
Talocrural joint	Ankle Joint, Right
	Ankle Joint, Left
Talofibular ligament	Ankle Bursa and Ligament, Right
	Ankle Bursa and Ligament, Left
Talus bone	Tarsal, Right
	Tarsal, Left
Tarsometatarsal ligament	Foot Bursa and Ligament, Right
	Foot Bursa and Ligament, Left
Temporal lobe	Cerebral Hemisphere
Temporalis muscle	Head Muscle
Temporoparietalis muscle	Head Muscle
Tensor fasciae latae muscle	Hip Muscle, Right
	Hip Muscle, Left
Tensor veli palatini muscle	Tongue, Palate, Pharynx Muscle
Tenth cranial nerve	Vagus Nerve
Tentorium cerebelli	Dura Mater
Teres major muscle	Shoulder Muscle, Right
	Shoulder Muscle, Left
Teres minor muscle	Shoulder Muscle, Right
	Shoulder Muscle, Left
Testicular artery	Abdominal Aorta
Thenar muscle	Hand Muscle, Right
	Hand Muscle, Left
Third cranial nerve	Oculomotor Nerve
Third occipital nerve	Cervical Nerve
Third ventricle	Cerebral Ventricle
Thoracic aortic plexus	Thoracic Sympathetic Nerve

Term	ICD-10-PCS Value
Thoracic esophagus	Esophagus, Middle
Thoracic facet joint	Thoracic Vertebral Joint
Thoracic ganglion	Thoracic Sympathetic Nerve
Thoracoacromial artery	Axillary Artery, Right
	Axillary Artery, Left
Thoracolumbar facet joint	Thoracolumbar Vertebral Joint
Thymus gland	Thymus
Thyroarytenoid muscle	Neck Muscle, Right
	Neck Muscle, Left
Thyrocervical trunk	Thyroid Artery, Right
	Thyroid Artery, Left
Thyroid cartilage	Larynx
Tibialis anterior muscle	Lower Leg Muscle, Right
	Lower Leg Muscle, Left
Tibialis posterior muscle	Lower Leg Muscle, Right
	Lower Leg Muscle, Left
Tibiofemoral joint	Knee Joint, Right
	Knee Joint, Left
	Knee Joint, Tibial Surface, Right
	Knee Joint, Tibial Surface, Left
Tibioperoneal trunk	Popliteal Artery, Right
	Popliteal Artery, Left
Tongue, base of	Pharynx
Tracheobronchial lymph node	Lymphatic, Thorax
Tragus	External Ear, Right
	External Ear, Left
	External Ear, Bilateral
Transversalis fascia	Subcutaneous Tissue and Fascia, Trunk
Transverse acetabular ligament	Hip Bursa and Ligament, Right
	Hip Bursa and Ligament, Left
Transverse (cutaneous) cervical nerve	Cervical Plexus
Transverse facial artery	Temporal Artery, Right
	Temporal Artery, Left
Transverse foramen	Cervical Vertebra
Transverse humeral ligament	Shoulder Bursa and Ligament, Right
	Shoulder Bursa and Ligament, Left
Transverse ligament of atlas	Head and Neck Bursa and Ligament
Transverse process	Cervical Vertebra
	Thoracic Vertebra
	Lumbar Vertebra
Transverse scapular ligament	Shoulder Bursa and Ligament, Right
	Shoulder Bursa and Ligament, Left
Transverse thoracis muscle	Thorax Muscle, Right
	Thorax Muscle, Left
Transversospinalis muscle	Trunk Muscle, Right
	Trunk Muscle, Left
Transversus abdominis muscle	Abdomen Muscle, Right
	Abdomen Muscle, Left
Trapezium bone	Carpal, Right
	Carpal, Left
Trapezius muscle	Trunk Muscle, Right
	Trunk Muscle, Left

Term	ICD-10-PCS Value
Trapezoid bone	Carpal, Right
	Carpal, Left
Triceps brachii muscle	Upper Arm Muscle, Right
	Upper Arm Muscle, Left
Tricuspid annulus	Tricuspid Valve
Trifacial nerve	Trigeminal Nerve
Trigone of bladder	Bladder
Triquetral bone	Carpal, Right
	Carpal, Left
Trochantericbursa	Hip Bursa and Ligament, Right
	Hip Bursa and Ligament, Left
Twelfth cranial nerve	Hypoglossal Nerve
Tympanic cavity	Middle Ear, Right
	Middle Ear, Left
Tympanic nerve	Glossopharyngeal Nerve
Tympanic part of temoporal bone	Temporal Bone, Right
	Temporal Bone, Left
Ulnar collateral carpal ligament	Wrist Bursa and Ligament, Right
	Wrist Bursa and Ligament, Left
Ulnar collateral ligament	Elbow Bursa and Ligament, Right
	Elbow Bursa and Ligament, Left
Ulnar notch	Radius, Right
	Radius, Left
Ulnar vein	Brachial Vein, Right
	Brachial Vein, Left
Umbilical artery	Internal Iliac Artery, Right
	Internal Iliac Artery, Left
	Lower Artery
Ureteral orifice	Ureter, Right
	Ureter, Left
	Ureters, Bilateral
	Ureter
Ureteropelvic junction (UPJ)	Kidney Pelvis, Right
	Kidney Pelvis, Left
Ureterovesical orifice	Ureter, Right
	Ureter, Left
	Ureters, Bilateral
	Ureter
Uterine artery	Internal Iliac Artery, Right
	Internal Iliac Artery, Left
Uterine cornu	Uterus
Uterine tube	Fallopian Tube, Right
	Fallopian Tube, Left
Uterine vein	Hypogastric Vein, Right
	Hypogastric Vein, Left
Vaginal artery	Internal Iliac Artery, Right
	Internal Iliac Artery, Left
Vaginal vein	Hypogastric Vein, Right
	Hypogastric Vein, Left
Vastus intermedius muscle	Upper Leg Muscle, Right
	Upper Leg Muscle, Left
Vastus lateralis muscle	Upper Leg Muscle, Right
	Upper Leg Muscle, Left
Vastus medialis muscle	Upper Leg Muscle, Right
	Upper Leg Muscle, Left

Term	ICD-10-PCS Value
Ventricular fold	Larynx
Vermiform appendix	Appendix
Vermilion border	Upper Lip
	Lower Lip
Vertebral arch	Cervical Vertebra
	Lumbar Vertebra
	Thoracic Vertebra
Vertebral body	Cervical Vertebra
	Lumbar Vertebra
	Thoracic Vertebra
Vertebral canal	Spinal Canal
Vertebral foramen	Cervical Vertebra
	Lumbar Vertebra
	Thoracic Vertebra
Vertebral lamina	Cervical Vertebra
	Lumbar Vertebra
	Thoracic Vertebra
Vertebral pedicle	Cervical Vertebra
	Lumbar Vertebra
	Thoracic Vertebra
Vesical vein	Hypogastric Vein, Right
	Hypogastric Vein, Left
Vestibular (Scarpa's) ganglion	Acoustic Nerve
Vestibular nerve	Acoustic Nerve
Vestibulocochlear nerve	Acoustic Nerve
Virchow's (supraclavicular) lymph node	Lymphatic, Right Neck
	Lymphatic, Left Neck
Vitreous body	Vitreous, Right
	Vitreous, Left
Vocal fold	Vocal Cord, Right
	Vocal Cord, Left
Volar (palmar) digital vein	Hand Vein, Right
	Hand Vein, Left
Volar (palmar) metacarpal vein	Hand Vein, Right
	Hand Vein, Left
Vomer bone	Nasal Septum
Vomer of nasal septum	Nasal Bone
Xiphoid process	Sternum
Zonule of Zinn	Lens, Right
	Lens, Left
Zygomatic process of frontal bone	Frontal Bone
Zygomatic process of temporal bone	Temporal Bone, Right
	Temporal Bone, Left
Zygomaticus muscle	Facial Muscle

Appendix E: Body Part Definitions

ICD-10-PCS Value	Definition
1st Toe, Left 1st Toe, Right	**Includes:** Hallux
Abdomen Muscle, Left Abdomen Muscle, Right	**Includes:** External oblique muscle Internal oblique muscle Pyramidalis muscle Rectus abdominis muscle Transversus abdominis muscle
Abdominal Aorta	**Includes:** Inferior phrenic artery Lumbar artery Median sacral artery Middle suprarenal artery Ovarian artery Testicular artery
Abdominal Sympathetic Nerve	**Includes:** Abdominal aortic plexus Auerbach's (myenteric) plexus Celiac (solar) plexus Celiac ganglion Gastric plexus Hepatic plexus Inferior hypogastric plexus Inferior mesenteric ganglion Inferior mesenteric plexus Meissner's (submucous) plexus Myenteric (Auerbach's) plexus Pancreatic plexus Pelvic splanchnic nerve Renal nerve Renal plexus Solar (celiac) plexus Splenic plexus Submucous (Meissner's) plexus Superior hypogastric plexus Superior mesenteric ganglion Superior mesenteric plexus Suprarenal plexus
Abducens Nerve	**Includes:** Sixth cranial nerve
Accessory Nerve	**Includes:** Eleventh cranial nerve
Acoustic Nerve	**Includes:** Cochlear nerve Eighth cranial nerve Scarpa's (vestibular) ganglion Spiral ganglion Vestibular (Scarpa's) ganglion Vestibular nerve Vestibulocochlear nerve
Adenoids	**Includes:** Pharyngeal tonsil
Adrenal Gland Adrenal Gland, Left Adrenal Gland, Right Adrenal Glands, Bilateral	**Includes:** Suprarenal gland
Ampulla of Vater	**Includes:** Duodenal ampulla Hepatopancreatic ampulla
Anal Sphincter	**Includes:** External anal sphincter Internal anal sphincter

ICD-10-PCS Value	Definition
Ankle Bursa and Ligament, Left Ankle Bursa and Ligament, Right	**Includes:** Calcaneofibular ligament Deltoid ligament Ligament of the lateral malleolus Talofibular ligament
Ankle Joint, Left Ankle Joint, Right	**Includes:** Inferior tibiofibular joint Talocrural joint
Anterior Chamber, Left Anterior Chamber, Right	**Includes:** Aqueous humour
Anterior Tibial Artery, Left Anterior Tibial Artery, Right	**Includes:** Anterior lateral malleolar artery Anterior medial malleolar artery Anterior tibial recurrent artery Dorsalis pedis artery Posterior tibial recurrent artery
Anus	**Includes:** Anal orifice
Aortic Valve	**Includes:** Aortic annulus
Appendix	**Includes:** Vermiform appendix
Atrial Septum	**Includes:** Interatrial septum
Atrium, Left	**Includes:** Atrium pulmonale Left auricular appendix
Atrium, Right	**Includes:** Atrium dextrum cordis Right auricular appendix Sinus venosus
Auditory Ossicle, Left Auditory Ossicle, Right	**Includes:** Incus Malleus Stapes
Axillary Artery, Left Axillary Artery, Right	**Includes:** Anterior circumflex humeral artery Lateral thoracic artery Posterior circumflex humeral artery Subscapular artery Superior thoracic artery Thoracoacromial artery
Azygos Vein	**Includes:** Right ascending lumbar vein Right subcostal vein
Basal Ganglia	**Includes:** Basal nuclei Claustrum Corpus striatum Globus pallidus Substantia nigra Subthalamic nucleus
Basilic Vein, Left Basilic Vein, Right	**Includes:** Median antebrachial vein Median cubital vein
Bladder	**Includes:** Trigone of bladder
Brachial Artery, Left Brachial Artery, Right	**Includes:** Inferior ulnar collateral artery Profunda brachii Superior ulnar collateral artery

ICD-10-PCS Value	Definition
Brachial Plexus	**Includes:** Axillary nerve Dorsal scapular nerve First intercostal nerve Long thoracic nerve Musculocutaneous nerve Subclavius nerve Suprascapular nerve
Brachial Vein, Left Brachial Vein, Right	**Includes:** Radial vein Ulnar vein
Brain	**Includes:** Cerebrum Corpus callosum Encephalon
Breast, Bilateral Breast, Left Breast, Right	**Includes:** Mammary duct Mammary gland
Buccal Mucosa	**Includes:** Buccal gland Molar gland Palatine gland
Carotid Bodies, Bilateral Carotid Body, Left Carotid Body, Right	**Includes:** Carotid glomus
Carpal Joint, Left Carpal Joint, Right	**Includes:** Intercarpal joint Midcarpal joint
Carpal, Left Carpal, Right	**Includes:** Capitate bone Hamate bone Lunate bone Pisiform bone Scaphoid bone Trapezium bone Trapezoid bone Triquetral bone
Celiac Artery	**Includes:** Celiac trunk
Cephalic Vein, Left Cephalic Vein, Right	**Includes:** Accessory cephalic vein
Cerebellum	**Includes:** Culmen
Cerebral Hemisphere	**Includes:** Frontal lobe Occipital lobe Parietal lobe Temporal lobe
Cerebral Meninges	**Includes:** Arachnoid mater, intracranial Leptomeninges, intracranial Pia mater, intracranial
Cerebral Ventricle	**Includes:** Aqueduct of Sylvius Cerebral aqueduct (Sylvius) Choroid plexus Ependyma Foramen of Monro (intraventricular) Fourth ventricle Interventricular foramen (Monro) Left lateral ventricle Right lateral ventricle Third ventricle

ICD-10-PCS Value	Definition
Cervical Nerve	**Includes:** Greater occipital nerve Spinal nerve, cervical Suboccipital nerve Third occipital nerve
Cervical Plexus	**Includes:** Ansa cervicalis Cutaneous (transverse) cervical nerve Great auricular nerve Lesser occipital nerve Supraclavicular nerve Transverse (cutaneous) cervical nerve
Cervical Vertebra	**Includes:** Dens Odontoid process Spinous process Transverse foramen Transverse process Vertebral arch Vertebral body Vertebral foramen Vertebral lamina Vertebral pedicle
Cervical Vertebral Joint	**Includes:** Atlantoaxial joint Cervical facet joint
Cervical Vertebral Joints, 2 or more	**Includes:** Cervical facet joint
Cervicothoracic Vertebral Joint	**Includes:** Cervicothoracic facet joint
Cisterna Chyli	**Includes:** Intestinal lymphatic trunk Lumbar lymphatic trunk
Coccygeal Glomus	**Includes:** Coccygeal body
Colic Vein	**Includes:** Ileocolic vein Left colic vein Middle colic vein Right colic vein
Conduction Mechanism	**Includes:** Atrioventricular node Bundle of His Bundle of Kent Sinoatrial node
Conjunctiva, Left Conjunctiva, Right	**Includes:** Plica semilunaris
Dura Mater	**Includes:** Diaphragma sellae Dura mater, intracranial Falx cerebri Tentorium cerebelli
Elbow Bursa and Ligament, Left Elbow Bursa and Ligament, Right	**Includes:** Annular ligament Olecranon bursa Radial collateral ligament Ulnar collateral ligament
Elbow Joint, Left Elbow Joint, Right	**Includes:** Distal humerus, involving joint Humeroradial joint Humeroulnar joint Proximal radioulnar joint
Epidural Space, Intracranial	**Includes:** Extradural space, intracranial

ICD-10-PCS Value	Definition
Epiglottis	**Includes:** Glossoepiglottic fold
Esophagogastric Junction	**Includes:** Cardia Cardioesophageal junction Gastroesophageal (GE) junction
Esophagus, Lower	**Includes:** Abdominal esophagus
Esophagus, Middle	**Includes:** Thoracic esophagus
Esophagus, Upper	**Includes:** Cervical esophagus
Ethmoid Bone, Left Ethmoid Bone, Right	**Includes:** Cribriform plate
Ethmoid Sinus, Left Ethmoid Sinus, Right	**Includes:** Ethmoidal air cell
Eustachian Tube, Left Eustachian Tube, Right	**Includes:** Auditory tube Pharyngotympanic tube
External Auditory Canal, Left External Auditory Canal, Right	**Includes:** External auditory meatus
External Carotid Artery, Left External Carotid Artery, Right	**Includes:** Ascending pharyngeal artery Internal maxillary artery Lingual artery Maxillary artery Occipital artery Posterior auricular artery Superior thyroid artery
External Ear, Bilateral External Ear, Left External Ear, Right	**Includes:** Antihelix Antitragus Auricle Earlobe Helix Pinna Tragus
External Iliac Artery, Left External Iliac Artery, Right	**Includes:** Deep circumflex iliac artery Inferior epigastric artery
External Jugular Vein, Left External Jugular Vein, Right	**Includes:** Posterior auricular vein
Extraocular Muscle, Left Extraocular Muscle, Right	**Includes:** Inferior oblique muscle Inferior rectus muscle Lateral rectus muscle Medial rectus muscle Superior oblique muscle Superior rectus muscle
Eye, Left Eye, Right	**Includes:** Ciliary body Posterior chamber
Face Artery	**Includes:** Angular artery Ascending palatine artery External maxillary artery Facial artery Inferior labial artery Submental artery Superior labial artery

ICD-10-PCS Value	Definition
Face Vein, Left Face Vein, Right	**Includes:** Angular vein Anterior facial vein Common facial vein Deep facial vein Frontal vein Posterior facial (retromandibular) vein Supraorbital vein
Facial Muscle	**Includes:** Buccinator muscle Corrugator supercilii muscle Depressor anguli oris muscle Depressor labii inferioris muscle Depressor septi nasi muscle Depressor supercilii muscle Levator anguli oris muscle Levator labii superioris alaeque nasi muscle Levator labii superioris muscle Mentalis muscle Nasalis muscle Occipitofrontalis muscle Orbicularis oris muscle Procerus muscle Risorius muscle Zygomaticus muscle
Facial Nerve	**Includes:** Chorda tympani Geniculate ganglion Greater superficial petrosal nerve Nerve to the stapedius Parotid plexus Posterior auricular nerve Seventh cranial nerve Submandibular ganglion
Fallopian Tube, Left Fallopian Tube, Right	**Includes:** Oviduct Salpinx Uterine tube
Femoral Artery, Left Femoral Artery, Right	**Includes:** Circumflex iliac artery Deep femoral artery Descending genicular artery External pudendal artery Superficial epigastric artery
Femoral Nerve	**Includes:** Anterior crural nerve Saphenous nerve
Femoral Shaft, Left Femoral Shaft, Right	**Includes:** Body of femur
Femoral Vein, Left Femoral Vein, Right	**Includes:** Deep femoral (profunda femoris) vein Popliteal vein Profunda femoris (deep femoral) vein
Fibula, Left Fibula, Right	**Includes:** Body of fibula Head of fibula Lateral malleolus
Finger Nail	**Includes:** Nail bed Nail plate

ICD-10-PCS Value	Definition
Finger Phalangeal Joint, Left **Finger Phalangeal Joint, Right**	**Includes:** Interphalangeal (IP) joint
Foot Artery, Left **Foot Artery, Right**	**Includes:** Arcuate artery Dorsal metatarsal artery Lateral plantar artery Lateral tarsal artery Medial plantar artery
Foot Bursa and Ligament, Left **Foot Bursa and Ligament, Right**	**Includes:** Calcaneocuboid ligament Cuneonavicular ligament Intercuneiform ligament Interphalangeal ligament Metatarsal ligament Metatarsophalangeal ligament Subtalar ligament Talocalcaneal ligament Talocalcaneonavicular ligament Tarsometatarsal ligament
Foot Muscle, Left **Foot Muscle, Right**	**Includes:** Abductor hallucis muscle Adductor hallucis muscle Extensor digitorum brevis muscle Extensor hallucis brevis muscle Flexor digitorum brevis muscle Flexor hallucis brevis muscle Quadratus plantae muscle
Foot Vein, Left **Foot Vein, Right**	**Includes:** Common digital vein Dorsal metatarsal vein Dorsal venous arch Plantar digital vein Plantar metatarsal vein Plantar venous arch
Frontal Bone	**Includes:** Zygomatic process of frontal bone
Gastric Artery	**Includes:** Left gastric artery Right gastric artery
Glenoid Cavity, Left **Glenoid Cavity, Right**	**Includes:** Glenoid fossa (of scapula)
Glomus Jugulare	**Includes:** Jugular body
Glossopharyngeal Nerve	**Includes:** Carotid sinus nerve Ninth cranial nerve Tympanic nerve
Hand Artery, Left **Hand Artery, Right**	**Includes:** Deep palmar arch Princeps pollicis artery Radialis indicis Superficial palmar arch
Hand Bursa and Ligament, Left **Hand Bursa and Ligament, Right**	**Includes:** Carpometacarpal ligament Intercarpal ligament Interphalangeal ligament Lunotriquetral ligament Metacarpal ligament Metacarpophalangeal ligament Pisohamate ligament Pisometacarpal ligament Scaphotrapezium ligament
Hand Muscle, Left **Hand Muscle, Right**	**Includes:** Hypothenar muscle Palmar interosseous muscle Thenar muscle
Hand Vein, Left **Hand Vein, Right**	**Includes:** Dorsal metacarpal vein Palmar (volar) digital vein Palmar (volar) metacarpal vein Superficial palmar venous arch Volar (palmar) digital vein Volar (palmar) metacarpal vein
Head and Neck Bursa and Ligament	**Includes:** Alar ligament of axis Cervical interspinous ligament Cervical intertransverse ligament Cervical ligamentum flavum Interspinous ligament, cervical Intertransverse ligament, cervical Lateral temporomandibular ligament Ligamentum flavum, cervical Sphenomandibular ligament Stylomandibular ligament Transverse ligament of atlas
Head and Neck Sympathetic Nerve	**Includes:** Cavernous plexus Cervical ganglion Ciliary ganglion Internal carotid plexus Otic ganglion Pterygopalatine (sphenopalatine) ganglion Sphenopalatine (pterygopalatine) ganglion Stellate ganglion Submandibular ganglion Submaxillary ganglion
Head Muscle	**Includes:** Auricularis muscle Masseter muscle Pterygoid muscle Splenius capitis muscle Temporalis muscle Temporoparietalis muscle
Heart, Left	**Includes:** Left coronary sulcus Obtuse margin
Heart, Right	**Includes:** Right coronary sulcus
Hemiazygos Vein	**Includes:** Left ascending lumbar vein Left subcostal vein
Hepatic Artery	**Includes:** Common hepatic artery Gastroduodenal artery Hepatic artery proper
Hip Bursa and Ligament, Left **Hip Bursa and Ligament, Right**	**Includes:** Iliofemoral ligament Ischiofemoral ligament Pubofemoral ligament Transverse acetabular ligament Trochanteric bursa
Hip Joint, Left **Hip Joint, Right**	**Includes:** Acetabulofemoral joint

ICD-10-PCS Value	Definition
Hip Muscle, Left Hip Muscle, Right	**Includes:** Gemellus muscle Gluteus maximus muscle Gluteus medius muscle Gluteus minimus muscle Iliacus muscle Obturator muscle Piriformis muscle Psoas muscle Quadratus femoris muscle Tensor fasciae latae muscle
Humeral Head, Left Humeral Head, Right	**Includes:** Greater tuberosity Lesser tuberosity Neck of humerus (anatomical)(surgical)
Humeral Shaft, Left Humeral Shaft, Right	**Includes:** Distal humerus Humerus, distal Lateral epicondyle of humerus Medial epicondyle of humerus
Hypogastric Vein, Left Hypogastric Vein, Right	**Includes:** Gluteal vein Internal iliac vein Internal pudendal vein Lateral sacral vein Middle hemorrhoidal vein Obturator vein Uterine vein Vaginal vein Vesical vein
Hypoglossal Nerve	**Includes:** Twelfth cranial nerve
Hypothalamus	**Includes:** Mammillary body
Inferior Mesenteric Artery	**Includes:** Sigmoid artery Superior rectal artery
Inferior Mesenteric Vein	**Includes:** Sigmoid vein Superior rectal vein
Inferior Vena Cava	**Includes:** Postcava Right inferior phrenic vein Right ovarian vein Right second lumbar vein Right suprarenal vein Right testicular vein
Inguinal Region, Bilateral Inguinal Region, Left Inguinal Region, Right	**Includes:** Inguinal canal Inguinal triangle
Inner Ear, Left Inner Ear, Right	**Includes:** Bony labyrinth Bony vestibule Cochlea Round window Semicircular canal
Innominate Artery	**Includes:** Brachiocephalic artery Brachiocephalic trunk
Innominate Vein, Left Innominate Vein, Right	**Includes:** Brachiocephalic vein Inferior thyroid vein
Internal Carotid Artery, Left Internal Carotid Artery, Right	**Includes:** Caroticotympanic artery Carotid sinus

ICD-10-PCS Value	Definition
Internal Iliac Artery, Left Internal Iliac Artery, Right	**Includes:** Deferential artery Hypogastric artery Iliolumbar artery Inferior gluteal artery Inferior vesical artery Internal pudendal artery Lateral sacral artery Middle rectal artery Obturator artery Superior gluteal artery Umbilical artery Uterine artery Vaginal artery
Internal Mammary Artery, Left Internal Mammary Artery, Right	**Includes:** Anterior intercostal artery Internal thoracic artery Musculophrenic artery Pericardiophrenic artery Superior epigastric artery
Intracranial Artery	**Includes:** Anterior cerebral artery Anterior choroidal artery Anterior communicating artery Basilar artery Circle of Willis Internal carotid artery, intracranial portion Middle cerebral artery Ophthalmic artery Posterior cerebral artery Posterior communicating artery Posterior inferior cerebellar artery (PICA)
Intracranial Vein	**Includes:** Anterior cerebral vein Basal (internal) cerebral vein Dural venous sinus Great cerebral vein Inferior cerebellar vein Inferior cerebral vein Internal (basal) cerebral vein Middle cerebral vein Ophthalmic vein Superior cerebellar vein Superior cerebral vein
Jejunum	**Includes:** Duodenojejunal flexure
Kidney	**Includes:** Renal calyx Renal capsule Renal cortex Renal segment
Kidney Pelvis, Left Kidney Pelvis, Right	**Includes:** Ureteropelvic junction (UPJ)
Kidney, Left Kidney, Right Kidneys, Bilateral	**Includes:** Renal calyx Renal capsule Renal cortex Renal segment

ICD-10-PCS Value	Definition	ICD-10-PCS Value	Definition
Knee Bursa and Ligament, Left **Knee Bursa and Ligament, Right**	**Includes:** Anterior cruciate ligament (ACL) Lateral collateral ligament (LCL) Ligament of head of fibula Medial collateral ligament (MCL) Patellar ligament Popliteal ligament Posterior cruciate ligament (PCL) Prepatellar bursa	**Lower Leg Muscle, Left** **Lower Leg Muscle, Right**	**Includes:** Extensor digitorum longus muscle Extensor hallucis longus muscle Fibularis brevis muscle Fibularis longus muscle Flexor digitorum longus muscle Flexor hallucis longus muscle Gastrocnemius muscle Peroneus brevis muscle Peroneus longus muscle Popliteus muscle Soleus muscle Tibialis anterior muscle Tibialis posterior muscle
Knee Joint, Femoral Surface, Left **Knee Joint, Femoral Surface, Right**	**Includes:** Femoropatellar joint Patellofemoral joint	**Lower Leg Tendon, Left** **Lower Leg Tendon, Right**	**Includes:** Achilles tendon
Knee Joint, Left **Knee Joint, Right**	**Includes:** Femoropatellar joint Femorotibial joint Lateral meniscus Medial meniscus Patellofemoral joint Tibiofemoral joint	**Lower Lip**	**Includes:** Frenulum labii inferioris Labial gland Vermilion border
Knee Joint, Tibial Surface, Left **Knee Joint, Tibial Surface, Right**	**Includes:** Femorotibial joint Tibiofemoral joint	**Lower Spine Bursa and Ligament**	**Includes:** Iliolumbar ligament Interspinous ligament, lumbar Intertransverse ligament, lumbar Ligamentum flavum, lumbar Sacrococcygeal ligament Sacroiliac ligament Sacrospinous ligament Sacrotuberous ligament Supraspinous ligament
Knee Tendon, Left **Knee Tendon, Right**	**Includes:** Patellar tendon		
Lacrimal Duct, Left **Lacrimal Duct, Right**	**Includes:** Lacrimal canaliculus Lacrimal punctum Lacrimal sac Nasolacrimal duct	**Lumbar Nerve**	**Includes:** Lumbosacral trunk Spinal nerve, lumbar Superior clunic (cluneal) nerve
Larynx	**Includes:** Aryepiglottic fold Arytenoid cartilage Corniculate cartilage Cuneiform cartilage False vocal cord Glottis Rima glottidis Thyroid cartilage Ventricular fold	**Lumbar Plexus**	**Includes:** Accessory obturator nerve Genitofemoral nerve Iliohypogastric nerve Ilioinguinal nerve Lateral femoral cutaneous nerve Obturator nerve Superior gluteal nerve
Lens, Left **Lens, Right**	**Includes:** Zonule of Zinn	**Lumbar Spinal Cord**	**Includes:** Cauda equina Conus medullaris
Liver	**Includes:** Quadrate lobe	**Lumbar Sympathetic Nerve**	**Includes:** Lumbar ganglion Lumbar splanchnic nerve
Lower Arm and Wrist Muscle, Left **Lower Arm and Wrist Muscle, Right**	**Includes:** Anatomical snuffbox Brachioradialis muscle Extensor carpi radialis muscle Extensor carpi ulnaris muscle Flexor carpi radialis muscle Flexor carpi ulnaris muscle Flexor pollicis longus muscle Palmaris longus muscle Pronator quadratus muscle Pronator teres muscle	**Lumbar Vertebra**	**Includes:** Spinous process Transverse process Vertebral arch Vertebral body Vertebral foramen Vertebral lamina Vertebral pedicle
Lower Artery	**Includes:** Umbilical artery	**Lumbar Vertebral Joint**	**Includes:** Lumbar facet joint
Lower Eyelid, Left **Lower Eyelid, Right**	**Includes:** Inferior tarsal plate Medial canthus	**Lumbosacral Joint**	**Includes:** Lumbosacral facet joint
Lower Femur, Left **Lower Femur, Right**	**Includes:** Lateral condyle of femur Lateral epicondyle of femur Medial condyle of femur Medial epicondyle of femur		

ICD-10-PCS Value	Definition
Lymphatic, Aortic	**Includes:** Celiac lymph node Gastric lymph node Hepatic lymph node Lumbar lymph node Pancreaticosplenic lymph node Paraaortic lymph node Retroperitoneal lymph node
Lymphatic, Head	**Includes:** Buccinator lymph node Infraauricular lymph node Infraparotid lymph node Parotid lymph node Preauricular lymph node Submandibular lymph node Submaxillary lymph node Submental lymph node Subparotid lymph node Suprahyoid lymph node
Lymphatic, Left Axillary	**Includes:** Anterior (pectoral) lymph node Apical (subclavicular) lymph node Brachial (lateral) lymph node Central axillary lymph node Lateral (brachial) lymph node Pectoral (anterior) lymph node Posterior (subscapular) lymph node Subclavicular (apical) lymph node Subscapular (posterior) lymph node
Lymphatic, Left Lower Extremity	**Includes:** Femoral lymph node Popliteal lymph node
Lymphatic, Left Neck	**Includes:** Cervical lymph node Jugular lymph node Mastoid (postauricular) lymph node Occipital lymph node Postauricular (mastoid) lymph node Retropharyngeal lymph node Supraclavicular (Virchow's) lymph node Virchow's (supraclavicular) lymph node
Lymphatic, Left Upper Extremity	**Includes:** Cubital lymph node Deltopectoral (infraclavicular) lymph node Epitrochlear lymph node Infraclavicular (deltopectoral) lymph node Supratrochlear lymph node
Lymphatic, Mesenteric	**Includes:** Inferior mesenteric lymph node Pararectal lymph node Superior mesenteric lymph node
Lymphatic, Pelvis	**Includes:** Common iliac (subaortic) lymph node Gluteal lymph node Iliac lymph node Inferior epigastric lymph node Obturator lymph node Sacral lymph node Subaortic (common iliac) lymph node Suprainguinal lymph node

ICD-10-PCS Value	Definition
Lymphatic, Right Axillary	**Includes:** Anterior (pectoral) lymph node Apical (subclavicular) lymph node Brachial (lateral) lymph node Central axillary lymph node Lateral (brachial) lymph node Pectoral (anterior) lymph node Posterior (subscapular) lymph node Subclavicular (apical) lymph node Subscapular (posterior) lymph node
Lymphatic, Right Lower Extremity	**Includes:** Femoral lymph node Popliteal lymph node
Lymphatic, Right Neck	**Includes:** Cervical lymph node Jugular lymph node Mastoid (postauricular) lymph node Occipital lymph node Postauricular (mastoid) lymph node Retropharyngeal lymph node Right jugular trunk Right lymphatic duct Right subclavian trunk Supraclavicular (Virchow's) lymph node Virchow's (supraclavicular) lymph node
Lymphatic, Right Upper Extremity	**Includes:** Cubital lymph node Deltopectoral (infraclavicular) lymph node Epitrochlear lymph node Infraclavicular (deltopectoral) lymph node Supratrochlear lymph node
Lymphatic, Thorax	**Includes:** Intercostal lymph node Mediastinal lymph node Parasternal lymph node Paratracheal lymph node Tracheobronchial lymph node
Main Bronchus, Right	**Includes:** Bronchus intermedius Intermediate bronchus
Mandible, Left **Mandible, Right**	**Includes:** Alveolar process of mandible Condyloid process Mandibular notch Mental foramen
Mastoid Sinus, Left **Mastoid Sinus, Right**	**Includes:** Mastoid air cells
Maxilla	**Includes:** Alveolar process of maxilla
Maxillary Sinus, Left **Maxillary Sinus, Right**	**Includes:** Antrum of Highmore
Median Nerve	**Includes:** Anterior interosseous nerve Palmar cutaneous nerve
Mediastinum	**Includes:** Mediastinal cavity Mediastinal space
Medulla Oblongata	**Includes:** Myelencephalon
Mesentery	**Includes:** Mesoappendix Mesocolon

ICD-10-PCS Value	Definition
Metatarsal-Phalangeal Joint, Left **Metatarsal-Phalangeal Joint, Right**	**Includes:** Metatarsophalangeal (MTP) joint
Middle Ear, Left **Middle Ear, Right**	**Includes:** Oval window Tympanic cavity
Minor Salivary Gland	**Includes:** Anterior lingual gland
Mitral Valve	**Includes:** Bicuspid valve Left atrioventricular valve Mitral annulus
Nasal Bone	**Includes:** Vomer of nasal septum
Nasal Mucosa and Soft Tissue	**Includes:** Columella External naris Greater alar cartilage Internal naris Lateral nasal cartilage Lesser alar cartilage Nasal cavity Nostril
Nasal Septum	**Includes:** Quadrangular cartilage Septal cartilage Vomer bone
Nasal Turbinate	**Includes:** Inferior turbinate Middle turbinate Nasal concha Superior turbinate
Nasopharynx	**Includes:** Choana Fossa of Rosenmuller Pharyngeal recess Rhinopharynx
Neck Muscle, Left **Neck Muscle, Right**	**Includes:** Anterior vertebral muscle Arytenoid muscle Cricothyroid muscle Infrahyoid muscle Levator scapulae muscle Platysma muscle Scalene muscle Splenius cervicis muscle Sternocleidomastoid muscle Suprahyoid muscle Thyroarytenoid muscle
Nipple, Left **Nipple, Right**	**Includes:** Areola
Occipital Bone	**Includes:** Foramen magnum
Oculomotor Nerve	**Includes:** Third cranial nerve
Olfactory Nerve	**Includes:** First cranial nerve Olfactory bulb

ICD-10-PCS Value	Definition
Omentum	**Includes:** Gastrocolic ligament Gastrocolic omentum Gastrohepatic omentum Gastrophrenic ligament Gastrosplenic ligament Greater Omentum Hepatogastric ligament Lesser Omentum
Optic Nerve	**Includes:** Optic chiasma Second cranial nerve
Orbit, Left **Orbit, Right**	**Includes:** Bony orbit Orbital portion of ethmoid bone Orbital portion of frontal bone Orbital portion of lacrimal bone Orbital portion of maxilla Orbital portion of palatine bone Orbital portion of sphenoid bone Orbital portion of zygomatic bone
Pancreatic Duct	**Includes:** Duct of Wirsung
Pancreatic Duct, Accessory	**Includes:** Duct of Santorini
Parotid Duct, Left **Parotid Duct, Right**	**Includes:** Stensen's duct
Pelvic Bone, Left **Pelvic Bone, Right**	**Includes:** Iliac crest Ilium Ischium Pubis
Pelvic Cavity	**Includes:** Retropubic space
Penis	**Includes:** Corpus cavernosum Corpus spongiosum
Perineum Muscle	**Includes:** Bulbospongiosus muscle Cremaster muscle Deep transverse perineal muscle Ischiocavernosus muscle Levator ani muscle Superficial transverse perineal muscle
Peritoneum	**Includes:** Epiploic foramen
Peroneal Artery, Left **Peroneal Artery, Right**	**Includes:** Fibular artery
Peroneal Nerve	**Includes:** Common fibular nerve Common peroneal nerve External popliteal nerve Lateral sural cutaneous nerve
Pharynx	**Includes:** Base of Tongue Hypopharynx Laryngopharynx Lingual tonsil Oropharynx Piriform recess (sinus) Tongue, base of
Phrenic Nerve	**Includes:** Accessory phrenic nerve

ICD-10-PCS Value	Definition
Pituitary Gland	**Includes:** Adenohypophysis Hypophysis Neurohypophysis
Pons	**Includes:** Apneustic center Basis pontis Locus ceruleus Pneumotaxic center Pontine tegmentum Superior olivary nucleus
Popliteal Artery, Left Popliteal Artery, Right	**Includes:** Inferior genicular artery Middle genicular artery Superior genicular artery Sural artery Tibioperoneal trunk
Portal Vein	**Includes:** Hepatic portal vein
Prepuce	**Includes:** Foreskin Glans penis
Pudendal Nerve	**Includes:** Posterior labial nerve Posterior scrotal nerve
Pulmonary Artery, Left	**Includes:** Arterial canal (duct) Botallo's duct Pulmoaortic canal
Pulmonary Valve	**Includes:** Pulmonary annulus Pulmonic valve
Pulmonary Vein, Left	**Includes:** Left inferior pulmonary vein Left superior pulmonary vein
Pulmonary Vein, Right	**Includes:** Right inferior pulmonary vein Right superior pulmonary vein
Radial Artery, Left Radial Artery, Right	**Includes:** Radial recurrent artery
Radial Nerve	**Includes:** Dorsal digital nerve Musculospiral nerve Palmar cutaneous nerve Posterior interosseous nerve
Radius, Left Radius, Right	**Includes:** Ulnar notch
Rectum	**Includes:** Anorectal junction
Renal Artery, Left Renal Artery, Right	**Includes:** Inferior suprarenal artery Renal segmental artery
Renal Vein, Left	**Includes:** Left inferior phrenic vein Left ovarian vein Left second lumbar vein Left suprarenal vein Left testicular vein
Retina, Left Retina, Right	**Includes:** Fovea Macula Optic disc
Retroperitoneum	**Includes:** Retroperitoneal cavity Retroperitoneal space

ICD-10-PCS Value	Definition
Rib(s) Bursa and Ligament	**Includes:** Costotransverse ligament
Sacral Nerve	**Includes:** Spinal nerve, sacral
Sacral Plexus	**Includes:** Inferior gluteal nerve Posterior femoral cutaneous nerve Pudendal nerve
Sacral Sympathetic Nerve	**Includes:** Ganglion impar (ganglion of Walther) Pelvic splanchnic nerve Sacral ganglion Sacral splanchnic nerve
Sacrococcygeal Joint	**Includes:** Sacrococcygeal symphysis
Saphenous Vein, Left Saphenous Vein, Right	**Includes:** External pudendal vein Great(er) saphenous vein Lesser saphenous vein Small saphenous vein Superficial circumflex iliac vein Superficial epigastric vein
Scapula, Left Scapula, Right	**Includes:** Acromion (process) Coracoid process
Sciatic Nerve	**Includes:** Ischiatic nerve
Shoulder Bursa and Ligament, Left Shoulder Bursa and Ligament, Right	**Includes:** Acromioclavicular ligament Coracoacromial ligament Coracoclavicular ligament Coracohumeral ligament Costoclavicular ligament Glenohumeral ligament Interclavicular ligament Sternoclavicular ligament Subacromial bursa Transverse humeral ligament Transverse scapular ligament
Shoulder Joint, Left Shoulder Joint, Right	**Includes:** Glenohumeral joint Glenoid ligament (labrum)
Shoulder Muscle, Left Shoulder Muscle, Right	**Includes:** Deltoid muscle Infraspinatus muscle Subscapularis muscle Supraspinatus muscle Teres major muscle Teres minor muscle
Sigmoid Colon	**Includes:** Rectosigmoid junction Sigmoid flexure
Skin	**Includes:** Dermis Epidermis Sebaceous gland Sweat gland
Skin, Chest	**Includes:** Breast procedures, skin only
Sphenoid Bone	**Includes:** Greater wing Lesser wing Optic foramen Pterygoid process Sella turcica

ICD-10-PCS Value	Definition
Spinal Canal	**Includes:** Epidural space, spinal Extradural space, spinal Subarachnoid space, spinal Subdural space, spinal Vertebral canal
Spinal Meninges	**Includes:** Arachnoid mater, spinal Denticulate (dentate) ligament Dura mater, spinal Filum terminale Leptomeninges, spinal Pia mater, spinal
Spleen	**Includes:** Accessory spleen
Splenic Artery	**Includes:** Left gastroepiploic artery Pancreatic artery Short gastric artery
Splenic Vein	**Includes:** Left gastroepiploic vein Pancreatic vein
Sternum	**Includes:** Manubrium Suprasternal notch Xiphoid process
Sternum Bursa and Ligament	**Includes:** Costoxiphoid ligament Sternocostal ligament
Stomach, Pylorus	**Includes:** Pyloric antrum Pyloric canal Pyloric sphincter
Subclavian Artery, Left Subclavian Artery, Right	**Includes:** Costocervical trunk Dorsal scapular artery Internal thoracic artery
Subcutaneous Tissue and Fascia, Chest	**Includes:** Pectoral fascia
Subcutaneous Tissue and Fascia, Face	**Includes:** Masseteric fascia Orbital fascia Submandibular space
Subcutaneous Tissue and Fascia, Left Foot	**Includes:** Plantar fascia (aponeurosis)
Subcutaneous Tissue and Fascia, Left Hand	**Includes:** Palmar fascia (aponeurosis)
Subcutaneous Tissue and Fascia, Left Lower Arm	**Includes:** Antebrachial fascia Bicipital aponeurosis
Subcutaneous Tissue and Fascia, Left Neck	**Includes:** Deep cervical fascia Pretracheal fascia Prevertebral fascia
Subcutaneous Tissue and Fascia, Left Upper Arm	**Includes:** Axillary fascia Deltoid fascia Infraspinatus fascia Subscapular aponeurosis Supraspinatus fascia
Subcutaneous Tissue and Fascia, Left Upper Leg	**Includes:** Crural fascia Fascia lata Iliac fascia Iliotibial tract (band)

ICD-10-PCS Value	Definition
Subcutaneous Tissue and Fascia, Right Foot	**Includes:** Plantar fascia (aponeurosis)
Subcutaneous Tissue and Fascia, Right Hand	**Includes:** Palmar fascia (aponeurosis)
Subcutaneous Tissue and Fascia, Right Lower Arm	**Includes:** Antebrachial fascia Bicipital aponeurosis
Subcutaneous Tissue and Fascia, Right Neck	**Includes:** Deep cervical fascia Pretracheal fascia Prevertebral fascia
Subcutaneous Tissue and Fascia, Right Upper Arm	**Includes:** Axillary fascia Deltoid fascia Infraspinatus fascia Subscapular aponeurosis Supraspinatus fascia
Subcutaneous Tissue and Fascia, Right Upper Leg	**Includes:** Crural fascia Fascia lata Iliac fascia Iliotibial tract (band)
Subcutaneous Tissue and Fascia, Scalp	**Includes:** Galea aponeurotica
Subcutaneous Tissue and Fascia, Trunk	**Includes:** External oblique aponeurosis Transversalis fascia
Submaxillary Gland, Left Submaxillary Gland, Right	**Includes:** Submandibular gland
Superior Mesenteric Artery	**Includes:** Ileal artery Ileocolic artery Inferior pancreaticoduodenal artery Jejunal artery
Superior Mesenteric Vein	**Includes:** Right gastroepiploic vein
Superior Vena Cava	**Includes:** Precava
Tarsal Joint, Left Tarsal Joint, Right	**Includes:** Calcaneocuboid joint Cuboideonavicular joint Cuneonavicular joint Intercuneiform joint Subtalar (talocalcaneal) joint Talocalcaneal (subtalar) joint Talocalcaneonavicular joint
Tarsal, Left Tarsal, Right	**Includes:** Calcaneus Cuboid bone Intermediate cuneiform bone Lateral cuneiform bone Medial cuneiform bone Navicular bone Talus bone
Temporal Artery, Left Temporal Artery, Right	**Includes:** Middle temporal artery Superficial temporal artery Transverse facial artery
Temporal Bone, Left Temporal Bone, Right	**Includes:** Mastoid process Petrous part of temporal bone Tympanic part of temporal bone Zygomatic process of temporal bone

ICD-10-PCS Value	Definition
Thalamus	**Includes:** Epithalamus Geniculate nucleus Metathalamus Pulvinar
Thoracic Aorta, Ascending/Arch	**Includes:** Aortic arch Ascending aorta
Thoracic Duct	**Includes:** Left jugular trunk Left subclavian trunk
Thoracic Nerve	**Includes:** Intercostal nerve Intercostobrachial nerve Spinal nerve, thoracic Subcostal nerve
Thoracic Sympathetic Nerve	**Includes:** Cardiac plexus Esophageal plexus Greater splanchnic nerve Inferior cardiac nerve Least splanchnic nerve Lesser splanchnic nerve Middle cardiac nerve Pulmonary plexus Superior cardiac nerve Thoracic aortic plexus Thoracic ganglion
Thoracic Vertebra	**Includes:** Spinous process Transverse process Vertebral arch Vertebral body Vertebral foramen Vertebral lamina Vertebral pedicle
Thoracic Vertebral Joint	**Includes:** Costotransverse joint Costovertebral joint Thoracic facet joint
Thoracolumbar Vertebral Joint	**Includes:** Thoracolumbar facet joint
Thorax Muscle, Left Thorax Muscle, Right	**Includes:** Intercostal muscle Levatores costarum muscle Pectoralis major muscle Pectoralis minor muscle Serratus anterior muscle Subclavius muscle Subcostal muscle Transverse thoracis muscle
Thymus	**Includes:** Thymus gland
Thyroid Artery, Left Thyroid Artery, Right	**Includes:** Cricothyroid artery Hyoid artery Sternocleidomastoid artery Superior laryngeal artery Superior thyroid artery Thyrocervical trunk
Tibia, Left Tibia, Right	**Includes:** Lateral condyle of tibia Medial condyle of tibia Medial malleolus

ICD-10-PCS Value	Definition
Tibial Nerve	**Includes:** Lateral plantar nerve Medial plantar nerve Medial popliteal nerve Medial sural cutaneous nerve
Toe Nail	**Includes:** Nail bed Nail plate
Toe Phalangeal Joint, Left Toe Phalangeal Joint, Right	**Includes:** Interphalangeal (IP) joint
Tongue	**Includes:** Frenulum linguae
Tongue, Palate, Pharynx Muscle	**Includes:** Chondroglossus muscle Genioglossus muscle Hyoglossus muscle Inferior longitudinal muscle Levator veli palatini muscle Palatoglossal muscle Palatopharyngeal muscle Pharyngeal constrictor muscle Salpingopharyngeus muscle Styloglossus muscle Stylopharyngeus muscle Superior longitudinal muscle Tensor veli palatini muscle
Tonsils	**Includes:** Palatine tonsil
Trachea	**Includes:** Cricoid cartilage
Transverse Colon	**Includes:** Hepatic flexure Splenic flexure
Tricuspid Valve	**Includes:** Right atrioventricular valve Tricuspid annulus
Trigeminal Nerve	**Includes:** Fifth cranial nerve Gasserian ganglion Mandibular nerve Maxillary nerve Ophthalmic nerve Trifacial nerve
Trochlear Nerve	**Includes:** Fourth cranial nerve
Trunk Muscle, Left Trunk Muscle, Right	**Includes:** Coccygeus muscle Erector spinae muscle Interspinalis muscle Intertransversarius muscle Latissimus dorsi muscle Quadratus lumborum muscle Rhomboid major muscle Rhomboid minor muscle Serratus posterior muscle Transversospinalis muscle Trapezius muscle
Tympanic Membrane, Left Tympanic Membrane, Right	**Includes:** Pars flaccida
Ulna, Left Ulna, Right	**Includes:** Olecranon process Radial notch

ICD-10-PCS Value	Definition
Ulnar Artery, Left Ulnar Artery, Right	**Includes:** Anterior ulnar recurrent artery Common interosseous artery Posterior ulnar recurrent artery
Ulnar Nerve	**Includes:** Cubital nerve
Upper Arm Muscle, Left Upper Arm Muscle, Right	**Includes:** Biceps brachii muscle Brachialis muscle Coracobrachialis muscle Triceps brachii muscle
Upper Artery	**Includes:** Aortic intercostal artery Bronchial artery Esophageal artery Subcostal artery
Upper Eyelid, Left Upper Eyelid, Right	**Includes:** Lateral canthus Levator palpebrae superioris muscle Orbicularis oculi muscle Superior tarsal plate
Upper Femur, Left Upper Femur, Right	**Includes:** Femoral head Greater trochanter Lesser trochanter Neck of femur
Upper Leg Muscle, Left Upper Leg Muscle, Right	**Includes:** Adductor brevis muscle Adductor longus muscle Adductor magnus muscle Biceps femoris muscle Gracilis muscle Pectineus muscle Quadriceps (femoris) Rectus femoris muscle Sartorius muscle Semimembranosus muscle Semitendinosus muscle Vastus intermedius muscle Vastus lateralis muscle Vastus medialis muscle
Upper Lip	**Includes:** Frenulum labii superioris Labial gland Vermilion border
Upper Spine Bursa and Ligament	**Includes:** Interspinous ligament, thoracic Intertransverse ligament, thoracic Ligamentum flavum, thoracic Supraspinous ligament
Ureter Ureter, Left Ureter, Right Ureters, Bilateral	**Includes:** Ureteral orifice Ureterovesical orifice
Urethra	**Includes:** Bulbourethral (Cowper's) gland Cowper's (bulbourethral) gland External urethral sphincter Internal urethral sphincter Membranous urethra Penile urethra Prostatic urethra
Uterine Supporting Structure	**Includes:** Broad ligament Infundibulopelvic ligament Ovarian ligament Round ligament of uterus

ICD-10-PCS Value	Definition
Uterus	**Includes:** Fundus uteri Myometrium Perimetrium Uterine cornu
Uvula	**Includes:** Palatine uvula
Vagus Nerve	**Includes:** Anterior vagal trunk Pharyngeal plexus Pneumogastric nerve Posterior vagal trunk Pulmonary plexus Recurrent laryngeal nerve Superior laryngeal nerve Tenth cranial nerve
Vas Deferens Vas Deferens, Bilateral Vas Deferens, Left Vas Deferens, Right	**Includes:** Ductus deferens Ejaculatory duct
Ventricle, Right	**Includes:** Conus arteriosus
Ventricular Septum	**Includes:** Interventricular septum
Vertebral Artery, Left Vertebral Artery, Right	**Includes:** Anterior spinal artery Posterior spinal artery
Vertebral Vein, Left Vertebral Vein, Right	**Includes:** Deep cervical vein Suboccipital venous plexus
Vestibular Gland	**Includes:** Bartholin's (greater vestibular) gland Greater vestibular (Bartholin's) gland Paraurethral (Skene's) gland Skene's (paraurethral) gland
Vitreous, Left Vitreous, Right	**Includes:** Vitreous body
Vocal Cord, Left Vocal Cord, Right	**Includes:** Vocal fold
Vulva	**Includes:** Labia majora Labia minora
Wrist Bursa and Ligament, Left Wrist Bursa and Ligament, Right	**Includes:** Palmar ulnocarpal ligament Radial collateral carpal ligament Radiocarpal ligament Radioulnar ligament Scapholunate ligament Ulnar collateral carpal ligament
Wrist Joint, Left Wrist Joint, Right	**Includes:** Distal radioulnar joint Radiocarpal joint

Appendix F: Device Classification

In most PCS codes, the sixth character of the code classifies the device. The sixth character device value "defines the material or appliance used to accomplish the objective of the procedure that remains in or on the procedure site at the end of the procedure." If the device is the means by which the procedural objective is accomplished, then a specific device value is coded in the sixth character. If no device is used to accomplish the objective of the procedure, the device value No Device is coded in the sixth character. In limited root operations, the classification provides the qualifier values Temporary and Intraoperative, for specific procedures involving clinically significant devices whose purpose is brief use during the procedure or current inpatient stay.

Material that is classified as a PCS device is distinguished from material classified as a PCS substance by its having a specific location. A device is intended to maintain a fixed location at the procedure site where it was put, whereas a substance is intended to disperse or be absorbed in the body. There are circumstances in which a device does not stay where it was put and may need to be "revised" in a subsequent procedure to move the device back to its intended location.

Material classified as a PCS device is also distinguishable by the fact that it is removable. Although it may not be practical to remove some types of devices once they become established at the site, it is physically possible to remove a device for some time after the procedure. A skin graft, for example, once it "takes," may be nearly indistinguishable from the surrounding skin and so is no longer clearly identifiable as a device. Nevertheless, procedures that involve material coded as a device can for the most part be "reversed" by removing the device from the procedure site.

General Device Types

Device Type	Definition	Examples
Grafts	Biological or synthetic material that **takes the place of all or a portion of a body part.**	Full- or partial-thickness skin grafts: • Autologous • Nonautologous • Synthetic • Zooplastic Other tissue grafts: • Bone • Tendon • Vascular
Prosthesis	Biological or synthetic material that **takes the place of all or a portion of a body part.**	Joint prosthesis: • Autologous • Nonautologous • Synthetic
Implants	**Therapeutic** material that is not absorbed by, eliminated by, or incorporated into a body part.	External fixation device Internal fixation device: • Orthopaedic pins • Intramedullary rods Radioactive element implant Mesh
Simple or mechanical appliances	Biological or synthetic material that **assists or prevents a physiological function.**	Drainage device Extraluminal device Endobrachial device Fusion device Intraluminal device (can be temporary) Tracheostomy device IUD
Electronic appliances	Electronic appliances used to **assist, monitor, take the pace of, or prevent a physiological function.**	Cardiac leads Diaphragmatic pacemaker External heart assist system Short-term external heart assist system (Intraoperative) Fetal monitoring Hearing device Monitoring device Neurostimulator
External appliances	Performed without making an incision or a puncture, external appliances are used for the purpose of **protection, immobilization, stretching, compression, or packing.**	Bandage Cast Packing material Pressure dressing Traction apparatus

Transplant/Grafting Tissue Type Terminology

Tissue Type	Terminology
Tissue or organ transferred into a new position in **the body of the same individual**	Autograft Autologous Autoplastic
Having to do with individuals or tissues that have **identical genes**, such as identical twins	Isograft Isologous Syngeneic Syngraft
Tissue or organ taken from **different individuals** of the same species	Allogeneic Allograft Homologous Homograft
Tissue or organ from a **cadaver**	Nonautologous
Tissue or organ from individuals of **different species**	Heterogeneic Heterologous Xenogeneic Xenograft Zooplastic

Device Key

Term	ICD-10-PCS Value
3f (Aortic) Bioprosthesis valve	Zooplastic Tissue in Heart and Great Vessels
AbioCor® Total Replacement Heart	Synthetic Substitute
Absolute Pro Vascular (OTW) Self-Expanding Stent System	Intraluminal Device
Acculink (RX) Carotid Stent System	Intraluminal Device
Acellular Hydrated Dermis	Nonautologous Tissue Substitute
Acetabular cup	Liner in Lower Joints
Activa PC neurostimulator	Stimulator Generator, Multiple Array for Insertion in Subcutaneous Tissue and Fascia
Activa RC neurostimulator	Stimulator Generator, Multiple Array Rechargeable for Insertion in Subcutaneous Tissue and Fascia
Activa SC neurostimulator	Stimulator Generator, Single Array for Insertion in Subcutaneous Tissue and Fascia
ACUITY™ Steerable Lead	Cardiac Lead, Pacemaker for Insertion in Heart and Great Vessels Cardiac Lead, Defibrillator for Insertion in Heart and Great Vessels
Advisa (MRI)	Pacemaker, Dual Chamber for Insertion in Subcutaneous Tissue and Fascia
AFX® Endovascular AAA System	Intraluminal Device
AMPLATZER® Muscular VSD Occluder	Synthetic Substitute
AMS 800® Urinary Control System	Artificial Sphincter in Urinary System
AneuRx® AAA Advantage®	Intraluminal Device
Annuloplasty ring	Synthetic Substitute
Articulating Spacer (Antibiotic)	Articulating Spacer in Lower Joints
Artificial anal sphincter (AAS)	Artificial Sphincter in Gastrointestinal System
Artificial bowel sphincter (neosphincter)	Artificial Sphincter in Gastrointestinal System
Artificial urinary sphincter (AUS)	Artificial Sphincter in Urinary System
Ascenda Intrathecal Catheter	Infusion Device
Assurant (Cobalt) stent	Intraluminal Device
AtriClip LAA Exclusion System	Extraluminal Device
Attain Ability® Lead	Cardiac Lead, Pacemaker for Insertion in Heart and Great Vessels Cardiac Lead, Defibrillator for Insertion in Heart and Great Vessels
Attain StarFix® (OTW) Lead	Cardiac Lead, Pacemaker for Insertion in Heart and Great Vessels Cardiac Lead, Defibrillator for Insertion in Heart and Great Vessels
Autograft	Autologous Tissue Substitute

Term	ICD-10-PCS Value
Autologous artery graft	Autologous Arterial Tissue in Heart and Great Vessels Autologous Arterial Tissue in Upper Arteries Autologous Arterial Tissue in Lower Arteries Autologous Arterial Tissue in Upper Veins Autologous Arterial Tissue in Lower Veins
Autologous vein graft	Autologous Venous Tissue in Heart and Great Vessels Autologous Venous Tissue in Upper Arteries Autologous Venous Tissue in Lower Arteries Autologous Venous Tissue in Upper Veins Autologous Venous Tissue in Lower Veins
Axial Lumbar Interbody Fusion System	Interbody Fusion Device in Lower Joints
AxiaLIF® System	Interbody Fusion Device in Lower Joints
BAK/C® Interbody Cervical Fusion System	Interbody Fusion Device in Upper Joints
Bard® Composix® (E/X)(LP) mesh	Synthetic Substitute
Bard® Composix® Kugel® patch	Synthetic Substitute
Bard® Dulex™ mesh	Synthetic Substitute
Bard® Ventralex™ hernia patch	Synthetic Substitute
Baroreflex Activation Therapy® (BAT®)	Stimulator Lead in Upper Arteries Stimulator Generator in Subcutaneous Tissue and Fascia
Barricaid® Annular Closure Device (ACD)	Synthetic Substitute
Berlin Heart Ventricular Assist Device	Implantable Heart Assist System in Heart and Great Vessels
Bioactive embolization coil(s)	Intraluminal Device, Bioactive in Upper Arteries
Biventricular external heart assist system	Short-term External Heart Assist System in Heart and Great Vessels
Blood glucose monitoring system	Monitoring Device
Bone anchored hearing device	Hearing Device, Bone Conduction for Insertion in Ear, Nose, Sinus Hearing Device, in Head and Facial Bones
Bone bank bone graft	Nonautologous Tissue Substitute
Bone screw (interlocking)(lag)(pedicle) (recessed)	Internal Fixation Device in Head and Facial Bones Internal Fixation Device in Upper Bones Internal Fixation Device in Lower Bones
Bovine pericardial valve	Zooplastic Tissue in Heart and Great Vessels
Bovine pericardium graft	Zooplastic Tissue in Heart and Great Vessels
Brachytherapy seeds	Radioactive Element
BRYAN® Cervical Disc System	Synthetic Substitute
BVS 5000 Ventricular Assist Device	Short-term External Heart Assist System in Heart and Great Vessels

Term	ICD-10-PCS Value
Cardiac contractility modulation lead	Cardiac Lead in Heart and Great Vessels
Cardiac event recorder	Monitoring Device
Cardiac resynchronization therapy (CRT) lead	Cardiac Lead, Pacemaker for Insertion in Heart and Great Vessels Cardiac Lead, Defibrillator for Insertion in Heart and Great Vessels
CardioMEMS® pressure sensor	Monitoring Device, Pressure Sensor for Insertion in Heart and Great Vessels
Carotid (artery) sinus (baroreceptor) lead	Stimulator Lead in Upper Arteries
Carotid WALLSTENT® Monorail® Endoprosthesis	Intraluminal Device
Centrimag® Blood Pump	Short-term External Heart Assist System in Heart and Great Vessels
Ceramic on ceramic bearing surface	Synthetic Substitute, Ceramic for Replacement in Lower Joints
Cesium-131 Collagen Implant	Radioactive Element, Cesium-131 Collagen Implant for Insertion in Central Nervous System and Cranial Nerves
CivaSheet®	Radioactive Element
Clamp and rod internal fixation system (CRIF)	Internal Fixation Device in Upper Bones Internal Fixation Device in Lower Bones
COALESCE® radiolucent interbody fusion device	Interbody Fusion Device, Radiolucent Porous in New Technology
CoAxia NeuroFlo catheter	Intraluminal Device
Cobalt/chromium head and polyethylene socket	Synthetic Substitute, Metal on Polyethylene for Replacement in Lower Joints
Cobalt/chromium head and socket	Synthetic Substitute, Metal for Replacement in Lower Joints
Cochlear implant (CI), multiple channel (electrode)	Hearing Device, Multiple Channel Cochlear Prosthesis for Insertion in Ear, Nose, Sinus
Cochlear implant (CI), single channel (electrode)	Hearing Device, Single Channel Cochlear Prosthesis for Insertion in Ear, Nose, Sinus
COGNIS® CRT-D	Cardiac Resynchronization Defibrillator Pulse Generator for Insertion in Subcutaneous Tissue and Fascia
COHERE® radiolucent interbody fusion device	Interbody Fusion Device, Radiolucent Porous in New Technology
Colonic Z-Stent®	Intraluminal Device
Complete (SE) stent	Intraluminal Device
Concerto II CRT-D	Cardiac Resynchronization Defibrillator Pulse Generator for Insertion in Subcutaneous Tissue and Fascia
CONSERVE® PLUS Total Resurfacing Hip System	Resurfacing Device in Lower Joints
Consulta CRT-D	Cardiac Resynchronization Defibrillator Pulse Generator for Insertion in Subcutaneous Tissue and Fascia
Consulta CRT-P	Cardiac Resynchronization Pacemaker Pulse Generator for Insertion in Subcutaneous Tissue and Fascia
CONTAK RENEWAL® 3 RF (HE) CRT-D	Cardiac Resynchronization Defibrillator Pulse Generator for Insertion in Subcutaneous Tissue and Fascia
Contegra Pulmonary Valved Conduit	Zooplastic Tissue in Heart and Great Vessels

Term	ICD-10-PCS Value
Continuous Glucose Monitoring (CGM) device	Monitoring Device
Cook Biodesign® Fistula Plug(s)	Nonautologous Tissue Substitute
Cook Biodesign® Hernia Graft(s)	Nonautologous Tissue Substitute
Cook Biodesign® Layered Graft(s)	Nonautologous Tissue Substitute
Cook Zenapro™ Layered Graft(s)	Nonautologous Tissue Substitute
Cook Zenith AAA Endovascular Graft	Intraluminal Device
Cook Zenith® Fenestrated AAA Endovascular Graft	Intraluminal Device, Branched or Fenestrated, One or Two Arteries for Restriction in Lower Arteries Intraluminal Device, Branched or Fenestrated, Three or More Arteries for Restriction in Lower Arteries
CoreValve transcatheter aortic valve	Zooplastic Tissue in Heart and Great Vessels
Cormet Hip Resurfacing System	Resurfacing Device in Lower Joints
CoRoent® XL	Interbody Fusion Device in Lower Joints
Corox (OTW) Bipolar Lead	Cardiac Lead, Pacemaker for Insertion in Heart and Great Vessels Cardiac Lead, Defibrillator for Insertion in Heart and Great Vessels
Cortical strip neurostimulator lead	Neurostimulator Lead in Central Nervous System and Cranial Nerves
Corvia IASD®	Synthetic Substitute
Cultured epidermal cell autograft	Autologous Tissue Substitute
CYPHER® Stent	Intraluminal Device, Drug-eluting in Heart and Great Vessels
Cystostomy tube	Drainage Device
DBS lead	Neurostimulator Lead in Central Nervous System and Cranial Nerves
DeBakey Left Ventricular Assist Device	Implantable Heart Assist System in Heart and Great Vessels
Deep brain neurostimulator lead	Neurostimulator Lead in Central Nervous System and Cranial Nerves
Delta frame external fixator	External Fixation Device, Hybrid for Insertion in Upper Bones External Fixation Device, Hybrid for Reposition in Upper Bones External Fixation Device, Hybrid for Insertion in Lower Bones External Fixation Device, Hybrid for Reposition in Lower Bones
Delta III Reverse shoulder prosthesis	Synthetic Substitute, Reverse Ball and Socket for Replacement in Upper Joints
Diaphragmatic pacemaker generator	Stimulator Generator in Subcutaneous Tissue and Fascia
Direct Lateral Interbody Fusion (DLIF) device	Interbody Fusion Device in Lower Joints
Driver stent (RX) (OTW)	Intraluminal Device
DuraHeart Left Ventricular Assist System	Implantable Heart Assist System in Heart and Great Vessels
Durata® Defibrillation Lead	Cardiac Lead, Defibrillator for Insertion in Heart and Great Vessels
DynaNail®	Internal Fixation Device, Sustained Compression for Fusion in Lower Joints Internal Fixation Device, Sustained Compression for Fusion in Upper Joints

Term	ICD-10-PCS Value
DynaNail Mini®	Internal Fixation Device, Sustained Compression for Fusion in Lower Joints Internal Fixation Device, Sustained Compression for Fusion in Upper Joints
Dynesys® Dynamic Stabilization System	Spinal Stabilization Device, Pedicle-Based for Insertion in Upper Joints Spinal Stabilization Device, Pedicle-Based for Insertion in Lower Joints
E-Luminexx™ (Biliary)(Vascular) Stent	Intraluminal Device
EDWARDS INTUITY Elite valve system	Zooplastic Tissue, Rapid Deployment Technique in New Technology
Electrical bone growth stimulator (EBGS)	Bone Growth Stimulator in Head and Facial Bones Bone Growth Stimulator in Upper Bones Bone Growth Stimulator in Lower Bones
Electrical muscle stimulation (EMS) lead	Stimulator Lead in Muscles
Electronic muscle stimulator lead	Stimulator Lead in Muscles
Eluvia™ Drug-eluting Vascular Stent System	Intraluminal Device, Sustained Release Drug-eluting in New Technology Intraluminal Device, Sustained Release Drug-eluting, Two in New Technology Intraluminal Device, Sustained Release Drug-eluting, Three in New Technology Intraluminal Device, Sustained Release Drug-eluting, Four or More in New Technology
Embolization coil(s)	Intraluminal Device
Endeavor® (III)(IV) (Sprint) Zotarolimus-eluting Coronary Stent System	Intraluminal Device, Drug-eluting in Heart and Great Vessels
Endologix AFX® Endovascular AAA System	Intraluminal Device
EndoSure® sensor	Monitoring Device, Pressure Sensor for Insertion in Heart and Great Vessels
ENDOTAK RELIANCE® (G) Defibrillation Lead	Cardiac Lead, Defibrillator for Insertion in Heart and Great Vessels
Endotracheal tube (cuffed)(double-lumen)	Intraluminal Device, Endotracheal Airway in Respiratory System
Endurant® Endovascular Stent Graft	Intraluminal Device
Endurant® II AAA stent graft system	Intraluminal Device
EnRhythm	Pacemaker, Dual Chamber for Insertion in Subcutaneous Tissue and Fascia
Enterra gastric neurostimulator	Stimulator Generator, Multiple Array for Insertion in Subcutaneous Tissue and Fascia
Epic™ Stented Tissue Valve (aortic)	Zooplastic Tissue in Heart and Great Vessels
Epicel® cultured epidermal autograft	Autologous Tissue Substitute
Esophageal obturator airway (EOA)	Intraluminal Device, Airway in Gastrointestinal System
Esteem® implantable hearing system	Hearing Device in Ear, Nose, Sinus
Evera (XT)(S)(DR/VR)	Defibrillator Generator for Insertion in Subcutaneous Tissue and Fascia

Term	ICD-10-PCS Value
Everolimus-eluting coronary stent	Intraluminal Device, Drug-eluting in Heart and Great Vessels
Ex-PRESS™ mini glaucoma shunt	Synthetic Substitute
EXCLUDER® AAA Endoprosthesis	Intraluminal Device Intraluminal Device, Branched or Fenestrated, One or Two Arteries for Restriction in Lower Arteries Intraluminal Device, Branched or Fenestrated, Three or More Arteries for Restriction in Lower Arteries
EXCLUDER® IBE Endoprosthesis	Intraluminal Device, Branched or Fenestrated, One or Two Arteries for Restriction in Lower Arteries
Express® (LD) Premounted Stent System	Intraluminal Device
Express® Biliary SD Monorail® Premounted Stent System	Intraluminal Device
Express® SD Renal Monorail® Premounted Stent System	Intraluminal Device
External fixator	External Fixation Device in Head and Facial Bones External Fixation Device in Upper Bones External Fixation Device in Lower Bones External Fixation Device in Upper Joints External Fixation Device in Lower Joints
EXtreme Lateral Interbody Fusion (XLIF) device	Interbody Fusion Device in Lower Joints
Facet replacement spinal stabilization device	Spinal Stabilization Device, Facet Replacement for Insertion in Upper Joints Spinal Stabilization Device, Facet Replacement for Insertion in Lower Joints
FLAIR® Endovascular Stent Graft	Intraluminal Device
Flexible Composite Mesh	Synthetic Substitute
Flow Diverter embolization device	Intraluminal Device, Flow Diverter for Restriction in Upper Arteries
Foley catheter	Drainage Device
Formula™ Balloon-Expandable Renal Stent System	Intraluminal Device
Freestyle (Stentless) Aortic Root Bioprosthesis	Zooplastic Tissue in Heart and Great Vessels
Fusion screw (compression)(lag)(locking)	Internal Fixation Device in Upper Joints Internal Fixation Device in Lower Joints
GammaTile™	Radioactive Element, Cesium-131 Collagen Implant for Insertion in Central Nervous System and Cranial Nerves
Gastric electrical stimulation (GES) lead	Stimulator Lead in Gastrointestinal System
Gastric pacemaker lead	Stimulator Lead in Gastrointestinal System
GORE EXCLUDER® AAA Endoprosthesis	Intraluminal Device Intraluminal Device, Branched or Fenestrated, One or Two Arteries for Restriction in Lower Arteries Intraluminal Device, Branched or Fenestrated, Three or More Arteries for Restriction in Lower Arteries
GORE EXCLUDER® IBE Endoprosthesis	Intraluminal Device, Branched or Fenestrated, One or Two Arteries for Restriction in Lower Arteries

Term	ICD-10-PCS Value
GORE TAG® Thoracic Endoprosthesis	Intraluminal Device
GORE® DUALMESH®	Synthetic Substitute
Guedel airway	Intraluminal Device, Airway in Mouth and Throat
Hancock Bioprosthesis (aortic)(mitral) valve	Zooplastic Tissue in Heart and Great Vessels
Hancock Bioprosthetic Valved Conduit	Zooplastic Tissue in Heart and Great Vessels
HeartMate 3™ LVAS	Implantable Heart Assist System in Heart and Great Vessels
HeartMate II® Left Ventricular Assist Device (LVAD)	Implantable Heart Assist System in Heart and Great Vessels
HeartMate XVE® Left Ventricular Assist Device (LVAD)	Implantable Heart Assist System in Heart and Great Vessels
Herculink (RX) Elite Renal Stent System	Intraluminal Device
Hip (joint) liner	Liner in Lower Joints
Holter valve ventricular shunt	Synthetic Substitute
IASD® (InterAtrial Shunt Device), Corvia	Synthetic Substitute
Ilizarov external fixator	External Fixation Device, Ring for Insertion in Upper Bones External Fixation Device, Ring for Reposition in Upper Bones External Fixation Device, Ring for Insertion in Lower Bones External Fixation Device, Ring for Reposition in Lower Bones
Ilizarov-Vecklich device	External Fixation Device, Limb Lengthening for Insertion in Upper Bones External Fixation Device, Limb Lengthening for Insertion in Lower Bones
Impella® heart pump	Short-term External Heart Assist System in Heart and Great Vessels
Implantable cardioverter-defibrillator (ICD)	Defibrillator Generator for Insertion in Subcutaneous Tissue and Fascia
Implantable drug infusion pump (anti-spasmodic) (chemotherapy)(pain)	Infusion Device, Pump in Subcutaneous Tissue and Fascia
Implantable glucose monitoring device	Monitoring Device
Implantable hemodynamic monitor (IHM)	Monitoring Device, Hemodynamic for Insertion in Subcutaneous Tissue and Fascia
Implantable hemodynamic monitoring system (IHMS)	Monitoring Device, Hemodynamic for Insertion in Subcutaneous Tissue and Fascia
Implantable Miniature Telescope™ (IMT)	Synthetic Substitute, Intraocular Telescope for Replacement in Eye
Implanted (venous)(access) port	Vascular Access Device, Totally Implantable in Subcutaneous Tissue and Fascia
InDura, intrathecal catheter (1P) (spinal)	Infusion Device
Injection reservoir, port	Vascular Access Device, Totally Implantable in Subcutaneous Tissue and Fascia
Injection reservoir, pump	Infusion Device, Pump in Subcutaneous Tissue and Fascia

Term	ICD-10-PCS Value
InterAtrial Shunt Device IASD®, Corvia	Synthetic Substitute
Interbody fusion (spine) cage	Interbody Fusion Device in Upper Joints Interbody Fusion Device in Lower Joints
Interspinous process spinal stabilization device	Spinal Stabilization Device, Interspinous Process for Insertion in Upper Joints Spinal Stabilization Device, Interspinous Process for Insertion in Lower Joints
InterStim® Therapy lead	Neurostimulator Lead in Peripheral Nervous System
InterStim® Therapy neurostimulator	Stimulator Generator, Single Array for Insertion in Subcutaneous Tissue and Fascia
Intramedullary (IM) rod (nail)	Internal Fixation Device, Intramedullary in Upper Bones Internal Fixation Device, Intramedullary in Lower Bones
Intramedullary skeletal kinetic distractor (ISKD)	Internal Fixation Device, Intramedullary in Upper Bones Internal Fixation Device, Intramedullary in Lower Bones
Intrauterine Device (IUD)	Contraceptive Device in Female Reproductive System
INTUITY Elite valve system, EDWARDS	Zooplastic Tissue, Rapid Deployment Technique in New Technology
Itrel (3)(4) neurostimulator	Stimulator Generator, Single Array for Insertion in Subcutaneous Tissue and Fascia
Joint fixation plate	Internal Fixation Device in Upper Joints Internal Fixation Device in Lower Joints
Joint liner (insert)	Liner in Lower Joints
Joint spacer (antibiotic)	Spacer in Upper Joints Spacer in Lower Joints
Kappa	Pacemaker, Dual Chamber for Insertion in Subcutaneous Tissue and Fascia
Kirschner wire (K-wire)	Internal Fixation Device in Head and Facial Bones Internal Fixation Device in Upper Bones Internal Fixation Device in Lower Bones Internal Fixation Device in Upper Joints Internal Fixation Device in Lower Joints
Knee (implant) insert	Liner in Lower Joints
Kuntscher nail	Internal Fixation Device, Intramedullary in Upper Bones Internal Fixation Device, Intramedullary in Lower Bones
LAP-BAND® adjustable gastric banding system	Extraluminal Device
LifeStent® (Flexstar)(XL) Vascular Stent System	Intraluminal Device
LIVIAN™ CRT-D	Cardiac Resynchronization Defibrillator Pulse Generator for Insertion in Subcutaneous Tissue and Fascia
Loop recorder, implantable	Monitoring Device
MAGEC® Spinal Bracing and Distraction System	Magnetically Controlled Growth Rod(s) in New Technology
Mark IV Breathing Pacemaker System	Stimulator Generator in Subcutaneous Tissue and Fascia
Maximo II DR (VR)	Defibrillator Generator for Insertion in Subcutaneous Tissue and Fascia

Term	ICD-10-PCS Value
Maximo II DR CRT-D	Cardiac Resynchronization Defibrillator Pulse Generator for Insertion in Subcutaneous Tissue and Fascia
Medtronic Endurant® II AAA stent graft system	Intraluminal Device
Melody® transcatheter pulmonary valve	Zooplastic Tissue in Heart and Great Vessels
Metal on metal bearing surface	Synthetic Substitute, Metal for Replacement in Lower Joints
Micro-Driver stent (RX) (OTW)	Intraluminal Device
MicroMed HeartAssist	Implantable Heart Assist System in Heart and Great Vessels
Micrus CERECYTE microcoil	Intraluminal Device, Bioactive in Upper Arteries
MIRODERM™ Biologic Wound Matrix	Skin Substitute, Porcine Liver Derived in New Technology
MitraClip valve repair system	Synthetic Substitute
Mitroflow® Aortic Pericardial Heart Valve	Zooplastic Tissue in Heart and Great Vessels
Mosaic Bioprosthesis (aortic) (mitral) valve	Zooplastic Tissue in Heart and Great Vessels
MULTI-LINK (VISION)(MINI-VISION)(ULTRA) Coronary Stent System	Intraluminal Device
nanoLOCK™ interbody fusion device	Interbody Fusion Device, Nanotextured Surface in New Technology
Nasopharyngeal airway (NPA)	Intraluminal Device, Airway in Ear, Nose, Sinus
Neuromuscular electrical stimulation (NEMS) lead	Stimulator Lead in Muscles
Neurostimulator generator, multiple channel	Stimulator Generator, Multiple Array for Insertion in Subcutaneous Tissue and Fascia
Neurostimulator generator, multiple channel rechargeable	Stimulator Generator, Multiple Array Rechargeable for Insertion in Subcutaneous Tissue and Fascia
Neurostimulator generator, single channel	Stimulator Generator, Single Array for Insertion in Subcutaneous Tissue and Fascia
Neurostimulator generator, single channel rechargeable	Stimulator Generator, Single Array Rechargeable for Insertion in Subcutaneous Tissue and Fascia
Neutralization plate	Internal Fixation Device in Head and Facial Bones Internal Fixation Device in Upper Bones Internal Fixation Device in Lower Bones
Nitinol framed polymer mesh	Synthetic Substitute
Non-tunneled central venous catheter	Infusion Device
Novacor Left Ventricular Assist Device	Implantable Heart Assist System in Heart and Great Vessels
Novation® Ceramic AHS® (Articulation Hip System)	Synthetic Substitute, Ceramic for Replacement in Lower Joints
Omnilink Elite Vascular Balloon Expandable Stent System	Intraluminal Device
Open Pivot Aortic Valve Graft (AVG)	Synthetic Substitute
Open Pivot (mechanical) Valve	Synthetic Substitute
Optimizer™ III implantable pulse generator	Contractility Modulation Device for Insertion in Subcutaneous Tissue and Fascia

Term	ICD-10-PCS Value
Oropharyngeal airway (OPA)	Intraluminal Device, Airway in Mouth and Throat
Ovatio™ CRT-D	Cardiac Resynchronization Defibrillator Pulse Generator for Insertion in Subcutaneous Tissue and Fascia
OXINIUM	Synthetic Substitute, Oxidized Zirconium on Polyethylene for Replacement in Lower Joints
Paclitaxel-eluting coronary stent	Intraluminal Device, Drug-eluting in Heart and Great Vessels
Paclitaxel-eluting peripheral stent	Intraluminal Device, Drug-eluting in Upper Arteries Intraluminal Device, Drug-eluting in Lower Arteries
Partially absorbable mesh	Synthetic Substitute
Pedicle-based dynamic stabilization device	Spinal Stabilization Device, Pedicle-Based for Insertion in Upper Joints Spinal Stabilization Device, Pedicle-Based for Insertion in Lower Joints
Perceval sutureless valve	Zooplastic Tissue, Rapid Deployment Technique in New Technology
Percutaneous endoscopic gastrojejunostomy (PEG/J) tube	Feeding Device in Gastrointestinal System
Percutaneous endoscopic gastrostomy (PEG) tube	Feeding Device in Gastrointestinal System
Percutaneous nephrostomy catheter	Drainage Device
Peripherally inserted central catheter (PICC)	Infusion Device
Pessary ring	Intraluminal Device, Pessary in Female Reproductive System
Phrenic nerve stimulator generator	Stimulator Generator in Subcutaneous Tissue and Fascia
Phrenic nerve stimulator lead	Diaphragmatic Pacemaker Lead in Respiratory System
PHYSIOMESH™ Flexible Composite Mesh	Synthetic Substitute
Pipeline™ (Flex) embolization device	Intraluminal Device, Flow Diverter for Restriction in Upper Arteries
Polyethylene socket	Synthetic Substitute, Polyethylene for Replacement in Lower Joints
Polymethylmethacrylate (PMMA)	Synthetic Substitute
Polypropylene mesh	Synthetic Substitute
Porcine (bioprosthetic) valve	Zooplastic Tissue in Heart and Great Vessels
PRECICE intramedullary limb lengthening system	Internal Fixation Device, Intramedullary Limb Lengthening for Insertion in Upper Bones Internal Fixation Device, Intramedullary Limb Lengthening for Insertion in Lower Bones
PRESTIGE® Cervical Disc	Synthetic Substitute
PrimeAdvanced neurostimulator (SureScan)(MRI Safe)	Stimulator Generator, Multiple Array for Insertion in Subcutaneous Tissue and Fascia
PROCEED™ Ventral Patch	Synthetic Substitute
Prodisc-C	Synthetic Substitute
Prodisc-L	Synthetic Substitute

Term	ICD-10-PCS Value
PROLENE Polypropylene Hernia System (PHS)	Synthetic Substitute
Protecta XT CRT-D	Cardiac Resynchronization Defibrillator Pulse Generator for Insertion in Subcutaneous Tissue and Fascia
Protecta XT DR (XT VR)	Defibrillator Generator for Insertion in Subcutaneous Tissue and Fascia
Protégé® RX Carotid Stent System	Intraluminal Device
Pump reservoir	Infusion Device, Pump in Subcutaneous Tissue and Fascia
REALIZE® Adjustable Gastric Band	Extraluminal Device
Rebound HRD® (Hernia Repair Device)	Synthetic Substitute
RestoreAdvanced neurostimulator (SureScan)(MRI Safe)	Stimulator Generator, Multiple Array Rechargeable for Insertion in Subcutaneous Tissue and Fascia
RestoreSensor neurostimulator (SureScan)(MRI Safe)	Stimulator Generator, Multiple Array Rechargeable for Insertion in Subcutaneous Tissue and Fascia
RestoreUltra neurostimulator (SureScan)(MRI Safe)	Stimulator Generator, Multiple Array Rechargeable for Insertion in Subcutaneous Tissue and Fascia
Reveal (LINQ)(DX)(XT)	Monitoring Device
Reverse® Shoulder Prosthesis	Synthetic Substitute, Reverse Ball and Socket for Replacement in Upper Joints
Revo MRI™ SureScan® pacemaker	Pacemaker, Dual Chamber for Insertion in Subcutaneous Tissue and Fascia
Rheos® System device	Stimulator Generator in Subcutaneous Tissue and Fascia
Rheos® System lead	Stimulator Lead in Upper Arteries
RNS System lead	Neurostimulator Lead in Central Nervous System and Cranial Nerves
RNS system neurostimulator generator	Neurostimulator Generator in Head and Facial Bones
S-ICD™ lead	Subcutaneous Defibrillator Lead in Subcutaneous Tissue and Fascia
Sacral nerve modulation (SNM) lead	Stimulator Lead in Urinary System
Sacral neuromodulation lead	Stimulator Lead in Urinary System
SAPIEN transcatheter aortic valve	Zooplastic Tissue in Heart and Great Vessels
SAVAL below-the-knee (BTK) drug-eluting stent system	Intraluminal Device, Sustained Release Drug-eluting in New Technology Intraluminal Device, Sustained Release Drug-eluting, Two in New Technology Intraluminal Device, Sustained Release Drug-eluting, Three in New Technology Intraluminal Device, Sustained Release Drug-eluting, Four or More in New Technology
Secura (DR) (VR)	Defibrillator Generator for Insertion in Subcutaneous Tissue and Fascia
Sheffield hybrid external fixator	External Fixation Device, Hybrid for Insertion in Upper Bones External Fixation Device, Hybrid for Reposition in Upper Bones External Fixation Device, Hybrid for Insertion in Lower Bones External Fixation Device, Hybrid for Reposition in Lower Bones

Term	ICD-10-PCS Value
Sheffield ring external fixator	External Fixation Device, Ring for Insertion in Upper Bones External Fixation Device, Ring for Reposition in Upper Bones External Fixation Device, Ring for Insertion in Lower Bones External Fixation Device, Ring for Reposition in Lower Bones
Single lead pacemaker (atrium)(ventricle)	Pacemaker, Single Chamber for Insertion in Subcutaneous Tissue and Fascia
Single lead rate responsive pacemaker (atrium)(ventricle)	Pacemaker, Single Chamber Rate Responsive for Insertion in Subcutaneous Tissue and Fascia
Sirolimus-eluting coronary stent	Intraluminal Device, Drug-eluting in Heart and Great Vessels
SJM Biocor® Stented Valve System	Zooplastic Tissue in Heart and Great Vessels
Spacer, Articulating (Antibiotic)	Articulating Spacer in Lower Joints
Spacer, Static (Antibiotic)	Spacer in Lower Joints
Spinal cord neurostimulator lead	Neurostimulator Lead in Central Nervous System and Cranial Nerves
Spinal growth rods, magnetically controlled	Magnetically Controlled Growth Rod(s) in New Technology
SpineJack® system	Synthetic Substitute, Mechanically Expandable (Paired) in New Technology
Spiration IBV™ Valve System	Intraluminal Device, Endobronchial Valve in Respiratory System
Static Spacer (Antibiotic)	Spacer in Lower Joints
Stent, intraluminal (cardiovascular) (gastrointestinal) (hepatobiliary)(urinary)	Intraluminal Device
Stented tissue valve	Zooplastic Tissue in Heart and Great Vessels
Stratos LV	Cardiac Resynchronization Pacemaker Pulse Generator for Insertion in Subcutaneous Tissue and Fascia
Subcutaneous injection reservoir, port	Vascular Access Device, Totally Implantable in Subcutaneous Tissue and Fascia
Subcutaneous injection reservoir, pump	Infusion Device, Pump in Subcutaneous Tissue and Fascia
Subdermal progesterone implant	Contraceptive Device in Subcutaneous Tissue and Fascia
Surpass Streamline™ Flow Diverter	Intraluminal Device, Flow Diverter for Restriction in Upper Arteries
Sutureless valve, Perceval	Zooplastic Tissue, Rapid Deployment Technique in New Technology
SynCardia Total Artificial Heart	Synthetic Substitute
Synchra CRT-P	Cardiac Resynchronization Pacemaker Pulse Generator for Insertion in Subcutaneous Tissue and Fascia
SyncroMed Pump	Infusion Device, Pump in Subcutaneous Tissue and Fascia
Talent® Converter	Intraluminal Device
Talent® Occluder	Intraluminal Device
Talent® Stent Graft (abdominal)(thoracic)	Intraluminal Device
TandemHeart® System	Short-term External Heart Assist System in Heart and Great Vessels

Term	ICD-10-PCS Value
TAXUS® Liberté® Paclitaxel-eluting Coronary Stent System	Intraluminal Device, Drug-eluting in Heart and Great Vessels
Therapeutic occlusion coil(s)	Intraluminal Device
Thoracostomy tube	Drainage Device
Thoratec IVAD (Implantable Ventricular Assist Device)	Implantable Heart Assist System in Heart and Great Vessels
Thoratec Paracorporeal Ventricular Assist Device	Short-term External Heart Assist System in Heart and Great Vessels
Tibial insert	Liner in Lower Joints
Tissue bank graft	Nonautologous Tissue Substitute
Tissue expander (inflatable)(injectable)	Tissue Expander in Skin and Breast Tissue Expander in Subcutaneous Tissue and Fascia
Titanium Sternal Fixation System (TSFS)	Internal Fixation Device, Rigid Plate for Insertion in Upper Bones Internal Fixation Device, Rigid Plate for Reposition in Upper Bones
Total artificial (replacement) heart	Synthetic Substitute
Tracheostomy tube	Tracheostomy Device in Respiratory System
Trifecta™ Valve (aortic)	Zooplastic Tissue in Heart and Great Vessels
Tunneled central venous catheter	Vascular Access Device, Tunneled in Subcutaneous Tissue and Fascia
Tunneled spinal (intrathecal) catheter	Infusion Device
Two lead pacemaker	Pacemaker, Dual Chamber for Insertion in Subcutaneous Tissue and Fascia
Ultraflex™ Precision Colonic Stent System	Intraluminal Device
ULTRAPRO Hernia System (UHS)	Synthetic Substitute
ULTRAPRO Partially Absorbable Lightweight Mesh	Synthetic Substitute
ULTRAPRO Plug	Synthetic Substitute
Ultrasonic osteogenic stimulator	Bone Growth Stimulator in Head and Facial Bones Bone Growth Stimulator in Upper Bones Bone Growth Stimulator in Lower Bones
Ultrasound bone healing system	Bone Growth Stimulator in Head and Facial Bones Bone Growth Stimulator in Upper Bones Bone Growth Stimulator in Lower Bones
Uniplanar external fixator	External Fixation Device, Monoplanar for Insertion in Upper Bones External Fixation Device, Monoplanar for Reposition in Upper Bones External Fixation Device, Monoplanar for Insertion in Lower Bones External Fixation Device, Monoplanar for Reposition in Lower Bones
Urinary incontinence stimulator lead	Stimulator Lead in Urinary System
V-Wave Interatrial Shunt System	Synthetic Substitute
Vaginal pessary	Intraluminal Device, Pessary in Female Reproductive System
Valiant Thoracic Stent Graft	Intraluminal Device
Vectra® Vascular Access Graft	Vascular Access Device, Tunneled in Subcutaneous Tissue and Fascia

Term	ICD-10-PCS Value
Ventrio™ Hernia Patch	Synthetic Substitute
Versa	Pacemaker, Dual Chamber for Insertion in Subcutaneous Tissue and Fascia
Virtuoso (II) (DR) (VR)	Defibrillator Generator for Insertion in Subcutaneous Tissue and Fascia
Viva(XT)(S)	Cardiac Resynchronization Defibrillator Pulse Generator for Insertion in Subcutaneous Tissue and Fascia
WALLSTENT® Endoprosthesis	Intraluminal Device
X-STOP® Spacer	Spinal Stabilization Device, Interspinous Process for Insertion in Upper Joints Spinal Stabilization Device, Interspinous Process for Insertion in Lower Joints
Xact Carotid Stent System	Intraluminal Device
Xenograft	Zooplastic Tissue in Heart and Great Vessels
XIENCE Everolimus Eluting Coronary Stent System	Intraluminal Device, Drug-eluting in Heart and Great Vessels
XLIF® System	Interbody Fusion Device in Lower Joints
Zenith® Fenestrated AAA Endovascular Graft	Intraluminal Device, Branched or Fenestrated, One or Two Arteries for Restriction in Lower Arteries Intraluminal Device, Branched or Fenestrated, Three or More Arteries for Restriction in Lower Arteries Intraluminal Device
Zenith Flex® AAA Endovascular Graft	Intraluminal Device
Zenith TX2® TAA Endovascular Graft	Intraluminal Device
Zenith® Renu™ AAA Ancillary Graft	Intraluminal Device
Zilver® PTX® (paclitaxel) Drug-Eluting Peripheral Stent	Intraluminal Device, Drug-eluting in Upper Arteries Intraluminal Device, Drug-eluting in Lower Arteries
Zimmer® NexGen® LPS Mobile Bearing Knee	Synthetic Substitute
Zimmer® NexGen® LPS-Flex Mobile Knee	Synthetic Substitute
Zotarolimus-eluting coronary stent	Intraluminal Device, Drug-eluting in Heart and Great Vessels

Device Aggregation Table

This table crosswalks specific device character value definitions for specific root operations in a specific body system to the more general device character value to be used when the root operation covers a wide range of body parts and the device character represents an entire family of devices.

Specific Device	for Operation	in Body System	General Device	
Autologous Arterial Tissue (A)	All applicable	Heart and Great Vessels Lower Arteries Lower Veins Upper Arteries Upper Veins	7	Autologous Tissue Substitute
Autologous Venous Tissue (9)	All applicable	Heart and Great Vessels Lower Arteries Lower Veins Upper Arteries Upper Veins	7	Autologous Tissue Substitute
Cardiac Lead, Defibrillator (K)	Insertion	Heart and Great Vessels	M	Cardiac Lead
Cardiac Lead, Pacemaker (J)	Insertion	Heart and Great Vessels	M	Cardiac Lead
Cardiac Resynchronization Defibrillator Pulse Generator (9)	Insertion	Subcutaneous Tissue and Fascia	P	Cardiac Rhythm Related Device
Cardiac Resynchronization Pacemaker Pulse Generator (7)	Insertion	Subcutaneous Tissue and Fascia	P	Cardiac Rhythm Related Device
Contractility Modulation Device (A)	Insertion	Subcutaneous Tissue and Fascia	P	Cardiac Rhythm Related Device
Defibrillator Generator (8)	Insertion	Subcutaneous Tissue and Fascia	P	Cardiac Rhythm Related Device
Epiretinal Visual Prosthesis (5)	All applicable	Eye	J	Synthetic Substitute
External Fixation Device, Hybrid (D)	Insertion	Lower Bones Upper Bones	5	External Fixation Device
External Fixation Device, Hybrid (D)	Reposition	Lower Bones Upper Bones	5	External Fixation Device
External Fixation Device, Limb Lengthening (8)	Insertion	Lower Bones Upper Bones	5	External Fixation Device
External Fixation Device, Monoplanar (B)	Insertion	Lower Bones Upper Bones	5	External Fixation Device
External Fixation Device, Monoplanar (B)	Reposition	Lower Bones Upper Bones	5	External Fixation Device
External Fixation Device, Ring (C)	Insertion	Lower Bones Upper Bones	5	External Fixation Device
External Fixation Device, Ring (C)	Reposition	Lower Bones Upper Bones	5	External Fixation Device
Hearing Device, Bone Conduction (4)	Insertion	Ear, Nose, Sinus	S	Hearing Device
Hearing Device, Multiple Channel Cochlear Prosthesis (6)	Insertion	Ear, Nose, Sinus	S	Hearing Device
Hearing Device, Single Channel Cochlear Prosthesis (5)	Insertion	Ear, Nose, Sinus	S	Hearing Device
Internal Fixation Device, Intramedullary (6)	All applicable	Lower Bones Upper Bones	4	Internal Fixation Device
Internal Fixation Device, Intramedullary Limb Lengthening (7)	Insertion	Lower Bones Upper Bones	6	Internal Fixation Device, Intramedullary
Internal Fixation Device, Rigid Plate (Ø)	Insertion	Upper Bones	4	Internal Fixation Device
Internal Fixation Device, Rigid Plate (Ø)	Reposition	Upper Bones	4	Internal Fixation Device
Intraluminal Device, Airway (B)	All applicable	Ear, Nose, Sinus Gastrointestinal System Mouth and Throat	D	Intraluminal Device
Intraluminal Device, Bioactive (B)	All applicable	Upper Arteries	D	Intraluminal Device
Intraluminal Device, Branched or Fenestrated, One or Two Arteries (E)	Restriction	Heart and Great Vessels Lower Arteries	D	Intraluminal Device
Intraluminal Device, Branched or Fenestrated, Three or More Arteries (F)	Restriction	Heart and Great Vessels Lower Arteries	D	Intraluminal Device
Intraluminal Device, Drug-eluting (4)	All applicable	Heart and Great Vessels Lower Arteries Upper Arteries	D	Intraluminal Device
Intraluminal Device, Drug-eluting, Four or More (7)	All applicable	Heart and Great Vessels Lower Arteries Upper Arteries	D	Intraluminal Device

Specific Device	for Operation	in Body System	General Device	
Intraluminal Device, Drug-eluting, Three (6)	All applicable	Heart and Great Vessels Lower Arteries Upper Arteries	D	Intraluminal Device
Intraluminal Device, Drug-eluting, Two (5)	All applicable	Heart and Great Vessels Lower Arteries Upper Arteries	D	Intraluminal Device
Intraluminal Device, Endobronchial Valve (G)	All applicable	Respiratory System	D	Intraluminal Device
Intraluminal Device, Endotracheal Airway (E)	All applicable	Respiratory System	D	Intraluminal Device
Intraluminal Device, Flow Diverter (H)	Restriction	Upper Arteries	D	Intraluminal Device
Intraluminal Device, Four or More (G)	All applicable	Heart and Great Vessels Lower Arteries Upper Arteries	D	Intraluminal Device
Intraluminal Device, Pessary (G)	All applicable	Female Reproductive System	D	Intraluminal Device
Intraluminal Device, Radioactive (T)	All applicable	Heart and Great Vessels	D	Intraluminal Device
Intraluminal Device, Three (F)	All applicable	Heart and Great Vessels Lower Arteries Upper Arteries	D	Intraluminal Device
Intraluminal Device, Two (E)	All applicable	Heart and Great Vessels Lower Arteries Upper Arteries	D	Intraluminal Device
Monitoring Device, Hemodynamic (Ø)	Insertion	Subcutaneous Tissue and Fascia	2	Monitoring Device
Monitoring Device, Pressure Sensor (Ø)	Insertion	Heart and Great Vessels	2	Monitoring Device
Pacemaker, Dual Chamber (6)	Insertion	Subcutaneous Tissue and Fascia	P	Cardiac Rhythm Related Device
Pacemaker, Single Chamber (4)	Insertion	Subcutaneous Tissue and Fascia	P	Cardiac Rhythm Related Device
Pacemaker, Single Chamber Rate Responsive (5)	Insertion	Subcutaneous Tissue and Fascia	P	Cardiac Rhythm Related Device
Spinal Stabilization Device, Facet Replacement (D)	Insertion	Lower Joints Upper Joints	4	Internal Fixation Device
Spinal Stabilization Device, Interspinous Process (B)	Insertion	Lower Joints Upper Joints	4	Internal Fixation Device
Spinal Stabilization Device, Pedicle-Based (C)	Insertion	Lower Joints Upper Joints	4	Internal Fixation Device
Stimulator Generator, Multiple Array (D)	Insertion	Subcutaneous Tissue and Fascia	M	Stimulator Generator
Stimulator Generator, Multiple Array Rechargeable (E)	Insertion	Subcutaneous Tissue and Fascia	M	Stimulator Generator
Stimulator Generator, Single Array (B)	Insertion	Subcutaneous Tissue and Fascia	M	Stimulator Generator
Stimulator Generator, Single Array Rechargeable (C)	Insertion	Subcutaneous Tissue and Fascia	M	Stimulator Generator
Synthetic Substitute, Ceramic (3)	Replacement	Lower Joints	J	Synthetic Substitute
Synthetic Substitute, Ceramic on Polyethylene (4)	Replacement	Lower Joints	J	Synthetic Substitute
Synthetic Substitute, Intraocular Telescope (Ø)	Replacement	Eye	J	Synthetic Substitute
Synthetic Substitute, Metal (1)	Replacement	Lower Joints	J	Synthetic Substitute
Synthetic Substitute, Metal on Polyethylene (2)	Replacement	Lower Joints	J	Synthetic Substitute
Synthetic Substitute, Oxidized Zirconium on Polyethylene (6)	Replacement	Lower Joints	J	Synthetic Substitute
Synthetic Substitute, Polyethylene (Ø)	Replacement	Lower Joints	J	Synthetic Substitute
Synthetic Substitute, Reverse Ball and Socket (Ø)	Replacement	Upper Joints	J	Synthetic Substitute

Appendix H: Device Definitions

ICD-10-PCS Value	Definition
Articulating Spacer in Lower Joints	**Includes:** Articulating Spacer (Antibiotic) Spacer, Articulating (Antibiotic)
Artificial Sphincter in Gastrointestinal System	**Includes:** Artificial anal sphincter (AAS) Artificial bowel sphincter (neosphincter)
Artificial Sphincter in Urinary System	**Includes:** AMS 800® Urinary Control System Artificial urinary sphincter (AUS)
Autologous Arterial Tissue in Heart and Great Vessels	**Includes:** Autologous artery graft
Autologous Arterial Tissue in Lower Arteries	**Includes:** Autologous artery graft
Autologous Arterial Tissue in Lower Veins	**Includes:** Autologous artery graft
Autologous Arterial Tissue in Upper Arteries	**Includes:** Autologous artery graft
Autologous Arterial Tissue in Upper Veins	**Includes:** Autologous artery graft
Autologous Tissue Substitute	**Includes:** Autograft Cultured epidermal cell autograft Epicel® cultured epidermal autograft
Autologous Venous Tissue in Heart and Great Vessels	**Includes:** Autologous vein graft
Autologous Venous Tissue in Lower Arteries	**Includes:** Autologous vein graft
Autologous Venous Tissue in Lower Veins	**Includes:** Autologous vein graft
Autologous Venous Tissue in Upper Arteries	**Includes:** Autologous vein graft
Autologous Venous Tissue in Upper Veins	**Includes:** Autologous vein graft
Bone Growth Stimulator in Head and Facial Bones	**Includes:** Electrical bone growth stimulator (EBGS) Ultrasonic osteogenic stimulator Ultrasound bone healing system
Bone Growth Stimulator in Lower Bones	**Includes:** Electrical bone growth stimulator (EBGS) Ultrasonic osteogenic stimulator Ultrasound bone healing system
Bone Growth Stimulator in Upper Bones	**Includes:** Electrical bone growth stimulator (EBGS) Ultrasonic osteogenic stimulator Ultrasound bone healing system
Cardiac Lead in Heart and Great Vessels	**Includes:** Cardiac contractility modulation lead

ICD-10-PCS Value	Definition
Cardiac Lead, Defibrillator for Insertion in Heart and Great Vessels	**Includes:** ACUITY™ Steerable Lead Attain Ability® lead Attain StarFix® (OTW) lead Cardiac resynchronization therapy (CRT) lead Corox (OTW) Bipolar Lead Durata® Defibrillation Lead ENDOTAK RELIANCE® (G) Defibrillation Lead
Cardiac Lead, Pacemaker for Insertion in Heart and Great Vessels	**Includes:** ACUITY™ Steerable Lead Attain Ability® lead Attain StarFix® (OTW) lead Cardiac resynchronization therapy (CRT) lead Corox (OTW) Bipolar Lead
Cardiac Resynchronization Defibrillator Pulse Generator for Insertion in Subcutaneous Tissue and Fascia	**Includes:** COGNIS® CRT-D Concerto II CRT-D Consulta CRT-D CONTAK RENEWA® 3 RF (HE) CRT-D LIVIAN™ CRT-D Maximo II DR CRT-D Ovatio™ CRT-D Protecta XT CRT-D Viva (XT)(S)
Cardiac Resynchronization Pacemaker Pulse Generator for Insertion in Subcutaneous Tissue and Fascia	**Includes:** Consulta CRT-P Stratos LV Synchra CRT-P
Contraceptive Device in Female Reproductive System	**Includes:** Intrauterine device (IUD)
Contraceptive Device in Subcutaneous Tissue and Fascia	**Includes:** Subdermal progesterone implant
Contractility Modulation Device for Insertion in Subcutaneous Tissue and Fascia	**Includes:** Optimizer™ III implantable pulse generator
Defibrillator Generator for Insertion in Subcutaneous Tissue and Fascia	**Includes:** Evera (XT)(S)(DR/VR) Implantable cardioverter-defibrillator (ICD) Maximo II DR (VR) Protecta XT DR (XT VR) Secura (DR) (VR) Virtuoso (II) (DR) (VR)
Diaphragmatic Pacemaker Lead in Respiratory System	**Includes:** Phrenic nerve stimulator lead
Drainage Device	**Includes:** Cystostomy tube Foley catheter Percutaneous nephrostomy catheter Thoracostomy tube
External Fixation Device in Head and Facial Bones	**Includes:** External fixator
External Fixation Device in Lower Bones	**Includes:** External fixator
External Fixation Device in Lower Joints	**Includes:** External fixator

ICD-10-PCS Value	Definition
External Fixation Device in Upper Bones	**Includes:** External fixator
External Fixation Device in Upper Joints	**Includes:** External fixator
External Fixation Device, Hybrid for Insertion in Lower Bones	**Includes:** Delta frame external fixator Sheffield hybrid external fixator
External Fixation Device, Hybrid for Insertion in Upper Bones	**Includes:** Delta frame external fixator Sheffield hybrid external fixator
External Fixation Device, Hybrid for Reposition in Lower Bones	**Includes:** Delta frame external fixator Sheffield hybrid external fixator
External Fixation Device, Hybrid for Reposition in Upper Bones	**Includes:** Delta frame external fixator Sheffield hybrid external fixator
External Fixation Device, Limb Lengthening for Insertion in Lower Bones	**Includes:** Ilizarov-Vecklich device
External Fixation Device, Limb Lengthening for Insertion in Upper Bones	**Includes:** Ilizarov-Vecklich device
External Fixation Device, Monoplanar for Insertion in Lower Bones	**Includes:** Uniplanar external fixator
External Fixation Device, Monoplanar for Insertion in Upper Bones	**Includes:** Uniplanar external fixator
External Fixation Device, Monoplanar for Reposition in Lower Bones	**Includes:** Uniplanar external fixator
External Fixation Device, Monoplanar for Reposition in Upper Bones	**Includes:** Uniplanar external fixator
External Fixation Device, Ring for Insertion in Lower Bones	**Includes:** Ilizarov external fixator Sheffield ring external fixator
External Fixation Device, Ring for Insertion in Upper Bones	**Includes:** Ilizarov external fixator Sheffield ring external fixator
External Fixation Device, Ring for Reposition in Lower Bones	**Includes:** Ilizarov external fixator Sheffield ring external fixator
External Fixation Device, Ring for Reposition in Upper Bones	**Includes:** Ilizarov external fixator Sheffield ring external fixator
Extraluminal Device	**Includes:** AtriClip LAA Exclusion System LAP-BAND® adjustable gastric banding system REALIZE® Adjustable Gastric Band
Feeding Device in Gastrointestinal System	**Includes:** Percutaneous endoscopic gastrojejunostomy (PEG/J) tube Percutaneous endoscopic gastrostomy (PEG) tube
Hearing Device in Ear, Nose, Sinus	**Includes:** Esteem® implantable hearing system
Hearing Device in Head and Facial Bones	**Includes:** Bone anchored hearing device

ICD-10-PCS Value	Definition
Hearing Device, Bone Conduction for Insertion in Ear, Nose, Sinus	**Includes:** Bone anchored hearing device
Hearing Device, Multiple Channel Cochlear Prosthesis for Insertion in Ear, Nose, Sinus	**Includes:** Cochlear implant (CI), multiple channel (electrode)
Hearing Device, Single Channel Cochlear Prosthesis for Insertion in Ear, Nose, Sinus	**Includes:** Cochlear implant (CI), single channel (electrode)
Implantable Heart Assist System in Heart and Great Vessels	**Includes:** Berlin Heart Ventricular Assist Device DeBakey Left Ventricular Assist Device DuraHeart Left Ventricular Assist System HeartMate 3™ LVAS HeartMate II® Left Ventricular Assist Device (LVAD) HeartMate XVE® Left Ventricular Assist Device (LVAD) MicroMed HeartAssist Novacor Left Ventricular Assist Device Thoratec IVAD (Implantable Ventricular Assist Device)
Infusion Device	**Includes:** Ascenda Intrathecal Catheter InDura, intrathecal catheter (1P) (spinal) Non-tunneled central venous catheter Peripherally inserted central catheter (PICC) Tunneled spinal (intrathecal) catheter
Infusion Device, Pump in Subcutaneous Tissue and Fascia	**Includes:** Implantable drug infusion pump (anti-spasmodic)(chemotherapy) (pain) Injection reservoir, pump Pump reservoir Subcutaneous injection reservoir, pump SynchroMed pump
Interbody Fusion Device in Lower Joints	**Includes:** Axial Lumbar Interbody Fusion System AxiaLIF® System CoRoent® XL Direct Lateral Interbody Fusion (DLIF) device EXtreme Lateral Interbody Fusion (XLIF) device Interbody fusion (spine) cage XLIF® System
Interbody Fusion Device in Upper Joints	**Includes:** BAK/C® Interbody Cervical Fusion System Interbody fusion (spine) cage
Interbody Fusion Device, Nanotextured Surface in New Technology	Includes: nanoLOCK™ interbody fusion device

ICD-10-PCS Value	Definition	ICD-10-PCS Value	Definition
Interbody Fusion Device, Radiolucent Porous in New Technology	Includes: COALESCE® radiolucent interbody fusion device COHERE® radiolucent interbody fusion device	**Internal Fixation Device, Sustained Compression for Fusion in Upper Joints**	Includes: DynaNail® DynaNail Mini®
Internal Fixation Device in Head and Facial Bones	**Includes:** Bone screw (interlocking)(lag)(pedicle) (recessed) Kirschner wire (K-wire) Neutralization plate	**Intraluminal Device**	**Includes:** Absolute Pro Vascular (OTW) Self-Expanding Stent System Acculink (RX) Carotid Stent System AFX® Endovascular AAA System AneuRx® AAA Advantage® Assurant (Cobalt) stent Carotid WALLSTENT® Monorail® Endoprosthesis CoAxia NeuroFlo catheter Colonic Z-Stent® Complete (SE) stent Cook Zenith AAA Endovascular Graft Driver stent (RX) (OTW) E-Luminexx™ (Biliary)(Vascular) Stent Embolization coil(s) Endologix AFX® Endovascular AAA System Endurant® Endovascular Stent Graft Endurant® II AAA stent graft system EXCLUDER® AAA Endoprosthesis Express® (LD) Premounted Stent System Express® Biliary SD Monorail® Premounted Stent System Express® SD Renal Monorail® Premounted Stent System FLAIR® Endovascular Stent Graft Formula™ Balloon-Expandable Renal Stent System GORE EXCLUDER® AAA Endoprosthesis GORE TAG® Thoracic Endoprosthesis Herculink (RX) Elite Renal Stent System LifeStent® (Flexstar)(XL) Vascular Stent System Medtronic Endurant® II AAA stent graft system Micro-Driver stent (RX) (OTW) MULTI-LINK (VISION)(MINI-VISION)(ULTRA) Coronary Stent System Omnilink Elite Vascular Balloon Expandable Stent System Protege® RX Carotid Stent System Stent, intraluminal (cardiovascular) (gastrointestinal)(hepatobiliary) (urinary) Talent® Converter Talent® Occluder Talent® Stent Graft (abdominal)(thoracic) Therapeutic occlusion coil(s) Ultraflex™ Precision Colonic Stent System Valiant Thoracic Stent Graft WALLSTENT® Endoprosthesis Xact Carotid Stent System Zenith AAA Endovascular Graft Zenith Flex® AAA Endovascular Graft Zenith TX2® TAA Endovascular Graft Zenith® Renu™ AAA Ancillary Graft
Internal Fixation Device in Lower Bones	**Includes:** Bone screw (interlocking)(lag)(pedicle) (recessed) Clamp and rod internal fixation system (CRIF) Kirschner wire (K-wire) Neutralization plate		
Internal Fixation Device in Lower Joints	**Includes:** Fusion screw (compression)(lag)(locking) Joint fixation plate Kirschner wire (K-wire)		
Internal Fixation Device in Upper Bones	**Includes:** Bone screw (interlocking)(lag)(pedicle) (recessed) Clamp and rod internal fixation system (CRIF) Kirschner wire (K-wire) Neutralization plate		
Internal Fixation Device in Upper Joints	**Includes:** Fusion screw (compression)(lag)(locking) Joint fixation plate Kirschner wire (K-wire)		
Internal Fixation Device, Intramedullary in Lower Bones	**Includes:** Intramedullary (IM) rod (nail) Intramedullary skeletal kinetic distractor (ISKD) Kuntscher nail		
Internal Fixation Device, Intramedullary in Upper Bones	**Includes:** Intramedullary (IM) rod (nail) Intramedullary skeletal kinetic distractor (ISKD) Kuntscher nail		
Internal Fixation Device Intramedullary Limb Lengthening for Insertion in Lower Bones	**Includes:** PRECICE intramedullary limb lengthening system		
Internal Fixation Device Intramedullary Limb Lengthening for Insertion in Upper Bones	**Includes:** PRECICE intramedullary limb lengthening system		
Internal Fixation Device, Rigid Plate for Insertion in Upper Bones	**Includes:** Titanium Sternal Fixation System (TSFS)		
Internal Fixation Device, Rigid Plate for Reposition in Upper Bones	**Includes:** Titanium Sternal Fixation System (TSFS)		
Internal Fixation Device, Sustained Compression for Fusion in Lower Joints	**Includes:** DynaNail® DynaNail Mini®	**Intraluminal Device, Airway in Ear, Nose, Sinus**	**Includes:** Nasopharyngeal airway (NPA)

ICD-10-PCS Value	Definition
Intraluminal Device, Airway in Gastrointestinal System	**Includes:** Esophageal obturator airway (EOA)
Intraluminal Device, Airway in Mouth and Throat	**Includes:** Guedel airway Oropharyngeal airway (OPA)
Intraluminal Device, Bioactive in Upper Arteries	**Includes:** Bioactive embolization coil(s) Micrus CERECYTE microcoil
Intraluminal Device, Branched or Fenestrated, One or Two Arteries for Restriction in Lower Arteries	**Includes:** Cook Zenith® Fenestrated AAA Endovascular Graft EXCLUDER® AAA Endoprosthesis EXCLUDER® IBE Endoprosthesis GORE EXCLUDER® AAA Endoprosthesis GORE EXCLUDER®IBE Endoprosthesis Zenith® Fenestrated AAA Endovascular Graft
Intraluminal Device, Branched or Fenestrated, Three or More Arteries for Restriction in Lower Arteries	**Includes:** Cook Zenith® Fenestrated AAA Endovascular Graft EXCLUDER® AAA Endoprosthesis GORE EXCLUDER® AAA Endoprosthesis Zenith® Fenestrated AAA Endovascular Graft
Intraluminal Device, Drug-eluting in Heart and Great Vessels	**Includes:** CYPHER® Stent Endeavor® (III)(IV) (Sprint) Zotarolimus-eluting Coronary Stent System Everolimus-eluting coronary stent Paclitaxel-eluting coronary stent Sirolimus-eluting coronary stent TAXUS® Liberte® Paclitaxel-eluting Coronary Stent System XIENCE Everolimus Eluting Coronary Stent System Zotarolimus-eluting coronary stent
Intraluminal Device, Drug-eluting in Lower Arteries	**Includes:** Paclitaxel-eluting peripheral stent Zilver® PTX® (paclitaxel) Drug-Eluting Peripheral Stent
Intraluminal Device, Drug-eluting in Upper Arteries	**Includes:** Paclitaxel-eluting peripheral stent Zilver® PTX® (paclitaxel) Drug-Eluting Peripheral Stent
Intraluminal Device, Endobronchial Valve in Respiratory System	**Includes:** Spiration IBV™ Valve System
Intraluminal Device, Endotracheal Airway in Respiratory System	**Includes:** Endotracheal tube (cuffed)(double-lumen)
Intraluminal Device, Flow Diverter for Restriction in Upper Arteries	**Includes:** Flow Diverter embolization device Pipeline™ (Flex) embolization device Surpass Streamline™ Flow Diverter
Intraluminal Device, Pessary in Female Reproductive System	**Includes:** Pessary ring Vaginal pessary

ICD-10-PCS Value	Definition
Intraluminal Device, Sustained Release Drug-eluting in New Technology	**Includes:** Eluvia™ Drug-eluting Vascular Stent System SAVAL below-the-knee (BTK) drug-eluting stent system
Intraluminal Device, Sustained Release Drug-eluting, Four or More in New Technology	**Includes:** Eluvia™ Drug-eluting Vascular Stent System SAVAL below-the-knee (BTK) drug-eluting stent system
Intraluminal Device, Sustained Release Drug-eluting, Three in New Technology	**Includes:** Eluvia™ Drug-eluting Vascular Stent System SAVAL below-the-knee (BTK) drug-eluting stent system
Intraluminal Device, Sustained Release Drug-eluting, Two in New Technology	**Includes:** Eluvia™ Drug-eluting Vascular Stent System SAVAL below-the-knee (BTK) drug-eluting stent system
Liner in Lower Joints	**Includes:** Acetabular cup Hip (joint) liner Joint liner (insert) Knee (implant) insert Tibial insert
Magnetically Controlled Growth Rod(s) in New Technology	**Includes:** MAGEC® Spinal Bracing and Distraction System Spinal growth rods, magnetically controlled
Monitoring Device	**Includes:** Blood glucose monitoring system Cardiac event recorder Continuous Glucose Monitoring (CGM) device Implantable glucose monitoring device Loop recorder, implantable Reveal (LINQ)(DX)(XT)
Monitoring Device, Hemodynamic for Insertion in Subcutaneous Tissue and Fascia	**Includes:** Implantable hemodynamic monitor (IHM) Implantable hemodynamic monitoring system (IHMS)
Monitoring Device, Pressure Sensor for Insertion in Heart and Great Vessels	**Includes:** CardioMEMS® pressure sensor EndoSure® sensor
Neurostimulator Generator in Head and Facial Bones	**Includes:** RNS system neurostimulator generator
Neurostimulator Lead in Central Nervous System and Cranial Nerves	**Includes:** Cortical strip neurostimulator lead DBS lead Deep brain neurostimulator lead RNS System lead Spinal cord neurostimulator lead
Neurostimulator Lead in Peripheral Nervous System	**Includes:** InterStim® Therapy lead

ICD-10-PCS Value	Definition
Nonautologous Tissue Substitute	**Includes:** Acellular Hydrated Dermis Bone bank bone graft Cook Biodesign® Fistula Plug(s) Cook Biodesign® Hernia Graft(s) Cook Biodesign® Layered Graft(s) Cook Zenapro™ Layered Graft(s) Tissue bank graft
Pacemaker, Dual Chamber for Insertion in Subcutaneous Tissue and Fascia	**Includes:** Advisa (MRI) EnRhythm Kappa Revo MRI™ SureScan® pacemaker Two lead pacemaker Versa
Pacemaker, Single Chamber for Insertion in Subcutaneous Tissue and Fascia	**Includes:** Single lead pacemaker (atrium)(ventricle)
Pacemaker, Single Chamber Rate Responsive for Insertion in Subcutaneous Tissue and Fascia	**Includes:** Single lead rate responsive pacemaker (atrium)(ventricle)
Radioactive Element	**Includes:** Brachytherapy seeds CivaSheet®
Radioactive Element, Cesium-131 Collagen Implant for Insertion in Central Nervous System and Cranial Nerves	**Includes:** Cesium-131 Collagen Implant GammaTile™
Resurfacing Device in Lower Joints	**Includes:** CONSERVE® PLUS Total Resurfacing Hip System Cormet Hip Resurfacing System
Short-term External Heart Assist System in Heart and Great Vessels	**Includes:** Biventricular external heart assist system BVS 5000 Ventricular Assist Device Centrimag® Blood Pump Impella® heart pump TandemHeart® System Thoratec Paracorporeal Ventricular Assist Device
Skin Substitute, Porcine Liver Derived in New Technology	**Includes:** MIRODERM™ Biologic Wound Matrix
Spacer in Lower Joints	**Includes:** Joint spacer (antibiotic) Spacer, Static (Antibiotic) Static Spacer (Antibiotic)
Spacer in Upper Joints	**Includes:** Joint spacer (antibiotic)
Spinal Stabilization Device, Facet Replacement for Insertion in Lower Joints	**Includes:** Facet replacement spinal stabilization device
Spinal Stabilization Device, Facet Replacement for Insertion in Upper Joints	**Includes:** Facet replacement spinal stabilization device
Spinal Stabilization Device, Interspinous Process for Insertion in Lower Joints	**Includes:** Interspinous process spinal stabilization device X-STOP® Spacer

ICD-10-PCS Value	Definition
Spinal Stabilization Device, Interspinous Process for Insertion in Upper Joints	**Includes:** Interspinous process spinal stabilization device X-STOP® Spacer
Spinal Stabilization Device, Pedicle- Based for Insertion in Lower Joints	**Includes:** Dynesys® Dynamic Stabilization System Pedicle-based dynamic stabilization device
Spinal Stabilization Device, Pedicle-Based for Insertion in Upper Joints	**Includes:** Dynesys® Dynamic Stabilization System Pedicle-based dynamic stabilization device
Stimulator Generator in Subcutaneous Tissue and Fascia	**Includes:** Baroreflex Activation Therapy® (BAT®) Diaphragmatic pacemaker generator Mark IV Breathing Pacemaker System Phrenic nerve stimulator generator Rheos® System device
Stimulator Generator, Multiple Array for Insertion in Subcutaneous Tissue and Fascia	**Includes:** Activa PC neurostimulator Enterra gastric neurostimulator Neurostimulator generator, multiple channel PrimeAdvanced neurostimulator (SureScan)(MRI Safe)
Stimulator Generator, Multiple Array Rechargeable for Insertion in Subcutaneous Tissue and Fascia	**Includes:** Activa RC neurostimulator Neurostimulator generator, multiple channel rechargeable RestoreAdvanced neurostimulator (SureScan)(MRI Safe) RestoreSensor neurostimulator (SureScan)(MRI Safe) RestoreUltra neurostimulator (SureScan)(MRI Safe)
Stimulator Generator, Single Array for Insertion in Subcutaneous Tissue and Fascia	**Includes:** Activa SC neurostimulator InterStim® Therapy neurostimulator Itrel (3)(4) neurostimulator Neurostimulator generator, single channel
Stimulator Generator, Single Array Rechargeable for Insertion in Subcutaneous Tissue and Fascia	**Includes:** Neurostimulator generator, single channel rechargeable
Stimulator Lead in Gastrointestinal System	**Includes:** Gastric electrical stimulation (GES) lead Gastric pacemaker lead
Stimulator Lead in Muscles	**Includes:** Electrical muscle stimulation (EMS) lead Electronic muscle stimulator lead Neuromuscular electrical stimulation (NEMS) lead
Stimulator Lead in Upper Arteries	**Includes:** Baroreflex Activation Therapy® (BAT®) Carotid (artery) sinus (baroreceptor) lead Rheos® System lead

ICD-10-PCS Value	Definition
Stimulator Lead in Urinary System	**Includes:** Sacral nerve modulation (SNM) lead Sacral neuromodulation lead Urinary incontinence stimulator lead
Subcutaneous Defibrillator Lead in Subcutaneous Tissue and Fascia	**Includes:** S-ICD™ lead
Synthetic Substitute	**Includes:** AbioCor® Total Replacement Heart AMPLATZER® Muscular VSD Occluder Annuloplasty ring Bard® Composix® (E/X) (LP) mesh Bard® Composix® Kugel® patch Bard® Dulex™ mesh Bard® Ventralex™ hernia patch Barricaid® Annular Closure Device (ACD) BRYAN® Cervical Disc System Corvia IASD® Ex-PRESS™ mini glaucoma shunt Flexible Composite Mesh GORE® DUALMESH® Holter valve ventricular shunt IASD® (InterAtrial Shunt Device), Corvia InterAtrial Shunt Device IASD®, Corvia MitraClip valve repair system Nitinol framed polymer mesh Open Pivot (mechanical) valve Open Pivot Aortic Valve Graft (AVG) Partially absorbable mesh PHYSIOMESH™ Flexible Composite Mesh Polymethylmethacrylate (PMMA) Polypropylene mesh PRESTIGE® Cervical Disc PROCEED™ Ventral Patch Prodisc-C Prodisc-L PROLENE Polypropylene Hernia System (PHS) Rebound HRD® (Hernia Repair Device) SynCardia Total Artificial Heart Total artificial (replacement) heart ULTRAPRO Hernia System (UHS) ULTRAPRO Partially Absorbable Lightweight Mesh ULTRAPRO Plug V-Wave Interatrial Shunt System Ventrio™ Hernia Patch Zimmer® NexGen® LPS Mobile Bearing Knee Zimmer® NexGen® LPS-Flex Mobile Knee
Synthetic Substitute, Ceramic for Replacement in Lower Joints	**Includes:** Ceramic on ceramic bearing surface Novation® Ceramic AHS® (Articulation Hip System)
Synthetic Substitute, Intraocular Telescope for Replacement in Eye	**Includes:** Implantable Miniature Telescope™ (IMT)
Synthetic Substitute, Mechanically Expandable (Paired) in New Technology	**Includes:** SpineJack® system

ICD-10-PCS Value	Definition
Synthetic Substitute, Metal for Replacement in Lower Joints	**Includes:** Cobalt/chromium head and socket Metal on metal bearing surface
Synthetic Substitute, Metal on Polyethylene for Replacement in Lower Joints	**Includes:** Cobalt/chromium head and polyethylene socket
Synthetic Substitute, Oxidized Zirconium on Polyethylene for Replacement in Lower Joints	**Includes:** OXINIUM
Synthetic Substitute, Polyethylene for Replacement in Lower Joints	**Includes:** Polyethylene socket
Synthetic Substitute, Reverse Ball and Socket for Replacement in Upper Joints	**Includes:** Delta III Reverse shoulder prosthesis Reverse® Shoulder Prosthesis
Tissue Expander in Skin and Breast	**Includes:** Tissue expander (inflatable) (injectable)
Tissue Expander in Subcutaneous Tissue and Fascia	**Includes:** Tissue expander (inflatable) (injectable)
Tracheostomy Device in Respiratory System	**Includes:** Tracheostomy tube
Vascular Access Device, Totally Implantable in Subcutaneous Tissue and Fascia	**Includes:** Implanted (venous)(access) port Injection reservoir, port Subcutaneous injection reservoir, port
Vascular Access Device, Tunneled in Subcutaneous Tissue and Fascia	**Includes:** Tunneled central venous catheter Vectra® Vascular Access Graft
Zooplastic Tissue in Heart and Great Vessels	**Includes:** 3f (Aortic) Bioprosthesis valve Bovine pericardial valve Bovine pericardium graft Contegra Pulmonary Valved Conduit CoreValve transcatheter aortic valve Epic™ Stented Tissue Valve (aortic) Freestyle (Stentless) Aortic Root Bioprosthesis Hancock Bioprosthesis (aortic) (mitral) valve Hancock Bioprosthetic Valved Conduit Melody® transcatheter pulmonary valve Mitroflow® Aortic Pericardial Heart Valve Mosaic Bioprosthesis (aortic) (mitral) valve Porcine (bioprosthetic) valve SAPIEN transcatheter aortic valve SJM Biocor® Stented Valve System Stented tissue valve Trifecta™ Valve (aortic) Xenograft
Zooplastic Tissue, Rapid Deployment Technique in New Technology	**Includes:** EDWARDS INTUITY Elite valve system INTUITY Elite valve system, EDWARDS Perceval sutureless valve Sutureless valve, Perceval

Appendix I: Substance Key/Substance Definitions

Substance Key

This table crosswalks a specific substance, listed by trade name or synonym, to the PCS value that would be used to represent that substance in either the Administration or New Technology section. The ICD-10-PCS value may be located in either the 6th-character Substance column or the 7th-character Qualifier column depending on the section/table to which it is classified. The most specific character is listed in the table.

Trade Name or Synonym	ICD-10-PCS Value	PCS Section
AIGISRx Antibacterial Envelope	Anti-Infective Envelope (A)	Administration (3)
Andexanet Alfa, Factor Xa Inhibitor Reversal Agent	Coagulation Factor Xa, Inactivated (7)	New Technology (X)
Andexxa	Coagulation Factor Xa, Inactivated (7)	New Technology (X)
Angiotensin II	Synthetic Human Angiotensin II (H)	New Technology (X)
Antibacterial Envelope (TYRX) (AIGISRx)	Anti-Infective Envelope (A)	Administration (3)
Antimicrobial envelope	Anti-Infective Envelope (A)	Administration (3)
Axicabtagene Ciloeucel	Engineered Autologous Chimeric Antigen Receptor T-cell Immunotherapy (C)	New Technology (X)
AZEDRA®	Iobenguane I-131 Antineoplastic (S)	New Technology (X)
Bone morphogenetic protein 2 (BMP 2)	Recombinant Bone Morphogenetic Protein (B)	Administration (3)
Brexucabtagene Autoleucel	Brexucabtagene Autoleucel Immunotherapy (4)	New Technology (X)
CBMA (Concentrated Bone Marrow Aspirate)	Concentrated Bone Marrow Aspirate (Ø)	New Technology (X)
Clolar	Clofarabine (P)	Administration (3)
Coagulation Factor Xa, (Recombinant) Inactivated	Coagulation Factor Xa, Inactivated (7)	New Technology (X)
CONTEPO™	Fosfomycin Anti-infective (K)	New Technology (X)
Defitelio	Defibrotide Sodium Anticoagulant (9)	New Technology (X)
DuraGraft® Endothelial Damage Inhibitor	Endothelial Damage Inhibitor (8)	New Technology (X)
ELZONRIS™	Tagraxofusp-erzs Antineoplastic (Q)	New Technology (X)
ERLEADA™	Apalutamide Antineoplastic (J)	New Technology (X)
Factor Xa Inhibitor Reversal Agent, Andexanet Alfa	Coagulation Factor Xa, Inactivated (7)	New Technology (X)
FETROJA®	Cefiderocol Anti-infective (A)	New Technology (X)
Fosfomycin injection	Fosfomycin Anti-infective (K)	New Technology (X)
GIAPREZA™	Synthetic Human Angiotensin II (H)	New Technology (X)
Hemospray® Endoscopic Hemostat	Mineral-based Topical Hemostatic Agent (8)	New Technology (X)
Human angiotensin II, synthetic	Synthetic Human Angiotensin II (H)	New Technology (X)
IMFINZI®	Durvalumab Antineoplastic (3)	New Technology (X)
IMI/REL	Imipenem-cilastatin-relebactam Anti-infective (U)	New Technology (X)
Iobenguane I-131, High Specific Activity (HSA)	Iobenguane I-131 Antineoplastic (S)	New Technology (X)
Jakafi®	Ruxolitinib (T)	New Technology (X)
Kcentra	4-Factor Prothrombin Complex Concentrate (B)	Administration (3)
KYMRIAH	Engineered Autologous Chimeric Antigen Receptor T-cell Immunotherapy (C)	New Technology (X)
Lisocabtagene Maraleucel	Lisocabtagene Maraleucel Immunotherapy (7)	New Technology (X)
NA-1 (Nerinitide)	Nerinitide (2)	New Technology (X)
Nesiritide	Human B-type Natriuretic Peptide (H)	Administration (3)
NUZYRA™	Omadacycline Anti-infective (B)	New Technology (X)
OTL-101	Hematopoietic Stem/Progenitor Cells, Genetically Modified (C)	Administration (3)
rhBMP-2	Recombinant Bone Morphogenetic Protein (B)	Administration (3)
Seprafilm	Adhesion Barrier (5)	Administration (3)
Soliris®	Eculizumab (C)	New Technology (X)
SPRAVATO™	Esketamine Hydrochloride (M)	New Technology (X)
STELARA®	Other New Technology Therapeutic Substance (F)	New Technology (X)
TECENTRIQ®	Atezolizumab Antineoplastic (D)	New Technology (X)
Tisagenlecleucel	Engineered Autologous Chimeric Antigen Receptor T-cell Immunotherapy (C)	New Technology (X)
Tissue Plasminogen Activator (tPA)(r- tPA)	Other Thrombolytic (7)	Administration (3)
TYRX Antibacterial Envelope	Anti-Infective Envelope (A)	Administration (3)

Trade Name or Synonym	ICD-10-PCS Value	PCS Section
Ustekinumab	Other New Technology Therapeutic Substance (F)	New Technology (X)
Vabomere™	Meropenem-vaborbactam Anti-infective (N)	New Technology (X)
Venclexta®	Ventoclax Antineoplastic (R)	New Technology (X)
Vistogard®	Uridine Triacetate (8)	New Technology (X)
Voraxaze	Glucarpidase (Q)	Administration (3)
VYXEOS™	Cytarabine and Daunorubicin Liposome Antineoplastic (B)	New Technology (X)
XENLETA™	Lefamulin Anti-infective (6)	New Technology (X)
XOSPATA®	Gilteritinib Antineoplastic (V)	New Technology (X)
ZERBAXA®	Ceftolozane/Tazobactam Anti-infective (9)	New Technology (X)
ZINPLAVA™	Bezlotoxumab Monoclonal Antibody (A)	New Technology (X)
ZULRESSO™	Brexanolone (Ø)	New Technology (X)
Zyvox	Oxazolidinones (8)	Administration (3)

Substance Definitions

This table crosswalks a PCS value, used in the Administration or New Technology section, to a specific substance. The specific substances are listed by trade name or synonym. The ICD-10-PCS value may be located in either the 6th-character Substance column or the 7th-character Qualifier column depending on the section/table to which it is classified.

ICD-10-PCS Value	Trade Name or Synonym	PCS Section
4-Factor Prothrombin Complex Concentrate (B)	**Includes:** Kcentra	Administration (3)
Adhesion Barrier (5)	**Includes:** Seprafilm	Administration (3)
Anti-Infective Envelope (A)	**Includes:** AIGISRx Antibacterial Envelope Antimicrobial envelope Antibacterial Envelope (TYRX) (AIGISRx) TYRX Antibacterial Envelope	Administration (3)
Apalutamide Antineoplastic (J)	**Includes:** ERLEADA™	New Technology (X)
Atezolizumab Antineoplastic (D)	**Includes:** TECENTRIQ®	New Technology (X)
Bezlotoxumab Monoclonal Antibody (A)	**Includes:** ZINPLAVA™	New Technology (X)
Brexanolone (Ø)	**Includes:** ZULRESSO™	New Technology (X)
Brexucabtagene Autoleucel Immunotherapy (4)	**Includes:** Brexucabtagene Autoleucel	New Technology (X)
Cefiderocol Anti-infective (A)	**Includes:** FETROJA®	New Technology (X)
Ceftolozane/Tazobactam Anti- infective (9)	**Includes:** ZERBAXA®	New Technology (X)
Clofarabine (P)	**Includes:** Clolar	Administration (3)
Coagulation Factor Xa, Inactivated (7)	**Includes:** Andexanet Alfa, Factor Xa Inhibitor Reversal Agent Andexxa Coagulation Factor Xa, (Recombinant) Inactivated Factor Xa Inhibitor Reversal Agent, Andexanet Alfa	New Technology (X)
Concentrated Bone Marrow Aspirate (Ø)	**Includes:** CBMA (Concentrated Bone Marrow Aspirate)	New Technology (X)
Cytarabine and Daunorubicin Liposome Antineoplastic (B)	**Includes:** VYXEOS™	New Technology (X)
Defibrotide Sodium Anticoagulant (9)	**Includes:** Defitelio	New Technology (X)
Durvalumab Antineoplastic (3)	**Includes:** IMFINZI®	New Technology (X)
Eculizumab (C)	**Includes:** Soliris®	New Technology (X)
Endothelial Damage Inhibitor (8)	**Includes:** DuraGraft® Endothelial Damage Inhibitor	New Technology (X)
Engineered Autologous Chimeric Antigen Receptor T-cell Immunotherapy (C)	**Includes:** Axicabtagene Ciloeucel KYMRIAH Tisagenlecleucel	New Technology (X)
Esketamine Hydrochloride (M)	**Includes:** SPRAVATO™	New Technology (X)
Fosfomycin Anti-infective (K)	**Includes:** CONTEPO™ Fosfomycin injection	New Technology (X)
Gilteritinib Antineoplastic (V)	**Includes:** XOSPATA®	New Technology (X)
Glucarpidase (Q)	**Includes:** Voraxaze	Administration (3)
Hematopoietic Stem/Progenitor Cells, Genetically Modified (C)	**Includes:** OTL-1Ø1	Administration (3)
Human B-type Natriuretic Peptide (H)	**Includes:** Nesiritide	Administration (3)

ICD-10-PCS Value	Trade Name or Synonym	PCS Section
Imipenem-cilastatin-relebactam Anti-infective (U)	**Includes:** IMI/REL	New Technology (X)
Iobenguane I-131 Antineoplastic (S)	**Includes:** AZEDRA® Iobenguane I-131, High Specific Activity (HSA)	New Technology (X)
Lefamulin Anti-infective (6)	**Includes:** XENLETA™	New Technology (X)
Lisocabtagene Maraleucel Immunotherapy (7)	**Includes:** Lisocabtagene Maraleucel	New Technology (X)
Meropenem-vaborbactam Anti-infective (N)	**Includes:** Vabomere™	New Technology (X)
Mineral-based Topical Hemostatic Agent (8)	**Includes:** Hemospray® Endoscopic Hemostat	New Technology (X
Nerinitide (2)	**Includes:** NA-1 (Nerinitide)	New Technology (X
Omadacycline Anti-infective (B)	**Includes:** NUZYRA™	New Technology (X
Other New Technology Therapeutic Substance (F)	**Includes:** STELARA® Ustekinumab	New Technology (X)
Other Thrombolytic (7)	**Includes:** Tissue Plasminogen Activator (tPA)(r-tPA)	Administration (3)
Oxazolidinones (8)	**Includes:** Zyvox	Administration (3)
Recombinant Bone Morphogenetic Protein (B)	**Includes:** Bone morphogenetic protein 2 (BMP 2) rhBMP-2	Administration (3)
Ruxolitinib (T)	**Includes:** Jakafi®	New Technology (X)
Synthetic Human Angiotensin II (H)	**Includes:** Angiotensin II GIAPREZA™ Human angiotensin II, synthetic	New Technology (X)
Tagraxofusp-erzs Antineoplastic (Q)	**Includes:** ELZONRIS™	New Technology (X)
Uridine Triacetate (8)	**Includes:** Vistogard®	New Technology (X)
Venetoclax Antineoplastic (R)	**Includes:** Venclexta®	New Technology (X)

Appendix J: Sections B–H Character Definitions

Sections B-H (Imaging through Substance Abuse Treatment) do not include root operations. Instead, the character 3 value represents the type of procedure performed with additional details about that procedure provided by the character 4 or 5 value, when appropriate. This resource provides the specific ICD-10-PCS value and its associated definition for the character 3, character 4, and character 5 values in the ancillary sections of B-H.

Section B–Imaging

ICD-10-PCS Value (Character 3)	Definition
Computerized Tomography (CT Scan) (2)	Computer reformatted digital display of multiplanar images developed from the capture of multiple exposures of external ionizing radiation
Fluoroscopy (1)	Single plane or bi-plane real time display of an image developed from the capture of external ionizing radiation on a fluorescent screen. The image may also be stored by either digital or analog means.
Magnetic Resonance Imaging (MRI) (3)	Computer reformatted digital display of multiplanar images developed from the capture of radiofrequency signals emitted by nuclei in a body site excited within a magnetic field
Other Imaging (5)	Other specified modality for visualizing a body part
Plain Radiography (Ø)	Planar display of an image developed from the capture of external ionizing radiation on photographic or photoconductive plate
Ultrasonography (4)	Real time display of images of anatomy or flow information developed from the capture of reflected and attenuated high frequency sound waves

Section C–Nuclear Medicine

ICD-10-PCS Value (Character 3)	Definition
Nonimaging Nuclear Medicine Assay (6)	Introduction of radioactive materials into the body for the study of body fluids and blood elements, by the detection of radioactive emissions
Nonimaging Nuclear Medicine Probe (5)	Introduction of radioactive materials into the body for the study of distribution and fate of certain substances by the detection of radioactive emissions; or, alternatively, measurement of absorption of radioactive emissions from an external source
Nonimaging Nuclear Medicine Uptake (4)	Introduction of radioactive materials into the body for measurements of organ function, from the detection of radioactive emissions
Planar Nuclear Medicine Imaging (1)	Introduction of radioactive materials into the body for single plane display of images developed from the capture of radioactive emissions
Positron Emission Tomographic (PET) Imaging (3)	Introduction of radioactive materials into the body for three dimensional display of images developed from the simultaneous capture, 18Ø degrees apart, of radioactive emissions
Systemic Nuclear Medicine Therapy (7)	Introduction of unsealed radioactive materials into the body for treatment
Tomographic (Tomo) Nuclear Medicine Imaging (2)	Introduction of radioactive materials into the body for three dimensional display of images developed from the capture of radioactive emissions

Section F–Physical Rehabilitation and Diagnostic Audiology

ICD-10-PCS Value (Character 3)	Definition
Activities of Daily Living Assessment (2)	Measurement of functional level for activities of daily living
Activities of Daily Living Treatment (8)	Exercise or activities to facilitate functional competence for activities of daily living
Caregiver Training (F)	Training in activities to support patient's optimal level of function
Cochlear Implant Treatment (B)	Application of techniques to improve the communication abilities of individuals with cochlear implant
Device Fitting (D)	Fitting of a device designed to facilitate or support achievement of a higher level of function
Hearing Aid Assessment (4)	Measurement of the appropriateness and/or effectiveness of a hearing device
Hearing Assessment (3)	Measurement of hearing and related functions
Hearing Treatment (9)	Application of techniques to improve, augment, or compensate for hearing and related functional impairment
Motor and/or Nerve Function Assessment (1)	Measurement of motor, nerve, and related functions

Continued on next page

Section F–Physical Rehabilitation and Diagnostic Audiology

Continued from previous page

ICD-10-PCS Value (Character 3)	Definition
Motor Treatment (7)	Exercise or activities to increase or facilitate motor function
Speech Assessment (Ø)	Measurement of speech and related functions
Speech Treatment (6)	Application of techniques to improve, augment, or compensate for speech and related functional impairment
Vestibular Assessment (5)	Measurement of the vestibular system and related functions
Vestibular Treatment (C)	Application of techniques to improve, augment, or compensate for vestibular and related functional impairment

Section F–Physical Rehabilitation and Diagnostic Audiology

ICD-10-PCS Value Qualifier (Character 5)	Definition
Acoustic Reflex Decay (J)	Measures reduction in size/strength of acoustic reflex over time Includes/Examples: Includes site of lesion test
Acoustic Reflex Patterns (G)	Defines site of lesion based upon presence/absence of acoustic reflexes with ipsilateral vs. contralateral stimulation
Acoustic Reflex Threshold (H)	Determines minimal intensity that acoustic reflex occurs with ipsilateral and/or contralateral stimulation
Aerobic Capacity and Endurance (7)	Measures autonomic responses to positional changes; perceived exertion, dyspnea or angina during activity; performance during exercise protocols; standard vital signs; and blood gas analysis or oxygen consumption
Alternate Binaural or Monaural Loudness Balance (7)	Determines auditory stimulus parameter that yields the same objective sensation Includes/Examples: Sound intensities that yield same loudness perception
Anthropometric Characteristics (B)	Measures edema, body fat composition, height, weight, length and girth
Aphasia (Assessment) (C)	Measures expressive and receptive speech and language function including reading and writing
Aphasia (Treatment) (3)	Applying techniques to improve, augment, or compensate for receptive/ expressive language impairments
Articulation/Phonology (Assessment) (9)	Measures speech production
Articulation/Phonology (Treatment) (4)	Applying techniques to correct, improve, or compensate for speech productive impairment
Assistive Listening Device (5)	Assists in use of effective and appropriate assistive listening device/system
Assistive Listening System/Device Selection (4)	Measures the effectiveness and appropriateness of assistive listening systems/devices
Assistive, Adaptive, Supportive or Protective Devices (9)	Explanation: Devices to facilitate or support achievement of a higher level of function in wheelchair mobility; bed mobility; transfer or ambulation ability; bath and showering ability; dressing; grooming; personal hygiene; play or leisure
Auditory Evoked Potentials (L)	Measures electric responses produced by the VIIIth cranial nerve and brainstem following auditory stimulation
Auditory Processing (Assessment) (Q)	Evaluates ability to receive and process auditory information and comprehension of spoken language
Auditory Processing (Treatment) (2)	Applying techniques to improve the receiving and processing of auditory information and comprehension of spoken language
Augmentative/Alternative Communication System (Assessment) (L)	Determines the appropriateness of aids, techniques, symbols, and/or strategies to augment or replace speech and enhance communication Includes/Examples: Includes the use of telephones, writing equipment, emergency equipment, and TDD
Augmentative/Alternative Communication System (Treatment) (3)	Includes/Examples: Includes augmentative communication devices and aids
Aural Rehabilitation (5)	Applying techniques to improve the communication abilities associated with hearing loss
Aural Rehabilitation Status (P)	Measures impact of a hearing loss including evaluation of receptive and expressive communication skills

Continued on next page

Section F–Physical Rehabilitation and Diagnostic Audiology

Continued from previous page

ICD-10-PCS Value Qualifier (Character 5)	Definition
Bathing/Showering (Ø)	Includes/Examples: Includes obtaining and using supplies; soaping, rinsing, and drying body parts; maintaining bathing position; and transferring to and from bathing positions
Bathing/Showering Techniques (Ø)	Activities to facilitate obtaining and using supplies, soaping, rinsing and drying body parts, maintaining bathing position, and transferring to and from bathing positions
Bed Mobility (Assessment) (B)	Transitional movement within bed
Bed Mobility (Treatment) (5)	Exercise or activities to facilitate transitional movements within bed
Bedside Swallowing and Oral Function (H)	Includes/Examples: Bedside swallowing includes assessment of sucking, masticating, coughing, and swallowing. Oral function includes assessment of musculature for controlled movements, structures, and functions to determine coordination and phonation.
Bekesy Audiometry (3)	Uses an instrument that provides a choice of discrete or continuously varying pure tones; choice of pulsed or continuous signal
Binaural Electroacoustic Hearing Aid Check (6)	Determines mechanical and electroacoustic function of bilateral hearing aids using hearing aid test box
Binaural Hearing Aid (Assessment) (3)	Measures the candidacy, effectiveness, and appropriateness of a hearing aid Explanation: Measures bilateral fit
Binaural Hearing Aid (Treatment) (2)	Explanation: Assists in achieving maximum understanding and performance
Bithermal, Binaural Caloric Irrigation (Ø)	Measures the rhythmic eye movements stimulated by changing the temperature of the vestibular system
Bithermal, Monaural Caloric Irrigation (1)	Measures the rhythmic eye movements stimulated by changing the temperature of the vestibular system in one ear
Brief Tone Stimuli (R)	Measures specific central auditory process
Cerumen Management (3)	Includes examination of external auditory canal and tympanic membrane and removal of cerumen from external ear canal
Cochlear Implant (Ø)	Measures candidacy for cochlear implant
Cochlear Implant Rehabilitation (Ø)	Applying techniques to improve the communication abilities of individuals with cochlear implant; includes programming the device, providing patients/families with information
Communicative/Cognitive Integration Skills (Assessment) (G)	Measures ability to use higher cortical functions Includes/Examples: Includes orientation, recognition, attention span, initiation and termination of activity, memory, sequencing, categorizing, concept formation, spatial operations, judgment, problem solving, generalization and pragmatic communication
Communicative/Cognitive Integration Skills (Treatment) (6)	Activities to facilitate the use of higher cortical functions Includes/Examples: Includes level of arousal, orientation, recognition, attention span, initiation and termination of activity, memory sequencing, judgment and problem solving, learning and generalization, and pragmatic communication
Computerized Dynamic Posturography (6)	Measures the status of the peripheral and central vestibular system and the sensory/motor component of balance; evaluates the efficacy of vestibular rehabilitation
Conditioned Play Audiometry (4)	Behavioral measures using nonspeech and speech stimuli to obtain frequency-specific and ear-specific information on auditory status from the patient Explanation: Obtains speech reception threshold by having patient point to pictures of spondaic words
Coordination/Dexterity (Assessment) (3)	Measures large and small muscle groups for controlled goal-directed movements Explanation: Dexterity includes object manipulation
Coordination/Dexterity (Treatment) (2)	Exercise or activities to facilitate gross coordination and fine coordination
Cranial Nerve Integrity (9)	Measures cranial nerve sensory and motor functions, including tastes, smell and facial expression
Dichotic Stimuli (T)	Measures specific central auditory process
Distorted Speech (S)	Measures specific central auditory process
Dix-Hallpike Dynamic (5)	Measures nystagmus following Dix-Hallpike maneuver

Continued on next page

Section F–Physical Rehabilitation and Diagnostic Audiology

Continued from previous page

ICD-10-PCS Value Qualifier (Character 5)	Definition
Dressing (1)	Includes/Examples: Includes selecting clothing and accessories, obtaining clothing from storage, dressing, fastening and adjusting clothing and shoes, and applying and removing personal devices, prosthesis or orthosis
Dressing Techniques (1)	Activities to facilitate selecting clothing and accessories, dressing and undressing, adjusting clothing and shoes, applying and removing devices, prostheses or orthoses
Dynamic Orthosis (6)	Includes/Examples: Includes customized and prefabricated splints, inhibitory casts, spinal and other braces, and protective devices; allows motion through transfer of movement from other body parts or by use of outside forces
Ear Canal Probe Microphone (1)	Real ear measures
Ear Protector Attentuation (7)	Measures ear protector fit and effectiveness
Electrocochleography (K)	Measures the VIIIth cranial nerve action potential
Environmental, Home, Work Barriers (B)	Measures current and potential barriers to optimal function, including safety hazards, access problems and home or office design
Ergonomics and Body Mechanics (C)	Ergonomic measurement of job tasks, work hardening or work conditioning needs; functional capacity; and body mechanics
Eustachian Tube Function (F)	Measures eustachian tube function and patency of eustachian tube
Evoked Otoacoustic Emissions, Diagnostic (N)	Measures auditory evoked potentials in a diagnostic format
Evoked Otoacoustic Emissions, Screening (M)	Measures auditory evoked potentials in a screening format
Facial Nerve Function (7)	Measures electrical activity of the VIIth cranial nerve (facial nerve)
Feeding/Eating (Assessment) (2)	Includes/Examples: Includes setting up food, selecting and using utensils and tableware, bringing food or drink to mouth, cleaning face, hands, and clothing, and management of alternative methods of nourishment
Feeding/Eating (Treatment) (3)	Exercise or activities to facilitate setting up food, selecting and using utensils and tableware, bringing food or drink to mouth, cleaning face, hands, and clothing, and management of alternative methods of nourishment
Filtered Speech (0)	Uses high or low pass filtered speech stimuli to assess central auditory processing disorders, site of lesion testing
Fluency (Assessment) (D)	Measures speech fluency or stuttering
Fluency (Treatment) (7)	Applying techniques to improve and augment fluent speech
Gait and/or Balance (D)	Measures biomechanical, arthrokinematic and other spatial and temporal characteristics of gait and balance
Gait Training/Functional Ambulation (9)	Exercise or activities to facilitate ambulation on a variety of surfaces and in a variety of environments
Grooming/Personal Hygiene (Assessment) (3)	Includes/Examples: Includes ability to obtain and use supplies in a sequential fashion, general grooming, oral hygiene, toilet hygiene, personal care devices, including care for artificial airways
Grooming/Personal Hygiene (Treatment) (2)	Activities to facilitate obtaining and using supplies in a sequential fashion: general grooming, oral hygiene, toilet hygiene, cleaning body, and personal care devices, including artificial airways
Hearing and Related Disorders Counseling (0)	Provides patients/families/caregivers with information, support, referrals to facilitate recovery from a communication disorder Includes/Examples: Includes strategies for psychosocial adjustment to hearing loss for clients and families/caregivers
Hearing and Related Disorders Prevention (1)	Provides patients/families/caregivers with information and support to prevent communication disorders
Hearing Screening (0)	Pass/refer measures designed to identify need for further audiologic assessment
Home Management (Assessment) (4)	Obtaining and maintaining personal and household possessions and environment Includes/Examples: Includes clothing care, cleaning, meal preparation and cleanup, shopping, money management, household maintenance, safety procedures, and childcare/parenting

Continued on next page

Section F–Physical Rehabilitation and Diagnostic Audiology

Continued from previous page

ICD-10-PCS Value Qualifier (Character 5)	Definition
Home Management (Treatment) (4)	Activities to facilitate obtaining and maintaining personal household possessions and environment Includes/Examples: Includes clothing care, cleaning, meal preparation and clean-up, shopping, money management, household maintenance, safety procedures, childcare/parenting
Instrumental Swallowing and Oral Function (J)	Measures swallowing function using instrumental diagnostic procedures Explanation: Methods include videofluoroscopy, ultrasound, manometry, endoscopy
Integumentary Integrity (1)	Includes/Examples: Includes burns, skin conditions, ecchymosis, bleeding, blisters, scar tissue, wounds and other traumas, tissue mobility, turgor and texture
Manual Therapy Techniques (7)	Techniques in which the therapist uses his/her hands to administer skilled movements Includes/Examples: Includes connective tissue massage, joint mobilization and manipulation, manual lymph drainage, manual traction, soft tissue mobilization and manipulation
Masking Patterns (W)	Measures central auditory processing status
Monaural Electroacoustic Hearing Aid Check (8)	Determines mechanical and electroacoustic function of one hearing aid using hearing aid test box
Monaural Hearing Aid (Assessment) (2)	Measures the candidacy, effectiveness, and appropriateness of a hearing aid Explanation: Measures unilateral fit
Monaural Hearing Aid (Treatment) (1)	Explanation: Assists in achieving maximum understanding and performance
Motor Function (Assessment) (4)	Measures the body's functional and versatile movement patterns Includes/Examples: Includes motor assessment scales, analysis of head, trunk and limb movement, and assessment of motor learning
Motor Function (Treatment) (3)	Exercise or activities to facilitate crossing midline, laterality, bilateral integration, praxis, neuromuscular relaxation, inhibition, facilitation, motor function and motor learning
Motor Speech (Assessment) (B)	Measures neurological motor aspects of speech production
Motor Speech (Treatment) (8)	Applying techniques to improve and augment the impaired neurological motor aspects of speech production
Muscle Performance (Assessment) (Ø)	Measures muscle strength, power and endurance using manual testing, dynamometry or computer-assisted electromechanical muscle test; functional muscle strength, power and endurance; muscle pain, tone, or soreness; or pelvic-floor musculature Explanation: Muscle endurance refers to the ability to contract a muscle repeatedly over time
Muscle Performance (Treatment) (1)	Exercise or activities to increase the capacity of a muscle to do work in terms of strength, power, and/or endurance Explanation: Muscle strength is the force exerted to overcome resistance in one maximal effort. Muscle power is work produced per unit of time, or the product of strength and speed. Muscle endurance is the ability to contract a muscle repeatedly over time.
Neuromotor Development (D)	Measures motor development, righting and equilibrium reactions, and reflex and equilibrium reactions
Non-invasive Instrumental Status (N)	Instrumental measures of oral, nasal, vocal, and velopharyngeal functions as they pertain to speech production
Nonspoken Language (Assessment) (7)	Measures nonspoken language (print, sign, symbols) for communication
Nonspoken Language (Treatment) (Ø)	Applying techniques that improve, augment, or compensate spoken communication
Oral Peripheral Mechanism (P)	Structural measures of face, jaw, lips, tongue, teeth, hard and soft palate, pharynx as related to speech production
Orofacial Myofunctional (Assessment) (K)	Measures orofacial myofunctional patterns for speech and related functions
Orofacial Myofunctional (Treatment) (9)	Applying techniques to improve, alter, or augment impaired orofacial myofunctional patterns and related speech production errors
Oscillating Tracking (3)	Measures ability to visually track
Pain (F)	Measures muscle soreness, pain and soreness with joint movement, and pain perception Includes/Examples: Includes questionnaires, graphs, symptom magnification scales or visual analog scales
Perceptual Processing (Assessment) (5)	Measures stereognosis, kinesthesia, body schema, right-left discrimination, form constancy, position in space, visual closure, figure-ground, depth perception, spatial relations and topographical orientation

Continued on next page

Section F–Physical Rehabilitation and Diagnostic Audiology

Continued from previous page

ICD-10-PCS Value Qualifier (Character 5)	Definition
Perceptual Processing (Treatment) (1)	Exercise and activities to facilitate perceptual processing Explanation: Includes stereognosis, kinesthesia, body schema, right-left discrimination, form constancy, position in space, visual closure, figure-ground, depth perception, spatial relations, and topographical orientation Includes/Examples: Includes stereognosis, kinesthesia, body schema, right-left discrimination, form constancy, position in space, visual closure, figure-ground, depth perception, spatial relations, and topographical orientation
Performance Intensity Phonetically Balanced Speech Discrimination (Q)	Measures word recognition over varying intensity levels
Postural Control (3)	Exercise or activities to increase postural alignment and control
Prosthesis (8)	Explanation: Artificial substitutes for missing body parts that augment performance or function Includes/Examples: Limb prosthesis, ocular prosthesis
Psychosocial Skills (Assessment) (6)	The ability to interact in society and to process emotions Includes/Examples: Includes psychological (values, interests, self-concept); social (role performance, social conduct, interpersonal skills, self expression); self-management (coping skills, time management, self-control)
Psychosocial Skills (Treatment) (6)	The ability to interact in society and to process emotions Includes/Examples: Includes psychological (values, interests, self-concept); social (role performance, social conduct, interpersonal skills, self expression); self-management (coping skills, time management, self-control)
Pure Tone Audiometry, Air (1)	Air-conduction pure tone threshold measures with appropriate masking
Pure Tone Audiometry, Air and Bone (2)	Air-conduction and bone-conduction pure tone threshold measures with appropriate masking
Pure Tone Stenger (C)	Measures unilateral nonorganic hearing loss based on simultaneous presentation of pure tones of differing volume
Range of Motion and Joint Integrity (5)	Measures quantity, quality, grade, and classification of joint movement and/or mobility Explanation: Range of Motion is the space, distance or angle through which movement occurs at a joint or series of joints. Joint integrity is the conformance of joints to expected anatomic, biomechanical and kinematic norms.
Range of Motion and Joint Mobility (Ø)	Exercise or activities to increase muscle length and joint mobility
Receptive/Expressive Language (Assessment) (8)	Measures receptive and expressive language
Receptive/Expressive Language (Treatment) (B)	Applying techniques to improve and augment receptive/expressive language
Reflex Integrity (G)	Measures the presence, absence, or exaggeration of developmentally appropriate, pathologic or normal reflexes
Select Picture Audiometry (5)	Establishes hearing threshold levels for speech using pictures
Sensorineural Acuity Level (4)	Measures sensorineural acuity masking presented via bone conduction
Sensory Aids (5)	Determines the appropriateness of a sensory prosthetic device, other than a hearing aid or assistive listening system/device
Sensory Awareness/ Processing/ Integrity (6)	Includes/Examples: Includes light touch, pressure, temperature, pain, sharp/dull, proprioception, vestibular, visual, auditory, gustatory, and olfactory
Short Increment Sensitivity Index (9)	Measures the ear's ability to detect small intensity changes; site of lesion test requiring a behavioral response
Sinusoidal Vertical Axis Rotational (4)	Measures nystagmus following rotation
Somatosensory Evoked Potentials (9)	Measures neural activity from sites throughout the body
Speech/Language Screening (6)	Identifies need for further speech and/or language evaluation
Speech Threshold (1)	Measures minimal intensity needed to repeat spondaic words

Continued on next page

Section F–Physical Rehabilitation and Diagnostic Audiology

Continued from previous page

ICD-10-PCS Value Qualifier (Character 5)	Definition
Speech-Language Pathology and Related Disorders Counseling (1)	Provides patients/families with information, support, referrals to facilitate recovery from a communication disorder
Speech-Language Pathology and Related Disorders Prevention (2)	Applying techniques to avoid or minimize onset and/or development of a communication disorder
Speech/Word Recognition (2)	Measures ability to repeat/identify single syllable words; scores given as a percentage; includes word recognition/speech discrimination
Staggered Spondaic Word (3)	Measures central auditory processing site of lesion based upon dichotic presentation of spondaic words
Static Orthosis (7)	Includes/Examples: Includes customized and prefabricated splints, inhibitory casts, spinal and other braces, and protective devices; has no moving parts, maintains joint(s) in desired position
Stenger (B)	Measures unilateral nonorganic hearing loss based on simultaneous presentation of signals of differing volume
Swallowing Dysfunction (D)	Activities to improve swallowing function in coordination with respiratory function Includes/Examples: Includes function and coordination of sucking, mastication, coughing, swallowing
Synthetic Sentence Identification (5)	Measures central auditory dysfunction using identification of third order approximations of sentences and competing messages
Temporal Ordering of Stimuli (V)	Measures specific central auditory process
Therapeutic Exercise (6)	Exercise or activities to facilitate sensory awareness, sensory processing, sensory integration, balance training, conditioning, reconditioning Includes/Examples: Includes developmental activities, breathing exercises, aerobic endurance activities, aquatic exercises, stretching and ventilatory muscle training
Tinnitus Masker (Assessment) (7)	Determines candidacy for tinnitus masker
Tinnitus Masker (Treatment) (Ø)	Explanation: Used to verify physical fit, acoustic appropriateness, and benefit; assists in achieving maximum benefit
Tone Decay (8)	Measures decrease in hearing sensitivity to a tone; site of lesion test requiring a behavioral response
Transfer (C)	Transitional movement from one surface to another
Transfer Training (8)	Exercise or activities to facilitate movement from one surface to another
Tympanometry (D)	Measures the integrity of the middle ear; measures ease at which sound flows through the tympanic membrane while air pressure against the membrane is varied
Unithermal Binaural Screen (2)	Measures the rhythmic eye movements stimulated by changing the temperature of the vestibular system in both ears using warm water, screening format
Ventilation/Respiration/Circulation (G)	Measures ventilatory muscle strength, power and endurance, pulmonary function and ventilatory mechanics Includes/Examples: Includes ability to clear airway, activities that aggravate or relieve edema, pain, dyspnea or other symptoms, chest wall mobility, cardiopulmonary response to performance of ADL and IAD, cough and sputum, standard vital signs
Vestibular (Ø)	Applying techniques to compensate for balance disorders; includes habituation, exercise therapy, and balance retraining
Visual Motor Integration (Assessment) (2)	Coordinating the interaction of information from the eyes with body movement during activity
Visual Motor Integration (Treatment) (2)	Exercise or activities to facilitate coordinating the interaction of information from eyes with body movement during activity
Visual Reinforcement Audiometry (6)	Behavioral measures using nonspeech and speech stimuli to obtain frequency/ear-specific information on auditory status Includes/Examples: Includes a conditioned response of looking toward a visual reinforcer (e.g., lights, animated toy) every time auditory stimuli are heard
Vocational Activities and Functional Community or Work Reintegration Skills (Assessment) (H)	Measures environmental, home, work (job/school/play) barriers that keep patients from functioning optimally in their environment Includes/Examples: Includes assessment of vocational skills and interests, environment of work (job/school/play), injury potential and injury prevention or reduction, ergonomic stressors, transportation skills, and ability to access and use community resources

Continued on next page

Section F–Physical Rehabilitation and Diagnostic Audiology   *Continued from previous page*

ICD-10-PCS Value Qualifier (Character 5)	Definition
Vocational Activities and Functional Community or Work Reintegration Skills (Treatment) (7)	Activities to facilitate vocational exploration, body mechanics training, job acquisition, and environmental or work (job/school/play) task adaptation Includes/Examples: Includes injury prevention and reduction, ergonomic stressor reduction, job coaching and simulation, work hardening and conditioning, driving training, transportation skills, and use of community resources
Voice (Assessment) (F)	Measures vocal structure, function and production
Voice (Treatment) (C)	Applying techniques to improve voice and vocal function
Voice Prosthetic (Assessment) (M)	Determines the appropriateness of voice prosthetic/adaptive device to enhance or facilitate communication
Voice Prosthetic (Treatment) (4)	Includes/Examples: Includes electrolarynx, and other assistive, adaptive, supportive devices
Wheelchair Mobility (Assessment) (F)	Measures fit and functional abilities within wheelchair in a variety of environments
Wheelchair Mobility (Treatment) (4)	Management, maintenance and controlled operation of a wheelchair, scooter or other device, in and on a variety of surfaces and environments
Wound Management (5)	Includes/Examples: Includes non-selective and selective debridement (enzymes, autolysis, sharp debridement), dressings (wound coverings, hydrogel, vacuum-assisted closure), topical agents, etc.

Section G–Mental Health

ICD-10-PCS Value (Character 3)	Definition
Biofeedback (C)	Provision of information from the monitoring and regulating of physiological processes in conjunction with cognitive-behavioral techniques to improve patient functioning or well-being Includes/Examples: Includes EEG, blood pressure, skin temperature or peripheral blood flow, ECG, electrooculogram, EMG, respirometry or capnometry, GSR/EDR, perineometry to monitor/regulate bowel/bladder activity, electrogastrogram to monitor/regulate gastric motility
Counseling (6)	The application of psychological methods to treat an individual with normal developmental issues and psychological problems in order to increase function, improve well-being, alleviate distress, maladjustment or resolve crises
Crisis Intervention (2)	Treatment of a traumatized, acutely disturbed or distressed individual for the purpose of short-term stabilization Includes/Examples: Includes defusing, debriefing, counseling, psychotherapy and/or coordination of care with other providers or agencies
Electroconvulsive Therapy (B)	The application of controlled electrical voltages to treat a mental health disorder Includes/Examples: Includes appropriate sedation and other preparation of the individual
Family Psychotherapy (7)	Treatment that includes one or more family members of an individual with a mental health disorder by behavioral, cognitive, psychoanalytic, psychodynamic or psychophysiological means to improve functioning or well-being Explanation: Remediation of emotional or behavioral problems presented by one or more family members in cases where psychotherapy with more than one family member is indicated
Group Psychotherapy (H)	Treatment of two or more individuals with a mental health disorder by behavioral, cognitive, psychoanalytic, psychodynamic or psychophysiological means to improve functioning or well-being
Hypnosis (F)	Induction of a state of heightened suggestibility by auditory, visual and tactile techniques to elicit an emotional or behavioral response
Individual Psychotherapy (5)	Treatment of an individual with a mental health disorder by behavioral, cognitive, psychoanalytic, psychodynamic or psychophysiological means to improve functioning or well-being
Light Therapy (J)	Application of specialized light treatments to improve functioning or well-being
Medication Management (3)	Monitoring and adjusting the use of medications for the treatment of a mental health disorder
Narcosynthesis (G)	Administration of intravenous barbiturates in order to release suppressed or repressed thoughts
Psychological Tests (1)	The administration and interpretation of standardized psychological tests and measurement instruments for the assessment of psychological function

Continued on next page

Section G–Mental Health

ICD-10-PCS Value Qualifier (Character 4)	Definition
Behavioral (1)	Primarily to modify behavior Includes/Examples: Includes modeling and role playing, positive reinforcement of target behaviors, response cost, and training of self-management skills
Cognitive (2)	Primarily to correct cognitive distortions and errors
Cognitive-Behavioral (8)	Combining cognitive and behavioral treatment strategies to improve functioning Explanation: Maladaptive responses are examined to determine how cognitions relate to behavior patterns in response to an event. Uses learning principles and information-processing models.
Developmental (Ø)	Age-normed developmental status of cognitive, social and adaptive behavior skills
Intellectual and Psychoeducational (2)	Intellectual abilities, academic achievement and learning capabilities (including behaviors and emotional factors affecting learning)
Interactive (Ø)	Uses primarily physical aids and other forms of non-oral interaction with a patient who is physically, psychologically or developmentally unable to use ordinary language for communication Includes/Examples: Includes the use of toys in symbolic play
Interpersonal (3)	Helps an individual make changes in interpersonal behaviors to reduce psychological dysfunction Includes/Examples: Includes exploratory techniques, encouragement of affective expression, clarification of patient statements, analysis of communication patterns, use of therapy relationship and behavior change techniques
Neurobehavioral and Cognitive Status (4)	Includes neurobehavioral status exam, interview(s), and observation for the clinical assessment of thinking, reasoning and judgment, acquired knowledge, attention, memory, visual spatial abilities, language functions, and planning
Neuropsychological (3)	Thinking, reasoning and judgment, acquired knowledge, attention, memory, visual spatial abilities, language functions, planning
Personality and Behavioral (1)	Mood, emotion, behavior, social functioning, psychopathological conditions, personality traits and characteristics
Psychoanalysis (4)	Methods of obtaining a detailed account of past and present mental and emotional experiences to determine the source and eliminate or diminish the undesirable effects of unconscious conflicts Explanation: Accomplished by making the individual aware of their existence, origin, and inappropriate expression in emotions and behavior
Psychodynamic (5)	Exploration of past and present emotional experiences to understand motives and drives using insight-oriented techniques to reduce the undesirable effects of internal conflicts on emotions and behavior Explanation: Techniques include empathetic listening, clarifying self-defeating behavior patterns, and exploring adaptive alternatives
Psychophysiological (9)	Monitoring and alteration of physiological processes to help the individual associate physiological reactions combined with cognitive and behavioral strategies to gain improved control of these processes to help the individual cope more effectively
Supportive (6)	Formation of therapeutic relationship primarily for providing emotional support to prevent further deterioration in functioning during periods of particular stress Explanation: Often used in conjunction with other therapeutic approaches
Vocational (1)	Exploration of vocational interests, aptitudes and required adaptive behavior skills to develop and carry out a plan for achieving a successful vocational placement Includes/Examples: Includes enhancing work related adjustment and/or pursuing viable options in training education or preparation

Section H–Substance Abuse Treatment

ICD-10-PCS Value (Character 3)	Definition
Detoxification Services (2)	Detoxification from alcohol and/or drugs Explanation: Not a treatment modality, but helps the patient stabilize physically and psychologically until the body becomes free of drugs and the effects of alcohol
Family Counseling (6)	The application of psychological methods that includes one or more family members to treat an individual with addictive behavior Explanation: Provides support and education for family members of addicted individuals. Family member participation is seen as a critical area of substance abuse treatment.
Group Counseling (4)	The application of psychological methods to treat two or more individuals with addictive behavior Explanation: Provides structured group counseling sessions and healing power through the connection with others
Individual Counseling (3)	The application of psychological methods to treat an individual with addictive behavior Explanation: Comprised of several different techniques, which apply various strategies to address drug addiction
Individual Psychotherapy (5)	Treatment of an individual with addictive behavior by behavioral, cognitive, psychoanalytic, psychodynamic or psychophysiological means
Medication Management (8)	Monitoring and adjusting the use of replacement medications for the treatment of addiction
Pharmacotherapy (9)	The use of replacement medications for the treatment of addiction

Appendix K: Hospital Acquired Conditions

Hospital acquired conditions (HACs) are conditions considered reasonably preventable through the application of evidence-based guidelines. Although it is the ICD-10-CM diagnosis code that drives a HAC designation, in some cases a specific ICD-10-PCS procedure code must also be present before that diagnosis code can be considered a HAC. This resource provides only those HAC categories that require both an ICD-10-PCS code and an ICD-10-CM diagnosis code. The official descriptions for each code are also provided. To see all 14 HAC categories and their corresponding codes, refer to Optum360's *ICD-10-CM Expert for Hospitals*.

Note: The resource used to compile this list is the proposed, version 38, MS-DRG Grouper software and Definitions Manual files published with the fiscal 2021 IPPS proposed rule. For the final, version 38, MS-DRG Grouper software and Definitions Manual files, refer to the following: https://www.cms.gov/Medicare/Medicare-Fee-for-Service-Payment/AcuteInpatientPPS/MS-DRG-Classifications-and-Software.

HAC 08: Surgical Site Infection of Mediastinitis After Coronary Bypass Graft (CABG) Procedures
Secondary diagnosis not POA:
- J98.51 Mediastinitis
- J98.59 Other diseases of mediastinum, not elsewhere classified

AND

Any of the following procedures:
- 0210083 Bypass Coronary Artery, One Artery from Coronary Artery with Zooplastic Tissue, Open Approach
- 0210088 Bypass Coronary Artery, One Artery from Right Internal Mammary with Zooplastic Tissue, Open Approach
- 0210089 Bypass Coronary Artery, One Artery from Left Internal Mammary with Zooplastic Tissue, Open Approach
- 021008C Bypass Coronary Artery, One Artery from Thoracic Artery with Zooplastic Tissue, Open Approach
- 021008F Bypass Coronary Artery, One Artery from Abdominal Artery with Zooplastic Tissue, Open Approach
- 021008W Bypass Coronary Artery, One Artery from Aorta with Zooplastic Tissue, Open Approach
- 0210093 Bypass Coronary Artery, One Artery from Coronary Artery with Autologous Venous Tissue, Open Approach
- 0210098 Bypass Coronary Artery, One Artery from Right Internal Mammary with Autologous Venous Tissue, Open Approach
- 0210099 Bypass Coronary Artery, One Artery from Left Internal Mammary with Autologous Venous Tissue, Open Approach
- 021009C Bypass Coronary Artery, One Artery from Thoracic Artery with Autologous Venous Tissue, Open Approach
- 021009F Bypass Coronary Artery, One Artery from Abdominal Artery with Autologous Venous Tissue, Open Approach
- 021009W Bypass Coronary Artery, One Artery from Aorta with Autologous Venous Tissue, Open Approach
- 02100A3 Bypass Coronary Artery, One Artery from Coronary Artery with Autologous Arterial Tissue, Open Approach
- 02100A8 Bypass Coronary Artery, One Artery from Right Internal Mammary with Autologous Arterial Tissue, Open Approach
- 02100A9 Bypass Coronary Artery, One Artery from Left Internal Mammary with Autologous Arterial Tissue, Open Approach
- 02100AC Bypass Coronary Artery, One Artery from Thoracic Artery with Autologous Arterial Tissue, Open Approach
- 02100AF Bypass Coronary Artery, One Artery from Abdominal Artery with Autologous Arterial Tissue, Open Approach
- 02100AW Bypass Coronary Artery, One Artery from Aorta with Autologous Arterial Tissue, Open Approach
- 02100J3 Bypass Coronary Artery, One Artery from Coronary Artery with Synthetic Substitute, Open Approach
- 02100J8 Bypass Coronary Artery, One Artery from Right Internal Mammary with Synthetic Substitute, Open Approach
- 02100J9 Bypass Coronary Artery, One Artery from Left Internal Mammary with Synthetic Substitute, Open Approach
- 02100JC Bypass Coronary Artery, One Artery from Thoracic Artery with Synthetic Substitute, Open Approach
- 02100JF Bypass Coronary Artery, One Artery from Abdominal Artery with Synthetic Substitute, Open Approach
- 02100JW Bypass Coronary Artery, One Artery from Aorta with Synthetic Substitute, Open Approach
- 02100K3 Bypass Coronary Artery, One Artery from Coronary Artery with Nonautologous Tissue Substitute, Open Approach
- 02100K8 Bypass Coronary Artery, One Artery from Right Internal Mammary with Nonautologous Tissue Substitute, Open Approach
- 02100K9 Bypass Coronary Artery, One Artery from Left Internal Mammary with Nonautologous Tissue Substitute, Open Approach
- 02100KC Bypass Coronary Artery, One Artery from Thoracic Artery with Nonautologous Tissue Substitute, Open Approach
- 02100KF Bypass Coronary Artery, One Artery from Abdominal Artery with Nonautologous Tissue Substitute, Open Approach
- 02100KW Bypass Coronary Artery, One Artery from Aorta with Nonautologous Tissue Substitute, Open Approach
- 02100Z3 Bypass Coronary Artery, One Artery from Coronary Artery, Open Approach
- 02100Z8 Bypass Coronary Artery, One Artery from Right Internal Mammary, Open Approach
- 02100Z9 Bypass Coronary Artery, One Artery from Left Internal Mammary, Open Approach
- 02100ZC Bypass Coronary Artery, One Artery from Thoracic Artery, Open Approach
- 02100ZF Bypass Coronary Artery, One Artery from Abdominal Artery, Open Approach
- 0210483 Bypass Coronary Artery, One Artery from Coronary Artery with Zooplastic Tissue, Percutaneous Endoscopic Approach
- 0210488 Bypass Coronary Artery, One Artery from Right Internal Mammary with Zooplastic Tissue, Percutaneous Endoscopic Approach
- 0210489 Bypass Coronary Artery, One Artery from Left Internal Mammary with Zooplastic Tissue, Percutaneous Endoscopic Approach
- 021048C Bypass Coronary Artery, One Artery from Thoracic Artery with Zooplastic Tissue, Percutaneous Endoscopic Approach
- 021048F Bypass Coronary Artery, One Artery from Abdominal Artery with Zooplastic Tissue, Percutaneous Endoscopic Approach
- 021048W Bypass Coronary Artery, One Artery from Aorta with Zooplastic Tissue, Percutaneous Endoscopic Approach
- 0210493 Bypass Coronary Artery, One Artery from Coronary Artery with Autologous Venous Tissue, Percutaneous Endoscopic Approach
- 0210498 Bypass Coronary Artery, One Artery from Right Internal Mammary with Autologous Venous Tissue, Percutaneous Endoscopic Approach
- 0210499 Bypass Coronary Artery, One Artery from Left Internal Mammary with Autologous Venous Tissue, Percutaneous Endoscopic Approach
- 021049C Bypass Coronary Artery, One Artery from Thoracic Artery with Autologous Venous Tissue, Percutaneous Endoscopic Approach
- 021049F Bypass Coronary Artery, One Artery from Abdominal Artery with Autologous Venous Tissue, Percutaneous Endoscopic Approach
- 021049W Bypass Coronary Artery, One Artery from Aorta with Autologous Venous Tissue, Percutaneous Endoscopic Approach
- 02104A3 Bypass Coronary Artery, One Artery from Coronary Artery with Autologous Arterial Tissue, Percutaneous Endoscopic Approach
- 02104A8 Bypass Coronary Artery, One Artery from Right Internal Mammary with Autologous Arterial Tissue, Percutaneous Endoscopic Approach
- 02104A9 Bypass Coronary Artery, One Artery from Left Internal Mammary with Autologous Arterial Tissue, Percutaneous Endoscopic Approach
- 02104AC Bypass Coronary Artery, One Artery from Thoracic Artery with Autologous Arterial Tissue, Percutaneous Endoscopic Approach

HAC 08: Surgical Site Infection of Mediastinitis After Coronary Bypass Graft (CABG) Procedures (continued)

02104AF   Bypass Coronary Artery, One Artery from Abdominal Artery with Autologous Arterial Tissue, Percutaneous Endoscopic Approach

02104AW   Bypass Coronary Artery, One Artery from Aorta with Autologous Arterial Tissue, Percutaneous Endoscopic Approach

02104J3   Bypass Coronary Artery, One Artery from Coronary Artery with Synthetic Substitute, Percutaneous Endoscopic Approach

02104J8   Bypass Coronary Artery, One Artery from Right Internal Mammary with Synthetic Substitute, Percutaneous Endoscopic Approach

02104J9   Bypass Coronary Artery, One Artery from Left Internal Mammary with Synthetic Substitute, Percutaneous Endoscopic Approach

02104JC   Bypass Coronary Artery, One Artery from Thoracic Artery with Synthetic Substitute, Percutaneous Endoscopic Approach

02104JF   Bypass Coronary Artery, One Artery from Abdominal Artery with Synthetic Substitute, Percutaneous Endoscopic Approach

02104JW   Bypass Coronary Artery, One Artery from Aorta with Synthetic Substitute, Percutaneous Endoscopic Approach

02104K3   Bypass Coronary Artery, One Artery from Coronary Artery with Nonautologous Tissue Substitute, Percutaneous Endoscopic Approach

02104K8   Bypass Coronary Artery, One Artery from Right Internal Mammary with Nonautologous Tissue Substitute, Percutaneous Endoscopic Approach

02104K9   Bypass Coronary Artery, One Artery from Left Internal Mammary with Nonautologous Tissue Substitute, Percutaneous Endoscopic Approach

02104KC   Bypass Coronary Artery, One Artery from Thoracic Artery with Nonautologous Tissue Substitute, Percutaneous Endoscopic Approach

02104KF   Bypass Coronary Artery, One Artery from Abdominal Artery with Nonautologous Tissue Substitute, Percutaneous Endoscopic Approach

02104KW   Bypass Coronary Artery, One Artery from Aorta with Nonautologous Tissue Substitute, Percutaneous Endoscopic Approach

02104Z3   Bypass Coronary Artery, One Artery from Coronary Artery, Percutaneous Endoscopic Approach

02104Z8   Bypass Coronary Artery, One Artery from Right Internal Mammary, Percutaneous Endoscopic Approach

02104Z9   Bypass Coronary Artery, One Artery from Left Internal Mammary, Percutaneous Endoscopic Approach

02104ZC   Bypass Coronary Artery, One Artery from Thoracic Artery, Percutaneous Endoscopic Approach

02104ZF   Bypass Coronary Artery, One Artery from Abdominal Artery, Percutaneous Endoscopic Approach

0211083   Bypass Coronary Artery, Two Arteries from Coronary Artery with Zooplastic Tissue, Open Approach

0211088   Bypass Coronary Artery, Two Arteries from Right Internal Mammary with Zooplastic Tissue, Open Approach

0211089   Bypass Coronary Artery, Two Arteries from Left Internal Mammary with Zooplastic Tissue, Open Approach

021108C   Bypass Coronary Artery, Two Arteries from Thoracic Artery with Zooplastic Tissue, Open Approach

021108F   Bypass Coronary Artery, Two Arteries from Abdominal Artery with Zooplastic Tissue, Open Approach

021108W   Bypass Coronary Artery, Two Arteries from Aorta with Zooplastic Tissue, Open Approach

0211093   Bypass Coronary Artery, Two Arteries from Coronary Artery with Autologous Venous Tissue, Open Approach

0211098   Bypass Coronary Artery, Two Arteries from Right Internal Mammary with Autologous Venous Tissue, Open Approach

0211099   Bypass Coronary Artery, Two Arteries from Left Internal Mammary with Autologous Venous Tissue, Open Approach

021109C   Bypass Coronary Artery, Two Arteries from Thoracic Artery with Autologous Venous Tissue, Open Approach

021109F   Bypass Coronary Artery, Two Arteries from Abdominal Artery with Autologous Venous Tissue, Open Approach

021109W   Bypass Coronary Artery, Two Arteries from Aorta with Autologous Venous Tissue, Open Approach

02110A3   Bypass Coronary Artery, Two Arteries from Coronary Artery with Autologous Arterial Tissue, Open Approach

02110A8   Bypass Coronary Artery, Two Arteries from Right Internal Mammary with Autologous Arterial Tissue, Open Approach

02110A9   Bypass Coronary Artery, Two Arteries from Left Internal Mammary with Autologous Arterial Tissue, Open Approach

02110AC   Bypass Coronary Artery, Two Arteries from Thoracic Artery with Autologous Arterial Tissue, Open Approach

02110AF   Bypass Coronary Artery, Two Arteries from Abdominal Artery with Autologous Arterial Tissue, Open Approach

02110AW   Bypass Coronary Artery, Two Arteries from Aorta with Autologous Arterial Tissue, Open Approach

02110J3   Bypass Coronary Artery, Two Arteries from Coronary Artery with Synthetic Substitute, Open Approach

02110J8   Bypass Coronary Artery, Two Arteries from Right Internal Mammary with Synthetic Substitute, Open Approach

02110J9   Bypass Coronary Artery, Two Arteries from Left Internal Mammary with Synthetic Substitute, Open Approach

02110JC   Bypass Coronary Artery, Two Arteries from Thoracic Artery with Synthetic Substitute, Open Approach

02110JF   Bypass Coronary Artery, Two Arteries from Abdominal Artery with Synthetic Substitute, Open Approach

02110JW   Bypass Coronary Artery, Two Arteries from Aorta with Synthetic Substitute, Open Approach

02110K3   Bypass Coronary Artery, Two Arteries from Coronary Artery with Nonautologous Tissue Substitute, Open Approach

02110K8   Bypass Coronary Artery, Two Arteries from Right Internal Mammary with Nonautologous Tissue Substitute, Open Approach

02110K9   Bypass Coronary Artery, Two Arteries from Left Internal Mammary with Nonautologous Tissue Substitute, Open Approach

02110KC   Bypass Coronary Artery, Two Arteries from Thoracic Artery with Nonautologous Tissue Substitute, Open Approach

02110KF   Bypass Coronary Artery, Two Arteries from Abdominal Artery with Nonautologous Tissue Substitute, Open Approach

02110KW   Bypass Coronary Artery, Two Arteries from Aorta with Nonautologous Tissue Substitute, Open Approach

02110Z3   Bypass Coronary Artery, Two Arteries from Coronary Artery, Open Approach

02110Z8   Bypass Coronary Artery, Two Arteries from Right Internal Mammary, Open Approach

02110Z9   Bypass Coronary Artery, Two Arteries from Left Internal Mammary, Open Approach

02110ZC   Bypass Coronary Artery, Two Arteries from Thoracic Artery, Open Approach

02110ZF   Bypass Coronary Artery, Two Arteries from Abdominal Artery, Open Approach

0211483   Bypass Coronary Artery, Two Arteries from Coronary Artery with Zooplastic Tissue, Percutaneous Endoscopic Approach

0211488   Bypass Coronary Artery, Two Arteries from Right Internal Mammary with Zooplastic Tissue, Percutaneous Endoscopic Approach

0211489   Bypass Coronary Artery, Two Arteries from Left Internal Mammary with Zooplastic Tissue, Percutaneous Endoscopic Approach

021148C   Bypass Coronary Artery, Two Arteries from Thoracic Artery with Zooplastic Tissue, Percutaneous Endoscopic Approach

021148F   Bypass Coronary Artery, Two Arteries from Abdominal Artery with Zooplastic Tissue, Percutaneous Endoscopic Approach

021148W   Bypass Coronary Artery, Two Arteries from Aorta with Zooplastic Tissue, Percutaneous Endoscopic Approach

0211493   Bypass Coronary Artery, Two Arteries from Coronary Artery with Autologous Venous Tissue, Percutaneous Endoscopic Approach

0211498   Bypass Coronary Artery, Two Arteries from Right Internal Mammary with Autologous Venous Tissue, Percutaneous Endoscopic Approach

0211499   Bypass Coronary Artery, Two Arteries from Left Internal Mammary with Autologous Venous Tissue, Percutaneous Endoscopic Approach

021149C   Bypass Coronary Artery, Two Arteries from Thoracic Artery with Autologous Venous Tissue, Percutaneous Endoscopic Approach

HAC 08: Surgical Site Infection of Mediastinitis After Coronary Bypass Graft (CABG) Procedures (continued)

021149F　Bypass Coronary Artery, Two Arteries from Abdominal Artery with Autologous Venous Tissue, Percutaneous Endoscopic Approach

021149W　Bypass Coronary Artery, Two Arteries from Aorta with Autologous Venous Tissue, Percutaneous Endoscopic Approach

02114A3　Bypass Coronary Artery, Two Arteries from Coronary Artery with Autologous Arterial Tissue, Percutaneous Endoscopic Approach

02114A8　Bypass Coronary Artery, Two Arteries from Right Internal Mammary with Autologous Arterial Tissue, Percutaneous Endoscopic Approach

02114A9　Bypass Coronary Artery, Two Arteries from Left Internal Mammary with Autologous Arterial Tissue, Percutaneous Endoscopic Approach

02114AC　Bypass Coronary Artery, Two Arteries from Thoracic Artery with Autologous Arterial Tissue, Percutaneous Endoscopic Approach

02114AF　Bypass Coronary Artery, Two Arteries from Abdominal Artery with Autologous Arterial Tissue, Percutaneous Endoscopic Approach

02114AW　Bypass Coronary Artery, Two Arteries from Aorta with Autologous Arterial Tissue, Percutaneous Endoscopic Approach

02114J3　Bypass Coronary Artery, Two Arteries from Coronary Artery with Synthetic Substitute, Percutaneous Endoscopic Approach

02114J8　Bypass Coronary Artery, Two Arteries from Right Internal Mammary with Synthetic Substitute, Percutaneous Endoscopic Approach

02114J9　Bypass Coronary Artery, Two Arteries from Left Internal Mammary with Synthetic Substitute, Percutaneous Endoscopic Approach

02114JC　Bypass Coronary Artery, Two Arteries from Thoracic Artery with Synthetic Substitute, Percutaneous Endoscopic Approach

02114JF　Bypass Coronary Artery, Two Arteries from Abdominal Artery with Synthetic Substitute, Percutaneous Endoscopic Approach

02114JW　Bypass Coronary Artery, Two Arteries from Aorta with Synthetic Substitute, Percutaneous Endoscopic Approach

02114K3　Bypass Coronary Artery, Two Arteries from Coronary Artery with Nonautologous Tissue Substitute, Percutaneous Endoscopic Approach

02114K8　Bypass Coronary Artery, Two Arteries from Right Internal Mammary with Nonautologous Tissue Substitute, Percutaneous Endoscopic Approach

02114K9　Bypass Coronary Artery, Two Arteries from Left Internal Mammary with Nonautologous Tissue Substitute, Percutaneous Endoscopic Approach

02114KC　Bypass Coronary Artery, Two Arteries from Thoracic Artery with Nonautologous Tissue Substitute, Percutaneous Endoscopic Approach

02114KF　Bypass Coronary Artery, Two Arteries from Abdominal Artery with Nonautologous Tissue Substitute, Percutaneous Endoscopic Approach

02114KW　Bypass Coronary Artery, Two Arteries from Aorta with Nonautologous Tissue Substitute, Percutaneous Endoscopic Approach

02114Z3　Bypass Coronary Artery, Two Arteries from Coronary Artery, Percutaneous Endoscopic Approach

02114Z8　Bypass Coronary Artery, Two Arteries from Right Internal Mammary, Percutaneous Endoscopic Approach

02114Z9　Bypass Coronary Artery, Two Arteries from Left Internal Mammary, Percutaneous Endoscopic Approach

02114ZC　Bypass Coronary Artery, Two Arteries from Thoracic Artery, Percutaneous Endoscopic Approach

02114ZF　Bypass Coronary Artery, Two Arteries from Abdominal Artery, Percutaneous Endoscopic Approach

0212083　Bypass Coronary Artery, Three Arteries from Coronary Artery with Zooplastic Tissue, Open Approach

0212088　Bypass Coronary Artery, Three Arteries from Right Internal Mammary with Zooplastic Tissue, Open Approach

0212089　Bypass Coronary Artery, Three Arteries from Left Internal Mammary with Zooplastic Tissue, Open Approach

021208C　Bypass Coronary Artery, Three Arteries from Thoracic Artery with Zooplastic Tissue, Open Approach

021208F　Bypass Coronary Artery, Three Arteries from Abdominal Artery with Zooplastic Tissue, Open Approach

021208W　Bypass Coronary Artery, Three Arteries from Aorta with Zooplastic Tissue, Open Approach

0212093　Bypass Coronary Artery, Three Arteries from Coronary Artery with Autologous Venous Tissue, Open Approach

0212098　Bypass Coronary Artery, Three Arteries from Right Internal Mammary with Autologous Venous Tissue, Open Approach

0212099　Bypass Coronary Artery, Three Arteries from Left Internal Mammary with Autologous Venous Tissue, Open Approach

021209C　Bypass Coronary Artery, Three Arteries from Thoracic Artery with Autologous Venous Tissue, Open Approach

021209F　Bypass Coronary Artery, Three Arteries from Abdominal Artery with Autologous Venous Tissue, Open Approach

021209W　Bypass Coronary Artery, Three Arteries from Aorta with Autologous Venous Tissue, Open Approach

02120A3　Bypass Coronary Artery, Three Arteries from Coronary Artery with Autologous Arterial Tissue, Open Approach

02120A8　Bypass Coronary Artery, Three Arteries from Right Internal Mammary with Autologous Arterial Tissue, Open Approach

02120A9　Bypass Coronary Artery, Three Arteries from Left Internal Mammary with Autologous Arterial Tissue, Open Approach

02120AC　Bypass Coronary Artery, Three Arteries from Thoracic Artery with Autologous Arterial Tissue, Open Approach

02120AF　Bypass Coronary Artery, Three Arteries from Abdominal Artery with Autologous Arterial Tissue, Open Approach

02120AW　Bypass Coronary Artery, Three Arteries from Aorta with Autologous Arterial Tissue, Open Approach

02120J3　Bypass Coronary Artery, Three Arteries from Coronary Artery with Synthetic Substitute, Open Approach

02120J8　Bypass Coronary Artery, Three Arteries from Right Internal Mammary with Synthetic Substitute, Open Approach

02120J9　Bypass Coronary Artery, Three Arteries from Left Internal Mammary with Synthetic Substitute, Open Approach

02120JC　Bypass Coronary Artery, Three Arteries from Thoracic Artery with Synthetic Substitute, Open Approach

02120JF　Bypass Coronary Artery, Three Arteries from Abdominal Artery with Synthetic Substitute, Open Approach

02120JW　Bypass Coronary Artery, Three Arteries from Aorta with Synthetic Substitute, Open Approach

02120K3　Bypass Coronary Artery, Three Arteries from Coronary Artery with Nonautologous Tissue Substitute, Open Approach

02120K8　Bypass Coronary Artery, Three Arteries from Right Internal Mammary with Nonautologous Tissue Substitute, Open Approach

02120K9　Bypass Coronary Artery, Three Arteries from Left Internal Mammary with Nonautologous Tissue Substitute, Open Approach

02120KC　Bypass Coronary Artery, Three Arteries from Thoracic Artery with Nonautologous Tissue Substitute, Open Approach

02120KF　Bypass Coronary Artery, Three Arteries from Abdominal Artery with Nonautologous Tissue Substitute, Open Approach

02120KW　Bypass Coronary Artery, Three Arteries from Aorta with Nonautologous Tissue Substitute, Open Approach

02120Z3　Bypass Coronary Artery, Three Arteries from Coronary Artery, Open Approach

02120Z8　Bypass Coronary Artery, Three Arteries from Right Internal Mammary, Open Approach

02120Z9　Bypass Coronary Artery, Three Arteries from Left Internal Mammary, Open Approach

02120ZC　Bypass Coronary Artery, Three Arteries from Thoracic Artery, Open Approach

02120ZF　Bypass Coronary Artery, Three Arteries from Abdominal Artery, Open Approach

0212483　Bypass Coronary Artery, Three Arteries from Coronary Artery with Zooplastic Tissue, Percutaneous Endoscopic Approach

0212488　Bypass Coronary Artery, Three Arteries from Right Internal Mammary with Zooplastic Tissue, Percutaneous Endoscopic Approach

0212489　Bypass Coronary Artery, Three Arteries from Left Internal Mammary with Zooplastic Tissue, Percutaneous Endoscopic Approach

021248C　Bypass Coronary Artery, Three Arteries from Thoracic Artery with Zooplastic Tissue, Percutaneous Endoscopic Approach

HAC 08: Surgical Site Infection of Mediastinitis After Coronary Bypass Graft (CABG) Procedures (continued)

021248F   Bypass Coronary Artery, Three Arteries from Abdominal Artery with Zooplastic Tissue, Percutaneous Endoscopic Approach

021248W   Bypass Coronary Artery, Three Arteries from Aorta with Zooplastic Tissue, Percutaneous Endoscopic Approach

0212493   Bypass Coronary Artery, Three Arteries from Coronary Artery with Autologous Venous Tissue, Percutaneous Endoscopic Approach

0212498   Bypass Coronary Artery, Three Arteries from Right Internal Mammary with Autologous Venous Tissue, Percutaneous Endoscopic Approach

0212499   Bypass Coronary Artery, Three Arteries from Left Internal Mammary with Autologous Venous Tissue, Percutaneous Endoscopic Approach

021249C   Bypass Coronary Artery, Three Arteries from Thoracic Artery with Autologous Venous Tissue, Percutaneous Endoscopic Approach

021249F   Bypass Coronary Artery, Three Arteries from Abdominal Artery with Autologous Venous Tissue, Percutaneous Endoscopic Approach

021249W   Bypass Coronary Artery, Three Arteries from Aorta with Autologous Venous Tissue, Percutaneous Endoscopic Approach

02124A3   Bypass Coronary Artery, Three Arteries from Coronary Artery with Autologous Arterial Tissue, Percutaneous Endoscopic Approach

02124A8   Bypass Coronary Artery, Three Arteries from Right Internal Mammary with Autologous Arterial Tissue, Percutaneous Endoscopic Approach

02124A9   Bypass Coronary Artery, Three Arteries from Left Internal Mammary with Autologous Arterial Tissue, Percutaneous Endoscopic Approach

02124AC   Bypass Coronary Artery, Three Arteries from Thoracic Artery with Autologous Arterial Tissue, Percutaneous Endoscopic Approach

02124AF   Bypass Coronary Artery, Three Arteries from Abdominal Artery with Autologous Arterial Tissue, Percutaneous Endoscopic Approach

02124AW   Bypass Coronary Artery, Three Arteries from Aorta with Autologous Arterial Tissue, Percutaneous Endoscopic Approach

02124J3   Bypass Coronary Artery, Three Arteries from Coronary Artery with Synthetic Substitute, Percutaneous Endoscopic Approach

02124J8   Bypass Coronary Artery, Three Arteries from Right Internal Mammary with Synthetic Substitute, Percutaneous Endoscopic Approach

02124J9   Bypass Coronary Artery, Three Arteries from Left Internal Mammary with Synthetic Substitute, Percutaneous Endoscopic Approach

02124JC   Bypass Coronary Artery, Three Arteries from Thoracic Artery with Synthetic Substitute, Percutaneous Endoscopic Approach

02124JF   Bypass Coronary Artery, Three Arteries from Abdominal Artery with Synthetic Substitute, Percutaneous Endoscopic Approach

02124JW   Bypass Coronary Artery, Three Arteries from Aorta with Synthetic Substitute, Percutaneous Endoscopic Approach

02124K3   Bypass Coronary Artery, Three Arteries from Coronary Artery with Nonautologous Tissue Substitute, Percutaneous Endoscopic Approach

02124K8   Bypass Coronary Artery, Three Arteries from Right Internal Mammary with Nonautologous Tissue Substitute, Percutaneous Endoscopic Approach

02124K9   Bypass Coronary Artery, Three Arteries from Left Internal Mammary with Nonautologous Tissue Substitute, Percutaneous Endoscopic Approach

02124KC   Bypass Coronary Artery, Three Arteries from Thoracic Artery with Nonautologous Tissue Substitute, Percutaneous Endoscopic Approach

02124KF   Bypass Coronary Artery, Three Arteries from Abdominal Artery with Nonautologous Tissue Substitute, Percutaneous Endoscopic Approach

02124KW   Bypass Coronary Artery, Three Arteries from Aorta with Nonautologous Tissue Substitute, Percutaneous Endoscopic Approach

02124Z3   Bypass Coronary Artery, Three Arteries from Coronary Artery, Percutaneous Endoscopic Approach

02124Z8   Bypass Coronary Artery, Three Arteries from Right Internal Mammary, Percutaneous Endoscopic Approach

02124Z9   Bypass Coronary Artery, Three Arteries from Left Internal Mammary, Percutaneous Endoscopic Approach

02124ZC   Bypass Coronary Artery, Three Arteries from Thoracic Artery, Percutaneous Endoscopic Approach

02124ZF   Bypass Coronary Artery, Three Arteries from Abdominal Artery, Percutaneous Endoscopic Approach

0213083   Bypass Coronary Artery, Four or More Arteries from Coronary Artery with Zooplastic Tissue, Open Approach

0213088   Bypass Coronary Artery, Four or More Arteries from Right Internal Mammary with Zooplastic Tissue, Open Approach

0213089   Bypass Coronary Artery, Four or More Arteries from Left Internal Mammary with Zooplastic Tissue, Open Approach

021308C   Bypass Coronary Artery, Four or More Arteries from Thoracic Artery with Zooplastic Tissue, Open Approach

021308F   Bypass Coronary Artery, Four or More Arteries from Abdominal Artery with Zooplastic Tissue, Open Approach

021308W   Bypass Coronary Artery, Four or More Arteries from Aorta with Zooplastic Tissue, Open Approach

0213093   Bypass Coronary Artery, Four or More Arteries from Coronary Artery with Autologous Venous Tissue, Open Approach

0213098   Bypass Coronary Artery, Four or More Arteries from Right Internal Mammary with Autologous Venous Tissue, Open Approach

0213099   Bypass Coronary Artery, Four or More Arteries from Left Internal Mammary with Autologous Venous Tissue, Open Approach

021309C   Bypass Coronary Artery, Four or More Arteries from Thoracic Artery with Autologous Venous Tissue, Open Approach

021309F   Bypass Coronary Artery, Four or More Arteries from Abdominal Artery with Autologous Venous Tissue, Open Approach

021309W   Bypass Coronary Artery, Four or More Arteries from Aorta with Autologous Venous Tissue, Open Approach

02130A3   Bypass Coronary Artery, Four or More Arteries from Coronary Artery with Autologous Arterial Tissue, Open Approach

02130A8   Bypass Coronary Artery, Four or More Arteries from Right Internal Mammary with Autologous Arterial Tissue, Open Approach

02130A9   Bypass Coronary Artery, Four or More Arteries from Left Internal Mammary with Autologous Arterial Tissue, Open Approach

02130AC   Bypass Coronary Artery, Four or More Arteries from Thoracic Artery with Autologous Arterial Tissue, Open Approach

02130AF   Bypass Coronary Artery, Four or More Arteries from Abdominal Artery with Autologous Arterial Tissue, Open Approach

02130AW   Bypass Coronary Artery, Four or More Arteries from Aorta with Autologous Arterial Tissue, Open Approach

02130J3   Bypass Coronary Artery, Four or More Arteries from Coronary Artery with Synthetic Substitute, Open Approach

02130J8   Bypass Coronary Artery, Four or More Arteries from Right Internal Mammary with Synthetic Substitute, Open Approach

02130J9   Bypass Coronary Artery, Four or More Arteries from Left Internal Mammary with Synthetic Substitute, Open Approach

02130JC   Bypass Coronary Artery, Four or More Arteries from Thoracic Artery with Synthetic Substitute, Open Approach

02130JF   Bypass Coronary Artery, Four or More Arteries from Abdominal Artery with Synthetic Substitute, Open Approach

02130JW   Bypass Coronary Artery, Four or More Arteries from Aorta with Synthetic Substitute, Open Approach

02130K3   Bypass Coronary Artery, Four or More Arteries from Coronary Artery with Nonautologous Tissue Substitute, Open Approach

02130K8   Bypass Coronary Artery, Four or More Arteries from Right Internal Mammary with Nonautologous Tissue Substitute, Open Approach

02130K9   Bypass Coronary Artery, Four or More Arteries from Left Internal Mammary with Nonautologous Tissue Substitute, Open Approach

02130KC   Bypass Coronary Artery, Four or More Arteries from Thoracic Artery with Nonautologous Tissue Substitute, Open Approach

02130KF   Bypass Coronary Artery, Four or More Arteries from Abdominal Artery with Nonautologous Tissue Substitute, Open Approach

HAC 08: Surgical Site Infection of Mediastinitis After Coronary Bypass Graft (CABG) Procedures (continued)

Ø213ØKW	Bypass Coronary Artery, Four or More Arteries from Aorta with Nonautologous Tissue Substitute, Open Approach
Ø213ØZ3	Bypass Coronary Artery, Four or More Arteries from Coronary Artery, Open Approach
Ø213ØZ8	Bypass Coronary Artery, Four or More Arteries from Right Internal Mammary, Open Approach
Ø213ØZ9	Bypass Coronary Artery, Four or More Arteries from Left Internal Mammary, Open Approach
Ø213ØZC	Bypass Coronary Artery, Four or More Arteries from Thoracic Artery, Open Approach
Ø213ØZF	Bypass Coronary Artery, Four or More Arteries from Abdominal Artery, Open Approach
Ø213483	Bypass Coronary Artery, Four or More Arteries from Coronary Artery with Zooplastic Tissue, Percutaneous Endoscopic Approach
Ø213488	Bypass Coronary Artery, Four or More Arteries from Right Internal Mammary with Zooplastic Tissue, Percutaneous Endoscopic Approach
Ø213489	Bypass Coronary Artery, Four or More Arteries from Left Internal Mammary with Zooplastic Tissue, Percutaneous Endoscopic Approach
Ø21348C	Bypass Coronary Artery, Four or More Arteries from Thoracic Artery with Zooplastic Tissue, Percutaneous Endoscopic Approach
Ø21348F	Bypass Coronary Artery, Four or More Arteries from Abdominal Artery with Zooplastic Tissue, Percutaneous Endoscopic Approach
Ø21348W	Bypass Coronary Artery, Four or More Arteries from Aorta with Zooplastic Tissue, Percutaneous Endoscopic Approach
Ø213493	Bypass Coronary Artery, Four or More Arteries from Coronary Artery with Autologous Venous Tissue, Percutaneous Endoscopic Approach
Ø213498	Bypass Coronary Artery, Four or More Arteries from Right Internal Mammary with Autologous Venous Tissue, Percutaneous Endoscopic Approach
Ø213499	Bypass Coronary Artery, Four or More Arteries from Left Internal Mammary with Autologous Venous Tissue, Percutaneous Endoscopic Approach
Ø21349C	Bypass Coronary Artery, Four or More Arteries from Thoracic Artery with Autologous Venous Tissue, Percutaneous Endoscopic Approach
Ø21349F	Bypass Coronary Artery, Four or More Arteries from Abdominal Artery with Autologous Venous Tissue, Percutaneous Endoscopic Approach
Ø21349W	Bypass Coronary Artery, Four or More Arteries from Aorta with Autologous Venous Tissue, Percutaneous Endoscopic Approach
Ø2134A3	Bypass Coronary Artery, Four or More Arteries from Coronary Artery with Autologous Arterial Tissue, Percutaneous Endoscopic Approach
Ø2134A8	Bypass Coronary Artery, Four or More Arteries from Right Internal Mammary with Autologous Arterial Tissue, Percutaneous Endoscopic Approach
Ø2134A9	Bypass Coronary Artery, Four or More Arteries from Left Internal Mammary with Autologous Arterial Tissue, Percutaneous Endoscopic Approach
Ø2134AC	Bypass Coronary Artery, Four or More Arteries from Thoracic Artery with Autologous Arterial Tissue, Percutaneous Endoscopic Approach
Ø2134AF	Bypass Coronary Artery, Four or More Arteries from Abdominal Artery with Autologous Arterial Tissue, Percutaneous Endoscopic Approach
Ø2134AW	Bypass Coronary Artery, Four or More Arteries from Aorta with Autologous Arterial Tissue, Percutaneous Endoscopic Approach
Ø2134J3	Bypass Coronary Artery, Four or More Arteries from Coronary Artery with Synthetic Substitute, Percutaneous Endoscopic Approach
Ø2134J8	Bypass Coronary Artery, Four or More Arteries from Right Internal Mammary with Synthetic Substitute, Percutaneous Endoscopic Approach
Ø2134J9	Bypass Coronary Artery, Four or More Arteries from Left Internal Mammary with Synthetic Substitute, Percutaneous Endoscopic Approach
Ø2134JC	Bypass Coronary Artery, Four or More Arteries from Thoracic Artery with Synthetic Substitute, Percutaneous Endoscopic Approach
Ø2134JF	Bypass Coronary Artery, Four or More Arteries from Abdominal Artery with Synthetic Substitute, Percutaneous Endoscopic Approach
Ø2134JW	Bypass Coronary Artery, Four or More Arteries from Aorta with Synthetic Substitute, Percutaneous Endoscopic Approach
Ø2134K3	Bypass Coronary Artery, Four or More Arteries from Coronary Artery with Nonautologous Tissue Substitute, Percutaneous Endoscopic Approach
Ø2134K8	Bypass Coronary Artery, Four or More Arteries from Right Internal Mammary with Nonautologous Tissue Substitute, Percutaneous Endoscopic Approach
Ø2134K9	Bypass Coronary Artery, Four or More Arteries from Left Internal Mammary with Nonautologous Tissue Substitute, Percutaneous Endoscopic Approach
Ø2134KC	Bypass Coronary Artery, Four or More Arteries from Thoracic Artery with Nonautologous Tissue Substitute, Percutaneous Endoscopic Approach
Ø2134KF	Bypass Coronary Artery, Four or More Arteries from Abdominal Artery with Nonautologous Tissue Substitute, Percutaneous Endoscopic Approach
Ø2134KW	Bypass Coronary Artery, Four or More Arteries from Aorta with Nonautologous Tissue Substitute, Percutaneous Endoscopic Approach
Ø2134Z3	Bypass Coronary Artery, Four or More Arteries from Coronary Artery, Percutaneous Endoscopic Approach
Ø2134Z8	Bypass Coronary Artery, Four or More Arteries from Right Internal Mammary, Percutaneous Endoscopic Approach
Ø2134Z9	Bypass Coronary Artery, Four or More Arteries from Left Internal Mammary, Percutaneous Endoscopic Approach
Ø2134ZC	Bypass Coronary Artery, Four or More Arteries from Thoracic Artery, Percutaneous Endoscopic Approach
Ø2134ZF	Bypass Coronary Artery, Four or More Arteries from Abdominal Artery, Percutaneous Endoscopic Approach

HAC 10: Deep Vein Thrombosis (DVT) or Pulmonary Embolism (PE) with Total Knee or Hip Replacement

Secondary diagnosis not POA:

I26.Ø2	Saddle embolus of pulmonary artery with acute cor pulmonale
I26.Ø9	Other pulmonary embolism with acute cor pulmonale
I26.92	Saddle embolus of pulmonary artery without acute cor pulmonale
I26.93	Single subsegmental pulmonary embolism without acute cor pulmonale
I26.94	Multiple subsegmental pulmonary emboli without acute cor pulmonale
I26.99	Other pulmonary embolism without acute cor pulmonale
I82.4Ø1	Acute embolism and thrombosis of unspecified deep veins of right lower extremity
I82.4Ø2	Acute embolism and thrombosis of unspecified deep veins of left lower extremity
I82.4Ø3	Acute embolism and thrombosis of unspecified deep veins of lower extremity, bilateral
I82.4Ø9	Acute embolism and thrombosis of unspecified deep veins of unspecified lower extremity
I82.411	Acute embolism and thrombosis of right femoral vein
I82.412	Acute embolism and thrombosis of left femoral vein
I82.413	Acute embolism and thrombosis of femoral vein, bilateral
I82.419	Acute embolism and thrombosis of unspecified femoral vein
I82.421	Acute embolism and thrombosis of right iliac vein
I82.422	Acute embolism and thrombosis of left iliac vein
I82.423	Acute embolism and thrombosis of iliac vein, bilateral
I82.429	Acute embolism and thrombosis of unspecified iliac vein
I82.431	Acute embolism and thrombosis of right popliteal vein
I82.432	Acute embolism and thrombosis of left popliteal vein
I82.433	Acute embolism and thrombosis of popliteal vein, bilateral
I82.439	Acute embolism and thrombosis of unspecified popliteal vein
I82.441	Acute embolism and thrombosis of right tibial vein
I82.442	Acute embolism and thrombosis of left tibial vein
I82.443	Acute embolism and thrombosis of tibial vein, bilateral
I82.449	Acute embolism and thrombosis of unspecified tibial vein
I82.451	Acute embolism and thrombosis of right peroneal vein
I82.452	Acute embolism and thrombosis of left peroneal vein
I82.453	Acute embolism and thrombosis of peroneal vein, bilateral

HAC 10: Deep Vein Thrombosis (DVT) or Pulmonary Embolism (PE) with Total Knee or Hip Replacement (continued)

I82.459	Acute embolism and thrombosis of unspecified peroneal vein
I82.491	Acute embolism and thrombosis of other specified deep vein of right lower extremity
I82.492	Acute embolism and thrombosis of other specified deep vein of left lower extremity
I82.493	Acute embolism and thrombosis of other specified deep vein of lower extremity, bilateral
I82.499	Acute embolism and thrombosis of other specified deep vein of unspecified lower extremity
I82.4Y1	Acute embolism and thrombosis of unspecified deep veins of right proximal lower extremity
I82.4Y2	Acute embolism and thrombosis of unspecified deep veins of left proximal lower extremity
I82.4Y3	Acute embolism and thrombosis of unspecified deep veins of proximal lower extremity, bilateral
I82.4Y9	Acute embolism and thrombosis of unspecified deep veins of unspecified proximal lower extremity
I82.4Z1	Acute embolism and thrombosis of unspecified deep veins of right distal lower extremity
I82.4Z2	Acute embolism and thrombosis of unspecified deep veins of left distal lower extremity
I82.4Z3	Acute embolism and thrombosis of unspecified deep veins of distal lower extremity, bilateral
I82.4Z9	Acute embolism and thrombosis of unspecified deep veins of unspecified distal lower extremity

AND

Any of the following procedures:

0SR9019	Replacement of Right Hip Joint with Metal Synthetic Substitute, Cemented, Open Approach
0SR901A	Replacement of Right Hip Joint with Metal Synthetic Substitute, Uncemented, Open Approach
0SR901Z	Replacement of Right Hip Joint with Metal Synthetic Substitute, Open Approach
0SR9029	Replacement of Right Hip Joint with Metal on Polyethylene Synthetic Substitute, Cemented, Open Approach
0SR902A	Replacement of Right Hip Joint with Metal on Polyethylene Synthetic Substitute, Uncemented, Open Approach
0SR902Z	Replacement of Right Hip Joint with Metal on Polyethylene Synthetic Substitute, Open Approach
0SR9039	Replacement of Right Hip Joint with Ceramic Synthetic Substitute, Cemented, Open Approach
0SR903A	Replacement of Right Hip Joint with Ceramic Synthetic Substitute, Uncemented, Open Approach
0SR903Z	Replacement of Right Hip Joint with Ceramic Synthetic Substitute, Open Approach
0SR9049	Replacement of Right Hip Joint with Ceramic on Polyethylene Synthetic Substitute, Cemented, Open Approach

0SR904A	Replacement of Right Hip Joint with Ceramic on Polyethylene Synthetic Substitute, Uncemented, Open Approach
0SR904Z	Replacement of Right Hip Joint with Ceramic on Polyethylene Synthetic Substitute, Open Approach
0SR9069	Replacement of Right Hip Joint with Oxidized Zirconium on Polyethylene Synthetic Substitute, Cemented, Open Approach
0SR906A	Replacement of Right Hip Joint with Oxidized Zirconium on Polyethylene Synthetic Substitute, Uncemented, Open Approach
0SR906Z	Replacement of Right Hip Joint with Oxidized Zirconium on Polyethylene Synthetic Substitute, Open Approach
0SR907Z	Replacement of Right Hip Joint with Autologous Tissue Substitute, Open Approach
0SR90EZ	Replacement of Right Hip Joint with Articulating Spacer, Open Approach
0SR90J9	Replacement of Right Hip Joint with Synthetic Substitute, Cemented, Open Approach
0SR90JA	Replacement of Right Hip Joint with Synthetic Substitute, Uncemented, Open Approach
0SR90JZ	Replacement of Right Hip Joint with Synthetic Substitute, Open Approach
0SR90KZ	Replacement of Right Hip Joint with Nonautologous Tissue Substitute, Open Approach
0SRA009	Replacement of Right Hip Joint, Acetabular Surface with Polyethylene Synthetic Substitute, Cemented, Open Approach
0SRA00A	Replacement of Right Hip Joint, Acetabular Surface with Polyethylene Synthetic Substitute, Uncemented, Open Approach
0SRA00Z	Replacement of Right Hip Joint, Acetabular Surface with Polyethylene Synthetic Substitute, Open Approach
0SRA019	Replacement of Right Hip Joint, Acetabular Surface with Metal Synthetic Substitute, Cemented, Open Approach
0SRA01A	Replacement of Right Hip Joint, Acetabular Surface with Metal Synthetic Substitute, Uncemented, Open Approach
0SRA01Z	Replacement of Right Hip Joint, Acetabular Surface with Metal Synthetic Substitute, Open Approach
0SRA039	Replacement of Right Hip Joint, Acetabular Surface with Ceramic Synthetic Substitute, Cemented, Open Approach
0SRA03A	Replacement of Right Hip Joint, Acetabular Surface with Ceramic Synthetic Substitute, Uncemented, Open Approach
0SRA03Z	Replacement of Right Hip Joint, Acetabular Surface with Ceramic Synthetic Substitute, Open Approach
0SRA07Z	Replacement of Right Hip Joint, Acetabular Surface with Autologous Tissue Substitute, Open Approach
0SRA0J9	Replacement of Right Hip Joint, Acetabular Surface with Synthetic Substitute, Cemented, Open Approach
0SRA0JA	Replacement of Right Hip Joint, Acetabular Surface with Synthetic Substitute, Uncemented, Open Approach

0SRA0JZ	Replacement of Right Hip Joint, Acetabular Surface with Synthetic Substitute, Open Approach
0SRA0KZ	Replacement of Right Hip Joint, Acetabular Surface with Nonautologous Tissue Substitute, Open Approach
0SRB019	Replacement of Left Hip Joint with Metal Synthetic Substitute, Cemented, Open Approach
0SRB01A	Replacement of Left Hip Joint with Metal Synthetic Substitute, Uncemented, Open Approach
0SRB01Z	Replacement of Left Hip Joint with Metal Synthetic Substitute, Open Approach
0SRB029	Replacement of Left Hip Joint with Metal on Polyethylene Synthetic Substitute, Cemented, Open Approach
0SRB02A	Replacement of Left Hip Joint with Metal on Polyethylene Synthetic Substitute, Uncemented, Open Approach
0SRB02Z	Replacement of Left Hip Joint with Metal on Polyethylene Synthetic Substitute, Open Approach
0SRB039	Replacement of Left Hip Joint with Ceramic Synthetic Substitute, Cemented, Open Approach
0SRB03A	Replacement of Left Hip Joint with Ceramic Synthetic Substitute, Uncemented, Open Approach
0SRB03Z	Replacement of Left Hip Joint with Ceramic Synthetic Substitute, Open Approach
0SRB049	Replacement of Left Hip Joint with Ceramic on Polyethylene Synthetic Substitute, Cemented, Open Approach
0SRB04A	Replacement of Left Hip Joint with Ceramic on Polyethylene Synthetic Substitute, Uncemented, Open Approach
0SRB04Z	Replacement of Left Hip Joint with Ceramic on Polyethylene Synthetic Substitute, Open Approach
0SRB069	Replacement of Left Hip Joint with Oxidized Zirconium on Polyethylene Synthetic Substitute, Cemented, Open Approach
0SRB06A	Replacement of Left Hip Joint with Oxidized Zirconium on Polyethylene Synthetic Substitute, Uncemented, Open Approach
0SRB06Z	Replacement of Left Hip Joint with Oxidized Zirconium on Polyethylene Synthetic Substitute, Open Approach
0SRB07Z	Replacement of Left Hip Joint with Autologous Tissue Substitute, Open Approach
0SRB0EZ	Replacement of Left Hip Joint with Articulating Spacer, Open Approach
0SRB0J9	Replacement of Left Hip Joint with Synthetic Substitute, Cemented, Open Approach
0SRB0JA	Replacement of Left Hip Joint with Synthetic Substitute, Uncemented, Open Approach
0SRB0JZ	Replacement of Left Hip Joint with Synthetic Substitute, Open Approach
0SRB0KZ	Replacement of Left Hip Joint with Nonautologous Tissue Substitute, Open Approach
0SRC069	Replacement of Right Knee Joint with Oxidized Zirconium on Polyethylene Synthetic Substitute, Cemented, Open Approach

HAC 10: Deep Vein Thrombosis (DVT) or Pulmonary Embolism (PE) with Total Knee or Hip Replacement (continued)

ØSRC06A Replacement of Right Knee Joint with Oxidized Zirconium on Polyethylene Synthetic Substitute, Uncemented, Open Approach

ØSRC06Z Replacement of Right Knee Joint with Oxidized Zirconium on Polyethylene Synthetic Substitute, Open Approach

ØSRC07Z Replacement of Right Knee Joint with Autologous Tissue Substitute, Open Approach

ØSRC0EZ Replacement of Right Knee Joint with Articulating Spacer, Open Approach

ØSRC0J9 Replacement of Right Knee Joint with Synthetic Substitute, Cemented, Open Approach

ØSRC0JA Replacement of Right Knee Joint with Synthetic Substitute, Uncemented, Open Approach

ØSRC0JZ Replacement of Right Knee Joint with Synthetic Substitute, Open Approach

ØSRC0KZ Replacement of Right Knee Joint with Nonautologous Tissue Substitute, Open Approach

ØSRC0L9 Replacement of Right Knee Joint with Medial Unicondylar Synthetic Substitute, Cemented, Open Approach

ØSRC0LA Replacement of Right Knee Joint with Medial Unicondylar Synthetic Substitute, Uncemented, Open Approach

ØSRC0LZ Replacement of Right Knee Joint with Medial Unicondylar Synthetic Substitute, Open Approach

ØSRC0M9 Replacement of Right Knee Joint with Lateral Unicondylar Synthetic Substitute, Cemented, Open Approach

ØSRC0MA Replacement of Right Knee Joint with Lateral Unicondylar Synthetic Substitute, Uncemented, Open Approach

ØSRC0MZ Replacement of Right Knee Joint with Lateral Unicondylar Synthetic Substitute, Open Approach

ØSRC0N9 Replacement of Right Knee Joint with Patellofemoral Synthetic Substitute, Cemented, Open Approach

ØSRC0NA Replacement of Right Knee Joint with Patellofemoral Synthetic Substitute, Uncemented, Open Approach

ØSRC0NZ Replacement of Right Knee Joint with Patellofemoral Synthetic Substitute, Open Approach

ØSRD069 Replacement of Left Knee Joint with Oxidized Zirconium on Polyethylene Synthetic Substitute, Cemented, Open Approach

ØSRD06A Replacement of Left Knee Joint with Oxidized Zirconium on Polyethylene Synthetic Substitute, Uncemented, Open Approach

ØSRD06Z Replacement of Left Knee Joint with Oxidized Zirconium on Polyethylene Synthetic Substitute, Open Approach

ØSRD07Z Replacement of Left Knee Joint with Autologous Tissue Substitute, Open Approach

ØSRD0EZ Replacement of Left Knee Joint with Articulating Spacer, Open Approach

ØSRD0J9 Replacement of Left Knee Joint with Synthetic Substitute, Cemented, Open Approach

ØSRD0JA Replacement of Left Knee Joint with Synthetic Substitute, Uncemented, Open Approach

ØSRD0JZ Replacement of Left Knee Joint with Synthetic Substitute, Open Approach

ØSRD0KZ Replacement of Left Knee Joint with Nonautologous Tissue Substitute, Open Approach

ØSRD0L9 Replacement of Left Knee Joint with Medial Unicondylar Synthetic Substitute, Cemented, Open Approach

ØSRD0LA Replacement of Left Knee Joint with Medial Unicondylar Synthetic Substitute, Uncemented, Open Approach

ØSRD0LZ Replacement of Left Knee Joint with Medial Unicondylar Synthetic Substitute, Open Approach

ØSRD0M9 Replacement of Left Knee Joint with Lateral Unicondylar Synthetic Substitute, Cemented, Open Approach

ØSRD0MA Replacement of Left Knee Joint with Lateral Unicondylar Synthetic Substitute, Uncemented, Open Approach

ØSRD0MZ Replacement of Left Knee Joint with Lateral Unicondylar Synthetic Substitute, Open Approach

ØSRD0N9 Replacement of Left Knee Joint with Patellofemoral Synthetic Substitute, Cemented, Open Approach

ØSRD0NA Replacement of Left Knee Joint with Patellofemoral Synthetic Substitute, Uncemented, Open Approach

ØSRD0NZ Replacement of Left Knee Joint with Patellofemoral Synthetic Substitute, Open Approach

ØSRE009 Replacement of Left Hip Joint, Acetabular Surface with Polyethylene Synthetic Substitute, Cemented, Open Approach

ØSRE00A Replacement of Left Hip Joint, Acetabular Surface with Polyethylene Synthetic Substitute, Uncemented, Open Approach

ØSRE00Z Replacement of Left Hip Joint, Acetabular Surface with Polyethylene Synthetic Substitute, Open Approach

ØSRE019 Replacement of Left Hip Joint, Acetabular Surface with Metal Synthetic Substitute, Cemented, Open Approach

ØSRE01A Replacement of Left Hip Joint, Acetabular Surface with Metal Synthetic Substitute, Uncemented, Open Approach

ØSRE01Z Replacement of Left Hip Joint, Acetabular Surface with Metal Synthetic Substitute, Open Approach

ØSRE039 Replacement of Left Hip Joint, Acetabular Surface with Ceramic Synthetic Substitute, Cemented, Open Approach

ØSRE03A Replacement of Left Hip Joint, Acetabular Surface with Ceramic Synthetic Substitute, Uncemented, Open Approach

ØSRE03Z Replacement of Left Hip Joint, Acetabular Surface with Ceramic Synthetic Substitute, Open Approach

ØSRE07Z Replacement of Left Hip Joint, Acetabular Surface with Autologous Tissue Substitute, Open Approach

ØSRE0J9 Replacement of Left Hip Joint, Acetabular Surface with Synthetic Substitute, Cemented, Open Approach

ØSRE0JA Replacement of Left Hip Joint, Acetabular Surface with Synthetic Substitute, Uncemented, Open Approach

ØSRE0JZ Replacement of Left Hip Joint, Acetabular Surface with Synthetic Substitute, Open Approach

ØSRE0KZ Replacement of Left Hip Joint, Acetabular Surface with Nonautologous Tissue Substitute, Open Approach

ØSRR019 Replacement of Right Hip Joint, Femoral Surface with Metal Synthetic Substitute, Cemented, Open Approach

ØSRR01A Replacement of Right Hip Joint, Femoral Surface with Metal Synthetic Substitute, Uncemented, Open Approach

ØSRR01Z Replacement of Right Hip Joint, Femoral Surface with Metal Synthetic Substitute, Open Approach

ØSRR039 Replacement of Right Hip Joint, Femoral Surface with Ceramic Synthetic Substitute, Cemented, Open Approach

ØSRR03A Replacement of Right Hip Joint, Femoral Surface with Ceramic Synthetic Substitute, Uncemented, Open Approach

ØSRR03Z Replacement of Right Hip Joint, Femoral Surface with Ceramic Synthetic Substitute, Open Approach

ØSRR07Z Replacement of Right Hip Joint, Femoral Surface with Autologous Tissue Substitute, Open Approach

ØSRR0J9 Replacement of Right Hip Joint, Femoral Surface with Synthetic Substitute, Cemented, Open Approach

ØSRR0JA Replacement of Right Hip Joint, Femoral Surface with Synthetic Substitute, Uncemented, Open Approach

ØSRR0JZ Replacement of Right Hip Joint, Femoral Surface with Synthetic Substitute, Open Approach

ØSRR0KZ Replacement of Right Hip Joint, Femoral Surface with Nonautologous Tissue Substitute, Open Approach

ØSRS019 Replacement of Left Hip Joint, Femoral Surface with Metal Synthetic Substitute, Cemented, Open Approach

ØSRS01A Replacement of Left Hip Joint, Femoral Surface with Metal Synthetic Substitute, Uncemented, Open Approach

ØSRS01Z Replacement of Left Hip Joint, Femoral Surface with Metal Synthetic Substitute, Open Approach

ØSRS039 Replacement of Left Hip Joint, Femoral Surface with Ceramic Synthetic Substitute, Cemented, Open Approach

ØSRS03A Replacement of Left Hip Joint, Femoral Surface with Ceramic Synthetic Substitute, Uncemented, Open Approach

ØSRS03Z Replacement of Left Hip Joint, Femoral Surface with Ceramic Synthetic Substitute, Open Approach

ØSRS07Z Replacement of Left Hip Joint, Femoral Surface with Autologous Tissue Substitute, Open Approach

ØSRS0J9 Replacement of Left Hip Joint, Femoral Surface with Synthetic Substitute, Cemented, Open Approach

ØSRS0JA Replacement of Left Hip Joint, Femoral Surface with Synthetic Substitute, Uncemented, Open Approach

ØSRS0JZ Replacement of Left Hip Joint, Femoral Surface with Synthetic Substitute, Open Approach

HAC 10: Deep Vein Thrombosis (DVT) or Pulmonary Embolism (PE) with Total Knee or Hip Replacement (continued)

ØSRSØKZ	Replacement of Left Hip Joint, Femoral Surface with Nonautologous Tissue Substitute, Open Approach
ØSRTØ7Z	Replacement of Right Knee Joint, Femoral Surface with Autologous Tissue Substitute, Open Approach
ØSRTØJ9	Replacement of Right Knee Joint, Femoral Surface with Synthetic Substitute, Cemented, Open Approach
ØSRTØJA	Replacement of Right Knee Joint, Femoral Surface with Synthetic Substitute, Uncemented, Open Approach
ØSRTØJZ	Replacement of Right Knee Joint, Femoral Surface with Synthetic Substitute, Open Approach
ØSRTØKZ	Replacement of Right Knee Joint, Femoral Surface with Nonautologous Tissue Substitute, Open Approach
ØSRUØ7Z	Replacement of Left Knee Joint, Femoral Surface with Autologous Tissue Substitute, Open Approach
ØSRUØJ9	Replacement of Left Knee Joint, Femoral Surface with Synthetic Substitute, Cemented, Open Approach
ØSRUØJA	Replacement of Left Knee Joint, Femoral Surface with Synthetic Substitute, Uncemented, Open Approach
ØSRUØJZ	Replacement of Left Knee Joint, Femoral Surface with Synthetic Substitute, Open Approach
ØSRUØKZ	Replacement of Left Knee Joint, Femoral Surface with Nonautologous Tissue Substitute, Open Approach
ØSRVØ7Z	Replacement of Right Knee Joint, Tibial Surface with Autologous Tissue Substitute, Open Approach
ØSRVØJ9	Replacement of Right Knee Joint, Tibial Surface with Synthetic Substitute, Cemented, Open Approach
ØSRVØJA	Replacement of Right Knee Joint, Tibial Surface with Synthetic Substitute, Uncemented, Open Approach
ØSRVØJZ	Replacement of Right Knee Joint, Tibial Surface with Synthetic Substitute, Open Approach
ØSRVØKZ	Replacement of Right Knee Joint, Tibial Surface with Nonautologous Tissue Substitute, Open Approach
ØSRWØ7Z	Replacement of Left Knee Joint, Tibial Surface with Autologous Tissue Substitute, Open Approach
ØSRWØJ9	Replacement of Left Knee Joint, Tibial Surface with Synthetic Substitute, Cemented, Open Approach
ØSRWØJA	Replacement of Left Knee Joint, Tibial Surface with Synthetic Substitute, Uncemented, Open Approach
ØSRWØJZ	Replacement of Left Knee Joint, Tibial Surface with Synthetic Substitute, Open Approach
ØSRWØKZ	Replacement of Left Knee Joint, Tibial Surface with Nonautologous Tissue Substitute, Open Approach
ØSU9ØBZ	Supplement Right Hip Joint with Resurfacing Device, Open Approach
ØSUAØBZ	Supplement Right Hip Joint, Acetabular Surface with Resurfacing Device, Open Approach
ØSUBØBZ	Supplement Left Hip Joint with Resurfacing Device, Open Approach

ØSUEØBZ	Supplement Left Hip Joint, Acetabular Surface with Resurfacing Device, Open Approach
ØSURØBZ	Supplement Right Hip Joint, Femoral Surface with Resurfacing Device, Open Approach
ØSUSØBZ	Supplement Left Hip Joint, Femoral Surface with Resurfacing Device, Open Approach

HAC 11: Surgical Site Infection-Bariatric Surgery

Principal diagnosis of:

E66.Ø1	Morbid (severe) obesity due to excess calories

AND

Secondary diagnosis not POA:

K68.11	Postprocedural retroperitoneal abscess
K95.Ø1	Infection due to gastric band procedure
K95.81	Infection due to other bariatric procedure
T81.4ØXA	Infection following a procedure, unspecified, initial encounter
T81.41XA	Infection following a procedure, superficial incisional surgical site, initial encounter
T81.42XA	Infection following a procedure, deep incisional surgical site, initial encounter
T81.43XA	Infection following a procedure, organ and space surgical site, initial encounter
T81.44XA	Sepsis following a procedure, initial encounter
T81.49XA	Infection following a procedure, other surgical site, initial encounter

AND

Any of the following procedures:

ØD16Ø79	Bypass Stomach to Duodenum with Autologous Tissue Substitute, Open Approach
ØD16Ø7A	Bypass Stomach to Jejunum with Autologous Tissue Substitute, Open Approach
ØD16Ø7B	Bypass Stomach to Ileum with Autologous Tissue Substitute, Open Approach
ØD16Ø7L	Bypass Stomach to Transverse Colon with Autologous Tissue Substitute, Open Approach
ØD16ØJ9	Bypass Stomach to Duodenum with Synthetic Substitute, Open Approach
ØD16ØJA	Bypass Stomach to Jejunum with Synthetic Substitute, Open Approach
ØD16ØJB	Bypass Stomach to Ileum with Synthetic Substitute, Open Approach
ØD16ØJL	Bypass Stomach to Transverse Colon with Synthetic Substitute, Open Approach
ØD16ØK9	Bypass Stomach to Duodenum with Nonautologous Tissue Substitute, Open Approach
ØD16ØKA	Bypass Stomach to Jejunum with Nonautologous Tissue Substitute, Open Approach
ØD16ØKB	Bypass Stomach to Ileum with Nonautologous Tissue Substitute, Open Approach
ØD16ØKL	Bypass Stomach to Transverse Colon with Nonautologous Tissue Substitute, Open Approach
ØD16ØZ9	Bypass Stomach to Duodenum, Open Approach
ØD16ØZA	Bypass Stomach to Jejunum, Open Approach
ØD16ØZB	Bypass Stomach to Ileum, Open Approach

ØD16ØZL	Bypass Stomach to Transverse Colon, Open Approach
ØD16479	Bypass Stomach to Duodenum with Autologous Tissue Substitute, Percutaneous Endoscopic Approach
ØD1647A	Bypass Stomach to Jejunum with Autologous Tissue Substitute, Percutaneous Endoscopic Approach
ØD1647B	Bypass Stomach to Ileum with Autologous Tissue Substitute, Percutaneous Endoscopic Approach
ØD1647L	Bypass Stomach to Transverse Colon with Autologous Tissue Substitute, Percutaneous Endoscopic Approach
ØD164J9	Bypass Stomach to Duodenum with Synthetic Substitute, Percutaneous Endoscopic Approach
ØD164JA	Bypass Stomach to Jejunum with Synthetic Substitute, Percutaneous Endoscopic Approach
ØD164JB	Bypass Stomach to Ileum with Synthetic Substitute, Percutaneous Endoscopic Approach
ØD164JL	Bypass Stomach to Transverse Colon with Synthetic Substitute, Percutaneous Endoscopic Approach
ØD164K9	Bypass Stomach to Duodenum with Nonautologous Tissue Substitute, Percutaneous Endoscopic Approach
ØD164KA	Bypass Stomach to Jejunum with Nonautologous Tissue Substitute, Percutaneous Endoscopic Approach
ØD164KB	Bypass Stomach to Ileum with Nonautologous Tissue Substitute, Percutaneous Endoscopic Approach
ØD164KL	Bypass Stomach to Transverse Colon with Nonautologous Tissue Substitute, Percutaneous Endoscopic Approach
ØD164Z9	Bypass Stomach to Duodenum, Percutaneous Endoscopic Approach
ØD164ZA	Bypass Stomach to Jejunum, Percutaneous Endoscopic Approach
ØD164ZB	Bypass Stomach to Ileum, Percutaneous Endoscopic Approach
ØD164ZL	Bypass Stomach to Transverse Colon, Percutaneous Endoscopic Approach
ØD16879	Bypass Stomach to Duodenum with Autologous Tissue Substitute, Via Natural or Artificial Opening Endoscopic
ØD1687A	Bypass Stomach to Jejunum with Autologous Tissue Substitute, Via Natural or Artificial Opening Endoscopic
ØD1687B	Bypass Stomach to Ileum with Autologous Tissue Substitute, Via Natural or Artificial Opening Endoscopic
ØD1687L	Bypass Stomach to Transverse Colon with Autologous Tissue Substitute, Via Natural or Artificial Opening Endoscopic
ØD168J9	Bypass Stomach to Duodenum with Synthetic Substitute, Via Natural or Artificial Opening Endoscopic
ØD168JA	Bypass Stomach to Jejunum with Synthetic Substitute, Via Natural or Artificial Opening Endoscopic
ØD168JB	Bypass Stomach to Ileum with Synthetic Substitute, Via Natural or Artificial Opening Endoscopic
ØD168JL	Bypass Stomach to Transverse Colon with Synthetic Substitute, Via Natural or Artificial Opening Endoscopic
ØD168K9	Bypass Stomach to Duodenum with Nonautologous Tissue Substitute, Via Natural or Artificial Opening Endoscopic
ØD168KA	Bypass Stomach to Jejunum with Nonautologous Tissue Substitute, Via Natural or Artificial Opening Endoscopic

HAC 11: Surgical Site Infection-Bariatric Surgery (continued)

ØD168KB	Bypass Stomach to Ileum with Nonautologous Tissue Substitute, Via Natural or Artificial Opening Endoscopic
ØD168KL	Bypass Stomach to Transverse Colon with Nonautologous Tissue Substitute, Via Natural or Artificial Opening Endoscopic
ØD168Z9	Bypass Stomach to Duodenum, Via Natural or Artificial Opening Endoscopic
ØD168ZA	Bypass Stomach to Jejunum, Via Natural or Artificial Opening Endoscopic
ØD168ZB	Bypass Stomach to Ileum, Via Natural or Artificial Opening Endoscopic
ØD168ZL	Bypass Stomach to Transverse Colon, Via Natural or Artificial Opening Endoscopic
ØDV64CZ	Restriction of Stomach with Extraluminal Device, Percutaneous Endoscopic Approach

HAC 12: Surgical Site Infection-Certain Orthopedic Procedures of the Spine, Shoulder, and Elbow

Secondary diagnosis not POA:

K68.11	Postprocedural retroperitoneal abscess
T81.40XA	Infection following a procedure, unspecified, initial encounter
T81.41XA	Infection following a procedure, superficial incisional surgical site, initial encounter
T81.42XA	Infection following a procedure, deep incisional surgical site, initial encounter
T81.43XA	Infection following a procedure, organ and space surgical site, initial encounter
T81.44XA	Sepsis following a procedure, initial encounter
T81.49XA	Infection following a procedure, other surgical site, initial encounter
T84.60XA	Infection and inflammatory reaction due to internal fixation device of unspecified site, initial encounter
T84.610A	Infection and inflammatory reaction due to internal fixation device of right humerus, initial encounter
T84.611A	Infection and inflammatory reaction due to internal fixation device of left humerus, initial encounter
T84.612A	Infection and inflammatory reaction due to internal fixation device of right radius, initial encounter
T84.613A	Infection and inflammatory reaction due to internal fixation device of left radius, initial encounter
T84.614A	Infection and inflammatory reaction due to internal fixation device of right ulna, initial encounter
T84.615A	Infection and inflammatory reaction due to internal fixation device of left ulna, initial encounter
T84.619A	Infection and inflammatory reaction due to internal fixation device of unspecified bone of arm, initial encounter
T84.63XA	Infection and inflammatory reaction due to internal fixation device of spine, initial encounter
T84.69XA	Infection and inflammatory reaction due to internal fixation device of other site, initial encounter
T84.7XXA	Infection and inflammatory reaction due to other internal orthopedic prosthetic devices, implants and grafts, initial encounter

AND

Any of the following procedures:

ØRG0070	Fusion of Occipital-cervical Joint with Autologous Tissue Substitute, Anterior Approach, Anterior Column, Open Approach
ØRG0071	Fusion of Occipital-cervical Joint with Autologous Tissue Substitute, Posterior Approach, Posterior Column, Open Approach
ØRG007J	Fusion of Occipital-cervical Joint with Autologous Tissue Substitute, Posterior Approach, Anterior Column, Open Approach
ØRG00A0	Fusion of Occipital-cervical Joint with Interbody Fusion Device, Anterior Approach, Anterior Column, Open Approach
ØRG00AJ	Fusion of Occipital-cervical Joint with Interbody Fusion Device, Posterior Approach, Anterior Column, Open Approach
ØRG00J0	Fusion of Occipital-cervical Joint with Synthetic Substitute, Anterior Approach, Anterior Column, Open Approach
ØRG00J1	Fusion of Occipital-cervical Joint with Synthetic Substitute, Posterior Approach, Posterior Column, Open Approach
ØRG00JJ	Fusion of Occipital-cervical Joint with Synthetic Substitute, Posterior Approach, Anterior Column, Open Approach
ØRG00K0	Fusion of Occipital-cervical Joint with Nonautologous Tissue Substitute, Anterior Approach, Anterior Column, Open Approach
ØRG00K1	Fusion of Occipital-cervical Joint with Nonautologous Tissue Substitute, Posterior Approach, Posterior Column, Open Approach
ØRG00KJ	Fusion of Occipital-cervical Joint with Nonautologous Tissue Substitute, Posterior Approach, Anterior Column, Open Approach
ØRG0370	Fusion of Occipital-cervical Joint with Autologous Tissue Substitute, Anterior Approach, Anterior Column, Percutaneous Approach
ØRG0371	Fusion of Occipital-cervical Joint with Autologous Tissue Substitute, Posterior Approach, Posterior Column, Percutaneous Approach
ØRG037J	Fusion of Occipital-cervical Joint with Autologous Tissue Substitute, Posterior Approach, Anterior Column, Percutaneous Approach
ØRG03A0	Fusion of Occipital-cervical Joint with Interbody Fusion Device, Anterior Approach, Anterior Column, Percutaneous Approach
ØRG03AJ	Fusion of Occipital-cervical Joint with Interbody Fusion Device, Posterior Approach, Anterior Column, Percutaneous Approach
ØRG03J0	Fusion of Occipital-cervical Joint with Synthetic Substitute, Anterior Approach, Anterior Column, Percutaneous Approach
ØRG03J1	Fusion of Occipital-cervical Joint with Synthetic Substitute, Posterior Approach, Posterior Column, Percutaneous Approach
ØRG03JJ	Fusion of Occipital-cervical Joint with Synthetic Substitute, Posterior Approach, Anterior Column, Percutaneous Approach
ØRG03K0	Fusion of Occipital-cervical Joint with Nonautologous Tissue Substitute, Anterior Approach, Anterior Column, Percutaneous Approach
ØRG03K1	Fusion of Occipital-cervical Joint with Nonautologous Tissue Substitute, Posterior Approach, Posterior Column, Percutaneous Approach
ØRG03KJ	Fusion of Occipital-cervical Joint with Nonautologous Tissue Substitute, Posterior Approach, Anterior Column, Percutaneous Approach
ØRG0470	Fusion of Occipital-cervical Joint with Autologous Tissue Substitute, Anterior Approach, Anterior Column, Percutaneous Endoscopic Approach
ØRG0471	Fusion of Occipital-cervical Joint with Autologous Tissue Substitute, Posterior Approach, Posterior Column, Percutaneous Endoscopic Approach
ØRG047J	Fusion of Occipital-cervical Joint with Autologous Tissue Substitute, Posterior Approach, Anterior Column, Percutaneous Endoscopic Approach
ØRG04A0	Fusion of Occipital-cervical Joint with Interbody Fusion Device, Anterior Approach, Anterior Column, Percutaneous Endoscopic Approach
ØRG04AJ	Fusion of Occipital-cervical Joint with Interbody Fusion Device, Posterior Approach, Anterior Column, Percutaneous Endoscopic Approach
ØRG04J0	Fusion of Occipital-cervical Joint with Synthetic Substitute, Anterior Approach, Anterior Column, Percutaneous Endoscopic Approach
ØRG04J1	Fusion of Occipital-cervical Joint with Synthetic Substitute, Posterior Approach, Posterior Column, Percutaneous Endoscopic Approach
ØRG04JJ	Fusion of Occipital-cervical Joint with Synthetic Substitute, Posterior Approach, Anterior Column, Percutaneous Endoscopic Approach
ØRG04K0	Fusion of Occipital-cervical Joint with Nonautologous Tissue Substitute, Anterior Approach, Anterior Column, Percutaneous Endoscopic Approach
ØRG04K1	Fusion of Occipital-cervical Joint with Nonautologous Tissue Substitute, Posterior Approach, Posterior Column, Percutaneous Endoscopic Approach
ØRG04KJ	Fusion of Occipital-cervical Joint with Nonautologous Tissue Substitute, Posterior Approach, Anterior Column, Percutaneous Endoscopic Approach
ØRG1070	Fusion of Cervical Vertebral Joint with Autologous Tissue Substitute, Anterior Approach, Anterior Column, Open Approach
ØRG1071	Fusion of Cervical Vertebral Joint with Autologous Tissue Substitute, Posterior Approach, Posterior Column, Open Approach
ØRG107J	Fusion of Cervical Vertebral Joint with Autologous Tissue Substitute, Posterior Approach, Anterior Column, Open Approach
ØRG10A0	Fusion of Cervical Vertebral Joint with Interbody Fusion Device, Anterior Approach, Anterior Column, Open Approach
ØRG10AJ	Fusion of Cervical Vertebral Joint with Interbody Fusion Device, Posterior Approach, Anterior Column, Open Approach

HAC 12: Surgical Site Infection-Certain Orthopedic Procedures of the Spine, Shoulder, and Elbow (continued)

ØRG10J0 Fusion of Cervical Vertebral Joint with Synthetic Substitute, Anterior Approach, Anterior Column, Open Approach

ØRG10J1 Fusion of Cervical Vertebral Joint with Synthetic Substitute, Posterior Approach, Posterior Column, Open Approach

ØRG10JJ Fusion of Cervical Vertebral Joint with Synthetic Substitute, Posterior Approach, Anterior Column, Open Approach

ØRG10K0 Fusion of Cervical Vertebral Joint with Nonautologous Tissue Substitute, Anterior Approach, Anterior Column, Open Approach

ØRG10K1 Fusion of Cervical Vertebral Joint with Nonautologous Tissue Substitute, Posterior Approach, Posterior Column, Open Approach

ØRG10KJ Fusion of Cervical Vertebral Joint with Nonautologous Tissue Substitute, Posterior Approach, Anterior Column, Open Approach

ØRG1370 Fusion of Cervical Vertebral Joint with Autologous Tissue Substitute, Anterior Approach, Anterior Column, Percutaneous Approach

ØRG1371 Fusion of Cervical Vertebral Joint with Autologous Tissue Substitute, Posterior Approach, Posterior Column, Percutaneous Approach

ØRG137J Fusion of Cervical Vertebral Joint with Autologous Tissue Substitute, Posterior Approach, Anterior Column, Percutaneous Approach

ØRG13A0 Fusion of Cervical Vertebral Joint with Interbody Fusion Device, Anterior Approach, Anterior Column, Percutaneous Approach

ØRG13AJ Fusion of Cervical Vertebral Joint with Interbody Fusion Device, Posterior Approach, Anterior Column, Percutaneous Approach

ØRG13J0 Fusion of Cervical Vertebral Joint with Synthetic Substitute, Anterior Approach, Anterior Column, Percutaneous Approach

ØRG13J1 Fusion of Cervical Vertebral Joint with Synthetic Substitute, Posterior Approach, Posterior Column, Percutaneous Approach

ØRG13JJ Fusion of Cervical Vertebral Joint with Synthetic Substitute, Posterior Approach, Anterior Column, Percutaneous Approach

ØRG13K0 Fusion of Cervical Vertebral Joint with Nonautologous Tissue Substitute, Anterior Approach, Anterior Column, Percutaneous Approach

ØRG13K1 Fusion of Cervical Vertebral Joint with Nonautologous Tissue Substitute, Posterior Approach, Posterior Column, Percutaneous Approach

ØRG13KJ Fusion of Cervical Vertebral Joint with Nonautologous Tissue Substitute, Posterior Approach, Anterior Column, Percutaneous Approach

ØRG1470 Fusion of Cervical Vertebral Joint with Autologous Tissue Substitute, Anterior Approach, Anterior Column, Percutaneous Endoscopic Approach

ØRG1471 Fusion of Cervical Vertebral Joint with Autologous Tissue Substitute, Posterior Approach, Posterior Column, Percutaneous Endoscopic Approach

ØRG147J Fusion of Cervical Vertebral Joint with Autologous Tissue Substitute, Posterior Approach, Anterior Column, Percutaneous Endoscopic Approach

ØRG14A0 Fusion of Cervical Vertebral Joint with Interbody Fusion Device, Anterior Approach, Anterior Column, Percutaneous Endoscopic Approach

ØRG14AJ Fusion of Cervical Vertebral Joint with Interbody Fusion Device, Posterior Approach, Anterior Column, Percutaneous Endoscopic Approach

ØRG14J0 Fusion of Cervical Vertebral Joint with Synthetic Substitute, Anterior Approach, Anterior Column, Percutaneous Endoscopic Approach

ØRG14J1 Fusion of Cervical Vertebral Joint with Synthetic Substitute, Posterior Approach, Posterior Column, Percutaneous Endoscopic Approach

ØRG14JJ Fusion of Cervical Vertebral Joint with Synthetic Substitute, Posterior Approach, Anterior Column, Percutaneous Endoscopic Approach

ØRG14K0 Fusion of Cervical Vertebral Joint with Nonautologous Tissue Substitute, Anterior Approach, Anterior Column, Percutaneous Endoscopic Approach

ØRG14K1 Fusion of Cervical Vertebral Joint with Nonautologous Tissue Substitute, Posterior Approach, Posterior Column, Percutaneous Endoscopic Approach

ØRG14KJ Fusion of Cervical Vertebral Joint with Nonautologous Tissue Substitute, Posterior Approach, Anterior Column, Percutaneous Endoscopic Approach

ØRG2070 Fusion of 2 or more Cervical Vertebral Joints with Autologous Tissue Substitute, Anterior Approach, Anterior Column, Open Approach

ØRG2071 Fusion of 2 or more Cervical Vertebral Joints with Autologous Tissue Substitute, Posterior Approach, Posterior Column, Open Approach

ØRG207J Fusion of 2 or more Cervical Vertebral Joints with Autologous Tissue Substitute, Posterior Approach, Anterior Column, Open Approach

ØRG20A0 Fusion of 2 or more Cervical Vertebral Joints with Interbody Fusion Device, Anterior Approach, Anterior Column, Open Approach

ØRG20AJ Fusion of 2 or more Cervical Vertebral Joints with Interbody Fusion Device, Posterior Approach, Anterior Column, Open Approach

ØRG20J0 Fusion of 2 or more Cervical Vertebral Joints with Synthetic Substitute, Anterior Approach, Anterior Column, Open Approach

ØRG20J1 Fusion of 2 or more Cervical Vertebral Joints with Synthetic Substitute, Posterior Approach, Posterior Column, Open Approach

ØRG20JJ Fusion of 2 or more Cervical Vertebral Joints with Synthetic Substitute, Posterior Approach, Anterior Column, Open Approach

ØRG20K0 Fusion of 2 or more Cervical Vertebral Joints with Nonautologous Tissue Substitute, Anterior Approach, Anterior Column, Open Approach

ØRG20K1 Fusion of 2 or more Cervical Vertebral Joints with Nonautologous Tissue Substitute, Posterior Approach, Posterior Column, Open Approach

ØRG20KJ Fusion of 2 or more Cervical Vertebral Joints with Nonautologous Tissue Substitute, Posterior Approach, Anterior Column, Open Approach

ØRG2370 Fusion of 2 or more Cervical Vertebral Joints with Autologous Tissue Substitute, Anterior Approach, Anterior Column, Percutaneous Approach

ØRG2371 Fusion of 2 or more Cervical Vertebral Joints with Autologous Tissue Substitute, Posterior Approach, Posterior Column, Percutaneous Approach

ØRG237J Fusion of 2 or more Cervical Vertebral Joints with Autologous Tissue Substitute, Posterior Approach, Anterior Column, Percutaneous Approach

ØRG23A0 Fusion of 2 or more Cervical Vertebral Joints with Interbody Fusion Device, Anterior Approach, Anterior Column, Percutaneous Approach

ØRG23AJ Fusion of 2 or more Cervical Vertebral Joints with Interbody Fusion Device, Posterior Approach, Anterior Column, Percutaneous Approach

ØRG23J0 Fusion of 2 or more Cervical Vertebral Joints with Synthetic Substitute, Anterior Approach, Anterior Column, Percutaneous Approach

ØRG23J1 Fusion of 2 or more Cervical Vertebral Joints with Synthetic Substitute, Posterior Approach, Posterior Column, Percutaneous Approach

ØRG23JJ Fusion of 2 or more Cervical Vertebral Joints with Synthetic Substitute, Posterior Approach, Anterior Column, Percutaneous Approach

ØRG23K0 Fusion of 2 or more Cervical Vertebral Joints with Nonautologous Tissue Substitute, Anterior Approach, Anterior Column, Percutaneous Approach

ØRG23K1 Fusion of 2 or more Cervical Vertebral Joints with Nonautologous Tissue Substitute, Posterior Approach, Posterior Column, Percutaneous Approach

ØRG23KJ Fusion of 2 or more Cervical Vertebral Joints with Nonautologous Tissue Substitute, Posterior Approach, Anterior Column, Percutaneous Approach

ØRG2470 Fusion of 2 or more Cervical Vertebral Joints with Autologous Tissue Substitute, Anterior Approach, Anterior Column, Percutaneous Endoscopic Approach

ØRG2471 Fusion of 2 or more Cervical Vertebral Joints with Autologous Tissue Substitute, Posterior Approach, Posterior Column, Percutaneous Endoscopic Approach

ØRG247J Fusion of 2 or more Cervical Vertebral Joints with Autologous Tissue Substitute, Posterior Approach, Anterior Column, Percutaneous Endoscopic Approach

ØRG24A0 Fusion of 2 or more Cervical Vertebral Joints with Interbody Fusion Device, Anterior Approach, Anterior Column, Percutaneous Endoscopic Approach

HAC 12: Surgical Site Infection-Certain Orthopedic Procedures of the Spine, Shoulder, and Elbow (continued)

ØRG24AJ Fusion of 2 or more Cervical Vertebral Joints with Interbody Fusion Device, Posterior Approach, Anterior Column, Percutaneous Endoscopic Approach

ØRG24JØ Fusion of 2 or more Cervical Vertebral Joints with Synthetic Substitute, Anterior Approach, Anterior Column, Percutaneous Endoscopic Approach

ØRG24J1 Fusion of 2 or more Cervical Vertebral Joints with Synthetic Substitute, Posterior Approach, Posterior Column, Percutaneous Endoscopic Approach

ØRG24JJ Fusion of 2 or more Cervical Vertebral Joints with Synthetic Substitute, Posterior Approach, Anterior Column, Percutaneous Endoscopic Approach

ØRG24KØ Fusion of 2 or more Cervical Vertebral Joints with Nonautologous Tissue Substitute, Anterior Approach, Anterior Column, Percutaneous Endoscopic Approach

ØRG24K1 Fusion of 2 or more Cervical Vertebral Joints with Nonautologous Tissue Substitute, Posterior Approach, Posterior Column, Percutaneous Endoscopic Approach

ØRG24KJ Fusion of 2 or more Cervical Vertebral Joints with Nonautologous Tissue Substitute, Posterior Approach, Anterior Column, Percutaneous Endoscopic Approach

ØRG4Ø7Ø Fusion of Cervicothoracic Vertebral Joint with Autologous Tissue Substitute, Anterior Approach, Anterior Column, Open Approach

ØRG4Ø71 Fusion of Cervicothoracic Vertebral Joint with Autologous Tissue Substitute, Posterior Approach, Posterior Column, Open Approach

ØRG4Ø7J Fusion of Cervicothoracic Vertebral Joint with Autologous Tissue Substitute, Posterior Approach, Anterior Column, Open Approach

ØRG4ØAØ Fusion of Cervicothoracic Vertebral Joint with Interbody Fusion Device, Anterior Approach, Anterior Column, Open Approach

ØRG4ØAJ Fusion of Cervicothoracic Vertebral Joint with Interbody Fusion Device, Posterior Approach, Anterior Column, Open Approach

ØRG4ØJØ Fusion of Cervicothoracic Vertebral Joint with Synthetic Substitute, Anterior Approach, Anterior Column, Open Approach

ØRG4ØJ1 Fusion of Cervicothoracic Vertebral Joint with Synthetic Substitute, Posterior Approach, Posterior Column, Open Approach

ØRG4ØJJ Fusion of Cervicothoracic Vertebral Joint with Synthetic Substitute, Posterior Approach, Anterior Column, Open Approach

ØRG4ØKØ Fusion of Cervicothoracic Vertebral Joint with Nonautologous Tissue Substitute, Anterior Approach, Anterior Column, Open Approach

ØRG4ØK1 Fusion of Cervicothoracic Vertebral Joint with Nonautologous Tissue Substitute, Posterior Approach, Posterior Column, Open Approach

ØRG4ØKJ Fusion of Cervicothoracic Vertebral Joint with Nonautologous Tissue Substitute, Posterior Approach, Anterior Column, Open Approach

ØRG437Ø Fusion of Cervicothoracic Vertebral Joint with Autologous Tissue Substitute, Anterior Approach, Anterior Column, Percutaneous Approach

ØRG4371 Fusion of Cervicothoracic Vertebral Joint with Autologous Tissue Substitute, Posterior Approach, Posterior Column, Percutaneous Approach

ØRG437J Fusion of Cervicothoracic Vertebral Joint with Autologous Tissue Substitute, Posterior Approach, Anterior Column, Percutaneous Approach

ØRG43AØ Fusion of Cervicothoracic Vertebral Joint with Interbody Fusion Device, Anterior Approach, Anterior Column, Percutaneous Approach

ØRG43AJ Fusion of Cervicothoracic Vertebral Joint with Interbody Fusion Device, Posterior Approach, Anterior Column, Percutaneous Approach

ØRG43JØ Fusion of Cervicothoracic Vertebral Joint with Synthetic Substitute, Anterior Approach, Anterior Column, Percutaneous Approach

ØRG43J1 Fusion of Cervicothoracic Vertebral Joint with Synthetic Substitute, Posterior Approach, Posterior Column, Percutaneous Approach

ØRG43JJ Fusion of Cervicothoracic Vertebral Joint with Synthetic Substitute, Posterior Approach, Anterior Column, Percutaneous Approach

ØRG43KØ Fusion of Cervicothoracic Vertebral Joint with Nonautologous Tissue Substitute, Anterior Approach, Anterior Column, Percutaneous Approach

ØRG43K1 Fusion of Cervicothoracic Vertebral Joint with Nonautologous Tissue Substitute, Posterior Approach, Posterior Column, Percutaneous Approach

ØRG43KJ Fusion of Cervicothoracic Vertebral Joint with Nonautologous Tissue Substitute, Posterior Approach, Anterior Column, Percutaneous Approach

ØRG447Ø Fusion of Cervicothoracic Vertebral Joint with Autologous Tissue Substitute, Anterior Approach, Anterior Column, Percutaneous Endoscopic Approach

ØRG4471 Fusion of Cervicothoracic Vertebral Joint with Autologous Tissue Substitute, Posterior Approach, Posterior Column, Percutaneous Endoscopic Approach

ØRG447J Fusion of Cervicothoracic Vertebral Joint with Autologous Tissue Substitute, Posterior Approach, Anterior Column, Percutaneous Endoscopic Approach

ØRG44AØ Fusion of Cervicothoracic Vertebral Joint with Interbody Fusion Device, Anterior Approach, Anterior Column, Percutaneous Endoscopic Approach

ØRG44AJ Fusion of Cervicothoracic Vertebral Joint with Interbody Fusion Device, Posterior Approach, Anterior Column, Percutaneous Endoscopic Approach

ØRG44JØ Fusion of Cervicothoracic Vertebral Joint with Synthetic Substitute, Anterior Approach, Anterior Column, Percutaneous Endoscopic Approach

ØRG44J1 Fusion of Cervicothoracic Vertebral Joint with Synthetic Substitute, Posterior Approach, Posterior Column, Percutaneous Endoscopic Approach

ØRG44JJ Fusion of Cervicothoracic Vertebral Joint with Synthetic Substitute, Posterior Approach, Anterior Column, Percutaneous Endoscopic Approach

ØRG44KØ Fusion of Cervicothoracic Vertebral Joint with Nonautologous Tissue Substitute, Anterior Approach, Anterior Column, Percutaneous Endoscopic Approach

ØRG44K1 Fusion of Cervicothoracic Vertebral Joint with Nonautologous Tissue Substitute, Posterior Approach, Posterior Column, Percutaneous Endoscopic Approach

ØRG44KJ Fusion of Cervicothoracic Vertebral Joint with Nonautologous Tissue Substitute, Posterior Approach, Anterior Column, Percutaneous Endoscopic Approach

ØRG6Ø7Ø Fusion of Thoracic Vertebral Joint with Autologous Tissue Substitute, Anterior Approach, Anterior Column, Open Approach

ØRG6Ø71 Fusion of Thoracic Vertebral Joint with Autologous Tissue Substitute, Posterior Approach, Posterior Column, Open Approach

ØRG6Ø7J Fusion of Thoracic Vertebral Joint with Autologous Tissue Substitute, Posterior Approach, Anterior Column, Open Approach

ØRG6ØAØ Fusion of Thoracic Vertebral Joint with Interbody Fusion Device, Anterior Approach, Anterior Column, Open Approach

ØRG6ØAJ Fusion of Thoracic Vertebral Joint with Interbody Fusion Device, Posterior Approach, Anterior Column, Open Approach

ØRG6ØJØ Fusion of Thoracic Vertebral Joint with Synthetic Substitute, Anterior Approach, Anterior Column, Open Approach

ØRG6ØJ1 Fusion of Thoracic Vertebral Joint with Synthetic Substitute, Posterior Approach, Posterior Column, Open Approach

ØRG6ØJJ Fusion of Thoracic Vertebral Joint with Synthetic Substitute, Posterior Approach, Anterior Column, Open Approach

ØRG6ØKØ Fusion of Thoracic Vertebral Joint with Nonautologous Tissue Substitute, Anterior Approach, Anterior Column, Open Approach

ØRG6ØK1 Fusion of Thoracic Vertebral Joint with Nonautologous Tissue Substitute, Posterior Approach, Posterior Column, Open Approach

ØRG6ØKJ Fusion of Thoracic Vertebral Joint with Nonautologous Tissue Substitute, Posterior Approach, Anterior Column, Open Approach

ØRG637Ø Fusion of Thoracic Vertebral Joint with Autologous Tissue Substitute, Anterior Approach, Anterior Column, Percutaneous Approach

ØRG6371 Fusion of Thoracic Vertebral Joint with Autologous Tissue Substitute, Posterior Approach, Posterior Column, Percutaneous Approach

ØRG637J Fusion of Thoracic Vertebral Joint with Autologous Tissue Substitute, Posterior Approach, Anterior Column, Percutaneous Approach

ØRG63AØ Fusion of Thoracic Vertebral Joint with Interbody Fusion Device, Anterior Approach, Anterior Column, Percutaneous Approach

HAC 12: Surgical Site Infection-Certain Orthopedic Procedures of the Spine, Shoulder, and Elbow (continued)

ØRG63AJ Fusion of Thoracic Vertebral Joint with Interbody Fusion Device, Posterior Approach, Anterior Column, Percutaneous Approach

ØRG63J0 Fusion of Thoracic Vertebral Joint with Synthetic Substitute, Anterior Approach, Anterior Column, Percutaneous Approach

ØRG63J1 Fusion of Thoracic Vertebral Joint with Synthetic Substitute, Posterior Approach, Posterior Column, Percutaneous Approach

ØRG63JJ Fusion of Thoracic Vertebral Joint with Synthetic Substitute, Posterior Approach, Anterior Column, Percutaneous Approach

ØRG63K0 Fusion of Thoracic Vertebral Joint with Nonautologous Tissue Substitute, Anterior Approach, Anterior Column, Percutaneous Approach

ØRG63K1 Fusion of Thoracic Vertebral Joint with Nonautologous Tissue Substitute, Posterior Approach, Posterior Column, Percutaneous Approach

ØRG63KJ Fusion of Thoracic Vertebral Joint with Nonautologous Tissue Substitute, Posterior Approach, Anterior Column, Percutaneous Approach

ØRG6470 Fusion of Thoracic Vertebral Joint with Autologous Tissue Substitute, Anterior Approach, Anterior Column, Percutaneous Endoscopic Approach

ØRG6471 Fusion of Thoracic Vertebral Joint with Autologous Tissue Substitute, Posterior Approach, Posterior Column, Percutaneous Endoscopic Approach

ØRG647J Fusion of Thoracic Vertebral Joint with Autologous Tissue Substitute, Posterior Approach, Anterior Column, Percutaneous Endoscopic Approach

ØRG64A0 Fusion of Thoracic Vertebral Joint with Interbody Fusion Device, Anterior Approach, Anterior Column, Percutaneous Endoscopic Approach

ØRG64AJ Fusion of Thoracic Vertebral Joint with Interbody Fusion Device, Posterior Approach, Anterior Column, Percutaneous Endoscopic Approach

ØRG64J0 Fusion of Thoracic Vertebral Joint with Synthetic Substitute, Anterior Approach, Anterior Column, Percutaneous Endoscopic Approach

ØRG64J1 Fusion of Thoracic Vertebral Joint with Synthetic Substitute, Posterior Approach, Posterior Column, Percutaneous Endoscopic Approach

ØRG64JJ Fusion of Thoracic Vertebral Joint with Synthetic Substitute, Posterior Approach, Anterior Column, Percutaneous Endoscopic Approach

ØRG64K0 Fusion of Thoracic Vertebral Joint with Nonautologous Tissue Substitute, Anterior Approach, Anterior Column, Percutaneous Endoscopic Approach

ØRG64K1 Fusion of Thoracic Vertebral Joint with Nonautologous Tissue Substitute, Posterior Approach, Posterior Column, Percutaneous Endoscopic Approach

ØRG64KJ Fusion of Thoracic Vertebral Joint with Nonautologous Tissue Substitute, Posterior Approach, Anterior Column, Percutaneous Endoscopic Approach

ØRG7070 Fusion of 2 to 7 Thoracic Vertebral Joints with Autologous Tissue Substitute, Anterior Approach, Anterior Column, Open Approach

ØRG7071 Fusion of 2 to 7 Thoracic Vertebral Joints with Autologous Tissue Substitute, Posterior Approach, Posterior Column, Open Approach

ØRG707J Fusion of 2 to 7 Thoracic Vertebral Joints with Autologous Tissue Substitute, Posterior Approach, Anterior Column, Open Approach

ØRG70A0 Fusion of 2 to 7 Thoracic Vertebral Joints with Interbody Fusion Device, Anterior Approach, Anterior Column, Open Approach

ØRG70AJ Fusion of 2 to 7 Thoracic Vertebral Joints with Interbody Fusion Device, Posterior Approach, Anterior Column, Open Approach

ØRG70J0 Fusion of 2 to 7 Thoracic Vertebral Joints with Synthetic Substitute, Anterior Approach, Anterior Column, Open Approach

ØRG70J1 Fusion of 2 to 7 Thoracic Vertebral Joints with Synthetic Substitute, Posterior Approach, Posterior Column, Open Approach

ØRG70JJ Fusion of 2 to 7 Thoracic Vertebral Joints with Synthetic Substitute, Posterior Approach, Anterior Column, Open Approach

ØRG70K0 Fusion of 2 to 7 Thoracic Vertebral Joints with Nonautologous Tissue Substitute, Anterior Approach, Anterior Column, Open Approach

ØRG70K1 Fusion of 2 to 7 Thoracic Vertebral Joints with Nonautologous Tissue Substitute, Posterior Approach, Posterior Column, Open Approach

ØRG70KJ Fusion of 2 to 7 Thoracic Vertebral Joints with Nonautologous Tissue Substitute, Posterior Approach, Anterior Column, Open Approach

ØRG7370 Fusion of 2 to 7 Thoracic Vertebral Joints with Autologous Tissue Substitute, Anterior Approach, Anterior Column, Percutaneous Approach

ØRG7371 Fusion of 2 to 7 Thoracic Vertebral Joints with Autologous Tissue Substitute, Posterior Approach, Posterior Column, Percutaneous Approach

ØRG737J Fusion of 2 to 7 Thoracic Vertebral Joints with Autologous Tissue Substitute, Posterior Approach, Anterior Column, Percutaneous Approach

ØRG73A0 Fusion of 2 to 7 Thoracic Vertebral Joints with Interbody Fusion Device, Anterior Approach, Anterior Column, Percutaneous Approach

ØRG73AJ Fusion of 2 to 7 Thoracic Vertebral Joints with Interbody Fusion Device, Posterior Approach, Anterior Column, Percutaneous Approach

ØRG73J0 Fusion of 2 to 7 Thoracic Vertebral Joints with Synthetic Substitute, Anterior Approach, Anterior Column, Percutaneous Approach

ØRG73J1 Fusion of 2 to 7 Thoracic Vertebral Joints with Synthetic Substitute, Posterior Approach, Posterior Column, Percutaneous Approach

ØRG73JJ Fusion of 2 to 7 Thoracic Vertebral Joints with Synthetic Substitute, Posterior Approach, Anterior Column, Percutaneous Approach

ØRG73K0 Fusion of 2 to 7 Thoracic Vertebral Joints with Nonautologous Tissue Substitute, Anterior Approach, Anterior Column, Percutaneous Approach

ØRG73K1 Fusion of 2 to 7 Thoracic Vertebral Joints with Nonautologous Tissue Substitute, Posterior Approach, Posterior Column, Percutaneous Approach

ØRG73KJ Fusion of 2 to 7 Thoracic Vertebral Joints with Nonautologous Tissue Substitute, Posterior Approach, Anterior Column, Percutaneous Approach

ØRG7470 Fusion of 2 to 7 Thoracic Vertebral Joints with Autologous Tissue Substitute, Anterior Approach, Anterior Column, Percutaneous Endoscopic Approach

ØRG7471 Fusion of 2 to 7 Thoracic Vertebral Joints with Autologous Tissue Substitute, Posterior Approach, Posterior Column, Percutaneous Endoscopic Approach

ØRG747J Fusion of 2 to 7 Thoracic Vertebral Joints with Autologous Tissue Substitute, Posterior Approach, Anterior Column, Percutaneous Endoscopic Approach

ØRG74A0 Fusion of 2 to 7 Thoracic Vertebral Joints with Interbody Fusion Device, Anterior Approach, Anterior Column, Percutaneous Endoscopic Approach

ØRG74AJ Fusion of 2 to 7 Thoracic Vertebral Joints with Interbody Fusion Device, Posterior Approach, Anterior Column, Percutaneous Endoscopic Approach

ØRG74J0 Fusion of 2 to 7 Thoracic Vertebral Joints with Synthetic Substitute, Anterior Approach, Anterior Column, Percutaneous Endoscopic Approach

ØRG74J1 Fusion of 2 to 7 Thoracic Vertebral Joints with Synthetic Substitute, Posterior Approach, Posterior Column, Percutaneous Endoscopic Approach

ØRG74JJ Fusion of 2 to 7 Thoracic Vertebral Joints with Synthetic Substitute, Posterior Approach, Anterior Column, Percutaneous Endoscopic Approach

ØRG74K0 Fusion of 2 to 7 Thoracic Vertebral Joints with Nonautologous Tissue Substitute, Anterior Approach, Anterior Column, Percutaneous Endoscopic Approach

ØRG74K1 Fusion of 2 to 7 Thoracic Vertebral Joints with Nonautologous Tissue Substitute, Posterior Approach, Posterior Column, Percutaneous Endoscopic Approach

ØRG74KJ Fusion of 2 to 7 Thoracic Vertebral Joints with Nonautologous Tissue Substitute, Posterior Approach, Anterior Column, Percutaneous Endoscopic Approach

ØRG8070 Fusion of 8 or More Thoracic Vertebral Joints with Autologous Tissue Substitute, Anterior Approach, Anterior Column, Open Approach

ØRG8071 Fusion of 8 or More Thoracic Vertebral Joints with Autologous Tissue Substitute, Posterior Approach, Posterior Column, Open Approach

ØRG807J Fusion of 8 or More Thoracic Vertebral Joints with Autologous Tissue Substitute, Posterior Approach, Anterior Column, Open Approach

ØRG80A0 Fusion of 8 or More Thoracic Vertebral Joints with Interbody Fusion Device, Anterior Approach, Anterior Column, Open Approach

ØRG80AJ Fusion of 8 or More Thoracic Vertebral Joints with Interbody Fusion Device, Posterior Approach, Anterior Column, Open Approach

HAC 12: Surgical Site Infection-Certain Orthopedic Procedures of the Spine, Shoulder, and Elbow (continued)

ØRG80JØ   Fusion of 8 or More Thoracic Vertebral Joints with Synthetic Substitute, Anterior Approach, Anterior Column, Open Approach

ØRG80J1   Fusion of 8 or More Thoracic Vertebral Joints with Synthetic Substitute, Posterior Approach, Posterior Column, Open Approach

ØRG80JJ   Fusion of 8 or More Thoracic Vertebral Joints with Synthetic Substitute, Posterior Approach, Anterior Column, Open Approach

ØRG80KØ   Fusion of 8 or More Thoracic Vertebral Joints with Nonautologous Tissue Substitute, Anterior Approach, Anterior Column, Open Approach

ØRG80K1   Fusion of 8 or More Thoracic Vertebral Joints with Nonautologous Tissue Substitute, Posterior Approach, Posterior Column, Open Approach

ØRG80KJ   Fusion of 8 or More Thoracic Vertebral Joints with Nonautologous Tissue Substitute, Posterior Approach, Anterior Column, Open Approach

ØRG837Ø   Fusion of 8 or More Thoracic Vertebral Joints with Autologous Tissue Substitute, Anterior Approach, Anterior Column, Percutaneous Approach

ØRG8371   Fusion of 8 or More Thoracic Vertebral Joints with Autologous Tissue Substitute, Posterior Approach, Posterior Column, Percutaneous Approach

ØRG837J   Fusion of 8 or More Thoracic Vertebral Joints with Autologous Tissue Substitute, Posterior Approach, Anterior Column, Percutaneous Approach

ØRG83AØ   Fusion of 8 or More Thoracic Vertebral Joints with Interbody Fusion Device, Anterior Approach, Anterior Column, Percutaneous Approach

ØRG83AJ   Fusion of 8 or More Thoracic Vertebral Joints with Interbody Fusion Device, Posterior Approach, Anterior Column, Percutaneous Approach

ØRG83JØ   Fusion of 8 or More Thoracic Vertebral Joints with Synthetic Substitute, Anterior Approach, Anterior Column, Percutaneous Approach

ØRG83J1   Fusion of 8 or More Thoracic Vertebral Joints with Synthetic Substitute, Posterior Approach, Posterior Column, Percutaneous Approach

ØRG83JJ   Fusion of 8 or More Thoracic Vertebral Joints with Synthetic Substitute, Posterior Approach, Anterior Column, Percutaneous Approach

ØRG83KØ   Fusion of 8 or More Thoracic Vertebral Joints with Nonautologous Tissue Substitute, Anterior Approach, Anterior Column, Percutaneous Approach

ØRG83K1   Fusion of 8 or More Thoracic Vertebral Joints with Nonautologous Tissue Substitute, Posterior Approach, Posterior Column, Percutaneous Approach

ØRG83KJ   Fusion of 8 or More Thoracic Vertebral Joints with Nonautologous Tissue Substitute, Posterior Approach, Anterior Column, Percutaneous Approach

ØRG847Ø   Fusion of 8 or More Thoracic Vertebral Joints with Autologous Tissue Substitute, Anterior Approach, Anterior Column, Percutaneous Endoscopic Approach

ØRG8471   Fusion of 8 or More Thoracic Vertebral Joints with Autologous Tissue Substitute, Posterior Approach, Posterior Column, Percutaneous Endoscopic Approach

ØRG847J   Fusion of 8 or More Thoracic Vertebral Joints with Autologous Tissue Substitute, Posterior Approach, Anterior Column, Percutaneous Endoscopic Approach

ØRG84AØ   Fusion of 8 or More Thoracic Vertebral Joints with Interbody Fusion Device, Anterior Approach, Anterior Column, Percutaneous Endoscopic Approach

ØRG84AJ   Fusion of 8 or More Thoracic Vertebral Joints with Interbody Fusion Device, Posterior Approach, Anterior Column, Percutaneous Endoscopic Approach

ØRG84JØ   Fusion of 8 or More Thoracic Vertebral Joints with Synthetic Substitute, Anterior Approach, Anterior Column, Percutaneous Endoscopic Approach

ØRG84J1   Fusion of 8 or More Thoracic Vertebral Joints with Synthetic Substitute, Posterior Approach, Posterior Column, Percutaneous Endoscopic Approach

ØRG84JJ   Fusion of 8 or More Thoracic Vertebral Joints with Synthetic Substitute, Posterior Approach, Anterior Column, Percutaneous Endoscopic Approach

ØRG84KØ   Fusion of 8 or More Thoracic Vertebral Joints with Nonautologous Tissue Substitute, Anterior Approach, Anterior Column, Percutaneous Endoscopic Approach

ØRG84K1   Fusion of 8 or More Thoracic Vertebral Joints with Nonautologous Tissue Substitute, Posterior Approach, Posterior Column, Percutaneous Endoscopic Approach

ØRG84KJ   Fusion of 8 or More Thoracic Vertebral Joints with Nonautologous Tissue Substitute, Posterior Approach, Anterior Column, Percutaneous Endoscopic Approach

ØRGAØ7Ø   Fusion of Thoracolumbar Vertebral Joint with Autologous Tissue Substitute, Anterior Approach, Anterior Column, Open Approach

ØRGAØ71   Fusion of Thoracolumbar Vertebral Joint with Autologous Tissue Substitute, Posterior Approach, Posterior Column, Open Approach

ØRGAØ7J   Fusion of Thoracolumbar Vertebral Joint with Autologous Tissue Substitute, Posterior Approach, Anterior Column, Open Approach

ØRGAØAØ   Fusion of Thoracolumbar Vertebral Joint with Interbody Fusion Device, Anterior Approach, Anterior Column, Open Approach

ØRGAØAJ   Fusion of Thoracolumbar Vertebral Joint with Interbody Fusion Device, Posterior Approach, Anterior Column, Open Approach

ØRGAØJØ   Fusion of Thoracolumbar Vertebral Joint with Synthetic Substitute, Anterior Approach, Anterior Column, Open Approach

ØRGAØJ1   Fusion of Thoracolumbar Vertebral Joint with Synthetic Substitute, Posterior Approach, Posterior Column, Open Approach

ØRGAØJJ   Fusion of Thoracolumbar Vertebral Joint with Synthetic Substitute, Posterior Approach, Anterior Column, Open Approach

ØRGAØKØ   Fusion of Thoracolumbar Vertebral Joint with Nonautologous Tissue Substitute, Anterior Approach, Anterior Column, Open Approach

ØRGAØK1   Fusion of Thoracolumbar Vertebral Joint with Nonautologous Tissue Substitute, Posterior Approach, Posterior Column, Open Approach

ØRGAØKJ   Fusion of Thoracolumbar Vertebral Joint with Nonautologous Tissue Substitute, Posterior Approach, Anterior Column, Open Approach

ØRGA37Ø   Fusion of Thoracolumbar Vertebral Joint with Autologous Tissue Substitute, Anterior Approach, Anterior Column, Percutaneous Approach

ØRGA371   Fusion of Thoracolumbar Vertebral Joint with Autologous Tissue Substitute, Posterior Approach, Posterior Column, Percutaneous Approach

ØRGA37J   Fusion of Thoracolumbar Vertebral Joint with Autologous Tissue Substitute, Posterior Approach, Anterior Column, Percutaneous Approach

ØRGA3AØ   Fusion of Thoracolumbar Vertebral Joint with Interbody Fusion Device, Anterior Approach, Anterior Column, Percutaneous Approach

ØRGA3AJ   Fusion of Thoracolumbar Vertebral Joint with Interbody Fusion Device, Posterior Approach, Anterior Column, Percutaneous Approach

ØRGA3JØ   Fusion of Thoracolumbar Vertebral Joint with Synthetic Substitute, Anterior Approach, Anterior Column, Percutaneous Approach

ØRGA3J1   Fusion of Thoracolumbar Vertebral Joint with Synthetic Substitute, Posterior Approach, Posterior Column, Percutaneous Approach

ØRGA3JJ   Fusion of Thoracolumbar Vertebral Joint with Synthetic Substitute, Posterior Approach, Anterior Column, Percutaneous Approach

ØRGA3KØ   Fusion of Thoracolumbar Vertebral Joint with Nonautologous Tissue Substitute, Anterior Approach, Anterior Column, Percutaneous Approach

ØRGA3K1   Fusion of Thoracolumbar Vertebral Joint with Nonautologous Tissue Substitute, Posterior Approach, Posterior Column, Percutaneous Approach

ØRGA3KJ   Fusion of Thoracolumbar Vertebral Joint with Nonautologous Tissue Substitute, Posterior Approach, Anterior Column, Percutaneous Approach

ØRGA47Ø   Fusion of Thoracolumbar Vertebral Joint with Autologous Tissue Substitute, Anterior Approach, Anterior Column, Percutaneous Endoscopic Approach

ØRGA471   Fusion of Thoracolumbar Vertebral Joint with Autologous Tissue Substitute, Posterior Approach, Posterior Column, Percutaneous Endoscopic Approach

ØRGA47J   Fusion of Thoracolumbar Vertebral Joint with Autologous Tissue Substitute, Posterior Approach, Anterior Column, Percutaneous Endoscopic Approach

HAC 12: Surgical Site Infection-Certain Orthopedic Procedures of the Spine, Shoulder, and Elbow (continued)

ØRGA4AØ   Fusion of Thoracolumbar Vertebral Joint with Interbody Fusion Device, Anterior Approach, Anterior Column, Percutaneous Endoscopic Approach

ØRGA4AJ   Fusion of Thoracolumbar Vertebral Joint with Interbody Fusion Device, Posterior Approach, Anterior Column, Percutaneous Endoscopic Approach

ØRGA4JØ   Fusion of Thoracolumbar Vertebral Joint with Synthetic Substitute, Anterior Approach, Anterior Column, Percutaneous Endoscopic Approach

ØRGA4J1   Fusion of Thoracolumbar Vertebral Joint with Synthetic Substitute, Posterior Approach, Posterior Column, Percutaneous Endoscopic Approach

ØRGA4JJ   Fusion of Thoracolumbar Vertebral Joint with Synthetic Substitute, Posterior Approach, Anterior Column, Percutaneous Endoscopic Approach

ØRGA4KØ   Fusion of Thoracolumbar Vertebral Joint with Nonautologous Tissue Substitute, Anterior Approach, Anterior Column, Percutaneous Endoscopic Approach

ØRGA4K1   Fusion of Thoracolumbar Vertebral Joint with Nonautologous Tissue Substitute, Posterior Approach, Posterior Column, Percutaneous Endoscopic Approach

ØRGA4KJ   Fusion of Thoracolumbar Vertebral Joint with Nonautologous Tissue Substitute, Posterior Approach, Anterior Column, Percutaneous Endoscopic Approach

ØRGE04Z   Fusion of Right Sternoclavicular Joint with Internal Fixation Device, Open Approach

ØRGE07Z   Fusion of Right Sternoclavicular Joint with Autologous Tissue Substitute, Open Approach

ØRGE0JZ   Fusion of Right Sternoclavicular Joint with Synthetic Substitute, Open Approach

ØRGE0KZ   Fusion of Right Sternoclavicular Joint with Nonautologous Tissue Substitute, Open Approach

ØRGE34Z   Fusion of Right Sternoclavicular Joint with Internal Fixation Device, Percutaneous Approach

ØRGE37Z   Fusion of Right Sternoclavicular Joint with Autologous Tissue Substitute, Percutaneous Approach

ØRGE3JZ   Fusion of Right Sternoclavicular Joint with Synthetic Substitute, Percutaneous Approach

ØRGE3KZ   Fusion of Right Sternoclavicular Joint with Nonautologous Tissue Substitute, Percutaneous Approach

ØRGE44Z   Fusion of Right Sternoclavicular Joint with Internal Fixation Device, Percutaneous Endoscopic Approach

ØRGE47Z   Fusion of Right Sternoclavicular Joint with Autologous Tissue Substitute, Percutaneous Endoscopic Approach

ØRGE4JZ   Fusion of Right Sternoclavicular Joint with Synthetic Substitute, Percutaneous Endoscopic Approach

ØRGE4KZ   Fusion of Right Sternoclavicular Joint with Nonautologous Tissue Substitute, Percutaneous Endoscopic Approach

ØRGF04Z   Fusion of Left Sternoclavicular Joint with Internal Fixation Device, Open Approach

ØRGF07Z   Fusion of Left Sternoclavicular Joint with Autologous Tissue Substitute, Open Approach

ØRGF0JZ   Fusion of Left Sternoclavicular Joint with Synthetic Substitute, Open Approach

ØRGF0KZ   Fusion of Left Sternoclavicular Joint with Nonautologous Tissue Substitute, Open Approach

ØRGF34Z   Fusion of Left Sternoclavicular Joint with Internal Fixation Device, Percutaneous Approach

ØRGF37Z   Fusion of Left Sternoclavicular Joint with Autologous Tissue Substitute, Percutaneous Approach

ØRGF3JZ   Fusion of Left Sternoclavicular Joint with Synthetic Substitute, Percutaneous Approach

ØRGF3KZ   Fusion of Left Sternoclavicular Joint with Nonautologous Tissue Substitute, Percutaneous Approach

ØRGF44Z   Fusion of Left Sternoclavicular Joint with Internal Fixation Device, Percutaneous Endoscopic Approach

ØRGF47Z   Fusion of Left Sternoclavicular Joint with Autologous Tissue Substitute, Percutaneous Endoscopic Approach

ØRGF4JZ   Fusion of Left Sternoclavicular Joint with Synthetic Substitute, Percutaneous Endoscopic Approach

ØRGF4KZ   Fusion of Left Sternoclavicular Joint with Nonautologous Tissue Substitute, Percutaneous Endoscopic Approach

ØRGG04Z   Fusion of Right Acromioclavicular Joint with Internal Fixation Device, Open Approach

ØRGG07Z   Fusion of Right Acromioclavicular Joint with Autologous Tissue Substitute, Open Approach

ØRGG0JZ   Fusion of Right Acromioclavicular Joint with Synthetic Substitute, Open Approach

ØRGG0KZ   Fusion of Right Acromioclavicular Joint with Nonautologous Tissue Substitute, Open Approach

ØRGG34Z   Fusion of Right Acromioclavicular Joint with Internal Fixation Device, Percutaneous Approach

ØRGG37Z   Fusion of Right Acromioclavicular Joint with Autologous Tissue Substitute, Percutaneous Approach

ØRGG3JZ   Fusion of Right Acromioclavicular Joint with Synthetic Substitute, Percutaneous Approach

ØRGG3KZ   Fusion of Right Acromioclavicular Joint with Nonautologous Tissue Substitute, Percutaneous Approach

ØRGG44Z   Fusion of Right Acromioclavicular Joint with Internal Fixation Device, Percutaneous Endoscopic Approach

ØRGG47Z   Fusion of Right Acromioclavicular Joint with Autologous Tissue Substitute, Percutaneous Endoscopic Approach

ØRGG4JZ   Fusion of Right Acromioclavicular Joint with Synthetic Substitute, Percutaneous Endoscopic Approach

ØRGG4KZ   Fusion of Right Acromioclavicular Joint with Nonautologous Tissue Substitute, Percutaneous Endoscopic Approach

ØRGH04Z   Fusion of Left Acromioclavicular Joint with Internal Fixation Device, Open Approach

ØRGH07Z   Fusion of Left Acromioclavicular Joint with Autologous Tissue Substitute, Open Approach

ØRGH0JZ   Fusion of Left Acromioclavicular Joint with Synthetic Substitute, Open Approach

ØRGH0KZ   Fusion of Left Acromioclavicular Joint with Nonautologous Tissue Substitute, Open Approach

ØRGH34Z   Fusion of Left Acromioclavicular Joint with Internal Fixation Device, Percutaneous Approach

ØRGH37Z   Fusion of Left Acromioclavicular Joint with Autologous Tissue Substitute, Percutaneous Approach

ØRGH3JZ   Fusion of Left Acromioclavicular Joint with Synthetic Substitute, Percutaneous Approach

ØRGH3KZ   Fusion of Left Acromioclavicular Joint with Nonautologous Tissue Substitute, Percutaneous Approach

ØRGH44Z   Fusion of Left Acromioclavicular Joint with Internal Fixation Device, Percutaneous Endoscopic Approach

ØRGH47Z   Fusion of Left Acromioclavicular Joint with Autologous Tissue Substitute, Percutaneous Endoscopic Approach

ØRGH4JZ   Fusion of Left Acromioclavicular Joint with Synthetic Substitute, Percutaneous Endoscopic Approach .

ØRGH4KZ   Fusion of Left Acromioclavicular Joint with Nonautologous Tissue Substitute, Percutaneous Endoscopic Approach

ØRGJ04Z   Fusion of Right Shoulder Joint with Internal Fixation Device, Open Approach

ØRGJ07Z   Fusion of Right Shoulder Joint with Autologous Tissue Substitute, Open Approach

ØRGJ0JZ   Fusion of Right Shoulder Joint with Synthetic Substitute, Open Approach

ØRGJ0KZ   Fusion of Right Shoulder Joint with Nonautologous Tissue Substitute, Open Approach

ØRGJ34Z   Fusion of Right Shoulder Joint with Internal Fixation Device, Percutaneous Approach

ØRGJ37Z   Fusion of Right Shoulder Joint with Autologous Tissue Substitute, Percutaneous Approach

ØRGJ3JZ   Fusion of Right Shoulder Joint with Synthetic Substitute, Percutaneous Approach

ØRGJ3KZ   Fusion of Right Shoulder Joint with Nonautologous Tissue Substitute, Percutaneous Approach

ØRGJ44Z   Fusion of Right Shoulder Joint with Internal Fixation Device, Percutaneous Endoscopic Approach

ØRGJ47Z   Fusion of Right Shoulder Joint with Autologous Tissue Substitute, Percutaneous Endoscopic Approach

ØRGJ4JZ   Fusion of Right Shoulder Joint with Synthetic Substitute, Percutaneous Endoscopic Approach

ØRGJ4KZ   Fusion of Right Shoulder Joint with Nonautologous Tissue Substitute, Percutaneous Endoscopic Approach

ØRGK04Z   Fusion of Left Shoulder Joint with Internal Fixation Device, Open Approach

ØRGK07Z   Fusion of Left Shoulder Joint with Autologous Tissue Substitute, Open Approach

ØRGK0JZ   Fusion of Left Shoulder Joint with Synthetic Substitute, Open Approach

ØRGK0KZ   Fusion of Left Shoulder Joint with Nonautologous Tissue Substitute, Open Approach

ØRGK34Z   Fusion of Left Shoulder Joint with Internal Fixation Device, Percutaneous Approach

HAC 12: Surgical Site Infection-Certain Orthopedic Procedures of the Spine, Shoulder, and Elbow (continued)

ØRGK37Z Fusion of Left Shoulder Joint with Autologous Tissue Substitute, Percutaneous Approach

ØRGK3JZ Fusion of Left Shoulder Joint with Synthetic Substitute, Percutaneous Approach

ØRGK3KZ Fusion of Left Shoulder Joint with Nonautologous Tissue Substitute, Percutaneous Approach

ØRGK44Z Fusion of Left Shoulder Joint with Internal Fixation Device, Percutaneous Endoscopic Approach

ØRGK47Z Fusion of Left Shoulder Joint with Autologous Tissue Substitute, Percutaneous Endoscopic Approach

ØRGK4JZ Fusion of Left Shoulder Joint with Synthetic Substitute, Percutaneous Endoscopic Approach

ØRGK4KZ Fusion of Left Shoulder Joint with Nonautologous Tissue Substitute, Percutaneous Endoscopic Approach

ØRGL04Z Fusion of Right Elbow Joint with Internal Fixation Device, Open Approach

ØRGL05Z Fusion of Right Elbow Joint with External Fixation Device, Open Approach

ØRGL07Z Fusion of Right Elbow Joint with Autologous Tissue Substitute, Open Approach

ØRGLØJZ Fusion of Right Elbow Joint with Synthetic Substitute, Open Approach

ØRGLØKZ Fusion of Right Elbow Joint with Nonautologous Tissue Substitute, Open Approach

ØRGL34Z Fusion of Right Elbow Joint with Internal Fixation Device, Percutaneous Approach

ØRGL35Z Fusion of Right Elbow Joint with External Fixation Device, Percutaneous Approach

ØRGL37Z Fusion of Right Elbow Joint with Autologous Tissue Substitute, Percutaneous Approach

ØRGL3JZ Fusion of Right Elbow Joint with Synthetic Substitute, Percutaneous Approach

ØRGL3KZ Fusion of Right Elbow Joint with Nonautologous Tissue Substitute, Percutaneous Approach

ØRGL44Z Fusion of Right Elbow Joint with Internal Fixation Device, Percutaneous Endoscopic Approach

ØRGL45Z Fusion of Right Elbow Joint with External Fixation Device, Percutaneous Endoscopic Approach

ØRGL47Z Fusion of Right Elbow Joint with Autologous Tissue Substitute, Percutaneous Endoscopic Approach

ØRGL4JZ Fusion of Right Elbow Joint with Synthetic Substitute, Percutaneous Endoscopic Approach

ØRGL4KZ Fusion of Right Elbow Joint with Nonautologous Tissue Substitute, Percutaneous Endoscopic Approach

ØRGM04Z Fusion of Left Elbow Joint with Internal Fixation Device, Open Approach

ØRGM05Z Fusion of Left Elbow Joint with External Fixation Device, Open Approach

ØRGM07Z Fusion of Left Elbow Joint with Autologous Tissue Substitute, Open Approach

ØRGMØJZ Fusion of Left Elbow Joint with Synthetic Substitute, Open Approach

ØRGMØKZ Fusion of Left Elbow Joint with Nonautologous Tissue Substitute, Open Approach

ØRGM34Z Fusion of Left Elbow Joint with Internal Fixation Device, Percutaneous Approach

ØRGM35Z Fusion of Left Elbow Joint with External Fixation Device, Percutaneous Approach

ØRGM37Z Fusion of Left Elbow Joint with Autologous Tissue Substitute, Percutaneous Approach

ØRGM3JZ Fusion of Left Elbow Joint with Synthetic Substitute, Percutaneous Approach

ØRGM3KZ Fusion of Left Elbow Joint with Nonautologous Tissue Substitute, Percutaneous Approach

ØRGM44Z Fusion of Left Elbow Joint with Internal Fixation Device, Percutaneous Endoscopic Approach

ØRGM45Z Fusion of Left Elbow Joint with External Fixation Device, Percutaneous Endoscopic Approach

ØRGM47Z Fusion of Left Elbow Joint with Autologous Tissue Substitute, Percutaneous Endoscopic Approach

ØRGM4JZ Fusion of Left Elbow Joint with Synthetic Substitute, Percutaneous Endoscopic Approach

ØRGM4KZ Fusion of Left Elbow Joint with Nonautologous Tissue Substitute, Percutaneous Endoscopic Approach

ØRQEØZZ Repair Right Sternoclavicular Joint, Open Approach

ØRQE3ZZ Repair Right Sternoclavicular Joint, Percutaneous Approach

ØRQE4ZZ Repair Right Sternoclavicular Joint, Percutaneous Endoscopic Approach

ØRQEXZZ Repair Right Sternoclavicular Joint, External Approach

ØRQFØZZ Repair Left Sternoclavicular Joint, Open Approach

ØRQF3ZZ Repair Left Sternoclavicular Joint, Percutaneous Approach

ØRQF4ZZ Repair Left Sternoclavicular Joint, Percutaneous Endoscopic Approach

ØRQFXZZ Repair Left Sternoclavicular Joint, External Approach

ØRQGØZZ Repair Right Acromioclavicular Joint, Open Approach

ØRQG3ZZ Repair Right Acromioclavicular Joint, Percutaneous Approach

ØRQG4ZZ Repair Right Acromioclavicular Joint, Percutaneous Endoscopic Approach

ØRQGXZZ Repair Right Acromioclavicular Joint, External Approach

ØRQHØZZ Repair Left Acromioclavicular Joint, Open Approach

ØRQH3ZZ Repair Left Acromioclavicular Joint, Percutaneous Approach

ØRQH4ZZ Repair Left Acromioclavicular Joint, Percutaneous Endoscopic Approach

ØRQHXZZ Repair Left Acromioclavicular Joint, External Approach

ØRQJØZZ Repair Right Shoulder Joint, Open Approach

ØRQJ3ZZ Repair Right Shoulder Joint, Percutaneous Approach

ØRQJ4ZZ Repair Right Shoulder Joint, Percutaneous Endoscopic Approach

ØRQJXZZ Repair Right Shoulder Joint, External Approach

ØRQKØZZ Repair Left Shoulder Joint, Open Approach

ØRQK3ZZ Repair Left Shoulder Joint, Percutaneous Approach

ØRQK4ZZ Repair Left Shoulder Joint, Percutaneous Endoscopic Approach

ØRQKXZZ Repair Left Shoulder Joint, External Approach

ØRQLØZZ Repair Right Elbow Joint, Open Approach

ØRQL3ZZ Repair Right Elbow Joint, Percutaneous Approach

ØRQL4ZZ Repair Right Elbow Joint, Percutaneous Endoscopic Approach

ØRQLXZZ Repair Right Elbow Joint, External Approach

ØRQMØZZ Repair Left Elbow Joint, Open Approach

ØRQM3ZZ Repair Left Elbow Joint, Percutaneous Approach

ØRQM4ZZ Repair Left Elbow Joint, Percutaneous Endoscopic Approach

ØRQMXZZ Repair Left Elbow Joint, External Approach

ØRUE07Z Supplement Right Sternoclavicular Joint with Autologous Tissue Substitute, Open Approach

ØRUEØJZ Supplement Right Sternoclavicular Joint with Synthetic Substitute, Open Approach

ØRUEØKZ Supplement Right Sternoclavicular Joint with Nonautologous Tissue Substitute, Open Approach

ØRUE37Z Supplement Right Sternoclavicular Joint with Autologous Tissue Substitute, Percutaneous Approach

ØRUE3JZ Supplement Right Sternoclavicular Joint with Synthetic Substitute, Percutaneous Approach

ØRUE3KZ Supplement Right Sternoclavicular Joint with Nonautologous Tissue Substitute, Percutaneous Approach

ØRUE47Z Supplement Right Sternoclavicular Joint with Autologous Tissue Substitute, Percutaneous Endoscopic Approach

ØRUE4JZ Supplement Right Sternoclavicular Joint with Synthetic Substitute, Percutaneous Endoscopic Approach

ØRUE4KZ Supplement Right Sternoclavicular Joint with Nonautologous Tissue Substitute, Percutaneous Endoscopic Approach

ØRUF07Z Supplement Left Sternoclavicular Joint with Autologous Tissue Substitute, Open Approach

ØRUFØJZ Supplement Left Sternoclavicular Joint with Synthetic Substitute, Open Approach

ØRUFØKZ Supplement Left Sternoclavicular Joint with Nonautologous Tissue Substitute, Open Approach

ØRUF37Z Supplement Left Sternoclavicular Joint with Autologous Tissue Substitute, Percutaneous Approach

ØRUF3JZ Supplement Left Sternoclavicular Joint with Synthetic Substitute, Percutaneous Approach

ØRUF3KZ Supplement Left Sternoclavicular Joint with Nonautologous Tissue Substitute, Percutaneous Approach

ØRUF47Z Supplement Left Sternoclavicular Joint with Autologous Tissue Substitute, Percutaneous Endoscopic Approach

ØRUF4JZ Supplement Left Sternoclavicular Joint with Synthetic Substitute, Percutaneous Endoscopic Approach

ØRUF4KZ Supplement Left Sternoclavicular Joint with Nonautologous Tissue Substitute, Percutaneous Endoscopic Approach

ØRUG07Z Supplement Right Acromioclavicular Joint with Autologous Tissue Substitute, Open Approach

HAC 12: Surgical Site Infection-Certain Orthopedic Procedures of the Spine, Shoulder, and Elbow (continued)

ØRUGØJZ   Supplement Right Acromioclavicular Joint with Synthetic Substitute, Open Approach

ØRUGØKZ   Supplement Right Acromioclavicular Joint with Nonautologous Tissue Substitute, Open Approach

ØRUG37Z   Supplement Right Acromioclavicular Joint with Autologous Tissue Substitute, Percutaneous Approach

ØRUG3JZ   Supplement Right Acromioclavicular Joint with Synthetic Substitute, Percutaneous Approach

ØRUG3KZ   Supplement Right Acromioclavicular Joint with Nonautologous Tissue Substitute, Percutaneous Approach

ØRUG47Z   Supplement Right Acromioclavicular Joint with Autologous Tissue Substitute, Percutaneous Endoscopic Approach

ØRUG4JZ   Supplement Right Acromioclavicular Joint with Synthetic Substitute, Percutaneous Endoscopic Approach

ØRUG4KZ   Supplement Right Acromioclavicular Joint with Nonautologous Tissue Substitute, Percutaneous Endoscopic Approach

ØRUHØ7Z   Supplement Left Acromioclavicular Joint with Autologous Tissue Substitute, Open Approach

ØRUHØJZ   Supplement Left Acromioclavicular Joint with Synthetic Substitute, Open Approach

ØRUHØKZ   Supplement Left Acromioclavicular Joint with Nonautologous Tissue Substitute, Open Approach

ØRUH37Z   Supplement Left Acromioclavicular Joint with Autologous Tissue Substitute, Percutaneous Approach

ØRUH3JZ   Supplement Left Acromioclavicular Joint with Synthetic Substitute, Percutaneous Approach

ØRUH3KZ   Supplement Left Acromioclavicular Joint with Nonautologous Tissue Substitute, Percutaneous Approach

ØRUH47Z   Supplement Left Acromioclavicular Joint with Autologous Tissue Substitute, Percutaneous Endoscopic Approach

ØRUH4JZ   Supplement Left Acromioclavicular Joint with Synthetic Substitute, Percutaneous Endoscopic Approach

ØRUH4KZ   Supplement Left Acromioclavicular Joint with Nonautologous Tissue Substitute, Percutaneous Endoscopic Approach

ØRUJØ7Z   Supplement Right Shoulder Joint with Autologous Tissue Substitute, Open Approach

ØRUJØJZ   Supplement Right Shoulder Joint with Synthetic Substitute, Open Approach

ØRUJØKZ   Supplement Right Shoulder Joint with Nonautologous Tissue Substitute, Open Approach

ØRUJ37Z   Supplement Right Shoulder Joint with Autologous Tissue Substitute, Percutaneous Approach

ØRUJ3JZ   Supplement Right Shoulder Joint with Synthetic Substitute, Percutaneous Approach

ØRUJ3KZ   Supplement Right Shoulder Joint with Nonautologous Tissue Substitute, Percutaneous Approach

ØRUJ47Z   Supplement Right Shoulder Joint with Autologous Tissue Substitute, Percutaneous Endoscopic Approach

ØRUJ4JZ   Supplement Right Shoulder Joint with Synthetic Substitute, Percutaneous Endoscopic Approach

ØRUJ4KZ   Supplement Right Shoulder Joint with Nonautologous Tissue Substitute, Percutaneous Endoscopic Approach

ØRUKØ7Z   Supplement Left Shoulder Joint with Autologous Tissue Substitute, Open Approach

ØRUKØJZ   Supplement Left Shoulder Joint with Synthetic Substitute, Open Approach

ØRUKØKZ   Supplement Left Shoulder Joint with Nonautologous Tissue Substitute, Open Approach

ØRUK37Z   Supplement Left Shoulder Joint with Autologous Tissue Substitute, Percutaneous Approach

ØRUK3JZ   Supplement Left Shoulder Joint with Synthetic Substitute, Percutaneous Approach

ØRUK3KZ   Supplement Left Shoulder Joint with Nonautologous Tissue Substitute, Percutaneous Approach

ØRUK47Z   Supplement Left Shoulder Joint with Autologous Tissue Substitute, Percutaneous Endoscopic Approach

ØRUK4JZ   Supplement Left Shoulder Joint with Synthetic Substitute, Percutaneous Endoscopic Approach

ØRUK4KZ   Supplement Left Shoulder Joint with Nonautologous Tissue Substitute, Percutaneous Endoscopic Approach

ØRULØ7Z   Supplement Right Elbow Joint with Autologous Tissue Substitute, Open Approach

ØRULØJZ   Supplement Right Elbow Joint with Synthetic Substitute, Open Approach

ØRULØKZ   Supplement Right Elbow Joint with Nonautologous Tissue Substitute, Open Approach

ØRUL37Z   Supplement Right Elbow Joint with Autologous Tissue Substitute, Percutaneous Approach

ØRUL3JZ   Supplement Right Elbow Joint with Synthetic Substitute, Percutaneous Approach

ØRUL3KZ   Supplement Right Elbow Joint with Nonautologous Tissue Substitute, Percutaneous Approach

ØRUL47Z   Supplement Right Elbow Joint with Autologous Tissue Substitute, Percutaneous Endoscopic Approach

ØRUL4JZ   Supplement Right Elbow Joint with Synthetic Substitute, Percutaneous Endoscopic Approach

ØRUL4KZ   Supplement Right Elbow Joint with Nonautologous Tissue Substitute, Percutaneous Endoscopic Approach

ØRUMØ7Z   Supplement Left Elbow Joint with Autologous Tissue Substitute, Open Approach

ØRUMØJZ   Supplement Left Elbow Joint with Synthetic Substitute, Open Approach

ØRUMØKZ   Supplement Left Elbow Joint with Nonautologous Tissue Substitute, Open Approach

ØRUM37Z   Supplement Left Elbow Joint with Autologous Tissue Substitute, Percutaneous Approach

ØRUM3JZ   Supplement Left Elbow Joint with Synthetic Substitute, Percutaneous Approach

ØRUM3KZ   Supplement Left Elbow Joint with Nonautologous Tissue Substitute, Percutaneous Approach

ØRUM47Z   Supplement Left Elbow Joint with Autologous Tissue Substitute, Percutaneous Endoscopic Approach

ØRUM4JZ   Supplement Left Elbow Joint with Synthetic Substitute, Percutaneous Endoscopic Approach

ØRUM4KZ   Supplement Left Elbow Joint with Nonautologous Tissue Substitute, Percutaneous Endoscopic Approach

ØSGØØ7Ø   Fusion of Lumbar Vertebral Joint with Autologous Tissue Substitute, Anterior Approach, Anterior Column, Open Approach

ØSGØØ71   Fusion of Lumbar Vertebral Joint with Autologous Tissue Substitute, Posterior Approach, Posterior Column, Open Approach

ØSGØØ7J   Fusion of Lumbar Vertebral Joint with Autologous Tissue Substitute, Posterior Approach, Anterior Column, Open Approach

ØSGØØAØ   Fusion of Lumbar Vertebral Joint with Interbody Fusion Device, Anterior Approach, Anterior Column, Open Approach

ØSGØØAJ   Fusion of Lumbar Vertebral Joint with Interbody Fusion Device, Posterior Approach, Anterior Column, Open Approach

ØSGØØJØ   Fusion of Lumbar Vertebral Joint with Synthetic Substitute, Anterior Approach, Anterior Column, Open Approach

ØSGØØJ1   Fusion of Lumbar Vertebral Joint with Synthetic Substitute, Posterior Approach, Posterior Column, Open Approach

ØSGØØJJ   Fusion of Lumbar Vertebral Joint with Synthetic Substitute, Posterior Approach, Anterior Column, Open Approach

ØSGØØKØ   Fusion of Lumbar Vertebral Joint with Nonautologous Tissue Substitute, Anterior Approach, Anterior Column, Open Approach

ØSGØØK1   Fusion of Lumbar Vertebral Joint with Nonautologous Tissue Substitute, Posterior Approach, Posterior Column, Open Approach

ØSGØØKJ   Fusion of Lumbar Vertebral Joint with Nonautologous Tissue Substitute, Posterior Approach, Anterior Column, Open Approach

ØSGØ37Ø   Fusion of Lumbar Vertebral Joint with Autologous Tissue Substitute, Anterior Approach, Anterior Column, Percutaneous Approach

ØSGØ371   Fusion of Lumbar Vertebral Joint with Autologous Tissue Substitute, Posterior Approach, Posterior Column, Percutaneous Approach

ØSGØ37J   Fusion of Lumbar Vertebral Joint with Autologous Tissue Substitute, Posterior Approach, Anterior Column, Percutaneous Approach

ØSGØ3AØ   Fusion of Lumbar Vertebral Joint with Interbody Fusion Device, Anterior Approach, Anterior Column, Percutaneous Approach

ØSGØ3AJ   Fusion of Lumbar Vertebral Joint with Interbody Fusion Device, Posterior Approach, Anterior Column, Percutaneous Approach

ØSGØ3JØ   Fusion of Lumbar Vertebral Joint with Synthetic Substitute, Anterior Approach, Anterior Column, Percutaneous Approach

HAC 12: Surgical Site Infection-Certain Orthopedic Procedures of the Spine, Shoulder, and Elbow (continued)

ØSG03J1 Fusion of Lumbar Vertebral Joint with Synthetic Substitute, Posterior Approach, Posterior Column, Percutaneous Approach

ØSG03JJ Fusion of Lumbar Vertebral Joint with Synthetic Substitute, Posterior Approach, Anterior Column, Percutaneous Approach

ØSG03KØ Fusion of Lumbar Vertebral Joint with Nonautologous Tissue Substitute, Anterior Approach, Anterior Column, Percutaneous Approach

ØSG03K1 Fusion of Lumbar Vertebral Joint with Nonautologous Tissue Substitute, Posterior Approach, Posterior Column, Percutaneous Approach

ØSG03KJ Fusion of Lumbar Vertebral Joint with Nonautologous Tissue Substitute, Posterior Approach, Anterior Column, Percutaneous Approach

ØSG0470 Fusion of Lumbar Vertebral Joint with Autologous Tissue Substitute, Anterior Approach, Anterior Column, Percutaneous Endoscopic Approach

ØSG0471 Fusion of Lumbar Vertebral Joint with Autologous Tissue Substitute, Posterior Approach, Posterior Column, Percutaneous Endoscopic Approach

ØSG047J Fusion of Lumbar Vertebral Joint with Autologous Tissue Substitute, Posterior Approach, Anterior Column, Percutaneous Endoscopic Approach

ØSG04AØ Fusion of Lumbar Vertebral Joint with Interbody Fusion Device, Anterior Approach, Anterior Column, Percutaneous Endoscopic Approach

ØSG04AJ Fusion of Lumbar Vertebral Joint with Interbody Fusion Device, Posterior Approach, Anterior Column, Percutaneous Endoscopic Approach

ØSG04JØ Fusion of Lumbar Vertebral Joint with Synthetic Substitute, Anterior Approach, Anterior Column, Percutaneous Endoscopic Approach

ØSG04J1 Fusion of Lumbar Vertebral Joint with Synthetic Substitute, Posterior Approach, Posterior Column, Percutaneous Endoscopic Approach

ØSG04JJ Fusion of Lumbar Vertebral Joint with Synthetic Substitute, Posterior Approach, Anterior Column, Percutaneous Endoscopic Approach

ØSG04KØ Fusion of Lumbar Vertebral Joint with Nonautologous Tissue Substitute, Anterior Approach, Anterior Column, Percutaneous Endoscopic Approach

ØSG04K1 Fusion of Lumbar Vertebral Joint with Nonautologous Tissue Substitute, Posterior Approach, Posterior Column, Percutaneous Endoscopic Approach

ØSG04KJ Fusion of Lumbar Vertebral Joint with Nonautologous Tissue Substitute, Posterior Approach, Anterior Column, Percutaneous Endoscopic Approach

ØSG1070 Fusion of 2 or More Lumbar Vertebral Joints with Autologous Tissue Substitute, Anterior Approach, Anterior Column, Open Approach

ØSG1071 Fusion of 2 or More Lumbar Vertebral Joints with Autologous Tissue Substitute, Posterior Approach, Posterior Column, Open Approach

ØSG107J Fusion of 2 or More Lumbar Vertebral Joints with Autologous Tissue Substitute, Posterior Approach, Anterior Column, Open Approach

ØSG10AØ Fusion of 2 or More Lumbar Vertebral Joints with Interbody Fusion Device, Anterior Approach, Anterior Column, Open Approach

ØSG10AJ Fusion of 2 or More Lumbar Vertebral Joints with Interbody Fusion Device, Posterior Approach, Anterior Column, Open Approach

ØSG10JØ Fusion of 2 or More Lumbar Vertebral Joints with Synthetic Substitute, Anterior Approach, Anterior Column, Open Approach

ØSG10J1 Fusion of 2 or More Lumbar Vertebral Joints with Synthetic Substitute, Posterior Approach, Posterior Column, Open Approach

ØSG10JJ Fusion of 2 or More Lumbar Vertebral Joints with Synthetic Substitute, Posterior Approach, Anterior Column, Open Approach

ØSG10KØ Fusion of 2 or More Lumbar Vertebral Joints with Nonautologous Tissue Substitute, Anterior Approach, Anterior Column, Open Approach

ØSG10K1 Fusion of 2 or More Lumbar Vertebral Joints with Nonautologous Tissue Substitute, Posterior Approach, Posterior Column, Open Approach

ØSG10KJ Fusion of 2 or More Lumbar Vertebral Joints with Nonautologous Tissue Substitute, Posterior Approach, Anterior Column, Open Approach

ØSG1370 Fusion of 2 or More Lumbar Vertebral Joints with Autologous Tissue Substitute, Anterior Approach, Anterior Column, Percutaneous Approach

ØSG1371 Fusion of 2 or More Lumbar Vertebral Joints with Autologous Tissue Substitute, Posterior Approach, Posterior Column, Percutaneous Approach

ØSG137J Fusion of 2 or More Lumbar Vertebral Joints with Autologous Tissue Substitute, Posterior Approach, Anterior Column, Percutaneous Approach

ØSG13AØ Fusion of 2 or More Lumbar Vertebral Joints with Interbody Fusion Device, Anterior Approach, Anterior Column, Percutaneous Approach

ØSG13AJ Fusion of 2 or More Lumbar Vertebral Joints with Interbody Fusion Device, Posterior Approach, Anterior Column, Percutaneous Approach

ØSG13JØ Fusion of 2 or More Lumbar Vertebral Joints with Synthetic Substitute, Anterior Approach, Anterior Column, Percutaneous Approach

ØSG13J1 Fusion of 2 or More Lumbar Vertebral Joints with Synthetic Substitute, Posterior Approach, Posterior Column, Percutaneous Approach

ØSG13JJ Fusion of 2 or More Lumbar Vertebral Joints with Synthetic Substitute, Posterior Approach, Anterior Column, Percutaneous Approach

ØSG13KØ Fusion of 2 or More Lumbar Vertebral Joints with Nonautologous Tissue Substitute, Anterior Approach, Anterior Column, Percutaneous Approach

ØSG13K1 Fusion of 2 or More Lumbar Vertebral Joints with Nonautologous Tissue Substitute, Posterior Approach, Posterior Column, Percutaneous Approach

ØSG13KJ Fusion of 2 or More Lumbar Vertebral Joints with Nonautologous Tissue Substitute, Posterior Approach, Anterior Column, Percutaneous Approach

ØSG1470 Fusion of 2 or More Lumbar Vertebral Joints with Autologous Tissue Substitute, Anterior Approach, Anterior Column, Percutaneous Endoscopic Approach

ØSG1471 Fusion of 2 or More Lumbar Vertebral Joints with Autologous Tissue Substitute, Posterior Approach, Posterior Column, Percutaneous Endoscopic Approach

ØSG147J Fusion of 2 or More Lumbar Vertebral Joints with Autologous Tissue Substitute, Posterior Approach, Anterior Column, Percutaneous Endoscopic Approach

ØSG14AØ Fusion of 2 or More Lumbar Vertebral Joints with Interbody Fusion Device, Anterior Approach, Anterior Column, Percutaneous Endoscopic Approach

ØSG14AJ Fusion of 2 or More Lumbar Vertebral Joints with Interbody Fusion Device, Posterior Approach, Anterior Column, Percutaneous Endoscopic Approach

ØSG14JØ Fusion of 2 or More Lumbar Vertebral Joints with Synthetic Substitute, Anterior Approach, Anterior Column, Percutaneous Endoscopic Approach

ØSG14J1 Fusion of 2 or More Lumbar Vertebral Joints with Synthetic Substitute, Posterior Approach, Posterior Column, Percutaneous Endoscopic Approach

ØSG14JJ Fusion of 2 or More Lumbar Vertebral Joints with Synthetic Substitute, Posterior Approach, Anterior Column, Percutaneous Endoscopic Approach

ØSG14KØ Fusion of 2 or More Lumbar Vertebral Joints with Nonautologous Tissue Substitute, Anterior Approach, Anterior Column, Percutaneous Endoscopic Approach

ØSG14K1 Fusion of 2 or More Lumbar Vertebral Joints with Nonautologous Tissue Substitute, Posterior Approach, Posterior Column, Percutaneous Endoscopic Approach

ØSG14KJ Fusion of 2 or More Lumbar Vertebral Joints with Nonautologous Tissue Substitute, Posterior Approach, Anterior Column, Percutaneous Endoscopic Approach

ØSG3070 Fusion of Lumbosacral Joint with Autologous Tissue Substitute, Anterior Approach, Anterior Column, Open Approach

ØSG3071 Fusion of Lumbosacral Joint with Autologous Tissue Substitute, Posterior Approach, Posterior Column, Open Approach

ØSG307J Fusion of Lumbosacral Joint with Autologous Tissue Substitute, Posterior Approach, Anterior Column, Open Approach

ØSG30AØ Fusion of Lumbosacral Joint with Interbody Fusion Device, Anterior Approach, Anterior Column, Open Approach

HAC 12: Surgical Site Infection-Certain Orthopedic Procedures of the Spine, Shoulder, and Elbow (continued)

0SG30AJ Fusion of Lumbosacral Joint with Interbody Fusion Device, Posterior Approach, Anterior Column, Open Approach

0SG30J0 Fusion of Lumbosacral Joint with Synthetic Substitute, Anterior Approach, Anterior Column, Open Approach

0SG30J1 Fusion of Lumbosacral Joint with Synthetic Substitute, Posterior Approach, Posterior Column, Open Approach

0SG30JJ Fusion of Lumbosacral Joint with Synthetic Substitute, Posterior Approach, Anterior Column, Open Approach

0SG30K0 Fusion of Lumbosacral Joint with Nonautologous Tissue Substitute, Anterior Approach, Anterior Column, Open Approach

0SG30K1 Fusion of Lumbosacral Joint with Nonautologous Tissue Substitute, Posterior Approach, Posterior Column, Open Approach

0SG30KJ Fusion of Lumbosacral Joint with Nonautologous Tissue Substitute, Posterior Approach, Anterior Column, Open Approach

0SG3370 Fusion of Lumbosacral Joint with Autologous Tissue Substitute, Anterior Approach, Anterior Column, Percutaneous Approach

0SG3371 Fusion of Lumbosacral Joint with Autologous Tissue Substitute, Posterior Approach, Posterior Column, Percutaneous Approach

0SG337J Fusion of Lumbosacral Joint with Autologous Tissue Substitute, Posterior Approach, Anterior Column, Percutaneous Approach

0SG33A0 Fusion of Lumbosacral Joint with Interbody Fusion Device, Anterior Approach, Anterior Column, Percutaneous Approach

0SG33AJ Fusion of Lumbosacral Joint with Interbody Fusion Device, Posterior Approach, Anterior Column, Percutaneous Approach

0SG33J0 Fusion of Lumbosacral Joint with Synthetic Substitute, Anterior Approach, Anterior Column, Percutaneous Approach

0SG33J1 Fusion of Lumbosacral Joint with Synthetic Substitute, Posterior Approach, Posterior Column, Percutaneous Approach

0SG33JJ Fusion of Lumbosacral Joint with Synthetic Substitute, Posterior Approach, Anterior Column, Percutaneous Approach

0SG33K0 Fusion of Lumbosacral Joint with Nonautologous Tissue Substitute, Anterior Approach, Anterior Column, Percutaneous Approach

0SG33K1 Fusion of Lumbosacral Joint with Nonautologous Tissue Substitute, Posterior Approach, Posterior Column, Percutaneous Approach

0SG33KJ Fusion of Lumbosacral Joint with Nonautologous Tissue Substitute, Posterior Approach, Anterior Column, Percutaneous Approach

0SG3470 Fusion of Lumbosacral Joint with Autologous Tissue Substitute, Anterior Approach, Anterior Column, Percutaneous Endoscopic Approach

0SG3471 Fusion of Lumbosacral Joint with Autologous Tissue Substitute, Posterior Approach, Posterior Column, Percutaneous Endoscopic Approach

0SG347J Fusion of Lumbosacral Joint with Autologous Tissue Substitute, Posterior Approach, Anterior Column, Percutaneous Endoscopic Approach

0SG34A0 Fusion of Lumbosacral Joint with Interbody Fusion Device, Anterior Approach, Anterior Column, Percutaneous Endoscopic Approach

0SG34AJ Fusion of Lumbosacral Joint with Interbody Fusion Device, Posterior Approach, Anterior Column, Percutaneous Endoscopic Approach

0SG34J0 Fusion of Lumbosacral Joint with Synthetic Substitute, Anterior Approach, Anterior Column, Percutaneous Endoscopic Approach

0SG34J1 Fusion of Lumbosacral Joint with Synthetic Substitute, Posterior Approach, Posterior Column, Percutaneous Endoscopic Approach

0SG34JJ Fusion of Lumbosacral Joint with Synthetic Substitute, Posterior Approach, Anterior Column, Percutaneous Endoscopic Approach

0SG34K0 Fusion of Lumbosacral Joint with Nonautologous Tissue Substitute, Anterior Approach, Anterior Column, Percutaneous Endoscopic Approach

0SG34K1 Fusion of Lumbosacral Joint with Nonautologous Tissue Substitute, Posterior Approach, Posterior Column, Percutaneous Endoscopic Approach

0SG34KJ Fusion of Lumbosacral Joint with Nonautologous Tissue Substitute, Posterior Approach, Anterior Column, Percutaneous Endoscopic Approach

0SG704Z Fusion of Right Sacroiliac Joint with Internal Fixation Device, Open Approach

0SG707Z Fusion of Right Sacroiliac Joint with Autologous Tissue Substitute, Open Approach

0SG70JZ Fusion of Right Sacroiliac Joint with Synthetic Substitute, Open Approach

0SG70KZ Fusion of Right Sacroiliac Joint with Nonautologous Tissue Substitute, Open Approach

0SG734Z Fusion of Right Sacroiliac Joint with Internal Fixation Device, Percutaneous Approach

0SG737Z Fusion of Right Sacroiliac Joint with Autologous Tissue Substitute, Percutaneous Approach

0SG73JZ Fusion of Right Sacroiliac Joint with Synthetic Substitute, Percutaneous Approach

0SG73KZ Fusion of Right Sacroiliac Joint with Nonautologous Tissue Substitute, Percutaneous Approach

0SG744Z Fusion of Right Sacroiliac Joint with Internal Fixation Device, Percutaneous Endoscopic Approach

0SG747Z Fusion of Right Sacroiliac Joint with Autologous Tissue Substitute, Percutaneous Endoscopic Approach

0SG74JZ Fusion of Right Sacroiliac Joint with Synthetic Substitute, Percutaneous Endoscopic Approach

0SG74KZ Fusion of Right Sacroiliac Joint with Nonautologous Tissue Substitute, Percutaneous Endoscopic Approach

0SG804Z Fusion of Left Sacroiliac Joint with Internal Fixation Device, Open Approach

0SG807Z Fusion of Left Sacroiliac Joint with Autologous Tissue Substitute, Open Approach

0SG80JZ Fusion of Left Sacroiliac Joint with Synthetic Substitute, Open Approach

0SG80KZ Fusion of Left Sacroiliac Joint with Nonautologous Tissue Substitute, Open Approach

0SG834Z Fusion of Left Sacroiliac Joint with Internal Fixation Device, Percutaneous Approach

0SG837Z Fusion of Left Sacroiliac Joint with Autologous Tissue Substitute, Percutaneous Approach

0SG83JZ Fusion of Left Sacroiliac Joint with Synthetic Substitute, Percutaneous Approach

0SG83KZ Fusion of Left Sacroiliac Joint with Nonautologous Tissue Substitute, Percutaneous Approach

0SG844Z Fusion of Left Sacroiliac Joint with Internal Fixation Device, Percutaneous Endoscopic Approach

0SG847Z Fusion of Left Sacroiliac Joint with Autologous Tissue Substitute, Percutaneous Endoscopic Approach

0SG84JZ Fusion of Left Sacroiliac Joint with Synthetic Substitute, Percutaneous Endoscopic Approach

0SG84KZ Fusion of Left Sacroiliac Joint with Nonautologous Tissue Substitute, Percutaneous Endoscopic Approach

XRG0092 Fusion of Occipital-cervical Joint using Nanotextured Surface Interbody Fusion Device, Open Approach, New Technology Group 2

XRG00F3 Fusion of Occipital-cervical Joint using Radiolucent Porous Interbody Fusion Device, Open Approach, New Technology Group 3

XRG1092 Fusion of Cervical Vertebral Joint using Nanotextured Surface Interbody Fusion Device, Open Approach, New Technology Group 2

XRG10F3 Fusion of Cervical Vertebral Joint using Radiolucent Porous Interbody Fusion Device, Open Approach, New Technology Group 3

XRG2092 Fusion of 2 or more Cervical Vertebral Joints using Nanotextured Surface Interbody Fusion Device, Open Approach, New Technology Group 2

XRG20F3 Fusion of 2 or more Cervical Vertebral Joints using Radiolucent Porous Interbody Fusion Device, Open Approach, New Technology Group 3

XRG4092 Fusion of Cervicothoracic Vertebral Joint using Nanotextured Surface Interbody Fusion Device, Open Approach, New Technology Group 2

XRG40F3 Fusion of Cervicothoracic Vertebral Joint using Radiolucent Porous Interbody Fusion Device, Open Approach, New Technology Group 3

XRG6092 Fusion of Thoracic Vertebral Joint using Nanotextured Surface Interbody Fusion Device, Open Approach, New Technology Group 2

HAC 12: Surgical Site Infection-Certain Orthopedic Procedures of the Spine, Shoulder, and Elbow (continued)

XRG60F3 Fusion of Thoracic Vertebral Joint using Radiolucent Porous Interbody Fusion Device, Open Approach, New Technology Group 3

XRG7092 Fusion of 2 to 7 Thoracic Vertebral Joints using Nanotextured Surface Interbody Fusion Device, Open Approach, New Technology Group 2

XRG70F3 Fusion of 2 to 7 Thoracic Vertebral Joints using Radiolucent Porous Interbody Fusion Device, Open Approach, New Technology Group 3

XRG8092 Fusion of 8 or more Thoracic Vertebral Joints using Nanotextured Surface Interbody Fusion Device, Open Approach, New Technology Group 2

XRG80F3 Fusion of 8 or more Thoracic Vertebral Joints using Radiolucent Porous Interbody Fusion Device, Open Approach, New Technology Group 3

XRGA092 Fusion of Thoracolumbar Vertebral Joint using Nanotextured Surface Interbody Fusion Device, Open Approach, New Technology Group 2

XRGA0F3 Fusion of Thoracolumbar Vertebral Joint using Radiolucent Porous Interbody Fusion Device, Open Approach, New Technology Group 3

XRGB092 Fusion of Lumbar Vertebral Joint using Nanotextured Surface Interbody Fusion Device, Open Approach, New Technology Group 2

XRGB0F3 Fusion of Lumbar Vertebral Joint using Radiolucent Porous Interbody Fusion Device, Open Approach, New Technology Group 3

XRGC092 Fusion of 2 or more Lumbar Vertebral Joints using Nanotextured Surface Interbody Fusion Device, Open Approach, New Technology Group 2

XRGC0F3 Fusion of 2 or more Lumbar Vertebral Joints using Radiolucent Porous Interbody Fusion Device, Open Approach, New Technology Group 3

XRGD092 Fusion of Lumbosacral Joint using Nanotextured Surface Interbody Fusion Device, Open Approach, New Technology Group 2

XRGD0F3 Fusion of Lumbosacral Joint using Radiolucent Porous Interbody Fusion Device, Open Approach, New Technology Group 3

HAC 13: Surgical Site Infection (SSI) Following Cardiac Implantable Electronic Device (CIED) Procedures

Secondary diagnosis not POA:

K68.11 Postprocedural retroperitoneal abscess

T81.40XA Infection following a procedure, unspecified, initial encounter

T81.41XA Infection following a procedure, superficial incisional surgical site, initial encounter

T81.42XA Infection following a procedure, deep incisional surgical site, initial encounter

T81.43XA Infection following a procedure, organ and space surgical site, initial encounter

T81.44XA Sepsis following a procedure, initial encounter

T81.49XA Infection following a procedure, other surgical site, initial encounter

T82.6XXA Infection and inflammatory reaction due to cardiac valve prosthesis, initial encounter

T82.7XXA Infection and inflammatory reaction due to other internal orthopedic prosthetic devices, implants and grafts, initial encounter

AND

Any of the following procedures:

02H43JZ Insertion of Pacemaker Lead into Coronary Vein, Percutaneous Approach

02H43KZ Insertion of Defibrillator Lead into Coronary Vein, Percutaneous Approach

02H43MZ Insertion of Cardiac Lead into Coronary Vein, Percutaneous Approach

02H63JZ Insertion of Pacemaker Lead into Right Atrium, Percutaneous Approach

02H63MZ Insertion of Cardiac Lead into Right Atrium, Percutaneous Approach

02H73JZ Insertion of Pacemaker Lead into Left Atrium, Percutaneous Approach

02H73MZ Insertion of Cardiac Lead into Left Atrium, Percutaneous Approach

02HK3JZ Insertion of Pacemaker Lead into Right Ventricle, Percutaneous Approach

02HL3JZ Insertion of Pacemaker Lead into Left Ventricle, Percutaneous Approach

02HN0JZ Insertion of Pacemaker Lead into Pericardium, Open Approach

02HN0MZ Insertion of Cardiac Lead into Pericardium, Open Approach

02HN3JZ Insertion of Pacemaker Lead into Pericardium, Percutaneous Approach

02HN3MZ Insertion of Cardiac Lead into Pericardium, Percutaneous Approach

02HN4JZ Insertion of Pacemaker Lead into Pericardium, Percutaneous Endoscopic Approach

02HN4MZ Insertion of Cardiac Lead into Pericardium, Percutaneous Endoscopic Approach

02PA0MZ Removal of Cardiac Lead from Heart, Open Approach

02PA3MZ Removal of Cardiac Lead from Heart, Percutaneous Approach

02PA4MZ Removal of Cardiac Lead from Heart, Percutaneous Endoscopic Approach

02PAXMZ Removal of Cardiac Lead from Heart, External Approach

02WA0MZ Revision of Cardiac Lead in Heart, Open Approach

02WA3MZ Revision of Cardiac Lead in Heart, Percutaneous Approach

02WA4MZ Revision of Cardiac Lead in Heart, Percutaneous Endoscopic Approach

0JH604Z Insertion of Pacemaker, Single Chamber into Chest Subcutaneous Tissue and Fascia, Open Approach

0JH605Z Insertion of Pacemaker, Single Chamber Rate Responsive into Chest Subcutaneous Tissue and Fascia, Open Approach

0JH606Z Insertion of Pacemaker, Dual Chamber into Chest Subcutaneous Tissue and Fascia, Open Approach

0JH607Z Insertion of Cardiac Resynchronization Pacemaker Pulse Generator into Chest Subcutaneous Tissue and Fascia, Open Approach

0JH608Z Insertion of Defibrillator Generator into Chest Subcutaneous Tissue and Fascia, Open Approach

0JH609Z Insertion of Cardiac Resynchronization Defibrillator Pulse Generator into Chest Subcutaneous Tissue and Fascia, Open Approach

0JH60PZ Insertion of Cardiac Rhythm Related Device into Chest Subcutaneous Tissue and Fascia, Open Approach

0JH634Z Insertion of Pacemaker, Single Chamber into Chest Subcutaneous Tissue and Fascia, Percutaneous Approach

0JH635Z Insertion of Pacemaker, Single Chamber Rate Responsive into Chest Subcutaneous Tissue and Fascia, Percutaneous Approach

0JH636Z Insertion of Pacemaker, Dual Chamber into Chest Subcutaneous Tissue and Fascia, Percutaneous Approach

0JH637Z Insertion of Cardiac Resynchronization Pacemaker Pulse Generator into Chest Subcutaneous Tissue and Fascia, Percutaneous Approach

0JH638Z Insertion of Defibrillator Generator into Chest Subcutaneous Tissue and Fascia, Percutaneous Approach

0JH639Z Insertion of Cardiac Resynchronization Defibrillator Pulse Generator into Chest Subcutaneous Tissue and Fascia, Percutaneous Approach

0JH63PZ Insertion of Cardiac Rhythm Related Device into Chest Subcutaneous Tissue and Fascia, Percutaneous Approach

0JH804Z Insertion of Pacemaker, Single Chamber into Abdomen Subcutaneous Tissue and Fascia, Open Approach

0JH805Z Insertion of Pacemaker, Single Chamber Rate Responsive into Abdomen Subcutaneous Tissue and Fascia, Open Approach

0JH806Z Insertion of Pacemaker, Dual Chamber into Abdomen Subcutaneous Tissue and Fascia, Open Approach

0JH807Z Insertion of Cardiac Resynchronization Pacemaker Pulse Generator into Abdomen Subcutaneous Tissue and Fascia, Open Approach

0JH808Z Insertion of Defibrillator Generator into Abdomen Subcutaneous Tissue and Fascia, Open Approach

0JH809Z Insertion of Cardiac Resynchronization Defibrillator Pulse Generator into Abdomen Subcutaneous Tissue and Fascia, Open Approach

0JH80PZ Insertion of Cardiac Rhythm Related Device into Abdomen Subcutaneous Tissue and Fascia, Open Approach

0JH834Z Insertion of Pacemaker, Single Chamber into Abdomen Subcutaneous Tissue and Fascia, Percutaneous Approach

0JH835Z Insertion of Pacemaker, Single Chamber Rate Responsive into Abdomen Subcutaneous Tissue and Fascia, Percutaneous Approach

0JH836Z Insertion of Pacemaker, Dual Chamber into Abdomen Subcutaneous Tissue and Fascia, Percutaneous Approach

0JH837Z Insertion of Cardiac Resynchronization Pacemaker Pulse Generator into Abdomen Subcutaneous Tissue and Fascia, Percutaneous Approach

0JH838Z Insertion of Defibrillator Generator into Abdomen Subcutaneous Tissue and Fascia, Percutaneous Approach

0JH839Z Insertion of Cardiac Resynchronization Defibrillator Pulse Generator into Abdomen Subcutaneous Tissue and Fascia, Percutaneous Approach

HAC 13: Surgical Site Infection (SSI) Following Cardiac Implantable Electronic Device (CIED) Procedures (continued)

ØJH83PZ	Insertion of Cardiac Rhythm Related Device into Abdomen Subcutaneous Tissue and Fascia, Percutaneous Approach
ØJPTØFZ	Removal of Subcutaneous Defibrillator Lead from Trunk Subcutaneous Tissue and Fascia, Open Approach
ØJPTØPZ	Removal of Cardiac Rhythm Related Device from Trunk Subcutaneous Tissue and Fascia, Open Approach
ØJPT3FZ	Removal of Subcutaneous Defibrillator Lead from Trunk Subcutaneous Tissue and Fascia, Percutaneous Approach
ØJPT3PZ	Removal of Cardiac Rhythm Related Device from Trunk Subcutaneous Tissue and Fascia, Percutaneous Approach
ØJWTØFZ	Revision of Subcutaneous Defibrillator Lead in Trunk Subcutaneous Tissue and Fascia, Open Approach
ØJWTØPZ	Revision of Cardiac Rhythm Related Device in Trunk Subcutaneous Tissue and Fascia, Open Approach
ØJWT3FZ	Revision of Subcutaneous Defibrillator Lead in Trunk Subcutaneous Tissue and Fascia, Percutaneous Approach
ØJWT3PZ	Revision of Cardiac Rhythm Related Device in Trunk Subcutaneous Tissue and Fascia, Percutaneous Approach

HAC 14: Iatrogenic Pneumothorax with Venous Catheterization

Secondary diagnosis not POA:

J95.811	Postprocedural pneumothorax

AND

Any of the following procedures:

02H633Z	Insertion of Infusion Device into Right Atrium, Percutaneous Approach
02HK33Z	Insertion of Infusion Device into Right Ventricle, Percutaneous Approach
02HS33Z	Insertion of Infusion Device into Right Pulmonary Vein, Percutaneous Approach
02HS43Z	Insertion of Infusion Device into Right Pulmonary Vein, Percutaneous Endoscopic Approach
02HT33Z	Insertion of Infusion Device into Left Pulmonary Vein, Percutaneous Approach
02HT43Z	Insertion of Infusion Device into Left Pulmonary Vein, Percutaneous Endoscopic Approach
02HV33Z	Insertion of Infusion Device into Superior Vena Cava, Percutaneous Approach
02HV43Z	Insertion of Infusion Device into Superior Vena Cava, Percutaneous Endoscopic Approach
05H033Z	Insertion of Infusion Device into Azygos Vein, Percutaneous Approach
05H043Z	Insertion of Infusion Device into Azygos Vein, Percutaneous Endoscopic Approach
05H133Z	Insertion of Infusion Device into Hemiazygos Vein, Percutaneous Approach
05H143Z	Insertion of Infusion Device into Hemiazygos Vein, Percutaneous Endoscopic Approach
05H333Z	Insertion of Infusion Device into Right Innominate Vein, Percutaneous Approach
05H343Z	Insertion of Infusion Device into Right Innominate Vein, Percutaneous Endoscopic Approach
05H433Z	Insertion of Infusion Device into Left Innominate Vein, Percutaneous Approach
05H443Z	Insertion of Infusion Device into Left Innominate Vein, Percutaneous Endoscopic Approach
05H533Z	Insertion of Infusion Device into Right Subclavian Vein, Percutaneous Approach
05H543Z	Insertion of Infusion Device into Right Subclavian Vein, Percutaneous Endoscopic Approach
05H633Z	Insertion of Infusion Device into Left Subclavian Vein, Percutaneous Approach
05H643Z	Insertion of Infusion Device into Left Subclavian Vein, Percutaneous Endoscopic Approach
05HM33Z	Insertion of Infusion Device into Right Internal Jugular Vein, Percutaneous Approach
05HN33Z	Insertion of Infusion Device into Left Internal Jugular Vein, Percutaneous Approach
05HP33Z	Insertion of Infusion Device into Right External Jugular Vein, Percutaneous Approach
05HQ33Z	Insertion of Infusion Device into Left External Jugular Vein, Percutaneous Approach
ØJH63XZ	Insertion of Vascular Access Device into Chest Subcutaneous Tissue and Fascia, Percutaneous Approach

Appendix L: Procedure Combination Tables

The tables below were developed to help simplify the relationship between ICD-10-PCS coding and MS-DRG assignment. The Centers for Medicare & Medicaid Services (CMS) has identified in the MS-DRG Definitions Manual certain procedure combinations that must occur in order to assign a specific MS-DRG. There are many factors influencing MS-DRG assignment, including principal and secondary diagnoses, MCC or CC use, sex of the patient, and discharge status. These tables should be used only as a guide. These tables were created based on the proposed, version 38, MS-DRG Grouper software and Definitions Manual files published with the fiscal 2021 IPPS proposed rule. To view the final, version 38, MS-DRG Grouper software and Definitions Manual files, refer to the following: https://www.cms.gov/Medicare/Medicare-Fee-for-Service-Payment/ AcuteInpatientPPS/MS-DRG-Classifications-and-Software.

DRG 001-002 Heart Transplant or Implant of Heart Assist System

Heart Transplant
Replacement of Right and Left Ventricle 02RK0JZ and 02RL0JZ

Insertion With Removal of Heart Assist System

Type of Heart Assist System	Code as appropriate Insertion by approach	Code also as appropriate Removal of Heart Assist System by approach
Biventricular External	02HA[0,3,4]RS	02PA[0,3,4]RZ
External	02HA[0,4]RZ	02PA[0,3,4]RZ

Revision With Removal of Heart Assist System

Type of Heart Assist System	Code as appropriate Revision by approach	Code also as appropriate Removal of Heart Assist System by approach
Implantable	02WA[0,3,4]QZ	02PA[0,3,4]RZ
External	02WA[0,3,4]RZ	02PA[0,3,4]RZ

DRG 008 Simultaneous Pancreas/Kidney Transplant

Transplanted Body Part	Code Transplant as appropriate by tissue type			Code also Pancreas Transplant as appropriate by tissue type		
	Allogeneic	Syngeneic	Zooplastic	Allogeneic	Syngeneic	Zooplastic
Kidney, Right	0TY00Z0	0TY00Z1	0TY00Z2	0FYG0Z0	0FYG0Z1	0FYG0Z2
Kidney, Left	0TY10Z0	0TY10Z1	0TY10Z2			

DRG 019 Simultaneous Pancreas/Kidney Transplant with Hemodialysis

Transplanted Body Part	Code Transplant as appropriate by tissue type			Code also Pancreas Transplant as appropriate by tissue type			Code also Hemodialysis		
	Allogeneic	Syngeneic	Zooplastic	Allogeneic	Syngeneic	Zooplastic	< 6 Hours	6-18 Hours	> 18 Hours
Kidney, Right	0TY00Z0	0TY00Z1	0TY00Z2	0FYG0Z0	0FYG0Z1	0FYG0Z2	5A1D07Z	5A1D80Z	5A1D90Z
Kidney, Left	0TY10Z0	0TY10Z1	0TY10Z2						

DRG 023-027 Craniotomy

Site of Neurostimulator Lead	Code as appropriate Insertion of Lead by approach	Code also as appropriate Insertion of Device by type and subcutaneous site						
		Neuro-stimulator Generator	Stimulator Multiple Array Code as appropriate by approach			Stimulator Multiple Array, Rechargeable Code as appropriate by approach		
		Skull	Chest	Back	Abdomen	Chest	Back	Abdomen
Brain	00H0[0,3,4]MZ	0NH00NZ	0JH6[0,3]DZ	0JH7[0,3]DZ	0JH8[0,3]DZ	0JH6[0,3]EZ	0JH7[0,3]EZ	0JH8[0,3]EZ
Cerebral Ventricle	00H6[0,3,4]MZ	0NH00NZ	0JH6[0,3]DZ	0JH7[0,3]DZ	0JH8[0,3]DZ	0JH6[0,3]EZ	0JH7[0,3]EZ	0JH8[0,3]EZ

DRG Ø28-Ø3Ø Spinal Procedures

Generator Type	Insertion of Generator by Site			Code also as appropriate Insertion of Neurostimulator Lead by approach	
	Chest	Abdomen	Back	Spinal Canal	Spinal Cord
Single Array	ØJH6[Ø,3]BZ	ØJH8[Ø,3]BZ	ØJH7[Ø,3]BZ	ØØHU[Ø,3,4]MZ	ØØHV[Ø,3,4]MZ
Single Array, Rechargeable	ØJH6[Ø,3]CZ	ØJH8[Ø,3]CZ	ØJH7[Ø,3]CZ	ØØHU[Ø,3,4]MZ	ØØHV[Ø,3,4]MZ
Multiple Array	ØJH6[Ø,3]DZ	ØJH8[Ø,3]DZ	ØJH7[Ø,3]DZ	ØØHU[Ø,3,4]MZ	ØØHV[Ø,3,4]MZ
Multiple Array, Rechargable	ØJH6[Ø,3]EZ	—	ØJH7[Ø,3]EZ	ØØHU[Ø,3,4]MZ	ØØHV[Ø,3,4]MZ
Multiple Array, Rechargable	—	ØJH8[Ø,3]EZ	—	ØØHU[Ø,3,4]MZ	ØØHV[Ø,3,4]MZ

DRG Ø4Ø-Ø42 Peripheral and Cranial Nerve and Other Nervous System Procedures

Insertion of Neurostimulator Lead With Device

Site of Neurostimulator Lead	Code as appropriate Insertion by approach	Code also as appropriate Insertion of Device by type and subcutaneous site					
		Stimulator Single Array Code as appropriate by approach			Stimulator Single Array, Rechargeable Code as appropriate by approach		
		Chest	Back	Abdomen	Chest	Back	Abdomen
Cranial Nerve	ØØHE[Ø,3,4]MZ	ØJH6[Ø,3]BZ	ØJH7[Ø,3]BZ	ØJH8[Ø,3]BZ	ØJH6[Ø,3]CZ	ØJH7[Ø,3]CZ	ØJH8[Ø,3]CZ
Peripheral Nerve	Ø1HY[Ø,3,4]MZ	ØJH6[Ø,3]BZ	ØJH7[Ø,3]BZ	ØJH8[Ø,3]BZ	ØJH6[Ø,3]CZ	ØJH7[Ø,3]CZ	ØJH8[Ø,3]CZ
Stomach	ØDH6[Ø,3,4]MZ	ØJH6[Ø,3]BZ	ØJH7[Ø,3]BZ	ØJH8[Ø,3]BZ	ØJH6[Ø,3]CZ	ØJH7[Ø,3]CZ	ØJH8[Ø,3]CZ
Azygos vein	Ø5HØ[Ø,3,4]MZ	ØJH6[Ø,3]BZ	ØJH7[Ø,S]BZ	ØJH8[Ø,3]BZ	ØJH6[Ø,3]CZ	ØJH7[Ø,S]CZ	ØJH8[Ø,3]CZ
Innominate Vein, Right	Ø5H3[Ø,3,4]MZ	ØJH6[Ø,3]BZ	ØJH7[Ø,S]BZ	ØJH8[Ø,3]BZ	ØJH6[Ø,3]CZ	ØJH7[Ø,S]CZ	ØJH8[Ø,3]CZ
Innominate Vein, Left	Ø5H4[Ø,3,4]MZ	ØJH6[Ø,3]BZ	ØJH7[Ø,S]BZ	ØJH8[Ø,3]BZ	ØJH6[Ø,3]CZ	ØJH7[Ø,S]CZ	ØJH8[Ø,3]CZ
		Stimulator Multiple Array Code as appropriate by approach			Stimulator Multiple Array, Rechargeable Code as appropriate by approach		
		Chest	Back	Abdomen	Chest	Back	Abdomen
Cranial Nerve	ØØHE[Ø,3,4]MZ	ØJH6[Ø,3]DZ	ØJH7[Ø,3]DZ	ØJH8[Ø,3]DZ	ØJH6[Ø,3]EZ	ØJH7[Ø,3]EZ	ØJH8[Ø,3]EZ
Peripheral Nerve	Ø1HY[Ø,3,4]MZ	ØJH6[Ø,3]DZ	ØJH7[Ø,3]DZ	ØJH8[Ø,3]DZ	ØJH6[Ø,3]EZ	ØJH7[Ø,3]EZ	ØJH8[Ø,3]EZ
Stomach	ØDH6[Ø,3,4]MZ	ØJH6[Ø,3]DZ	ØJH7[Ø,3]DZ	ØJH8[Ø,3]DZ	ØJH6[Ø,3]EZ	ØJH7[Ø,3]EZ	ØJH8[Ø,3]EZ
Azygos vein	Ø5HØ[Ø,3,4]MZ	ØJH6[Ø,3]DZ	ØJH7[Ø,S]DZ	ØJH8[Ø,3]DZ	ØJH6[Ø,3]EZ	ØJH7[Ø,S]EZ	ØJH8[Ø,3]EZ
Innominate Vein, Right	Ø5H3[Ø,3,4]MZ	ØJH6[Ø,3]DZ	ØJH7[Ø,S]DZ	ØJH8[Ø,3]DZ	ØJH6[Ø,3]EZ	ØJH7[Ø,S]EZ	ØJH8[Ø,3]EZ
Innominate Vein, Left	Ø5H4[Ø,3,4]MZ	ØJH6[Ø,3]DZ	ØJH7[Ø,S]DZ	ØJH8[Ø,3]DZ	ØJH6[Ø,3]EZ	ØJH7[Ø,S]EZ	ØJH8[Ø,3]EZ

DRG 222-227 Cardiac Defibrillator Implant

Insertion of Generator With Insertion of Lead(s) into Coronary Vein, Atrium or Ventricle

Generator Type	Insertion of Generator by Site		Code also as appropriate Insertion of Leads by site				
	Chest	Abdomen	Coronary Vein	Atrium		Ventricle	
				Right	Left	Right	Left
Defibrillator	ØJH6[Ø,3]8Z	ØJH8[Ø,3]8Z	Ø2H4[Ø,4]KZ	Ø2H6[Ø,3,4]KZ	Ø2H7[Ø,3,4]KZ	Ø2HK[Ø,3,4]KZ	Ø2HL[Ø,3,4]KZ
Cardiac Resynch Defibrillator Pulse Generator	ØJH6[Ø,3]9Z	ØJH8[Ø,3]9Z	Ø2H4[Ø,3,4]KZ or Ø2H43[J,M]Z	Ø2H6[Ø,3,4]KZ	Ø2H7[Ø,3,4]KZ	Ø2HK[Ø,3,4]KZ	Ø2HL[Ø,3,4]KZ
Contractility Modulation Device	ØJH6[Ø,3]AZ	ØJH8[Ø,3]AZ	—	Ø2H6[Ø,3,4]MZ	—	Ø2HK[Ø,3,4]MZ	—

Insertion of Generator with Insertion of Lead(s) into Pericardium or Chest

Generator Type	Insertion of Generator by Site		Code also as appropriate Insertion of Leads by Site and Type			
	Chest	Abdomen	Pericardium			Chest
			Pacemaker	Defibrillator	Cardiac	Subcutaneous
Defibrillator	ØJH6[Ø,3]8Z	ØJH8[Ø,3]8Z	02HN[Ø,3,4]JZ	02HN[Ø,3,4]KZ	02HN[Ø,3,4]MZ	ØJH6[Ø,3]FZ
Cardiac Resynch Defibrillator Pulse Generator	ØJH6[Ø,3]9Z	ØJH8[Ø,3]9Z	02HN[Ø,3,4]JZ	02HN[Ø,3,4]KZ	02HN[Ø,3,4]MZ	ØJH6[Ø,3]FZ

DRG 242-244 Permanent Cardiac Pacemaker Implant

Insertion of Generator and Lead(s) Only

Generator Type	Insertion of Generator by Site		Code also as appropriate Insertion of Leads by site					
	Chest	Abdomen	Coronary Vein	Atrium		Ventricle		Pericardium
				Right	Left	Right	Left	
Single Chamber	ØJH6[Ø,3]4Z	ØJH8[Ø,3]4Z	02H4[Ø,3,4][J,M]Z	02H6[Ø,3,4][J,M]Z	02H7[Ø,3,4][J,M]Z	02HK[Ø,3,4][J,M]Z	02HL[Ø,3,4][J,M]Z	02HN[Ø,3,4][J,M]Z
Single Chamber RR	ØJH6[Ø,3]5Z	ØJH8[Ø,3]5Z	02H4[Ø,3,4][J,M]Z	02H6[Ø,3,4][J,M]Z	02H7[Ø,3,4][J,M]Z	02HK[Ø,3,4][J,M]Z	02HL[Ø,3,4][J,M]Z	02HN[Ø,3,4][J,M]Z
Dual Chamber	ØJH6[Ø,3]6Z	ØJH8[Ø,3]6Z	02H4[Ø,3,4][J,M]Z	02H6[Ø,3,4][J,M]Z	02H7[Ø,3,4][J,M]Z	02HK[Ø,3,4][J,M]Z	02HL[Ø,3,4][J,M]Z	02HN[Ø,3,4][J,M]Z
Cardiac Resynch Pulse Generator	ØJH6[Ø,3]7Z	ØJH8[Ø,3]7Z	02H4[Ø,3,4][J,M]Z	02H6[Ø,3,4][J,M]Z	02H7[Ø,3,4][J,M]Z	02HK[Ø,3,4][J,M]Z	02HL[Ø,3,4][J,M]Z	02HN[Ø,3,4][J,M]Z
Cardiac Rhythm Related	ØJH6[Ø,3]PZ	ØJH8[Ø,3]PZ	02H4[Ø,3,4][J,M]Z	02H6[Ø,3,4][J,M]Z	02H7[Ø,3,4][J,M]Z	02HK[Ø,3,4][J,M]Z	02HL[Ø,3,4][J,M]Z	02HN[Ø,3,4][J,M]Z

DRG 326-328 Stomach, Esophageal and Duodenal Procedures

Site	Resection by Open Approach	Code also as appropriate Resection of Pancreas by Open Approach
Duodenum	ØDT9ØZZ	ØFTGØZZ

DRG 344-346 Minor Small and Large Bowel Procedures

Site	Repair by Open Approach	Code also as appropriate Repair by external approach of Abdominal Wall Stoma
Small Intestine	ØDQ8ØZZ	ØWQFXZ2
Duodenum	ØDQ9ØZZ	ØWQFXZ2
Jejunum	ØDQAØZZ	ØWQFXZ2
Ileum	ØDQBØZZ	ØWQFXZ2
Large Intestine	ØDQEØZZ	ØWQFXZ2
Large Intestine, Right	ØDQFØZZ	ØWQFXZ2
Large Intestine, Left	ØDQGØZZ	ØWQFXZ2
Cecum	ØDQHØZZ	ØWQFXZ2
Ascending Colon	ØDQKØZZ	ØWQFXZ2
Transverse Colon	ØDQLØZZ	ØWQFXZ2
Descending Colon	ØDQMØZZ	ØWQFXZ2
Sigmoid Colon	ØDQNØZZ	ØWQFXZ2

DRG 456-458 Spinal Fusion Except Cervical with Spinal Curvature/Malignancy/ Infection or Extensive Fusions

Fusion of Thoracic and Lumbar Vertebra, Anterior Column

2 to 7 Thoracic Vertebra		Code also 2 or more Lumbar Vertebra	
ØRG[Ø,3,4][7,A,J,K]Ø	XRG7ØF3	ØSG1[Ø,3,4][7,A,J,K]Ø	XRGCØF3

Fusion of Thoracic and Lumbar Vertebra, Posterior Column

2 to 7 Thoracic Vertebra			Code also 2 or more Lumbar Vertebra		
Posterior Approach	Anterior Approach	New Technology	Posterior Approach	Anterior Approach	New Technology
ØRG7[Ø,3,4][7,J,K]1	ØRG7[Ø,3,4][7,A,J,K]J	XRG7Ø92 XRG7ØF3	ØSG1[Ø,3,4][7,J,K]1	ØSG1[Ø,3,4][7,A,J,K]J	XRGCØ92 XRGCØF3

DRG 461-462 Bilateral or Multiple Major Joint Procedures of Lower Extremity

For procedures to qualify as bilateral or multiple joint procedures, at least one replacement code or combination removal and replacement code from two different lower extremity sites from the following table(s) must be reported.

Examples: Left hip and right hip codes (bilateral); left hip and left knee codes (multiple); left hip and right ankle codes (multiple); left knee and right knee codes (bilateral); right hip removal and replacement, with right knee replacement

Hip, RT	Hip, LT	Knee, RT	Knee, LT	Ankle, RT	Ankle, LT
ØSR9Ø19	ØSRBØ19	ØSRCØ69	ØSRDØ69	ØSRFØ7Z	ØSRGØ7Z
ØSR9Ø1A	ØSRBØ1A	ØSRCØ6A	ØSRDØ6A	ØSRFØJ9	ØSRGØJ9
ØSR9Ø1Z	ØSRBØ1Z	ØSRCØ6Z	ØSRDØ6Z	ØSRFØJA	ØSRGØJA
ØSR9Ø29	ØSRBØ29	ØSRCØ7Z	ØSRDØ7Z	ØSRFØJZ	ØSRGØJZ
ØSR9Ø2A	ØSRBØ2A	ØSRCØJ9	ØSRDØJ9	ØSRFØKZ	ØSRGØKZ
ØSR9Ø2Z	ØSRBØ2Z	ØSRCØJA	ØSRDØJA		
ØSR9Ø39	ØSRBØ39	ØSRCØJZ	ØSRDØJZ		
ØSR9Ø3A	ØSRBØ3A	ØSRCØKZ	ØSRDØKZ		
ØSR9Ø3Z	ØSRBØ3Z	ØSRCØL9	ØSRDØL9		
ØSR9Ø49	ØSRBØ49	ØSRCØLA	ØSRDØLA		
ØSR9Ø4A	ØSRBØ4A	ØSRCØLZ	ØSRDØLZ		
ØSR9Ø4Z	ØSRBØ4Z	ØSRCØM9	ØSRDØM9		
ØSR9Ø69	ØSRBØ69	ØSRCØMA	ØSRDØMA		
ØSR9Ø6A	ØSRBØ6A	ØSRCØMZ	ØSRDØMZ		
ØSR9Ø6Z	ØSRBØ6Z	ØSRCØN9	ØSRDØN9		
ØSR9Ø7Z	ØSRBØ7Z	ØSRCØNA	ØSRDØNA		
ØSR9ØJ9	ØSRBØJ9	ØSRCØNZ	ØSRDØNZ		
ØSR9ØJA	ØSRBØJA	ØSRTØ7Z	ØSRUØ7Z		
ØSR9ØJZ	ØSRBØJZ	ØSRTØJ9	ØSRUØJ9		
ØSR9ØKZ	ØSRBØKZ	ØSRTØJA	ØSRUØJA		
ØSRAØØ9	ØSREØØ9	ØSRTØJZ	ØSRUØJZ		
ØSRAØØA	ØSREØØA	ØSRTØKZ	ØSRUØKZ		
ØSRAØØZ	ØSREØØZ	ØSRVØ7Z	ØSRWØ7Z		
ØSRAØ19	ØSREØ19	ØSRVØJ9	ØSRWØJ9		
ØSRAØ1A	ØSREØ1A	ØSRVØJA	ØSRWØJA		
ØSRAØ1Z	ØSREØ1Z	ØSRVØJZ	ØSRWØJZ		
ØSRAØ39	ØSREØ39	ØSRVØKZ	ØSRWØKZ		
ØSRAØ3A	ØSREØ3A	ØSPCØJZ	ØSPDØJZ		
ØSRAØ3Z	ØSREØ3Z				
ØSRAØ7Z	ØSREØ7Z				
ØSRAØJ9	ØSREØJ9				
ØSRAØJA	ØSREØJA				
ØSRAØJZ	ØSREØJZ				
ØSRAØKZ	ØSREØKZ				
ØSRRØ19	ØSRSØ19				

Hip, RT	Hip, LT	Knee, RT	Knee, LT	Ankle, RT	Ankle, LT
ØSRRØ1A	ØSRSØ1A				
ØSRRØ1Z	ØSRSØ1Z				
ØSRRØ39	ØSRSØ39				
ØSRRØ3A	ØSRSØ3A				
ØSRRØ3Z	ØSRSØ3Z				
ØSRRØ7Z	ØSRSØ7Z				
ØSRRØJ9	ØSRSØJ9				
ØSRRØJA	ØSRSØJA				
ØSRRØJZ	ØSRSØJZ				
ØSRRØKZ	ØSRSØKZ				
ØSU9ØBZ	ØSUBØBZ				
ØSUAØBZ	ØSUEØBZ				
ØSURØBZ	ØSUSØBZ				
ØSP9ØJZ	ØSPBØJZ				

Hip Procedure Combinations

Open Removal of Hip Spacer with Replacement

Removal of Spacer		Code also as appropriate Replacement by Device Type					
		Metal	Metal on Poly	Ceramic	Ceramic on Poly	Oxidized Zirc on Poly	Synth Subst
Hip, RT	ØSP9Ø8Z	ØSR9Ø1[9,A,Z]	ØSR9Ø2[9,A,Z]	ØSR9Ø3[9,A,Z]	ØSR9Ø4[9,A,Z]	ØSR9Ø6[9,A,Z]	ØSR9ØJ[9,A,Z]
Hip, LT	ØSPBØ8Z	ØSRBØ1[9,A,Z]	ØSRBØ2[9,A,Z]	ØSRBØ3[9,A,Z]	ØSRBØ4[9,A,Z]	ØSRBØ6[9,A,Z]	ØSRBØJ[9,A,Z]

Open Removal of Hip Spacer with Replacement

Removal of Spacer		Code also as appropriate Replacement by Device Type						
		Acetabular Surface				Femoral Surface		
		Poly	Metal	Ceramic	Synthetic	Metal	Ceramic	Synth
Hip, RT	ØSP9Ø8Z	ØSRAØØ[9,A,Z]	ØSRAØ1[9,A,Z]	ØSRAØ3[9,A,Z]	ØSRAØJ[9,A,Z]	ØSRRØ1[9,A,Z]	ØSRRØ3[9,A,Z]	ØSRRØJ[9,A,Z]
Hip, LT	ØSPBØ8Z	ØSREØØ[9,A,Z]	ØSREØ1[9,A,Z]	ØSREØ3[9,A,Z]	ØSREØJ[9,A,Z]	ØSRSØ1[9,A,Z]	ØSRSØ3[9,A,Z]	ØSRSØJ[9,A,Z]

Open Removal of Hip Liner with Replacement

Removal of Liner		Code also as appropriate Replacement by Device Type					
		Metal	Metal on Poly	Ceramic	Ceramic on Poly	Oxidized Zirc on Poly	Synth Subst
Hip, RT	ØSP9Ø9Z	ØSR9Ø1[9,A,Z]	ØSR9Ø2[9,A,Z]	ØSR9Ø3[9,A,Z]	ØSR9Ø4[9,A,Z]	ØSR9Ø6[9,A,Z]	ØSR9ØJ[9,A,Z]
Hip, LT	ØSPBØ9Z	ØSRBØ1[9,A,Z]	ØSRBØ2[9,A,Z]	ØSRBØ3[9,A,Z]	ØSRBØ4[9,A,Z]	ØSRBØ6[9,A,Z]	ØSRBØJ[9,A,Z]

Open Removal of Hip Liner with Replacement

Removal of Liner		Code also as appropriate Replacement by Device Type						
		Acetabular Surface				Femoral Surface		
		Poly	Metal	Ceramic	Synthetic	Metal	Ceramic	Synth
Hip, RT	ØSP9Ø9Z	ØSRAØØ[9,A,Z]	ØSRAØ1[9,A,Z]	ØSRAØ3[9,A,Z]	ØSRAØJ[9,A,Z]	ØSRRØ1[9,A,Z]	ØSRRØ3[9,A,Z]	ØSRRØJ[9,A,Z]
Hip, LT	ØSPBØ9Z	ØSREØØ[9,A,Z]	ØSREØ1[9,A,Z]	ØSREØ3[9,A,Z]	ØSREØJ[9,A,Z]	ØSRSØ1[9,A,Z]	ØSRSØ3[9,A,Z]	ØSRSØJ[9,A,Z]

Open Removal of Hip Resurfacing Device with Replacement

Removal of Resurfacing Device		Code also as appropriate Replacement by Device Type					
		Metal	Metal on Poly	Ceramic	Ceramic on Poly	Oxidized Zirc on Poly	Synth Subst
Hip, RT	0SP90BZ	0SR901[9,A,Z]	0SR902[9,A,Z]	0SR903[9,A,Z]	0SR904[9,A,Z]	0SR906[9,A,Z]	0SR90J[9,A,Z]
Hip, LT	0SPB0BZ	0SRB01[9,A,Z]	0SRB02[9,A,Z]	0SRB03[9,A,Z]	0SRB04[9,A,Z]	0SRB06[9,A,Z]	0SRB0J[9,A,Z]

Open Removal of Hip Resurfacing Device with Replacement

Removal of Resurfacing Device		Code also as appropriate Replacement by Device Type						
		Acetabular Surface				Femoral Surface		
		Poly	Metal	Ceramic	Synthetic	Metal	Ceramic	Synth
Hip, RT	0SP90BZ	0SRA00[9,A,Z]	0SRA01[9,A,Z]	0SRA03[9,A,Z]	0SRA0J[9,A,Z]	0SRR01[9,A,Z]	0SRR03[9,A,Z]	0SRR0J[9,A,Z]
Hip, LT	0SPB0BZ	0SRE00[9,A,Z]	0SRE01[9,A,Z]	0SRE03[9,A,Z]	0SRE0J[9,A,Z]	0SRS01[9,A,Z]	0SRS03[9,A,Z]	0SRS0J[9,A,Z]

Open Removal of Hip Articulating Spacer with Replacement

Removal of Articulating Spacer		Code also as appropriate Replacement by Device Type					
		Metal	Metal on Poly	Ceramic	Ceramic on Poly	Oxidized Zirc on Poly	Synth Subst
Hip, RT	0SP90EZ	0SR901[9,A,Z]	0SR902[9,A,Z]	0SR903[9,A,Z]	0SR904[9,A,Z]	0SR906[9,A,Z]	0SR90J[9,A,Z]
Hip, LT	0SPB0EZ	0SRB01[9,A,Z]	0SRB02[9,A,Z]	0SRB03[9,A,Z]	0SRB04[9,A,Z]	0SRB06[9,A,Z]	0SRB0J[9,A,Z]

Open Removal of Hip Articulating Spacer with Replacement

Removal of Articulating Spacer		Code also as appropriate Replacement by Device Type						
		Acetabular Surface				Femoral Surface		
		Poly	Metal	Ceramic	Synthetic	Metal	Ceramic	Synth
Hip, RT	0SP90EZ	0SRA00[9,A,Z]	0SRA01[9,A,Z]	0SRA03[9,A,Z]	0SRA0J[9,A,Z]	0SRR01[9,A,Z]	0SRR03[9,A,Z]	0SRR0J[9,A,Z]
Hip, LT	0SPB0EZ	0SRE00[9,A,Z]	0SRE01[9,A,Z]	0SRE03[9,A,Z]	0SRE0J[9,A,Z]	0SRS01[9,A,Z]	0SRS03[9,A,Z]	0SRS0J[9,A,Z]

Open Removal of Hip Synthetic Substitute with Replacement

Removal of Synthetic Substitute		Code also as appropriate Replacement by Device Type					
		Metal	Metal on Poly	Ceramic	Ceramic on Poly	Oxidized Zirc on Poly	Synth Subst
Hip, RT	0SP[9,A,R]0JZ	0SR901[9,A,Z]	0SR902[9,A,Z]	0SR903[9,A,Z]	0SR904[9,A,Z]	0SR906[9,A,Z]	0SR90J[9,A,Z]
Hip, LT	0SP[B,E,S]0JZ	0SRB01[9,A,Z]	0SRB02[9,A,Z]	0SRB03[9,A,Z]	0SRB04[9,A,Z]	0SRB06[9,A,Z]	0SRB0J[9,A,Z]

Open Removal of Hip Synthetic Substitute with Replacement

Removal of Synthetic Substitute		Code also as appropriate Replacement by Device Type						
		Acetabular Surface				Femoral Surface		
		Poly	Metal	Ceramic	Synthetic	Metal	Ceramic	Synth
Hip, RT	0SP[9,A,R]0JZ	0SRA00[9,A,Z]	0SRA01[9,A,Z]	0SRA03[9,A,Z]	0SRA0J[9,A,Z]	0SRR01[9,A,Z]	0SRR03[9,A,Z]	0SRR0J[9,A,Z]
Hip, LT	0SP[B,E,S]0JZ	0SRE00[9,A,Z]	0SRE01[9,A,Z]	0SRE03[9,A,Z]	0SRE0J[9,A,Z]	0SRS01[9,A,Z]	0SRS03[9,A,Z]	0SRS0J[9,A,Z]

Percutaneous Endoscopic Removal of Hip Spacer with Open Replacement

Removal of Spacer		Code also as appropriate Replacement by Device Type					
		Metal	Metal on Poly	Ceramic	Ceramic on Poly	Oxidized Zirc on Poly	Synth Subst
Hip, RT	0SP948Z	0SR901[9,A,Z]	0SR902[9,A,Z]	0SR903[9,A,Z]	0SR904[9,A,Z]	0SR906[9,A,Z]	0SR90J[9,A,Z]
Hip, LT	0SPB48Z	0SRB01[9,A,Z]	0SRB02[9,A,Z]	0SRB03[9,A,Z]	0SRB04[9,A,Z]	0SRB06[9,A,Z]	0SRB0J[9,A,Z]

Percutaneous Endoscopic Removal of Hip Spacer with Open Replacement

Removal of Spacer		Code also as appropriate Replacement by Device Type						
		Acetabular Surface				Femoral Surface		
		Poly	Metal	Ceramic	Synthetic	Metal	Ceramic	Synth
Hip, RT	ØSP948Z	ØSRAØØ[9,A,Z]	ØSRAØ1[9,A,Z]	ØSRAØ3[9,A,Z]	ØSRAØJ[9,A,Z]	ØSRRØ1[9,A,Z]	ØSRRØ3[9,A,Z]	ØSRRØJ[9,A,Z]
Hip, LT	ØSPB48Z	ØSREØØ[9,A,Z]	ØSREØ1[9,A,Z]	ØSREØ3[9,A,Z]	ØSREØJ[9,A,Z]	ØSRSØ1[9,A,Z]	ØSRSØ3[9,A,Z]	ØSRSØJ[9,A,Z]

Percutaneous Endoscopic Removal of Hip Synthetic Substitute with Open Replacement

Removal of Synthetic Substitute		Code also as appropriate Replacement by Device Type					
		Metal	Metal on Poly	Ceramic	Ceramic on Poly	Oxidized Zirc on Poly	Synth Subst
Hip, RT	ØSP[9,A,R]4JZ	ØSR9Ø1[9,A,Z]	ØSR9Ø2[9,A,Z]	ØSR9Ø3[9,A,Z]	ØSR9Ø4[9,A,Z]	ØSR9Ø6[9,A,Z]	ØSR9ØJ[9,A,Z]
Hip, LT	ØSP[B,E,S]4JZ	ØSRBØ1[9,A,Z]	ØSRBØ2[9,A,Z]	ØSRBØ3[9,A,Z]	ØSRBØ4[9,A,Z]	ØSRBØ6[9,A,Z]	ØSRBØJ[9,A,Z]

Percutaneous Endoscopic Removal of Hip Synthetic Substitute with Open Replacement

Removal of Synthetic Substitute		Code also as appropriate Replacement by Device Type						
		Acetabular Surface				Femoral Surface		
		Poly	Metal	Ceramic	Synthetic	Metal	Ceramic	Synth
Hip, RT	ØSP[9,A,R]4JZ	ØSRAØØ[9,A,Z]	ØSRAØ1[9,A,Z]	ØSRAØ3[9,A,Z]	ØSRAØJ[9,A,Z]	ØSRRØ1[9,A,Z]	ØSRRØ3[9,A,Z]	ØSRRØJ[9,A,Z]
Hip, LT	ØSP[B,E,S]4JZ	ØSREØØ[9,A,Z]	ØSREØ1[9,A,Z]	ØSREØ3[9,A,Z]	ØSREØJ[9,A,Z]	ØSRSØ1[9,A,Z]	ØSRSØ3[9,A,Z]	ØSRSØJ[9,A,Z]

Knee Procedure Combinations

Open Removal of Knee Spacer with Synthetic Substitute Replacement

Removal of Spacer		Code also as appropriate Replacement by Type of Synthetic Substitute				
		Oxidized Zircon on Poly	Synth Subst	Patello-femoral	Femoral Surface	Tibial Surface
Knee, RT	ØSPC08Z	ØSRCØ6[9,A,Z]	ØSRCØJ[9,A,Z]	ØSRCØN[9,A,Z]	ØSRTØJ[9,A,Z]	ØSRVØJ[9,A,Z]
Knee, LT	ØSPD08Z	ØSRDØ6[9,A,Z]	ØSRDØJ[9,A,Z]	ØSRDØN[9,A,Z]	ØSRUØJ[9,A,Z]	ØSRWØJ[9,A,Z]

Open Removal of Knee Liner with Synthetic Substitute Replacement

Removal of Liner		Code also as appropriate Replacement by Type of Synthetic Substitute						
		Oxidized Zircon on Poly	Synth Subst	Medial Unicondylar	Lateral Unicondylar	Patello-femoral	Femoral Surface	Tibial Surface
Knee, RT	ØSPC09Z	ØSRCØ6[9,A,Z]	ØSRCØJ[9,A,Z]	ØSRCØL[9,A,Z]	ØSRCØM[9,A,Z]	ØSRCØN[9,A,Z]	ØSRTØJ[9,A,Z]	ØSRVØJ[9,A,Z]
Knee, LT	ØSPD09Z	ØSRDØ6[9,A,Z]	ØSRDØJ[9,A,Z]	ØSRDØL[9,A,Z]	ØSRDØM[9,A,Z]	ØSRDØN[9,A,Z]	ØSRUØJ[9,A,Z]	ØSRWØJ[9,A,Z]

Open Removal of Knee Articulating Spacer with Synthetic Substitute Replacement

Removal of Articulating Spacer		Code also as appropriate Replacement by Type of Synthetic Substitute			
		Oxidized Zircon on Poly	Synth Subst	Femoral Surface	Tibial Surface
Knee, RT	ØSPCØEZ	ØSRCØ6[9,A,Z]	ØSRCØJ[9,A,Z]	ØSRTØJ[9,A,Z]	ØSRVØJ[9,A,Z]
Knee, LT	ØSPDØEZ	ØSRDØ6[9,A,Z]	ØSRDØJ[9,A,Z]	ØSRUØJ[9,A,Z]	ØSRWØJ[9,A,Z]

Open Removal of Patellar Surface of Knee with Synthetic Substitute Replacement

Removal of Patellar Surface		Code also as appropriate Replacement by Type of Synthetic Substitute				
		Oxidized Zircon on Poly	Synth Subst	Patello-femoral	Femoral Surface	Tibial Surface
Knee, RT	ØSPCØJC	ØSRCØ6[9,A,Z]	ØSRCØJ[9,A,Z]	ØSRCØN[9,A,Z]	ØSRTØJ[9,A,Z]	ØSRVØJ[9,A,Z]
Knee, LT	ØSPDØJC	ØSRDØ6[9,A,Z]	ØSRDØJ[9,A,Z]	ØSRDØN[9,A,Z]	ØSRUØJ[9,A,Z]	ØSRWØJ[9,A,Z]

Open Removal of Knee Synthetic Substitute with Synthetic Substitute Replacement

Removal of Synthetic Substitute		Code also as appropriate Replacement by Type of Synthetic Substitute						
		Oxidized Zircon on Poly	Synth Subst	Medial Unicondylar	Lateral Unicondylar	Patello-femoral	Femoral Surface	Tibial Surface
Knee, RT	ØSPCØJZ	ØSRCØ6[9,A,Z]	ØSRCØJ[9,A,Z]	ØSRCØL[9,A,Z]	ØSRCØM[9,A,Z]	ØSRCØN[9,A,Z]	ØSRTØJ[9,A,Z]	ØSRVØJ[9,A,Z]
Knee, LT	ØSPDØJZ	ØSRDØ6[9,A,Z]	ØSRDØJ[9,A,Z]	ØSRDØL[9,A,Z]	ØSRDØM[9,A,Z]	ØSRDØN[9,A,Z]	ØSRUØJ[9,A,Z]	ØSRWØJ[9,A,Z]

Open Removal of Medial or Lateral Unicondylar Knee with Synthetic Substitute Replacement

Removal of Medial/Lateral Unicondylar Knee		Code also as appropriate Replacement by Type of Synthetic Substitute				
		Oxidized Zircon on Poly	Synth Subst	Medial Unicondylar	Femoral Surface	Tibial Surface
Knee, RT	ØSPCØ[L,M]Z	ØSRCØ6[9,A,Z]	ØSRCØJ[9,A,Z]	ØSRCØL[9,A,Z]	ØSRTØJ[9,A,Z]	ØSRVØJ[9,A,Z]
Knee, LT	ØSPDØ[L,M]Z	ØSRDØ6[9,A,Z]	ØSRDØJ[9,A,Z]	ØSRDØL[9,A,Z]	ØSRUØJ[9,A,Z]	ØSRWØJ[9,A,Z]

Open Removal of Patellofemoral Knee with Synthetic Substitute Replacement

Removal of Patellofemoral Knee		Code also as appropriate Replacement by Type of Synthetic Substitute				
		Oxidized Zircon on Poly	Synth Subst	Medial Unicondylar	Femoral Surface	Tibial Surface
Knee, RT	ØSPCØNZ	ØSRCØ6[9,A,Z]	ØSRCØJ[9,A,Z]	ØSRCØL[9,A,Z]	ØSRTØJ[9,A,Z]	ØSRVØJ[9,A,Z]
Knee, LT	ØSPDØNZ	ØSRDØ6[9,A,Z]	ØSRDØJ[9,A,Z]	ØSRDØL[9,A,Z]	ØSRUØJ[9,A,Z]	ØSRWØJ[9,A,Z]

Open Removal of Femoral/Tibial Surface of Knee with Synthetic Substitute Replacement

Removal of Femoral/Tibial Surface of Knee		Code also as appropriate Replacement by Type of Synthetic Substitute					
		Oxidized Zircon on Poly	Synth Subst	Articulating Spacer	Patello-femoral	Femoral Surface	Tibial Surface
Knee, RT	ØSP[T,V]ØJZ	ØSRCØ6[9,A,Z]	ØSRCØJ[9,A,Z]	ØSRCØEZ	ØSRCØN[9,A,Z]	ØSRTØJ[9,A,Z]	ØSRVØJ[9,A,Z]
Knee, LT	ØSP[U,W]ØJZ	ØSRDØ6[9,A,Z]	ØSRDØJ[9,A,Z]	ØSRDØEZ	ØSRDØN[9,A,Z]	ØSRUØJ[9,A,Z]	ØSRWØJ[9,A,Z]

Percutaneous/Percutaneous Endoscopic Removal of Knee Spacer with Open Synthetic Substitute Replacement

Removal of Spacer		Code also as appropriate Replacement by Type of Synthetic Substitute				
		Oxidized Zircon on Poly	Synth Subst	Patello-femoral	Femoral Surface	Tibial Surface
Knee, RT	ØSPC[3,4]8Z	ØSRCØ6[9,A,Z]	ØSRCØJ[9,A,Z]	ØSRCØN[9,A,Z]	ØSRTØJ[9,A,Z]	ØSRVØJ[9,A,Z]
Knee, LT	ØSPD[3,4]8Z	ØSRDØ6[9,A,Z]	ØSRDØJ[9,A,Z]	ØSRDØN[9,A,Z]	ØSRUØJ[9,A,Z]	ØSRWØJ[9,A,Z]

Percutaneous Endoscopic Removal of Patellar Surface of Knee with Synthetic Substitute Replacement

Removal of Patellar Surface		Code also as appropriate Replacement by Type of Synthetic Substitute				
		Oxidized Zircon on Poly	Synth Subst	Patello-femoral	Femoral Surface	Tibial Surface
Knee, RT	ØSPC4JC	ØSRCØ6[9,A,Z]	ØSRCØJ[9,A,Z]	ØSRCØN[9,A,Z]	ØSRTØJ[9,A,Z]	ØSRVØJ[9,A]
Knee, LT	ØSPD4JC	ØSRDØ6[9,A,Z]	ØSRDØJ[9,A,Z]	ØSRDØN[9,A,Z]	ØSRUØJ[9,A]	ØSRWØJ[9,A,Z]

Percutaneous Endoscopic Removal of Knee Synthetic Substitute with Synthetic Substitute Replacement

Removal of Synthetic Substitute		Code also as appropriate Replacement by Type of Synthetic Substitute						
		Oxidized Zircon on Poly	Synth Subst	Medial Unicondylar	Lateral Unicondylar	Patello-femoral	Femoral Surface	Tibial Surface
Knee, RT	ØSPC4JZ	ØSRCØ6[9,A,Z]	ØSRCØJ[9,A,Z]	ØSRCØL[9,A,Z]	ØSRCØM[9,A,Z]	ØSRCØN[9,A,Z]	ØSRTØJ[9,A,Z]	ØSRVØJ[9,A,Z]
Knee, LT	ØSPD4JZ	ØSRDØ6[9,A,Z]	ØSRDØJ[9,A,Z]	ØSRDØL[9,A,Z]	ØSRDØM[9,A,Z]	ØSRDØN[9,A,Z]	ØSRUØJ[9,A,Z]	ØSRWØJ[9,A,Z]

Percutaneous Endoscopic Removal of Medial or Lateral Unicondylar Knee with Synthetic Substitute Replacement

Removal of Medial/Lateral Unicondylar Knee		Code also as appropriate Replacement by Type of Synthetic Substitute				
		Oxidized Zircon on Poly	Synth Subst	Medial Unicondylar	Femoral Surface	Tibial Surface
Knee, RT	ØSPC4[L,M]Z	ØSRCØ6[9,A,Z]	ØSRCØJ[9,A,Z]	ØSRCØL[9,A,Z]	ØSRTØJ[9,A,Z]	ØSRVØJ[9,A,Z]
Knee, LT	ØSPD4[L,M]Z	ØSRDØ6[9,A,Z]	ØSRDØJ[9,A,Z]	ØSRDØL[9,A,Z]	ØSRUØJ[9,A,Z]	ØSRWØJ[9,A,Z]

Percutaneous Endoscopic Removal of Patellofemoral Knee with Synthetic Substitute Replacement

Removal of Patellofemoral Knee		Code also as appropriate Replacement by Type of Synthetic Substitute				
		Oxidized Zircon on Poly	Synth Subst	Medial Unicondylar	Femoral Surface	Tibial Surface
Knee, RT	ØSPC4NZ	ØSRCØ6[9,A,Z]	ØSRCØJ[9,A,Z]	ØSRCØL[9,A,Z]	ØSRTØJ[9,A,Z]	ØSRVØJ[9,A,Z]
Knee, LT	ØSPD4NZ	ØSRDØ6[9,A,Z]	ØSRDØJ[9,A,Z]	ØSRDØL[9,A,Z]	ØSRUØJ[9,A,Z]	ØSRWØJ[9,A,Z]

Percutaneous Endoscopic Removal of Femoral/Tibial Surface of Knee with Synthetic Substitute Replacement

Removal of Femoral/Tibial Surface of Knee		Code also as appropriate Replacement by Type of Synthetic Substitute					
		Oxidized Zircon on Poly	Synth Subst	Articulating Spacer	Patello-femoral	Femoral Surface	Tibial Surface
Knee, RT	ØSP[T,V]4JZ	ØSRCØ6[9,A,Z]	ØSRCØJ[9,A,Z]	ØSRCØEZ	ØSRCØN[9,A,Z]	ØSRTØJ[9,A,Z]	ØSRVØJ[9,A]
Knee, LT	ØSP[U,W]4JZ	ØSRDØ6[9,A,Z]	ØSRDØJ[9,A,Z]	ØSRDØEZ	ØSRDØN[9,A,Z]	ØSRUØJ[9,A,Z]	ØSRWØJ[9,A,Z]

466-468 Revision of Hip or Knee Replacement

Hip Procedures

Open Removal of Hip Spacer with Replacement

Removal of Spacer		Code also as appropriate Replacement by Device Type						
		Metal	Metal on Poly	Ceramic	Ceramic on Poly	Oxidized Zirc on Poly	Articulating Spacer	Synth Subst
Hip, RT	ØSP9Ø8Z	ØSR9Ø1[9,A,Z]	ØSR9Ø2[9,A,Z]	ØSR9Ø3[9,A,Z]	ØSR9Ø4[9,A,Z]	ØSR9Ø6[9,A,Z]	ØSR9ØEZ	ØSR9ØJ[9,A,Z]
Hip, LT	ØSPBØ8Z	ØSRBØ1[9,A,Z]	ØSRBØ2[9,A,Z]	ØSRBØ3[9,A,Z]	ØSRBØ4[9,A,Z]	ØSRBØ6[9,A,Z]	ØSRBØEZ	ØSRBØJ[9,A,Z]

Open Removal of Hip Spacer with Replacement

Removal of Spacer		Code also as appropriate Replacement by Device Type						
		Acetabular Surface				Femoral Surface		
		Poly	Metal	Ceramic	Synthetic	Metal	Ceramic	Synth
Hip, RT	ØSP9Ø8Z	ØSRAØØ[9,A,Z]	ØSRAØ1[9,A,Z]	ØSRAØ3[9,A,Z]	ØSRAØJ[9,A,Z]	ØSRRØ1[9,A,Z]	ØSRRØ3[9,A,Z]	ØSRRØJ[9,A,Z]
Hip, LT	ØSPBØ8Z	ØSREØØ[9,A,Z]	ØSREØ1[9,A,Z]	ØSREØ3[9,A,Z]	ØSREØJ[9,A,Z]	ØSRSØ1[9,A,Z]	ØSRSØ3[9,A,Z]	ØSRSØJ[9,A,Z]

Open Removal of Hip Spacer with Liner Insertion (supplement)

Removal of Spacer		Code also as appropriate Supplement of Body Part by Site		
		Joint	Acetabular Surface	Femoral Surface
Hip, RT	ØSP9Ø8Z	ØSU9Ø9Z	ØSUAØ9Z	ØSURØ9Z
Hip, LT	ØSPBØ8Z	ØSUBØ9Z	ØSUEØ9Z	ØSUSØ9Z

Open Removal of Hip Liner with Replacement

Removal of Liner		Code also as appropriate Replacement by Device Type						
		Metal	Metal on Poly	Ceramic	Ceramic on Poly	Oxidized Zirc on Poly	Articulating Spacer	Synth Subst
Hip, RT	ØSP9Ø9Z	ØSR9Ø1[9,A,Z]	ØSR9Ø2[9,A,Z]	ØSR9Ø3[9,A,Z]	ØSR9Ø4[9,A,Z]	ØSR9Ø6[9,A,Z]	ØSR9ØEZ	ØSR9ØJ[9,A,Z]
Hip, LT	ØSPBØ9Z	ØSRBØ1[9,A,Z]	ØSRBØ2[9,A,Z]	ØSRBØ3[9,A,Z]	ØSRBØ4[9,A,Z]	ØSRBØ6[9,A,Z]	ØSRBØEZ	ØSRBØJ[9,A,Z]

Open Removal of Hip Liner with Replacement

Removal of Liner		Code also as appropriate Replacement by Device Type						
		Acetabular Surface				Femoral Surface		
		Poly	Metal	Ceramic	Synthetic	Metal	Ceramic	Synth
Hip, RT	ØSP9Ø9Z	ØSRAØØ[9,A,Z]	ØSRAØ1[9,A,Z]	ØSRAØ3[9,A,Z]	ØSRAØJ[9,A,Z]	ØSRRØ1[9,A,Z]	ØSRRØ3[9,A,Z]	ØSRRØJ[9,A,Z]
Hip, LT	ØSPBØ9Z	ØSREØØ[9,A,Z]	ØSREØ1[9,A,Z]	ØSREØ3[9,A,Z]	ØSREØJ[9,A,Z]	ØSRSØ1[9,A,Z]	ØSRSØ3[9,A,Z]	ØSRSØJ[9,A,Z]

Open Removal of Hip Liner with Liner Insertion (supplement)

Removal of Liner		Code also as appropriate Supplement of Body Part by Site		
		Joint	Acetabular Surface	Femoral Surface
Hip, RT	ØSP9Ø9Z	ØSU9Ø9Z	ØSUAØ9Z	ØSURØ9Z
Hip, LT	ØSPBØ9Z	ØSUBØ9Z	ØSUEØ9Z	ØSUSØ9Z

Open Removal of Hip Resurfacing Device with Replacement

Removal of Resurfacing Device		Code also as appropriate Replacement by Device Type						
		Metal	Metal on Poly	Ceramic	Ceramic on Poly	Oxidized Zirc on Poly	Articulating Spacer	Synth Subst
Hip, RT	ØSP9ØBZ	ØSR9Ø1[9,A,Z]	ØSR9Ø2[9,A,Z]	ØSR9Ø3[9,A,Z]	ØSR9Ø4[9,A,Z]	ØSR9Ø6[9,A,Z]	ØSR9ØEZ	ØSR9ØJ[9,A,Z]
Hip, LT	ØSPBØBZ	ØSRBØ1[9,A,Z]	ØSRBØ2[9,A,Z]	ØSRBØ3[9,A,Z]	ØSRBØ4[9,A,Z]	ØSRBØ6[9,A,Z]	ØSRBØEZ	ØSRBØJ[9,A,Z]

Open Removal of Hip Resurfacing Device with Replacement

Removal of Resurfacing Device		Code also as appropriate Replacement by Device Type						
		Acetabular Surface				Femoral Surface		
		Poly	Metal	Ceramic	Synthetic	Metal	Ceramic	Synth
Hip, RT	ØSP9ØBZ	ØSRAØØ[9,A,Z]	ØSRAØ1[9,A,Z]	ØSRAØ3[9,A,Z]	ØSRAØJ[9,A,Z]	ØSRRØ1[9,A,Z]	ØSRRØ3[9,A,Z]	ØSRRØJ[9,A,Z]
Hip, LT	ØSPBØBZ	ØSREØØ[9,A,Z]	ØSREØ1[9,A,Z]	ØSREØ3[9,A,Z]	ØSREØJ[9,A,Z]	ØSRSØ1[9,A,Z]	ØSRSØ3[9,A,Z]	ØSRSØJ[9,A,Z]

Open Removal of Hip Resurfacing Device with Liner Insertion (supplement)

Removal of Resurfacing Device		Code also as appropriate Supplement of Body Part by Site		
		Joint	Acetabular Surface	Femoral Surface
Hip, RT	ØSP9ØBZ	ØSU9Ø9Z	ØSUAØ9Z	ØSURØ9Z
Hip, LT	ØSPBØBZ	ØSUBØ9Z	ØSUEØ9Z	ØSUSØ9Z

Open Removal of Hip Articulating Spacer with Replacement

Removal of Articulating Spacer		Code also as appropriate Replacement by Device Type					
		Metal	Metal on Poly	Ceramic	Ceramic on Poly	Oxidized Zirc on Poly	Synth Subst
Hip, RT	ØSP9ØEZ	ØSR9Ø1[9,A,Z]	ØSR9Ø2[9,A,Z]	ØSR9Ø3[9,A,Z]	ØSR9Ø4[9,A,Z]	ØSR9Ø6[9,A,Z]	ØSR9ØJ[9,A,Z]
Hip, LT	ØSPBØEZ	ØSRBØ1[9,A,Z]	ØSRBØ2[9,A,Z]	ØSRBØ3[9,A,Z]	ØSRBØ4[9,A,Z]	ØSRBØ6[9,A,Z]	ØSRBØJ[9,A,Z]

Open Removal of Hip Articulating Spacer with Replacement

Removal of Articulating Spacer		Code also as appropriate Replacement by Device Type						
		Acetabular Surface				Femoral Surface		
		Poly	Metal	Ceramic	Synthetic	Metal	Ceramic	Synth
Hip, RT	ØSP9ØEZ	ØSRAØØ[9,A,Z]	ØSRAØ1[9,A,Z]	ØSRAØ3[9,A,Z]	ØSRAØJ[9,A,Z]	ØSRRØ1[9,A,Z]	ØSRRØ3[9,A,Z]	ØSRRØJ[9,A,Z]
Hip, LT	ØSPBØEZ	ØSREØØ[9,A,Z]	ØSREØ1[9,A,Z]	ØSREØ3[9,A,Z]	ØSREØJ[9,A,Z]	ØSRSØ1[9,A,Z]	ØSRSØ3[9,A,Z]	ØSRSØJ[9,A,Z]

Open Removal of Hip Articulating Spacer with Liner Insertion (supplement)

Removal of Articulating Spacer		Code also as appropriate Supplement of Body Part by Site		
		Joint	Acetabular Surface	Femoral Surface
Hip, RT	ØSP9ØEZ	ØSU9Ø9Z	ØSUAØ9Z	ØSURØ9Z
Hip, LT	ØSPBØEZ	ØSUBØ9Z	ØSUEØ9Z	ØSUSØ9Z

Open Removal of Hip Synthetic Substitute with Replacement

Removal of Synthetic Substitute		Code also as appropriate Replacement by Device Type						
		Metal	Metal on Poly	Ceramic	Ceramic on Poly	Oxidized Zirc on Poly	Articulating Spacer	Synth Subst
Hip, RT	ØSP[9,A,R]ØJZ	ØSR9Ø1[9,A,Z]	ØSR9Ø2[9,A,Z]	ØSR9Ø3[9,A,Z]	ØSR9Ø4[9,A,Z]	ØSR9Ø6[9,A,Z]	ØSR9ØEZ	ØSR9ØJ[9,A,Z]
Hip, LT	ØSP[B,E,S]ØJZ	ØSRBØ1[9,A,Z]	ØSRBØ2[9,A,Z]	ØSRBØ3[9,A,Z]	ØSRBØ4[9,A,Z]	ØSRBØ6[9,A,Z]	ØSRBØEZ	ØSRBØJ[9,A,Z]

Open Removal of Hip Synthetic Substitute with Replacement

Removal of Synthetic Substitute		Code also as appropriate Replacement by Device Type						
		Acetabular Surface				Femoral Surface		
		Poly	Metal	Ceramic	Synthetic	Metal	Ceramic	Synth
Hip, RT	ØSP[9,A,R]ØJZ	ØSRAØØ[9,A,Z]	ØSRAØ1[9,A,Z]	ØSRAØ3[9,A,Z]	ØSRAØJ[9,A,Z]	ØSRRØ1[9,A,Z]	ØSRRØ3[9,A,Z]	ØSRRØJ[9,A,Z]
Hip, LT	ØSP[B,E,S]ØJZ	ØSREØØ[9,A,Z]	ØSREØ1[9,A,Z]	ØSREØ3[9,A,Z]	ØSREØJ[9,A,Z]	ØSRSØ1[9,A,Z]	ØSRSØ3[9,A,Z]	ØSRSØJ[9,A,Z]

Percutaneous Endoscopic Removal of Hip Spacer with Open Replacement

Removal of Spacer		Code also as appropriate Replacement by Device Type						
		Metal	Metal on Poly	Ceramic	Ceramic on Poly	Oxidized Zirc on Poly	Articulating Spacer	Synth Subst
Hip, RT	ØSP948Z	ØSR9Ø1[9,A,Z]	ØSR9Ø2[9,A,Z]	ØSR9Ø3[9,A,Z]	ØSR9Ø4[9,A,Z]	ØSR9Ø6[9,A,Z]	ØSR9ØEZ	ØSR9ØJ[9,A,Z]
Hip, LT	ØSPB48Z	ØSRBØ1[9,A,Z]	ØSRBØ2[9,A,Z]	ØSRBØ3[9,A,Z]	ØSRBØ4[9,A,Z]	ØSRBØ6[9,A,Z]	ØSRBØEZ	ØSRBØJ[9,A,Z]

Percutaneous Endoscopic Removal of Hip Spacer with Open Replacement

Removal of Spacer		Code also as appropriate Replacement by Device Type						
		Acetabular Surface				Femoral Surface		
		Poly	Metal	Ceramic	Synthetic	Metal	Ceramic	Synth
Hip, RT	ØSP948Z	ØSRAØØ[9,A,Z]	ØSRAØ1[9,A,Z]	ØSRAØ3[9,A,Z]	ØSRAØJ[9,A,Z]	ØSRRØ1[9,A,Z]	ØSRRØ3[9,A,Z]	ØSRRØJ[9,A,Z]
Hip, LT	ØSPB48Z	ØSREØØ[9,A,Z]	ØSREØ1[9,A,Z]	ØSREØ3[9,A,Z]	ØSREØJ[9,A,Z]	ØSRSØ1[9,A,Z]	ØSRSØ3[9,A,Z]	ØSRSØJ[9,A,Z]

Percutaneous Endoscopic Removal of Hip Spacer with Open Liner Insertion (supplement)

Removal of Spacer		Code also as appropriate Supplement of Body Part by Site		
		Joint	Acetabular Surface	Femoral Surface
Hip, RT	ØSP948Z	ØSU9Ø9Z	ØSUAØ9Z	ØSURØ9Z
Hip, LT	ØSPB48Z	ØSUBØ9Z	ØSUEØ9Z	ØSUSØ9Z

Percutaneous Endoscopic Removal of Hip Synthetic Substitute with Open Replacement

Removal of Synthetic Substitute		Code also as appropriate Replacement by Device Type						
		Metal	Metal on Poly	Ceramic	Ceramic on Poly	Oxidized Zirc on Poly	Articulating Spacer	Synth Subst
Hip, RT	ØSP[9,A,R]4JZ	ØSR9Ø1[9,A,Z]	ØSR9Ø2[9,A,Z]	ØSR9Ø3[9,A,Z]	ØSR9Ø4[9,A,Z]	ØSR9Ø6[9,A,Z]	ØSR9ØEZ	ØSR9ØJ[9,A,Z]
Hip, LT	ØSP[B,E,S]4JZ	ØSRBØ1[9,A,Z]	ØSRBØ2[9,A,Z]	ØSRBØ3[9,A,Z]	ØSRBØ4[9,A,Z]	ØSRBØ6[9,A,Z]	ØSRBØEZ	ØSRBØJ[9,A,Z]

Percutaneous Endoscopic Removal of Hip Synthetic Substitute with Open Replacement

Removal of Synthetic Substitute		Code also as appropriate Replacement by Device Type						
		Acetabular Surface				Femoral Surface		
		Poly	Metal	Ceramic	Synthetic	Metal	Ceramic	Synth
Hip, RT	ØSP[9,A,R]4JZ	ØSRAØØ[9,A,Z]	ØSRAØ1[9,A,Z]	ØSRAØ3[9,A,Z]	ØSRAØJ[9,A,Z]	ØSRRØ1[9,A,Z]	ØSRRØ3[9,A,Z]	ØSRRØJ[9,A,Z]
Hip, LT	ØSP[B,E,S]4JZ	ØSREØØ[9,A,Z]	ØSREØ1[9,A,Z]	ØSREØ3[9,A,Z]	ØSREØJ[9,A,Z]	ØSRSØ1[9,A,Z]	ØSRSØ3[9,A,Z]	ØSRSØJ[9,A,Z]

Percutaneous Endoscopic Removal of Hip Synthetic Substitute with Open Liner Insertion (supplement)

Removal of Synthetic Substitute		Code also as appropriate Supplement of Body Part by Site		
		Joint	Acetabular Surface	Femoral Surface
Hip, RT	ØSP[9,A,R]4JZ	ØSU9Ø9Z	ØSUAØ9Z	ØSURØ9Z
Hip, LT	ØSP[B,E,S]4JZ	ØSUBØ9Z	ØSUEØ9Z	ØSUSØ9Z

Knee Procedures

Open Removal of Knee Spacer with Articulating Spacer Replacement

Removal of Spacer		Code also as appropriate Replacement with Articulating Spacer
Knee, RT	ØSPCØ8Z	ØSRCØEZ
Knee, LT	ØSPDØ8Z	ØSRDØEZ

Open Removal of Knee Spacer with Synthetic Substitute Replacement

Removal of Spacer		Code also as appropriate Replacement by Type of Synthetic Substitute				
		Oxidized Zircon on Poly	Synth Subst	Patello-femoral	Femoral Surface	Tibial Surface
Knee, RT	ØSPCØ8Z	ØSRCØ6[9,A,Z]	ØSRCØJ[9,A,Z]	ØSRCØN[9,A,Z]	ØSRTØJ[9,A,Z]	ØSRVØJ[9,A,Z]
Knee, LT	ØSPDØ8Z	ØSRDØ6[9,A,Z]	ØSRDØJ[9,A,Z]	ØSRDØN[9,A,Z]	ØSRUØJ[9,A,Z]	ØSRWØJ[9,A,Z]

Open Removal of Knee Liner with Articulating Spacer Replacement

Removal of Liner		Code also as appropriate Replacement with Articulating Spacer
Knee, RT	ØSPCØ9Z	ØSRCØEZ
Knee, LT	ØSPDØ9Z	ØSRDØEZ

Open Removal of Knee Liner with Synthetic Substitute Replacement

Removal of Liner		Code also as appropriate Replacement by Type of Synthetic Substitute						
		Oxidized Zircon on Poly	Synth Subst	Medial Unicondylar	Lateral Unicondylar	Patello-femoral	Femoral Surface	Tibial Surface
Knee, RT	ØSPCØ9Z	ØSRCØ6[9,A,Z]	ØSRCØJ[9,A,Z]	ØSRCØL[9,A,Z]	ØSRCØM[9,A,Z]	ØSRCØN[9,A,Z]	ØSRTØJ[9,A,Z]	ØSRVØJ[9,A,Z]
Knee, LT	ØSPDØ9Z	ØSRDØ6[9,A,Z]	ØSRDØJ[9,A,Z]	ØSRDØL[9,A,Z]	ØSRDØM[9,A,Z]	ØSRDØN[9,A,Z]	ØSRUØJ[9,A,Z]	ØSRWØJ[9,A,Z]

Open Removal of Knee Articulating Spacer with Synthetic Substitute Replacement

Removal of Articulating Spacer		Code also as appropriate Replacement by Type of Synthetic Substitute			
		Oxidized Zircon on Poly	Synth Subst	Femoral Surface	Tibial Surface
Knee, RT	ØSPCØEZ	ØSRCØ6[9,A,Z]	ØSRCØJ[9,A,Z]	ØSRTØJ[9,A,Z]	ØSRVØJ[9,A,Z]
Knee, LT	ØSPDØEZ	ØSRDØ6[9,A,Z]	ØSRDØJ[9,A,Z]	ØSRUØJ[9,A,Z]	ØSRWØJ[9,A,Z]

Open Removal of Patellar Surface of Knee with Synthetic Substitute Replacement

Removal of Patellar Surface		Code also as appropriate Replacement by Type of Synthetic Substitute				
		Oxidized Zircon on Poly	Synth Subst	Patello-femoral	Femoral Surface	Tibial Surface
Knee, RT	ØSPCØJC	ØSRCØ6[9,A,Z]	ØSRCØJ[9,A,Z]	ØSRCØN[9,A,Z]	ØSRTØJ[9,A,Z]	ØSRVØJ[9,A,Z]
Knee, LT	ØSPDØJC	ØSRDØ6[9,A,Z]	ØSRDØJ[9,A,Z]	ØSRDØN[9,A,Z]	ØSRUØJ[9,A,Z]	ØSRWØJ[9,A,Z]

Open Removal of Patellar Surface of Knee with Articulating Spacer Replacement

Removal of Patellar Surface		Code also as appropriate Replacement with Articulating Spacer
Knee, RT	ØSPCØJC	ØSRCØEZ
Knee, LT	ØSPDØJC	ØSRDØEZ

Open Removal of Knee Synthetic Substitute with Synthetic Substitute Replacement

Removal of Synthetic Substitute		Code also as appropriate Replacement by Type of Synthetic Substitute						
		Oxidized Zircon on Poly	Synth Subst	Medial Unicondylar	Lateral Unicondylar	Patello-femoral	Femoral Surface	Tibial Surface
Knee, RT	ØSPCØJZ	ØSRCØ6[9,A,Z]	ØSRCØJ[9,A,Z]	ØSRCØL[9,A,Z]	ØSRCØM[9,A,Z]	ØSRCØN[9,A,Z]	ØSRTØJ[9,A,Z]	ØSRVØJ[9,A,Z]
Knee, LT	ØSPDØJZ	ØSRDØ6[9,A,Z]	ØSRDØJ[9,A,Z]	ØSRDØL[9,A,Z]	ØSRDØM[9,A,Z]	ØSRDØN[9,A,Z]	ØSRUØJ[9,A,Z]	ØSRWØJ[9,A,Z]

Open Removal of Knee Synthetic Substitute with Articulating Spacer Replacement

Removal of Synthetic Substitute		Code also as appropriate Replacement with Articulating Spacer
Knee, RT	ØSPCØJZ	ØSRCØEZ
Knee, LT	ØSPDØJZ	ØSRDØEZ

Open Removal of Medial or Lateral Unicondylar Knee with Synthetic Substitute Replacement

Removal of Medial/Lateral Unicondylar Knee		Code also as appropriate Replacement by Type of Synthetic Substitute				
		Oxidized Zircon on Poly	Synth Subst	Medial Unicondylar	Femoral Surface	Tibial Surface
Knee, RT	ØSPCØ[L,M]Z	ØSRCØ6[9,A,Z]	ØSRCØJ[9,A,Z]	ØSRCØL[9,A,Z]	ØSRTØJ[9,A,Z]	ØSRVØJ[9,A,Z]
Knee, LT	ØSPDØ[L,M]Z	ØSRDØ6[9,A,Z]	ØSRDØJ[9,A,Z]	ØSRDØL[9,A,Z]	ØSRUØJ[9,A,Z]	ØSRWØJ[9,A,Z]

Open Removal of Patellofemoral Knee with Synthetic Substitute Replacement

Removal of Patellofemoral Knee		Code also as appropriate Replacement by Type of Synthetic Substitute				
		Oxidized Zircon on Poly	Synth Subst	Medial Unicondylar	Femoral Surface	Tibial Surface
Knee, RT	ØSPCØNZ	ØSRCØ6[9,A,Z]	ØSRCØJ[9,A,Z]	ØSRCØL[9,A,Z]	ØSRTØJ[9,A,Z]	ØSRVØJ[9,A,Z]
Knee, LT	ØSPDØNZ	ØSRDØ6[9,A,Z]	ØSRDØJ[9,A,Z]	ØSRDØL[9,A,Z]	ØSRUØJ[9,A,Z]	ØSRWØJ[9,A,Z]

Open Removal of Femoral/Tibial Surface of Knee with Synthetic Substitute Replacement

Removal of Femoral/Tibial Surface of Knee		Code also as appropriate Replacement by Type of Synthetic Substitute					
		Oxidized Zircon on Poly	Synth Subst	Articulating Spacer	Patello-femoral	Femoral Surface	Tibial Surface
Knee, RT	ØSP[T,V]ØJZ	ØSRCØ6[9,A,Z]	ØSRCØJ[9,A,Z]	ØSRCØEZ	ØSRCØN[9,A,Z]	ØSRTØJ[9,A,Z]	ØSRVØJ[9,A,Z]
Knee, LT	ØSP[U,W]ØJZ	ØSRDØ6[9,A,Z]	ØSRDØJ[9,A,Z]	ØSRDØEZ	ØSRDØN[9,A,Z]	ØSRUØJ[9,A,Z]	ØSRWØJ[9,A,Z]

Percutaneous/Percutaneous Endoscopic Removal of Knee Spacer with Open Synthetic Substitute Replacement

Removal of Spacer		Code also as appropriate Replacement by Type of Synthetic Substitute				
		Oxidized Zircon on Poly	Synth Subst	Patello-femoral	Femoral Surface	Tibial Surface
Knee, RT	ØSPC[3,4]8Z	ØSRCØ6[9,A,Z]	ØSRCØJ[9,A,Z]	ØSRCØN[9,A,Z]	ØSRTØJ[9,A,Z]	ØSRVØJ[9,A,Z]
Knee, LT	ØSPD[3,4]8Z	ØSRDØ6[9,A,Z]	ØSRDØJ[9,A,Z]	ØSRDØN[9,A,Z]	ØSRUØJ[9,A,Z]	ØSRWØJ[9,A,Z]

Percutaneous/Percutaneous Endoscopic Removal of Knee Spacer with Open Articulating Spacer Replacement

Removal of Spacer		Code also as appropriate Replacement with Articulating Spacer
Knee, RT	ØSPC[3,4]8Z	ØSRCØEZ
Knee, LT	ØSPD[3,4]8Z	ØSRDØEZ

Percutaneous Endoscopic Removal of Patellar Surface of Knee with Synthetic Substitute Replacement

Removal of Patellar Surface		Code also as appropriate Replacement by Type of Synthetic Substitute				
		Oxidized Zircon on Poly	Synth Subst	Patello-femoral	Femoral Surface	Tibial Surface
Knee, RT	ØSPC4JC	ØSRCØ6[9,A,Z]	ØSRCØJ[9,A,Z]	ØSRCØN[9,A,Z]	ØSRTØJ[9,A,Z]	ØSRVØJ[9,A]
Knee, LT	ØSPD4JC	ØSRDØ6[9,A,Z]	ØSRDØJ[9,A,Z]	ØSRDØN[9,A,Z]	ØSRUØJ[9,A,Z]	ØSRWØJ[9,A,Z]

Percutaneous Endoscopic Removal of Patellar Surface of Knee with Articulating Spacer Replacement

Removal of Patellar Surface		Code also as appropriate Replacement with Articulating Spacer
Knee, RT	ØSPC4JC	ØSRCØEZ
Knee, LT	ØSPD4JC	ØSRDØEZ

Percutaneous Endoscopic Removal of Knee Synthetic Substitute with Synthetic Substitute Replacement

Removal of Synthetic Substitute		Code also as appropriate Replacement by Type of Synthetic Substitute						
		Oxidized Zircon on Poly	Synth Subst	Medial Unicondylar	Lateral Unicondylar	Patello-femoral	Femoral Surface	Tibial Surface
Knee, RT	ØSPC4JZ	ØSRCØ6[9,A,Z]	ØSRCØJ[9,A,Z]	ØSRCØL[9,A,Z]	ØSRCØM[9,A,Z]	ØSRCØN[9,A,Z]	ØSRTØJ[9,A,Z]	ØSRVØJ[9,A,Z]
Knee, LT	ØSPD4JZ	ØSRDØ6[9,A,Z]	ØSRDØJ[9,A,Z]	ØSRDØL[9,A,Z]	ØSRDØM[9,A,Z]	ØSRDØN[9,A,Z]	ØSRUØJ[9,A,Z]	ØSRWØJ[9,A,Z]

Percutaneous Endoscopic Removal of Knee Synthetic Substitute with Articulating Spacer Replacement

Removal of Synthetic Substitute		Code also as appropriate Replacement with Articulating Spacer
Knee, RT	ØSPC4JZ	ØSRCØEZ
Knee, LT	ØSPD4JZ	ØSRDØEZ

Percutaneous Endoscopic Removal of Medial or Lateral Unicondylar Knee with Synthetic Substitute Replacement

Removal of Medial/Lateral Unicondylar Knee		Code also as appropriate Replacement by Type of Synthetic Substitute				
		Oxidized Zircon on Poly	Synth Subst	Medial Unicondylar	Femoral Surface	Tibial Surface
Knee, RT	ØSPC4[L,M]Z	ØSRC06[9,A,Z]	ØSRCØJ[9,A,Z]	ØSRCØL[9,A,Z]	ØSRTØJ[9,A,Z]	ØSRVØJ[9,A,Z]
Knee, LT	ØSPD4[L,M]Z	ØSRD06[9,A,Z]	ØSRDØJ[9,A,Z]	ØSRDØL[9,A,Z]	ØSRUØJ[9,A,Z]	ØSRWØJ[9,A,Z]

Percutaneous Endoscopic Removal of Patellofemoral Knee with Synthetic Substitute Replacement

Removal of Patellofemoral Knee		Code also as appropriate Replacement by Type of Synthetic Substitute				
		Oxidized Zircon on Poly	Synth Subst	Medial Unicondylar	Femoral Surface	Tibial Surface
Knee, RT	ØSPC4NZ	ØSRC06[9,A,Z]	ØSRCØJ[9,A,Z]	ØSRCØL[9,A,Z]	ØSRTØJ[9,A,Z]	ØSRVØJ[9,A,Z]
Knee, LT	ØSPD4NZ	ØSRD06[9,A,Z]	ØSRDØJ[9,A,Z]	ØSRDØL[9,A,Z]	ØSRUØJ[9,A,Z]	ØSRWØJ[9,A,Z]

Percutaneous Endoscopic Removal of Femoral/Tibial Surface of Knee with Synthetic Substitute Replacement

Removal of Femoral/Tibial Surface of Knee		Code also as appropriate Replacement by Type of Synthetic Substitute					
		Oxidized Zircon on Poly	Synth Subst	Articulating Spacer	Patello-femoral	Femoral Surface	Tibial Surface
Knee, RT	ØSP[T,V]4JZ	ØSRC06[9,A,Z]	ØSRCØJ[9,A,Z]	ØSRCØEZ	ØSRCØN[9,A,Z]	ØSRTØJ[9,A,Z]	ØSRVØJ[9,A]
Knee, LT	ØSP[U,W]4JZ	ØSRD06[9,A,Z]	ØSRDØJ[9,A,Z]	ØSRDØEZ	ØSRDØN[9,A,Z]	ØSRUØJ[9,A,Z]	ØSRWØJ[9,A,Z]

DRG 485-489 Knee Procedures

Joint	Removal of Liner by open approach	Code also as appropriate Supplement of Tibial Surface by Site
Knee, RT	ØSPC09Z	ØSUV09Z
Knee, LT	ØSPD09Z	ØSUW09Z

DRG 515-517 Other Musculoskeletal System and Connective Tissue Procedures

Site	Reposition of Vertebra by percutaneous approach	Code also as appropriate Supplement With Synthetic Substitute by Percutaneous Approach at site of Repositioned Vertebra
Cervical	ØPS33ZZ	ØPU33JZ
Coccyx	ØQSS3ZZ	ØQUS3JZ
Lumbar	ØQS03ZZ	ØQU03JZ
Sacrum	ØQS13ZZ	ØQU13JZ
Thoracic	ØPS43ZZ	ØPU43JZ

DRG 518-52Ø Back and Neck Procedures, Except Spinal Fusion, or Disc Devices/Neurostimulators

Generator Type	Insertion of Generator by Site			Code also as appropriate Insertion Neurostimulator Lead by approach and Site	
	Chest	Abdomen	Back	Spinal Canal	Spinal Cord
Single Array	ØJH6[Ø,3]BZ	ØJH8[Ø,3]BZ	ØJH7[Ø,3]BZ	00HU[Ø,3,4]MZ	00HV[Ø,3,4]MZ
Single Array, Rechargeable	ØJH6[Ø,3]CZ	ØJH8[Ø,3]CZ	ØJH7[Ø,3]CZ	00HU[Ø,3,4]MZ	00HV[Ø,3,4]MZ
Multiple Array	ØJH6[Ø,3]DZ	ØJH8[Ø,3]DZ	ØJH7[Ø,3]DZ	00HU[Ø,3,4]MZ	00HV[Ø,3,4]MZ
Multiple Array, Rechargable	ØJH6[Ø,3]EZ	—	ØJH7[Ø,3]EZ	00HU[Ø,3,4]MZ	00HV[Ø,3,4]MZ
Multiple Array, Rechargable	—	ØJH8[Ø,3]EZ	—	00HU[Ø,3,4]MZ	00HV[Ø,3,4]MZ

DRG 582-583 Mastectomy for Malignancy

Site	Resection by Open approach	Code also as appropriate Resection of Lymph Nodes by Open approach by site			Code also as appropriate Resection of Thorax Muscle by Open approach	
		Axillary	Internal Mammary	Thorax	Right	Left
Breast, Right	ØHTTØZZ	07T50ZZ	07T80ZZ	07T70ZZ	ØKTHØZZ	—
Breast, Left	ØHTUØZZ	07T60ZZ	07T90ZZ	07T70ZZ	—	ØKTJØZZ
Breast, Bilateral	ØHTVØZZ	07T50ZZ and 07T60ZZ	07T80ZZ and 07T90ZZ	07T70ZZ	ØKTHØZZ	ØKTJØZZ

DRG 584-585 Breast Biopsy, Local Excision and Other Breast procedures

Resection of Breast With Resection of Lymph Nodes and Thorax Muscle

Site	Resection by Open approach	Code also as appropriate Resection of Lymph Nodes by Open approach by site			Code also as appropriate Resection of Thorax Muscle by Open approach	
		Axillary	Internal Mammary	Thorax	Right	Left
Breast, Right	ØHTTØZZ	07T50ZZ	07T80ZZ	07T70ZZ	ØKTHØZZ	—
Breast, Left	ØHTUØZZ	07T60ZZ	07T90ZZ	07T70ZZ	—	ØKTJØZZ
Breast, Bilateral	ØHTVØZZ	07T50ZZ and 07T60ZZ	07T80ZZ and 07T90ZZ	07T70ZZ	ØKTHØZZ	ØKTJØZZ

Replacement of Breast Tissue

Site	Replacement by Percutaneous approach with Autologous Tissue	Code also as appropriate Extraction of Subcutaneous Tissue by Percutaneous approach					
		Abdomen	Back	Buttock	Chest	Leg, Upper, Right	Leg, Upper, Left
Breast, Right	ØHRT37Z	ØJD83ZZ	ØJD73ZZ	ØJD93ZZ	ØJD63ZZ	ØJDL3ZZ	ØJDM3ZZ
Breast, Left	ØHRU37Z	ØJD83ZZ	ØJD73ZZ	ØJD93ZZ	ØJD63ZZ	ØJDL3ZZ	ØJDM3ZZ
Breast, Bilateral	ØHRV37Z	ØJD83ZZ	ØJD73ZZ	ØJD93ZZ	ØJD63ZZ	ØJDL3ZZ	ØJDM3ZZ

DRG 628-630 Other Endocrine, Nutritional and Metabolic Procedures

Hip Procedures

Open Removal of Hip Spacer with Replacement

Removal of Spacer		Code also as appropriate Replacement by Device Type					
		Metal	Metal on Poly	Ceramic	Ceramic on Poly	Oxidized Zirc on Poly	Synthetic Substitute
Hip, RT	ØSP908Z	ØSR901[9,A,Z]	ØSR902[9,A,Z]	ØSR903[9,A,Z]	ØSR904[9,A,Z]	ØSR906[9,A,Z]	ØSR90J[9,A,Z]
Hip, LT	ØSPBØ8Z	ØSRBØ1[9,A,Z]	ØSRBØ2[9,A,Z]	ØSRBØ3[9,A,Z]	ØSRBØ4[9,A,Z]	ØSRBØ6[9,A,Z]	ØSRBØJ[9,A,Z]

Open Removal of Hip Spacer with Replacement

Removal of Spacer		Code also as appropriate Replacement by Device Type						
		Acetabular Surface				Femoral Surface		
		Poly	Metal	Ceramic	Synthetic	Metal	Ceramic	Synthetic
Hip, RT	ØSP908Z	ØSRAØØ[9,A,Z]	ØSRAØ1[9,A,Z]	ØSRAØ3[9,A,Z]	ØSRAØJ[9,A,Z]	ØSRRØ1[9,A,Z]	ØSRRØ3[9,A,Z]	ØSRRØJ[9,A,Z]
Hip, LT	ØSPBØ8Z	ØSREØØ[9,A,Z]	ØSREØ1[9,A,Z]	ØSREØ3[9,A,Z]	ØSREØJ[9,A,Z]	ØSRSØ1[9,A,Z]	ØSRSØ3[9,A,Z]	ØSRSØJ[9,A,Z]

Open Removal of Hip Spacer with Liner Insertion (supplement)

Removal of Spacer		Code also as appropriate Supplement of Body Part by Site		
		Joint	Acetabular Surface	Femoral Surface
Hip, RT	ØSP908Z	ØSU909Z	ØSUAØ9Z	ØSURØ9Z
Hip, LT	ØSPBØ8Z	ØSUBØ9Z	ØSUEØ9Z	ØSUSØ9Z

Open Removal of Hip Liner with Replacement

Removal of Liner		Code also as appropriate Replacement by Device Type					
		Metal	Metal on Poly	Ceramic	Ceramic on Poly	Oxidized Zirc on Poly	Synthetic Substitute
Hip, RT	ØSP9Ø9Z	ØSR9Ø1[9,A,Z]	ØSR9Ø2[9,A,Z]	ØSR9Ø3[9,A,Z]	ØSR9Ø4[9,A,Z]	ØSR9Ø6[9,A,Z]	ØSR9ØJ[9,A,Z]
Hip, LT	ØSPBØ9Z	ØSRBØ1[9,A,Z]	ØSRBØ2[9,A,Z]	ØSRBØ3[9,A,Z]	ØSRBØ4[9,A,Z]	ØSRBØ6[9,A,Z]	ØSRBØJ[9,A,Z]

Open Removal of Hip Liner with Replacement

Removal of Liner		Code also as appropriate Replacement by Device Type						
		Acetabular Surface				Femoral Surface		
		Poly	Metal	Ceramic	Synthetic	Metal	Ceramic	Synthetic
Hip, RT	ØSP9Ø9Z	ØSRAØØ[9,A,Z]	ØSRAØ1[9,A,Z]	ØSRAØ3[9,A,Z]	ØSRAØJ[9,A,Z]	ØSRRØ1[9,A,Z]	ØSRRØ3[9,A,Z]	ØSRRØJ[9,A,Z]
Hip, LT	ØSPBØ9Z	ØSREØØ[9,A,Z]	ØSREØ1[9,A,Z]	ØSREØ3[9,A,Z]	ØSREØJ[9,A,Z]	ØSRSØ1[9,A,Z]	ØSRSØ3[9,A,Z]	ØSRSØJ[9,A,Z]

Open Removal of Hip Liner with Liner Insertion (supplement)

Removal of Liner		Code also as appropriate Supplement of Body Part by Site		
		Joint	Acetabular Surface	Femoral Surface
Hip, RT	ØSP9Ø9Z	ØSU9Ø9Z	ØSUAØ9Z	ØSURØ9Z
Hip, LT	ØSPBØ9Z	ØSUBØ9Z	ØSUEØ9Z	ØSUSØ9Z

Open Removal of Hip Resurfacing Device with Replacement

Removal of Resurfacing Device		Code also as appropriate Replacement by Device Type					
		Metal	Metal on Poly	Ceramic	Ceramic on Poly	Oxidized Zirc on Poly	Synthetic Substitute
Hip, RT	ØSP9ØBZ	ØSR9Ø1[9,A,Z]	ØSR9Ø2[9,A,Z]	ØSR9Ø3[9,A,Z]	ØSR9Ø4[9,A,Z]	ØSR9Ø6[9,A,Z]	ØSR9ØJ[9,A,Z]
Hip, LT	ØSPBØBZ	ØSRBØ1[9,A,Z]	ØSRBØ2[9,A,Z]	ØSRBØ3[9,A,Z]	ØSRBØ4[9,A,Z]	ØSRBØ6[9,A,Z]	ØSRBØJ[9,A,Z]

Open Removal of Hip Resurfacing Device with Replacement

Removal of Resurfacing Device		Code also as appropriate Replacement by Device Type						
		Acetabular Surface				Femoral Surface		
		Poly	Metal	Ceramic	Synthetic	Metal	Ceramic	Synthetic
Hip, RT	ØSP9ØBZ	ØSRAØØ[9,A,Z]	ØSRAØ1[9,A,Z]	ØSRAØ3[9,A,Z]	ØSRAØJ[9,A,Z]	ØSRRØ1[9,A,Z]	ØSRRØ3[9,A,Z]	ØSRRØJ[9,A,Z]
Hip, LT	ØSPBØBZ	ØSREØØ[9,A,Z]	ØSREØ1[9,A,Z]	ØSREØ3[9,A,Z]	ØSREØJ[9,A,Z]	ØSRSØ1[9,A,Z]	ØSRSØ3[9,A,Z]	ØSRSØJ[9,A,Z]

Open Removal of Hip Resurfacing Device with Liner Insertion (supplement)

Removal of Resurfacing Device		Code also as appropriate Supplement of Body Part by Site		
		Joint	Acetabular Surface	Femoral Surface
Hip, RT	ØSP9ØBZ	ØSU9Ø9Z	ØSUAØ9Z	ØSURØ9Z
Hip, LT	ØSPBØBZ	ØSUBØ9Z	ØSUEØ9Z	ØSUSØ9Z

Open Removal of Hip Synthetic Substitute with Replacement

Removal of Synthetic Substitute		Code also as appropriate Replacement by Device Type					
		Metal	Metal on Poly	Ceramic	Ceramic on Poly	Oxidized Zirc on Poly	Synthetic Substitute
Hip, RT	ØSP9ØJZ	ØSR9Ø1[9,A,Z]	ØSR9Ø2[9,A,Z]	ØSR9Ø3[9,A,Z]	ØSR9Ø4[9,A,Z]	ØSR9Ø6[9,A,Z]	ØSR9ØJ[9,A,Z]
Hip, LT	ØSPBØJZ	ØSRBØ1[9,A,Z]	ØSRBØ2[9,A,Z]	ØSRBØ3[9,A,Z]	ØSRBØ4[9,A,Z]	ØSRBØ6[9,A,Z]	ØSRBØJ[9,A,Z]

Open Removal of Hip Synthetic Substitute with Replacement

Removal of Synthetic Substitute		Code also as appropriate Replacement by Device Type						
		Acetabular Surface				Femoral Surface		
		Poly	Metal	Ceramic	Synthetic	Metal	Ceramic	Synthetic
Hip, RT	ØSP9ØJZ	ØSRAØØ[9,A,Z]	ØSRAØ1[9,A,Z]	ØSRAØ3[9,A,Z]	ØSRAØJ[9,A,Z]	ØSRRØ1[9,A,Z]	ØSRRØ3[9,A,Z]	ØSRRØJ[9,A,Z]
Hip, LT	ØSPBØJZ	ØSREØØ[9,A,Z]	ØSREØ1[9,A,Z]	ØSREØ3[9,A,Z]	ØSREØJ[9,A,Z]	ØSRSØ1[9,A,Z]	ØSRSØ3[9,A,Z]	ØSRSØJ[9,A,Z]

Open Removal of Hip Acetabular/Femoral Surface with Replacement

Removal of Acetabular/Femoral Surface		Code also as appropriate Replacement by Device Type					
		Metal	Metal on Poly	Ceramic	Ceramic on Poly	Oxidized Zirc on Poly	Synthetic Substitute
Hip, RT	ØSP[A,R]ØJZ	ØSR9Ø1[9,A,Z]	ØSR9Ø2[9,A,Z]	ØSR9Ø3[9,A,Z]	ØSR9Ø4[9,A,Z]	ØSR9Ø6[9,A,Z]	ØSR9ØJ[9,A,Z]
Hip, LT	ØSP[E,S]ØJZ	ØSRBØ1[9,A,Z]	ØSRBØ2[9,A,Z]	ØSRBØ3[9,A,Z]	ØSRBØ4[9,A,Z]	ØSRBØ6[9,A,Z]	ØSRBØJ[9,A,Z]

Open Removal of Hip Acetabular/Femoral Surface with Replacement

Removal of Acetabular/Femoral Surface		Code also as appropriate Replacement by Device Type						
		Acetabular Surface				Femoral Surface		
		Poly	Metal	Ceramic	Synthetic	Metal	Ceramic	Synthetic
Hip, RT	ØSP[A,R]ØJZ	ØSRAØØ[9,A,Z]	ØSRAØ1[9,A,Z]	ØSRAØ3[9,A,Z]	ØSRAØJ[9,A,Z]	ØSRRØ1[9,A,Z]	ØSRRØ3[9,A,Z]	ØSRRØJ[9,A,Z]
Hip, LT	ØSP[E,S]ØJZ	ØSREØØ[9,A,Z]	ØSREØ1[9,A,Z]	ØSREØ3[9,A,Z]	ØSREØJ[9,A,Z]	ØSRSØ1[9,A,Z]	ØSRSØ3[9,A,Z]	ØSRSØJ[9,A,Z]

Percutaneous Endoscopic Removal of Hip Spacer with Replacement

Removal of Spacer		Code also as appropriate Replacement by Device Type					
		Metal	Metal on Poly	Ceramic	Ceramic on Poly	Oxidized Zirc on Poly	Synthetic Substitute
Hip, RT	ØSP948Z	ØSR9Ø1[9,A,Z]	ØSR9Ø2[9,A,Z]	ØSR9Ø3[9,A,Z]	ØSR9Ø4[9,A,Z]	ØSR9Ø6[9,A,Z]	ØSR9ØJ[9,A,Z]
Hip, LT	ØSPB48Z	ØSRBØ1[9,A,Z]	ØSRBØ2[9,A,Z]	ØSRBØ3[9,A,Z]	ØSRBØ4[9,A,Z]	ØSRBØ6[9,A,Z]	ØSRBØJ[9,A,Z]

Percutaneous Endoscopic Removal of Hip Spacer with Replacement

Removal of Spacer		Code also as appropriate Replacement by Device Type						
		Acetabular Surface				Femoral Surface		
		Poly	Metal	Ceramic	Synthetic	Metal	Ceramic	Synthetic
Hip, RT	ØSP948Z	ØSRAØØ[9,A,Z]	ØSRAØ1[9,A,Z]	ØSRAØ3[9,A,Z]	ØSRAØJ[9,A,Z]	ØSRRØ1[9,A,Z]	ØSRRØ3[9,A,Z]	ØSRRØJ[9,A,Z]
Hip, LT	ØSPB48Z	ØSREØØ[9,A,Z]	ØSREØ1[9,A,Z]	ØSREØ3[9,A,Z]	ØSREØJ[9,A,Z]	ØSRSØ1[9,A,Z]	ØSRSØ3[9,A,Z]	ØSRSØJ[9,A,Z]

Percutaneous Endoscopic Removal of Hip Spacer with Liner Insertion (supplement)

Removal of Spacer		Code also as appropriate Supplement of Body Part by Site		
		Joint	Acetabular Surface	Femoral Surface
Hip, RT	ØSP948Z	ØSU9Ø9Z	ØSUAØ9Z	ØSURØ9Z
Hip, LT	ØSPB48Z	ØSUBØ9Z	ØSUEØ9Z	ØSUSØ9Z

Percutaneous Endoscopic Removal of Hip Synthetic Substitute with Replacement

Removal of Synthetic Substitute		Code also as appropriate Replacement by Device Type					
		Metal	Metal on Poly	Ceramic	Ceramic on Poly	Oxidized Zirc on Poly	Synthetic Substitute
Hip, RT	ØSP94JZ	ØSR9Ø1[9,A,Z]	ØSR9Ø2[9,A,Z]	ØSR9Ø3[9,A,Z]	ØSR9Ø4[9,A,Z]	ØSR9Ø6[9,A,Z]	ØSR9ØJ[9,A,Z]
Hip, LT	ØSPB4JZ	ØSRBØ1[9,A,Z]	ØSRBØ2[9,A,Z]	ØSRBØ3[9,A,Z]	ØSRBØ4[9,A,Z]	ØSRBØ6[9,A,Z]	ØSRBØJ[9,A,Z]

Percutaneous Endoscopic of Hip Synthetic Substitute with Replacement

Removal of Synthetic Substitute		Code also as appropriate Replacement by Device Type						
		Acetabular Surface				Femoral Surface		
		Poly	Metal	Ceramic	Synthetic	Metal	Ceramic	Synthetic
Hip, RT	0SP94JZ	0SRA00[9,A,Z]	0SRA01[9,A,Z]	0SRA03[9,A,Z]	0SRA0J[9,A,Z]	0SRR01[9,A,Z]	0SRR03[9,A,Z]	0SRR0J[9,A,Z]
Hip, LT	0SPB4JZ	0SRE00[9,A,Z]	0SRE01[9,A,Z]	0SRE03[9,A,Z]	0SRE0J[9,A,Z]	0SRS01[9,A,Z]	0SRS03[9,A,Z]	0SRS0J[9,A,Z]

Percutaneous Endoscopic Removal of Hip Synthetic Substitute with Liner Insertion (supplement)

Removal of Synthetic Substitute		Code also as appropriate Supplement of Body Part by Site		
		Joint	Acetabular Surface	Femoral Surface
Hip, RT	0SP94JZ	0SU909Z	0SUA09Z	0SUR09Z
Hip, LT	0SPB4JZ	0SUB09Z	0SUE09Z	0SUS09Z

Percutaneous Endoscopic Removal of Hip Acetabular/Femoral Surface with Replacement

Removal of Acetabular/Femoral Surface		Code also as appropriate Replacement by Device Type					
		Metal	Metal on Poly	Ceramic	Ceramic on Poly	Oxidized Zirc on Poly	Synthetic Substitute
Hip, RT	0SP[A,R]4JZ	0SR901[9,A,Z]	0SR902[9,A,Z]	0SR903[9,A,Z]	0SR904[9,A,Z]	0SR906[9,A,Z]	0SR90J[9,A,Z]
Hip, LT	0SP[E,S]4JZ	0SRB01[9,A,Z]	0SRB02[9,A,Z]	0SRB03[9,A,Z]	0SRB04[9,A,Z]	0SRB06[9,A,Z]	0SRB0J[9,A,Z]

Percutaneous Endoscopic of Hip Acetabular/Femoral Surface with Replacement

Removal of Acetabular/Femoral Surface		Code also as appropriate Replacement by Device Type						
		Acetabular Surface				Femoral Surface		
		Poly	Metal	Ceramic	Synthetic	Metal	Ceramic	Synthetic
Hip, RT	0SP[A,R]4JZ	0SRA00[9,A,Z]	0SRA01[9,A,Z]	0SRA03[9,A,Z]	0SRA0J[9,A,Z]	0SRR01[9,A,Z]	0SRR03[9,A,Z]	0SRR0J[9,A,Z]
Hip, LT	0SP[E,S]4JZ	0SRE00[9,A,Z]	0SRE01[9,A,Z]	0SRE03[9,A,Z]	0SRE0J[9,A,Z]	0SRS01[9,A,Z]	0SRS03[9,A,Z]	0SRS0J[9,A,Z]

Percutaneous Endoscopic Removal of Hip Acetabular/Femoral Surface with Liner Insertion (supplement)

Removal of Acetabular/Femoral Surface		Code also as appropriate Supplement of Body Part by Site		
		Joint	Acetabular Surface	Femoral Surface
Hip, RT	0SP[A,R]4JZ	0SU909Z	0SUA09Z	0SUR09Z
Hip, LT	0SP[E,S]4JZ	0SUB09Z	0SUE09Z	0SUS09Z

Knee Procedures

Open Removal of Knee Liner with Synthetic Substitute Replacement

Removal of Liner		Code also as appropriate Replacement by Type of Synthetic Substitute						
		Oxidized Zircon on Poly	Synthetic Substitute	Medial Unicondylar	Lateral Unicondylar	Patello-femoral	Femoral Surface	Tibial Surface
Knee, RT	0SPC09Z	0SRC06[9,A,Z]	0SRC0J[9,A,Z]	0SRC0L[9,A,Z]	0SRC0M[9,A,Z]	0SRC0N[9,A,Z]	0SRT0J[9,A,Z]	0SRV0J[9,A,Z]
Knee, LT	0SPD09Z	0SRD06[9,A,Z]	0SRD0J[9,A,Z]	0SRD0L[9,A,Z]	0SRD0M[9,A,Z]	0SRD0N[9,A,Z]	0SRU0J[9,A,Z]	0SRW0J[9,A,Z]

Open Removal of Patellar Surface of Knee with Synthetic Substitute Replacement

Removal of Patellar Surface		Code also as appropriate Replacement by Type of Synthetic Substitute	
		Femoral Surface	Tibial Surface
Knee, RT	0SPC0JC	0SRT0J[9,A]	0SRV0J[9,A]
Knee, LT	0SPD0JC	0SRU0J[9,A]	0SRW0J[9,A,Z]

Open Removal of Knee Synthetic Substitute with Synthetic Substitute Replacement

Removal of Synthetic Substitute		Code also as appropriate Replacement by Type of Synthetic Substitute	
		Femoral Surface	Tibial Surface
Knee, RT	ØSPCØJZ	ØSRTØJ[9,A]	ØSRVØJ[9,A]
Knee, LT	ØSPDØJZ	ØSRUØJ[9,A]	ØSRWØJ[9,A,Z]

Open Removal of Knee Medial/Lateral Unicondylar Device with Synthetic Substitute Replacement

Removal of Medial/Lateral Unicondylar Device		Code also as appropriate Replacement by Type of Synthetic Substitute	
		Femoral Surface	Tibial Surface
Knee, Medial Unicondylar, RT	ØSPCØLZ	ØSRTØJ[9,A]	ØSRVØJ[9,A]
Knee, Medial Unicondylar, LT	ØSPDØLZ	ØSRUØJ[9,A]	ØSRWØJ[9,A,Z]
Knee, Lateral Unicondylar, RT	ØSPCØMZ	ØSRTØJ[9,A]	ØSRVØJ[9,A]
Knee, Lateral Unicondylar, LT	ØSPDØMZ	ØSRUØJ[9,A]	ØSRWØJ[9,A,Z]

Open Removal of Knee Patellofemoral Device with Synthetic Substitute Replacement

Removal of Patellofemoral Device		Code also as appropriate Replacement by Type of Synthetic Substitute	
		Femoral Surface	Tibial Surface
Knee, RT	ØSPCØNZ	ØSRTØJ[9,A]	ØSRVØJ[9,A]
Knee, LT	ØSPDØNZ	ØSRUØJ[9,A]	ØSRWØJ[9,A,Z]

Open Removal of Femoral/Tibial Surface of Knee with Synthetic Substitute Replacement

Removal of Femoral/Tibial Surface		Code also as appropriate Replacement by Type of Synthetic Substitute	
		Femoral Surface	Tibial Surface
Knee, RT	ØSP[T,V]ØJZ	ØSRTØJ[9,A]	ØSRVØJ[9,A]
Knee, LT	ØSP[U,W]ØJZ	ØSRUØJ[9,A]	ØSRWØJ[9,A,Z]

Percutaneous Endoscopic Removal of Patellar Surface of Knee with Synthetic Substitute Replacement

Removal of Patellar Surface		Code also as appropriate Replacement by Type of Synthetic Substitute	
		Femoral Surface	Tibial Surface
Knee, RT	ØSPC4JC	ØSRTØJ[9,A]	ØSRVØJ[9,A]
Knee, LT	ØSPD4JC	ØSRUØJ[9,A]	ØSRWØJ[9,A,Z]

Percutaneous Endoscopic Removal of Knee Synthetic Substitute with Synthetic Substitute Replacement

Removal of Synthetic Substitute		Code also as appropriate Replacement by Type of Synthetic Substitute	
		Femoral Surface	Tibial Surface
Knee, RT	ØSPC4JZ	ØSRTØJ[9,A]	ØSRVØJ[9,A]
Knee, LT	ØSPD4JZ	ØSRUØJ[9,A]	ØSRWØJ[9,A,Z]

Percutaneous Endoscopic Removal of Knee Medial/Lateral Unicondylar Device with Synthetic Substitute Replacement

Removal of Medial/Lateral Unicondylar Device		Code also as appropriate Replacement by Type of Synthetic Substitute	
		Femoral Surface	**Tibial Surface**
Knee, Medial Unicondylar, RT	ØSPC4LZ	ØSRTØJ[9,A]	ØSRVØJ[9,A]
Knee, Medial Unicondylar, LT	ØSPD4LZ	ØSRUØJ[9,A]	ØSRWØJ[9,A,Z]
Knee, Lateral Unicondylar, RT	ØSPC4MZ	ØSRTØJ[9,A]	ØSRVØJ[9,A]
Knee, Lateral Unicondylar, LT	ØSPD4MZ	ØSRUØJ[9,A]	ØSRWØJ[9,A,Z]

Percutaneous Endoscopic Removal of Knee Patellofemoral Device with Synthetic Substitute Replacement

Removal of Patellofemoral Device		Code also as appropriate Replacement by Type of Synthetic Substitute	
		Femoral Surface	**Tibial Surface**
Knee, RT	ØSPC4NZ	ØSRTØJ[9,A]	ØSRVØJ[9,A]
Knee, LT	ØSPD4NZ	ØSRUØJ[9,A]	ØSRWØJ[9,A,Z]

Percutaneous Endoscopic Removal of Femoral/Tibial Surface of Knee with Synthetic Substitute Replacement

Removal of Femoral/Tibial Surface		Code also as appropriate Replacement by Type of Synthetic Substitute	
		Femoral Surface	**Tibial Surface**
Knee, RT	ØSP[T,V]4JZ	ØSRTØJ[9,A]	ØSRVØJ[9,A]
Knee, LT	ØSP[U,W]4JZ	ØSRUØJ[9,A]	ØSRWØJ[9,A,Z]

DRG 662-664 Minor Bladder Procedure

Repair of Bladder	Code also as appropriate Repair of Abdominal Wall	
	with Stoma	**without Stoma**
ØTQB[Ø,3,4]ZZ	ØWQFXZ2	ØWQFXZZ

DRG 665-667 Prostatectomy

Site	Resection by approach				Code also as appropriate Resection of Seminal Vesicles, Bilateral by approach	
	Open	**Percutaneous Endoscopic**	**Via Natural or Artificial Opening**	**Via Natural or Artificial Opening Endoscopic**	**Open**	**Percutaneous Endoscopic**
Prostate	ØVTØØZZ	ØVTØ4ZZ	ØVTØ7ZZ	ØVTØ8ZZ	ØVT3ØZZ	ØVT34ZZ

DRG 7Ø7-7Ø8 Major Male Pelvic Procedures

Site	Resection by approach				Code also as appropriate Resection of Seminal Vesicles, Bilateral by approach	
	Open	**Percutaneous Endoscopic**	**Via Natural or Artificial Opening**	**Via Natural or Artificial Opening Endoscopic**	**Open**	**Percutaneous Endoscopic**
Prostate	ØVTØØZZ	ØVTØ4ZZ	ØVTØ7ZZ	ØVTØ8ZZ	ØVT3ØZZ	ØVT34ZZ

DRG 734-735 Pelvic Evisceration, Radical Hysterectomy and Radical Vulvectomy

Pelvic Evisceration

Resection by Site						
Bladder	**Cervix**	**Fallopian Tubes, Bilateral**	**Ovaries, Bilateral**	**Urethra**	**Uterus**	**Vagina**
ØTTBØZZ	ØUTCØZZ	ØUT7ØZZ	ØUT2ØZZ	ØTTDØZZ	ØUT9ØZZ	ØUTGØZZ

Radical Hysterectomy

Approach	Resection by Site		
	Cervix	**Uterus**	**Uterine Support Structure**
Vaginal	ØUTC[7,8]ZZ	ØUT9[7,8]ZZ	ØUT4[7,8]ZZ
Abdominal, Endoscopic	ØUTC4ZZ	ØUT9[4,F]ZZ	ØUT44ZZ
Abdominal, Open	ØUTCØZZ	ØUT9ØZZ	ØUT4ØZZ

Radical Vulvectomy

Resection by Site	Code also as appropriate Excision of Inguinal Lymph Nodes by Approach	
Vulva	**Right**	**Left**
ØUTM[Ø,X]ZZ	Ø7BH[Ø,4]ZZ	Ø7BJ[Ø,4]ZZ

Non-OR procedure combinations

Note: The following table identifies procedure combinations that are considered Non-OR even though one or more procedures of the combination are considered valid DRG OR procedures

Insertion With Removal of Intraluminal Device

Code as appropriate Insertion of Intraluminal Device into Hepatobiliary Duct	Code also as appropriate Removal of Intraluminal Device by Approach and Site			
	Via Natural or Artificial Opening		External	
	Hepatobiliary Duct	**Pancreatic Duct**	**Hepatobiliary Duct**	**Pancreatic Duct**
ØFHB7DZ	ØFPB[7,8]DZ	ØFPD[7,8]DZ	ØFPBXDZ	ØFPDXDZ

Using the ICD-10-PCS tables construct the code that accurately represents the procedure performed.

Medical Surgical Section

Procedure	Code
1. Excision of malignant melanoma from skin of right ear	
2. Laparoscopy with excision of endometrial implant from left ovary	
3. Percutaneous needle core biopsy of right kidney	
4. EGD with gastric biopsy	
5. Open endarterectomy of left common carotid artery	
6. Excision of basal cell carcinoma of lower lip	
7. Open excision of tail of pancreas	
8. Percutaneous biopsy of right gastrocnemius muscle	
9. Sigmoidoscopy with sigmoid polypectomy	
10. Open excision of lesion from right Achilles tendon	
11. Open resection of cecum	
12. Total excision of pituitary gland, open	
13. Explantation of left failed kidney, open	
14. Open left axillary total lymphadenectomy	
15. Laparoscopic-assisted vaginal hysterectomy	
16. Right total mastectomy, open	
17. Open resection of papillary muscle	
18. Total retropubic prostatectomy, open	
19. Laparoscopic cholecystectomy	
20. Endoscopic bilateral total maxillary sinusectomy	
21. Amputation at right elbow level	
22. Right below-knee amputation, proximal tibia/fibula	
23. Fifth ray carpometacarpal joint amputation, left hand	
24. Right leg and hip amputation through ischium	
25. DIP joint amputation of right thumb	
26. Right wrist joint amputation	
27. Trans-metatarsal amputation of foot at left big toe	
28. Mid-shaft amputation, right humerus	
29. Left fourth toe amputation, mid-proximal phalanx	
30. Right above-knee amputation, distal femur	
31. Cryotherapy of wart on left hand	
32. Percutaneous radiofrequency ablation of right vocal cord lesion	
33. Left heart catheterization with laser destruction of arrhythmogenic focus, A-V node	
34. Cautery of nosebleed	
35. Transurethral endoscopic laser ablation of prostate	
36. Percutaneous cautery of oozing varicose vein, left calf	

Procedure	Code
37. Laparoscopy with destruction of endometriosis, bilateral ovaries	
38. Laser coagulation of right retinal vessel hemorrhage, percutaneous	
39. Thoracoscopic pleurodesis, left side	
40. Percutaneous insertion of Greenfield IVC filter	
41. Forceps total mouth extraction, upper and lower teeth	
42. Removal of left thumbnail	
43. Extraction of right intraocular lens without replacement, percutaneous	
44. Laparoscopy with needle aspiration of ova for in vitro fertilization	
45. Nonexcisional debridement of skin ulcer, right foot	
46. Open stripping of abdominal fascia, right side	
47. Hysteroscopy with D&C, diagnostic	
48. Liposuction for medical purposes, left upper arm	
49. Removal of tattered right ear drum fragments with tweezers	
50. Microincisional phlebectomy of spider veins, right lower leg	
51. Routine Foley catheter placement	
52. Incision and drainage of external anal abscess	
53. Percutaneous drainage of ascites	
54. Laparoscopy with left ovarian cystotomy and drainage	
55. Laparotomy and drain placement for liver abscess, right lobe	
56. Right knee arthrotomy with drain placement	
57. Thoracentesis of left pleural effusion	
58. Phlebotomy of left median cubital vein for polycythemia vera	
59. Percutaneous chest tube placement for right pneumothorax	
60. Endoscopic drainage of left ethmoid sinus	
61. External ventricular CSF drainage catheter placement via burr hole	
62. Removal of foreign body, right cornea	
63. Percutaneous mechanical thrombectomy, left brachial artery	
64. Esophagogastroscopy with removal of bezoar from stomach	
65. Foreign body removal, skin of left thumb	
66. Transurethral cystoscopy with removal of bladder stone	
67. Forceps removal of foreign body in right nostril	
68. Laparoscopy with excision of old suture from mesentery	
69. Incision and removal of right lacrimal duct stone	
70. Nonincisional removal of intraluminal foreign body from vagina	
71. Right common carotid endarterectomy, open	
72. Open excision of retained sliver, subcutaneous tissue of left foot	
73. Extracorporeal shockwave lithotripsy (ESWL), bilateral ureters	

Procedure	Code
74. Endoscopic retrograde cholangiopancreatography (ERCP) with lithotripsy of common bile duct stone	
75. Thoracotomy with crushing of pericardial calcifications	
76. Transurethral cystoscopy with fragmentation of bladder calculus	
77. Hysteroscopy with intraluminal lithotripsy of left fallopian tube calcification	
78. Division of right foot tendon, percutaneous	
79. Left heart catheterization with division of bundle of HIS	
80. Open osteotomy of capitate, left hand	
81. EGD with esophagotomy of esophagogastric junction	
82. Sacral rhizotomy for pain control, percutaneous	
83. Laparotomy with exploration and adhesiolysis of right ureter	
84. Incision of scar contracture, right elbow	
85. Frenulotomy for treatment of tongue-tie syndrome	
86. Right shoulder arthroscopy with coracoacromial ligament release	
87. Mitral valvulotomy for release of fused leaflets, open approach	
88. Percutaneous left Achilles tendon release	
89. Laparoscopy with lysis of peritoneal adhesions	
90. Manual rupture of right shoulder joint adhesions under general anesthesia	
91. Open posterior tarsal tunnel release	
92. Laparoscopy with freeing of left ovary and fallopian tube	
93. Liver transplant with donor matched liver	
94. Orthotopic heart transplant using porcine heart	
95. Right lung transplant, open, using organ donor match	
96. Transplant of large intestine, organ donor match	
97. Left kidney/pancreas organ bank transplant	
98. Replantation of avulsed scalp	
99. Reattachment of severed right ear	
100. Reattachment of traumatic left gastrocnemius avulsion, open	
101. Closed replantation of three avulsed teeth, lower jaw	
102. Reattachment of severed left hand	
103. Right open palmaris longus tendon transfer	
104. Endoscopic radial to median nerve transfer	
105. Fasciocutaneous flap closure of left thigh, open	
106. Transfer left index finger to left thumb position, open	
107. Percutaneous fascia transfer to fill defect, right neck	
108. Trigeminal to facial nerve transfer, percutaneous endoscopic	
109. Endoscopic left leg flexor hallucis longus tendon transfer	
110. Right scalp advancement flap to right temple	

Procedure	Code
111. Bilateral TRAM pedicle flap reconstruction status post mastectomy, muscle only, open	
112. Skin transfer flap closure of complex open wound, left lower back	
113. Open fracture reduction, right tibia	
114. Laparoscopy with gastropexy for malrotation	
115. Left knee arthroscopy with reposition of anterior cruciate ligament	
116. Open transposition of ulnar nerve	
117. Closed reduction with percutaneous internal fixation of right femoral neck fracture	
118. Trans-vaginal intraluminal cervical cerclage	
119. Cervical cerclage using Shirodkar technique	
120. Thoracotomy with banding of left pulmonary artery using extraluminal device	
121. Restriction of thoracic duct with intraluminal stent, percutaneous	
122. Craniotomy with clipping of cerebral aneurysm	
123. Nonincisional, transnasal placement of restrictive stent in right lacrimal duct	
124. Catheter-based temporary restriction of blood flow in abdominal aorta for treatment of cerebral ischemia	
125. Percutaneous ligation of esophageal vein	
126. Percutaneous embolization of left internal carotid-cavernous fistula	
127. Laparoscopy with bilateral occlusion of fallopian tubes using Hulka extraluminal clips	
128. Open suture ligation of failed AV graft, left brachial artery	
129. Percutaneous embolization of vascular supply, intracranial meningioma	
130. Percutaneous embolization of right uterine artery, using coils	
131. Open occlusion of left atrial appendage, using extraluminal pressure clips	
132. Percutaneous suture exclusion of left atrial appendage, via femoral artery access	
133. ERCP with balloon dilation of common bile duct	
134. PTCA of two coronary arteries, LAD with stent placement, RCA with no stent	
135. Cystoscopy with intraluminal dilation of bladder neck stricture	
136. Open dilation of old anastomosis, left femoral artery	
137. Dilation of upper esophageal stricture, direct visualization, with Bougie sound	
138. PTA of right brachial artery stenosis	
139. Transnasal dilation and stent placement in right lacrimal duct	
140. Hysteroscopy with balloon dilation of bilateral fallopian tubes	
141. Tracheoscopy with intraluminal dilation of tracheal stenosis	
142. Cystoscopy with dilation of left ureteral stricture, with stent placement	
143. Open gastric bypass with Roux-en-Y limb to jejunum	
144. Right temporal artery to intracranial artery bypass using Gore-Tex graft, open	

Procedure	Code
145. Tracheostomy formation with tracheostomy tube placement, percutaneous	
146. PICVA (percutaneous in situ coronary venous arterialization) of single coronary artery	
147. Open left femoral-popliteal artery bypass using cadaver vein graft	
148. Shunting of intrathecal cerebrospinal fluid to peritoneal cavity using synthetic shunt	
149. Colostomy formation, open, transverse colon to abdominal wall	
150. Open urinary diversion, left ureter, using ileal conduit to skin	
151. CABG of LAD using pedicled left internal mammary artery, open off-bypass	
152. Open pleuroperitoneal shunt, right pleural cavity, using synthetic device	
153. Percutaneous placement of ventriculoperitoneal shunt for treatment of hydrocephalus	
154. End-of-life replacement of spinal neurostimulator generator, multiple array, in lower abdomen	
155. Percutaneous insertion of spinal neurostimulator lead, lumbar spinal cord	
156. Percutaneous replacement of broken pacemaker lead in left atrium	
157. Open placement of dual chamber pacemaker generator in chest wall	
158. Percutaneous placement of venous central line in right internal jugular, with tip in superior vena cava	
159. Open insertion of multiple channel cochlear implant, left ear	
160. Percutaneous placement of Swan-Ganz catheter in pulmonary trunk	
161. Bronchoscopy with insertion of Low Dose, Pd-103 brachytherapy seeds, right lung	
162. Open insertion of interspinous process device into lumbar vertebral joint	
163. Open placement of bone growth stimulator, left femoral shaft	
164. Cystoscopy with placement of brachytherapy seeds in prostate gland	
165. Percutaneous insertion of Greenfield IVC filter	
166. Full-thickness skin graft to right lower arm, autograft (do not code graft harvest for this exercise)	
167. Excision of necrosed left femoral head with bone bank bone graft to fill the defect, open	
168. Penetrating keratoplasty of right cornea with donor matched cornea, percutaneous approach	
169. Excision of abdominal aorta with Gore-Tex graft replacement, open	
170. Total right knee arthroplasty with insertion of total knee prosthesis	
171. Tenonectomy with graft to right ankle using cadaver graft, open	
172. Mitral valve replacement using porcine valve, open	
173. Percutaneous phacoemulsification of right eye cataract with prosthetic lens insertion	
174. Transcatheter replacement of pulmonary valve using of bovine jugular vein valve	

Procedure	Code
175. Total left hip replacement using ceramic on ceramic prosthesis, without bone cement	
176. Aortic valve annuloplasty using ring, open	
177. Laparoscopic repair of left inguinal hernia with marlex plug	
178. Autograft nerve graft to right median nerve, percutaneous endoscopic (do not code graft harvest for this exercise)	
179. Exchange of liner in femoral component of previous left hip replacement, open approach	
180. Anterior colporrhaphy with polypropylene mesh reinforcement, open approach	
181. Implantation of CorCap cardiac support device, open approach	
182. Abdominal wall herniorrhaphy, open, using synthetic mesh	
183. Tendon graft to strengthen injured left shoulder using autograft, open (do not code graft harvest for this exercise)	
184. Onlay lamellar keratoplasty of left cornea using autograft, external approach	
185. Resurfacing procedure on right femoral head, open approach	
186. Exchange of drainage tube from right hip joint	
187. Tracheostomy tube exchange	
188. Change chest tube for left pneumothorax	
189. Exchange of cerebral ventriculostomy drainage tube	
190. Foley urinary catheter exchange	
191. Open removal of lumbar sympathetic neurostimulator lead	
192. Nonincisional removal of Swan-Ganz catheter from right pulmonary artery	
193. Laparotomy with removal of pancreatic drain	
194. Extubation, endotracheal tube	
195. Nonincisional PEG tube removal	
196. Transvaginal removal of brachytherapy seeds	
197. Transvaginal removal of extraluminal cervical cerclage	
198. Incision with removal of K-wire fixation, right first metatarsal	
199. Cystoscopy with retrieval of left ureteral stent	
200. Removal of nasogastric drainage tube for decompression	
201. Removal of external fixator, left radial fracture	
202. Trimming and reanastomosis of stenosed femorofemoral synthetic bypass graft, open	
203. Open revision of right hip replacement, with readjustment of prosthesis	
204. Adjustment of position, pacemaker lead in left ventricle, percutaneous	
205. External repositioning of Foley catheter to bladder	
206. Taking out loose screw and putting larger screw in fracture repair plate, left tibia	
207. Revision of totally implantable VAD port placement in chest wall, causing patient discomfort, open	
208. Thoracotomy with exploration of right pleural cavity	
209. Diagnostic laryngoscopy	

Procedure	Code
210. Exploratory arthrotomy of left knee	
211. Colposcopy with diagnostic hysteroscopy	
212. Digital rectal exam	
213. Diagnostic arthroscopy of right shoulder	
214. Endoscopy of maxillary sinus	
215. Laparotomy with palpation of liver	
216. Transurethral diagnostic cystoscopy	
217. Colonoscopy, discontinued at sigmoid colon	
218. Percutaneous mapping of basal ganglia	
219. Heart catheterization with cardiac mapping	
220. Intraoperative whole brain mapping via craniotomy	
221. Mapping of left cerebral hemisphere, percutaneous endoscopic	
222. Intraoperative cardiac mapping during open heart surgery	
223. Hysteroscopy with cautery of post-hysterectomy oozing and evacuation of clot	
224. Open exploration and ligation of post-op arterial bleeder, left forearm	
225. Control of post-operative retroperitoneal bleeding via laparotomy	
226. Reopening of thoracotomy site with drainage and control of post-op hemopericardium	
227. Arthroscopy with drainage of hemarthrosis at previous operative site, right knee	
228. Radiocarpal fusion of left hand with internal fixation, open	
229. Posterior approach spinal fusion at L1-L3 level with BAK cage interbody fusion device, open	
230. Intercarpal fusion of right hand with bone bank bone graft, open	
231. Sacrococcygeal fusion with bone graft from same operative site, open	
232. Interphalangeal fusion of left great toe, percutaneous pin fixation	
233. Suture repair of left radial nerve laceration	
234. Laparotomy with suture repair of blunt force duodenal laceration	
235. Perineoplasty with repair of old obstetric laceration, open	
236. Suture repair of right biceps tendon (upper arm) laceration, open	
237. Closure of abdominal wall stab wound	
238. Cosmetic face lift, open, no other information available	
239. Bilateral breast augmentation with silicone implants, open	
240. Cosmetic rhinoplasty with septal reduction and tip elevation using local tissue graft, open	
241. Abdominoplasty (tummy tuck), open	
242. Liposuction of bilateral thighs	
243. Creation of penis in female patient using tissue bank donor graft	
244. Creation of vagina in male patient using synthetic material	
245. Laparoscopic vertical (sleeve) gastrectomy	
246. Left uterine artery embolization with intraluminal biosphere injection	

Obstetrics

Procedure	Code
1. Abortion by dilation and evacuation following laminaria insertion	
2. Manually assisted spontaneous abortion	
3. Abortion by abortifacient insertion	
4. Bimanual pregnancy examination	
5. Extraperitoneal C-section, low transverse incision	
6. Fetal spinal tap, percutaneous	
7. Fetal kidney transplant, laparoscopic	
8. Open in utero repair of congenital diaphragmatic hernia	
9. Laparoscopy with total excision of tubal pregnancy	
10. Transvaginal removal of fetal monitoring electrode	

Placement

Procedure	Code
1. Placement of packing material, right ear	
2. Mechanical traction of entire left leg	
3. Removal of splint, right shoulder	
4. Placement of neck brace	
5. Change of vaginal packing	
6. Packing of wound, chest wall	
7. Sterile dressing placement to left groin region	
8. Removal of packing material from pharynx	
9. Placement of intermittent pneumatic compression device, covering entire right arm	
10. Exchange of pressure dressing to left thigh	

Administration

Procedure	Code
1. Peritoneal dialysis via indwelling catheter	
2. Transvaginal artificial insemination	
3. Infusion of total parenteral nutrition via central venous catheter	
4. Esophagogastroscopy with Botox injection into esophageal sphincter	
5. Percutaneous irrigation of knee joint	
6. Systemic infusion of recombinant tissue plasminogen activator (r-tPA) via peripheral venous catheter	
7. Transabdominal in vitro fertilization, implantation of donor ovum	
8. Autologous bone marrow transplant via central venous line	
9. Implantation of anti-microbial envelope with cardiac defibrillator placement, open	
10. Sclerotherapy of brachial plexus lesion, alcohol injection	
11. Percutaneous peripheral vein injection, glucarpidase	
12. Introduction of anti-infective envelope into subcutaneous tissue, open	

Measurement and Monitoring

Procedure	Code
1. Cardiac stress test, single measurement	
2. EGD with biliary flow measurement	
3. Right and left heart cardiac catheterization with bilateral sampling and pressure measurements	
4. Temperature monitoring, rectal	
5. Peripheral venous pulse, external, single measurement	
6. Holter monitoring	
7. Respiratory rate, external, single measurement	
8. Fetal heart rate monitoring, transvaginal	
9. Visual mobility test, single measurement	
10. Left ventricular cardiac output monitoring from pulmonary artery wedge (Swan-Ganz) catheter	
11. Olfactory acuity test, single measurement	

Extracorporeal or Systemic Assistance and Performance

Procedure	Code
1. Intermittent mechanical ventilation, 16 hours	
2. Liver dialysis, single encounter	
3. Cardiac countershock with successful conversion to sinus rhythm	
4. IPPB (intermittent positive pressure breathing) for mobilization of secretions, 22 hours	
5. Renal dialysis, 12 hours	
6. IABP (intra-aortic balloon pump) continuous	
7. Intra-operative cardiac pacing, continuous	
8. Intraoperative ECMO (extracorporeal membrane oxygenation), central	
9. Controlled mechanical ventilation (CMV), 45 hours	
10. Pulsatile compression boot with intermittent inflation	

Extracorporeal or Systemic Therapies

Procedure	Code
1. Donor thrombocytapheresis, single encounter	
2. Bili-lite phototherapy, series treatment	
3. Whole body hypothermia, single treatment	
4. Circulatory phototherapy, single encounter	
5. Shock wave therapy of plantar fascia, single treatment	
6. Antigen-free air conditioning, series treatment	
7. TMS (transcranial magnetic stimulation), series treatment	
8. Therapeutic ultrasound of peripheral vessels, single treatment	
9. Plasmapheresis, series treatment	
10. Extracorporeal electromagnetic stimulation (EMS) for urinary incontinence, single treatment	

Osteopathic

Procedure	Code
1. Isotonic muscle energy treatment of right leg	
2. Low velocity-high amplitude osteopathic treatment of head	
3. Lymphatic pump osteopathic treatment of left axilla	
4. Indirect osteopathic treatment of sacrum	
5. Articulatory osteopathic treatment of cervical region	

Other Procedures

Procedure	Code
1. Near infrared spectroscopy of leg vessels	
2. CT computer assisted sinus surgery	
3. Suture removal, abdominal wall	
4. Isolation after infectious disease exposure	
5. Robotic assisted open prostatectomy	
6. In vitro fertilization	

Chiropractic

Procedure	Code
1. Chiropractic treatment of lumbar region using long lever specific contact	
2. Chiropractic manipulation of abdominal region, indirect visceral	
3. Chiropractic extra-articular treatment of hip region	
4. Chiropractic treatment of sacrum using long and short lever specific contact	
5. Mechanically-assisted chiropractic manipulation of head	

Imaging

Procedure	Code
1. Noncontrast CT of abdomen and pelvis	
2. Intravascular ultrasound, left subclavian artery	
3. Fluoroscopic guidance for insertion of central venous catheter in SVC, low osmolar contrast	
4. Chest x-ray, AP/PA and lateral views	
5. Endoluminal ultrasound of gallbladder and bile ducts	
6. MRI of thyroid gland, contrast unspecified	
7. Esophageal videofluoroscopy study with oral barium contrast	
8. Portable x-ray study of right radius/ulna shaft, standard series	
9. Routine fetal ultrasound, second trimester twin gestation	
10. CT scan of bilateral lungs, high osmolar contrast with densitometry	
11. Fluoroscopic guidance for percutaneous transluminal angioplasty (PTA) of left common femoral artery, low osmolar contrast	

Nuclear Medicine

Procedure	Code
1. Tomo scan of right and left heart, unspecified radiopharmaceutical, qualitative gated rest	
2. Technetium pentetate assay of kidneys, ureters, and bladder	
3. Uniplanar scan of spine using technetium oxidronate, with first-pass study	
4. Thallous chloride tomographic scan of bilateral breasts	
5. PET scan of myocardium using rubidium	
6. Gallium citrate scan of head and neck, single plane imaging	
7. Xenon gas nonimaging probe of brain	
8. Upper GI scan, radiopharmaceutical unspecified, for gastric emptying	
9. Carbon 11 PET scan of brain with quantification	
10. Iodinated albumin nuclear medicine assay, blood plasma volume study	

Radiation Therapy

Procedure	Code
1. Plaque radiation of left eye, single port	
2. 8 MeV photon beam radiation to brain	
3. IORT of colon, 3 ports	
4. HDR brachytherapy of prostate using low dose palladium-103, unidirectional source	
5. Electron radiation treatment of right breast, with custom device	
6. Hyperthermia oncology treatment of pelvic region	
7. Contact radiation of tongue	
8. Heavy particle radiation treatment of pancreas, four risk sites	
9. LDR brachytherapy to spinal cord using iodine	
10. Whole body Phosphorus 32 administration with risk to hematopoetic system	

Physical Rehabilitation and Diagnostic Audiology

Procedure	Code
1. Bekesy assessment using audiometer	
2. Individual fitting of left eye prosthesis	
3. Physical therapy for range of motion and mobility, patient right hip, no special equipment	
4. Bedside swallow assessment using assessment kit	
5. Caregiver training in airway clearance techniques	
6. Application of short arm cast in rehabilitation setting	
7. Verbal assessment of patient's pain level	
8. Caregiver training in communication skills using manual communication board	
9. Group musculoskeletal balance training exercises, whole body, no special equipment	
10. Individual therapy for auditory processing using tape recorder	

Mental Health

Procedure	Code
1. Cognitive-behavioral psychotherapy, individual	
2. Narcosynthesis	
3. Light therapy	
4. ECT (electroconvulsive therapy), unilateral, multiple seizure	
5. Crisis intervention	
6. Neuropsychological testing	
7. Hypnosis	
8. Developmental testing	
9. Vocational counseling	
10. Family psychotherapy	

Substance Abuse Treatment

Procedure	Code
1. Naltrexone treatment for drug dependency	
2. Substance abuse treatment family counseling	
3. Medication monitoring of patient on methadone maintenance	
4. Individual interpersonal psychotherapy for drug abuse	
5. Patient in for alcohol detoxification treatment	
6. Group motivational counseling	
7. Individual 12-step psychotherapy for substance abuse	
8. Post-test infectious disease counseling for IV drug abuser	
9. Psychodynamic psychotherapy for drug dependent patient	
10. Group cognitive-behavioral counseling for substance abuse	

New Technology

Procedure	Code
1. Infusion of ceftazidime via peripheral venous catheter	
2. Transcatheter dilation of left peroneal artery with 2 SAVAL stents	

Answers to Coding Exercises

Medical Surgical Section

	Procedure	Code
1.	Excision of malignant melanoma from skin of right ear	0HB2XZZ
2.	Laparoscopy with excision of endometrial implant from left ovary	0UB14ZZ
3.	Percutaneous needle core biopsy of right kidney	0TB03ZX
4.	EGD with gastric biopsy	0DB68ZX
5.	Open endarterectomy of left common carotid artery	03CJ0ZZ
6.	Excision of basal cell carcinoma of lower lip	0CB1XZZ
7.	Open excision of tail of pancreas	0FBG0ZZ
8.	Percutaneous biopsy of right gastrocnemius muscle	0KBS3ZX
9.	Sigmoidoscopy with sigmoid polypectomy	0DBN8ZZ
10.	Open excision of lesion from right Achilles tendon	0LBN0ZZ
11.	Open resection of cecum	0DTH0ZZ
12.	Total excision of pituitary gland, open	0GT00ZZ
13.	Explantation of left failed kidney, open	0TT10ZZ
14.	Open left axillary total lymphadenectomy	07T60ZZ (RESECTION is coded for cutting out a chain of lymph nodes.)
15.	Laparoscopic-assisted vaginal hysterectomy	0UT9FZZ
16.	Right total mastectomy, open	0HTT0ZZ
17.	Open resection of papillary muscle	02TD0ZZ (The papillary muscle refers to the heart and is found in the *Heart and Great Vessels* body system.)
18.	Total retropubic prostatectomy, open	0VT00ZZ
19.	Laparoscopic cholecystectomy	0FT44ZZ
20.	Endoscopic bilateral total maxillary sinusectomy	09TQ8ZZ, 09TR8ZZ
21.	Amputation at right elbow level	0X6B0ZZ
22.	Right below-knee amputation, proximal tibia/fibula	0Y6H0Z1 (The qualifier *High* here means the portion of the tib/fib closest to the knee.)
23.	Fifth ray carpometacarpal joint amputation, left hand	0X6K0Z8 (A *complete* ray amputation is through the carpometacarpal joint.)
24.	Right leg and hip amputation through ischium	0Y620ZZ (The *Hindquarter* body part includes amputation along any part of the hip bone.)
25.	DIP joint amputation of right thumb	0X6L0Z3 (The qualifier *low* here means through the distal interphalangeal joint.)
26.	Right wrist joint amputation	0X6J0Z0 (Amputation at the wrist joint is actually complete amputation of the hand.)
27.	Trans-metatarsal amputation of foot at left big toe	0Y6N0Z9 (A *partial* amputation is through the shaft of the metatarsal bone.)
28.	Mid-shaft amputation, right humerus	0X680Z2
29.	Left fourth toe amputation, mid-proximal phalanx	0Y6W0Z1 (The qualifier *High* here means anywhere along the proximal phalanx.)
30.	Right above-knee amputation, distal femur	0Y6C0Z3
31.	Cryotherapy of wart on left hand	0H5GXZZ
32.	Percutaneous radiofrequency ablation of right vocal cord lesion	0C5T3ZZ
33.	Left heart catheterization with laser destruction of arrhythmogenic focus, A-V node	02583ZZ
34.	Cautery of nosebleed	095KXZZ
35.	Transurethral endoscopic laser ablation of prostate	0V508ZZ
36.	Percutaneous cautery of oozing varicose vein, left calf	065Y3ZZ
37.	Laparoscopy with destruction of endometriosis, bilateral ovaries	0U524ZZ
38.	Laser coagulation of right retinal vessel hemorrhage, percutaneous	085G3ZZ (The *Retinal Vessel* body-part values are in the *Eye* body system.)
39.	Thoracoscopic pleurodesis, left side	0B5P4ZZ
40.	Percutaneous insertion of Greenfield IVC filter	06H03DZ
41.	Forceps total mouth extraction, upper and lower teeth	0CDWXZ2, 0CDXXZ2
42.	Removal of left thumbnail	0HDQXZZ (No separate body-part value is given for thumbnail, so this is coded to *Fingernail*.)
43.	Extraction of right intraocular lens without replacement, percutaneous	08DJ3ZZ
44.	Laparoscopy with needle aspiration of ova for in vitro fertilization	0UDN4ZZ
45.	Nonexcisional debridement of skin ulcer, right foot	0HDMXZZ
46.	Open stripping of abdominal fascia, right side	0JD80ZZ
47.	Hysteroscopy with D&C, diagnostic	0UDB8ZX
48.	Liposuction for medical purposes, left upper arm	0JDF3ZZ (The *Percutaneous* approach is inherent in the liposuction technique.)
49.	Removal of tattered right ear drum fragments with tweezers	09D77ZZ
50.	Microincisional phlebectomy of spider veins, right lower leg	06DY3ZZ
51.	Routine Foley catheter placement	0T9B70Z
52.	Incision and drainage of external anal abscess	0D9QXZZ
53.	Percutaneous drainage of ascites	0W9G3ZZ (This is drainage of the cavity and not the peritoneal membrane itself.)
54.	Laparoscopy with left ovarian cystotomy and drainage	0U914ZZ
55.	Laparotomy and drain placement for liver abscess, right lobe	0F9100Z
56.	Right knee arthrotomy with drain placement	0S9C00Z
57.	Thoracentesis of left pleural effusion	0W9B3ZZ (This is drainage of the pleural cavity)
58.	Phlebotomy of left median cubital vein for polycythemia vera	059C3ZZ (The median cubital vein is a branch of the basilic vein)

Procedure	Code		Procedure	Code
59. Percutaneous chest tube placement for right pneumothorax	0W9930Z		84. Incision of scar contracture, right elbow	0HNDXZZ (The skin of the elbow region is coded to *Lower Arm*.)
60. Endoscopic drainage of left ethmoid sinus	099V4ZZ		85. Frenulotomy for treatment of tongue-tie syndrome	0CN7XZZ (The frenulum is coded to the body-part value *Tongue*.)
61. External ventricular CSF drainage catheter placement via burr hole	009630Z		86. Right shoulder arthroscopy with coracoacromial ligament release	0MN14ZZ
62. Removal of foreign body, right cornea	08C8XZZ		87. Mitral valvulotomy for release of fused leaflets, open approach	02NG0ZZ
63. Percutaneous mechanical thrombectomy, left brachial artery	03C83ZZ		88. Percutaneous left Achilles tendon release	0LNP3ZZ
64. Esophagogastroscopy with removal of bezoar from stomach	0DC68ZZ		89. Laparoscopy with lysis of peritoneal adhesions	0DNW4ZZ
65. Foreign body removal, skin of left thumb	0HCGXZZ (There is no specific value for thumb skin, so the procedure is coded to *Hand*.)		90. Manual rupture of right shoulder joint adhesions under general anesthesia	0RNJXZZ
66. Transurethral cystoscopy with removal of bladder stone	0TCB8ZZ		91. Open posterior tarsal tunnel release	01NG0ZZ (The nerve released in the posterior tarsal tunnel is the tibial nerve.)
67. Forceps removal of foreign body in right nostril	09CKXZZ (Nostril is coded to the *Nasal muscosa and soft tissue* body-part value.)		92. Laparoscopy with freeing of left ovary and fallopian tube	0UN14ZZ, 0UN64ZZ
68. Laparoscopy with excision of old suture from mesentery	0DCV4ZZ		93. Liver transplant with donor matched liver	0FY00Z0
69. Incision and removal of right lacrimal duct stone	08CX0ZZ		94. Orthotopic heart transplant using porcine heart	02YA0Z2 (The donor heart comes from an animal [pig], so the qualifier value is *Zooplastic.*)
70. Nonincisional removal of intraluminal foreign body from vagina	0UCG7ZZ (The approach *External* is also a possibility. It is assumed here that since the patient went to the doctor to have the object removed, that it was not in the vaginal orifice.)		95. Right lung transplant, open, using organ donor match	0BYK0Z0
			96. Transplant of large intestine, organ donor match	0DYE0Z0
			97. Left kidney/pancreas organ bank transplant	0FYG0Z0, 0TY10Z0
			98. Replantation of avulsed scalp	0HM0XZZ
71. Right common carotid endarterectomy, open	03CH0ZZ		99. Reattachment of severed right ear	09M0XZZ
72. Open excision of retained sliver, subcutaneous tissue of left foot	0JCR0ZZ		100. Reattachment of traumatic left gastrocnemius avulsion, open	0KMT0ZZ
73. Extracorporeal shockwave lithotripsy (ESWL), bilateral ureters	0TF6XZZ, 0TF7XZZ (The *Bilateral Ureter* body-part value is not available for the root operation FRAGMENTATION, so the procedures are coded separately.)		101. Closed replantation of three avulsed teeth, lower jaw	0CMXXZ1
			102. Reattachment of severed left hand	0XMK0ZZ
			103. Right open palmaris longus tendon transfer	0LX50ZZ
			104. Endoscopic radial to median nerve transfer	01X64Z5
74. Endoscopic retrograde cholangiopancreatography (ERCP) with lithotripsy of common bile duct stone	0FF98ZZ (ERCP is performed through the mouth to the biliary system via the duodenum, so the approach value is *Via Natural or Artificial Opening Endoscopic*.)		105. Fasciocutaneous flap closure of left thigh, open	0JXM0ZC (The qualifier identifies the body layers in addition to fascia included in the procedure.)
			106. Transfer left index finger to left thumb position, open	0XXP0ZM
			107. Percutaneous fascia transfer to fill defect, right neck	0JX43ZZ
75. Thoracotomy with crushing of pericardial calcifications	02FN0ZZ		108. Trigeminal to facial nerve transfer, percutaneous endoscopic	00XK4ZM
76. Transurethral cystoscopy with fragmentation of bladder calculus	0TFB8ZZ		109. Endoscopic left leg flexor hallucis longus tendon transfer	0LXP4ZZ
77. Hysteroscopy with intraluminal lithotripsy of left fallopian tube calcification	0UF68ZZ		110. Right scalp advancement flap to right temple	0HX0XZZ
78. Division of right foot tendon, percutaneous	0L8V3ZZ		111. Bilateral TRAM pedicle flap reconstruction status post mastectomy, muscle only, open	0KXK0Z6, 0KXL0Z6 (The transverse rectus abdominus muscle (TRAM) flap is coded for each flap developed.)
79. Left heart catheterization with division of bundle of HIS	02883ZZ			
80. Open osteotomy of capitate, left hand	0P8N0ZZ (The capitate is one of the carpal bones of the hand.)			
81. EGD with esophagotomy of esophagogastric junction	0D948ZZ		112. Skin transfer flap closure of complex open wound, left lower back	0HX6XZZ
82. Sacral rhizotomy for pain control, percutaneous	018R3ZZ		113. Open fracture reduction, right tibia	0QSG0ZZ
			114. Laparoscopy with gastropexy for malrotation	0DS64ZZ
83. Laparotomy with exploration and adhesiolysis of right ureter	0TN60ZZ		115. Left knee arthroscopy with reposition of anterior cruciate ligament	0MSP4ZZ

Procedure	Code
116. Open transposition of ulnar nerve	01S40ZZ
117. Closed reduction with percutaneous internal fixation of right femoral neck fracture	0QS634Z
118. Trans-vaginal intraluminal cervical cerclage	0UVC7DZ
119. Cervical cerclage using Shirodkar technique	0UVC7ZZ
120. Thoracotomy with banding of left pulmonary artery using extraluminal device	02VR0CZ
121. Restriction of thoracic duct with intraluminal stent, percutaneous	07VK3DZ
122. Craniotomy with clipping of cerebral aneurysm	03VG0CZ (The clip is placed lengthwise on the outside wall of the widened portion of the vessel.)
123. Nonincisional, transnasal placement of restrictive stent in right lacrimal duct	08VX7DZ
124. Catheter-based temporary restriction of blood flow in abdominal aorta for treatment of cerebral ischemia	04V03DJ
125. Percutaneous ligation of esophageal vein	06L33ZZ
126. Percutaneous embolization of left internal carotid-cavernous fistula	03LL3DZ
127. Laparoscopy with bilateral occlusion of fallopian tubes using Hulka extraluminal clips	0UL74CZ
128. Open suture ligation of failed AV graft, left brachial artery	03L80ZZ
129. Percutaneous embolization of vascular supply, intracranial meningioma	03LG3DZ
130. Percutaneous embolization of right uterine artery, using coils	04LE3DT
131. Open occlusion of left atrial appendage, using extraluminal pressure clips	02L70CK
132. Percutaneous suture exclusion of left atrial appendage, via femoral artery access	02L73ZK
133. ERCP with balloon dilation of common bile duct	0F798ZZ
134. PTCA of two coronary arteries, LAD with stent placement, RCA with no stent	02703DZ, 02703ZZ (A separate procedure is coded for each artery dilated, since the device value differs for each artery.)
135. Cystoscopy with intraluminal dilation of bladder neck stricture	0T7C8ZZ
136. Open dilation of old anastomosis, left femoral artery	047L0ZZ
137. Dilation of upper esophageal stricture, direct visualization, with Bougie sound	0D717ZZ
138. PTA of right brachial artery stenosis	03773ZZ
139. Transnasal dilation and stent placement in right lacrimal duct	087X7DZ
140. Hysteroscopy with balloon dilation of bilateral fallopian tubes	0U778ZZ
141. Tracheoscopy with intraluminal dilation of tracheal stenosis	0B718ZZ
142. Cystoscopy with dilation of left ureteral stricture, with stent placement	0T778DZ
143. Open gastric bypass with Roux-en-Y limb to jejunum	0D160ZA
144. Right temporal artery to intracranial artery bypass using Gore-Tex graft, open	031S0JG
145. Tracheostomy formation with tracheostomy tube placement, percutaneous	0B113F4
146. PICVA (percutaneous in situ coronary venous arterialization) of single coronary artery	02103D4

Procedure	Code
147. Open left femoral-popliteal artery bypass using cadaver vein graft	041L0KL
148. Shunting of intrathecal cerebrospinal fluid to peritoneal cavity using synthetic shunt	00160J6
149. Colostomy formation, open, transverse colon to abdominal wall	0D1L0Z4
150. Open urinary diversion, left ureter, using ileal conduit to skin	0T170ZC
151. CABG of LAD using pedicled left internal mammary artery, open off-bypass	02100Z9
152. Open pleuroperitoneal shunt, right pleural cavity, using synthetic device	0W190JG
153. Percutaneous placement of ventriculoperitoneal shunt for treatment of hydrocephalus	00163J6
154. End-of-life replacement of spinal neurostimulator generator, multiple array, in lower abdomen	0JH80DZ (Taking out of the old generator is coded separately to the root operation *Removal*)
155. Percutaneous insertion of spinal neurostimulator lead, lumbar spinal cord	00HV3MZ
156. Percutaneous replacement of broken pacemaker lead in left atrium	02H73JZ (Taking out the broken pacemaker lead is coded separately to the root operation *Removal*.)
157. Open placement of dual chamber pacemaker generator in chest wall	0JH606Z
158. Percutaneous placement of venous central line in right internal jugular, with tip in superior vena cava	02HV33Z
159. Open insertion of multiple channel cochlear implant, left ear	09HE06Z
160. Percutaneous placement of Swan-Ganz catheter in pulmonary trunk	02HP32Z (The Swan-Ganz catheter is coded to the device value *Monitoring Device* because it monitors pulmonary artery output.)
161. Bronchoscopy with insertion of Low Dose Pd-103 brachytherapy seeds, right lung	0BHK81Z, DB11BBZ
162. Open insertion of interspinous process device into lumbar vertebral joint	0SH00BZ
163. Open placement of bone growth stimulator, left femoral shaft	0QHY0MZ
164. Cystoscopy with placement of brachytherapy seeds in prostate gland	0VH081Z
165. Percutaneous insertion of Greenfield IVC filter	06H03DZ
166. Full-thickness skin graft to right lower arm, autograft (do not code graft harvest for this exercise)	0HRDX73
167. Excision of necrosed left femoral head with bone bank bone graft to fill the defect, open	0QR70KZ
168. Penetrating keratoplasty of right cornea with donor matched cornea, percutaneous approach	08R83KZ
169. Excision of abdominal aorta with Gore-Tex graft replacement, open	04R00JZ
170. Total right knee arthroplasty with insertion of total knee prosthesis	0SRC0JZ
171. Tenonectomy with graft to right ankle using cadaver graft, open	0LRS0KZ
172. Mitral valve replacement using porcine valve, open	02RG08Z
173. Percutaneous phacoemulsification of right eye cataract with prosthetic lens insertion	08RJ3JZ
174. Transcatheter replacement of pulmonary valve using of bovine jugular vein valve	02RH38Z

Procedure	Code
175. Total left hip replacement using ceramic on ceramic prosthesis, without bone cement	ØSRBØ3A
176. Aortic valve annuloplasty using ring, open	Ø2UFØJZ
177. Laparoscopic repair of left inguinal hernia with marlex plug	ØYU64JZ
178. Autograft nerve graft to right median nerve, percutaneous endoscopic (do not code graft harvest for this exercise)	Ø1U547Z
179. Exchange of liner in femoral component of previous left hip replacement, open approach	ØSUSØ9Z (Taking out of the old liner is coded separately to the root operation *Removal*)
180. Anterior colporrhaphy with polypropylene mesh reinforcement, open approach	ØJUCØJZ
181. Implantation of CorCap cardiac support device, open approach	Ø2UAØJZ
182. Abdominal wall herniorrhaphy, open, using synthetic mesh	ØWUFØJZ
183. Tendon graft to strengthen injured left shoulder using autograft, open (do not code graft harvest for this exercise)	ØLU2Ø7Z
184. Onlay lamellar keratoplasty of left cornea using autograft, external approach	Ø8U9X7Z
185. Resurfacing procedure on right femoral head, open approach	ØSURØBZ
186. Exchange of drainage tube from right hip joint	ØS2YXØZ
187. Tracheostomy tube exchange	ØB21XFZ
188. Change chest tube for left pneumothorax	ØW2BXØZ
189. Exchange of cerebral ventriculostomy drainage tube	ØØ2ØXØZ
190. Foley urinary catheter exchange	ØT2BXØZ (This is coded to *Drainage Device* because urine is being drained.)
191. Open removal of lumbar sympathetic neurostimulator lead	Ø1PYØMZ
192. Nonincisional removal of Swan-Ganz catheter from right pulmonary artery	Ø2PYX2Z
193. Laparotomy with removal of pancreatic drain	ØFPGØØZ
194. Extubation, endotracheal tube	ØBP1XDZ
195. Nonincisional PEG tube removal	ØDP6XUZ
196. Transvaginal removal of brachytherapy seeds	ØUPH71Z
197. Transvaginal removal of extraluminal cervical cerclage	ØUPD7CZ
198. Incision with removal of K-wire fixation, right first metatarsal	ØQPNØ4Z
199. Cystoscopy with retrieval of left ureteral stent	ØTP98DZ
200. Removal of nasogastric drainage tube for decompression	ØDP6XØZ
201. Removal of external fixator, left radial fracture	ØPPJX5Z
202. Trimming and reanastomosis of stenosed femorofemoral synthetic bypass graft, open	Ø4WYØJZ
203. Open revision of right hip replacement, with readjustment of prosthesis	ØSW9ØJZ
204. Adjustment of position, pacemaker lead in left ventricle, percutaneous	Ø2WA3MZ
205. External repositioning of Foley catheter to bladder	ØTWBXØZ
206. Taking out loose screw and putting larger screw in fracture repair plate, left tibia	ØQWHØ4Z
207. Revision of totally implantable VAD port placement in chest wall, causing patient discomfort, open	ØJWTØWZ
208. Thoracotomy with exploration of right pleural cavity	ØWJ9ØZZ

Procedure	Code
209. Diagnostic laryngoscopy	ØCJS8ZZ
210. Exploratory arthrotomy of left knee	ØSJDØZZ
211. Colposcopy with diagnostic hysteroscopy	ØUJD8ZZ
212. Digital rectal exam	ØDJD7ZZ
213. Diagnostic arthroscopy of right shoulder	ØRJJ4ZZ
214. Endoscopy of maxillary sinus	Ø9JY4ZZ
215. Laparotomy with palpation of liver	ØFJØØZZ
216. Transurethral diagnostic cystoscopy	ØTJB8ZZ
217. Colonoscopy, discontinued at sigmoid colon	ØDJD8ZZ
218. Percutaneous mapping of basal ganglia	ØØK83ZZ
219. Heart catheterization with cardiac mapping	Ø2K83ZZ
220. Intraoperative whole brain mapping via craniotomy	ØØKØØZZ
221. Mapping of left cerebral hemisphere, percutaneous endoscopic	ØØK74ZZ
222. Intraoperative cardiac mapping during open heart surgery	Ø2K8ØZZ
223. Hysteroscopy with cautery of post-hysterectomy oozing and evacuation of clot	ØW3R8ZZ
224. Open exploration and ligation of post-op arterial bleeder, left forearm	ØX3FØZZ
225. Control of post-operative retroperitoneal bleeding via laparotomy	ØW3HØZZ
226. Reopening of thoracotomy site with drainage and control of post-op hemopericardium	ØW3DØZZ
227. Arthroscopy with drainage of hemarthrosis at previous operative site, right knee	ØY3F4ZZ
228. Radiocarpal fusion of left hand with internal fixation, open	ØRGPØ4Z
229. Posterior approach spinal fusion at L1-L3 level with BAK cage interbody fusion device, open	ØSG1ØAJ
230. Intercarpal fusion of right hand with bone bank bone graft, open	ØRGQØKZ
231. Sacrococcygeal fusion with bone graft from same operative site, open	ØSG5Ø7Z
232. Interphalangeal fusion of left great toe, percutaneous pin fixation	ØSGQ34Z
233. Suture repair of left radial nerve laceration	Ø1Q6ØZZ (The approach value is *Open*, though the surgical exposure may have been created by the wound itself.)
234. Laparotomy with suture repair of blunt force duodenal laceration	ØDQ9ØZZ
235. Perineoplasty with repair of old obstetric laceration, open	ØWQNØZZ
236. Suture repair of right biceps tendon (upper arm) laceration, open	ØLQ3ØZZ
237. Closure of abdominal wall stab wound	ØWQFØZZ
238. Cosmetic face lift, open, no other information available	ØWØ2ØZZ
239. Bilateral breast augmentation with silicone implants, open	ØHØVØJZ
240. Cosmetic rhinoplasty with septal reduction and tip elevation using local tissue graft, open	Ø9ØKØ7Z
241. Abdominoplasty (tummy tuck), open	ØWØFØZZ
242. Liposuction of bilateral thighs	ØJØL3ZZ, ØJØM3ZZ
243. Creation of penis in female patient using tissue bank donor graft	ØW4NØK1
244. Creation of vagina in male patient using synthetic material	ØW4MØJØ

Procedure	Code
245. Laparoscopic vertical (sleeve) gastrectomy	0DB64Z3
246. Left uterine artery embolization with intraluminal biosphere injection	04LF3DU

Obstetrics

Procedure	Code
1. Abortion by dilation and evacuation following laminaria insertion	10A07ZW
2. Manually assisted spontaneous abortion	10E0XZZ (Since the pregnancy was not artificially terminated, this is coded to *Delivery* because it captures the procedure objective. The fact that it was an abortion will be identified in the diagnosis code.)
3. Abortion by abortifacient insertion	10A07ZX
4. Bimanual pregnancy examination	10J07ZZ
5. Extraperitoneal C-section, low transverse incision	10D00Z1
6. Fetal spinal tap, percutaneous	10903ZA
7. Fetal kidney transplant, laparoscopic	10Y04ZS
8. Open in utero repair of congenital diaphragmatic hernia	10Q00ZK (Diaphragm is classified to the *Respiratory* body system in the *Medical and Surgical* section.)
9. Laparoscopy with total excision of tubal pregnancy	10T24ZZ
10. Transvaginal removal of fetal monitoring electrode	10P073Z

Placement

Procedure	Code
1. Placement of packing material, right ear	2Y42X5Z
2. Mechanical traction of entire left leg	2W6MX0Z
3. Removal of splint, right shoulder	2W5AX1Z
4. Placement of neck brace	2W32X3Z
5. Change of vaginal packing	2Y04X5Z
6. Packing of wound, chest wall	2W44X5Z
7. Sterile dressing placement to left groin region	2W27X4Z
8. Removal of packing material from pharynx	2Y50X5Z
9. Placement of intermittent pneumatic compression device, covering entire right arm	2W18X7Z
10. Exchange of pressure dressing to left thigh	2W0PX6Z

Administration

Procedure	Code
1. Peritoneal dialysis via indwelling catheter	3E1M39Z
2. Transvaginal artificial insemination	3E0P7LZ
3. Infusion of total parenteral nutrition via central venous catheter	3E0436Z
4. Esophagogastroscopy with Botox injection into esophageal sphincter	3E0G8GC (Botulinum toxin is a paralyzing agent with temporary effects; it does not sclerose or destroy the nerve.)
5. Percutaneous irrigation of knee joint	3E1U38Z
6. Systemic infusion of recombinant tissue plasminogen activator (r-tPA) via peripheral venous catheter	3E03317
7. Transabdominal in vitro fertilization, implantation of donor ovum	3E0P3Q1
8. Autologous bone marrow transplant via central venous line	30243G0
9. Implantation of anti-microbial envelope with cardiac defibrillator placement, open	3E0102A
10. Sclerotherapy of brachial plexus lesion, alcohol injection	3E0T3TZ
11. Percutaneous peripheral vein injection, glucarpidase	3E033GQ
12. Introduction of anti-infective envelope into subcutaneous tissue, open	3E0102A

Measurement and Monitoring

Procedure	Code
1. Cardiac stress test, single measurement	4A02XM4
2. EGD with biliary flow measurement	4A0C85Z
3. Right and left heart cardiac catheterization with bilateral sampling and pressure measurements	4A023N8
4. Temperature monitoring, rectal	4A1Z7KZ
5. Peripheral venous pulse, external, single measurement	4A04XJ1
6. Holter monitoring	4A12X45
7. Respiratory rate, external, single measurement	4A09XCZ
8. Fetal heart rate monitoring, transvaginal	4A1H7CZ
9. Visual mobility test, single measurement	4A07X7Z
10. Left ventricular cardiac output monitoring from pulmonary artery wedge (Swan-Ganz) catheter	4A1239Z
11. Olfactory acuity test, single measurement	4A08X0Z

Extracorporeal or Systemic Assistance and Performance

	Procedure	Code
1.	Intermittent mechanical ventilation, 16 hours	5A1935Z
2.	Liver dialysis, single encounter	5A1C00Z
3.	Cardiac countershock with successful conversion to sinus rhythm	5A2204Z
4.	IPPB (intermittent positive pressure breathing) for mobilization of secretions, 22 hours	5A09358
5.	Renal dialysis, 12 hours	5A1D80Z
6.	IABP (intra-aortic balloon pump) continuous	5A02210
7.	Intra-operative cardiac pacing, continuous	5A1223Z
8.	Intraoperative ECMO (extracorporeal membrane oxygenation), central	5A15A2F
9.	Controlled mechanical ventilation (CMV), 45 hours	5A1945Z
10.	Pulsatile compression boot with intermittent inflation	5A02115 (This is coded to the function value *Cardiac Output*, because the purpose of such compression devices is to return blood to the heart faster.)

Extracorporeal or Systemic Therapies

	Procedure	Code
1.	Donor thrombocytapheresis, single encounter	6A550Z2
2.	Bili-lite phototherapy, series treatment	6A601ZZ
3.	Whole body hypothermia, single treatment	6A4Z0ZZ
4.	Circulatory phototherapy, single encounter	6A650ZZ
5.	Shock wave therapy of plantar fascia, single treatment	6A930ZZ
6.	Antigen-free air conditioning, series treatment	6A0Z1ZZ
7.	TMS (transcranial magnetic stimulation), series treatment	6A221ZZ
8.	Therapeutic ultrasound of peripheral vessels, single treatment	6A750Z6
9.	Plasmapheresis, series treatment	6A551Z3
10.	Extracorporeal electromagnetic stimulation (EMS) for urinary incontinence, single treatment	6A210ZZ

Osteopathic

	Procedure	Code
1.	Isotonic muscle energy treatment of right leg	7W06X8Z
2.	Low velocity-high amplitude osteopathic treatment of head	7W00X5Z
3.	Lymphatic pump osteopathic treatment of left axilla	7W07X6Z
4.	Indirect osteopathic treatment of sacrum	7W04X4Z
5.	Articulatory osteopathic treatment of cervical region	7W01X0Z

Other Procedures

	Procedure	Code
1.	Near infrared spectroscopy of leg vessels	8E023DZ
2.	CT computer assisted sinus surgery	8E09XBG (The primary procedure is coded separately.)
3.	Suture removal, abdominal wall	8E0WXY8
4.	Isolation after infectious disease exposure	8E0ZXY6
5.	Robotic assisted open prostatectomy	8E0W0CZ (The primary procedure is coded separately.)
6.	In vitro fertilization	8E0ZXY1

Chiropractic

	Procedure	Code
1.	Chiropractic treatment of lumbar region using long lever specific contact	9WB3XGZ
2.	Chiropractic manipulation of abdominal region, indirect visceral	9WB9XCZ
3.	Chiropractic extra-articular treatment of hip region	9WB6XDZ
4.	Chiropractic treatment of sacrum using long and short lever specific contact	9WB4XJZ
5.	Mechanically-assisted chiropractic manipulation of head	9WB0XKZ

Imaging

	Procedure	Code
1.	Noncontrast CT of abdomen and pelvis	BW21ZZZ
2.	Intravascular ultrasound, left subclavian artery	B342ZZ3
3.	Fluoroscopic guidance for insertion of central venous catheter in SVC, low osmolar contrast	B5181ZA
4.	Chest x-ray, AP/PA and lateral views	BW03ZZZ
5.	Endoluminal ultrasound of gallbladder and bile ducts	BF43ZZZ
6.	MRI of thyroid gland, contrast unspecified	BG34YZZ
7.	Esophageal videofluoroscopy study with oral barium contrast	BD11YZZ
8.	Portable x-ray study of right radius/ulna shaft, standard series	BP0JZZZ
9.	Routine fetal ultrasound, second trimester twin gestation	BY4DZZZ
10.	CT scan of bilateral lungs, high osmolar contrast with densitometry	BB240ZZ
11.	Fluoroscopic guidance for percutaneous transluminal angioplasty (PTA) of left common femoral artery, low osmolar contrast	B41G1ZZ

Nuclear Medicine

	Procedure	Code
1.	Tomo scan of right and left heart, unspecified radiopharmaceutical, qualitative gated rest	C226YZZ
2.	Technetium pentetate assay of kidneys, ureters, and bladder	CT631ZZ
3.	Uniplanar scan of spine using technetium oxidronate, with first-pass study	CP151ZZ
4.	Thallous chloride tomographic scan of bilateral breasts	CH22SZZ
5.	PET scan of myocardium using rubidium	C23GQZZ
6.	Gallium citrate scan of head and neck, single plane imaging	CW1BLZZ
7.	Xenon gas nonimaging probe of brain	C050VZZ
8.	Upper GI scan, radiopharmaceutical unspecified, for gastric emptying	CD15YZZ
9.	Carbon 11 PET scan of brain with quantification	C030BZZ
10.	Iodinated albumin nuclear medicine assay, blood plasma volume study	C763HZZ

Radiation Therapy

	Procedure	Code
1.	Plaque radiation of left eye, single port	D8Y0FZZ
2.	8 MeV photon beam radiation to brain	D0011ZZ
3.	IORT of colon, 3 ports	DDY5CZZ
4.	HDR brachytherapy of prostate using low dose palladium-103, unidirectional source	DV10BB1
5.	Electron radiation treatment of right breast, with custom device	DM013ZZ
6.	Hyperthermia oncology treatment of pelvic region	DWY68ZZ
7.	Contact radiation of tongue	D9Y57ZZ
8.	Heavy particle radiation treatment of pancreas, four risk sites	DF034ZZ
9.	LDR brachytherapy to spinal cord using iodine	D016B9Z
10.	Whole body Phosphorus 32 administration with risk to hematopoetic system	DWY5GFZ

Physical Rehabilitation and Diagnostic Audiology

	Procedure	Code
1.	Bekesy assessment using audiometer	F13Z31Z
2.	Individual fitting of left eye prosthesis	F0DZ8UZ
3.	Physical therapy for range of motion and mobility, patient right hip, no special equipment	F07L0ZZ
4.	Bedside swallow assessment using assessment kit	F00ZHYZ
5.	Caregiver training in airway clearance techniques	F0FZ8ZZ
6.	Application of short arm cast in rehabilitation setting	F0DZ7EZ (Inhibitory cast is listed in the equipment reference table under E, *Orthosis*.)
7.	Verbal assessment of patient's pain level	F02ZFZZ

	Procedure	Code
8.	Caregiver training in communication skills using manual communication board	F0FZJMZ (Manual communication board is listed in the equipment reference table under M, *Augmentative/ Alternative Communication*.)
9.	Group musculoskeletal balance training exercises, whole body, no special equipment	F07M6ZZ (Balance training is included in the motor treatment reference table under *Therapeutic Exercise*.)
10.	Individual therapy for auditory processing using tape recorder	F09Z2KZ (Tape recorder is listed in the equipment reference table under *Audiovisual Equipment*.)

Mental Health

	Procedure	Code
1.	Cognitive-behavioral psychotherapy, individual	GZ58ZZZ
2.	Narcosynthesis	GZGZZZZ
3.	Light therapy	GZJZZZZ
4.	ECT (electroconvulsive therapy), unilateral, multiple seizure	GZB1ZZZ
5.	Crisis intervention	GZ2ZZZZ
6.	Neuropsychological testing	GZ13ZZZ
7.	Hypnosis	GZFZZZZ
8.	Developmental testing	GZ10ZZZ
9.	Vocational counseling	GZ61ZZZ
10.	Family psychotherapy	GZ72ZZZ

Substance Abuse Treatment

	Procedure	Code
1.	Naltrexone treatment for drug dependency	HZ94ZZZ
2.	Substance abuse treatment family counseling	HZ63ZZZ
3.	Medication monitoring of patient on methadone maintenance	HZ81ZZZ
4.	Individual interpersonal psychotherapy for drug abuse	HZ54ZZZ
5.	Patient in for alcohol detoxification treatment	HZ2ZZZZ
6.	Group motivational counseling	HZ47ZZZ
7.	Individual 12-step psychotherapy for substance abuse	HZ53ZZZ
8.	Post-test infectious disease counseling for IV drug abuser	HZ3CZZZ
9.	Psychodynamic psychotherapy for drug dependent patient	HZ5CZZZ
10.	Group cognitive-behavioral counseling for substance abuse	HZ42ZZZ

New Technology

	Procedure	Code
1.	Infusion of ceftazidime via peripheral venous catheter	XW03321
2.	Transcatheter dilation of left peroneal artery with 2 SAVAL stents	X27U395